英汉双解医学词典

Dictionary of Medicine

编者:P.H.Collin
审订:韩宗萸
译者:陈育红　胜　利

外语教学与研究出版社
FOREIGN LANGUAGE TEACHING AND RESEARCH PRESS

(京)新登字 155 号

京权图字：01－1997－1145
图书在版编目(CIP)数据

英汉双解医学词典/(英)柯林(Collin，P.H.)编；陈育红，胜利译. －北京：外语教学与研究出版社，2001
ISBN 7－5600－2187－5

Ⅰ.英… Ⅱ.①何… ②陈… ③胜… Ⅲ.医学－双解词典－英、汉 Ⅳ.R-61

中国版本图书馆 CIP 数据核字(2001)第 13548 号

First published in Great Britain by Peter Collin Publishing Ltd. with the title Dictionary of Medicine 1994.

英汉双解医学词典
编者：P. H. Collin
审订：韩宗荻
译者：陈育红 胜 利
* * *
责任编辑：吴 静
出版发行：外语教学与研究出版社
社 址：北京市西三环北路 19 号 (100089)
网 址：http://www.fltrp.com.cn
印 刷：北京外国语大学印刷厂
开 本：850×1168 1/32
印 张：21.25
版 次：2001 年 3 月第 1 版 2001 年 3 月第 1 次印刷
印 数：1—20000 册
书 号：ISBN 7－5600－2187－5/H·1167
定 价：28.90 元
* * *
如有印刷、装订质量问题出版社负责调换

译者前言

本词典根据英国彼德科林出版公司(Peter Collin Publishing)第二版翻译,采取英汉双解的形式,一般词条均给出汉语对应词,读者可同时借助英语解释理解词条的含义。本词典的解释用英语控制在500词以内,例句丰富,读者可据此学习该词条的具体用法。另有大量选自国外著名刊物的注释(Comment)和引文(Quote),有助于读者在实际工作中运用、掌握。语法注释(Note)则告诉读者该词有无复数、特殊的复数拼法、动词的不同变化形式和美国英语与英国英语的区别等。本书的附录则给出了人体结构图、食物热量表、人名术语一览表和其他一些有用的信息。

本词典收词多,词汇新,共收集了12,000余词条,涵盖的领域也极其广泛,包含了内、外、妇、儿等临床医学,病理、解剖等基础医学以及护理、制药等领域的词汇。本词典的编排亦很有特色,把由多个词组成的词条和它的缩略语分别作为词条列出并加以解释,方便读者查阅。本词典的翻译力求译名的规范化、标准化。在翻译过程中译者参考了国内最新的、权威的词典,如青岛出版社出版的《英中医学辞海》、学苑出版社出版的《英汉汉英医学大词典》、上海科学技术出版社的《英汉医学辞典》、在此译者表示衷心谢意。

本词典是一本为医护专业的学生及从业人员编写的医学英语学习词典,内容实用,便于学习与更深入地理解医学英语常用术语,对于一般的读者也有一定的帮助,在翻译过程中译者也受益匪浅。由于时间紧张,资料有限,译文可能有疏漏之处,敬请读者指正。

译者

2000年10月

目　录

Aa

A & E = ACCIDENT AND EMERGENCY 创伤与急诊；**A & E department** 创伤急诊科；**an A & E ward** 创伤急诊病房；**A & E nurses** 创伤急诊护士

Vitamin A *noun* retinol, a vitamin which is soluble in fat and can be formed in the body from precursors but is mainly found in food, such as liver, vegetables, eggs and cod liver oil 维生素A,视黄醇，可以由机体从前体合成的一种脂溶性维生素，但主要来源于食物，如肝、蔬菜、蛋类和鱼肝油

> COMMENT: Lack of Vitamin A affects the body's growth and resistance to disease and can cause night blindness or xerophthalmia. Carotene (the yellow substance in carrots) is a precursor of Vitamin A, which accounts for the saying that eating carrots helps you to see in the dark.
> 注释：缺乏维生素 A 会影响机体的生长和机体对疾病的抵抗力，导致夜盲症和干眼病。胡萝卜素（胡萝卜中的黄色物质）是合成维生素 A 的前体物质，所以说多吃胡萝卜帮助维持黑暗中的视力。

A band *noun* part of the pattern in muscle tissue, seen through a microscope as a dark band A 带，肌肉组织在显微镜下呈黑色条带的部分

ABC *abbreviation for*（缩写）Airway, Breathing and Circulation: the basic initial checks of a casualty's condition 气道、呼吸和循环状况，对伤亡患者首要的基本检查

abdomen *noun* space in front of the body below the diaphragm and above the pelvis, containing the stomach, intestines, liver and other vital organs 腹部，躯体前部横膈以下骨盆以上的部分，内含胃、肠道、肝和其它重要器官；**acute abdomen** = any serious condition of the abdomen which requires surgery 急腹症，需要外科治疗的严重腹部疾患

◇ **abdomin-** *prefix* referring to the abdomen 腹的

◇ **abdominal** *adjective* referring to the abdomen 腹部的；**abdominal aorta** 腹主动脉 *see* 见 AORTA；**abdominal cavity** = space in the body below the chest 腹腔，位于胸部以下；**abdominal distension** = condition where the abdomen is stretched (because of gas *or* fluid) 腹胀，多由气或液体引起；**abdominal pain** = pain in the abdomen caused by indigestion or more serious disorders 腹痛，由于消化不良或其它更严重疾病导致；**abdominal viscera** = organs contained in the abdomen (such as the stomach, liver, etc.) 腹腔脏器，如胃、肝等位于腹腔内的器官；**abdominal wall** = muscular tissue which surrounds the abdomen 腹壁，围绕腹腔的肌组织

◇ **abdominoperineal excision** *noun* cutting out of tissue in both the abdomen and the perineum 腹会阴切除术

◇ **abdominoscopy** *noun* internal examination of the abdomen, usually with an endoscope 腹腔镜检查，用内窥镜对腹腔内部进行检查

◇ **abdominothoracic** *adjective* referring to the abdomen and thorax 胸腹的 (NOTE: for other terms referring to the abdomen, see words beginning with **coeli-**)

> COMMENT: The abdomen is divided for medical purposes into nine regions: at the top, the right and left hypochondriac regions with the epigastrium between them; in the centre, the right and left lumbar regions with the umbilical between them; and at the bottom, the right and left iliac regions with the hypogastrium between them.
> 注释：腹部在医学上分为 9 个区域：上部的左、右季肋区及中间的腹上区，中部的左、右腰区及中间的脐区，下部的左、右髂区及中间的腹下区。

abducens *or* **abducent nerve** *noun* sixth cranial nerve, which controls the muscle which makes the eyeball turn outwards 外展神经，第6对颅神经，控制眼肌使眼球向外转

abduct *verb* to pull away from the centre line of the body 外展，偏离身体中线；**vocal folds abducted** = normal condition of the vocal cords in quiet breathing 声带外展，平静呼吸时声带的正常位置

◇ **abduction** *noun* movement of part of the body away from the midline or away from a neighbouring part 外展，远离身体中线或相邻部位

◇ **abductor (muscle)** *noun* muscle which pulls a part of the body away from the midline of the body or from a neighbouring part 外展肌，使身体的一部分远离中线或远离临近部位的肌肉（NOTE: opposites are **adducted**, **adduction**, **adductor**）

> QUOTE: Mary was nursed in a position of not more than 90°upright with her legs in abduction.
> 引文：使玛丽的下肢处于外展位，抬高低于90°。
> **British Journal of Nursing** 英国护理杂志

aberrant *adjective* not normal 异常的

◇ **aberration** *noun* action *or* growth which is not normal 异常，指动作或生长不正常；**chromosome** *or* **chromosomal aberration** = abnormality in the number, arrangement, etc. of chromosomes 染色体异常，指染色体数目、排列等的异常；**mental aberration** = slight forgetfulness *or* slightly abnormal mental process 精神失常，指轻度的健忘或精神活动异常

ablation *noun* removal of an organ *or* of part of the body by surgery 部分切除，手术去除机体的部分器官；**segmental ablation** = surgical removal of part of a nail, as treatment for an ingrowing toenail 分节段切除，手术切除部分趾甲，治疗嵌甲

able *adjective* 能：**After the injection he was able to breathe more easily.** = He could breathe more easily. 经注射后他的呼吸顺畅多了。（NOTE: *opposite is* **unable**. *Note also that* **able** is used with **to** *and a verb*）

◇ **ability** *noun* being able to do something 能力

abnormal *adjective* not normal 不正常，异常；**abnormal behaviour** = conduct which is different from the way normal people behave 行为异常，行为异于常人；**abnormal motion** *or* **abnormal stool** = faeces which are different in colour, which are very liquid 便异常，稀便，颜色不正常大便

◇ **abnormality** *noun* form *or* action which is not normal 反常，形式或举止不正常

◇ **abnormally** *adverb* in a way which is not normal 反常地：***He had an abnormally fast pulse.*** 他的脉搏异常地快。***Her periods were abnormally frequent.*** 她的经期异常频繁。（NOTE: for other terms referring to abnormality, see words beginning with **terat-**）

> QUOTE: The synovium produces an excess of synovial fluid, which is abnormal and becomes thickened. This causes pain, swelling and immobility of the affected joint.
> 引文：滑膜产生大量异常的粘稠滑液，导致受累关节疼痛、肿胀和僵化。
> **Nursing Times** 护理时代

> QUOTE: Even children with the milder forms of sickle-cell disease have an increased frequency of pneumococcal infection. The reason for this susceptibility is a profound abnormality of the immune system in children with SCD.
> 引文：即使是患轻度镰刀状贫血的儿童也易并发肺炎球菌感染，原因是此类患儿的免疫系统严重受损。
> **Lancet** 柳叶刀

ABO system *noun* system of classifying blood groups *ABO* 血型系统 *see* 见 *note at* BLOOD GROUP

abort *verb* (i) to eject the embryo *or* fetus and so end a pregnancy before the fetus is fully developed 流产，将胚胎或胎儿排出体外以致在胚胎完全成熟前即终止妊娠 (ii) to have an abortion 使流产：***The doctors decided to abort the fetus.*** 医生

决定实行流产。***The tissue will be aborted spontaneously.*** 组织将自然退化。

◊ **abortifacient** *noun* drug which provokes an abortion 堕胎药,可导致流产的药物

◊ **abortion** *noun* situation where an unborn baby leaves the womb before the end of pregnancy, especially during the first twenty-eight weeks of pregnancy when it is not likely to survive birth 流产,妊娠结束前胎儿离开子宫,特别是发生在妊娠前 28 周,此时胎儿不易成活; **to have an abortion** = to have an operation to make a fetus leave the womb during the first period of pregnancy 人工流产,在妊娠早期通过手术终止妊娠: ***The girl asked the clinic if she could have an abortion.*** 这姑娘问大夫她能否进行人工流产。***She had two abortions before her first child was born.*** 在她生第一个孩子前有过两次流产。**complete abortion** = abortion where the whole contents of the uterus are expelled 完全流产,流产时宫内物全部娩出; **criminal abortion** *or* **illegal abortion** = abortion which is carried out illegally 非法堕胎,非法进行流产; **habitual abortion** *or* **recurrent abortion** = condition where a woman has several abortions with successive pregnancies 习惯性流产,连续几次妊娠均发生流产; **incomplete abortion** = abortion where part of the contents of the uterus is not expelled 不全流产,流产时部分宫内物未娩出; **induced abortion** = abortion which is produced by drugs *or* by surgery 人工流产,用药物或手术方法进行流产; **legal abortion** = abortion which is carried out legally 合法堕胎,法律允许的堕胎; **spontaneous abortion** = MISCARRIAGE 自发流产; **therapeutic abortion** = abortion which is carried out because the health of the mother is in danger 治疗性流产,妊娠危及孕妇生命时进行的人工流产; **threatened abortion** = possible abortion in the early stages of pregnancy, indicated by bleeding 先兆流产,妊娠早期出现流产的征兆,多表现为阴道出血

◊ **abortionist** *noun* person who makes a woman abort, usually a person who performs an illegal abortion 堕胎师,做人工流产的人,多指非法堕胎师

◊ **abortive** *adjective* which does not succeed 失败的,不成功的; **abortive poliomyelitis** = mild form of polio which only affects the throat and intestines 顿挫型脊髓灰质炎,一种轻型的脊髓灰质炎,仅影响咽喉和肠道

> COMMENT: In the UK an abortion can be carried out legally if two doctors agree that the mother's life is in danger or that the fetus is likely to be born with severe handicaps.
> 注释:在英国,当两位医生一致认为孕妇存在生命危险或娩出的胎儿有严重生理缺陷时可进行合法流产。

abortus fever *noun* brucellosis, a disease which can be caught from cattle, or from drinking infected milk, spread by a species of the bacterium Brucella 流产儿热,布氏热,布氏杆菌病,一种经牛或污染的奶制品传播的由布氏杆菌引起的疾病

> COMMENT: Symptoms include tiredness, arthritis, headaches, sweating and swelling of the spleen.
> 注释:症状包括乏力、关节炎、头痛、出汗和脾肿大。

above *preposition & adverb* higher than 高于: ***His temperature was above 100 degrees.*** 他的体温超过了(华氏)100 度。**Her pulse rate was far above normal.** 她的脉搏大大高于正常值。**babies aged six months and above** 6 个月及 6 个月以上的婴儿

abrasion *noun* condition where the surface of the skin has been rubbed off by a rough surface and bleeds 擦伤,皮肤被粗糙表面磨破出血

> COMMENT: As the intact skin is an efficient barrier to bacteria, even minor abrasions can allow infection to enter the body and thus should be cleaned and treated with an antiseptic.
> 注释:完整的皮肤是有效抵抗细菌的屏障,即使是轻微的损伤也会导致感染侵入体内,因此,需要清创和抗感染治疗。

abreaction *noun* (*in psychology*) treatment of a neurotic patient by making him think again about past bad experiences 精神疏泄疗法,(在精神病学上)让神经症患者回忆过去不愉快的经历

abscess *noun* painful swollen area where pus forms, often accompanied by high temperature 脓肿,(皮肤)痛性肿胀,有脓液形成,常伴发热: ***He had an abscess under a tooth.*** 他齿下有脓肿。***The doctor decided to lance the abscess.*** 医生决定切开脓肿(进行引流)。**acute abscess** = abscess which develops rapidly 急性脓肿,迅速发展的脓肿; **chronic abscess** = abscess which develops slowly over a period of time 慢性脓肿,一段时间内缓慢发展的脓肿 (NOTE: plural is **abscesses**)

> COMMENT: An acute abscess can be dealt with by opening and draining when it has reached the stage where sufficient pus has been formed; a chronic abscess is usually treated with drugs.
> 注释:急性脓肿成熟(脓液形成充分)后可切开引流,慢性脓肿常需药物治疗。

absence *noun* not being here *or* there 没有,无; **in the absence of any other symptoms** = because no other symptoms are present 无其他任何症状

◇ **absent** *adjective* not here, not there 没有的,缺席的: ***Normal symptoms of malaria are absent in this form of the disease.*** 此型病例缺乏疟疾的常有症状。***Three children are absent because they are ill.*** 三名儿童因病缺席。

absolutely *adverb* really, completely 真的,完全的: ***He's still not absolutely fit after his operation.*** 他手术后还未完全复原。***The patient must remain absolutely still while the scan is taking place.*** 扫描时患者必须保持绝对静止不动。

absorb *verb* to take in (a liquid) 吸收(液体): ***Cotton wads are used to absorb the discharge from the wound.*** 棉垫用来吸收伤口的分泌物。

◇ **absorbable suture** *noun* suture which will eventually be absorbed into the body, and does not need to be removed 可吸收缝线,能被机体吸收的不需拆除的缝线

◇ **absorbent** *adjective* which absorbs 有吸收力的; **absorbent cotton** = soft white stuff used as a dressing to put on wounds 吸水棉,一种松软的用来覆盖伤口的白色敷料

◇ **absorption** *noun* (i) action of taking a liquid into a solid 吸收,将液体吸入固相的过程 (ii) taking substances into the body, such as proteins or fats which have been digested from food and are taken into the bloodstream from the stomach and intestines 吸收,食物消化为蛋白或脂肪后经胃肠道进入血液; **absorption rate** = rate at which a liquid is absorbed by a solid 吸收率,液体吸入固相的速度; **percutaneous absorption** = absorbing a substance through the skin 经皮吸收,物质通过皮肤吸收 (NOTE: the spellings: **absorb but absorption**)

abstain *verb* not to do something voluntarily 戒除,戒断,自觉地不做某事: ***He abstained from taking any drugs for two months.*** 他已经戒毒两个多月了。***They decided to abstain from sexual intercourse.*** 他们决定停止性交往。

◇ **abstainer** *noun* person who does not drink alcohol 忌酒者,不饮酒的人

◇ **abstinence** *noun* not doing something voluntarily 戒绝,自愿不做某事: ***The clinic recommended total abstinence from alcohol*** *or* ***from drugs.*** 临床医生建议严禁一切酒类或毒品。

abulia *noun* lack of willpower 意志缺乏,丧失意志力

abuse 1 *noun* (**a**) using something wrongly 滥用,错误应用; **alcohol abuse** *or* ***amphetamine abuse*** *or* ***drug abuse*** *or* ***solvent abuse*** = being mentally and physically dependent on regularly taking alcohol *or* amphetamines *or* drugs *or* inhaling solvents 滥用酒精、安非他明、药物和溶媒,心理上或生理上依赖定期服用酒精、安非他明、药物和溶媒 (**b**) bad treatment of a person 虐待,粗暴对待某人; ***child abuse*** *or* ***sexual abuse of children*** 虐待儿童或对儿童进行性虐待 (NOTE: no plural)

2 *verb* (**a**) to use something wrongly 滥用: ***Heroin and cocaine are commonly abused drugs***. 海洛因和可卡因是常被滥用的麻醉药。**to abuse one's authority** = to use one's powers in an illegal or harmful way 滥用职权,非法或恶意使用某人的权力 (**b**) to treat someone badly 虐待,粗暴对待某人: ***He had sexually abused small children***. 他曾对幼儿进行性虐待。

a. c. *abbreviation of* (缩写) 'ante cibum': meaning 'before food' (used on prescriptions) 饭前(用于处方书写)

acanthosis *noun* disease of the prickle cell layer of the skin, where warts appear on the skin or inside the mouth 棘皮症,皮肤棘皮细胞层的疾病,导致皮肤或口腔内出现疣

acaricide *noun* substance which kills mites 杀螨剂

acatalasia *noun* inherited condition which results in a defect of catalase in all tissue 过氧化氢酶缺乏症,遗传性疾病,所有组织中均缺乏过氧化氢酶

accelerate *verb* to go faster, make something go faster 加速,使加速

◇ **acceleration** *noun* going faster, making something go faster 加速: ***The nurse noticed an acceleration in the patient's pulse rate***. 护士注意到患者的脉搏加快了。

accentuate *verb* to make stronger 强调,着重; ***to accentuate pain*** 加重疼痛

accessory *adjective* (thing) which helps, without being most important 附属的,辅助的; **accessory nerve** = eleventh cranial nerve which supplies the muscles in the neck and shoulders 副神经,第十一对颅神经,支配颈部和肩部的肌肉运动; **accessory organ** = organ which has a function which is controlled by another organ 从属器官

accident *noun* (**a**) something which happens by chance 偶发事件: ***I met her by accident at the bus stop***. 我意外地在车站遇见她。(**b**) unpleasant event which happens suddenly and harms someone's health 不幸的意外事故: ***She had an accident in the kitchen and had to go to hospital***. 她在厨房发生意外,不得不去医院。***Three people were killed in the accident on the motorway***. 在车祸中有 3 人死亡。**accident and emergency department** (**A & E**) = department of a hospital which deals with accidents and emergency cases 创伤急诊科; **accident prevention** = taking steps to prevent accidents from happening 事故预防; **accident ward** = ward in a hospital for victims of accidents 创伤病区

◇ **accidentally** *adverb* (**a**) by chance 偶然地,意外地: ***I found the missing watch accidentally***. 我意外地发现了丢失的手表。(**b**) in an accident 意外,横祸: ***He was killed accidentally***. 他意外被害。

◇ **accident-prone** *adjective* (person) who has awkward movements and frequently has *or* causes minor accidents 笨拙的,易出轻微事故的(人)

accommodation *noun* (*of the lens of the eye*) ability to focus on objects at different distances, using the ciliary muscle (对眼球晶状体的)调节,利用睫状肌聚焦于不同距离目标的能力

◇ **accommodative squint** *noun* squint when the eye is trying to focus on an object which is very close 调节性斜视,眼睛试图聚焦于很近的目标时出现的斜视

accompany *verb* to go with 陪伴,伴有: ***He accompanied his wife to hospital***. 他陪妻子去医院。***The pain was accompanied by high temperature***. 疼痛伴有高热。

according to *preposition* as someone says or writes 据,根据: ***According to the dosage on the bottle, the medicine can be given to very young children***. 根据瓶上的剂量,此药可以给幼儿服用。

accretion *noun* growth of a substance which sticks to an object 增长,堆积: ***An accretion of calcium round the joint***. 关节周围有钙质增生。

accumulate *verb* to grow together in a group 加,积累: ***Large quantities of fat accumulated in the arteries***. 大量脂肪沉积于动脉。

◇ **accumulation** *noun* (i) act of accumulating 积累 (ii) material which has accumulated 累积物: ***The drug aims at clearing the accumulation of fatty deposits in the arteries.*** 此药可清除动脉内沉积的脂肪。

accurate *adjective* very correct 准确的,精确的: ***The sphygmomanometer does not seem to be giving an accurate reading.*** 这台血压计读数不准。***The scan helped to give an accurate location for the operation site.*** 扫描有助于手术的准确定位。***The results of the lab tests should help the consultant make an accurate diagnosis.*** 实验结果有助于会诊医生作出正确诊断。

◇ **accurately** *adverb* very correctly 准确地,精确地: ***The GP accurately diagnosed a brain tumour.*** 这位全科医生准确诊断出了脑瘤。

acephalus *noun* fetus born without a head 无脑儿

acetabulum *or* **cotyloid cavity** *noun* part of the pelvic bone, shaped like a cup, into which the head of the femur fits to form the hip joint 髋臼,是盆骨的一部分,形如茶杯,使股骨头嵌入以形成髋关节 (NOTE: plural is **acetabula**)

◇ **acetabuloplasty** *noun* surgical operation to repair or rebuild the acetabulum 髋成形术

acetic acid *noun* acid which turns wine into vinegar 醋酸

> COMMENT: A weak solution of acetic acid can be used to cool the body in hot weather; a strong solution can be used to burn away warts.
> 注释:低浓度的醋酸可以在热天用来降温;高浓度的醋酸可以烧除疣子。

acetone *noun* colourless, volatile substance, used in nail varnish, also formed in the body after vomiting or during diabetes 丙酮,无色的挥发性物质,用于指甲上光;呕吐或糖尿病时也可在体内形成

◇ **acetonuria** *noun* presence of acetone in the urine, giving off a sweet smell 酮尿

acetylcholine *noun* substance released from nerve endings, which allows nerve impulses to move from one nerve to another or from a nerve to the organ it controls 乙酰胆碱,神经末梢释放的物质,使神经冲动从一根神经传递到另一根神经,或由神经传递到它所控制的器官

acetylsalicylic acid *noun* 乙酰水杨酸 *see* 见 ASPIRIN

achalasia *noun* being unable to relax the muscles 失弛缓,肌肉不能放松; **cardiac achalasia** *or* **achalasia of the cardia** = being unable to relax the cardia (the muscle at the entrance to the stomach), with the result that food cannot enter the stomach 贲门失弛缓,贲门不能松弛,结果是食物不能进入胃中 *see also* 参见 CARDIOMYOTOMY

ache 1 *noun* pain which goes on for a time, but is not very acute 疼,疼痛: ***He complained of various aches and pains.*** 他主诉有各种疼痛。(NOTE: used with other words to show where the pain is situated *see* 见 BACKACHE, HEADACHE, STOMACH ACHE, TOOTHACHE) **2** *verb* to have a pain in part of the body 使疼痛: ***Reading in bad light can make the eyes ache.*** 在光线暗的情况下阅读会引起眼睛疼痛。***His tooth ached so much he went to the dentist.*** 他牙疼得厉害必须去看大夫。

◇ **aching** *adjective* with a continuous pain 持续疼痛的

Achilles tendon *noun* tendon at the back of the ankle which connects the calf muscles to the heel and which acts to pull up the heel when the calf muscle is contracted 跟腱,脚踝背侧的肌腱,将小腿肌连在跟骨上,小腿肌收缩时可以使足跟抬起

◇ **achillorrhaphy** *noun* surgical operation to stitch a torn Achilles tendon 跟腱缝合术

◇ **achillotomy** *noun* act of dividing the Achilles tendon 跟腱切断术

achlorhydria *noun* condition where the gastric juices do not contain hydrochloric acid, a symptom of stomach cancer or pernicious anaemia 无酸,乏酸,胃液内不含盐酸,是胃癌或恶性贫血的症状之一

acholia *noun* absence of bile 无胆汁

◇ **acholuria** *noun* absence of bile colouring in the urine 无胆色素尿

◇ **acholuric jaundice** *noun* hereditary spherocytosis, a disease where abnormally round red blood cells form, leading to anaemia, enlarged spleen and the formation of gallstones 无胆色素尿性黄疸,即遗传性球形细胞增多症,导致贫血、脾大和胆石形成

achondroplasia *noun* hereditary condition where the long bones in the arms and legs do not grow fully, while the rest of the bones in the body do so, producing dwarfism 软骨发育不全,是一种遗传疾病,造成侏儒

acid *noun* (**a**) chemical compound containing hydrogen, which reacts with an alkali to form a salt and water 酸,含氢的化合物,与碱作用形成盐和水: ***Hydrochloric acid is secreted in the stomach and forms part of the gastric juices.*** 盐酸由胃分泌,是胃液的组成成份。 **bile acids** = acids (such as cholic acid) found in the bile 胆汁酸; **inorganic acids** = acids which come from minerals, used in dilute form to help indigestion 无机酸; **organic acids** = acids which come from plants, taken to stimulate the production of urine 有机酸 (**b**) any bitter juice 任何有苦味儿的液体

◇ **acidity** *noun* (**a**) level of acid in a liquid 酸度: ***The alkaline solution may help to reduce acidity.*** 碱性液体有助于减低酸度。(**b**) acid stomach, a form of indigestion where the patient has a burning feeling in his stomach caused by too much acid forming there 返酸,胃酸过多

◇ **acidosis** *noun* (**a**) condition when there are more acid waste products (such as urea) than normal in the blood because of a lack of alkali 酸中毒,血液中酸性废物(如尿素)过多; **metabolic acidosis** = acidosis caused by a defect in the body's metabolism 代谢性酸中毒 (**b**) = ACIDITY 酸度

◇ **acid stomach** = ACIDITY 返酸,胃酸过多

acinus *noun* (i) tiny alveolus which forms part of a gland 腺泡 (ii) part of a lobule in the lung 肺泡 (NOTE: plural is **acini**)

acne *or* **acne vulgaris** *noun* inflammation of the sebaceous glands during puberty, which makes blackheads appear on the skin, usually on the face, neck and shoulders, and these then become infected 痤疮,寻常性痤疮: ***He suffers from acne.*** 他患有痤疮。 ***She is using a cream to clear up her acne.*** 她用洗面奶来清除痤疮。

acoustic *adjective* referring to sound or hearing 有关听的,听觉的; **acoustic nerve** 听神经 *see* 见 NERVE; **acoustic neurofibroma** *or* **acoustic neuroma** = tumour in the sheath of the auditory nerve, causing deafness 听神经纤维瘤,听神经瘤,可导致耳聋

acquired *adjective* (condition) which is neither congenital nor hereditary and which a person develops after birth in reaction to his environment 获得性的,后天的; **acquired immunity** = immunity which a body acquires and which is not congenital 获得性免疫; **acquired immunodeficiency syndrome** = AIDS 获得性免疫缺陷综合症,即艾滋病 *see also* 参见 CONGENITAL, HEREDITARY

acro- *prefix* referring to a point *or* tip 顶点,最高点

◇ **acrocyanosis** *noun* blue colour of the extremities (fingers, toes, ears and nose) due to bad circulation 肢端紫绀,手足发绀,身体端点(手指、脚趾、耳和鼻)由于循环不良而颜色发紫

◇ **acrodynia** *noun* pink disease, a children's disease where the child's hands, feet and face swell and become pink, with a fever and loss of appetite, caused by allergy to mercury 肢痛症,粉红病,儿科疾病,患儿的手、足和面部肿胀,呈粉红色,伴有发热和食欲减退,是由对汞过敏引起的

◇ **acromegaly** *noun* disease caused by

excessive quantities of growth hormone produced by the pituitary gland, causing a slow enlargement of the hands, feet and jaws in adults 肢端肥大症,垂体分泌的生长激素过多,造成成人手、足和下巴缓慢增大

◇ **acromial** *adjective* referring to the acromion 肩峰的; **coraco-acromial** = referring to both the coracoid process and the acromion 喙突和肩峰

◇ **acromion** *noun* pointed top of the scapula, which forms the tip of the shoulder 肩峰 ◊ 见图 SHOULDER, SKELETON

acronyx *noun* (*of a nail*) growing into the flesh 嵌甲,指甲(趾甲)长到肉里

acroparaesthesia *noun* condition where the patient suffers sharp pains in the arms and numbness in the fingers after sleep 肢端感觉异常,患者在睡醒后感双臂刺痛和手指麻木

acrophobia *noun* fear of heights 恐高症

acrosclerosis *noun* sclerosis which affects the extremities 肢端硬化

act *verb* to do something, to have the effect of 做,起作用: ***The connecting tissue acts as a supporting framework.*** 结缔组织起支架作用。***He had to act quickly to save his sister.*** 他必须快速行动以救他姐姐。

◇ **act on** *or* **upon** *verb* (**a**) to do something as the result of something which has been said 按照…行动: ***He acted upon your suggestion.*** 他按你的建议去做。(**b**) to have an effect on 对…发挥作用: ***The antibiotic acted quickly on the infection.*** 抗生素很快针对感染发挥效用。

ACTH = ADRENOCORTICOTROPHIC HORMONE 促肾上腺皮质激素

actin *noun* protein which, with myosin, forms the contractile tissue of muscle 肌动蛋白,与肌球旦白一起形成肌肉的可收缩组织

◇ **actinomycosis** *noun* disease transmitted by cattle, where the patient is infected with fungus which forms abscesses in the mouth and lungs (pulmonary actinomycosis) or in the ileum (intestinal actinomycosis) 放线菌病,经牛传播的真菌病,在口腔、肺或回肠中形成脓肿

action *noun* thing which is done, effect 作用,效应: ***The injection will speed up the action of the antibiotic.*** 注射可加快抗生素起效。

◇ **activate** *verb* to make something start to work 使活动,活化: ***The muscle activates the heart.*** 心肌的收缩使心脏跳动。***Hormones from the pituitary gland activate other glands.*** 垂体分泌的激素可以激活其他腺体。

◇ **active** *adjective* (**a**) (*of person*) lively, energetic(人)有活力的: ***Although he is over eighty he is still very active.*** 尽管年过八旬,他仍精力充沛。**active movement** = movement made by a patient using his own willpower and muscles 病人的自主运动 (**b**) (*of disease*) which affects a patient, which is not dormant(疾病)活动的: ***after two years of active rheumatoid disease*** 患活动性类风湿疾病两年后 (**c**) which acts, does something 有效的,起作用的; **active ingredient** = main medicinal ingredient of an ointment or lotion (as opposed to the base) 软膏或洗液的有效成分; **active principle** = main medicinal ingredient of a drug which makes it have the required effect on a patient 活性成分,药物中赋与疗效的成分

◇ **activity** *noun* what something does 活性,活力: ***The drug's activity did not last more than a few hours.*** 此药的活性仅能保持几个小时。**antibacterial activity** = effective action against bacteria 抗菌活性

actomyosin *noun* combination of actin and myosin, which forms the contractile tissue of muscle 肌动肌球蛋白,肌动蛋白和肌球蛋白的联合体,是肌肉中的可收缩组织

actual *adjective* real 实际的: ***What are the actual figures for the number of children in school?*** 学校内学生的实际人数是多少?

◇ **actually** *adverb* really 实际,事实上: ***Is he actually going to discharge***

himself from the hospital？他真的打算出院吗？

acuity *noun* sharpness 敏锐；**visual acuity** = being able to see objects clearly 视觉敏锐

acupuncture *noun* treatment originating in China, where needles are inserted through the skin into nerve centres in order to relieve pain or treat a disorder, etc. 针灸

◇ **acupuncturist** *noun* person who practises acupuncture 针灸师

acute *adjective* (i) (disease) which comes on rapidly and can be dangerous (疾病)急性的(ii) (pain) which is sharp and intense (疼痛)剧烈的，严重的：***She had an acute attack of shingles.*** 他患了急性带状疱疹。***He felt acute chest pains.*** 他感觉剧烈胸痛。***After the acute stage of the illness had passed he felt very weak.*** 当疾病的急性期过去后，他感觉很虚弱。**acute abdomen** = any serious condition of the abdomen which may require surgery 急腹症；**acute bed** = hospital bed reserved for acute cases 急诊床(NOTE: the opposite is **chronic**)

◇ **acute yellow atrophy** 急性黄色萎缩 *see* 见 YELLOW

> QUOTE: Twenty-seven adult patients admitted to hospital with acute abdominal pains were referred for study.
> 引文：对27例因急腹症入院的患者进行了研究。
> **Lancet** 柳叶刀

> QUOTE: The survey shows a reduction in acute beds in the last six years. The bed losses forced one hospital to send acutely ill patients to hospitals up to sixteen miles away.
> 引文：调查显示最近6年急诊床位减少。床位的减少迫使一家医院将急性病人送到16英里外的医院去。
> **Nursing Times** 护理时代

acystia *noun* congenital defect, where a baby is born without a bladder 无膀胱，是一种先天缺陷

Adam's apple *noun* piece of the thyroid cartilage surrounding the voice box, which projects from the neck below the chin in a man and moves up and down when he speaks or swallows 喉结

adapt *verb* to change to fit a new situation 适应：***She has adapted very well to her new job in the children's hospital.*** 她很适应在儿童医院的新工作。***The brace has to be adapted to fit the patient.*** 支架必须调整使之适合病人。

◇ **adaptation** *noun* (i) changing something so that it fits a new situation 适合，适应 (ii) process by which sensory receptors become accustomed to a sensation which is repeated 适应过程；**dark adaptation** *or* **light adaptation** = changes in the eye in response to changes in light conditions 暗适应或光适应，眼睛对光线变化的反应

addict *noun* 有瘾的人，瘾君子；**drug addict** = person who is physically and mentally dependent on taking drugs regularly 药瘾者，肉体和精神长期依赖药物的人；***a heroin addict*** 对海洛因成瘾者；***a morphine addict*** 吗啡成瘾者

◇ **addicted** *adjective* 成瘾的；**addicted to alcohol** *or* **drugs** = being unable to live without taking alcohol *or* drugs regularly 对酒精或药物成瘾的，离开酒精或药物不能生活的

◇ **addiction** *noun* 成瘾；**drug addiction** *or* **drug dependence** = being mentally and physically dependent on taking a drug regularly 药瘾或药物依赖

◇ **addictive** *adjective* (drug) which is habit-forming *or* which people can become addicted to 使成瘾的：***Certain narcotic drugs are addictive.*** 某些麻醉药有成瘾性。

> QUOTE: Three quarters of patients, aged 35 – 64 on GPs' lists have at least one major risk factor: high cholesterol, high blood pressure or addiction to tobacco.

引文:在全科医生那里登记的 35-64 岁患者中有 3/4 的病人至少有以下一种危险因素:高胆固醇、高血压或烟瘾。
Health Services Journal 健康服务杂志

Addison's anaemia = PERNICIOUS ANAEMIA 恶性贫血

◇ **Addison's disease** *noun* disease of the adrenal glands, resulting in general weakness, anaemia, low blood pressure and wasting away 阿狄森氏病,表现虚弱、贫血、低血压和消瘦

COMMENT: The most noticeable symptom of the disease is the change in skin colour to yellow and then to dark brown. Treatment consists of corticosteroid injections.
注释:本病最常见的症状是皮肤颜色变黄进而变成深棕色。治疗包括注射可的松。

additive *noun* chemical substance which is added, especially one which is added to food to improve its appearance or to prevent it going bad 添加剂: ***The tin of beans contains a number of additives.*** 豆罐头中含有大量添加剂。***Asthmatic and allergic reactions to additives are frequently found in workers in food processing factories.*** 在食品加工厂工作的工人中常有对添加剂发生哮喘和过敏反应的人。

adducted *adjective* brought towards the middle of the body 内收的; **vocal folds adducted** = position of the vocal cords for speaking 声带处于内收状态,声带在说话时的位置

◇ **adduction** *noun* movement of part of the body towards the midline or towards a neighbouring part 内收,身体的某一部分向中线靠近或向临近部位靠近

◇ **adductor (muscle)** *noun* muscle which pulls a part of the body towards the midline of the body 内收肌,使身体的一部分向中线运动的肌肉 (NOTE: opposites are **abducted**, **abduction**, **abductor**)

aden- *or* **adeno-** *prefix* referring to glands 腺体的

◇ **adenectomy** *noun* surgical removal of a gland 腺体切除术

◇ **adenine** *noun* one of the four basic elements in DNA 腺嘌呤,形成脱氧核糖核酸的 4 种碱基之一

◇ **adenitis** *noun* inflammation of the lymph glands 淋巴结炎, 腺炎

◇ **adenocarcinoma** *noun* malignant tumour of a gland 腺癌

◇ **adenohypophysis** *noun* front lobe of the pituitary gland which secretes several hormones which themselves stimulate the adrenal and thyroid glands, or which stimulate the production of sex hormones, melanin and milk 腺垂体,垂体前叶,分泌若干种激素,刺激肾上腺和甲状腺,或性激素、黑色素和乳汁的分泌

adenoid *adjective* like a gland 腺体样的

◇ **adenoids** *plural noun* condition where growths form on the glands at the back of the throat where the passages from the nose join the throat, which prevent the patient breathing through the nose 腺样增殖体,喉后部经鼻到喉通道上腺体增生,使病人难于用鼻呼吸; **enlargement of the adenoids** *or* **adenoid vegetation** = condition in children where the adenoidal tissue is covered with growths and can block the nasal passages or the Eustachian tubes 腺样增殖体,小孩腺样增生,可阻塞鼻道或咽鼓管: ***Removal of the adenoids is sometimes indicated.*** 有时需切除腺样增殖体。

◇ **adenoidal** *adjective* referring to adenoids 腺样的; **adenoidal expression** = common symptom of child suffering from adenoids, where his mouth is always open, the nose is narrow and the top teeth appear to project forward 腺样增殖面容,腺样增殖儿童的常见症状,口总张着,鼻道狭窄,上牙外龇; **adenoidal tissue** = the pharyngeal tonsils, glands at the back of the throat where the passages from the nose join the throat 腺样组织,咽扁桃体,喉后部从鼻到喉的通道上的腺体

◇ **adenoidectomy** *noun* surgical removal of the adenoids 增埴腺切除术

◇ **adenoidism** *noun* condition of a person with adenoids 增殖腺病: ***The***

little boy suffers from adenoidism. 这个小男孩患有增埴腺病。

adenoma *noun* benign tumour of a gland 腺瘤,腺体的良性肿瘤

◇ **adenomyoma** *noun* benign tumour made up of glands and muscle 腺肌瘤,由腺体和肌肉组织组成的良性肿瘤

◇ **adenopathy** *noun* disease of a gland 腺体病

◇ **adenosclerosis** *noun* hardening of a gland 腺硬化

◇ **adenosine triphosphate** (**ATP**) *noun* chemical which occurs in all cells, but mainly in muscle, where it forms the energy reserve 三磷酸腺苷,存在于所有细胞中,但更多见于肌肉,是肌肉中的能量储存物质

◇ **adenosis** *noun* any disease or disorder of the glands 腺体疾病

◇ **adenovirus** *noun* virus which produces upper respiratory infections and sore throats and can cause fatal pneumonia in infants 腺病毒,造成上呼吸道感染和嗓子疼,对婴儿可以造成致命的肺炎

adequate *adjective* enough 充足的,足够的: ***The brain must have an adequate supply of blood.*** 大脑必须有充足的供血。***Does the children's diet provide them with an adequate quantity of iron?*** 儿童的膳食是否提供了足量的铁?

ADH = ANTIDIURETIC HORMONE 抗利尿激素

adhesion *noun* abnormal connection between two surfaces in the body which should not be connected 粘连

◇ **adhesive** *adjective* which sticks 粘附的; **adhesive dressing** *or* **adhesive plaster** *or* **adhesive tape** = dressing with a sticky substance on the back so that it can stick to the skin 胶带,橡皮膏; **adhesive strapping** = overlapping strips of adhesive plaster used to protect a lesion 创可贴

adipose *adjective* containing fat, made of fat 多脂的; **adipose tissue** = body fat, tissue where the cells contain fat 脂肪组织; **adipose degeneration** 脂肪变性 *see* 见 DEGENERATION

COMMENT: Normal fibrous tissue is replaced by adipose tissue when more food is eaten than is necessary. 注释:摄食过多可导致正常的纤维组织被脂肪组织替代。

◇ **adiposis dolorosa** *noun* Dercum's disease, a disease of middle-aged women where painful lumps of fatty substance form in the body 痛性肥胖病,即德尔肯氏病,侵及中年妇女,体内形成由脂肪物质构成的痛性团块

◇ **adiposogenitalis** = DYSTROPHIA ADIPOSOGENITALIS 肥胖性生殖器退化综合症 *see* 见 FRÖHLICH'S SYNDROME

◇ **adiposuria** *noun* fat in the urine 脂肪尿

◇ **adiposus**脂的 *see* 见 PANNICULUS

aditus *noun* opening or entrance to a passage 口,入口

adjuvant 1 *adjective* (treatment) which uses drugs, radiation therapy, etc. following surgery for cancer 辅助的,癌症手术后进行的诸如药物、放疗等辅助性的(治疗) **2** *noun* substance added to a drug to enhance the effect of the main ingredient 佐剂,辅药

administer *verb* to give (a medicine) to a patient 给病人用药; **to administer orally** = to give a medicine by mouth 口服给药

◇ **administration** *noun* (**a**) giving of a medicine 给药: ***Administration of drugs must be supervised by a qualified doctor or nurse.*** 用药必须有合格的医护人员的监管。(**b**) management, running of a hospital, service, etc. 管理,经营; **medical administration** = running of hospitals and other health services 医院管理: ***She started her career in medical administration.*** 她最初从事的职业是医院管理。

◇ **administrative** *adjective* referring to administration 管理的,行政的: ***Most of the GP's spare time is taken up with administrative work.*** 大部分全科医生的业余时间用于管理工作。

◇ **administrator** *noun* person who

runs (a hospital, district health authority,etc.)(对医院、地区卫生局)进行管理的行政管理人员

admit *verb* to allow (someone) to go in; to register a patient in a hospital 接纳,入院: ***Children are admitted free.*** 儿童免费入院。***He was admitted (to hospital) this morning.*** 他今晨住院了。

◇ **admission** *noun* being allowed into a place 允许进入; **admission to the hospital** = official registering of a patient in a hospital 住院,入院

> QUOTE: 80% of elderly patients admitted to geriatric units are on medication.
> 引文:老年病区中80%的患者需药物治疗。
> **Nursing Times** 护理时代

> QUOTE: Ten patients were admitted to the ICU before operation, the main indications being the need for evaluation of patients with a history of severe heart disease.
> 引文:10名患者在手术前被送入ICU,评估的主要指征是有严重心脏病史。
> **Southern Medical Journal** 南方医学杂志

adnexa *plural noun* structures attached to an organ 附件,附器

adolescence *noun* period of life when a child is developing into an adult 青春期

◇ **adolescent** *noun & adjective* (person) who is at the stage of life when he is developing into an adult 青少年,青春期的

adopt *verb* to become the legal parent of a child who was born to other parents 收养

◇ **adoption** *noun* act of becoming the legal parent of a child who was born to other parents 收养; **adoption order** = order by a court which legally transfers the rights of the natural parents to the adoptive parents 收养令,法庭判定合法收养的命令; **adoption proceedings** = court action to adopt someone 收养程序,收养某人的法庭行为

◇ **adoptive** *adjective* 收养的; **adoptive child** *or* **son** *or* **daughter** = child *or* son *or* daughter who has been adopted 养子或养女; **adoptive parent** = person who has adopted a child 养父母

> COMMENT: If a child's parents are divorced or if one parent dies, the child may be adopted by a step-father or step-mother.
> 注释:如果一个儿童的父母离婚了或一方死亡,他可被养父或养母收养。

◇ **adoptive immunotherapy** *noun* treatment for cancer in which the patient's own white blood cells are used to attack cancer cells 过继免疫疗法

> COMMENT: This technique was discovered in 1980 and can halt the growth of cancer cells in the body. Much of the more recent research has examined ways of minimizing the distressing toxic side-effects of the substances used.
> 注释:此技术发明于1980年,它可以延缓机体肿瘤细胞的生长。最近的研究大部分在探讨减少其毒副作用的方法。

adrenal *adjective* situated near the kidney 肾脏附近的,肾上腺的; **adrenal body** = an adrenal gland 肾上腺; **adrenal cortex** = firm outside layer of an adrenal gland, which secretes a series of hormones affecting the metabolism of carbohydrates and water 肾上腺皮质,肾上腺较坚硬的外层,分泌影响碳水化合物和水代谢的一系列激素; **adrenal glands** *or* **suprarenal glands** *US* **the adrenals** = two endocrine glands at the top of the kidneys, which secrete cortisone, adrenaline and other hormones 肾上腺,肾上的两个内分泌腺,分泌皮质素、肾上腺素和其他激素; **adrenal medulla** = soft inner part of the adrenal gland which secretes adrenaline and noradrenaline 肾上腺髓质,肾上腺内部的较软的部分,分泌肾上腺素和去甲肾上腺素 ◊ 见图 KIDNEY

◇ **adrenalectomy** *noun* surgical removal of one of the adrenal glands 肾上腺切除术; **bilateral adrenalectomy** = surgical removal of both adrenal glands

双侧肾上腺切除

◇ **adrenaline** *noun* hormone secreted by the medulla of the adrenal glands which has an effect similar to stimulation of the sympathetic nervous system 肾上腺素,肾上腺髓质分泌的激素,作用与刺激交感系统相类似 (NOTE: US English is **epinephrine**)

> COMMENT: Adrenaline is produced when a person experiences surprise, shock, fear, excitement; it speeds up the heartbeat and raises blood pressure.
> 注释:当人处于惊讶、震惊、恐惧或兴奋状态时,会分泌肾上腺素使心跳加速、血压升高。

◇ **adrenergic receptors** *plural noun* nerves which are stimulated by adrenaline 肾上腺素能受体

> COMMENT: Three types of adrenergic receptor act in different ways when stimulated by adrenaline. Alpha receptors constrict the bronchi, beta 1 receptors speed up the heartbeat and beta 2 receptors dilate the bronchi. see also 参见 BETA BLOCKER
> 注释:肾上腺素可激活 3 种受体而发挥不同的作用。α 受体收缩支气管,$β_1$ 受体使心跳加速,$β_2$ 舒张支气管。

adrenocortical *adjective* referring to the cortex of the adrenal glands 肾上腺皮质的

◇ **adrenocorticotrophin** *or* **adrenocorticotrophic hormone** (**ACTH**) *noun* corticotrophin, a hormone secreted by the pituitary gland, which makes the cortex of the adrenal glands produce corticosteroids 促肾上腺皮质激素,由垂体分泌的激素,促使肾上腺皮质产生皮质醇

◇ **adrenogenital syndrome** *noun* condition caused by overproduction of male sex hormones, where boys show rapid sexual development and females show virilization 肾上腺(性)性征综合征,雄性激素产生过多所致,男孩表现为性发育加速,女子表现为男性化

◇ **adrenolytic** *adjective* acting against the secretion of adrenaline 抗肾上腺素的,对抗肾上腺素分泌的

adsorbent *adjective* capable of adsorption 有吸附力的

◇ **adsorption** *noun* bonding of a solid with a gas or vapour which touches its surface 吸附,气体或蒸汽与固体表面接触时与之结合

adult *noun & adjective* grown-up (person, animal) 成人,成熟: ***Adolescents reach the adult stage about the age of eighteen or twenty.*** 青少年在 18 或 20 岁时跨入成人阶段。

advanced *adjective* which has developed 进展的; ***the advanced stages of a disease*** 疾病的进展期: ***He is suffering from advanced syphilis.*** 他得了进展期梅毒。

adventitia *noun* 外膜; (**tunica**) **adventitia** = outer layer of the wall of an artery or vein 动脉或静脉壁的外层,外膜

◇ **adventitious** *adjective* which is on the outside 外层的,异位的; **adventitious bursa** 外膜囊,磨擦囊,偶发性粘液囊 *see* 见 BURSA

adverse *adjective* harmful, unfavourable 敌对的,不利的: **The treatment had an adverse effect on his dermatitis.** = It made it worse. 这种治疗有恶化他的皮炎的副作用。**adverse reaction from a drug** = situation where a patient suffers harmful effects from the application of a drug 药物引起的不良反应

advice *noun* suggestion about what should be done 建议: ***He went to the psychiatrist for advice on how to cope with his problem.*** 他去看精神科医生寻求解决自己问题的建议。***She would not listen to my advice.*** 他不听我的忠告。***The doctor's advice was that he should take a long holiday.*** 医生建议他休个长假。***The doctor's advice was to stay in bed.*** 医生建议卧床休息。***He took the doctor's advice and went to bed.*** 他听从医生的建议上床休息。(NOTE: no plural: **some advice** or **a piece of advice**)

advise *verb* to suggest what should be done 劝告,建议: ***The doctor advised him to stay in bed.*** 医生劝他卧床休息。***She***

advised me to have a checkup. 她劝我去做次体检。***I would advise you not to drink alcohol.*** 我劝你不要再喝酒了。

◇ **advise against** *verb* to suggest that something should not be done 忠告：***He wanted to leave hospital but the consultant advised against it.*** 他想出院，但会诊医生不同意。***The doctor advised against going to bed late.*** 医生建议不要晚睡。

adynamic ileus *noun* obstruction in the ileum caused by paralysis of the muscles of the intestine 麻痹性肠梗阻，肠道肌肉瘫痪造成的肠梗阻

aegophony *noun* high sound of the voice heard through a stethoscope, where there is fluid in the pleural cavity 羊鸣音，当胸膜腔积液时从听诊器听到的高调声音

aeroba *or* **aerobe** *noun* tiny organism which needs oxygen to survive 需氧生物

◇ **aerobic** *adjective* needing oxygen to live 需氧的；**aerobic respiration** = process where the oxygen which is breathed in is used to conserve energy as ATP 需氧呼吸，吸入氧气以供将能量储存为 ATP

◇ **aerobics** *plural noun* exercises which aim to increase the amount of oxygen taken into the body 有氧运动，旨在增加氧气摄入量的运动

aerogenous *adjective* (bacterium) which produces gas（细菌）产气的 **aerophagy** *or* **aerophagia** *noun* habit of swallowing air when suffering from indigestion, so making the stomach pains worse 吞气症，消化不良时因咽下空气导致胃疼加重

aerosol *noun* (**a**) tiny particles of liquid suspended in a gas under pressure, sprayed from a container and used as a medicine, sterilizing agent, etc. 气雾剂，在一定压力下悬浮在气体中的小液滴，可从贮存罐中喷出，用作药物或消毒剂 (**b**) **aerosol** *or* **aerosol dispenser** = container, device from which liquid can be sprayed in tiny particles 气雾器

aetiology *or US* **etiology** *noun* (study of) the cause *or* origin of a disease 病因学

◇ **aetiological agent** *noun* agent which causes a disease 病因，致病因素

> QUOTE: Wide variety of organs or tissues may be infected by the Salmonella group of organisms, presenting symptoms which are not immediately recognised as being of Salmonella aetiology.
> 引文：很多器官和组织都会被沙门氏菌感染，凭症状不易判定病原菌。
> **Indian Journal of Medical Sciences** 印度医学科学杂志

afebrile *adjective* with no fever 不发热的，无热的

affect *verb* to make something change 影响：***Some organs are rapidly affected if the patient lacks oxygen for even a short time.*** 一些器官即使缺氧很短时间，其功能也会受影响。

◇ **affection** *or* **affect** *noun* type of feeling; general state of a person's emotions 感情，情感

> QUOTE: Depression has degrees of severity, ranging from sadness, through flatness of affect or feeling, to suicide and psychosis.
> 引文：抑郁有不同程度，从难过、情感平淡到自杀和精神病。
> **British Journal of Nursing**
> 英国护理杂志

◇ **affective** *adjective* concerning the emotions 情感的；**affective disorder** = condition which changes the mood of a patient, making him or her depressed or excited 情感障碍，改变病人心境的疾病，使他或她抑郁或兴奋

afferent *adjective* which conducts liquid *or* impulses towards the inside 传入的 (NOTE: opposite is **efferent**)

affinity *noun* attraction between two substances 亲和，吸引

afford *verb* to have enough money to pay for something 担负得起：***I can't afford to go to hospital.*** 我负不起医药费。***How can you afford this expensive***

treatment？你如何能负得起如此昂贵的治疗费？

after- *prefix* which comes later, which take place later 在…之后

◇ **afterbirth** *noun* tissues (including the placenta and umbilical cord) which are present in the uterus during pregnancy and are expelled after the birth of the baby 胞衣，胎盘，胎膜，孕期存在于子宫中，胎儿娩出后排除的组织，包括胎盘和脐带 *see also* 参见 PLACENTA

◇ **aftercare** *noun* care of a person who has had an operation; care of a mother who has just given birth 术后护理或产后护理：***Aftercare treatment involves changing dressings and helping the patient to look after himself again.*** 术后护理包括更换敷料，帮助患者重新学会照顾自己。

◇ **after-effects** *plural noun* changes which appear only some time after the cause 后遗症：***The operation had some unpleasant after-effects.*** 手术有一些令人不快的后遗症。

◇ **after-image** *noun* image of an object which remains in a person's sight after the object itself has gone 视觉后像，当物体已经移开后留在人视觉上的图像

◇ **afterpains** *plural noun* regular pains in the uterus which are sometimes experienced after childbirth 产后痛

◇ **aftertaste** *noun* taste which remains in the mouth after the substance which caused it has been removed 余味，引起味觉的物质去除后留在口腔里的味道：***The linctus leaves an unpleasant aftertaste.*** 舔膏剂有一种难闻的余味。

Ag *chemical symbol for* silver 银的化学元素符号

agalactia *noun* (*of mother after childbirth*) being unable to produce milk 无乳的产妇

agammaglobulinaemia *noun* deficiency or absence of gamma globulin in the blood, which results in a reduced ability to provide immune responses 无丙种球蛋白血症，导致免疫反应能力低下

agar *or* **agar agar** *noun* jelly made from seaweed, used to cultivate bacterial cultures in laboratories and also as a laxative 琼脂，用作细菌培养基，也可用来作导泻剂

age 1 *noun* number of years which a person has lived 年龄：***What's your age on your next birthday?*** 明年您多大年纪？***He was sixty years of age.*** 他60岁了。***She looks younger than her age.*** 她比实际年龄显得年轻。***The size varies according to age.*** 大小随年龄而改变。**mental age** = age of a person's mental state, measured by intelligence tests (usually compared to that of a normal person of the same chronological age) 智力年龄，即智力水平与通常多大年龄者相当；**old age** = period when a person is old (usually taken to be after the age of sixty-five) 老年(通常指65岁以上) **2** *verb* to grow old 变老，老化

◇ **aged** *adjective* (**a**) with a certain age…岁的：***a boy aged twelve*** 12岁的男孩儿；***He died last year, aged 64.*** 他去年去世，享年64岁。(**b**) very old 老的：***an aged man*** 老人

◇ **ageing** *noun* growing old 变老；**the ageing process** = the physical changes which take place in a person as he grows older 衰老

> COMMENT: Changes take place in almost every part of the body as the person ages. Bones become more brittle, skin is less elastic. The most important changes affect the blood vessels which are less elastic, making thrombosis more likely. This also reduces the supply of blood to the brain, which in turn reduces the mental faculties.
>
> 注释：人衰老时身体的各部分都会发生变化，骨质变脆，皮肤弹性减弱。最明显的是血管弹性降低，易形成血栓，导致脑供血不足，最终影响智力。

agent *noun* (**a**) person who acts for another, often in another country 代理人：***He is the agent for an American pharmaceutical firm.*** 他是一家美国药厂的代理人。(**b**) chemical substance which makes another substance react 试剂 (**c**) substance or organism which causes a disease or condition 致病物质,病原

◇ **agency** *noun* (**a**) action of causing something to happen 媒介: ***The disease develops through the agency of certain bacteria present in the bloodstream.*** 此病是由血液中的某种细菌介导发生的。(**b**) office, organization which provides nurses for temporary work in hospitals, clinics, in private houses(介绍临时护士的)代理机构

> QUOTE: The cost of employing agency nurses should be no higher than the equivalent full-time staff.
> 引文:由代理机构介绍的护士,其费用不能高于同等的全日制员工。
> **Nursing Times** 护理时代

> QUOTE: Growing numbers of nurses are choosing agency careers, which pay more and provide more flexible schedules than hospitals.
> 引文:越来越多的护士选择代理机构,因为它提供的报酬比医院高,且工作时间更灵活。
> **American Journal of Nursing** 美国护理杂志

agglutinate *verb* to form into groups or clusters 粘连,聚集

◇ **agglutination** *noun* action of grouping together of cells (as of bacteria cells in the presence of serum *or* blood cells when blood of different types is mixed) 细胞凝集; **agglutination test** = (i) test to identify bacteria (ii) test to identify if a woman is pregnant 凝集实验,用于鉴别细菌或确定妊娠

◇ **agglutinin** *noun* factor in a serum which makes cells group together 凝集素,血清中使细胞凝集的因子

◇ **agglutinogen** *noun* factor in red blood cells which reacts with a specific agglutinin in serum 凝集原,红细胞中的因子,与血清中特异性凝集素起反应 *see also* 参见 PAUL-BUNNELL, WEIL-FELIX, WIDAL

aggravate *verb* to make worse 使加重,使恶化: ***Playing football only aggravates his knee injury.*** 踢足球只会加重他的膝伤。***The treatment seems to aggravate the disease.*** 治疗似乎加重了病情。

aggression *noun* state of feeling violently angry towards someone, something 攻击性,敌意

◇ **aggressive** *adjective* (treatment) involving frequent high doses of medication(治疗)加强的,强化的

agitated *adjective* moving about or twitching nervously (because of worry or other psychological state) 焦躁不安的: ***The patient became agitated and had to be given a sedative.*** 患者变得焦躁不安,不得不给予镇静药。

◇ **agitans** 震颤 *see* 见 PARALYSIS

agnosia *noun* brain disorder where the patient cannot understand what his senses tell him and so fails to recognize places, people *or* tastes, smells which he used to know well 失认,是一种脑功能障碍,病人不能理解听到言语的意义,不能识别以前能分辨的地点、人、味及嗅。

agony *noun* very severe pain 极度痛苦: ***He lay in agony on the floor.*** 他痛苦地躺在地板上。***She suffered agonies until her condition was diagnosed.*** 在确诊前她忍受了极大的痛苦。

agoraphobia *noun* fear of being in open spaces 广场恐惧症(精神病的一种)

◇ **agoraphobic** *noun & adjective* (person) suffering from agoraphobia 患有广场恐惧症的(人)(NOTE: opposite is **claustrophobia**)

agranulocytosis *noun* usually fatal disease where the number of granulocytes (white blood cells) falls sharply because of a defect in the bone marrow 粒细胞缺乏症,粒性白血球缺乏症,由于骨髓缺陷导致粒细胞(白细胞)数量急剧下降,通常是致命的

agraphia *noun* being unable to put ideas in writing 失写,不能写出有意义的词句

agree with *verb* (**a**) to say that you think the same way as someone; to say yes 同意: ***The consultant agreed with***

***the GP's diagnosis*.** 会诊医生同意全科大夫的诊断。(**b**) to be easily digested by someone 易消化的: ***This rich food does not agree with me*.** 我不易消化这种油腻食物。

◇ **agreement** *noun* action of agreeing 同意: **They are in agreement with our plan.** = They agree with it. 他们同意我们的计划。

aid **1** *noun* (**a**) help 帮助; **medical aid** = treatment of someone who is ill or injured, given by a doctor 医疗救助 *see also* 参见 FIRST (**b**) machine or tool or drug which helps someone do something 辅助物: ***He uses a walking frame as an aid to exercising his legs*.** 他利用拐杖进行腿部锻炼。**2** *verb* to help 帮助: ***The reason for the procedure is to aid repair of tissues after surgery*.** 此过程用来帮助术后组织的修复。

◇ **aider** *noun* person who helps 提供帮助的人; **first-aider** = person who gives first aid to someone who is suddenly ill *or* injured 第一救护者,当某人突然病倒或受伤时第一个提供紧急救助的人

AID = ARTIFICIAL INSEMINATION BY DONOR 人工受精

AIDS *or* **Aids** *noun* (= ACQUIRED IMMUNODEFICIENCY SYNDROME) viral infection which breaks down the body's immune system 艾滋病,获得性免疫缺陷综合症: ***There are two patients with AIDS or two AIDS patients in the clinic*.** 诊所有两位艾滋病患者。**AIDS-related condition** *or* **complex** (**ARC**) = early symptom or illness, such as loss of weight, fever, herpes zoster, etc., exhibited by a patient infected with the HIVvirus 艾滋病相关症状,体重下降、发热、带状疱疹等爱滋病患者的早期症状或伴发疾病

> COMMENT: AIDS is a virus disease, spread by the HIV virus. It is spread mostly by sexual intercourse and although at first associated with male homosexuals, it is now known to affect anyone. It is also transmitted through infected blood and plasma transfusions, through using unsterilized needles for injections, and can be passed from a mother to a fetus. The disease takes a long time, even years, to show symptoms, so there are many carriers. It causes a breakdown of the body's immune system, making the patient susceptible to any infection and often results in the development of rare skin cancers. It is not curable.
> 注释:艾滋病是由 HIV 病毒引起的一种病毒性疾病,多由性传播。早期主要是男性同性恋者,现认为任何人均可累及。它还可通过输注污染的血制品、未经消毒的注射器及母婴传播。此病的潜伏期很长,甚至几年,所以有很多带毒者。它可以导致机体的抵抗力下降,患者易患感染及少见的皮肤肿瘤,它是不治之症。

AIH = ARTIFICIAL INSEMINATION BY HUSBAND 亲夫人工受精

ailing *adjective* not well for a period of time 患病的: ***He stayed at home to look after his ailing parents*.** 他在家照顾患病的父母。

◇ **ailment** *noun* illness, though not generally a very serious one 疾病,小恙: ***Measles is one of the common childhood ailments*.** 麻疹是一种常见的儿童疾病。

ailurophobia *noun* fear of cats 恐猫症

aim *verb* (**a**) to point at 针对,对准: ***The X-ray beam is aimed at the patient's jaw*.** X 射线对准患者的下颌。(**b**) to intend to do something 目的在于: ***We aim to eradicate tuberculosis by the end of the century*.** 我们计划在本世纪末消灭结核。

air *noun* mixture of gases (mainly oxygen and nitrogen) which cannot be seen, but which exists all around us and which is breathed 空气: ***The air in the mountains felt cold*.** 山中的空气有点凉。***He breathed the polluted air into his lungs*.** 他呼吸着受污染的空气。**air bed** = mattress which is filled with air, used to prevent the formation of bedsores 气

褥,用于防止褥疮的产生 *see also* 参见 CONDUCTION; **air embolism** = interference with blood flow caused by air bubbles 空气栓塞,气泡妨碍血流; **air hunger** = condition where the patient needs air because of lack of oxygen in the tissues 缺氧; **air passages** = tubes, formed of the nose, pharynx, larynx, trachea and bronchi, which take air to the lungs 气道; **air sac** *or* **alveolus** = small sac in the lungs which contains air 气囊,肺泡囊

◇ **airsick** *adjective* feeling sick because of the movement of an aircraft 晕机的

◇ **airsickness** *noun* sickness caused by the movement of an aircraft 晕机

◇ **airway** *noun* passage through which air passes, especially the trachea 气道; **airway clearing** = making sure that the airways in a newborn baby or an unconscious person are free of any obstruction 清理气道; **airway obstruction** = something which blocks the air passages 气道阻塞

akinesia *noun* lack of voluntary movement (as in Parkinson's disease) 运动不能,不能自主运动,如帕金森氏病

◇ **akinetic** *adjective* without movement 运动不能

alactasia *noun* condition where there is a deficiency of lactase in the intestine, making the patient incapable of digesting milk sugar(lactose) 乳糖酶缺乏症,小肠缺乏此酶病人不能消化乳糖

alanine *noun* amino acid in protein 丙氨酸

alar cartilage *noun* cartilage in the outer wings of the nose 翼状软骨,鼻软骨之一

alba 脑白质 *see* 见 LINEA

Albee's operation *noun* (i) surgical operation to fuse two or more vertebrae 脊椎椎体融合术 (ii) surgical operation to fuse the femur to the pelvis 阿尔比氏手术,股骨头髋臼融和术

albicans 白色的 *see* 见 CANDIDA ALBICANS, CORPUS ALBICANS

albino *noun* person who is deficient in melanin, with little or no pigmentation in skin, hair or eyes 白化病人,缺乏黑色素的人,皮肤、头发和眼睛几乎没有色素

◇ **albinism** *noun* condition where the patient lacks melanin and so has pink skin and eyes and white hair 白化病,病人缺乏黑色素,皮肤、眼睛呈粉红色,头发白色 *see also* 参见 VITILIGO

> COMMENT: Albinism is hereditary and cannot be treated.
> 注释:白化病是一种遗传性的不治之症。

albuginea *noun* layer of white tissue covering a part of the body 白膜; **albuginea oculi** = sclera, the white outer covering of the eyeball 巩膜

albumin *noun* common protein, soluble in water and found in plant and animal tissue and digested in the intestine 白蛋白; **serum albumin** = major protein in blood plasma 血清白蛋白

◇ **albuminometer** *noun* instrument for measuring the level of albumin in the urine 白蛋白测量计

◇ **albuminuria** *noun* condition where albumin is found in the urine, usually a sign of kidney disease, but also sometimes of heart failure 白蛋白尿,见于肾病和心衰时

◇ **albumose** *noun* intermediate product in the digestion of protein 蛋白䏡,蛋白质消化的中间产物

alcohol *noun* pure colourless liquid, which forms part of drinks such as wine and whisky, and which is formed by the action of yeast on sugar solutions 酒精; **alcohol abuse** *or* **alcohol addiction** = condition where a patient is addicted to drinking alcohol and cannot stop 滥用酒精,酗酒; **alcohol poisoning** = poisoning and disease caused by excessive drinking of alcohol 酒精中毒; **pure alcohol** *or* **ethyl alcohol** *or* **ethanol** = colourless liquid, which is the basis of drinking alcohols(whisky, gin, vodka, etc.) and which is also used in medicines and as a disinfectant 乙醇,食用酒精中的基本物质,医学上用于制剂或消毒; **denatured alcohol** = ethyl alcohol (such as methylated spirit, rubbingalcohol, surgical spirit) with an additive (usually methyl-alcohol) to make it unpleasant to drink 变性醇; **methyl alcohol** = wood alcohol (poisonous alcohol used for heating) 甲醇; **alcohol rub** = rubbing a bedridden patient with alcohol to help protect against bedsores and as a tonic 酒精擦浴

◇ **alcohol-fast** *adjective* (organ stained for testing) which is not discoloured by alcohol 抗酒精脱色的

◇ **alcoholic 1** *adjective* (i) containing alcohol 含酒精的 (ii) caused by alcoholism 酒精中毒的: ***Children should not be encouraged to take alcoholic drinks.*** 儿童不能喝含酒精的饮料。***alcoholic poisoning*** 酒精中毒; **alcoholic cirrhosis** = cirrhosis of the liver caused by alcoholism 酒精性肝硬化 **2** *noun* person who is addicted to drinking alcohol and shows changes in behaviour and personality 酗酒者

◇ **Alcoholics Anonymous** *noun* organization of former alcoholics which helps sufferers from alcoholism to overcome their dependence on alcohol by encouraging them to talk about their problems in group therapy 匿名者酒协会,由曾对酒精成瘾的人组成,旨在帮助酒瘾者脱离对酒精依赖的组织,主要靠在集体治疗中鼓励倾诉问题达到治疗效果。

◇ **alcoholicum**谵妄 *see* 见 DELIRIUM

◇ **alcoholism** *noun* excessive drinking of alcohol which becomes addictive 酒精中毒,酗酒

◇ **alcoholuria** *noun* condition where alcohol is present in the urine (the level of alcohol in the urine is used as a test for drunken drivers) 醇尿

> COMMENT: Alcohol is used medicinally to dry wounds or harden the skin. When drunk, alcohol is rapidly absorbed into the bloodstream. It is a source of energy, so any carbohydrates taken at the same time are not used by the body and are stored as fat. Alcohol is adepressant, not a stimulant, and affects the mental faculties.
> 注释:酒精在医学上用于干燥伤口,硬化皮肤。喝酒后,酒精会很快进入血液并产生能量,而同时摄入的碳水化合物将会转化为脂肪。酒精对大脑活动是抑制剂而不是兴奋剂,并会影响心智。

aldosterone *noun* hormone secreted by the cortex of the adrenal gland and which regulates the balance of sodium and potassium in the body and the amount of body fluid 醛固酮,肾上腺皮质分泌的一种激素,调节体内钠、钾平衡和体液量

alert *adjective* (person) who takes an intelligent interest in his surroundings 警觉的,清醒的,警醒的: ***The patient is still alert, though in great pain.*** 尽管疼痛剧烈,患者仍保持清醒。

aleukaemic *adjective* (i) (state) where leukaemia is not present 非白血病的 (ii) (state) where leucocytes are not normal 白细胞异常的

alexia *noun* word blindness, a condition where the patient cannot understand printed words 失读,字盲,不能理解书写的词句

algae *plural noun* class of lower plants, many of which are seaweeds 海藻,水藻

algesimeter *noun* instrument to measure the sensitivity of the skin to pain 痛觉测定仪

algid *adjective* cold, (stage in an attack of cholera or malaria) where the body becomes cold 发冷的(尤指生疟疾和霍乱时发冷)

alimentary canal *noun* tube in the body going from the mouth to the anus and including the throat, stomach, intestine, etc., through which food passes and is digested 消化道

◇ **alimentary system** *noun* arrangement of tubes and organs, including the alimentary canal, salivary glands, liver, etc., through which food passes and is digested 消化系统

◇ **alimentation** *noun* feeding, taking

in food 供给食物

alive *adjective* living, not dead 活着的: ***The patient was still alive, even though he had been in the sea for two days.*** 尽管在海水里泡了两天,那病人仍然活着。(NOTE: alive cannot be used in front of a noun: **The patient is alive but a living patient**; Note also that live can be used in front of a noun: **The patient was injected with live vaccine**)

alkalaemia *noun* excess of alkali in the blood 碱血症

◇ **alkali** *noun* one of many substances which neutralize acids and form salts 碱 (NOTE: British English plural is **alkalis**, but US English is **alkalies**)

◇ **alkaline** *adjective* containing more alkali than acid 碱的,碱性的

◇ **alkalinity** *noun* level of alkali in a body 碱度,碱性: ***Hyperventilation causes fluctuating carbon dioxide levels in the blood, resulting in an increase of blood alkalinity.*** 过度通气使血中的二氧化碳水平波动,血的碱度增高。

◇ **alkaloid 1** *adjective* similar to an alkali 似碱的,碱样的 **2** *noun* one of many poisonous substances (such as atropine, morphine or quinine) found in plants and used as medicines 生物碱,如阿托品、吗啡或奎宁之类从植物中提取的物质,可以作药

◇ **alkalosis** *noun* condition where the alkali level in the body tissue is high, producing cramps 碱中毒,体内碱水平过高,可导致痉挛; **metabolic alkalosis** = alkalosis caused by a defect in the body's metabolism 代谢性碱中毒

> COMMENT: Alkalinity and acidity are measured according to the pH scale. pH7 is neutral, and pH8 and upwards are alkaline. Alkaline solutions are used to counteract the effects of acid poisoning and also of bee stings. If strong alkali (such as ammonia) is swallowed, the patient should drink water and an acid such as orange juice. Alkalosis can be caused by vomiting.
>
> 注释:酸碱度由 pH 值来衡量,pH 7 是中性,pH 8 以上是碱性。碱性液可用来对抗酸中毒,治疗蜂蜇伤。喝入强碱(如氨)后,病人需喝水或酸性液体如橘汁等中和。碱中毒可由呕吐引起。

alkaptonuria *noun* hereditary condition where dark pigment is present in the urine 尿黑酸尿,尿中有暗色的色素,是一种遗传疾病

allantoin *noun* powder from the herb comfrey, used to treat skin disorders 尿囊素,从草药西门肺草中提取,用于治疗皮肤病

allantois *noun* one of the membranes in the embryo, shaped like a sac, which grows out of the embryonic hindgut 尿囊,胚胎的一层膜,形如囊状,由胚胎的后肠发育而来

allergen *noun* substance which produces hypersensitivity 过敏原,变应原; **food allergen** = substance in food which produces an allergy 食物中的过敏原

◇ **allergenic** *adjective* which produces an allergy 过敏原的,变应原的; ***the allergenic properties of fungal spores*** 霉菌孢子的过敏原性; **allergenic agent** = substance which produces an allergy 过敏物质,过敏原

◇ **allergic** *adjective* suffering from an allergy 过敏性的,变应性的: ***She is allergic to cats.*** 她对猫过敏。***I'm allergic to penicillin.*** 我对青霉素过敏。***He showed an allergic reaction to chocolate.*** 他对巧克力过敏。**allergic agent** = substance which produces an allergic reaction 过敏原,引起过敏的物质; **allergic person** = person who has an allergy to something 对…过敏的人; **allergic reaction** = effect (such as a skin rash or sneezing) produced by a substance to which a person has an allergy 过敏反应

◇ **allergist** *noun* doctor who specializes in the treatment of allergies 过敏症专家

◇ **allergy** *noun* sensitivity to certain substances such as pollen or dust, which cause a physical reaction 过敏性,反应性: ***She has an allergy to household dust.***

她对室内灰尘过敏。***He has a penicillin allergy*.**他对青霉素过敏。**drug allergy** = reaction to a certain drug 药物过敏; **respiratory allergy** = allergy caused by a substance which is inhaled 吸入过敏,呼吸道过敏 *see also* 参见 ALVEOLITIS, FOOD (NOTE: you have an allergy or you are allergic **to** something)

> COMMENT: Allergens are usually proteins, and include foods, dust, hair of animals, as well as pollen from flowers. Allergic reaction to serum is known as anaphylaxis. Treatment of allergies depends on correctly identifying the allergen to which the patient is sensitive. This is done by patch tests in which drops of different allergens are placed on scratches in the skin. Food allergens discovered in this way can be avoided, but other allergens (such as dust and pollen) can hardly be avoided and have to be treated by a course of desensitizing injections.
> 注释:过敏原常是蛋白质,包括食物、尘埃、动物的毛发及花粉。血清过敏称为过敏反应。治疗过敏反应在于正确识别过敏原,可通过将不同的过敏原置于皮肤划痕上的斑片实验获得。食物中的过敏原可以避免,但其他过敏原(如灰尘、花粉)很难回避,只能通过一系列的脱敏注射来治疗。

alleviate *verb* to make (a pain) less, to relieve (a pain) 减轻,缓解: ***He was given injections to alleviate the pain*.** 给他注射药物缓解疼痛。***The nurses tried to alleviate the suffering of the injured*.** 护士设法减轻伤员的痛苦。

allo- *prefix* different 不同的

◇ **allograft** *or* **homograft** *noun* graft of an organ or tissue from a donor to a recipient of the same species (as from one person to another) 异体移植 *compare* 比较 AUTOGRAFT

◇ **allopathy** *noun* treatment of a condition using drugs which produce opposite symptoms to those of the condition 对抗疗法,用产生与原发病相反症状的药物来治疗 *compare with* 比较 HOMEOPATHY

all or none law *noun* rule that the heart muscle either contracts fully or does not contract at all 全或无法则

all over (**a**) everywhere 浑身,到处: ***There were red marks all over the child's body*.** 此患儿全身布满红斑。***She poured water all over the patient's head*.** 她将水泼了患者一头。(**b**) finished 结束: ***When it was all over we went home*.** 当一切都结束后我们回家。

◇ **all right** *adjective* fine, well, not ill 行,好: ***He's feeling very sick at the moment, but he will be all right in a few hours*.** 现在他觉得很难受,几个小时后就会好多了。***My mother had flu but she is all right now*.** 我母亲患了流感,但她现在已经好了。***His hearing is all right, but his sight is failing*.** 他的听力很好,但视力在下降。

allow *verb* to say that someone can do something 允许,同意: ***The consultant allowed him to watch the operation*.** 会诊医生同意他观看手术。***Patients are not allowed to go outside the hospital*.** 患者不允许走出医院。***He is allowed to eat certain types of food*.** 他被允许吃某几种食物。

almoner *noun* formerly a person working in a hospital, looking after the welfare of patients and the families of patients (now called medical social worker) 医院的社会服务人员

alopecia *noun* baldness 脱发; **alopecia areata** = condition where the hair falls out in patches 斑秃

> COMMENT: Baldness in men is hereditary; it can also occur in men and women as a reaction to an illness or to a drug.
> 注释:男人脱发有遗传性,但某些疾病或药物引起的脱发在男女中都可发生。

alpha *noun* first letter of the Greek alphabet 希腊字母表的第一个字母; **alpha cell** = one of the types of cells in glands (such as the pancreas) which have more than one type of cell 阿尔法细胞,α 细胞 某些腺体细胞,如胰腺细胞的一种

◇ **alpha-fetoprotein** *noun* protein found in the amniotic fluid when the fetus has an open neurological deficiency such as meningomyelocele 胎甲球蛋白

ALS = ANTILYMPHOCYTIC SERUM 抗淋巴细胞血清

altitude sickness = MOUNTAIN SICKNESS 高空病

aluminium hydroxide *or US* **aluminum hydroxide** (**$Al(OH)_3$** *or* **$Al_2O_{33}H_2O$**) *noun* chemical substance used as an antacid to treat indigestion 氢氧化铝,用作抗酸剂治疗消化不良

alveolus *noun* small cavity, such as one of the air sacs in the lungs or the socket into which a tooth fits 泡,槽,小窝 (NOTE: plural is **alveoli**) ◇ 见图 LUNGS

◇ **alveolar** *adjective* referring to alveoli 小泡的,窝的; **alveolar bone** = part of the jawbone to which the teeth are attached 牙槽; **alveolar duct** = duct in the lung which leads from the respiratory bronchioles to the alveoli 肺泡管; **alveolar walls** = walls which separate the alveoli in the lungs 肺泡壁

◇ **alveolitis** *noun* inflammation of an alveolus in the lungs or the socket of a tooth 肺泡炎或牙槽炎; **extrinsic allergic alveolitis** = condition where the lungs are allergic to fungus and other allergens 外源性过敏性肺泡炎

Alzheimer's disease *noun* condition where a patient suffers from presenile dementia in middle age, caused when areas of the brain atrophy, making the ventricles expand 阿尔茨海默氏病,中年人发生的早老性痴呆,因脑萎缩使脑室扩张

> COMMENT: No cause has been identified for the disease, although it is more prevalent in certain families than in others. It appears to be linked to a mutant gene on chromosome 21 (which is itself linked to Down's syndrome). It is thought that there may be a connection between Alzheimer's disease and absorption by the body of aluminium. 注释:尽管此病在某些家族中发生率高,但病因未明,可能与 21 号染色体上基因突变有关(此异常与 Down 氏综合症亦有关)。现认为本病与机体摄入铝有关。

amalgam *noun* mixture of metals (based on mercury and tin) used by dentists to fill holes in teeth 汞合金,由汞和锡组成,牙医用来补牙齿上的洞

amaurosis *noun* blindness where there is no visible defect in the eye, caused by a defect in the optic nerves 黑朦,无可见的眼缺陷,由视神经缺损引起; **amaurosis fugax** = temporary blindness on one eye, caused by problems of circulation 一时性黑朦,单眼暂时失明,由循环障碍引起

◇ **amaurotic familial idiocy** = TAY-SACHS DISEASE 家族黑朦性白痴,即泰-萨氏病

ambi- *prefix* meaning both 二,两者

◇ **ambidextrous** *adjective* (person) who can use both hands equally well and who is not right- or left-handed 左右手都善用的

◇ **ambisexual** *or* **bisexual** *adjective* (person) who is sexually attracted to both males and females 双性恋的,男性、女性对其都有性吸引力

amblyopia *noun* partial blindness, leading to blindness, for which no cause seems to exist, although it may be caused by the cyanide in tobacco smoke or by drinking methylated spirits (toxic amblyopia) 弱视

◇ **amblyopic** *adjective* suffering from amblyopia 弱视的

◇ **amblyoscope** *noun* surgical instrument for training an amblyopic eye 弱视镜,训练弱视眼的外科仪器

ambulance *noun* van for taking sick or injured people to hospital 救护车: ***The injured man was taken away in an ambulance.*** 伤员被救护车接走了。 ***The telephone number of the local ambulance***

service is in the telephone book. 本地的救护服务号码在电话簿里。*see also* 参见 ST JOHN

◇ **ambulanceman** *noun* man who drives or assists in an ambulance 救护人员 (NOTE: plural is **ambulancemen**)

ambulant *adjective* (patient) who can walk 非卧床的,可走动的

ambulation *noun* walking 行走: ***Early ambulation is recommended.*** = Patients should try to get out of bed and walk about as soon as possible after the operation. 建议术后尽早下床行走。

◇ **ambulatory** *adjective* (patient) who is able to walk 可走动的; **ambulatory fever** = mild fever (such as the early stages of typhoid fever) where the patient can walk about and can therefore act as a carrier 轻度发热,病人仍能到处走动,还能做搬运工

> QUOTE: Ambulatory patients with essential hypertension were evaluated and followed up at the hypertension clinic.
> 引文:患有原发性高血压,行动方便的患者在高血压诊所就诊和随访。
> **British Medical Journal** 英国医学杂志

ameba *US* = AMOEBA 阿米巴

amelia *noun* congenital absence of a limb, condition where a limb is congenitally short 无肢畸形,短肢畸形

amelioration *noun* improvement, getting better 改进,改善

ameloblastoma *noun* tumour in the jaw, usually in the lower jaw 成釉细胞瘤,下颌的肿瘤

amenity bed *noun* bed (usually in a separate room) in an NHS hospital, for which the patient pays extra 温馨病床,国立医院中的特殊病床,病人需额外付钱

amenorrhoea *noun* absence of one or more menstrual periods, normal during pregnancy and after the menopause, but otherwise abnormal in adult women 闭经,停经; **primary amenorrhoea** = condition where a woman has never had menstrual periods 原发性闭经,从来没有来过月经; **secondary amenorrhoea** = situation where a woman's menstrual periods have stopped 继发性闭经,曾有月经,后来停经

amentia *noun* being mentally subnormal 精神失常

ametropia *noun* condition where the eye cannot focus light correctly onto the retina, as in astigmatism, hypermetropia and myopia 屈光不正 *compare with* 比较 EMMETROPIA

amino acid *noun* chemical compound which is broken down from proteins in the digestive system and then used by the body to form its own protein 氨基酸: ***Proteins are first broken down into amino acids.*** 蛋白先降解为氨基酸。**essential amino acids** = eight amino acids which are essential for growth, but which cannot be synthesized and so must be obtained from food or medicinal substances 必需氨基酸,8 种生长所必须的氨基酸,身体不能合成,只能由食物或药物中摄取

> COMMENT: Amino acids all contain carbon, hydrogen, nitrogen and oxygen, as well as other elements. Some amino acids are produced in the body itself, but others have to be absorbed from food. The eight essential amino acids are: isoleucine, leucine, lysine, methionine, phenylalanine, threonine, tryptophan and valine.
> 注释:所有的氨基酸都含有碳、氢、氮、氧及其他元素。部分氨基酸可由机体合成,但其余的必须从食物中获得。8 种必需氨基酸是:异亮氨酸、亮氨酸、赖氨酸、蛋氨酸、苯丙氨酸、苏氨酸、色氨酸和缬氨酸。

aminobutyric acid 氨基丁酸 *see* 见 GAMMA

amitosis *noun* multiplication of a cell by splitting the nucleus 有丝分裂

ammonia (NH_3) *noun* gas with a strong smell, a compound of nitrogen and hydrogen, which is a normal product of human metabolism 氨气,有强烈的气味,是人体正常代谢的产物

ammonium *noun* ion formed from ammonia 铵

amnesia *noun* loss of memory 记忆丧失,健忘; **general amnesia** = loss of all memory, a state where a person does not even remember who he is 记忆完全丧失,甚至记不起自己是谁; **partial amnesia** = being unable to remember certain facts, such as names of people 部分遗忘

amniocentesis *noun* taking a test sample of the amniotic fluid during pregnancy using a hollow needle and syringe 羊膜穿刺

◇ **amnion** *noun* thin sac (containing the amniotic fluid) which covers an unborn baby in the womb 羊膜,子宫内未出生胎儿的薄被囊

◇ **amnioscopy** *noun* examination of the amniotic fluid during pregnancy 羊膜镜检查

◇ **amniotic** *adjective* referring to the amnion 羊膜的; **amniotic cavity** = space formed by the amnion, full of amniotic fluid 羊膜腔; **amniotic fluid** = fluid contained in the amnion, which surrounds an unborn baby 羊水; **amniotic sac** = AMNION 羊膜

◇ **amniotomy** *noun* puncture of the amnion to help induce labour 人工破水

> COMMENT: Amniocentesis and amnioscopy are the examination and testing of the amniotic fluid, giving information about possible congenital abnormalities in the fetus and also the sex of the unborn baby.
> 注释:羊膜穿刺和羊水检查是对羊水进行化验、检查,确定胎儿有无遗传性缺陷和胎儿性别。

amoeba *noun* form of animal life, made up of a single cell 阿米巴,一种单细胞生物 (NOTE: plural is **amoebae.** Note also the US spelling **ameba**)

◇ **amoebiasis** *noun* infection caused by amoeba, which can result in amoebic dysentery in the large intestine (intestinal amoebiasis) and can sometimes infect the lungs (pulmonary amoebiasis) 阿米巴病,阿米巴感染导致痢疾(肠阿米巴病),有时还可侵及肺脏(肺阿米巴病)

◇ **amoebic** *adjective* referring to an amoeba 阿米巴的; **amoebic dysentery** = mainly tropical form of dysentery which is caused by *Entamoeba histolytica* which enters the body through contaminated water or unwashed food 阿米巴痢疾,热带地区的痢疾多由溶组织性肠阿米巴引起,通过喝了污染的水或未清洗的食物进入人体

◇ **amoebicide** *noun* substance which kills amoebae 杀阿米巴的物质

amorphous *adjective* with no regular shape 无定型的

amount 1 *noun* quantity 数量: ***He is not allowed to drink a large amount of water.*** 不允许他喝大量的水。***She should not eat large amounts of fried food.*** 她不能吃大量的油炸食品。**2** *verb* to be equal (to) 相当于: ***The bill for surgery amounted to 1,000.*** 手术费高达1,000英镑。

amphetamine *noun* addictive drug, similar to adrenaline, used to give a feeling of well being and wakefulness 安非他明,与肾上腺素类似的一种药物,有成瘾性,用药后感觉良好并较警醒; **amphetamine abuse** = repeated addictive use of amphetamines which in the end affects the mental faculties 滥用安非他明,重复地成瘾性地使用安非他明,最终会影响智力

amphiarthrosis *noun* joint which only has limited movement (such as the joints in the spine) 微动关节

amphotericin *noun* antifungal agent, used against *Candida* 两性霉素(抗真菌药)

ampicillin *noun* type of penicillin, used as an antibiotic 氨苄青霉素

ampoule *or* **ampule** *noun* small glass container, closed at the neck, used to contain sterile drugs for use in injections 安钵

◇ **ampulla** *noun* swelling of a canal or duct, shaped like a bottle 壶腹,腔道或导管的膨大部分,形如瓶子 (NOTE: plural is **ampullae**)

amputate *verb* to remove a limb or part of a limb in a surgical operation 截肢：***a patient whose leg needs to be amputated below the knee*** 一个需截去膝盖以下部分的患者：***After gangrene set in, surgeons had to amputate her toes.*** 因坏疽，她的脚趾需切除。

◇ **amputation** *noun* surgical removal of a limb or part of a limb 截肢手术

◇ **amputee** *noun* patient who has had a limb or part of a limb removed in a surgical operation 被截肢者

amuse *verb* to make someone happy 给…娱乐：***The nurses amused the children at Christmas.*** 护士在圣诞节同儿童玩耍。

◇ **amusement** *noun* being made happy 娱乐，消遣：***Father Christmas gave out presents to the great amusement of the children in the ward.*** 圣诞老人的礼物给患儿带来了欢乐。

◇ **amusing** *adjective* which makes you happy 可笑的，逗人发笑的

amygdala *or* **amygdaloid body** *noun* almond-shaped body in the brain, at the end of the caudate nucleus of the thalamus 杏仁核，位于丘脑尾核的末端

amyl- *prefix* starch 淀粉的

◇ **amylase** *noun* enzyme which converts starch into maltose 淀粉酶

◇ **amyloid disease** *or* **amyloidosis** *noun* disease of the kidneys and liver, where the tissues are filled with amyloid, a wax-like protein 淀粉样变，肾或肝的疾病，组织中充满淀粉样、蜡样蛋白沉积

◇ **amylopsin** *noun* enzyme which converts starch into maltose 胰淀粉酶，将淀粉转化成麦芽糖的酶

◇ **amylose** *noun* carbohydrate of starch 直链淀粉

amyotonia *noun* lack of muscle tone 肌无力，肌张力缺乏；**amyotonia congenita** *or* **floppy baby syndrome** = congenital disease of children, where the muscles lack tone 遗传性肌无力

◇ **amyotrophia** *noun* wasting away of a muscle 肌萎缩

◇ **amyotrophic lateral sclerosis** *noun* Gehrig's disease, a motor neurone disease, similar to muscular sclerosis, where the limbs twitch and the muscles gradually waste away 萎缩性侧索硬化，是一种运动神经原病，与肌肉硬化症相似，肢体痉挛，肌肉逐渐萎缩。

an- *prefix* without or lacking 无

anabolic *adjective* (substance) which synthesizes protein 合成的；**anabolic steroid** = drug which encourages the synthesis of new living tissue(especially muscle) from nutrients 同化激素，促进营养物质合成新的活体组织的药物

◇ **anabolism** *noun* process of building up complex chemical substances on the basis of simpler ones 合成反应，合成代谢

> QUOTE: Insulin, secreted by the islets of Langerhans, is the body's major anabolic hormone, regulating the metabolism of all body fuels and substrates.
> 引文：由胰岛的朗格旱细胞分泌的胰岛素是体内最主要的同化激素，调节所有机体燃料和物质的代谢。
>
> **Nursing Times** 护理时代

anae 厌-(NOTE: words beginning with **anae**-are spelt **ane**-in US English)

anaemia *or US* **anemia** *noun* condition where the level of red blood cells is less than normal or where the haemoglobin is less, making it more difficult for the blood to carry oxygen 贫血，红细胞数量少于正常或血红蛋白少于正常，使血液携带氧气的能力下降；**haemolytic anaemia** = anaemia caused by the destruction of red blood cells 溶血性贫血，红细胞破坏过多造成的贫血；**iron-deficiency anaemia** = anaemia caused by lack of iron in red blood cells 缺铁性贫血；**pernicious anaemia** *or* **Addison's anaemia** = disease where an inability to absorb vitamin B_{12} prevents the production of red blood cells and damages the spinal cord 恶性贫血，不能吸收维生素 B_{12}，从而阻碍红细胞的生成，并有破坏脊髓的作用；**splenic anaemia** = type of anaemia where the patient has portal hypertension, an enlarged spleen and haemorrhages, caused by cirrhosis of the liver 脾亢性贫血,肝硬化时门脉高压、脾脏增大、出血导致的贫血 *see also* 参见 APLASTIC, SICKLE-CELL

◇ **anaemic** *adjective* suffering from anaemia 贫血的

> COMMENT: Symptoms of anaemia are tiredness and pale colour especially pale lips, nails and the inside of the eyelids. The condition can be fatal if not treated.
> 注释:贫血常见的症状是乏力、面色苍白,尤其是嘴唇、甲床和眼睑。如不经治疗可以致命。

anaerobe *noun* microorganism (such as the tetanus bacillus) which lives without oxygen 厌氧菌

◇ **anaerobic respiration** *noun* biochemical processes which lead to the formation of ATP without oxygen 无氧呼吸,无氧状况下生成三磷酸腺酐

anaesthesia *or US* **anesthesia** *noun* loss of the feeling of pain 麻醉; **epidural anaesthesia** = local anaesthesia (used in childbirth) in which anaesthetic is injected into the space between the vertebral canal and the dura mater 硬膜外麻醉; **general anaesthesia** = loss of feeling and loss of consciousness 全麻; **local anaesthesia** = loss of feeling in a certain part of the body 局部麻醉; **spinal anaesthesia** = local anaesthesia in which an anaesthetic is injected into the cerebrospinal fluid 脊髓麻醉

◇ **anaesthesiologist** *noun* specialist in the study of anaesthetics 麻醉学家

◇ **anaesthesiology** *noun* study of anaesthetics 麻醉学

◇ **anaesthetic 1** *adjective* which produces loss of feeling 麻醉的; **anaesthetic induction** = methods of inducing anaesthesia in a patient 诱导麻醉; **anaesthetic risk** = risk that an anaesthetic may cause serious unwanted side effects 麻醉危险 **2** *noun* substance given to a patient to remove feeling, so that he can undergo an operation without feeling pain 麻醉剂; **caudal anaesthetic** = anaesthetic often used in childbirth, where the drug is injected into the base of the spine to remove feeling in the lower part of the trunk 马尾麻醉剂,用于分娩时,将药物注入脊髓底部,以去掉躯干下段的感觉; **general anaesthetic** = substance given to make a patient lose consciousness so that a major surgical operation can be carried out 全麻剂; **local anaesthetic** = substance which removes the feeling in a certain part of the body only 局麻药; **spinal anaesthetic** = anaesthetic given by injection into the spine, which results in large parts of the body losing the sense of feeling 脊髓麻醉药

◇ **anaesthetist** *noun* specialist who administers anaesthetics 麻醉师

◇ **anaesthetize** *verb* to produce a loss of feeling in a patient or in part of the body 使麻醉: ***The patient was anaesthetized before the operation.*** 患者在手术前被麻醉了。

> QUOTE: Spinal and epidural anaesthetics can also cause gross vasodilation, leading to heat loss.
> 引文:脊髓和硬膜外麻醉还可引起显著的血管扩张,导致热量散失。
> **British Journal of Nursing** 英国护理杂志

anal *adjective* referring to the anus 肛门的; **anal canal** = passage leading from the rectum to the anus 肛管; **anal fissure** = crack in the mucous membrane of the wall of the anal canal 肛裂; **anal fistula** *or* **fistula in ano** = fistula which develops between the rectum and the outside of the body after an abscess near the anus 肛瘘,肛周脓肿后直肠和体表间形成的瘘道; **anal sphincter** = strong ring of muscle which closes the anus 肛门括约肌; **anal triangle** *or* **rectal triangle** = posterior part of the perineum 直肠三角

◇ **anally** *adverb* through the anus 通过肛门地: ***The patient is not able to pass faeces anally.*** 患者不能通过肛门排便。

analeptic *noun* drug used to make someone regain consciousness or to stimulate a patient 兴奋剂,回苏剂

analgesia *noun* reduction of the feeling of pain without loss of consciousness 止痛; **caudal analgesia** = technique often used in childbirth, where an analgesic is injected into the extradural space at the base of the spine to remove feeling in the lower part of the trunk 马尾止痛,用于分娩中的一项技术,将镇痛药注射到脊髓底部的硬膜外腔,以去掉躯干下段的感觉

◇ **analgesic 1** *adjective* referring to analgesia 止痛的 **2** *noun* pain killing drug which produces analgesia 止痛剂

> COMMENT: Analgesics are commonly used as local anaesthetics, for example in dentistry.
> 注释:止痛剂常用于局部麻醉,如牙科。

analyse *or US* **analyze** *verb* to examine something in detail 分析: ***The laboratory is analysing the blood samples.*** 此实验室正进行血样分析。***When the food was analysed it was found to contain traces of bacteria.*** 经分析发现此食物含有微量细菌。

◇ **analyser** *or US* **analyzer** *noun* machine which analyses blood or tissue samples automatically 分析仪

◇ **analysis** *noun* examination of a substance to find out what it is made of 分析 (NOTE: plural is **analyses**)

◇ **analyst** *noun* (**a**) person who examines samples of substances or tissue, to find out what they are made of 分析者 (**b**) = PSYCHOANALYST 精神分析学家

anaphase *noun* stage in cell division, after the metaphase and before the telophase(细胞)分裂间期

anaphylaxis *noun* reaction, similar to an allergic reaction, to an injection *or* to a bee sting 过敏反应

◇ **anaphylactic shock** *noun* sudden allergic reaction to an allergen such as an injection, which can be fatal 过敏性休克

anaplasia *noun* loss of a cell's characteristics, caused by cancer 退行性变,由癌变引起

◇ **anaplastic** *adjective* referring to anaplasia 退行性变的; **anaplastic neoplasm** = cancer where the cells are not similar to those of the tissue from which they come 退行性变的新生物

anasarca *noun* dropsy, presence of fluid in the body tissues 水肿

anastomose *verb* to attach two arteries or tubes together 吻合

◇ **anastomosis** *noun* connection made between two vessels or two tubes, either naturally or by surgery 吻合术

anatomy *noun* (i) structure of the body 机体结构(ii) study of the structure of the body 解剖学: ***He is studying anatomy.*** 他在学习解剖学。***She failed her anatomy examination.*** 她没有通过解剖学考试。**human anatomy** = structure, shape and functions of the human body 人体解剖; **the anatomy of a bone** = description of the structure and shape of a bone 骨骼解剖

◇ **anatomical** *adjective* referring to anatomy 解剖的; ***the anatomical features of a fetus*** 胎儿的解剖特点

◇ **anatomist** *noun* scientist who specializes in the study of anatomy 解剖学家

ancestor *noun* person from whom someone is descended, usually a person who lived a long time ago 祖先

ancillary staff *noun* staff in a hospital who are not administrators, doctors or nurses (such as cleaners, porters, kitchen staff, etc.) 辅助人员,后勤人员

anconeus *noun* small triangular muscle at the back of the elbow 肘后肌

Ancylostoma *or* **Ankylostoma** *noun* *Ancylostoma duodenale*, the hookworm, a parasitic worm in the intestine, that holds onto the wall of the intestine with its teeth and lives on the blood and protein of the carrier 十二指肠钩口线虫

◇ **ancylostomiasis** *noun* hookworm disease, a disease of which the symptoms are weakness and anaemia, caused by a hookworm which lives on the blood of the host. In severe cases the patient may die 钩虫病，主要症状是虚弱和贫血，严重病例可导致患者死亡 *see also* 参见 NECATOR

androgen *noun* male sex hormone (testosterone and androsterone), the hormone which increases the male characteristics of the body 雄性激素

◇ **androgenic** *adjective* which produces male characteristics 雄性激素的

androsterone *noun* one of the male sex hormones 雄甾酮

anemia *US* = ANAEMIA 贫血

anencephalous *adjective* having no brain 无脑的

◇ **anencephaly** *noun* absence of a brain, which causes a fetus to die a few hours after birth 无脑儿

anergy *noun* (i) being weak, lacking energy 虚弱，无活力 (ii) lack of immunity 无免疫力

anesthesia *US* = ANAESTHESIA 麻醉

aneurine *noun* thiamine *or* vitamin B_1 盐酸硫胺素，维生素 B_1

aneurysm *or* **aneurism** *noun* swelling caused by the weakening of a wall of a blood vessel 动脉瘤; **congenital aneurysm** = weakening of the arteries at the base of the brain, occurring in a baby from birth 遗传性动脉瘤，脑底部动脉壁薄弱所致，出生后的婴儿即可发生

> COMMENT: Aneurysm usually occurs in the wall of the aorta, ('aortic aneurysm') and is often due to atherosclerosis, and sometimes to syphilis.
> 注释：动脉瘤常发生于主动脉壁(主动脉瘤)，多由动脉硬化，有时是梅毒引起。

angiectasis *noun* swelling of the blood vessels 血管扩张

angiitis *noun* inflammation of a blood vessel 血管炎

angina (pectoris) *noun* pain in the chest caused by inadequate supply of blood to the heart muscles, following exercise or eating, because of narrowing of the arteries 心绞痛，运动或进食后心肌供血不足导致的胸痛，由动脉狭窄所致; **stable angina** = angina which has not changed for a long time 稳定性心绞痛; **unstable angina** = angina which has suddenly become worse 不稳定心绞痛

◇ **anginal** *adjective* referring to angina 心绞痛的: ***He suffered anginal pains.*** 他患心绞痛。

angio- *prefix* referring to a blood vessel 血管的

◇ **angiocardiography** *noun* X-ray examination of the cardiac system after injection with an opaque dye so that the organs show up clearly on the film 心血管造影

◇ **angiogram** *noun* X-ray picture of blood vessels 血管像

◇ **angiography** *noun* X-ray examination of blood vessels after injection with an opaque dye so that they show up clearly on the film 血管造影

◇ **angioma** *noun* benign tumour (such as a naevus) formed of blood vessels 良性血管瘤

◇ **angioneurotic oedema** *noun* sudden accumulation of liquid under the skin, similar to nettle rash 血管神经性水肿

◇ **angioplasty** *noun* plastic surgery to repair a blood vessel, such as a narrowed coronary artery 血管成型术; **percutaneous angioplasty** = repair of a narrowed artery by passing a balloon into the artery through a catheter and then inflating it 经皮血管成型术

◇ **angiosarcoma** *noun* malignant tumour in a blood vessel 恶性血管肉瘤

◇ **angiospasm** *noun* spasm which constricts blood vessels 血管痉挛

◇ **angiotensin** *noun* one of the factors responsible for high blood pressure 血管紧张素(导致高血压的因素之一)

angle *noun* bend, corner 角 *see also* 参见 STERNOCLAVICULAR

◇ **angular vein** *noun* vein which

continues the facial vein at the side of the nose 角静脉

anhidrosis *noun* condition where the amount of sweat is reduced or there is no sweat at all 无汗症

◇ **anhidrotic** *adjective* drug which reduces sweating 止汗的,止汗药

anhydraemia *noun* lack of sufficient fluid in the blood 脱水

anidrosis *noun* = ANHIDROSIS 无汗症

animal *noun* living organism which can feel sensation and move voluntarily 动物: ***Dogs and cats are animals and man is also an animal***. 狗和猫是动物,人也是动物。**animal bite** = bite from an animal 动物咬伤

> COMMENT: Bites from animals should be cleaned immediately. The main danger from animal bites is the possibility of catching Rabies.
> 注释:被动物咬伤后,应立即清洗伤口,其最主要的危险是感染狂犬病。

aniridia *noun* congenital absence of the iris 先天无虹膜

anisometropia *noun* state where the refraction in the two eyes is different 屈光参差

ankle *noun* part of the body where the foot is connected to the leg 踝: **He twisted his ankle** *or* **he sprained his ankle.** = He hurt it by stretching it *or* bending it. 他把脚踝扭了。**anklebone** *or* **talus** = bone which is part of the tarsus and links the bones of the lower leg to the calcaneus 距骨; **ankle fracture** = break in any of the bones in the ankle 踝骨骨折; **ankle jerk** = sudden jerk as a reflex action of the foot when the back of the ankle is tapped 踝反射; **ankle joint** = joint which connects the bones of the lower leg (the tibia and fibula) to the talus 踝关节

ankyloblepharon *noun* state where the edges of the eyelids are stuck together 睑缘粘连

ankylosis *noun* condition where the bones of a joint fuse together 关节僵硬,骨融合

◇ **ankylose** *verb* (*of bones*) to fuse together (使骨)长合 *see also* 参见 SPONDYLITIS

Ankylostoma *or* **ankylostomiasis** 钩虫病 *see* 见 ANCYLOSTOMA, ANCYLOSTOMIASIS

annulus *noun* ring, structure shaped like a ring 环状,环

◇ **annular** *adjective* shaped like a ring 环状的

anococcygeal *adjective* referring to both the anus and coccyx 肛门尾骨的

anomaly *noun* something which is different from the usual 畸形

◇ **anomalous** *adjective* different from what is usual 反常的; **anomalous pulmonary venous drainage** = condition where oxygenated blood from the lungs drains into the right atrium instead of the left 肺静脉异常引流,指氧合的血流入右心房而不是左心房

anonychia *noun* congenital absence of one or more nails 无甲症

anopheles *noun* mosquito which carries the malaria parasite 疟蚊

anorchism *noun* congenital absence of testicles 无睾症

anorectal *adjective* referring to both the anus and rectum 肛门直肠的

anorexia *noun* loss of appetite 食欲缺乏,厌食; **anorexia nervosa** = psychological condition (usually found in girls) where the patient refuses to eat because of a fear of becoming fat 神经性厌食

◇ **anorexic** *adjective* referring to anorexia; (person) suffering from anorexia 食欲不振的,厌食的: ***The school has developed a programme of counselling for anorexic students***. 学校为厌食的学生开设了咨询课。

anosmia *noun* lack of the sense of smell 嗅觉丧失

anovular bleeding *noun* bleeding from the uterus when ovulation has not taken place 非排卵性阴道出血

anoxaemia *noun* reduction of the amount of oxygen in the blood 缺氧血症,低氧血症

◇ **anoxia** *noun* lack of oxygen in body tissue 缺氧症

◇ **anoxic** *noun* referring to anoxia; lacking oxygen 缺氧的,乏氧的

anserina 鹅肌肽 *see* 见 CUTIS

answer 1 *noun* reply, words spoken or written when someone has spoken to you or asked you a question 回答,答案: ***He phoned the laboratory but there was no answer***. 他给实验室打电话,但没有人接。***Have the tests provided an answer to the problem*** ? 通过此实验找到问题的答案了吗? **2** *verb* to reply or speak or write words when someone has spoken to you or asked you a question 答复,回答: ***When asked if the patient would survive, the consultant did not answer***. 当问到患者是否能活下去时,会诊医生没有回答。**to answer an emergency call** = to go to the place where the call came from to bring help 应对急诊求救电话

antacid *adjective & noun* (substance, such as a medicine) that stops too much acid forming in the stomach or alters the amount of acid in the stomach 抗酸的,抗酸剂

ante- *prefix* meaning before …前

◇ **ante cibum** *Latin phrase meaning* 'before food' (used in prescriptions) 饭前(用于处方)

◇ **anteflexion** *noun* abnormal bending forward, especially of the uterus 前屈位

◇ **antemortem** *noun* period before death 临终

◇ **antenatal** *adjective* during the period between conception and childbirth 出生前的; **antenatal diagnosis** *or* **prenatal diagnosis** = medical examination of a pregnant woman to see if the fetus is developing normally 产前诊断 *see also* 参见 CLINIC

◇ **antepartum** *noun & adjective* period of three months before childbirth 产前,分娩前

anterior *adjective* in front 以前的,前面的; **anterior aspect** = view of the front of the body, of part of the body 前面; **anterior superior iliac spine** = projection at the front end of the iliac crest of the pelvis 髂前上棘; **anterior jugular** = small jugular vein in the neck 颈前静脉; **anterior synechia** = condition of the eye, where the iris sticks to the cornea 虹膜前粘连(NOTE: opposite is **posterior**)

anteversion *noun* leaning forward of an organ, especially of the uterus 前倾位

anthelmintic *noun & adjective* (substance) which removes worms from the intestine 驱虫剂,驱虫的

anthracosis *noun* lung disease caused by breathing coal dust 尘肺

anthrax *noun* disease of cattle and sheep which can be transmitted to humans 炭疽病

> COMMENT: Caused by Bacillus anthracis, anthrax can be transmitted by touching infected skin, meat or other parts of an animal (including bone meal used as a fertilizer). It causes pustules on the skin or in the lungs(woolsorter's disease).
> 注释:由炭疽杆菌引起,通过接触污染的皮肤、肉或动物的其他部分(包括用作肥料的骨粉)而传播。本病可引起皮肤或肺的小脓肿(分拣羊毛工人中常见的病)。

anti- *prefix* meaning against 反对,反,抗

◇ **antiallergenic** *adjective* (cosmetic, etc.) which will not aggravate an allergy 抗过敏的

◇ **anti-arrhythmic** *adjective* (drug) which corrects an irregular heartbeat 抗心率失常的

◇ **antibacterial** *adjective* which destroys bacteria 抗菌的

◇ **antibiogram** *noun* laboratory technique which establishes to what degree an organism is sensitive to an antibiotic 药敏实验

◇ **antibiotic 1** *adjective* which stops the spread of bacteria 抗菌的 **2** *noun* drug (such as penicillin) which is developed from living substances and which stops the spread of microorganisms 抗菌素，抗生素：***He was given a course of antibiotics***；***antibiotics have no use against virus diseases.*** 他接受了一周的抗菌素治疗，抗菌素对病毒感染无效。**broad-spectrum antibiotic** = antibiotic used to control many types of bacteria 广谱抗生素

> COMMENT：Penicillin is one of the commonest antibiotics, together with streptomycin, tetracycline, erythromycin and many others. Although antibiotics are widely and successfully used, new forms of bacteria have developed which are resistant to them.
>
> 注释：青霉素是应用最普遍的抗菌素之一，除青霉素之外，还有链霉素、四环素、红霉素及许多其他抗菌素。尽管抗菌素已经被广泛而有效的应用，仍不断有新的耐药细菌出现。

◇ **antibody** *noun* substance which is naturally present in the body and which attacks foreign substances (such as bacteria) 抗体：***Tests showed that he was antibody-positive.*** 检查显示他抗体呈阳性。

◇ **anti-cancer drug** *noun* drug which can control or destroy cancer cells 抗肿瘤药

◇ **anticoagulant** *noun & adjective* (drug) which slows down or stops the clotting of blood 抗凝剂，抗凝的

◇ **anti-convulsant** *noun & adjective* (drug) used to control convulsions, as in the treatment of epilepsy 抗惊厥药

◇ **anti D immunoglobulin** *noun* immunoglobulin administered to Rh-negative mothers after the birth of a Rh-positive baby, to prevent haemolytic disease of the newborn in the next pregnancy 抗D抗原的免疫球蛋白

antidepressant *noun & adjective* (drug) used to treat depression 抗抑郁药，抗抑郁的

◇ **antidiuretic** *adjective & noun* (substance) which stops the production of excessive amounts of urine 抗利尿的，抗利尿剂；***hormones which have an antidiuretic effect on the kidneys*** 对肾脏有抗利尿作用的激素；**antidiuretic hormone** (**ADH**) *or* **vasopressin** = hormone secreted by the pituitary gland which acts on the kidneys to regulate the quantity of salt in body fluids and the amount of urine excreted by the kidneys 抗利尿激素或血管加压素

◇ **antidote** *noun* substance which counteracts the effect of a poison 解毒剂：***There is no satisfactory antidote to cyanide.*** 对氰化物无有效的解毒剂。

◇ **antiemetic** *noun & adjective* (drug) which prevents sickness, vomiting 止吐药，止吐的

◇ **antifungal** *adjective* (substance) which kills or controls fungi 抗真菌的

◇ **antigen** *noun* substance (such as a virus or germ) in the body which makes the body produce antibodies to attack it 抗原

◇ **antigenic** *adjective* (substance) which stimulates the formation of antibodies 抗原的

◇ **antihaemophilic factor** *noun* factor VIII (used to encourage clotting in haemophiliacs) 抗血友病因子

◇ **antihistamine** (**drug**) *noun* drug used to control the effects of an allergy which releases histamine 抗组胺药(用以治疗伤风或过敏性疾病)

◇ **anti-HIV antibodies** *noun* antibodies which attack HIV 抗HIV抗体

◇ **antihypertensive** *adjective & noun* (drug) used to reduce high blood pressure 抗高血压的，抗高血压药

◇ **anti-inflammatory** *adjective* (drug) which reduces inflammation, as in a joint, etc. 消炎的

◇ **antilymphocytic serum** (**ALS**) *noun* serum used to produce immunosuppression in transplants 抗淋巴细胞血清

◇ **antimalarial** *adjective & noun* (drug) used to treat malaria 抗疟疾的，抗疟药

◇ **antimetabolite** *noun* substance which can replace a cell metabolism but which is not active 抗代谢剂

◇ **antimitotic** *adjective* which prevents the division of a cell by mitosis 抗有丝分裂的

◇ **antimycotic** *adjective* which destroys fungi 抗霉菌的

◇ **antiperistalsis** *noun* movement in the oesophagus or intestine where the contents are moved in the opposite direction to normal peristalsis, so leading to vomiting 逆蠕动

◇ **antiperspirant** *noun* & *adjective* (substance) which prevents sweating 止汗药,止汗的

◇ **antipruritic** *noun* & *adjective* (substance) which prevents itching 止痒药,止痒的

◇ **antipyretic** *noun* & *adjective* (drug) which helps to reduce a fever 退热药,退热的

◇ **anti Rh body** *noun* antibody formed in the mother's blood in reaction to a Rhesusantigen in the blood of the fetus 抗 Rh 抗体

◇ **antisepsis** *noun* preventing sepsis 消毒

◇ **antiseptic** 1 *adjective* which prevents germs spreading 消毒的: ***She gargled with an antiseptic mouthwash.*** 她用口腔消毒水漱口。2 *noun* substance which prevents germs growing or spreading 消毒剂: ***The nurse painted the wound with antiseptic.*** 护士用消毒剂涂抹伤口。

◇ **antiserum** *noun* serum taken from an animal which has developed antibodies to bacteria and used to give temporary immunity to a disease 抗血清 (NOTE: plural is **antisera**)

◇ **antisocial** *adjective* (behaviour) which is harmful to other people 反社会的; **antisocial hours** = hours of work (such as night duty) which can disrupt the worker's family life 与生物钟不一致的工作时间(如夜班),常打破员工及其家庭的日常生活规律

◇ **antispasmodic** *noun* drug used to prevent spasms 镇痉药

◇ **antitetanus serum** (**ATS**) *noun* serum which protects a patient against tetanus 抗破伤风血清

◇ **antithrombin** *noun* substance present in the blood which prevents clotting 抗凝血酶

◇ **antitoxic serum** *noun* immunizing agent, formed of serum taken from an animal which has developed antibodies to a disease, used to protect a person from that disease 抗毒血清

◇ **antitoxin** *noun* antibody produced by the body to counteract a poison in the body 抗毒素(中和体内毒素的物质)

◇ **antitragus** *noun* small projection on the outer ear opposite the tragus 对耳屏

◇ **antituberculous drug** *noun* drug used to treat tuberculosis 抗结核药

◇ **antitussive** *noun* drug used to reduce coughing 止咳药

◇ **antivenene** *or* **antivenom** (**serum**) *noun* serum which is used to counteract the poison from snake *or* insect bites 抗蛇毒素或抗昆虫毒素血清

◇ **antiviral drug** *noun* drug which is effective against a virus 抗病毒药

antral *adjective* referring to an antrum 窦的,房的; **antral puncture** = making a hole in the wall of the maxillary sinus to remove fluid 上颌窦穿刺

◇ **antrectomy** *noun* surgical removal of an antrum in the stomach to prevent gastrin being formed 胃窦切除术

◇ **antrostomy** *noun* surgical operation to make an opening in the maxillary sinus 上颌窦造口术

◇ **antrum** *noun* any cavity inside the body, especially one in bone 窦,房; **mastoid antrum** = cavity linking the air cells of the mastoid process with the middle ear 乳突窦; **maxillary antrum** *or* **antrum of Highmore** = one of two sinuses behind the cheekbones in the upper jaw 上颌窦; **pyloric antrum** = space at the bottom of the stomach, before the pyloric sphincter 幽门窦

anuria *noun* condition where the patient does not make urine, either because of a deficiency in the kidneys or because the urinary tract is blocked 无尿

anus *noun* opening at the end of the rectum between the buttocks, leading outside the body and through which faeces are passed 肛门 ◊ 见图 DIGESTIVE SYSTEM, UROGENITAL SYSTEM

(NOTE: for terms referring to the anus, see also **anal and words beginning with ano-**)

anvil *noun* incus, one of the three ossicles in the middle ear 砧骨 ◊ 见图 EAR

anxious *adjective* (**a**) very worried and afraid 担心的: ***My sister is ill, I am anxious about her.*** 我姐姐生病了,我很担心。(**b**) eager 急切的: ***She was anxious to get home.*** 她急着回家。***I was anxious to see the doctor.*** 我焦急地等待着医生。

◊ **anxiety** *noun* state of being very worried and afraid 焦急,忧虑; **anxiety disorder** = mental disorder (such as a phobia) where the patient is very worried and afraid 焦虑症

aorta *noun* large artery which takes blood away from the left side of the heart and carries it to other arteries 主动脉 ◊ 见图 HEART **abdominal aorta** = part of the aorta between the diaphragm and the point where it divides into the iliac arteries 腹主动脉 ◊ 见图 KIDNEY **ascending aorta** *or* **descending aorta** = first two sections of the aorta as it leaves the heart, first rising and then turning downwards 升主动脉或降主动脉; **thoracic aorta** = part of the aorta which crosses the thorax 胸主动脉

◊ **aortic** *adjective* referring to the aorta 主动脉的; **aortic arch** = bend in the aorta which links the ascending aorta to the descending 主动脉弓; **aortic aneurysm** = serious aneurysm of the aorta, associated with atherosclerosis 主动脉瘤; **aortic hiatus** = opening in the diaphragm through which the aorta passes 主动脉裂孔; **aortic incompetence** = defective aortic valve, causing regurgitation 主动脉瓣关闭不全; **aortic regurgitation** = backwards flow of blood caused by a defective aortic valve 主动脉反流; **aortic sinuses** = swellings in the aorta from which the coronary arteries leadback into the heart itself 主动脉窦; **aortic stenosis** = condition where the aortic valve is narrow, caused by rheumatic fever 主动脉瓣狭窄; **aortic valve** = valve with three flaps, situated at the opening into the aorta 主动脉瓣

◊ **aortitis** *noun* inflammation of the aorta 主动脉炎

◊ **aortography** *noun* X-ray examination of the aorta after an opaque substance has been injected into it 主动脉造影

> COMMENT: The aorta is about 45 centimetres long. It leaves the left ventricle rises (where the carotid arteries branch off), then goes downwards through the abdomen and divides into the two iliac arteries. The aorta is the blood vessel which carries all arterial blood from the heart.
> 注释:主动脉大约有 45 厘米长。从左心室发出先上升(此处分出颈动脉)后下降过腹腔,分为两条髂动脉。主动脉含有所有从心脏出来的动脉血。

apathetic *adjective* (patient) who takes no interest in anything 淡漠的

aperient *noun* & *adjective* (substance, such as a laxative or purgative) which causes a bowel movement 泻药,泻的

aperistalsis *noun* lack of the peristaltic movement in the bowel 肠蠕动消失

aperture *noun* hole 孔,洞

apex *noun* top of the heart or lung; end of the root of a tooth 顶端,尖端; **apex beat** = heartbeat which can be felt if the hand is placed on the heart 心尖搏动

Apgar score *noun* method of judging the condition of a newborn baby 阿普伽新生儿评分,评定新生儿状况的方法

> QUOTE: The baby is given a maximum of two points on each of five criteria: colour of the skin, heartbeat, breathing, muscle tone and reaction to stimuli in this study, babies having an Apgar score of four or less had 100% mortality. The lower the Apgar score, the poorer the chance of survival.
> 引文:对婴儿的以下五个项目进行评分,每项最高分为2分:皮肤颜色、心率、呼吸、肌张力和对刺激的反应。Apgar评分≤4,婴儿的死亡率为100%。Apgar评分越低,存活率越小。
> **Indian Journal of Medical Sciences** 印度医学科学杂志

aphagia *noun* being unable to swallow 吞咽不能

aphakia *noun* absence of the crystalline lens in the eye 无晶状体

◇ **aphakic** *adjective* referring to aphakia 无晶状体的

aphasia *noun* being unable to speak or write or understand speech or writing because of damage to the brain centres controlling speech 失语症

aphonia *noun* being unable to make sounds 失音症

aphrodisiac *noun & adjective* (substance) which increases sexual urges 促欲剂,刺激性欲的

aphthae *or* **aphthous ulcers** *plural noun* ulcers in the mouth 阿夫达溃疡,口腔多发溃疡

apical abscess *noun* abscess in the socket around the root of a tooth (牙根)冠状脓肿

◇ **apicectomy** *noun* surgical removal of the root of a tooth(牙)根尖切除术

aplasia *noun* lack of growth of tissue 发育不全,先天萎缩

aplastic anaemia *noun* anaemia caused by bone marrow failure which stops the formation of red blood cells 再生障碍性贫血

apnoea *noun* stopping of breathing 呼吸暂停

◇ **apnoeic** *adjective* where breathing has stopped 呼吸暂停的

apocrine gland *noun* gland, such as a sweat gland producing body odour, where part of the gland's cells breaks off with the secretions 顶泌腺

aponeurosis *noun* band of tissue which attaches muscles to each other 腱膜

apophysis *noun* growth of bone, not at a joint 骨突

◇ **apophyseal** *adjective* referring to apophysis 骨突的

◇ **apophysitis** *noun* inflammation of an apophysis 骨突炎

apoplexy *noun* stroke, the sudden loss of consciousness caused by a cerebral haemorrhage or blood clot in the brain 脑卒中

◇ **apoplectic** *adjective* (person) suffering from apoplexy, likely to have a stroke 脑卒中的

apparatus *noun* equipment used in a laboratory or hospital 设备: ***The hospital has installed new apparatus in the physiotherapy department.*** 医院为理疗科安装了新设备。***The blood sample was tested in a special piece of apparatus.*** 血样经一特殊装置检查。(NOTE: no plural: **a piece of apparatus; some new apparatus**)

appear *verb* (**a**) to start being seen 出现: ***A rash suddenly appeared on the upper part of the body.*** 上半身突然出现了皮疹。(**b**) to seem 显得: ***He appears to be seriously ill.*** 他好像病得很厉害。

◇ **appearance** *noun* how a person or thing looks 外貌: ***You could tell from her appearance that she was suffering from anaemia.*** 从外表你可以看出她患有贫血。

appendage *noun* part of the body or piece of tissue which hangs down from another part 配件,悬挂物

appendix *noun* (**a**) any small tube or

sac hanging from an organ 附属物 (**b**) (vermiform) appendix = small tube shaped like a worm, attached to the caecum, which serves no function but can become infected, causing appendicitis 阑尾: ***She had her appendix removed.*** 她已经切除了阑尾。***an operation to remove the appendix*** 阑尾切除手术; **grumbling appendix** = chronic appendicitis 慢性阑尾炎 (NOTE: plural is **appendices**) ◊ 见图 DIGESTIVE SYSTEM

◊ **appendectomy** *noun US* = APPENDICECTOMY 阑尾切除术,

◊ **appendiceal** *adjective* referring to the appendix 阑尾的: ***There is a risk of appendiceal infection.*** 有阑尾感染的危险。**appendiceal colic** = colic caused by a grumbling appendix 阑尾绞痛

◊ **appendicectomy** *noun* surgical removal of an appendix 阑尾切除术

◊ **appendicitis** *noun* inflammation of the vermiform appendix 阑尾炎

> COMMENT: Appendicitis takes several forms, the main ones being: acute appendicitis, which is a sudden attack of violent pain in the right lower part of the abdomen, accompanied by a fever. Acute appendicitis normally requires urgent surgery. A second form is chronic appendicitis, where the appendix is continually slightly inflamed, giving a permanent dull pain or a feeling of indigestion.
> 注释:阑尾炎发作有几种形式,最主要的是:急性阑尾炎,表现为突发的右下腹剧烈疼痛伴有发热,常需急诊手术。第二种是慢性阑尾炎,阑尾长期轻度发炎,有持续性钝痛及消化不良。

◊ **appendicular skeleton** *noun* part of the skeleton, formed of the pelvic girdle, pectoral girdle and the bones of the arms and legs 四肢骨骼 *compare with* 比较 AXIAL SKELETON

appetite *noun* wanting food 食欲; **good appetite** = interest in eating food 食欲良好; **loss of appetite** = becoming uninterested in eating food 无食欲; **poor appetite** = lack of interest in eating food 食欲不振

appliance *noun* piece of apparatus used on the body 器具,器械: ***He wore a surgical appliance to support his neck.*** 他颈子上戴着外科器具以支撑他的脖子。

application *noun* (**a**) asking for a job (usually in writing) 请求,申请: ***If you are applying for the job, you must fill in an application form.*** 如果你申请此工作,必须先填申请表。(**b**) putting a substance on 应用: ***Two applications of the lotion should be made each day.*** 每天需涂两次洗液。

◊ **applicator** *noun* instrument for applying a substance 涂药器

apply *verb* (**a**) to ask for a job 申请: ***She applied for a job in a teaching hospital.*** 她申请在一所教学医院工作。(**b**) to refer to 适用: ***This order applies to all medical staff.*** 此规定适于全体医护人员。***The rule applies to visitors only.*** 此条例仅针对探视者。(**c**) to put (a substance) on 敷,擦; ***to apply a dressing to a wound*** 包扎伤口; ***The ointment should not be applied to the face.*** 药膏不能擦在脸上。(**d**) to carry out a treatment 应用,运用; ***to apply traction*** 施行牵引

appoint *verb* to give someone a job 指派: ***She was appointed night sister.*** 她被指派夜间护理。

◊ **appointment** *noun* (**a**) giving someone a job 任命; **on his appointment as head of the clinical department** = when he was made head of the clinical department 被任命为门诊部主任时 (**b**) arrangement to see someone at a particular time 约会: ***I have an appointment with the doctor*** *or* ***to see the doctor on Tuesday*** *or* ***I have a doctor's appointment on Tuesday.*** 我约好了周二看大夫。***Can I make an appointment to see Dr Jones?*** 我可以预约 Jones 大夫的号吗? ***I'm very busy, I've got appointments all day.*** 我很忙,全天都约满了。

appreciate *verb* to notice how good

something is 感激: ***The patients always appreciate a talk with the ward sister.*** 患者很感激病区护士和他们聊天。

approach 1 *noun* (**a**) way of dealing with a problem 手段,方法: ***The authority has adopted a radical approach to the problem of patient waiting lists.*** 当局针对患者排队问题采取了有力措施。(**b**) (*in surgery*) path used by a surgeon when carrying out an operation 入路,通道; **posterior approach** = (operation) carried out from the back 后入路; **transdiaphragmatic approach** = (operation) carried out through the diaphragm 经横膈路径 **2** *verb* to go, come nearer 走近: ***As the consultant approached, all the patients looked at him.*** 当会诊医生走近时,所有的患者都看着他。

approve *verb* **to approve of something** = to think that something is good 同意,赞同: ***I don't approve of patients staying in bed.*** 我不同意患者卧床。***The Medical Council does not approve of this new treatment.*** 医学委员会不同意这项新的治疗技术。***The drug has been approved by the Department of Health.*** 此药已经卫生部批准。

apraxia *noun* being unable to make proper movements 运动不能

apron *noun* cloth or plastic cover which you wear in front of your clothes to stop them getting dirty 围裙,围腰布: ***The surgeon was wearing a green apron.*** 术者穿着绿色的围腰。

apyrexia *noun* absence of fever 不发热

◇ **apyrexial** *adjective* no longer having any fever 不发热的

aqua *noun* water 水

aqueduct *noun* canal, tube which carries fluid from one part of the body to another 输水道,引流管,导管; **cerebral aqueduct** *or* **aqueduct of Sylvius** = canal connecting the third and fourth ventricles in the brain 大脑导水管,连接第三和第四脑室的通道

aqueous *adjective* (solution) made with water 水的,似水的

◇ **aqueous (humour)** *noun* fluid in the eye between the lens and the cornea 房水,(眼球的)水状液 (NOTE: usually referred to as 'the aqueous)

aquiline nose *noun* nose which is large and strongly curved 鹰钩鼻

arachidonic acid *noun* essential fatty acid 花生四烯酸

arachnidism *noun* poisoning by the bite of a spider 蜘蛛咬伤中毒

arachnodactyly *noun* one of the conditions of Marfan's syndrome, a congenital condition where the fingers and toes are long and thin 蜘蛛样指或趾

arachnoid mater *or* **arachnoid membrane** *noun* middle membrane covering the brain 蛛网膜

◇ **arachnoiditis** *noun* inflammation of the arachnoid membrane 蛛网膜炎

arbor vitae *noun* structure of the cerebellum or of the womb which looks like a tree 小脑活树,小脑或子宫里的树状结构

◇ **arborization** *noun* (i) branching ends of some nerve fibres or of a motor nerve in muscle fibre 树突 (ii) normal tree-like appearance of venules, capillaries and arterioles 树状血管 (iii) branching of capillaries when inflamed 发炎时毛细血管长出的新分支

arbovirus *noun* virus transmitted by blood-sucking insects 树木病毒,由吸血昆虫传播的病毒

arc *noun* (i) nerve pathway 弧,神经通道 (ii) part of a curved structure in the body 弧; **arc eye** *or* **snow blindness** = temporary painful blindness caused by ultraviolet rays, especially in arc welding or by bright sunlight shining on snow 电光性眼炎,雪盲; **reflex arc** = nerve pathway of a reflex action 反射弧

ARC = AIDS-RELATED CONDITION *or* COMPLEX 艾滋病相关症群

arch *noun* curved part of the body, especially under the foot 弧形的,拱状的,如脚弓; **aortic arch** = bend in the aorta which links the ascending aorta to the descending 主动脉弓; **deep plantar arch** = curved artery crossing the sole of the foot 足弓; **palmar arch** = one of two arches in the palm of the hand, formed by two arteries which link together 掌弓; **longitudinal arch** *or* **plantar arch** = curved part of the sole of the foot running along the length of the foot 纵向足弓; **metatarsal arch** *or* **transverse arch** = arched part of the sole of the foot, running across the sole of the foot from side to side 横向足弓; **zygomatic arch** = ridge of bone across the temporal bone, running between the ear and the bottom of the eye socket 颧弓; **fallen arches** = condition where the arches in the sole of the foot are not high 平足

arcus *noun* arch 弓; **arcus senilis** = grey ring round the cornea, found in old people(角膜上的)老人弓,老人环

◊ **arcuate** *adjective* arched 拱状的; **medial arcuate ligament** = fibrous arch to which the diaphragm is attached 内侧弓形韧带 *see also* 参见 ARTERY

area *noun* (**a**) measurement of the space occupied by something 面积: ***To measure the area of a room you must multiply the length by the width.*** 测量房屋面积必须将长度乘以宽度。***The area of the ward is 250 square metres.*** 病区面积是250平方米。(**b**) space occupied by something 范围,地区: ***There is a small area of affected tissue in the right lung.*** 右肺有一小块感染组织。***Treat the infected area with antiseptic.*** 对感染部位进行抗生素治疗。**bare area of the liver** = large triangular part of the liver, not covered with peritoneum 肝脏的裸区; **visual area** = part of the cerebral cortex which is concerned with sight 视区

areata 脱发,秃顶 *see* 见 ALOPECIA

areola *noun* (i) coloured part round the nipple 乳晕 (ii) part of the iris closest to the pupil 虹膜近瞳孔处的部分

◊ **areolar tissue** *noun* type of connective tissue 蜂窝组织

arginine *noun* amino acid which helps the liver form urea 精氨酸

Argyll Robertson pupil *noun* condition of the eye, where the lens is able to focus but the pupil does not react to light 阿罗氏瞳孔,晶状体可以聚焦但瞳孔不再有对光反射

> COMMENT: A symptom of general paralysis of the insane or of locomotor ataxia.
> 注释:这是麻痹性痴呆或局部运动共济失调的症状。

arise *verb* (i) to begin in, come from (a place) 从…开始,来自…(ii) to start to happen 出现,开始; ***a muscle arising in the scapula*** 附着于肩胛骨的肌肉; ***Two problems have arisen concerning the removal of the geriatric patients to the other hospital.*** 将老年患者转到其它医院会产生两个问题(NOTE: **arises - arising - arose - has arisen**)

> QUOTE: The target cells for adult myeloid leukaemia are located in the bone marrow, and there is now evidence that a substantial proportion of childhood leukaemias also arise in bone marrow.
> 引文:成人髓性白血病的肿瘤细胞位于骨髓,现有证据表明绝大部分儿童白血病也起于骨髓。
> **British Medical Journal** 英国医学杂志

> QUOTE: One issue has consistently arisen - the amount of time and effort which nurses need to put into the writing of detailed care plans.
> 引文:有一个常会遇到的问题-护士书写详细的护理计划所花费的时间及精力。
> **Nursing Times** 护理时代

arm *noun* one of the limbs, the part of the body which goes from the shoulder to the hand, formed of the upper arm, the elbow and the forearm 上肢,手臂: ***She broke her arm skiing.*** 她滑雪时摔断了胳膊。***Lift your arms up above your head.*** 将你的手臂高举过头。**arm bones** = the humerus, the ulna and the radius 上肢骨; **arm sling** = bandage attached round the neck, used to support an injured arm and prevent it from moving 悬臂带: ***He had his arm in a sling.*** 他戴着悬臂带。

◇ **armpit** *noun* the axilla, the hollow under the shoulder, between the upper arm and the body, where the upper arm joins the shoulder 腋窝 (NOTE: for other terms referring to the arm see words beginning with **brachi-**)

Arnold-Chiari malformation *noun* congenital condition where the base of the skull is malformed, allowing parts of the cerebellum into the spinal canal 阿-希氏畸形,颅底畸形,由于颅底畸形使得小脑部分进入椎管

aromatherapy *noun* treatment to relieve tension, etc., in which fragrant oils and creams containing plant extracts are massaged into the skin 涂擦按摩

◇ **aromatherapist** *noun* person specializing in aromatherapy 涂擦按摩治疗师

arrange *verb* (**a**) to put in order 整理,排列: ***The beds are arranged in rows.*** 床铺排列成行。***The patients' records are arranged in alphabetical order.*** 病历按字母顺序排列。(**b**) to organize 组织,安排: ***He arranged the appointment for 6 o'clock.*** 他定了6点的约会。

◇ **arrangement** *noun* way in which something is put in order; way in which something is organized 排列,整理,安排

arrector pili muscle *noun* small muscle attached to a hair follicle, which makes the hair stand upright and also forms goose pimples 立毛肌,竖毛肌 ◊ 见图 SKIN & SENSORY RECEPTORS

arrest *noun* stopping of a bodily function 阻止,抑制 *see also* 参见 CARDIAC

arrhythmia *noun* variation in the rhythm of the heartbeat 心律不齐 *see also* 参见 ANTI-ARRHYTHMIC

> QUOTE: Cardiovascular effects may include atrial arrhythmias but at 30°C there is the possibility of spontaneous ventricular fibrillation.
> 引文:心血管作用包括房性心律失常,但在30摄氏度时可能发生自发性室颤。
> **British Journal of Nursing** 英国护理杂志

arsenic *noun* chemical element which forms poisonous compounds, such as arsenic trioxide, and which was once used in some medicines 砷,某些毒物的成分,如三氧化砷,一度用作某些药物的成分 (NOTE: chemical symbol is **As**)

artefact *noun* something which is made or introduced artificially 人工制品 *see also* 参见 DERMATITIS

artery *noun* blood vessel taking blood from the heart to the tissues of the body 动脉; **arcuate artery** = curved artery in the foot or kidney 弓形动脉; **axillary artery** = artery leading from the subclavian artery in the armpit 腋动脉; **basilar artery** = artery which lies at the base of the brain 基底动脉; **brachial artery** = artery running down the arm from the axillary artery to the elbow, where it divides into the radial and ulnar arteries 肱动脉; **brachiocephalic artery** = INNOMINATE ARTERY 头臂动脉; **cerebral arteries** = main arteries which take blood into the brain 脑动脉; **common carotid artery** = main artery running up each side of the lower part of the neck 颈总动脉; **communicating arteries** = arteries which connect the blood supply from each side of the brain, forming part of the circle of Willis 交通动脉; **coronary arteries** = arteries which supply blood to the heart muscles 冠状动脉; **facial artery** = artery which branches off the external carotid into the face and mouth 面动脉; **femoral artery** = continuation of the external iliac artery, which runs down the front of the thigh and then crosses to the back 股动脉; **gastric artery** = artery leading from the coeliac trunk to the stomach 胃动脉; **hardened arteries** *or* **hardening of the arteries** = arteriosclerosis, a condition (mainly found in old people) where the walls of arteries become thicker and more rigid because of deposits of fats and minerals, making it more difficult for the blood to pass and so causing high blood pressure, strokes and coronary thrombosis 动脉硬化,脂肪和矿物质沉积使动脉壁变厚变硬,使得血流通过困难,因而引起高血压、中风和冠脉血栓形成; **hepatic artery** = artery which takes the blood to the liver 肝动脉; **common iliac artery** = one of two arteries which branch from the aorta in the abdomen and in turn divide into the internal iliac artery(leading to the pelvis) and the external iliac artery (leading to the leg) 髂总动脉; **ileocolic artery** = branch of the superior mesenteric artery 回结肠动脉; **innominate artery** = largest branch of the arch of the aorta, which continues as the right common carotid and right subclavian arteries 无名动脉; **interlobar artery** = artery running towards the cortex on each side of a renal pyramid 叶间动脉; **interlobular arteries** = arteries running to the glomeruli of the kidneys 小叶间动脉; **lingual artery** = artery which supplies blood to the tongue 舌动脉; **lumbar artery** = one of four arteries which supply blood to the back muscles and skin 腰动脉; **mesenteric artery** = one of two arteries ('superior and inferior mesenteri carteries') which supply the small intestine or the transverse colon and rectum 肠系膜动脉; **popliteal artery** = artery which branches from the femoral artery behind the knee and leads into the tibial arteries 腘动脉; **pulmonary arteries** = arteries which take deoxygenated blood from the heart to the lungs for oxygenation 肺动脉; **radial artery** = artery which branches from the brachial artery, running near the radius, from the elbow to the palm of the hand 桡动脉; **renal arteries** = pair of arteries running from the abdominal aorta to the kidneys 肾动脉; **retinal artery** = sole artery of the retina (it accompanies the optic nerve) 视网膜动脉; **subclavian artery** = one of two arteries branching from the aorta on the left and from the innominate artery on the right, continuing into the brachial arteries and supplying blood to each arm 锁骨下动脉; **tibial arteries** = two arteries which run down the front and back of the lower leg 胫动脉; **ulnar artery** = artery which branches from the brachial artery at the elbow and runs down the inside of the forearm to join the radial artery in the palm of the hand 尺动脉; **vertebral arteries** = two arteries which go up the back of the neck into the brain 椎动脉 *compare with* 比较 VEIN

COMMENT: In most arteries the blood has been oxygenated in the lungs and is bright red in colour. In the pulmonary artery, the blood is deoxygenated and so is darker. The arterial system begins with the aorta which leaves the heart and from which all the arteries branch.
注释:大多数动脉的血液在肺进行氧和,是鲜红色。而在肺动脉血液去氧,颜色变深。动脉系统开始于从心脏发出的主动脉,由主动脉分出所有的动脉分支。

◇ **arterial** *adjective* referring to arteries 动脉的; **arterial bleeding** = bleeding from an artery 动脉出血; **arterial block** = blocking of an artery by a blood clot 动脉栓塞; **arterial blood** = oxygenated blood, bright red blood in an artery which has received oxygen in the lungs and is being taken to the tissues 动脉血; **arterial supply to the brain** = supply of blood to the brain by the internal carotid arteries and the vertebral arteries 脑的动脉血供

◇ **arteriectomy** *noun* surgical removal of an artery or part of an artery 动脉切除术

◇ **arterio-** *prefix* referring to arteries 动脉的

◇ **arteriogram** *noun* X-ray photograph of an artery, taken after injection with an opaque dye 动脉造影片

◇ **arteriography** *noun* taking of X-ray photographs of arteries after injection with an opaque dye 动脉造影

◇ **arteriole** *noun* very small artery 小动脉

◇ **arteriopathy** *noun* disease of an artery 动脉病变

◇ **arterioplasty** *noun* plastic surgery to make good a damaged or blocked artery 动脉成形术

◇ **arteriorrhaphy** *noun* stitching of an artery 动脉缝合术

◇ **arteriosclerosis** *noun* hardening of the arteries, condition (mainly found in old people) where the walls of arteries become thicker and more rigid because of deposits of fats and minerals, making it more difficult for the blood to pass and so causing high blood pressure, strokes and coronary thrombosis 动脉粥样硬化,脂肪和矿物质沉积使动脉壁变厚变硬,使得血流通过困难,因而引起高血压、中风和冠脉血栓形成,主要见于老年人

◇ **arteriosus** 动脉的 *see* 见 DUCTUS

◇ **arteriotomy** *noun* puncture made in the wall of an artery 动脉穿刺

◇ **arteriovenous** *adjective* referring to both an artery and a vein 动静脉的

◇ **arteritis** *noun* inflammation of the walls of an artery 动脉炎; **giant-cell arteritis** = disease of old people, which often affects the arteries in the scalp 巨细胞动脉炎

arthr- *prefix* referring to a joint 关节的

◇ **arthralgia** *noun* pain in a joint 关节痛

◇ **arthrectomy** *noun* surgical removal of a joint 关节切除术

◇ **arthritis** *noun* painful inflammation of a joint 关节炎; **reactive arthritis** = arthritis caused by a reaction to something 反应性关节炎; **rheumatoid arthritis** = general painful disabling collagen disease affecting any joint, but especially the hands, feet, and hips, making them swollen and inflamed 类风湿性关节炎 *see also* 参见 OSTEOARTHRITIS

◇ **arthritic** 1 *adjective* referring to arthritis 关节炎的: ***He has an arthritic hip.*** 他患髋关节炎。2 *noun* person suffering from arthritis 关节炎患者

◇ **arthroclasia** *noun* removal of ankylosis in a joint 关节活动术

◇ **arthrodesis** *noun* surgical operation where a joint is fused in a certain position so preventing pain from movement 关节固定术

◇ **arthrodynia** *noun* pain in a joint 关节痛

◇ **arthrography** *noun* X-ray photography of a joint 关节造影

◇ **arthropathy** *noun* disease in a joint 关节病

◇ **arthroplasty** *noun* surgical operation to repair a joint, to replace a joint 关节成形术; **total hip arthroplasty** = replacing both the head of the femur and the acetabulum with an artificial joint 全髋关节成形术

◇ **arthroscope** *noun* instrument which is inserted into the cavity of a joint to inspect it 关节镜

◇ **arthroscopy** *noun* examining the inside of a joint by means of an arthroscope 关节镜检查

◇ **arthrosis** *noun* degeneration of a joint 关节病

◇ **arthrotomy** *noun* cutting into a joint to drain pus 关节切开术

articulation *noun* joint or series of joints 关节

◇ **articular** *adjective* referring to joints 关节的; **articular cartilage** = layer of cartilage at the end of a bone where it forms a joint with another bone 关节软骨 ◇ 见图 BONE STRUCTURE; **articular facet of a rib** = point at which a rib articulates with the spine 肋关节面

◇ **articulate** *verb* to be linked with another bone in a joint 关节联接; **articulating bones** = bones which form a joint 关节骨; **articulating process** = piece of bone which sticks out of the neural arch in a vertebra and links with the next vertebra 关节突

artificial *adjective* which is made by

man, which is not a natural part of the body 人造的; ***artificial cartilage*** 人造软骨; ***artificial kidney*** 人工肾; ***artificial lung*** 人工肺; ***artificial leg*** 人造腿; **artificial insemination** = introduction of semen into a woman's womb by artificial means 人工受精 *see also* 参见 AID, AIH; **artificial respiration** = way of reviving someone who has stopped breathing (as by mouth-to-mouth resuscitation) 人工呼吸; **artificial ventilation** = breathing which is assisted or controlled by a machine 机械通气

◇ **artificially** *adverb* in an artificial way 人工地,人造地

arytenoid *adjective* (cartilage) at the back of the larynx 杓状软骨

As *chemical symbol for* arsenic 砷的化学元素符号

asbestosis *noun* disease of the lungs caused by inhaling asbestos dust 石棉肺

COMMENT: Asbestos was formerly widely used in cement and cladding and other types of fireproof construction materials; it is now recognized that asbestos dust can cause many lung diseases, leading in some cases to forms of cancer.

注释:石棉曾被广泛地用于水泥、包层及其他防火建材。现认为石棉粉尘可引起肺病,部分病例甚至癌变。

ascariasis *noun* disease of the intestine and sometimes the lungs, caused by infestation with *Ascaris lumbricoides* 蛔虫病

◇ **Ascaris lumbricoides** *noun* type of large roundworm which is a parasite in the human intestine 人肠道寄生的蛔虫

ascending *adjective* going upwards 上升的,升高的; **ascending aorta** = first part of the aorta which goes up from the heart until it turns at the aortic arch 升主动脉; **ascending colon** = first part of the colon which goes up the right side of the body from the caecum 升结肠 ➪见图 DIGESTIVE SYSTEM

Aschoff nodules *plural noun* nodules which are formed mainly in or near the heart in rheumatic fever 阿少夫结节,风湿热时心脏内或心脏旁形成的小结节

ascites *noun* abnormal accumulation of liquid from the blood in the peritoneal cavity, occurring in dropsy 腹水,血管内的液体异常多的渗入腹腔而致

ascorbic acid *noun* vitamin C 抗坏血酸,维生素 C

COMMENT: Ascorbic acid is found in fresh fruit (especially oranges and lemons) and in vegetables. Lack of Vitamin C can cause anaemia and scurvy.

注释:维生素 C 在新鲜的水果和蔬菜(尤其是橙和柠檬)中含量丰富。缺乏维生素 C 可引起贫血和坏血病。

-ase *suffix* meaning an enzyme 酶

asepsis *noun* state of being sterilized, having no infection 无菌,无毒

◇ **aseptic** *adjective* referring to asepsis 无菌的: ***It is important that aseptic techniques should be used in microbiological experiments.*** 在微生物实验中保持无菌相当重要。**aseptic meningitis** = relatively mild viral form of meningitis 无菌性脑膜炎; **aseptic surgery** = surgery using sterilized equipment, rather than relying on killing germs with antiseptic drugs 无菌手术 *compare* 比较 ANTISEPTIC

asexual *adjective* not sexual, not involving sexual intercourse 无性的; **asexual reproduction** = reproduction of a cell by cloning 无性繁殖

Asian flu 亚洲流感 *see* 见 FLU

asleep *adjective* sleeping 睡着的,熟睡的: ***The patient is asleep and must not be disturbed.*** 患者入睡了,不要打扰。***She fell asleep.*** = She began to sleep. 她睡着了。**fast asleep** = sleeping deeply 熟睡: ***The babies are all fast asleep.*** 婴儿都熟睡了。(NOTE: **asleep** cannot be used in front of a noun **the patient is asleep** but **a sleeping patient**)

asparagine *nouns* amino acid found in protein 天门冬氨酰胺

aspartic acid *nouns* amino acid found in sugar 天门冬氨酸

aspect *noun* way of looking at a patient 面,方面; **anterior aspect** = view of the front of the body *or* of the front of part of the body 前面; **posterior aspect** = view of the back of the body *or* of the back of part of the body 后面

aspergillosis *noun* infection of the lungs with *Aspergillus*, a type of fungus 曲霉菌病

aspermia *noun* absence of sperm in semen 无精子

asphyxia *noun* suffocation, condition where someone is prevented from breathing and therefore cannot take oxygen into the bloodstream 呼吸困难,窒息; **asphyxia neonatorum** = failure to breathe in a newborn baby 新生儿窒息

> COMMENT: Asphyxia can be caused by strangulation or by breathing poisonous gas or by having the head in a plastic bag, etc.
> 注释:呼吸困难可因勒扼、吸入有毒气体或将头置于塑料袋中引起。

◇ **asphyxiate** *verb* to prevent someone from breathing or to be prevented from breathing 使窒息: ***The baby caught his head in a plastic bag and was asphyxiated.*** 婴儿的头被套在塑料袋里,造成了呼吸困难。***An unconscious patient may become asphyxiated or may asphyxiate if left lying on his back.*** 昏迷病人平躺会或可能会发生窒息。

◇ **asphyxiation** *noun* being prevented from breathing 窒息

aspiration *noun* removing fluid from a cavity in the body (often using a hollow needle) 吸出; **aspiration pneumonia** = form of pneumonia where infected matter is inhaled from the bronchi or oesophagus 吸入性肺炎

◇ **aspirator** *noun* instrument to suck fluid out of a cavity, out of the mouth in dentistry, from an operation site 吸管

aspirin *noun* (i) common pain-killing drug, acetylsalicylic acid 氨基水杨酸 (ii) tablet of this drug 阿斯匹林片: ***He took two aspirin tablets or two aspirins before going to bed.*** 他睡前吃了两片阿斯匹林。

> COMMENT: Aspirin can have an irritating effect on the lining of the stomach and can cause bleeding.
> 注释:阿斯匹林对胃粘膜有刺激作用,可引起胃出血。

assay *noun* testing of a substance 分析,化验 *see also* 参见 BIOASSAY, IMMUNOASSAY

assimilate *verb* to take into the body's tissues substances which have been absorbed into the blood from digested food 消化吸收

◇ **assimilation** *noun* action of assimilating food substances 吸收

assist *verb* to help 帮助; **assisted respiration** = breathing with the help of a machine 辅助呼吸

◇ **assistance** *noun* help 帮助; **medical assistance** = help provided by a nurse *or* by an ambulanceman *or* by a member of the Red Cross, etc., to a person who is ill or injured 医疗帮助

◇ **assistant** *noun* person who helps 助手: ***Six assistants helped the consultant.*** 会诊医生有6个助手。

associate *verb* to be related to *or* to be connected with 由…联想到…, 把…同…联系起来: ***The condition is often associated with diabetes.*** 这些症状常与糖尿病有关。***side effects which may be associated with the drug*** 可能与药物有关的副作用

◇ **association** *noun* (**a**) relating one thing to another in the mind 联想; **association area** = area of the cortex of the brain which is concerned with relating stimuli coming from different sources 联想区; **association neurone** = neurone which links an association area to the main parts of the cortex 联络神经原; **association tracts** = tracts which link areas of the cortex in the same cerebral hemisphere 联络束 (**b**) group of people in the same profession, with similar interests社团，学会，协会 *see also* 参见 BRITISH MEDICAL ASSOCIATION

aster *noun* structure shaped like a star, seen around the centrosome during cell division 星状体

asthenia *noun* being weak, not having any strength 虚弱

◇ **asthenic** *adjective* (general condition) where the patient has no strength and no interest in things 虚弱的

asthenopia *noun* = EYESTRAIN 眼疲劳

asthma *noun* narrowing of the bronchial tubes, where the muscles go into spasm and the patient has difficulty breathing 哮喘; **cardiac asthma** = difficulty in breathing caused by heart failure 心源性哮喘; **occupational asthma** = asthma caused by materials with which one comes into contact at work (such as asthma in farmworkers, caused by hay) 职业性哮喘

◇ **asthmatic 1** *adjective* referring to asthma 哮喘的: ***He has an asthmatic attack every spring.*** 每到春季他的哮喘都要发作。**acute asthmatic attack** = sudden attack of asthma 哮喘急性发作; **asthmatic bronchitis** = asthma associated with bronchitis 喘息性支气管炎 **2** *noun* person suffering from asthma 哮喘病人

◇ **asthmaticus**哮喘的 *see* 见 STATUS

astigmatism *noun* defect in the eye, which prevents the eye from focusing correctly 散光

◇ **astigmatic** *adjective* referring to astigmatism 散光的: **He is astigmatic.** = He suffers from astigmatism. 他有散光。

> COMMENT: In astigmatism, horizontal and vertical objects are not both in correct focus.
> 注释：散光时，水平和垂直物体不能同时被正确聚焦。

astonish *verb* to surprise 使吃惊，使惊讶: ***I was astonished to hear that she had recovered.*** 我很吃惊她竟然康复了。

◇ **astonishing** *adjective* which surprises 令人惊讶的: ***It's astonishing how many people catch flu in the winter.*** 真让人惊讶，这个冬季有那么多的人患流感。

◇ **astonishment** *noun* great surprise 惊奇: ***To the doctor's great astonishment, she suddenly started to walk.*** 她突然开始行走令医生大吃一惊。

astragalus *noun* old name for the talus, anklebone 距骨

astringent *noun & adjective* (substance) which stops bleeding and makes the skin tissues contract and harden 收敛的，止血的(药)

astrocyte *noun* star-shaped brain cell 星形胶质细胞

◇ **astrocytoma** *noun* type of brain tumour, consisting of star-shaped cells which develop slowly in the brain and spinal cord 星形胶质细胞瘤

asymmetry *noun* state where two sides of the body, of an organ are not closely similar to each other 不对称，不平衡

asymptomatic *adjective* which does not show any symptoms of disease 无症状的

asynclitism *noun* situation at childbirth, where the head of the baby enters the vagina at an angle 头盆倾势不均，分娩时胎儿的头进入阴道时与产道成角

asynergia *noun* awkward movements and bad coordination, caused by a disorder of the cerebellum 协同不能，动作笨拙，共济不良，由小脑障碍引起 (NOTE: also called **dyssynergia**)

asystole *noun* state where the heart has stopped beating 心脏停搏

ataraxia *noun* being calm, not worrying 平静，心平气和

◇ **ataractic** *or* **ataraxic** *adjective & noun* (drug) which calms a patient 镇静剂(的)，安定药(的)

atavism *noun* situation where a patient suffers from a condition which an ancestor was known to have suffered from, but not his immediate parents 隔代遗传，反祖

ataxia *noun* lack of control of movements due to defects in the nervous system 运动技能失调，共济失调；**cerebellar ataxia** = disorder where the patient staggers and cannot speak clearly, due to a disease of the cerebellum 小脑性共济失调，病人口吃，不能清晰地说话；**locomotor ataxia** = TABES DORSALIS 运动性共济失调，脊髓痨

◇ **ataxic** *adjective* referring to ataxia 共济失调的 *see also* 参见 GAIT

atelectasis *noun* collapse of a lung, where the lung fails to expand properly 肺不张

atherogenic *adjective* which may produce atheroma 致动脉粥样化的

◇ **atheroma** *noun* thickening of the walls of an artery by deposits of a fatty substance such as cholesterol 动脉粥样化

◇ **atherosclerosis** *noun* condition where deposits of fats and minerals form on the walls of an artery (especially the aorta, the coronary arteries and the cerebral arteries) and prevent blood from flowing easily 动脉粥样硬化

◇ **atherosclerotic** *adjective* referring to atherosclerosis 动脉粥样硬化的；**atherosclerotic plaque** = deposit on the walls of arteries 动脉粥样硬化斑

athetosis *noun* repeated slow movements of the limbs, caused by a brain disorder such as cerebral palsy 由大脑障碍(如中风)引起的手足徐动症

athlete's foot = TINEA PEDIS 脚气，脚癣

atlas *noun* top vertebra in the spine, which supports the skull and pivots on the axis or second vertebra 寰椎 ◊ 见图 VERTEBRAL COLUMN

atmospheric pressure *noun* normal pressure of the air 大气压

> COMMENT: Disorders due to variations in atmospheric pressure include mountain sickness and caisson diseases.
> 注释：大气压的改变可导致高原病和沉箱病。

atomizer *noun* instrument which sprays liquid in the form of very small drops like mist 喷雾器 (NOTE: also called **a nebulizer**)

atony *noun* lack of tone or tension in the muscles 肌张力缺乏，肌弛缓

atopen *noun* allergen which causes an atopy 特异反应原，引起特异反应性的变应原

◇ **atopic eczema** *or* **atopic dermatitis** *noun* type of eczema often caused by hereditary allergy 遗传性过敏引起的异位性皮炎，异位性湿疹

◇ **atopy** *noun* hereditary allergic reaction 特异反应性，遗传性过敏反应

ATP = ADENOSINE TRIPHOSPHATE 三磷酸腺苷

atresia *noun* abnormal closing or absence of a tube in the body 闭锁

◇ **atretic** *adjective* referring to atresia 闭锁的；**atretic follicle** = scarred remains of an ovarian follicle 闭锁卵泡，卵泡排卵后的瘢痕残留

atrium *noun* (i) one of the two upper chambers in the heart 心房 (ii) cavity in the ear behind the eardrum 鼓室 ◊ 见图 HEART (NOTE: plural is **atria**)

> COMMENT: The two atria in the heart both receive blood from veins; the right atrium receives venous blood from the superior and inferior vena cavae and the left atrium receives oxygenated blood from the pulmonary veins.
> 注释：两心房均接受来自静脉的血液，右心房接受上、下腔静脉的静脉血，左心房接受肺静脉已氧和的动脉血。

◇ **atrial** *adjective* referring to the heart 房的；**atrial fibrillation** = rapid uncoordinated fluttering of the atria of the heart, causing an irregular heartbeat 心房纤颤

◇ **atrioventricular** *adjective* referring to the atria and ventricles 房室的；**atrioventricular bundle** *or* **AV bundle** *or* **bundle of His** = bundle of modified cardiac muscle which conducts impulses from the atrioventricular node to the septum and then divides to connect with the ventricles 房室束; **atrioventricular groove** = groove round the outside of the heart, showing the division between the atria and ventricles 房室沟; **atrioventricular node** *or* **AV node** = mass of conducting tissue in the right atrium, which continues as the bundle of His and passes impulses from the atria to the ventricles 房室结

atrophy 1 *noun* wasting of an organ or part of the body 萎缩 2 *verb* (of an organ or part of the body) to waste away, become smaller 使萎缩

atropine *noun* alkaloid substance derived from belladonna, a poisonous plant, used, among other things, to enlarge the pupil of the eye 阿托品

ATS = ANTITETANUS SERUM 抗破伤风血清

attach *verb* to fix, fasten 固定,附上: ***The stomach is attached to the other organs by the greater and lesser omenta.*** 胃通过大、小网膜附着于其它器官上。

◇ **attachment** *noun* (i) something which is attached 附着物,附件(ii) arrangement where a home nurse is attached to a particular general practice 为特定全科医师行医配备家庭护理的机构

attack *noun* sudden illness 发作,发病: ***He had an attack of fever.*** 他发烧了。 ***She had two attacks of laryngitis during the winter.*** 这个冬天她的喉炎发作了两次。**heart attack** = condition where the heart suffers from defective blood supply because one of the arteries becomes blocked by a blood clot(coronary thrombosis), causing myocardial ischaemia and myocardial infarction 冠心病发作

attempt 1 *noun* try 尝试: ***They made an attempt to treat the disease with antibiotics.*** 他们试着用抗生素治疗此病。2 *verb* to try 试,努力: ***The surgeons attempted to sew the finger back on.*** 术者努力将手指缝合上。

attend *verb* (**a**) to be present at 出席,参加: ***Will you attend the meeting tomorrow?*** 你参加明天的会议吗? ***Seventeen patients are attending the antenatal clinic.*** 有17名患者经产前门诊检查。(**b**) to look after (a patient) 看护,照料: ***He was attended by two doctors.*** 两名医生负责他的治疗。**attending physician** = doctor who is looking after a certain patient 主治医师: ***He was referred to the hypertension unit by his attending physician.*** 他的主治医师把他转到了高血压病房。

◇ **attend to** *verb* to deal with 照料: ***The doctor is attending to his patients.*** 医生正在看病人。

attention *noun* care in looking after a patient 照料,看护: ***He has had the best medical attention.*** 他受到了最好的医治。 ***She needs urgent medical attention.*** 她需要急诊治疗。

attract *verb* to make something come nearer 吸引,吸附: ***The solid attracts the gas to its surface.*** 固体将气体吸附于它的表面。 ***The patient is sexually attracted to both males and females.*** 这个患者对男女两性都有性吸引力。

◇ **attraction** *noun* act of attracting 吸引; **sexual attraction** = feeling of wanting to have sexual intercourse with someone 性吸引

attrition *noun* wearing away, as may be caused by friction 磨擦: ***Examination showed attrition of two extensor tendons.*** 检查显示两个伸肌腱间有磨擦。

Au *chemical symbol for* gold 金的化学符号

audi- *prefix* referring to hearing, sound 听

◇ **audible** *adjective* which can be heard 可听到的; **audible limits** = upper and lower limits of sound frequencies which can be heard by humans 听觉阈

◇ **audiogram** *noun* graph drawn by an audiometer 听力图

◇ **audiometer** *noun* apparatus for testing hearing, for testing the range of sounds that the human ear can detect 听力计

◇ **audiometry** *noun* science of testing hearing 听力测定

audit *noun* (i) analysis of the accounts of a hospital or doctor's practice to see if they are correct 审计,对医院的账目或医生的工作进行检查(ii) analysis of statistics relating to a doctor's practice (as numbers of patients *or* incidence of disease, numbers of patients referred to specialists, etc.) for research purposes 为研究目地对医生的工作进行统计调查

auditory *adjective* referring to hearing 听觉的; **external auditory canal** *or* **external auditory meatus** = tube in the skull leading from the outer ear to the eardrum 外耳道; **internal auditory meatus** = channel which takes the auditory nerve through the temporal bone 内耳道; **auditory nerve** = the vestibulocochlear nerve, the eighth cranial nerve which governs hearing and balance 听神经 ◊ 见图 EAR

Auerbach's plexus *noun* group of nerve fibres in the intestine wall 奥尔巴赫神经丛,肠壁内神经丛

aura *noun* warning sensation of varying kinds which is experienced before an attack of epilepsy, migraine, asthma 先兆,预兆,癫痫、周期性偏头痛、哮喘等病发作前的预感

aural *adjective* (i) referring to the ear 耳的(ii) like an aura 预兆的; **aural polyp** = polyp in the middle ear 耳息肉; **aural surgery** = surgery on the ear 耳手术

auricle *noun* tip of each atrium in the heart 心耳

◊ **auriculae**耳廓,心耳 *see* 见 CONCHA

◊ **auricular** *adjective* (i) referring to the ear 耳的 (ii) referring to an auricle 心耳的; **auricular veins** = veins which lead into the posterior facial vein 耳静脉,通向面后静脉的静脉

auriscope *noun* instrument for examining the ear and eardrum 耳镜 (NOTE: also called **otoscope**)

auscultation *noun* listening to the sounds of the body using a stethoscope 听诊

◊ **auscultatory** *adjective* referring to auscultation 听诊的

authority *noun* (**a**) power to act 权威; **to abuse one's authority** = to use powers in an illegal, harmful way 滥用职权 (**b**) official body which controls an area, region 当局,权力机关 *see also* 参见 DISTRICT, HEALTH, REGIONAL

autism *noun* condition of children and adolescents where the patient is completely absorbed in himself, pays no attention to others and does not communicate with anyone 孤独症,自闭症

◊ **autistic** *adjective* (i) referring to autism 孤独症的(ii) suffering from autism 孤僻的

auto- *prefix* meaning self 自身

◊ **autoantibody** *noun* antibody formed to attack the body's own cells 自身抗体

◊ **autoclave 1** *noun* equipment for sterilizing surgical instruments using heat under high pressure 高压消毒锅 **2** *verb* to sterilize using heat under high pressure 高压消毒: ***Autoclaving is the best method of sterilization.*** 高压消毒是最好的消毒方法。***Waste should be put into autoclavable plastic bags.*** 废弃物应放入可高压消毒的塑料袋内。

◊ **autograft** *noun* graft, transplant made using parts of the patient's own body 自体移植

◊ **autoimmune** *adjective* referring to an immune reaction in a person to antigens in his own tissue 自身免疫的; **autoimmune disease** = disease where the patient's own cells are attacked by autoantibodies 自身免疫性疾病: ***Rheumatoid arthritis is thought to be an autoimmune disease.*** 类风湿性关节炎被认为是自身免疫性疾病。

◊ **autoimmunity** *noun* state where an organism produces autoantibodies to attack its own cells 自身免疫性

◊ **autoinfection** *noun* infection by a germ already in the body; infection of one part of the body by another 自体感染

◊ **autointoxication** *noun* poisoning of the body by toxins produced in the body itself 自体中毒

◇ **autologous** *adjective* (graft, material) coming from the same source 自体的

◇ **autolysis** *noun* action of cells destroying themselves with their own enzymes 自溶

◇ **automatic** *adjective* which works by itself, without anyone giving instructions 自动的

◇ **automatically** *adverb* by itself, without anyone giving instructions 自动地: ***The heart beats automatically.*** 心脏呈自主跳动。

◇ **automatism** *noun* state where a person acts without consciously knowing that he is acting 自动症

> COMMENT: Automatic acts can take place after concussion or epileptic fits. In law, automatism can be a defence to a criminal charge when the accused states that he acted without knowing what he was doing.
> 注释:自动行为可在脑震荡或癫痫发作后发生。在法律上,自动症可用来为犯罪进行辩护,被告可申明自己不知在做什么。

◇ **autonomic** *adjective* which governs itself independently 自主的; **autonomic nervous system** = nervous system formed of ganglia linked to the spinal column, which regulates the automatic functioning of the main organs of the body, such as the heart and lungs, and which works when a person is asleep or even unconscious 自主神经系统 *see also* 参见 PARASYMPATHETIC SYSTEM, SYMPATHETIC SYSTEM

◇ **autonomy** *noun* being free to act as one wishes 自主,自治

◇ **autopsy** *or* **post mortem** *noun* examination of a dead body by a pathologist to find out the cause of death 尸检: ***The autopsy showed that he had been poisoned.*** 尸检证实他中毒了。

◇ **autosome** *noun* one of a pair of similar chromosomes 常染色体

◇ **autotransfusion** *noun* infusion into a patient of his own blood 自体输血

auxiliary 1 *adjective* which helps 辅助的: ***The hospital has an auxiliary power supply in case the electricity supply breaks down.*** 当电力供应中断时,医院有辅助发电系统备用。**2** *noun* assistant 助手; **nursing auxiliary** = helper who does general work in a hospital, clinic 护理助手

AV bundle = ATRIOVENTRICULAR BUNDLE 房室束

AV node = ATRIOVENTRICULAR NODE 房室结

available *adjective* which can be got 可得到的: ***The drug is available only on prescription.*** 此药只能有处方才能得到。***All available ambulances were rushed to the scene of the accident.*** 所有能动用的救护车都赶到了事故现场。

avascular *adjective* with no blood vessels, with a deficient blood supply 无血管的,缺血的; **avascular necrosis** = condition where tissue cells die because their supply of blood has been cut 缺血性坏死

average 1 *noun* (**a**) usual amount, size, rate, etc. 一般水平: ***Her weight is above (the) average.*** 他体重超过平均水平。(**b**) value calculated by adding together several quantities and then dividing the total by the number of quantities 平均数 **2** *adjective* (**a**) usual, ordinary 一般的: ***Their son is of above average weight.*** 他们的儿子超重。(**b**) calculated by adding together several quantities and then dividing the total by the number of quantities 平均的: ***Their average age is 25.*** 他们的平均年龄是25岁。

aversion to *noun* great dislike of 嫌恶; **aversion therapy** = treatment where the patient is cured of a type of behaviour by making him develop a great dislike for it 厌恶疗法

avitaminosis *noun* disorder caused by lack of vitamins 维生素缺乏症

avoid *verb* to try not to do something such as not to eat a particular food 回避,避免: ***You must try to avoid overexert-***

ing yourself*.** 你要避免过度劳累。A patient on this diet should avoid alcohol*.** 吃这种食谱的患者应避免饮酒。

avulse *verb* to tear away 撕开

◇ **avulsion** *noun* pulling away tissue by force 撕开; **nail avulsion** = pulling away an ingrowing toenail 拔甲治疗; **phrenic avulsion** = surgical removal of part of the phrenic nerve in order to paralyse the diaphragm 膈神经切除; **avulsion fracture** = fracture where a tendon pulls away part of the bone to which it is attached 撕脱骨折

awake 1 *verb* (**a**) to wake somebody up 唤醒: ***He was awoken by pains in his chest*.** 他被胸痛疼醒。(**b**) to wake up 醒: ***After the accident he awoke to find himself in hospital*.** 事故后,他醒来发现自己在医院里。(NOTE: **awakes - awaking - awoke - has awoken**) **2** *adjective* not asleep 清醒的: ***He was still awake at 2 o'clock in the morning*.** 凌晨2点他还醒着。***The patients were kept awake by shouts in the next ward*.** 患者因隔壁病房的叫嚷声一直不能入睡。***The baby is wide awake*** = very awake. 婴儿醒了。(NOTE: **awake** cannot be used in front of a noun)

◇ **awaken** *verb* to wake somebody up; to stimulate someone's senses 使觉醒,唤醒

aware *adjective* knowing, conscious enough to know what is happening 知道,了解: ***She is not aware of what is happening around her*.** 她一点儿也不知道周围发生了什么。***The surgeon became aware of a problem with the heart-lung machine*.** 术者意识到心肺机出了问题。

◇ **awareness** *noun* being aware (especially of a problem) 知道,觉醒

> QUOTE: Doctors should use the increased public awareness of whooping cough during epidemics to encourage parents to vaccinate children.
> 引文:医生应利用百日咳流行期间公众对此病了解程度的提高,鼓励父母让儿童注射疫苗。
>
> **Health Visitor** 健康咨询杂志

awkward *adjective* difficult to reach or to find or to deal with 棘手的,困难的: ***The tumour is in a very awkward position for surgery*.** 肿瘤生长的位置给手术切除造成很大困难。

◇ **awkwardly** *adverb* in a way which is difficult to reach, to find, to deal with 困难地,难办地: ***The tumour is awkwardly placed and not easy to reach*.** 肿瘤生长的位置很难触及。

axial *adjective* referring to an axis 轴的; **axial skeleton** = trunk, the main part of the skeleton, formed of the spine, skull, ribs and breastbone 躯干骨,中轴骨胳 *compare* 比较 APPENDICULAR SKELETON; **computerized axial tomography (CAT)** = system of scanning a patient's body, where a narrow X-ray beam, guided by a computer, can photograph a thin section of the body or of an organ from several angles, using the computer to build up an image of the section 电子计算机体轴断层扫描

axilla *noun* armpit, the hollow under the shoulder, between the upper arm and the body, where the upper arm joins the shoulder 腋窝 (NOTE: plural is **axillae**)

◇ **axillary** *adjective* referring to the armpit 腋窝的; **axillary artery** = artery leading from the subclavian artery in the armpit 腋动脉; **axillary nodes** = part of the lymphatic system in the arm 腋窝淋巴结; **axillary temperature** = temperature in the armpit 腋表体温

> COMMENT: The armpit contains several important blood vessels, lymph nodes and sweat glands.
> 注释:腋窝内含几条重要血管、淋巴结和汗腺。

axis *noun* (**a**) imaginary line through the centre of the body 轴线,轴 (**b**) central vessel which divides into other vessels 中心血管 (**c**) second vertebra on which the atlas sits 枢椎 ◊见图 VERTEBRAL COLUMN (NOTE: plural is **axes**)

axodendrite *noun* appendage like a

fibril on the axon of a nerve 轴索旁支

◊ **axon** *noun* nerve fibre which sends impulses from one neurone to another, linking with the dendrites of the other neurone 轴突; **axon covering** = myelin sheath which covers a nerve 轴突被膜,覆盖神经的髓鞘; **postsynaptic axon** *or* **presynaptic axon** = nerves on either side of a synapse 突触后轴突或突触前轴突 ◊见图 NEURONE

azidothymidine (**AZT**) *noun* zidovudine, a drug used in the treatment of AIDS 叠氮胸腺嘧啶,一种治疗艾滋病的药物

> COMMENT: There is no cure for AIDS but this drug may help to slow its progress.
> 注释:对艾滋病尚无治愈方法,但此药可延缓疾病的进程。

azo dyes *plural noun* artificial colouring additives derived from coal tar, added to food to give it colour 偶氮染料

> COMMENT: Many of the azo dyes (such as tartrazine) provoke allergic reactions; some are believed to be carcinogenic.
> 注释:许多偶氮染料可引起变态反应,其中有一些被认为是致癌剂。

azoospermia *noun* absence of sperm 无精子

azotaemia *noun* presence of urea or other nitrogen compounds in the blood 氮质血症

◊ **azoturia** *noun* presence of urea or other nitrogen compounds in the urine, caused by kidney disease 氮尿

AZT = AZIDOTHYMIDINE 叠氮胸腺嘧啶

azygos *adjective* single, not one of a pair 单一的, 不成对的; **azygos vein** = vein which brings blood back into the vena cava from the abdomen 奇静脉

Bb

B *chemical symbol for* boron 硼的化学元素符号

Vitamin B *noun* 维生素 B; **Vitamin B complex** = group of vitamins which are soluble in water, including folic acid, pyridoxine, riboflavine and many others 复合维生素 B; **Vitamin B_1** *or* **thiamine** = vitamin found in yeast, liver, cereals and pork 维生素 B_1,硫胺; **Vitamin B_2** *or* **riboflavine** = vitamin found in eggs, liver, green vegetables, milk and yeast 维生素 B_2,核黄素; **Vitamin B_6** *or* **pyridoxine** = vitamin found in meat, cereals and molasses 维生素 B_6,吡多醇; **Vitamin B_{12}** *or* **cyanocobalamin** = vitamin found in liver and kidney, but not present in vegetables 维生素 B_{12},氰钴胺

COMMENT: Lack of vitamins from the B complex can have different results: lack of thiamine causes beriberi; lack of riboflavine affects a child's growth, and can cause anaemia and inflammation of the tongue and mouth; lack of pyridoxine causes convulsions and vomiting in babies; lack of vitamin B_{12} causes anaemia.
注释:缺乏某种维生素 B 可导致疾病:缺维生素 B_1 致脚气病;缺维生素 B_2 影响儿童的生长,导致贫血、口炎和舌炎;缺维生素 B_6 可致婴儿惊厥和呕吐;缺维生素 B_{12} 致贫血。

Ba *chemical symbol for* barium 钡的化学符号

Babinski reflex *or* **Babinski test** *noun* abnormal response of the toes to running a finger lightly across the sole of the foot 巴宾斯基反射(试验) *see* 见 PLANTAR REFLEX

COMMENT: The normal response is for all the toes to turn down but in the case of the Babinski reflex, the big toe turns up while the others turn down and spread out, a sign of hemiplegia and pyramidal tract disease.
注释:正常的反应是所有的脚趾向下弯曲,但在阳性反应中拇趾上翘,其他四趾展开向下弯曲,这是脑偏瘫和椎体束疾病的症状。

baby *noun* very young child 婴儿: ***Babies start to walk when they are about 12 months old.*** 婴儿12月时开始走路。**baby care** = looking after babies 照看婴儿; **baby clinic** = special clinic which deals with babies 婴儿诊所 (NOTE: if you do not know the sex of a baby you can use **it**: '**the baby was sucking its thumb**')

bacillaemia *noun* infection of the blood by bacilli 杆菌血症

◇ **bacillary** *adjective* referring to bacillus 杆菌的; **bacillary dysentery** = dysentery caused by the bacillus *Shigella* in contaminated food 杆菌性痢疾

bacille Calmette-Guérin (**BCG**) *noun* vaccine which immunizes against tuberculosis 卡介苗

bacillus *noun* bacterium shaped like a rod 杆菌 (NOTE: plural is **bacilli**)

◇ **bacilluria** *noun* presence of bacilli in the urine 杆菌尿

back *noun* (**a**) dorsum, the part of the body from the neck downwards to the waist, which is made up of the spine and the bones attached to it 背: ***He complained of a pain in the back.*** 他主诉背痛。***He hurt his back lifting the piece of wood.*** 他搬木头时伤了后背。***She strained her back working in the garden.*** 她在花园劳动时拉伤了背。**back muscles** = strong muscles in the back which help hold the body upright 背肌; **back pain** = pain in the back 背痛; **back strain** = condition where the muscles or ligaments in the back have been strained 背肌劳损 (**b**) other side to the front 后面的: ***She has a swelling on the back of her hand.*** 她的手背肿了。***The calf muscles are at the back of the lower leg.*** 腓肠肌位于小腿后部。

◇ **backache** *noun* pain in the back 后

背痛

> COMMENT: Backache can result from bad posture, a soft bed or muscle strain, but it can also be caused by rheumatism (lumbago), fevers such as typhoid fever, and osteoarthritis. Pains in the back can also be referred pains from gallstones or kidney disease.
> 注释:背痛可因错误的姿式、睡软床或肌劳损引起,有时也可因风湿病(腰痛)、发热如伤寒、骨关节炎导致,背痛也可能是胆结石或肾病引起的牵涉痛。

◇ **backbone** *noun* rachis or spine, a series of bones (the vertebrae) linked together to form a flexible column running from the pelvis to the skull 脊柱 *see also* 参见 SPINE, SPINAL COLUMN, VERTEBRAL COLUMN (NOTE: for other terms referring to the back, see words beginning with **dors**)

baclofen *noun* drug which is a muscle relaxant 巴氯酚,氯氨丁酸

bacteria *plural noun* microscopic organisms, some of which are permanently present in the gut and can break down food tissue; many of them can cause disease 细菌 (NOTE: the singular is **bacterium**)

> COMMENT: Bacteria can be shaped like rods (bacilli), like balls (cocci) or have a spiral form (such as spirochaetes). Bacteria, especially bacilli and spirochaetes, can move and reproduce very rapidly.
> 注释:细菌可为杆状(杆菌)、球状(球菌)或螺旋状(螺旋菌)。细菌尤其是杆菌和螺旋菌可以快速运动和繁殖。

◇ **bacteraemia** *noun* blood poisoning, having bacteria in the blood 菌血症

◇ **bacterial** *adjective* referring to bacteria or caused by bacteria 细菌的: ***Children with sickle-cell anaemia are susceptible to bacterial infection.*** 镰状细胞贫血的患儿易患细菌感染。(**subacute**) **bacterial endocarditis** = infection of the endocardium (the membrane covering the inner surfaces of the heart) by bacteria(亚急性)细菌性心内膜炎; **bacterial strain** = distinct variety of bacteria 菌株

◇ **bactericidal** *adjective* (substance) which destroys bacteria 杀菌的

◇ **bactericide** *noun* substance which destroys bacteria 杀菌剂

◇ **bacteriological** *adjective* referring to bacteriology 细菌学的; **bacteriological warfare** = war where one side tries to kill or affect the people of the enemy side by infecting them with bacteria 细菌战

◇ **bacteriologist** *noun* doctor who specializes in the study of bacteria 细菌学家

◇ **bacteriology** *noun* scientific study of bacteria 细菌学

◇ **bacteriolysin** *noun* protein, usually an immunoglobulin, which destroys bacterial cells 溶菌素

◇ **bacteriolysis** *noun* destruction of bacterial cells 溶菌作用

◇ **bacteriophage** *noun* virus which affects bacteria 噬菌体

◇ **bacteriostasis** *noun* action of stopping bacteria from multiplying 抑菌作用

◇ **bacteriostatic** *adjective* (substance) which does not kill bacteria but stops them from multiplying 抑菌的

◇ **bacterium** *noun see* 见 BACTERIA 细菌

◇ **bacteriuria** *noun* having bacteria in the urine 菌尿

bad *adjective* (**a**) not good, not well 坏的,不好的: ***He has a bad leg and can't walk fast.*** 他腿不好,不能走得很快。***Eating too much fat is bad for you.*** = It will make you ill. 吃太多脂肪对你不好。**bad breath** = halitosis, condition where a person has breath which smells unpleasant 口臭; **bad tooth** = tooth which has caries 龋齿 (**b**) unpleasant or quite serious 严重的,重的: ***She has got a bad cold.*** 她患了重感冒。***He had a bad attack of bronchitis.*** 他患严重支气管炎。(NOTE: **bad - worse - worst**)

bag *noun* something made of paper,

cloth, plastic or tissue which can contain things 袋，兜；**colostomy bag** *or* **ileostomy bag** = bag attached to the opening made by a colostomy *or* an ileostomy, to collect faeces as they are passed out of the body 结肠(或回肠)造瘘袋；**sleeping bag** = comfortable warm bag for sleeping in 睡袋；**bag of waters** = part of the amnion which covers an unborn baby in the womb and contains the amniotic fluid 羊膜囊

Baghdad boil *or* **Baghdad sore** *noun* Leishmaniasis *or* oriental sore, a skin disease of tropical countries caused by the parasite *Leishmania* 利什曼病或东方病,利什曼原虫感染所致的皮肤病

Baker's cyst *noun* swelling filled with synovial fluid, at the back of the knee, caused by weakness of the joint membrane 贝克氏囊肿,因关节膜薄弱引起的膝部囊肿

baker's itch *or* **baker's dermatitis** *noun* irritation of the skin caused by handling yeast 面包师皮炎,由酵母引起的皮炎

BAL = BRITISH ANTI-LEWISITE 二巯基丙醇,抗路易药

balance 1 *noun* (**a**) device for weighing, made with springs or weights 天平：***He weighed the powder in a spring balance.*** 他用弹簧天平称粉的重量。(**b**) staying upright, not falling 平衡；**sense of balance** = feeling that keeps someone upright, governed by the fluid in the inner ear balance mechanism 平衡感：***He stood on top of the fence and kept his balance.*** = He did not fall off. 他站在围墙上,保持平衡,没有摔下来。(**c**) **balance of mind** = good mental state 神志正常；**disturbed balance of mind** = state of mind when someone is for a time incapable of reasoned action (because of illness or depression) 神经错乱 (**d**) proportions of substances as, for example, in the diet 平衡；***to maintain a healthy balance of vitamins in the diet*** 保持饮食中维生素的平衡；**water balance** = state where the water lost by the body (in urine or perspiration, etc.) is made up by water absorbed from food and drink 水平衡 **2** *verb* to stand on something narrow without falling 保持平衡：***He was balancing on top of the fence.*** 他稳稳地站在围墙顶上。***How long can you balance on one foot?*** 你一只脚独立能保持多长时间?

◇ **balanced diet** *noun* diet which provides all the nutrients needed in the correct proportions 平衡膳食

balanus *noun* glans, the round end of the penis 阴茎头,龟头

◇ **balanitis** *noun* inflammation of the glans of the penis 龟头炎

◇ **balanoposthitis** *noun* inflammation of the foreskin and the end of the penis 龟头包皮炎

balantidiasis *noun* infestation of the large intestine by a parasite *Balantidium coli*, which causes ulceration of the wall of the intestine, giving diarrhoea and finally dysentery 小袋虫病(大肠感染了结肠小袋虫,发生肠壁溃疡,伴有腹泻,最终成为痢疾)

bald *adjective* with no hair, (person) who has no hair 无发的,秃头的：***He is going bald or he is becoming bald.*** = He is beginning to lose his hair. 他开始秃顶。***He went bald when he was still young.*** 他还年轻的时候就已秃顶了。***After the operation she became quite bald.*** 手术后她完全脱发了。

◇ **balding** *adjective* (man) who is losing his hair 秃头的

◇ **baldness** *noun* alopecia, the state of not having any hair 秃,无发

Balkan frame *or* **Balkan beam** *noun* frame fitted above a bed to which a leg in plaster can be attached 巴尔干夹板

ball *noun* (i) round object 球 (ii) soft part of the hand below the thumb; soft part of the foot below the big toe 趾(指)肚

◇ **ball and socket joint** *noun* joint where the round end of a long bone is attached to a cup-shaped hollow in another bone in such a way that the long bone can move in almost any direction 杵臼关节

balloon *noun* bag of light material inflated with air or a gas (used to unblock arteries) 气球 *see also* 参见 ANGIOPLASTY

ballottement *noun* method of examining the body by tapping or moving a part, especially during pregnancy 冲击触诊法

balneotherapy *noun* treatment of diseases by bathing in hot water *or* water containing certain chemicals 药浴疗法

balsam *noun* mixture of resin and oil, used to rub on sore joints or to put in hot water and use as an inhalant 香脂 *see also* 参见 FRIAR'S BALSAM

ban *verb* to forbid or to say that something should not be done 禁止: ***Alcohol has been banned by his doctor*** *or* ***he has been banned alcohol by his doctor.*** 医生禁止他喝酒。***Smoking is banned in most restaurants.*** 在许多饭馆禁止抽烟。

band *noun* thin piece of material for tying things together 带子: ***The papers were held together with a rubber band.*** 用橡皮筋把纸捆在一起。

bandage 1 *noun* piece of cloth which is wrapped around a wound or an injured limb 绷带: ***His head was covered with bandages.*** 他的头包着绷带。***Put a bandage round your knee.*** 用绷带把你的膝盖包扎一下。**elastic bandage** = stretch bandage used to support a weak joint or for treatment of a varicose vein 弹性绷带; **pressure bandage** = bandage which presses on a part of the body 压迫绷带; **rolled bandage** *or* **roller bandage** = bandage in the form of a long strip of cloth which is rolled up from one or both ends 成卷绷带; **spiral bandage** = bandage which is wrapped round a limb, each turn overlapping the one before 螺旋绷带; **T bandage** = bandage shaped like the letter T, used for bandaging the area between the legs T字带; **triangular bandage** = bandage made of a triangle of cloth, used to make a sling for the arm 三角巾; **tubular bandage** = bandage made of a tube of elastic cloth 管形绷带 *see also* 参见 ESMARCH'S **2** *verb* to wrap a piece of cloth around a wound 包扎: ***She bandaged his leg.*** 她给他的腿进行了包扎。***His arm is bandaged up.*** 他的胳膊被绷带包了起来。

Bandl's ring = RETRACTION RING 班都氏环,子宫收缩环

bank *noun* place where blood or organs from donors can be stored until needed 库 *see also* 亦见 BLOOD BANK, EYE BANK, SPERM BANK

Bankart's operation *noun* operation to repair a recurrent dislocation of the shoulder 拜恩卡特手术,治疗反复发作的肩关节脱位

Banti's syndrome *or* **Banti's disease** *noun* splenic anaemia, type of anaemia where the patient has portal hypertension, an enlarged spleen and haemorrhages, caused by cirrhosis of the liver 班替氏综合症(脾性贫血,因肝硬化引起门脉高压、脾大和出血所致)

Barbados leg *noun* form of elephantiasis, a large swelling due to a Filaria worm 象皮腿

barber's itch *or* **barber's rash** = SYCOSIS 须疮,须癣

barbitone *noun* type of barbiturate 巴比妥(二乙基丙二酰脲)

barbiturate *noun* sleeping pill, a drug which is used to make people sleep and which may become addictive if taken frequently 巴比妥酸盐; **barbiturate abuse** = repeated addictive use of barbiturates which in the end affects the brain 滥用巴比妥酸盐; **barbiturate dependence** = being dependent on regularly taking barbiturate tablets 巴比妥酸盐依赖; **barbiturate poisoning** = poisoning caused by an overdose of barbiturates 巴比妥酸盐中毒

◇ **barbiturism** *noun* addiction to barbiturates 巴比妥中毒

barbotage *noun* method of spinal analgesia where cerebrospinal fluid is withdrawn and reinjected 往返吸注，一种脊髓麻醉法

bare *adjective* (**a**) not covered by clothes 裸露的: ***The children had bare feet.*** 小孩子们光着脚。***Her dress left her arms bare.*** 她的衣服露着胳膊。(**b**) **bare area of the liver** = large triangular part of the liver not covered with peritoneum 肝裸区

barium *noun* chemical element, forming poisonous compounds, used as a contrast when taking X-ray photographs of soft tissue 钡; **barium enema** = liquid solution containing barium sulphate which is put into the rectum so that an X-ray can be taken of the lower intestine 钡灌肠; **barium meal** *or* **barium solution** = liquid solution containing barium sulphate which a patient drinks to increase the contrast of an X-ray of the alimentary tract 钡餐; **barium sulphate** (**$BaSO_4$**) = salt of barium not soluble in water and which shows as opaque in X-ray photographs 硫酸钡 (NOTE: chemical symbol is **Ba**)

Barlow's disease *noun* scurvy in children, caused by lack of vitamin C 巴洛氏病，婴儿坏血病，维生素 C 缺乏引起

baroreceptor *noun* one of a group of nerves near the carotid artery and aortic arch, which sense changes in blood pressure 压力感受器

barotrauma *noun* injury caused by a sharp increase in pressure 气压伤

Barr body 巴氏小体，性染色体 *see* 见 CHROMATIN

barrier *noun* thing which prevents contact 屏障; **barrier cream** = cream put on the skin to prevent the skin coming into contact with irritating substances 防护霜; **barrier nursing** = nursing of a patient suffering from an infectious disease, while keeping him away from other patients and making sure that faeces and soiled bedclothes do not carry the infection to other patients 隔离护理

> QUOTE: Those affected by salmonella poisoning are being nursed in five isolation wards and about forty suspected sufferers are being barrier nursed in other wards.
> 引文:沙门氏菌感染患者住在 5 间隔离病房内,大约 40 名可能感染者在其他病房被隔离护理。
>
> **Nursing Times** 护理时代

Bartholin's glands *plural noun* vestibular glands, two glands at the side of the vagina and between it and the vulva, which secrete a lubricating substance 巴氏腺，前庭大腺

◇ **bartholinitis** *noun* inflammation of the Bartholin's glands 前庭大腺炎

basal *adjective* extremely important; which affects a base 基础的; **basal cell carcinoma** = RODENT ULCER 基底细胞癌; **basal ganglia** = masses of grey matter at the base of each cerebral hemisphere which receive impulses from the thalamus and influence the motor impulses from the frontal cortex 基底神经节; **basal metabolic rate** (**BMR**) = amount of energy used by a body in exchanging oxygen and carbon dioxide when at rest, i. e. energy needed to keep the body functioning and the temperature normal (formerly used as away of testing the thyroid gland) 基础代谢率; **basal metabolism** = minimum amount of energy needed to keep the body functioning and the temperature normal when at rest 基础代谢; **basal narcosis** = making a patient completely unconscious by administering a narcotic before a general anaesthetic 基础麻醉; **basal nuclei** = masses of grey matter at the bottom of each cerebral hemisphere 基底核

◇ **basale** 基底 *see* 见 STRATUM

◇ **basalis** 基底的 *see* 见 DECIDUA

base 1 *noun* (**a**) bottom part 底部; ***the base of the spine*** 脊髓底部; **base of the brain** = bottom surface of the cerebrum 脑底 (**b**) main ingredient of an ointment, as opposed to the active ingredient 主剂 (**c**) substance which reacts with an acid to form a salt 碱 **2** *verb* to make, using a substance as a main ingredient 用…作主剂; **cream based on zinc oxide** = cream which uses zinc oxide as a base 霜剂的主剂是氧化锌

Basedow's disease = THYROTOXICOSIS 巴塞多氏病,突眼性甲状腺肿

basement membrane *noun* membrane at the base of an epithelium 基膜

basic *adjective* (**a**) very simple, from which everything else comes 基本的: ***You should know basic maths if you want to work in a shop.*** 如果你想在商店工作,你应该掌握基础数学知识。**basic structure of the skin** = the two layers of skin (the inner dermis and the outer epidermis) 皮肤的基本结构,真皮和表皮 (**b**) (chemical substance) which reacts with an acid to form a salt 碱的; **basic salt** = chemical compound formed when an acid reacts with a base 碱盐

basilar *adjective* referring to a base 基底的; **basilar artery** = artery which lies at the base of the brain 基底动脉; **basilar membrane** = membrane in the cochlea which transmits nerve impulses from sound vibrations to the auditory nerve 基底层(耳蜗)

basilic *adjective* important *or* prominent 重要的; **basilic vein** = large vein running along the inside of the arm 贵要静脉

basin *noun* large bowl 盆

basis *noun* (**a**) main part of which something is formed 基础: ***Water forms the basis of the solution.*** 水是溶液的主要组成成分。***The basis of the treatment is quiet and rest.*** 治疗原则是静养。(**b**) main reason for deciding 依据: ***The basis for the diagnosis is the result of the test for the patient's blood sugar.*** 诊断的依据是患者的血糖结果。

basophil *or* **basophilic granulocyte** *noun* type of leucocyte *or* white blood cell which contains granules 嗜碱性粒细胞; **basophil leucocyte** = blood cell which carries histamines 嗜碱性白细胞

◇ **basophilia** *noun* increase in the number of basophils in the blood 嗜碱性粒细胞增多症

Batchelor plaster *noun* plaster cast which keeps both legs apart 巴切勒氏石膏托,使双腿分开

bath 1 *noun* (**a**) large container for water, in which you can wash your whole body 浴盆: ***There's a shower and a bath in the bathroom.*** 浴室里有喷头和浴盆。**hip bath** = small low bath in which a person can sit but not lie down 坐浴盆 (**b**) washing the whole body 沐浴: ***The patient was given a hot bath.*** 患者热水澡。***He believes that a cold bath every morning is good for you.*** 他认为每天早晨冲个冷水澡对你有好处。**blanket bath** = washing a patient who is confined to bed. 给卧床病人洗澡; **medicinal bath** = treatment where the patient lies in a bath of hot water containing certain chemicals *or* in hot mud *or* in other substances 药浴; **sponge bath** = washing a patient in bed, using a sponge *or* damp cloth 擦浴: ***The nurse gave her a sponge bath.*** 护士给她擦浴。(**c**) **eye bath** = small dish into which a solution can be placed for bathing the eye 洗眼杯 **2** *verb* to wash with a lot of liquid 给…洗澡: ***He's bathing the baby.*** 他在给婴儿洗澡。

◇ **bathroom** *noun* small room with a bath or shower and usually a toilet 浴室

bathe *verb* to wash (a wound) 冲洗: ***He bathed his knee with boiled water.*** 他用沸水冲洗膝盖。

battered baby syndrome *or* **battered child syndrome** *noun* condition where a baby or small child is frequently beaten by one or both of its parents, sustaining injuries such as multiple fractures 婴儿或儿童经常被父母责打致伤的综合症

battledore placenta *noun* placenta where the umbilical cord is attached at the edge and not the centre 球拍状胎盘

Bazin's disease = ERYTHEMA INDURATUM 巴赞氏病，硬红斑

BC = BONE CONDUCTION 骨传导 *see* 见 CONDUCTION

BCG = BACILLE CALMETTE-GUERIN 卡介苗：***The baby had a BCG vaccination.*** 这婴儿注射了卡介苗。***We need some more BCG vaccine.*** 我们需药更多的卡介苗。

BCh = BACHELOR OF SURGERY 外科学士

BDA = BRITISH DENTAL ASSOCIATION 英国牙科协会

Be *chemical symbol for* beryllium 铍的化学元素符号

beam *noun* line of light or rays 光束：***The X-ray beam is directed at the patient's jaw.*** X 光光束对准了患者的下颌。

bearing down *noun* (*of a woman giving birth*) stage in childbirth when the woman starts to push out the baby from the uterus 分娩时屏气

beat 1 *noun* regular sound which forms a rhythm 搏动：***The patient's heart had an irregular beat.*** 患者的心跳不规则。**2** *verb* (**a**) to hit 打；**beat joint** (**beat elbow** *or* **beat knee**) = inflammation of a joint (such as the elbow *or* knee) caused by frequent sharp blows or other pressure 因为经常受打击或受压引起的关节(肘或膝)炎症 (**b**) to make a regular sound 跳动：***His heart was beating fast.*** 他的心跳快。(NOTE：**beats - beating - beat - has beaten**)

becquerel *noun* SI unit of measurement of radiation：1 becquerel is the amount of radioactivity in a substance where one nucleus decays per second 贝克勒耳，放射剂量单位 (NOTE：now used in place of the **curie.** See also **rad.** Becquerel is written **Bq** with figures：**200Bq**)

bed *noun* piece of furniture for sleeping on 床：***Lie down on the bed if you're tired.*** 如果累了就躺在床上。***She always goes to bed at 9 o'clock.*** 她总是 9 点钟上床。***He was sitting up in bed drinking a cup of coffee.*** 他正坐在床上喝咖啡。***She's in bed with a cold.*** 她感冒了躺在床上。***ward with twenty beds*** 有 20 张床的病房；a 250-bed *or* ***250-bedded hospital*** 有 250 张床位的医院；**hospital bed** = (i) special type of bed used in hospitals；病床(ii) place in a hospital which can be occupied by a patient 床位：***Hospital bed is needed if the patient has to have traction.*** 如果患者要作牵引必须要有病床。***There will be no reduction in the number of hospital beds.*** 医院床位不会减少。**bed occupancy rate** = number of beds occupied in a hospital shown as a percentage of all the beds in the hospital 床位使用率

◇ **bedbug** *noun* small insect which lives in dirty bedclothes and sucks blood 臭虫

◇ **bedclothes** *plural noun* sheets and blankets which cover a bed 被褥

◇ **bedpan** *noun* dish into which a patient can urinate or defecate without getting out of bed 便盆

◇ **bedridden** *adjective* (patient) who cannot get out of bed 卧床不起的：***He is bedridden and has to be looked after by a nurse.*** 他卧床，必须由护士照顾。***She stayed at home to look after her bedridden mother.*** 她在家照顾卧床不起的母亲。

◇ **bedroom** *noun* room where you sleep 卧室

◇ **bedside manner** *noun* way in which a doctor behaves towards a patient, especially a patient who is in bed 临床态度；**doctor with a good bedside manner** = doctor who comforts and reassures patients, especially those patients who are in bed 临床态度良好的医生

◇ **bedsore** *noun* decubitus ulcer, inflamed patch of skin on a bony part of the body, which develops into an ulcer, caused by pressure of the part on the mattress after lying for some time in one position 褥疮

COMMENT: Special types of mattresses can be used to try to prevent the formation of bedsores. See AIR BED, RIPPLE BED, WATERBED.
注释:有多种特殊的床垫可用来防止褥疮的形成,见 AIR BED, RIPPLE BED, WATER BED。

◇ **bedtime** *noun* time when someone (usually) goes to bed 就寝时间: ***9 o'clock is the patients' bedtime.*** 9点是患者的就寝时间。***Go to bed — it's past your bedtime.*** 上床,已经过了就寝时间。

◇ **bedwetting** *noun* nocturnal enuresis, passing urine when asleep in bed at night (especially used of children) 遗尿

Beer's knife *noun* knife with a triangular blade, used in eye operations 贝尔刀,内障刀

bee sting *noun* sting by a bee 蜂蜇

COMMENT: Because a bee injects acid into the body, relief can be obtained by dabbing an alkaline solution onto a sting.
注释:蜂蜇时有酸性物质进入体内,可用碱性液体涂抹伤口缓解症状。

behave *verb* to act 行动: ***After she was ill she started to behave in a very strange way.*** 生病后她的举动很奇怪。***The children behaved (themselves) or behaved very well when the doctor visited the ward.*** 医生查房时患儿们表现很好。

◇ **behaviour** *or US* **behavior** *noun* way of acting. 举止: ***His behaviour was very strange.*** 他的举止很奇怪。***The behaviour of the patients in the mental ward is causing concern.*** 精神病房患者的举动引起了关注。**behaviour therapy** = psychiatric treatment where the patient learns to improve his condition 行为疗法

◇ **behavioural** *adjective* referring to behaviour 行为的; **behavioural scientist** = person who specializes in the study of behaviour 行为学家

◇ **behaviourism** *noun* psychological theory that only the patient's behaviour should be studied to discover his psychological problems 行为主义

◇ **behaviourist** *noun* psychologist who follows behaviourism 行为主义者

Behçet's syndrome *noun* viral condition with no known cause, in which the patient has mouth ulcers and inflamed eyes accompanied by polyarthritis 贝切特综合症,病因未明的病毒性疾病,表现为口腔溃疡,眼色素层炎和多发性关节炎

bejel *noun* endemic syphilis, non-venereal form of syphilis which is endemic among children in some areas of the Middle East and elsewhere and is caused by a spirochaete strain of bacteria 非性病性梅毒

belch 1 *noun* eructation, allowing air in the stomach to come up through the mouth 嗳气,打嗝 **2** *verb* to make air in the stomach come up through the mouth 嗳气 (NOTE: with babies the word **burp** is used)

belladonna *or* **deadly nightshade** *noun* poisonous plant which produces atropine 颠茄,一种茄科有毒的植物,可制成阿托品

belle indifférence *noun* excessively calm state of a patient, when normally he should show emotion 快意淡漠

Bellocq's cannula *or* **Bellocq's sound** *noun* instrument used to control a nosebleed 贝洛克氏套管,止鼻血用

Bell's palsy *noun* facial paralysis, paralysis of one side of the face, preventing the patient from closing one eye, caused by a defect in the facial nerve 贝耳氏麻痹,面神经麻痹

◇ **Bell's mania** *noun* form of acute mania with delirium 贝耳氏躁狂,一种急性伴有谵妄的躁狂

belly *noun* (**a**) abdomen, the space in the front of the body below the diaphragm and above the pelvis, containing the stomach 腹部 (**b**) fatter central part of a muscle 肌腹

◇ **bellyache** *noun* pain in the abdomen *or* stomach 腹痛

◇ **belly button** *noun* (*used mainly by children*) navel 脐

belt *noun* long piece of leather *or* plastic, etc. which goes around the waist to keep trousers, etc. up or to attach a coat 带子; **seat belt** = belt in a car *or* in an aeroplane which holds someone safely in his seat 座位安全带; **surgical belt** = fitted covering, worn to support part of the back *or* chest *or* abdomen 手术带

Bence Jones protein *noun* protein found in the urine of patients suffering from myelomatosis, lymphoma, leukaemia and some other cancers 本－周氏蛋白,骨髓瘤、淋巴瘤、白血病和其他癌症患者尿液中发现的蛋白

bend 1 *noun* (**a**) curved shape 弯曲: ***The pipe under the washbasin has two bends in it.*** 水盆下的管子有两个弯儿。(**b**) **the bends** = CAISSON DISEASE 沉箱病 **2** *verb* (**a**) to make something curved; to be curved 使弯曲: ***He bent the pipe into the shape of an S.*** 他将管子弯成 S 形。(**b**) to lean towards the ground 弯腰: ***He bent down to tie up his shoe.*** 他弯腰去系鞋带。***She was bending over the table.*** 她弯腰到桌子的另一侧。(NOTE: **bends - bending - bent - has bent**)

Benedict's test *noun* test to see if sugar is present in the urine 本尼迪特试验,检测尿糖

◇ **Benedict's solution** *noun* solution used to carry out Benedict's test 本尼迪特溶液,本尼迪特试验用的试剂

benign *adjective* generally harmless 良性的; **benign tumour** *or* **benign growth** = tumour which will not grow again or spread to other parts of the body if it is removed surgically, but which can be fatal if not treated 良性肿瘤,良性生长 (NOTE: opposite is **malignant**)

Bennett's fracture *noun* fracture of the first metacarpal, the bone between the thumb and the wrist 贝奈特骨折,第一掌骨纵折

benorylate *noun* drug used as a painkiller in treatment of arthritis 贝诺酯,缓解关节炎疼痛的药物

benzoin *noun* resin used to make friar's balsam 安息香

benzyl penicillin *noun* penicillin G 青霉素 G

bereavement *noun* loss of someone you know, especially a close relative, through death 丧亲

beriberi *noun* disease of the nervous system caused by lack of vitamin B_1 脚气病; **dry beriberi** = beriberi where the patient suffers loss of feeling and paralysis 干性脚气病; **wet beriberi** = beriberi where the patient's body swells with oedema 湿性脚气病

> COMMENT: Beriberi is prevalent in tropical countries where the diet is mainly formed of white rice which is deficient in thiamine.
> 注释:脚气病在热带常见,因当地的饮食以白米为主,缺乏硫胺。

beryllium *noun* chemical element 铍 (NOTE: chemical symbol is **Be**)

◇ **berylliosis** *noun* poisoning caused by breathing in particles of beryllium oxide 铍中毒

Besnier's prurigo 贝尼埃氏痒疹 *see* 见 PRURIGO Besnier

beta *noun* second letter of the Greek alphabet 希腊字母表的第二个字母; **beta blocker** = drug which blocks the beta-adrenergic receptors and so reduces the activity of the heart β受体阻滞剂; **beta cell** = cell which produces insulin β细胞,生成胰导素的细胞

◇ **betamethasone** *noun* very strong corticosteroid drug 倍他米松

better *adjective* & *adverb* healthy again *or* not as ill as before 好的,好转地: ***I had a cold last week but now I'm better.*** 上周我感冒了,但现在已经好些了。***I hope you're better soon.*** 我希望你很快康复。***She had flu but now she's feeling better.*** 她患了流感,但现在好多了。***Veg-***

etables are better for you than sweets. = Vegetables make you healthier. 蔬菜比糖有利于健康。

Bi *chemical symbol for* bismuth 铋的化学元素符号

bi- *prefix meaning* two or twice 双,两

bicarbonate of soda ($NaHCO_3$) *noun* sodium salt used to treat acidity in the stomach 碳酸氢钠

bicellular *adjective* which has two cells 两个细胞的

biceps *noun* any muscle formed of two parts joined to form one tendon, especially the muscles in the front of the upper arm and the back of the thigh 二头肌; **biceps femoris** = extensor muscle in the back of the thigh 股二头肌; *compare* 比较 TRICEPS 三头肌 (NOTE: plural is **biceps**)

◇ **bicipital** *adjective* (i) referring to a biceps muscle 二头肌的 (ii) with two parts 两部分的

biconcave *adjective* (lens) which is concave on both sides 双凹形的

◇ **biconvex** *adjective* (lens) which is convex on both sides 双凸形的

◇ **bicornuate** *adjective* which is divided into two parts (sometimes applied to a malformation of the uterus) 双角的

◇ **bicuspid 1** *adjective* with two points 有两个尖的; **bicuspid valve** = mitral valve, the valve in the heart which allows blood to flow from the left atrium to the left ventricle but not in the opposite direction 二尖瓣 ◇ 见图 HEART **2** *noun* premolar tooth 双尖牙

b.i.d. *or* **bis in die** *Latin phrase meaning* twice daily 一天两次

bifid *adjective* in two parts 对裂的,两叉的

◇ **bifida** 裂 *see* 见 SPINA BIFIDA

bifocal lenses *or* **bifocals** *plural noun* type of spectacles where two lenses are combined in the same piece of glass, the top lens being for seeing at a distance and the lower lens for reading 双焦镜 *see also* 参见 TRIFOCAL

bifurcation *noun* place where something divides into two parts 叉,分叉点

big toe *noun* largest of the five toes, on the inside of the foot 拇趾

bigeminy *or* **pulsus bigeminus** *noun* double pulse, with an extra ectopic beat 二联律

bilateral *adjective* which affects both sides 两侧的; **bilateral pneumonia** = pneumonia affecting both lungs 双侧肺炎; **bilateral vasectomy** = surgical operation to cut both vasa deferentia and so make the patient sterile 双侧输精管切除术

bile *noun* thick bitter brownish yellow fluid produced by the liver, stored in the gall bladder and used to digest fatty substances and to neutralize acids 胆汁; **bile acids** = acids (such as cholic acid) found in bile 胆汁酸; **bile canal** = very small vessel leading from a hepatic cell to the bile duct 肝管; **bile duct** = tube which links the cystic duct and the hepatic duct to the duodenum 胆管; **common bile duct** = duct leading to the duodenum, formed of the hepatic and cystic ducts together 胆总管; **bile pigment** = colouring matter in bile 胆色素; **bile salts** = sodium salts of bile acids 胆盐 (NOTE: for other terms referring to bile, see words beginning with **chol-**)

> COMMENT: In jaundice, excess bile pigments flow into the blood and cause the skin to turn yellow. 注释:黄疸时,过多的胆红素进入血液,使皮肤变为黄色。

Bilharzia *noun* Schistosoma, genus of fluke which enters the patient's bloodstream and causes bilharziasis 血吸虫

◇ **bilharziasis** *noun* schistosomiasis, tropical disease caused by flukes in the intestine or bladder 血吸虫病 (NOTE: although strictly speaking, Bilharzia is the name of the fluke, it is also generally used for the name of the disease: **bilharzia patients; six cases of bilharzia**)

COMMENT: The larvae of the fluke enter the skin through the feet and lodge in the walls of the intestine or bladder. They are passed out of the body in stools or urine and return to water, where they lodge and develop in the water snail, the secondary host, before going back into humans. Patients suffer from fever and anaemia.
注释:吸虫的蚴虫通过脚部的皮肤进入人体,寄居于肠壁或膀胱,经粪便和尿返回水中,在第二宿主水螺体内寄居、发育直至返回人体。血吸虫病患者伴有发热、贫血。

biliary *adjective* referring to bile 胆汁的; **primary biliary cirrhosis** = cirrhosis of the liver caused by autoimmune disease 原发性胆汁性肝硬化; **secondary biliary cirrhosis** = cirrhosis of the liver caused by an obstruction of the bile ducts 继发性胆汁性肝硬化; **biliary colic** = pain in the abdomen caused by gallstones in the bile duct *or* by inflammation of the gall bladder 胆绞痛; **biliary fistula** = opening which discharges bile onto the surface of the skin from the gall bladder, bile duct or liver 胆瘘

◇ **bilious** *adjective* (condition) caused by bile or where bile is brought up in to the mouth; (any condition) where the patient suffers nausea 胆汁的,恶心的: ***He had a bilious attack***. = He had indigestion together with nausea. 他感到恶心。

◇ **biliousness** *noun* feeling of indigestion and nausea 消化不良,恶心

◇ **bilirubin** *noun* red pigment in bile 胆红素; **serum bilirubin** = bilirubin in serum, converted from haemoglobin as red blood cells are destroyed 血清胆红素

◇ **bilirubinaemia** *noun* excess of bilirubin in the blood 胆红素血症

◇ **biliuria** *noun* presence of bile in the urine 胆汁尿 *see* 见 CHOLURIA

◇ **biliverdin** *noun* green pigment in bile, produced by oxidation of bilirubin 胆绿素 (NOTE: for other terms referring to bile, see words beginning with **chol-**)

billion *noun* number equal to one thousand million *or* one million million 十亿 (NOTE: in the US it has always meant one thousand million, but in GB it formerly meant one million million, and it is still sometimes used with this meaning. With figures it is usually written **bn**: **$5bn** say 'five billion dollars')

Billroth's operations *plural noun* surgical operations where the lower part of the stomach is removed and the part which is left is linked to the duodenum or jejunum 比罗特手术,幽门切除术

bilobate *adjective* with two lobes 二叶的

bimanual *adjective* done with two hands, needing both hands to be done 需双手作的

binary *adjective* (i) made of two parts 两部分的 (ii) (compound) made of two elements 两种成分的; **binary fission** = splitting into two parts (in some types of cell division) 二分裂

binaural *adjective* referring to both ears; using both ears 双耳的

bind *verb* to tie; to fasten 系: ***She bound his sprained wrist with a wet cloth***. 她把湿巾系在他扭伤的腕上。(NOTE: **binds - binding - bound - has bound**)

◇ **binder** *noun* bandage which is wrapped round a limb to support it 肢带

Binet's test *noun* intelligence test for children 比内氏测验,查儿童智力

binocular *adjective* referring to the two eyes 双眼的; **binocular vision** = ability to see with both eyes at the same time, which gives a stereoscopic effect and allows a person to judge distances 双眼视力 *compare* 比较 MONOCULAR

◇ **binovular** *adjective* (twins) which come from two different ova 双卵的

◇ **binucleate** *adjective* with two nuclei 双核的

bio- *prefix* referring to living organisms 生物的

◊ **bioassay** *noun* test of the strength of a drug *or* hormone *or* vitamin *or* serum, by examining the effect it has on living animals *or* tissue 生物鉴定

◊ **bioavailability** *noun* extent to which a nutrient *or* medicine can be taken up by the body 生物利用度

◊ **biochemical** *adjective* referring to biochemistry 生物化学的

◊ **biochemist** *noun* scientist who specializes in biochemistry 生物化学家

◊ **biochemistry** *noun* chemistry of living tissues 生物化学

◊ **biocide** *noun* substance which kills living organisms 杀生物的

◊ **bioengineering** *noun* science of manipulating and combining different genetic material to produce living organisms with particular characteristics 生物工程

◊ **biofeedback** *noun* control of the autonomic nervous system by the patient's conscious thought (as he sees the results of tests or scans) 生物反馈

◊ **biogenesis** *noun* theory that living organisms can only develop from other living organisms 生物起源的

biology *noun* study of living organisms 生物学

◊ **biological** *adjective* referring to biology 生物学的; **biological clock** = circadian rhythm, the rhythm of daily activities and bodily processes (eating, defecating, sleeping, etc.) frequently controlled by hormones, which repeats every twenty-four hours 生物钟; **biological warfare** = war where one side tries to kill or to affect the people of the enemy side by infecting them with living organisms or poison derived from living organisms 生物战

◊ **biologist** *noun* scientist who specializes in biology 生物学家

biomaterial *noun* synthetic material which can be used as an implant in living tissue 生物材料

◊ **bionics** *noun* applying knowledge of biological systems to mechanical and electronic devices 仿生学

◊ **biopsy** *noun* taking a small piece of living tissue for examination and diagnosis 活检: ***The biopsy of the tissue from the growth showed that it was benign.*** 赘生物的活检显示它是良性的。

◊ **biorhythms** *plural noun* recurring cycles of different lengths which some people believe affect a person's behaviour, sensitivity and intelligence 生物节律

◊ **biostatistics** *plural noun* statistics used in medicine and the study of disease 生物统计学

biotechnology *noun* use of technology to manipulate and combine different genetic materials to produce living organisms with particular characteristics 生物技术: ***A biotechnology company is developing a range of new pesticides based on naturally occurring toxins.*** 生物技术公司在天然毒素的基础上研制了一系列新的杀虫剂。***Artificial insemination of cattle was one of the first examples of biotechnology.*** 牛的人工授精是应用生物技术的先例之一。

biotin *noun* type of vitamin B, found in egg yolks, liver and yeast 生物素,维生素B的一种,来源于蛋黄、肝和酵母

bipara *noun* woman who has been pregnant twice and each time has given birth normally 二产妇

◊ **biparietal** *adjective* referring to the two parietal bones 双顶骨的

◊ **biparous** *adjective* which produces twins 产双胎的

◊ **bipennate** *adjective* (muscle) with fibres which rise from either side of the tendon 双羽(肌)

◊ **bipolar** *adjective* with two poles 两极的; **bipolar disorder** = mental disorder where the patient moves from mania to depression 两极精神障碍; **bipolar neurone** = nerve cell with two processes, a dendrite and an axon (found in the retina) 双极神经元 ◊ 见图 NEURONE

birth *noun* being born 出生; **date of birth** = date when a person was born 出生日期; **to give birth** = to have a baby 生孩子: ***She gave birth to twins.*** 她生了个双胞胎。**breech birth** = birth where the baby's buttocks appear first 臀先露; **premature birth** = birth of a baby earlier than 37 weeks from conception 早产; **birth canal** = uterus, vagina and vulva 产道; **birth certificate** = official document giving details of a person's date and place of birth and parents 出生证; **birth control** = restricting the number of children born by using contraception 计划生育; **birth defect** = congenital defect, a malformation which exists in a person's body from birth 先天性缺陷; **birth injury** = injury (such as brain damage) which a baby suffers during a difficult birth 产伤; **birth rate** = number of births per year, shown per thousand of the population 出生率: ***A birth rate of 15 per thousand.*** 出生率是15‰。***There has been a severe decline in the birth rate.*** 出生率有明显下降。

◇ **birthing chair** *noun* special chair in which a mother sits to give birth 产床

◇ **birthmark** *noun* naevus, a mark on the skin which a baby has at birth and which cannot be removed 胎记

bisexual *adjective* (i) (person) who is sexually attracted to both males and females 双性恋的 (ii) (person) who has both male and female physical characteristics 两性的

◇ **bisexuality** *noun* (i) being sexually attracted to both males and females 双性恋 (ii) having both male and female physical characteristics 两性人 *compare with* 比较 AMBISEXUAL, HETEROSEXUAL, HOMOSEXUAL

bis in die 一日两次 *see* 见 B.I.D.

bismuth *noun* chemical element 铋; **bismuth salts** = salts used to treat acid stomach and formerly used in the treatment of syphilis 铋剂 (NOTE: chemical symbol is **Bi**)

bistoury *noun* sharp, thin surgical knife 外科用的一种细长小刀

bite 1 *verb* to cut into something with the teeth 咬: ***The dog bit the postman.*** 那狗咬了邮递员。***He bit a piece out of the apple.*** 他咬了口苹果。***She was bitten by an insect.*** 她被虫子咬了。**to bite on something** = to hold onto something with the teeth 用牙咬住: ***The dentist told him to bite on the bite wing.*** 牙医让他咬住咬合翼片。(NOTE: **bites - biting - bit - has bitten**) **2** *noun* action of biting or of being bitten; place where someone has been bitten 咬, 被咬的伤口; **animal bite** 动物咬伤; **dog bite** 狗咬伤; **insect bite** 虫咬伤; ***Her arm was covered with bites.*** 她的胳膊上布满了被咬的伤痕。

◇ **bite wing** *noun* holder for dental X-ray film, which the patient holds between the teeth, so allowing an X-ray of both upper and lower teeth to be taken 咬合翼片(牙科照像时用)

Bitot's spots *plural noun* small white spots on the conjunctiva, caused by vitamin A deficiency 比托斑, 结膜上的小白斑, 由维生素A缺乏引起

bitter *adjective* one of the four tastes, not sweet, sour or salt 苦的: ***Quinine is bitter but oranges are sweet.*** 奎宁是苦的, 橘子是甜的。◇见图 TONGUE

bivalve *noun & adjective* (organ) which has two valves 两瓣(的)

black *adjective & noun* having the very darkest colour which is the opposite of white 黑的, 黑: ***The surgeon was wearing a black coat.*** 术者穿着黑衣。**black coffee** = coffee with no milk in it (无奶)清咖啡; **Black Death** = violent form of bubonic plague, a pandemic during the Middle Ages 黑死病; **black eye** = bruising and swelling of the tissues round an eye, caused by a blow 眼圈青肿: ***He got a black eye in the fight.*** 他被打得眼圈青肿。(NOTE: **black - blacker - blackest**)

◇ **blackhead** *noun* comedo, a small point of dark, hard matter in a sebaceous follicle, often found associated with acne on the skin of adolescents 黑头粉刺 *see* 见 ACNE

◇ **blackout** *noun* fainting fit *or* sudden loss of consciousness 一时性黑蒙: ***He must have had a blackout while driving***. 他驾车时一定发作了一时性黑蒙。

◇ **black out** *verb* to have a fainting fit *or* sudden loss of consciousness 晕厥: ***I suddenly blacked out and I can't remember anything more***. 我突然晕厥不记得任何事了。

◇ **blackwater fever** *noun* tropical disease, a form of malaria, where haemoglobin from red blood cells is released into plasma and makes the urine dark 黑水热(疟疾的一种,血红蛋白进入血浆,使尿色变黑)

bladder *noun* any sac in the body, especially the sac where the urine collects before being passed out of the body 囊,膀胱: ***He is suffering from bladder trouble***. 他患膀胱疾病。***She is taking antibiotics for a bladder infection***. 她在服用抗生素治疗膀胱感染。**gall bladder** = sac situated underneath the liver, in which bile produced by the liver is stored 胆囊 ◊ 见图 DIGESTIVE SYSTEM **neurogenic bladder** = any disturbance of the bladder function caused by lesions in the nerve supply to the bladder 神经原性膀胱; **urinary bladder** = sac where the urine collects from the kidneys through the ureters, before being passed out of the body through the urethra 膀胱 ◊ 见图 KIDNEY, UROGENITAL SYSTEM (NOTE: for other terms referring to the bladder, see words beginning with **cyst-**, **vesico-**)

◇ **bladder worm** *noun* cysticercus, the larva of a tapeworm found in pork, which is enclosed in a cyst, typical of *Taenia* 囊尾蚴

blade *noun* thin flat piece of metal 刀片: ***This bistoury has a very sharp blade***. 这把细长刀的刀片很锋利。

Blalock's operation *or* **Blalock-Taussig operation** *noun* surgical operation to connect the pulmonary artery to the subclavian artery, in order to increase blood flow to the lungs in a patient suffering from tetralogy of Fallot 布氏手术,锁骨下动脉肺动脉吻合术

bland *adjective* (food) which is not spicy *or* not irritating *or* not acid 温和的; **bland diet** = diet in which the patient eats mainly milk-based foods, boiled vegetables and white meat, as a treatment for peptic ulcers 软食

blank *adjective* (paper) with nothing written on it 空的: ***The doctor took out a blank prescription form***. 医生拿了张空白处方。

blanket *noun* thick woollen cover which is put over a person to keep him warm when asleep or lying still 毯子: ***He woke up when his blankets fell off***. 毯子掉地上时他醒了。**blanket bath** = washing a patient who is confined to bed 给卧床病人洗澡

blast *noun* (**a**) immature form of a cell before definite characteristics develop 幼稚细胞 (**b**) wave of air pressure from an explosion, which can cause concussion 冲击波; **blast injury** = severe injury to the chest following a blast 冲击伤

-blast *suffix* referring to a very early stage in the development of a cell 成…母细胞

blasto- *prefix* referring to a germ cell 芽,胚

blastocoele *noun* cavity filled with fluid in a morula 囊胚腔

◇ **blastocyst** *noun* early stage in the development of an embryo 胚泡

◇ **Blastomyces** *noun* type of parasitic fungus which affects the skin 芽生菌属

◇ **blastomycosis** *noun* infection caused by Blastomyces 芽生菌病

◇ **blastula** *noun* first stage of the development of an embryo in animals 囊胚

bleb *noun* small blister 疱,小疱 *compare* 比较 BULLA

bled 出血 *see* 见 BLEED

bleed *verb* to lose blood 失血: ***His knee was bleeding.*** 他的膝盖在流血。***His nose began to bleed.*** 他鼻子开始出血。***When she cut her finger it bled.*** 她切伤了手,流血了。***He was bleeding from a cut on the head.*** 他头上的伤口在流血。(NOTE: **bleeds - bleeding - bled - has bled**)

◇ **bleeder** *noun* person who suffers from haemophilia 血友病患者,易出血者

◇ **bleeding** *noun* abnormal loss of blood from the body through the skin or through an orifice or internally 出血; **internal bleeding** = loss of blood inside the body (as from a wound in the intestine) 内出血; **control of bleeding** = ways of stopping bleeding by applying pressure to blood vessels 止血; **bleeding point** *or* **bleeding site** = place in the body where bleeding is taking place 出血部位; **bleeding time** = test of clotting of a patient's blood, by timing the length of time it takes for the blood to congeal 出血时间

> COMMENT: Blood lost through bleeding from an artery is bright red and can rush out because it is under pressure. Blood from a vein is darker red and flows more slowly.
> 注释:动脉出血为鲜红色,因动脉压可呈喷射状,静脉出血是暗红色,流出缓慢。

blenno- *prefix* referring to mucus 粘液的

◇ **blennorrhagia** *noun* (i) discharge of mucus 粘液溢出(ii) gonorrhoea 淋病

◇ **blennorrhoea** *noun* (i) discharge of watery mucus 水样粘液溢出(ii) gonorrhoea 淋病

blephar- *prefix* referring to the eyelid 眼睑的

◇ **blepharitis** *noun* inflammation of the eyelid 睑炎

◇ **blepharon** *noun* eyelid 眼睑

◇ **blepharoptosis** *noun* condition where the upper eyelid is half closed because of paralysis of the muscle or nerve 睑下垂

◇ **blepharospasm** *noun* sudden contraction of the eyelid, as when a tiny piece of dust gets in the eye 睑痉挛

blind 1 *adjective* not able to see 盲的; ***a blind man with a white stick*** 拄着白拐杖的盲人; ***After her illness she became blind.*** 病后她的眼就瞎了。**colour blind** = not able to tell the difference between certain colours, especially red and green 色盲; **blind loop syndrome** 盲袢综合症 *see* 见 LOOP; **blind spot** = point in the retina where the optic nerve joins it, which does not register light 盲点 **2** *plural noun* **the blind** = people who are blind 盲人; **blind register** = official list of blind people 盲人登记 **3** *verb* to make someone blind 使盲,致盲: ***He was blinded in the accident.*** 他因事故致盲。

◇ **blindness** *noun* not being able to see 盲; **colour blindness** = being unable to tell the difference between certain colours 色盲; **day blindness** = hemeralopia, being able to see better in bad light than in ordinary daylight (usually a congenital condition) 昼盲; **night blindness** = nyctalopia, being unable to see in bad light 夜盲; **snow blindness** = temporary painful blindness caused by bright sunlight shining on snow 雪盲; **sun blindness** = PHOTORETINITIS 光照性视网膜炎

blink *verb* to close and open the eyelids rapidly several times or once 眨眼: ***He blinked in the bright light.*** 他在强光下眨眼。

blister 1 *noun* (i) swelling on the skin containing serous liquid 水泡(ii) substance which acts as a counterirritant 发疱剂 **2** *verb* to have blisters 起泡: ***After the fire his hands and face were badly blistered.*** 火灾后他的手和脸起了很多水泡。

> COMMENT: Blisters contain serum or watery liquid from the blood. They can be caused by rubbing, burning or by a disease such as chickenpox. Blood blisters contain

blood which has passed from broken blood vessels under the skin. Water blisters contain lymph.
注释:水泡中含有从血管流出的血清或水样液体。可因摩擦、烧伤、或水痘等疾病引起。血泡含有从皮下破裂的血管流出的血液,水泡含有的是淋巴液。

block 1 *noun* (**a**) stopping of a function 阻滞;**caudal block** = local analgesia of the cauda equina nerves in the lower spine 骶管阻滞; **epidural block** = analgesia produced by injecting an analgesic solution into the space between the vertebral canal and the dura mater 硬膜外阻滞; **heart block** = slowing of the action of the heart because the impulses from the SA node to the ventricles are delayed or interrupted 心传导阻滞; **mental block** = temporary inability to remember something, caused by the effect of nervous stress on the mental processes 精神阻滞; **nerve block** = stopping the function of a nerve by injecting an anaesthetic 神经阻滞; **speech block** = temporary inability to speak, caused by the effect of nervous stress on the mental processes 言语阻滞; **spinal block** analgesia produced by injecting the spinal cord with an anaesthetic 脊髓阻滞 (**b**) large piece 大块: ***A block of wood fell on his foot.*** 一大块木头砸在他的脚上。(**c**) one of the different buildings forming a section of a hospital 病区: ***The patient is in Block 2, Ward 7.*** 病人在2病区7病房。***She is having treatment in the physiotherapy block.*** 她在理疗病区接受治疗。**2** *verb* to obstruct 阻断: ***The artery was blocked by a clot.*** 这动脉被血块阻塞了。***He swallowed a piece of plastic which blocked his oesophagus.*** 他吞下了一大块塑料,堵住了食管。

◇ **blockage** *noun* something which obstructs; being obstructed 阻滞: ***There is a blockage in the rectum.*** 直肠梗阻。***The blockage of the artery was caused by a blood clot.*** 这动脉受阻是因为血凝块。

◇ **blocker** *noun* substance which blocks 阻滞剂; **beta blocker** = drug which blocks the beta-adrenergic receptors and so reduces the activity of the heart β受体阻滞剂

◇ **blocking** *noun* psychiatric disorder, where the patient suddenly stops one train of thought and switches to another 思维中断

blood *noun* red liquid in the body 血液: ***The police followed the spots of blood to find the wounded man.*** 警察沿着血迹找到了受伤的人。***Blood was pouring from the cut in his hand.*** 血从他手上的伤口涌出。***He suffered serious loss of blood*** *or* ***blood loss in the accident.*** 他在事故中严重失血。**blood bank** = section of a hospital where blood given by donors is stored for use in transfusions 血库; **blood casts** = pieces of blood cells which are secreted by the kidneys in kidney disease 血细胞管型; **blood cell** *or* **blood corpuscle** = red blood cell *or* white blood cell which is one of the parts of blood 血细胞; **blood chemistry** *or* **chemistry of the blood** = (i) substances which make up blood, which can be analysed in blood tests, the results of which are useful in diagnosing disease 血液化学成分 (ii) record of changes which take place in blood during disease and treatment 血液成分变化; **blood clot** = thrombus, a soft mass of coagulated blood in a vein or an artery 血块; **blood clotting** *or* **blood coagulation** = process where blood changes from being liquid to being semi-solid and so stops flowing 凝血过程; **blood count** = test to count the number and types of different blood cells in a certain tiny sample of blood, to give an indication of the condition of the patient's blood as a whole 血细胞计数; **blood culture** = putting a sample of blood into a culture medium to see if foreign organisms in it grow 血培养; **blood donor** = person who gives blood which is then used in transfusions to other patients 供

血者,献血者; **blood formation** = haemopoiesis, the continual production of blood cells and blood platelets by the bone marrow 造血; **blood-letting** = phlebotomy *or* venesection, an operation where a vein or an artery is cut so that blood can be removed 血管切开术; **blood loss** = loss of blood from the body by bleeding 失血; **blood plasma** = yellow watery liquid which makes up the main part of blood 血浆; **blood platelet** = small blood cell which releases thromboplastin and which multiplies rapidly after an injury, encouraging the coagulation of blood 血小板; **blood poisoning** = septicaemia, a condition where bacteria are present in blood and cause illness 败血症; **blood sample** = sample of blood, taken for testing 血样; **blood serum** = yellowish watery liquid which separates from (whole) blood when the blood clots 血清; **blood sugar level** = amount of glucose in the blood 血糖水平; **blood test** = laboratory test of a blood sample to analyse its chemical composition 血液检查; **blood transfusion** = transferring blood from another person into a patient's vein 输血; **blood type** = BLOOD GROUP 血型; **blood urea** = urea present in the blood (a high level occurs following heart failure or kidney disease) 血尿; **blood vessel** = any tube (artery, vein, capillary) which carries blood round the body 血管 (NOTE: for other terms referring to blood, see words beginning with **haem-**, **haemato-**)

COMMENT: Blood is formed of red and white corpuscles, platelets and plasma. It circulates round the body, going from the heart and lungs along arteries and returns to the heart through the veins. As it moves round the body it takes oxygen to the tissues and removes waste material which is cleaned out through the kidneys or exhaled through the lungs. It also carries hormones produced by glands to the various organs which need them. Each adult person has about six litres or ten pints of blood in his body.
注释:血液由红白细胞、血小板及血浆组成。从心、肺经动脉流到全身,再经静脉回心脏。在此过程中将氧携带至组织,而将废物从肾、肺排出。它还将腺体产生的激素运到不同的器官。每一个成人的体内大约有6升或10品脱的血液。

◇ **blood-brain barrier** *noun* process by which certain substances are held back by the endothelium of cerebral capillaries (where in other parts of the body the same substances will diffuse from capillaries) so preventing these substances from getting into contact with the fluids round the brain 血脑屏障

◇ **blood group** *noun* one of the different types of blood by which groups of people are identified 血型

COMMENT: Blood is classified in various ways. The most common classifications are by the agglutinogens in red blood corpuscles (factors A and B) and by the Rhesus factor. Blood can therefore have either factor (Group A and Group B) or both factors (GroupAB) or neither (Group O) and each of these groups can be Rhesus negative or positive.
注释:血可分为不同的类型。最常用的是根据红细胞上的凝集原(A,B)或Rh因子进行分型。根据前者分为A型(含A凝集原),B型(含B凝集原),AB型(含A,B两种凝集原)和O型(不含任何凝集原);据后者分Rh阴性和阳性两类。

◇ **blood pressure** *noun* pressures (measured in millimetres of mercury) at which the blood is pumped round the body by the heart 血压; **high blood pressure** *or* **raised blood pressure** = level of blood pressure which is higher than normal 高血压: ***She suffers from high blood pressure.*** 她患有高血压病。

COMMENT: Blood pressure is mea

sured using a sphygmomanometer, where a rubber tube is wrapped round the patient's arm and inflated. Two readings of blood pressure are taken: the systolic pressure, when the heart is contracting and so pumping out, and the diastolic pressure (which is always a lower figure) when the heart relaxes.
注释:量血压要使用血压计,测量时,将血压计的袖带缚于患者胳膊上然后充气。测定采用两声法,心脏收缩泵出血液时为收缩压、当心脏舒张时为舒张压。

QUOTE: Raised blood pressure may account for as many as 70% of all strokes. The risk of stroke rises with both systolic and diastolic blood pressure in the normotensive and hypertensive ranges. Blood pressure control reduces the incidence of first stroke and aspirin appears to reduce the risk of stroke after TIAs.
引文:70%的卒中发作是因血压升高引起。在正常或高于正常血压的范围内发生卒中的危险度随收缩压,舒张压的升高而升高。而控制血压可以减少卒中的发生率,阿司匹林可减少短暂脑缺血后卒中的发生。

British Journal of Hospital Medicine 英国医院医学杂志

◇ **bloodshot** *adjective* (eye) with small specks of blood in it 充血的
◇ **bloodstained** *adjective* having blood in or on it 血迹: ***He coughed up bloodstained sputum.*** 他咳血痰。***The nurses took away the bloodstained sheets.*** 护士将沾有血迹的床单拿走。
◇ **bloodstream** *noun* blood flowing round the body 血流: ***The antibiotics are injected into the bloodstream.*** 抗生素注入血流。***Hormones are secreted by the glands into the bloodstream.*** 激素由腺体分泌入血。

blot 印迹 *see* 见 RORSCHACH TEST

blue *adjective* & *noun* (of a) colour such as that of a clear unclouded sky in the daytime 蓝色的,蓝色: ***The sister was dressed in a blue uniform.*** 护士身穿蓝色制服。**blue baby** = baby suffering from congenital cyanosis, born either with a congenital heart defect or with atelectasis (a collapsed lung), which prevents an adequate supply of oxygen reaching the tissues, giving the baby's skin a bluish colour 患先天性紫绀的婴儿(因先天性心脏病或肺不张引起组织缺氧,皮肤发紫) (NOTE: **blue - bluer - bluest**)
◇ **Blue Cross** *or* **Blue Shield** *noun US* systems of private medical insurance 蓝十字
◇ **blueness** *or* **blue disease** *noun* cyanosis, the blue colour of the skin, a symptom of lack of oxygen in the blood 紫绀(血中缺氧的症状)

blunt *adjective* not sharp or which does not cut well 钝的: ***He hurt his hand with a blunt knife.*** 他用一把钝刀伤了自己的手。***The surgeon's instruments must not be blunt.*** 手术器械不能发钝。(NOTE: **blunt - blunter - bluntest**)

blurred *adjective* not clear 不清楚的; **blurred vision** = condition where the patient does not see objects clearly 视力模糊
◇ **blurring of vision** *noun* condition where a patient does not see objects clearly, caused by loss of blood or sometimes by inadequate diet 视力模糊

blush 1 *noun* rush of red colour to the skin of the face (caused by emotion) 潮红 **2** *verb* to go red in the face because of emotion 变红

BM = BACHELOR OF MEDICINE 医学学士

BMA = BRITISH MEDICAL ASSOCIATION 英国医学会

BMR = BASAL METABOLIC RATE 基础代谢率; **BMR test** = test of thyroid function 基础代谢率试验

BO = BODY ODOUR 体臭

board of directors *noun* group of people (usually, consultants, heads of nursing staff and administrators) chosen to run a hospital trust 董事会

body *noun* (**a**) the trunk, the main

part of a person, not including the head or arms and legs 躯干 (**b**) all of a person (as opposed to the mind) 身体: ***The dead man's body was found several days later.*** 尸体几天后才被发现。**body fat** = adipose tissue, tissue where the cells contain fat, which replaces the normal fibrous tissue when too much food is eaten 脂肪组织; **body fluids** = liquid in the body, including mainly water and blood 体液; **body image** *or* **body schema** = mental image which a person has of his own body 体像; **body odour** = unpleasant smell caused by perspiration 体臭; **body scan** = examination of the whole of a patient's body using ultrasound or other scanning techniques 全身扫描; **body temperature** = internal temperature of the human body (normally about 37°C) 体温 (**c**) mass *or* piece of material (of any size) 物体; **cell body** = part of a nerve cell which surrounds the nucleus and from which the axon and dendrites begin 胞体; **ciliary body** = part of the eye which connects the iris to the choroid 睫状体; **inclusion bodies** = very small particles found in cells infected by virus 内涵体; **Nissl bodies** *or* **Nissl granules** = coarse granules surrounding the nucleus in the cytoplasm of nerve cells 尼斯尔氏小体,虎斑小体; **pineal body** *or* **pineal gland** = small cone-shaped gland situated below the corpus callosum in the brain, which produces melatonin and is believed to be associated with the circadian rhythm 松果体 ◊ 见图 BRAIN (**d**) main part of something 主体; **body of sternum** = main central part of the breastbone 胸骨体; **body of vertebra** = main part of a vertebra which supports the weight of the body 椎体; **body of the stomach** = main part of the stomach between the fundus and the pylorus 胃体 ◊ 见图 STOMACH (**e**) **foreign body** = piece of material which is not part of the surrounding tissue and should not be there (such as sand in a cut *or* dust in the eye *or* pin which has been swallowed) 异物: ***The X-ray showed the presence of a foreign body.*** X线显示有异物存在。**swallowed foreign bodies** = anything (a pin *or* coin *or* button) which should not have been swallowed 被吞咽的异物

◊ **bodily** *adjective* referring to the body 机体的: ***The main bodily functions are controlled by the sympathetic nervous system.*** 身体的主要机能由交感神经支配。***He suffered from several minor bodily disorders.*** 他患有几种轻微疾病。

Boeck's disease *or* **Boeck's sarcoid** = SARCOIDOSIS 伯克氏肉样瘤,结节病

Bohn's nodules *or* **Bohn's epithelial pearls** *plural noun* tiny cysts found in the mouths of healthy infants 博恩氏小结

boil 1 *noun* furuncle, a tender raised mass of infected tissue and skin, usually caused by infection of a hair follicle by the bacterium *Staphylococcus aureus* 疖 2 *verb* to heat water (or another liquid) until it changes into gas (*of water, etc.*) to change into a gas because of heating 煮;沸腾: ***Can you boil some water so we can sterilize the instruments?*** 你能煮些水来消毒器械吗?

bolus *noun* food which has been chewed and is ready to be swallowed; mass of food passing along the intestine 食团

bonding *noun* making a psychological link between the baby and its mother 母婴依附: ***In autistic children bonding is difficult.*** 自闭症患儿母婴依附有困难。

bone *noun* (**a**) one of the calcified pieces of connective tissue which make the skeleton 骨: ***He fell over and broke a bone in his ankle.*** 他摔下来,摔断了踝骨。***There are several small bones in the human ear.*** 人耳内有几块小骨。**cranial bones** = bones in the skull 颅骨 ◊ 见图 SKULL; **metacarpal bone** = one of the five bones in the hand 掌骨 ◊ 见图

HAND (**b**) hard substance which forms a bone 骨质; **cancellous bone** *or* **spongy bone** = light spongy bone tissue which forms the inner core of a bone and also the ends of long bones 松质骨; **compact bone** *or* **dense bone** = type of bone tissue which forms the hard outer layer of a bone 密质骨◊见图 BONE STRUCTURE; **bone conduction** 骨传导 *see* 见 CONDUCTION; **bone graft** = piece of bone taken from one part of the body to repair a defect in another bone 骨移植; **bone structure** = (i) system of jointed bones forming the body 骨骼(ii) arrangement of the various components of a bone (NOTE: for other terms referring to bone, see words beginning with **ost-**, **osteo-**)

COMMENT: Bones are formed of a hard outer layer (compact bone) which is made up of a series of layers of tissue (Haversian systems) and a softer inner part (cancellous bone *or* spongy bone) which contains bone marrow.

注释:骨由坚硬的外层(密质骨)和松软的内层(松质骨)组成。外层有多层组织(Haversian 系统),内层含有骨髓。

◊ **bone marrow** *noun* soft tissue in cancellous bone 骨髓; **bone marrow transplant** = transplant of marrow from a donor to a recipient 骨髓移植◊见图 BONE STRUCTURE (NOTE: for other terms referring to bone marrow, see words beginning with **myel-**, **myelo-**)

COMMENT: Two types of bone marrow are to be found: red bone marrow or myeloid tissue, which forms red blood cells and is found in cancellous bone in the vertebrae, the sternum and other flat bones; as a person gets older, fatty yellow bone marrow develops in the central cavity of long bones。

注释:骨髓有两类,红骨髓或髓样组织,主要位于椎体、胸骨和其他扁骨的松质骨内,可形成红细胞。随着年龄的增长黄骨髓逐渐出现于长骨的骨腔。

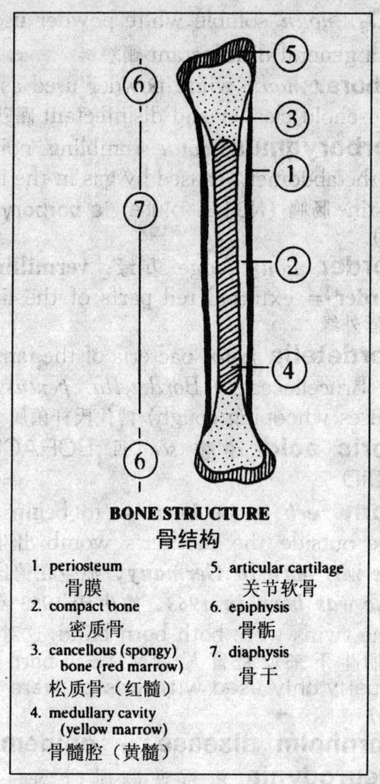

BONE STRUCTURE
骨结构

1. periosteum 骨膜
2. compact bone 密质骨
3. cancellous (spongy) bone (red marrow) 松质骨(红髓)
4. medullary cavity (yellow marrow) 骨髓腔(黄髓)
5. articular cartilage 关节软骨
6. epiphysis 骨骺
7. diaphysis 骨干

◊ **bony** *adjective* (i) referring to bones 骨的(ii) (part of the body) where the structure of the bones underneath can be seen 可见骨的,露骨的: ***She has long bony hands.*** 她的手又长又瘦。**bony labyrinth** = hard part of the temporal bone surrounding the membranous labyrinth in the inner ear 骨迷路

Bonney's blue *noun* blue dye used as a disinfectant 邦尼蓝,用于消毒的染料

booster (injection) *noun* repeat injection of vaccine given some time after the first injection so as to keep the immunizing effect 强化免疫辅助药剂

boot *noun* strong shoe which goes above the ankle 靴; **surgical boot** = specially made boot for a person who has a deformed foot; boot made to correct a deformity 矫形鞋

boracic acid *or* **boric acid** (H_3BO_3) *noun* soluble white powder used as a general disinfectant 硼酸
◇ **borax** *noun* white powder used as a household cleaner and disinfectant 硼砂

borborygmus *noun* rumbling noise in the abdomen, caused by gas in the intestine 肠鸣(NOTE: plural is **borborygmi**)

border *noun* edge 边缘; **vermillion border** = external red parts of the lips 红唇外缘

Bordetella *noun* bacteria of the family Brucellaceae (*Bordetella pertussis* causes whooping cough) 博代氏杆菌属

boric acid 硼酸 *see* 见 BORACIC ACID

born *verb* **to be born** = to begin to live outside the mother's womb 出生: ***He was born in Germany.*** 他生在德国。***She was born in 1963.*** 她生于1963年。The twins were both born blind. 这对双胞胎生下来就是盲人。(NOTE: **born** is usually only used with **was** or **were** or **be**)

Bornholm disease *or* **epidemic pleurodynia** 流行性胸肌痛 *see* 见 PLEURODYNIA

bother 1 *noun* thing which is annoying or worrying 麻烦: ***The accident has caused a lot of bother.*** 这起意外引起了很多麻烦。**2** *verb* (i) to take trouble to do something 烦扰 (ii) to worry about something 操心: ***She didn't bother to send a telegram.*** 她懒得发电报。***Don't bother about cleaning the room.*** 不要为打扫房间操心。***Smoke bothers him because he has asthma.*** 烟雾使他心烦,因为他有哮喘。

bottle *noun* glass container for liquids 瓶: ***He drinks a bottle of milk a day.*** 他一天喝一瓶牛奶。***Open another bottle of orange juice.*** 再开一瓶橘子汁。**baby's (feeding) bottle** = special bottle with a rubber teat, used for giving milk (or other liquids) to babies 奶瓶; **bottle feeding** = giving a baby milk from a bottle, as opposed to breast feeding 用奶瓶喂养 *compare* 比较 BREAST FEEDING
◇ **bottle-fed** *adjective* (baby) which is fed from a bottle 用奶瓶喂养的: ***She was bottle-fed after the first two months.*** 2月后她开始用奶瓶喂养。*compare* 比较 BREASTFED

bottom *noun* (**a**) lowest part 基底部: ***There was some jam left in the bottom of the jar.*** 在罐子的底部还留有些果酱。(**b**) part of the body on which you sit 臀 *see also* 参见 BUTTOCKS

botulism *noun* type of food poisoning caused by a toxin of *Clostridium botulinum* in badly canned or preserved food 肉毒中毒

> COMMENT: Symptoms include paralysis of the muscles, vomiting and hallucinations. Botulism is often fatal.
> 注释:症状包括肌麻痹、呕吐和幻觉,肉毒中毒常为致命的。

bougie *noun* thin tube which can be inserted into passages in the body (such as the oesophagus or rectum) either to allow liquid to be introduced or simply to dilate the passage 探条

bout *noun* sudden attack of a disease, especially one which recurs 发作: ***He is recovering from a bout of flu.*** 他流感康复了。***She has recurrent bouts of malarial fever.*** 她因疟疾反复发热。

bowel *or* **bowels** *noun* the intestine, especially the large intestine 肠; **to open the bowels** = to defecate, to have a bowel movement 排便; **bowel movement** = defecation, the evacuation of solid waste matter from the bowel through the anus 排便: ***The patient had a bowel movement this morning.*** 患者今晨排便一次。**irritable bowel syndrome** = MUCOUS COLITIS 肠易激惹综合症

bowl *noun* (**a**) wide container with higher sides than a plate, used for semi-liquids 碗; ***a bowl of soup*** *or* ***of cream*** 一碗汤(奶); **soup bowl** = bowl specially made for soup 汤碗（**b**）the part of a sink *or* washbasin *or* toilet which contains water 碗状物

bow legs *noun* genu varum, state where the ankles touch and the knees area part when a person is standing straight 弓形腿 *compare* 比较 KNOCK KNEE

◇ **bow-legged** *adjective* with bow legs 弓形腿的

Bowman's capsule *noun* Malpighian glomerulus, expanded end of a renal tubule, surrounding a glomerular tuft 鲍曼氏囊,肾小球囊

boy *noun* male child 男孩：***They have three children - two boys and a girl.*** 他们有3个孩子,2个男孩和1个女孩。The boys were playing in the field. 男孩们在田地里玩耍。

BP = BLOOD PRESSURE 血压, BRITISH PHARMACOPOEIA 英国药典

Bq = BECQUEREL 贝克(勒尔)

Br *chemical symbol for* bromine 溴的化学元素符号

brace *noun* any type of splint or appliance worn for support, such as a metal support used on children's legs to make the bones straight or on teeth which are forming badly 支架：***She wore a brace on her front teeth.*** 她戴着牙箍。

bracelet *noun* chain *or* band which is worn around the wrist 手镯；**identity bracelet** = label attached to the wrist of a newborn baby *or* patient in hospital so that he can be identified 戴在新生儿腕上用来识别的标签

brachi- *prefix* referring to the arm 臂的

◇ **brachial** *adjective* referring to the arm, especially the upper arm 臂的；**brachial artery** = artery running down the arm from the axillary artery to the elbow, where it divides into the radial and ulnar arteries 臂动脉；**brachial plexus** = group of nerves at the armpit and base of the neck which lead to the nerves in the arms and hands; injury to the brachial plexus at birth leads to Erb's palsy 臂丛；**brachial pressure point** = point on the arm where pressure will stop bleeding from the brachial artery 臂动脉压迫止血点；**brachial veins** = veins accompanying the brachial artery, draining into the axillary vein 臂静脉

◇ **brachialis muscle** *noun* flexor of the elbow 肱肌

◇ **brachiocephalic artery** *noun* largest branch of the arch of the aorta, which continues as the right common carotid and right subclavian arteries 头臂动脉

◇ **brachiocephalic veins** *plural noun* innominate veins, two veins which continue the subclavian and jugular veins to the superior vena cava 头臂静脉

◇ **brachium** *noun* arm, especially the upper arm between the elbow and the shoulder 臂,上臂（NOTE: plural is **brachia**）

brachy- *prefix meaning* short 短的

◇ **brachycephaly** *noun* condition where the skull is shorter than normal 短头畸形

Bradford's frame *noun* frame of metal and cloth, used to support a patient 布莱德福氏支架

brady- *prefix meaning* slow 慢的

◇ **bradycardia** *noun* slow rate of heart contraction, shown by a slow pulse rate (less than 70 per minute) 心跳过缓

◇ **bradykinesia** *noun* walking slowly *or* making slow movements (because of disease) 运动徐缓

◇ **bradypnoea** *noun* abnormally slow breathing 呼吸徐缓

Braille *noun* system of writing using raised dots on the paper to indicate letters, which allows a blind person to read by passing his fingers over the page 点字法,盲文：***She was reading a Braille book.*** 她在阅读盲文书。***The book has been published in Braille.*** 这本书是用盲文出版的。

brain *noun* encephalon, cranial part of the central nervous system, situated inside the skull 脑; **brain death** = condition where the nerves in the brain stem have died, and the patient can be certified as dead, although the heart may not have stopped beating 脑死亡; **brain haemorrhage** = bleeding inside the brain from a cerebral artery 脑出血 *see also* 参见 FOREBRAIN, HINDBRAIN, MIDBRAIN (NOTE: for other terms referring to the brain, see words beginning with **cerebr-**, **encephal-**)

> COMMENT: The main part of the brain is the cerebrum, formed of two sections or hemispheres, which relate to thought and to sensations from either side of the body; at the back of the head and beneath the cerebrum is the cerebellum which coordinates muscle reaction and balance. Also in the brain are the hypothalamus which governs body temperature, hunger, thirst and sexual urges, and the tiny pituitary gland which is the most important endocrine gland in the body.
> 注释:脑的主要部分是大脑,由两个半球组成,支配思想和对侧身体的感觉。头的后部,大脑下部是小脑,支配肌肉运动和保持平衡。脑内还有下丘脑,控制体温、饥饿感、渴感和性欲,小小的垂体是体内最重要的内分泌腺。

◇ **brain damage** *noun* damage caused to the brain in an accident 脑损伤: ***He suffered brain damage in the car crash.*** 他在车祸中损伤了脑。

◇ **brain-damaged** *adjective* (person) who has suffered brain damage 有脑损伤的: ***She was brain-damaged from birth.*** 她一出生就有脑损伤。

◇ **brain fever** *noun* non-medical term for an infection which affects the brain (such as encephalitis *or* meningitis) 中枢系统感染引起的发热

◇ **brain stem** *noun* lower part of the brain, shaped like a stem, which connects the brain to the spinal cord 脑干

◇ **brain tumour** *noun* tumour which grows in the brain 脑瘤

> COMMENT: Tumours may grow in any part of the brain. The symptoms of brain tumour are usually headaches and dizziness, and as the tumour grows it may affect the senses or mental faculties. Operations to remove brain tumours can be very successful.
> 注释:肿瘤可发生于脑的任何部位。常见症状是头疼、眩晕,随着肿瘤的生长会影响脑的感觉和智力活动。手术切除脑瘤疗效显著。

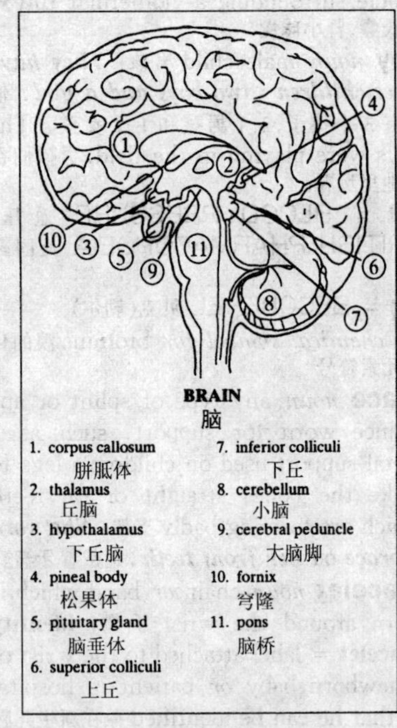

bran *noun* outside covering of the wheat seed, removed to make white flour, but an important source of roughage, hence used in breakfast cereals 糠,麸

branch 1 *noun* (i) part of a tree growing out of the main trunk 树支(ii) any part which grows out of a main part 分支 2 *verb* to split out into smaller parts 分支: ***The radial artery branches from***

the brachial artery at the elbow. 桡动脉在肘部从臂动脉处分出。

branchial cyst *or* **branchial fistula** *noun* cyst on the side of the neck of an embryo 鳃裂囊肿

◇ **branchial pouch** *noun* pouch on the side of the neck of an embryo 鳃囊

Braun's frame *or* **Braun's splint** *noun* metal splint and frame to which pulleys are attached, used for holding up a fractured leg while a patient is lying in bed 布朗氏支架

bread *noun* food made by baking flour and yeast 面包

break 1 *noun* point at which a bone has broken 断裂点; **clean break** = break in a bone which is not complicated *or* where the two parts will join again easily 简单骨折 **2** *verb* to make something go to pieces; to go to pieces 打碎,断裂: *She fell off the wall and broke her leg*. 她从墙上摔下来,摔断了腿。*He can't play football with a broken leg*. 他腿断了不能踢球。(NOTE: **breaks - breaking - broke - has broken**)

◇ **breakbone fever** = DENGUE 登革热

◇ **breakdown** *noun* (**a**) (**nervous**) **breakdown** = non-medical term for a sudden illness where a patient becomes so depressed *or* worried that he is incapable of doing anything 精神崩溃 (**b**) **breakdown product** = substance which is produced when a compound is broken down into its parts 分解物

◇ **break down** *verb* (**a**) to reduce a compound to its parts 分解 (**b**) to collapse in a nervous state 崩溃: *She broke down and cried as she described the symptoms to the doctor*. 她完全崩溃了,哭着向医生诉说症状。

◇ **breakfast** *noun* first meal of the day 早餐: *The patient had a boiled egg for breakfast*. 患者早餐吃的是煮鸡蛋。*She didn't have any breakfast because she was due to have surgery later in the day*. 因为她当天晚些时候要手术,所以没有吃早餐。*We have breakfast at 7.30 every day*. 我们每天 7:30 吃早餐。

breast *noun* mamma, one of two glands in a woman which secrete milk 乳腺; **breast cancer** = malignant tumour in the breast 乳腺癌; **breast feeding** = feeding a baby from the mother's breast as opposed to from a bottle 母乳喂养 *compare* 比较 BOTTLE FEEDING (NOTE: for other terms referring to the breast, see words beginning with **mamm-**, **mast-**)

◇ **breastbone** *noun* sternum, bone which is in the centre of the front of the thorax and to which the ribs are connected 胸骨

◇ **breastfed** *adjective* (baby) which is fed from the mother's breast 母乳喂养的: *She was breastfed for the first two months*. 她头两个月是靠母乳喂养。

breath *noun* air which goes in and out of the body when you breathe 气息: *He ran so fast he was out of breath*. 他跑得太快了,上气不接下气。*Stop for a moment to get your breath back*. 歇一会儿,让你的呼吸平静下来。*She took a deep breath and dived into the water*. 她深吸一口气潜入水中。**to hold your breath** = to stop breathing out, after having inhaled deeply 屏气; **short of breath** = unable to breathe quickly enough to supply the oxygen needed 气短; **bad breath** = HALITOSIS 口臭; **breath sounds** = hollow sounds made by the lungs and heard through a stethoscope placed on a patient's chest, used in diagnosis 呼吸音

◇ **breathe** *verb* to inhale and exhale *or* to take air in and blow air out through the nose or mouth 呼吸: *He could not breathe under water*. 他在水下不能呼吸。*He breathed in the smoke from the fire and it made him cough*. 他在烟雾中呼吸,熏得直咳嗽。*The patient has begun to breathe normally*. 患者呼吸开始正常。*The doctor told him to take a deep breath and breathe out slowly*. 医

生让他深吸气再缓慢呼出。

◇ **breathing** *noun* respiration, taking air into the lungs and blowing it out again through the mouth or nose 呼吸: ***If breathing is difficult or has stopped, begin artificial ventilation immediately.*** 如果发生呼吸困难或呼吸停止,应立刻进行人工呼吸。**breathing rate** = number of times a person breathes in and out 呼吸频率 (NOTE: for other terms referring to breathing, see words beginning with **pneumo-**)

◇ **breathless** *adjective* (patient) who finds it difficult to breathe enough air 呼吸困难的: ***After running upstairs she became breathless and had to sit down.*** 她爬上楼后呼吸困难,不得不坐下来休息。

◇ **breathlessness** *noun* difficulty in breathing enough air 呼吸困难

> COMMENT: Children breathe about 20 to 30 times per minute, men 16–18 per minute, and women slightly faster. The breathing rate increases if the person is taking exercise or has a fever. Some babies hold their breath and go blue in the face, especially when crying or during a temper tantrum.
> 注释:儿童的呼吸频率是每分钟 20–30 次,男性为 16–18 次,女性略快。运动或发热时可加快。一些婴儿屏住呼吸,面色会青紫,尤其在哭闹或发怒时。

> QUOTE: 26 patients were selected from the outpatient department on grounds of disabling breathlessness present for at least five years.
> 引文:从门诊选择了 26 例有呼吸困难 5 年以上病史的患者。
>
> **Lancet** 柳叶刀

breech *noun* buttocks 臀; **breech birth** *or* **breech delivery** = birth where the baby's buttocks appear first 臀位分娩; **breech presentation** = position of the baby in the womb, where the buttocks will appear first 臀先露

breed *verb* to reproduce and spread 繁殖: ***The bacteria breed in dirty water.*** 细菌在污水中繁殖。***Insanitary conditons help to breed disease.*** 不良的卫生条件有助于疾病的传播。

bregma *noun* point at the top of the head where the soft gap between the bones of a baby's skull (the anterior fontanelle) hardens 前囟

bridge *noun* (**a**) top part of the nose where it joins the forehead 鼻梁 (**b**) (*for teeth*) artificial tooth (or teeth) which is joined to natural teeth which hold it in place 义齿 (**c**) a part joining two or more other parts 桥梁

Bright's disease *noun* glomerulonephritis, inflammation of the kidney, characterized by albuminuria and high blood pressure 布赖特肾病,肾小球肾炎

brim *noun* edge 边; **pelvic brim** = line on the ilium which separates the false pelvis from the true pelvis 骨盆上口

bring up *verb* (**a**) to look after and educate a child 抚养: ***He was brought up by his uncle in Scotland.*** 他由叔叔在苏格兰养大。***I was brought up in the country.*** 我在乡村长大。***She has been badly brought up.*** 她的成长条件不好。(**b**) (i) to vomit, to force material from the stomach back into the mouth 呕吐 (ii) to cough up material such as mucus from the lungs *or* throat 咳出: ***He was bringing up mucus.*** 他咳的是粘液。

British *adjective* referring to Great Britain 英国

◇ **British anti-lewisite** (**BAL**) *noun* antidote for blister gases, but also used to treat cases of poisoning, such as mercury poisoning 二巯基丙醇

◇ **British Dental Association** (**BDA**) *noun* professional association of dentists 英国牙科协会

◇ **British Medical Association** (**BMA**) *noun* professional association of doctors 英国医学会

◇ **British Pharmacopoeia** (**BP**) *noun* book listing approved drugs and their dosages 英国药典

> COMMENT: Drugs listed in the British Pharmacopoeia have the let-

ters BP written after them on labels.
注释：凡英国药典中的药物在商标上均有 BP 字样。

brittle *adjective* which breaks easily 脆的：***The bones of old people become brittle.*** 老年人的骨质开始发脆。（NOTE：the opposite is **ductile**）

◇ **brittle bone disease** 脆骨病 *see* 见 OSTEOGENESIS，OSTEOPOROSIS

broad *adjective* wide in relation to length 宽的；**broad ligament** = peritoneal folds supporting the uterus on either side 阔韧带；**broad-spectrum antibiotic** = antibiotic used to control many types of bacteria 广谱抗生素（NOTE：**broad - broader - broadest**；opposite is **narrow**）

Broadbent's sign *noun* movement of a patient's left side near the lower ribs at each beat of the heart, indicating adhesion between the diaphragm and pericardium in cases of pericarditis 布罗德本症，患者左肋下部随心跳而动，提示心包炎时膈肌和心包粘连

Broca's aphasia *noun* being unable to speak or write, caused by damage to Broca's area 布罗卡氏失语，因 Broca 区受损导致言语、书写不能

◇ **Broca's area** *noun* area on the left side of the brain which governs the motor aspects of speaking 布罗卡氏区，旁嗅区，位于左脑，主管说话运动

Brodie's abscess *noun* abscess of a bone, caused by staphylococcal osteomyelitis 布罗迪氏脓肿，葡萄球菌骨髓炎引起的骨脓肿

bromhidrosis *noun* condition where the perspiration has an unpleasant smell 腋臭，狐臭

bromides *plural noun* bromine salts, formerly used as depressants or sedatives 溴化物

◇ **bromine** *noun* chemical element 溴（NOTE：chemical symbol is **Br**）

◇ **bromism** *or* **bromide poisoning** *noun* chronic ill health caused by excessive use of bromides 溴中毒

bronch- *prefix* referring to the windpipe 气管的

◇ **bronchi** *plural noun* air passages leading from the trachea into the lungs, where they split into many bronchioles 支气管；**lobar bronchi** *or* **secondary bronchi** = air passages supplying a lobe of a lung 叶支气管；**main** *or* **primary bronchi** = two main air passages which branch from the trachea outside the lung 主支气管；**segmental bronchi** *or* **tertiary bronchi** = air passages supplying a segment of a lung 段支气管 ◊ 见图 LUNGS（NOTE：singular is **bronchus**）

◇ **bronchial** *adjective* referring to the bronchi 支气管的；**bronchial asthma** = type of asthma mainly caused by an allergen or by exertion 支气管哮喘；**bronchial breath sounds** = distinctive breath sounds from the lungs which help diagnosis 支气管呼吸音；**bronchial pneumonia** = BRONCHOPNEUMONIA 支气管肺炎；**bronchial tree** = system of tubes (bronchi and bronchioles) which take the air from the trachea into the lungs 支气管树；**bronchial tubes** = bronchi, air tubes leading from the windpipe into the lungs 支气管

◇ **bronchiectasis** *noun* disorder of the bronchi which become wide, infected and filled with pus; the disorder can lead to pneumonia 支气管扩张症

◇ **bronchiolar** *adjective* referring to the bronchioles 细支气管的

◇ **bronchiole** *noun* very small air tube in the lungs leading from a bronchus to the alveoli 细支气管 ◊ 见图 LUNGS

◇ **bronchiolitis** *noun* inflammation of the bronchioles 细支气管炎

◇ **bronchitis** *noun* inflammation of the mucous membrane of the bronchi 支气管炎；**acute bronchitis** = attack of bronchitis caused by a virus or by exposure to cold and wet 急性支气管炎；**chronic bronchitis** = long-lasting form of bronchial inflammation 慢性支气管炎

◇ **bronchitic** *adjective* (i) referring to bronchitis 支气管炎的(ii)(patient) suffering from bronchitis 患支气管炎的

◇ **bronchoconstrictor** *noun* drug which narrows the bronchi 支气管收缩药

◇ **bronchodilator** *noun* drug which makes the bronchi wider 支气管扩张剂

◇ **bronchogram** *noun* X-ray picture of the bronchial tubes after an opaque substance has been put into them 支气管造影片

◇ **bronchography** *noun* X-ray examination of the lungs after an opaque substance has been put into the bronchi 支气管造影术

◇ **bronchomediastinal trunk** *noun* lymph nodes draining part of the chest 支气管纵隔干

◇ **bronchomycosis** *noun* infection of the bronchi by a fungus 支气管真菌病

◇ **bronchophony** *noun* vibrations of the voice heard when the consolidation of the lungs produces a loud sound 支气管音

◇ **bronchopleural** *adjective* referring to a bronchus and pleura 支气管胸膜的

◇ **bronchopneumonia** *noun* infectious inflammation of the bronchioles, which may lead to general infection of the lungs 支气管肺炎

◇ **bronchopulmonary** *adjective* referring to the bronchi and the lungs 支气管肺的

◇ **bronchoscope** *noun* instrument which is passed down the trachea into the lungs, which a doctor can use to inspect the inside passages of the lungs 支气管镜

◇ **bronchoscopy** *noun* examination of a patient's bronchi using a bronchoscope 支气管镜检查

◇ **bronchospasm** *noun* tightening of the bronchial muscles which causes the tubes to contract 支气管痉挛

◇ **bronchospirometer** *noun* instrument for measuring the volume of the lungs 支气管肺量仪

◇ **bronchospirometry** *noun* measuring the volume of the lungs 支气管肺量测定

◇ **bronchostenosis** *noun* abnormal constriction of the bronchial tubes 支气管狭窄

◇ **bronchotracheal** *adjective* referring to the bronchi and the trachea 气管支气管的

◇ **bronchus** *noun* air passage leading from the trachea into the lungs, where it splits into many bronchioles 支气管 (NOTE: plural is **bronchi**)

QUOTE: 19 children with mild to moderately severe perennial bronchial asthma were selected. These children gave a typical history of exercise-induced asthma and their symptoms were controlled with oral or aerosol bronchodilators.
引文:选择了 19 例患轻至中度支气管哮喘多年的儿童。这些儿童都有典型的运动诱发哮喘的病史,且通过口服或吸入支气管扩张剂可缓解症状。

Lancet 柳叶刀

bronze diabetes = HAEMOCHROMATOSIS 血色素沉着症,青铜色糖尿病

broth *noun* (i) light soup made from meat 肉汤(ii) medium in which bacteria can be cultivated 肉汤培养基

brother *noun* male who has the same mother and father as another child 兄弟: ***He's my brother.*** 他是我的兄弟。***That girl has three brothers.*** 那个女孩有三个兄弟。***His brother is a doctor.*** 他兄弟是名医生。

brow *noun* (i) forehead, the part of the face above the eyes 额(ii) eyebrow, the line of hair above the eye 睫毛

brown *adjective* & *noun* (of a) colour like the colour of earth or wood 棕色,棕色的: ***He has brown hair and blue eyes.*** 他有棕色的头发和蓝色的眼睛。***You're very brown — you must have been sitting in the sun.*** 你晒黑了,一定是坐在太阳下了。**brown bread** = bread made with flour which has not been refined 黑面包: ***Brown bread is better for you than white.*** 黑面包比白面包对你更有益处。

brown fat = animal fat which can easily be converted to energy and is believed to offset the effects of ordinary white fat 棕色脂肪（NOTE：**brown - browner - brownest**）

Brown-Séquard syndrome *noun* condition of a patient where the spinal cord has been partly severed or compressed, with the result that the lower half of the body is paralysed on one side and loses feeling in the other side 布朗·塞卡综合症,脊索部分离断或受压,导致一侧下肢瘫痪和对侧感觉丧失

Brucella *noun* type of rod-shaped bacterium 布氏杆菌

◇ **brucellosis** *noun* disease which can be caught from cattle or goats or from drinking infected milk, spread by a species of the bacterium *Brucella* 布氏杆菌病（NOTE：also called **undulant fever** *or* **Malta fever** *or* **mountain fever**）

> COMMENT：Symptoms include tiredness, arthritis, headache, sweating, irritability and swelling of the spleen.
> 注释：症状有疲劳、关节炎、头痛、出汗、易激动和脾大。

bruise 1 *noun* contusion, dark painful area on the skin, where blood has escaped under the skin following a blow 青紫 *see also* 参见 BLACK EYE **2** *verb* to make a bruise 擦伤,碰伤：***She bruised her knee on the corner of the table.*** 她被桌角碰伤了膝盖。***The nurse put a compress on his bruised leg.*** 护士拿了块敷料盖在伤腿上。**She bruises easily.** = Even a soft blow will give her a bruise. 她很容易出现瘀癍。

◇ **bruising** *noun* area of bruises 瘀癍,青紫：***The baby has bruising on the back and legs.*** 婴儿的背和腿上都是瘀癍。

bruit *noun* abnormal noise heard through a stethoscope 杂音

Brunner's glands *plural noun* glands in the duodenum and jejunum 布伦内氏腺

brush 1 *noun* stiff hairs or wire set in a hard base, used for cleaning 刷子：***You need a stiff brush to remove the dandruff from the scalp.*** 你需要把硬刷子去头皮屑。**2** *verb* to clean with a brush. 用刷子刷：***Have you brushed your hair?*** 你梳头了吗？***Remember to brush your teeth after a meal.*** 别忘了饭后刷牙。

bubble *noun* small amount of air or gas surrounded by a liquid 气泡：***Air bubbles formed in the blood vessel, causing embolism.*** 血中的气泡可导致栓塞。

bubo *noun* swelling of a lymph node in the groin or armpit 腹股沟或腋窝淋巴结肿

◇ **bubonic plague** *noun* fatal disease caused by *Pasteurella pestis* in the lymph system transmitted to humans by fleas from rats 淋巴腺鼠疫

> COMMENT：Bubonic plague was the Black Death of the Middle Ages; its symptoms are fever, delirium, vomiting and swelling of the lymph nodes.
> 注释：淋巴腺鼠疫即中世纪的黑死病,症状为发热、谵妄、呕吐和淋巴结肿。

buccal *adjective* referring to the cheek 颊的; **buccal cavity** = the mouth 口腔; **buccal fat** = pad of fat separating the buccinator muscle from the masseter 颊垫

buccinator（muscle） *noun* cheek muscle which helps the jaw to move when chewing 颊肌

bud *noun* small appendage 蕾; **taste bud** = tiny sensory receptor in the vallate and fungiform papillae of the tongue and in part of the back of the mouth 味蕾

Budd-Chiari syndrome *noun* disease of the liver, where thrombosis has occurred in the hepatic veins 布-希综合症(肝静脉血栓形成引起的肝病)

Buerger's disease = THROMBOANGIITIS OBLITERANS 伯格氏病,血栓闭塞性脉管炎

buffer 1 *noun* (i) substance that keeps a constant balance between acid and alkali 缓冲剂(ii) solution where the pH is not changed by adding acid or alkali

缓冲液；**buffer action** = balancing between acid and alkali 缓冲作用 **2** *verb* to prevent a solution from becoming acid 缓冲；***buffered aspirin*** 缓冲型阿司匹林

bug *noun* (*informal* 非正式) infectious disease 感染性疾病：***He caught a bug on holiday.*** 度假时，他患了感染性疾病。***Half the staff are sick with a stomach bug.*** 有一半的人员患了胃炎。

build *noun* general size of a person's body 体格：***He has a heavy or strong build for his height.*** 就身高来说，他体格强壮。***The girl has a slight build, but she can run very fast.*** 那女孩弱小，但跑得很快。

◇ **built** *adjective & suffix* referring to the general size of a person's body 体格的：***She's slightly built.*** 她体型瘦弱。***a heavily-built man*** 体格健壮的男人

◇ **build-up** *noun* gradual accumulation 组成，积累；***a build-up of fatty deposits on the walls of the arteries*** 动脉壁上脂肪组织沉积

◇ **build up** *verb* to form gradually by accumulation 积累（NOTE：**builds - building - built - has built**）

bulb *noun* round part at the end of an organ or bone 球；**olfactory bulb** = end of the olfactory tract, where the processes of the sensory cells in the nose are linked to the fibres of the olfactory nerve 嗅球；**bulb of the penis** *or* **glans penis** = round end of the penis 尿道球

◇ **bulbar** *adjective* referring to a bulb; referring to the medulla oblongata 球的，延髓的；**bulbar paralysis** *or* **bulbar palsy** = form of motor neurone disease which affects the muscles of the mouth, jaw and throat 球麻痹；**bulbar poliomyelitis** = type of polio affecting the brain stem, which makes it difficult for a patient to swallow or breathe 延髓型脊髓灰质炎

◇ **bulbospongiosus muscle** *noun* muscle in the perineum behind the penis 球海绵体肌

◇ **bulbourethral glands** *or* **Cowper's glands** 尿道球腺 *see* 见 GLAND

bulge *verb* to swell out *or* to push out 膨出：***The wall of the abdomen becomes weak and part of the intestine bulges through.*** 腹壁薄弱，部分肠子膨出。

bulimia (nervosa) *noun* psychological condition where the patient eats too much and is incapable of controlling his eating 食欲过盛

◇ **bulimic** *adjective* referring to bulimia; (person) suffering from bulimia 食欲过盛的

> COMMENT：Although the patient eats a large quantity of food, this is followed by vomiting which is induced by the patient himself, so that the patient does not in fact become overweight.
> 注释：尽管患者吃了大量的食物，但他都主动吐了出来，所以没有超重。

bulla *noun* large blister 大疱（NOTE：plural is **bullae**）

bump 1 *noun* (**a**) slight knock against something 碰撞：***The plane landed with a bump.*** 飞机颠簸着着陆。(**b**) slightly swollen part on the skin, caused by a blow *or* sting, etc. 泡，肿：***She has a bump on the back of her head where the door hit her.*** 门撞得她后脑勺起了个包。***The vaccination has left a little bump on her left arm.*** 疫苗接种在她的左臂上留了个小包。**2** *verb* to knock slightly 撞：***She bumped her head on the door.*** 他的头撞在了门上。

bumper fracture *noun* fracture in the upper part of the tibia (so called, because it can be caused by a blow from the bumper of a car) 车撞骨折

bundle *noun* (i) collection of things roughly fastened together 束(ii) group of nerves running in the same direction 束支；**bundle branch block** = defect in the heart's conduction tissue 束支阻滞；**bundle of His** = atrioventricular bundle, bundle of modified cardiac muscle which conducts impulses from the atrioventricular node to the septum and then divides to connect with the ventricles 希斯束

bunion *noun* inflammation and swelling of the big toe, caused by tight shoes which force the toe sideways with a callus developing over the joint between the toe and the metatarsal 踇囊肿

buphthalmos *noun* type of congenital glaucoma occurring in infants 牛眼,水眼

burial *noun* putting a dead person's body into the ground 埋葬: ***He died on Monday and the burial took place on Friday***. 他周一去世,周五下葬。

Burkitt's tumour *or* **Burkitt's lymphoma** *noun* malignant tumour, usually on the maxilla 伯基特氏瘤,上颌骨的恶性肿瘤

> COMMENT: Burkitt's tumour is found especially in children in Africa.
> 注释:伯基特淋巴瘤在非洲儿童中多见。

burn 1 *noun* injury to skin and tissue caused by light, heat, radiation, electricity or chemicals 灼伤; **cold burn** = injury to the skin caused by exposure to extreme cold or by touching a very cold surface 低温灼伤; **deep dermal burn** *or* **full thickness burn** = burn which is so severe that a graft will be necessary to repair the skin damage 真皮深层灼伤; **dry burn** = injury to the skin caused by touching a very hot dry surface 干热灼伤; **partial thickness burn** *or* **superficial thickness burn** = burn which leaves enough tissue for the skin to grow again 表浅灼伤; **wet burn** = scald, an injury to the skin caused by touching a very hot liquid or steam 湿热灼伤; **first-degree burn** = burn where the skin turns red because the epidermis has been affected 一度烧伤; **second-degree burn** = burn where the skin becomes very red and blisters 二度烧伤; **burns unit** = special department in a hospital which deals with burns 烧伤科 **2** *verb* to destroy by fire 烧,灼: ***She burnt her hand on the hot frying pan***. 热煎锅烧伤了她的手。***Most of his hair or*** **his skin was burnt off**. 他大部分的皮毛被烧掉了。(NOTE: **burns - burning - burnt/burned - has burnt/burned**)

◇ **burning** *adjective* (sensation) similar to that of being hurt by fire 烧灼的: ***He had a burning pain in his foot***. 他的脚灼痛。

> COMMENT: Burns were formerly classified by degrees and are still often referred to in this way. The modern classification is into two categories: deep and superficial.
> 注释:以前烧伤根据程度分类,目前还常用。但现代医学将其分为两类:浅表和深部烧伤。

burp 1 *noun* allowing air in the stomach to come up through the mouth 嗳气 **2** *verb* to allow air in the stomach to come up through the mouth 嗳气,打嗝; **to burp a baby** = to pat a baby on the back until it burps 轻拍婴儿使其打嗝 (NOTE: used particularly of babies. For adults the word **belch** is used)

burr *noun* bit used with a drill to make holes in a bone (as in the cranium) or in a tooth 牙钻

bursa *noun* sac containing fluid, forming part of the normal structure of a joint such as the knee and elbow, where it protects against frequent pressure and rubbing 粘液囊; **adventitious bursa** = abnormal bursa which develops as a result of continued pressure or rubbing 摩擦囊 (NOTE: plural is **bursae**)

◇ **bursitis** *noun* inflammation of a bursa, especially in the shoulder 粘液囊炎; **prepatellar bursitis** = housemaid's knee, a condition where the bursa in the knee becomes inflamed, caused by kneeling on hard surfaces 髌前粘液囊炎

burst *verb* (*of a sac or blister*) to break open 破裂: ***Never use a needle to burst a blister***. 绝不要用针挑破水泡。***He was rushed to hospital with a burst appendix***. 他阑尾破裂被急送入医院。(NOTE: **bursts - bursting - burst - has burst**)

bury *verb* to put a dead person's body into the ground 埋葬: ***He died on Monday and was buried on Friday.*** 他周一去世,周五下葬。

butter *noun* solid yellow edible fat made from cream 黄油,酪: ***He was spreading butter on a piece of bread.*** 他将黄油涂在面包上。***Fry the onions in butter.*** 将洋葱在黄油里煎。

buttock *noun* one of the two fleshy parts below the back, on which a person sits, made up mainly of the gluteal muscles 臀: ***He had a boil on his right buttock.*** 他右臀上有一个疖子。(NOTE: the buttocks are also called **nates**)

bypass *noun* act of going round an obstruction 旁道; **cardiopulmonary bypass** = machine or method for artificially circulating the patient's blood during open-heart surgery, where the heart and lungs are cut off from the circulation and replaced by a pump 心肺分流术(体外循环); **heart bypass operation** *or* **coronary bypass surgery** = surgical operation to treat angina by grafting pieces of vein to go around the diseased part of a coronary artery 冠状动脉搭桥手术

byssinosis *noun* lung disease (a form of pneumoconiosis) caused by inhaling cotton dust 棉屑肺

Cc

C 1 *abbreviation for* (缩写) Celsius 摄氏度的简写 2 *chemical symbol for* carbon 碳的化学元素符号 3 *noun* **vitamin C** = ascorbic acid, vitamin which is soluble in water and is found in fresh fruit (especially oranges and lemons) and in raw vegetables, liver and milk 维生素 C

> COMMENT: Lack of vitamin C can cause anaemia and scurvy.
> 注释:缺乏维生素 C 可导致贫血和坏血病。

c *symbol for* centi- 百分

Ca *chemical symbol for* calcium 钙的化学元素符号

CABG = CORONARY ARTERY BYPASS GRAFT 冠状动脉旁路移植

cabinet *noun* cupboard 柜子: ***The drugs cabinet must be kept locked.*** 药柜一定要锁好。

cachet *noun* quantity of a drug wrapped in paper, to be swallowed 扁囊剂

cachexia *noun* state of ill health with wasting and general weakness 恶液质

cadaver *noun* dead body, especially one used for dissection (解剖用的)尸体 ◊ **cadaveric** *or* **cadaverous** *adjective* (person who is) thin or wasting away 尸体的,尸体似的

cadmium *noun* metallic element, which if present in soil can make plants poisonous 镉 (NOTE: chemical symbol is **Cd**)

caecum *or US* **cecum** *noun* wider part of the large intestine in the lower right-hand side of the abdomen at the point where the small intestine joins it and which has the appendix attached to it 盲肠 ◊ 见图 DIGESTIVE SYSTEM ◊ **caecostomy** *noun* surgical operation to make an opening between the caecum and the abdominal wall to allow faeces to be passed without going through the rectum and anus 盲肠造口术

Caesarean section *or* **caesarean** *or US* **Cesarean section** *or* **cesarean** *noun* surgical operation to deliver a baby by cutting through the abdominal wall into the uterus 剖宫产术 (NOTE: the operation is correctly called **Caesarean section** but informally most people use **caesarean**: **'she had her baby by Caesarean section** *or* **she had a caesarean; the baby was delivered by caesarean'**)

> COMMENT: Caesarean section is performed only when it appears that normal childbirth is impossible or might endanger mother or child, and only after the 28th week of gestation.
> 注释:剖宫产术只有在不能进行正常分娩,或正常分娩对母婴有危险并且妊娠超过 28 周时才能进行。

caesium *or US* **cesium** *noun* radioactive element, used in treatment by radiation 铯 (NOTE: chemical symbol is **Cs**)

caffeine *noun* alkaloid found in coffee, tea and chocolate, which acts as a stimulant 咖啡因

> COMMENT: Apart from acting as a stimulant, caffeine also helps in the production of urine. It can be addictive, and exists in both tea and coffee in about the same percentages as well as in chocolate and other drinks.
> 注释:咖啡因除有刺激作用外,还有利尿作用。它有成瘾性,在茶、咖啡以及巧克力和其他饮料中有相似的含量。

caisson disease *noun* condition where the patient suffers pains in the joints and stomach, and dizziness caused by nitrogen in the blood 潜水员病 (NOTE: also called **decompression sickness** *or* **compressed air sickness**)

> COMMENT: Found when a person has moved rapidly from high atmospheric pressure to a lower pressure area, especially in divers who come

back to the surface too quickly after a deep dive. The first symptoms, pains in the joints, are known as 'the bends'. The disease can be fatal.
注释：在人迅速从高气压区进入低压区时发生，尤其是当潜水员从深的水底快速浮出水面时。首发症状是关节疼痛，称为'减压病'，本病可为致命的。

cal *abbreviation for* (缩写) calorie 卡路里

Cal *abbreviation for* (缩写) Calorie *or* kilocalorie 卡路里或千卡

calamine (lotion) *noun* lotion, based on zinc oxide, which helps relieve skin irritation (such as that caused by sunburn or chickenpox) 炉甘石(洗剂)，由氧化锌组成，能缓解阳光灼伤或水痘等皮肤病造成的皮肤瘙痒

calc- *or* **calci-** *prefix* referring to calcium 钙

◇ **calcaemia** *noun* condition where the blood contains an abnormally large amount of calcium 高钙血症

calcaneal *adjective* referring to the calcaneus 跟骨的; **calcaneal tendon** = Achilles tendon, the tendon at the back of the ankle which connects the calf muscles to the heel and which acts to pull up the heel when the calf muscle is contracted 跟腱

◇ **calcaneus** *noun* heel bone, situated underneath the talus 跟骨 ◊ 见图 FOOT

calcareous degeneration *noun* formation of calcium on bones or at joints in old age 钙化；石灰变性

calciferol *noun* vitamin D_2 骨化醇，维生素 D_2

calcification *noun* hardening by forming deposits of calcium salts 钙化 *see also* 参见 PELLEGRINI-STIEDA'S DISEASE

COMMENT: Calcification can be normal in the formation of bones, but can occur abnormally in joints, muscles and organs, where it is known as calcinosis.
注释：钙化在骨的形成中是正常现象，但也可不正常地发生于关节、肌肉和其他器官，此时称为钙质沉着。

◇ **calcified** *adjective* made hard 钙化的: ***Bone is calcified connective tissue.*** 骨是钙化了的结缔组织。

◇ **calcinosis** *noun* abnormal condition where deposits of calcium salts form in joints, muscles and organs 钙质沉着

◇ **calcitonin** *or* **thyrocalcitonin** *noun* hormone, produced by the thyroid gland, which is believed to regulate the level of calcium in the blood 降钙素

calcium *noun* metallic chemical element which is a major component of bones and teeth and which is essential for various bodily processes such as blood clotting 钙; **calcium deficiency** = lack of calcium in the bloodstream 缺钙; **calcium phosphate** ($Ca_3(PO_4)_2$) = main constituent of bones 磷酸钙; **calcium supplement** = addition of calcium to the diet, or as injections, to improve the level of calcium in the bloodstream 钙的补充，补钙 (NOTE: chemical symbol is **Ca**)

COMMENT: Calcium is an important element in a balanced diet. Milk, cheese, eggs and certain vegetables are its main sources. Calcium deficiency can be treated by injections of calcium salts.
注释：钙是平衡膳食中的重要成分。牛奶、奶酪、鸡蛋和某些蔬菜是钙的主要来源。钙缺乏可通过注射钙盐补充。

calculus *noun* stone, a hard mass like a little piece of stone, which forms inside the body 结石; **renal calculus** = stone in the kidney 肾结石 (NOTE: plural is **calculi**)

COMMENT: Calculi are formed of cholesterol and various inorganic substances, and are commonly found in the bladder, the gall bladder (gallstones) and various parts of the kidney.
注释：结石由胆固醇和其它无机物组成，多位于膀胱、胆囊和肾脏。

◇ **calculosis** *noun* condition where

calculi exist in an organ 结石病

Caldwell-Luc operation *noun* surgical operation to drain the maxillary sinus by making an incision above the canine tooth 考-路二氏手术

calf *noun* muscular fleshy part at the back of the lower leg, formed by the gastrocnemius muscles 小腿 (NOTE: plural is **calves**)

calibrate *verb* (**a**) to measure the inside diameter of a tube or passage 测量管径 (**b**) (*in surgery*) to measure the sizes of two parts of the body to be joined together (术中)测量将要吻合的两部分组织的大小 (**c**) to adjust an instrument or piece of equipment against a known standard 校准

◇ **calibrator** *noun* (i) instrument used to enlarge a tube or passage 扩张器 (ii) instrument for measuring the diameter of a tube or passage 测径器

caliper *noun* (**a**) instrument with two legs, used for measuring the width of the pelvic cavity 双脚规(测量骨盆的宽度) (**b**) instrument with two sharp points which are put into a fractured bone and weights attached to cause traction 重力牵引器 (**c**) metal splints used to support an injured leg, made of a pair of rods attached to the thigh and to a special boot 骨折固定支架

call 1 *noun* (**a**) speaking by telephone 打电话: ***I want to make a (phone) call to Canada.*** 我要给加拿大去个电话。***There were three calls for you while you were out.*** 你出去后有3个电话找你。**on call** = ready to be called for duty 待命: ***Three nurses are on call during the night.*** 夜间有3个护士当班。(**b**) visit 访问: ***The district nurse makes a regular call every Thursday.*** 地区护士每周四都要做例行走访。**2** *verb* (**a**) to telephone 打电话: ***If he comes, tell him I'll call him when I'm at the surgery.*** 如果他来了,告诉他我做手术时会给他打电话。***Mr Smith is out, shall I ask him to call you back?*** 斯密恩先生出去了,我让他给你回电话好吗?(**b**) to visit 访问: ***The district nurse called at the house, but there was no one there.*** 地区护士进行家访,但家中没人。***She called on the patient for the last time on Tuesday.*** 她最后一次走访这位患者是星期二。

calliper = CALIPER

callosity *or* **callus** *noun* hard patch on the skin (such as a corn) resulting from frequent pressure or rubbing 胼胝

callosum 胼胝体 *see* 见 CORPUS

callus *noun* (**a**) = CALLOSITY 胼胝 (**b**) tissue which forms round a broken bone as it starts to mend, leading to consolidation 骨痂: ***Callus formation is more rapid in children and young adults than in elderly patients.*** 儿童和年轻人骨痂的形成要快于老年人。

calm *adjective* quiet, not upset 平静: ***The patient was delirious but became calm after the injection.*** 这患者处于谵妄状态,但打针后变得平静了。

◇ **calm down** *verb* to become quiet; to make someone quiet 使平静: ***He was soon calmed down*** *or* ***he soon calmed down when the nurse gave him an injection.*** 护士给他打针后,他很快就平静了下来。

calomel (Hg_2Cl_2) *noun* mercurous chloride, poisonous substance used to treat pinworms in the intestine 甘汞,氯化汞,有毒物质,曾用于治疗肠道蛲虫感染

calor *noun* heat 热

◇ **caloric** *adjective* referring to calories 热的; **caloric energy** = amount of energy shown as a number of calories 热能; **caloric requirement** = amount of energy (shown in calories) which a person needs each day 人每天所需要的热卡

◇ **calorie** *or* **gram calorie** *or* **small calorie** *noun* unit of measurement of heat or energy (the heat needed to raise the temperature of 1g of water by 1°C) 卡,克卡,小卡(使1克水升温1度所需要的热能) (NOTE: the **joule** is now more usual; also written **cal** after figures: **2,500 cal**)

◇ **Calorie** *or* **large calorie** *noun* kilocalorie *or* 1,000 calories (the heat needed to raise the temperature of 1kg of water by 1℃) 千卡,大卡(使1公斤水升温1度所需要的热能)(NOTE: spelt with a capital; also written **Cal** and **kcal** after figures: **250 Cal**, **360 kcal**)

◇ **calorific value** *noun* heat value of a substance, the number of Calories which a certain amount of a substance (such as a certain food) contains 热量价: ***The tin of beans has 250 calories or has a calorific value of 250 calories.*** 一罐豆子热量价为250卡。

> COMMENT: One calorie is the amount of heat needed to raise the temperature of one gram of water by one degree Celsius. A Calorie or kilocalorie is the amount of heat needed to raise the temperature of one kilogram of water by one degree Celsius. The Calorie is also used as a measurement of the energy content of food and to show the caloric requirement or amount of energy needed by an average person. The average adult in an office job requires about 3,000 Calories per day, supplied by carbohydrates and fats to give energy and proteins to replace tissue. More strenuous physical work needs more Calories. If a person eats more than the number of Calories needed by his energy output or for his growth, the extra Calories are stored in the body as fat.
> 注释:1卡的热能是使1克的水升温1摄氏度所需要的能量。1千卡是使1公斤水升温1度所需要的热能。千卡也被用来描述食物中所含的能量,以及平均每人所需的热能。办公室的工作人员平均每天需3,000千卡的热能,主要由碳水化合物和脂肪提供,蛋白质用来修补组织。更剧烈的体力工作需要更高的热能。如果某人的摄入量超过了他消耗和生长所需,剩余的热能将转变为脂肪在体内储存。

calvaria *or* **calvarium** *noun* top part of the skull 颅盖

calyx *noun* part of the body shaped like a cup especially the tube leading to a renal pyramid(肾)盏 (NOTE: plural is **calyces**) ◊ 见图 KIDNEY

> COMMENT: The renal pelvis is formed of three major calyces, which themselves are formed of several smaller minor calyces.
> 注释:肾盂由3个大肾盏组成,每个肾盏又由更小的肾小盏形成。

camphor *noun* white crystals with a strong smell, made from a tropical tree, used to keep insects away or as a liniment 樟脑; **camphor oil** *or* **camphorated oil** = mixture of 20% camphor and oil, used as a rub 樟脑油

canal *noun* tube along which something flows 管道; **alimentary canal** = tube in the body going from the mouth to the anus and including the throat, stomach, intestine, etc., through which food passes and is digested 消化道; **anal canal** = passage leading from the rectum to the anus 肛管; **auditory canals** = external and internal passages of the ear 耳道; **bile canal** = very small vessel leading from a hepatic cell to the bile duct 胆小管; **central canal** = thin tube in the centre of the spinal cord containing cerebrospinal fluid 中央管; **cervical canal** *or* **cervicouterine canal** = tube running through the cervix from the point where the uterus joins the vagina to the entrance of the uterine cavity 宫颈管; **Eustachian canal** = passage through the porous bone forming the outside part of the Eustachian tube 咽鼓管; **femoral canal** = inner tube of the sheath surrounding the femoral artery and vein 股管; **Haversian canal** = fine canal which runs vertically through the Haversian systems in compact bone, containing blood vessels and lymph ducts Haversian(哈弗)管; **inguinal canal** = passage in the lower abdominal wall, carrying the spermatic cord in the male and the round ligament of the uterus in the female 腹股沟管; **root canal** = canal in the root of a tooth through which the nerves and blood vessels pass 牙根管 ◊ 见图 TOOTH; **canal of Schlemm** *or* **Schlemm's canal** = circular canal in the sclera of the eye, which drains the aqueous humour 施累姆氏管(巩膜静脉管); **semicircular canals** = three canals in the inner ear partly filled with fluid and which regulate the sense of balance 半规管 ◊ 见图 EAR; **vertebral canal** = channel formed of the holes in the centre of each vertebra, through which the spinal cord passes 椎管; **Volkmann's canal** = canal running horizontally through compact bone, carrying blood to the Haversian systems 福耳克曼氏管(骨板小管)

◊ **canaliculotomy** *noun* surgical operation to open up a little canal 小管切开术

◊ **canaliculus** *noun* little canal, such as a canal leading to the Haversian systems in compact bone, or a canal leading to the lacrimal duct 小管 (NOTE: plural is **canaliculi**)

cancellous bone *noun* light spongy bone tissue which forms the inner core of a bone and also the ends of long bones 网状骨 ◊ 见图 BONE STRUCTURE

cancer *noun* malignant growth, a tumour which develops in tissue and destroys it, which can spread by metastasis to other parts of the body and cannot be controlled by the body itself 癌症: ***Cancer cells developed in the lymph.*** 癌细胞已侵及淋巴结。***He has been diagnosed as having lung cancer*** *or* ***as having cancer of the lung.*** 他被确诊患有肺癌。(NOTE: used with **the** or **a** to indicate one particular tumour, and without **the** or **a** to indicate the disease: **doctors removed a cancer from her breast; she has breast cancer.** For other terms referring to cancer, see words beginning with **carcin-**)

◊ **cancerophobia** *noun* fear of cancer 恐癌症

◊ **cancerous** *adjective* referring to cancer 癌症的: ***The X-ray revealed a cancerous growth in the breast.*** X线显示乳腺上有一癌性增生物。

> COMMENT: Cancers can be divided into cancers of the skin (carcinomas) or cancers of connective tissue, such as bone or muscle (sarcomas). Cancer can be caused by tobacco, radiation and many other factors. Many cancers are curable by surgery, by chemotherapy or by radiation, especially if they are detected early.
> 注释:癌分为皮肤肿瘤(癌)和结缔组织如骨、肌肉肿瘤(肉瘤)。肿瘤的发生与烟草、放射线及许多其他因素有关。很多肿瘤,尤其当早期发现时可通过手术、化疗或放疗进行治疗。

cancrum oris *noun* noma, severe ulcers in the mouth, leading to gangrene 坏疽性口炎

Candida *noun* Monilia, a type of fungus which causes mycosis 念珠菌属; **Candida albicans** = one type of Candida which is normally present in the mouth and throat without causing any illness, but which can cause thrush 白色念珠菌

◊ **candidiasis** *or* **candidosis** *noun* moniliasis, infection with Candida 念珠菌病

> COMMENT: When the infection occurs in the vagina or mouth it is known as 'thrush'. Thrush in the mouth usually affects small children.
> 注释:当感染发生于阴道和口腔时称为鹅口疮,鹅口疮多累及幼儿。

> QUOTE: It is incorrect to say that oral candida is an infection. Candida is easily isolated from the mouths of up to 50% of healthy adults and is a normal commensal.
> 引文:认为口腔中有念珠菌即为感染是不正确的。从高达50%的健康成人口腔中很容易分离出念珠菌,它是一种正常的共生菌。
>
> **Nursing Times** 护理时代

candidate *noun* (i) person who is applying for a job or for a promotion 候选

人(ii)patient who could have an operation 可手术治疗的患者: ***The board is interviewing the candidates for the post of administrator.*** 委员会接见了竟选理事的候选人。***These types of patients may be candidates for embolization.*** 这些类型的患者可接受栓塞治疗。**candidate vaccine** = vaccine which is being tested for use in immunization 待选疫苗

canicola fever *noun* form of leptospirosis, giving high fever and jaundice 犬钩端螺旋体病

canine (tooth) *noun* pointed tooth next to an incisor 尖牙 ◊ 见图 TEETH

> COMMENT: There are four canines in all, two in the upper jaw and two in the lower; those in the upper jaw are referred to as the 'eyeteeth'
> 注释:共有 4 颗尖牙,两颗在上颌,两颗在下颌。上面的两颗也称为上尖牙。

canities *noun* loss of pigments, which makes the hair turn white 白发

canker *noun* lesion of the skin 溃疡

cannabis *or* **(Indian) hemp** *noun* **(a)** tropical plant from whose leaves or flowers an addictive drug is produced 大麻(植物) **(b)** marijuana, an addictive drug made from the dried leaves or flowers of the Indian hemp plant 大麻; **cannabis resin** = addictive drug, a purified extract made from the flowers of the Indian hemp plant 纯化大麻

cannula *noun* tube with a trocar or blunt needle inside, inserted into the body to introduce fluids 套管

canthus *noun* corner of the eye 眦,眼角

◊ **canthal** *adjective* referring to the corner of the eye 眼角的

cap *noun* **(a)** type of hat which fits tightly on the head 帽子: ***The surgeons were wearing white caps.*** 术者戴着白帽子。**(b)** top which covers something 帽儿,盖子: ***Screw the cap back on the bottle.*** 把瓶盖儿拧上。**child-proof cap** = special top on a bottle containing a potentially dangerous substance, designed so that a young child cannot open it 防儿童误开盖 **(c)** covering which protects something 隔; **Dutch cap** = vaginal diaphragm, a contraceptive device for women, which is placed over the cervix uteri before sexual intercourse 阴道隔 **(d)** artificial hard covering for a damaged or broken tooth 人工牙冠

capacity *noun* (of a person) ability to do something; (of an organ) ability to contain or absorb a substance 能力,容量

capillary *noun* (i) tiny blood vessel between the arterioles and the venules, which carries blood and nutrients into the tissues 毛细血管(ii) any tiny tube carrying a liquid in the body 细管,小管; **capillary bleeding** = bleeding where blood oozes out from small blood vessels 毛细血管出血

capitate (bone) *noun* largest of the eight small carpal bones in the wrist 头状骨 ◊ 见图 HAND

capitis 头 *see* 见 CORONA

capitulum *noun* round end of a bone, such as the distal end of the humerus, which articulates with another bone 小头(NOTE: plural is **capitula**)

capsular *adjective* referring to a capsule 囊的

◊ **capsularis** 包的 *see* 见 DECIDUA

◊ **capsule** *noun* **(a)** membrane round an organ or joint 囊; **fibrous capsule** *or* **renal capsule** = fibrous tissue surrounding a kidney 纤维囊,肾囊; **joint capsule** = white fibrous tissue which surrounds and holds a joint together 关节囊; **Tenon's capsule** = tissue which lines the orbit of the eye 特农氏囊,眼球囊 **(b)** **internal capsule** = bundle of fibres linking the cerebral cortex and other parts of the brain 内囊 **(c)** small hollow digestible case, filled with a drug to be swallowed by the patient 胶囊: ***She swallowed three capsules of painkiller.*** 她吃了 3 粒止痛胶囊。The doctor prescribed the drug in capsule form. 医生开的是这药的胶囊剂。*see also* 参见 BOW-

MAN'S CAPSULE

◇ **capsulectomy** *noun* surgical removal of the capsule round a joint 囊切除术

◇ **capsulitis** *noun* inflammation of a capsule 囊炎

caput *noun* (i) the head 头(ii) top of part of the body 顶部 (NOTE: plural is **capita**)

carbohydrates *plural noun* organic compounds which derive from sugar and which are the main ingredients of many types of food 碳水化合物

> COMMENT: Carbohydrates are compounds of carbon, hydrogen and oxygen. They are found in particular in sugar and starch, and provide the body with energy.
> 注释:碳水化合物由碳,氢和氧组成。主要存在于糖和淀粉中,提供机体所需的能量。

carbolic acid = PHENOL 石炭酸

carbon *noun* one of the common non-metallic elements, an essential component of living matter and organic chemical compounds 碳 (NOTE: chemical symbol is **C**)

◇ **carbonated** *adjective* (drink) with bubbles in it, because carbon dioxide has been added 含碳酸盐的(饮料)

◇ **carbon dioxide** (CO_2) *noun* colourless gas produced by the body's metabolism as the tissues burn carbon, and breathed out by the lungs as waste 二氧化碳

> COMMENT: Carbon dioxide can be solidified at low temperatures and is known as 'dry ice' or 'carbon dioxide snow', being used to remove growths on the skin.
> 注释:二氧化碳在低温下可固化,形成所谓的干冰或二氧化碳雪,用来去除皮肤上的赘生物。

◇ **carbon monoxide** (CO) *noun* poisonous gas found in fumes from car engines, from burning gas and cigarette smoke 一氧化碳; **carbon monoxide poisoning** = poisoning caused by breathing carbon monoxide 一氧化碳中毒

> COMMENT: Carbon monoxide exists in tobacco smoke and in car exhaust fumes and is dangerous because it is easily absorbed into the blood and takes the place of the oxygen in the blood, combining with haemoglobin to form carboxyhaemoglobin, which has the effect of starving the tissues of oxygen. Carbon monoxide has no smell and people do not realize that they are being poisoned by it until they become unconscious. The treatment for carbon monoxide poisoning is very rapid inhalation of fresh air together with carbon dioxide if this can be provided.
> 注释:一氧化碳存在于烟雾和汽车的尾气中,它易溶于血,取代血内的氧,和血红蛋白结合,形成碳氧血红蛋白,使组织缺氧,对人体造成损害。一氧化碳是无味的,中毒早期不易被发觉,直至昏迷。治疗原则是如果可能的话尽快吸入新鲜空气和二氧化碳。

◇ **carboxyhaemoglobin** *noun* compound of carbon monoxide and haemoglobin formed when a person breathes in carbon monoxide from tobacco smoke or car exhaust fumes 碳氧血红蛋白; **background carboxyhaemoglobin level** = level of carboxyhaemoglobin in the blood of a person living a normal existence without exposure to particularly high levels of carbon monoxide 基础碳氧血红蛋白水平

carbuncle *noun* localized staphylococcal infection, which goes deep into the tissue 痈

carcin- *prefix* referring to carcinoma *or* cancer 癌

◇ **carcinogen** *noun* substance which produces carcinoma 致癌物

> COMMENT: Carcinogens are found in pesticides such as DDT, in asbestos, aromatic compounds such as benzene, and radioactive substances.

注释：致癌物存在于一些杀虫剂如DDT、石棉、芳香化合物如苯以及放射活性物质中。

◇ **carcinogenesis** *noun* process of forming carcinoma in tissue 致癌过程，癌发生

◇ **carcinogenic** *adjective* which produces carcinoma 致癌的

◇ **carcinoid** (**tumour**) *noun* type of intestinal tumour (especially in the appendix), which causes diarrhoea 类癌; **carcinoid syndrome** = group of symptoms which are associated with a carcinoid tumour 类癌综合症

◇ **carcinoma** *noun* cancer of the epithelium or glands 癌; **carcinoma-in-situ** = first stage in the development of a cancer, where the epithelial cells begin to change 原位癌

◇ **carcinomatosis** *noun* carcinoma which has spread to many sites in the body 癌转移

◇ **carcinomatous** *adjective* referring to carcinoma 癌的

card *noun* stiff piece of paper which can carry information on it for reference 卡片; **filing card** = card with information written on it, used to classify information in correct order 登记卡片; **index card** = card used to make a card index 索引卡; **punched card** = card with holes punched in it which a computer can read 打孔卡

◇ **card index** *noun* series of cards with information written on them, kept in special order so that the information can be found easily 卡片式索引: ***The hospital records used to be kept on a card index, but have been transferred to the computer.*** 病历记录以前是保存在索引卡上，现在是储存在计算机内。**card-index file** = information kept on filing cards 卡片式文件

◇ **card-index** *verb* to put information onto a card index 制作卡片索引

cardi- *or* **cardio-** *prefix* referring to the heart 心的

cardia *noun* (i) opening at the top of the stomach which joins it to the gullet 贲门 (ii) the heart 心脏 ◇ 见图 STOMACH

cardiac *adjective* (i) referring to the heart 心的 (ii) referring to the cardia 贲门的; **cardiac achalasia** = being unable to relax the cardia (the muscle at the entrance to the stomach), with the result that food cannot enter the stomach 贲门失弛缓症 *see also* 参见 CARDIOMYOTOMY; **cardiac arrest** = stopping of the heart, a condition where the heart muscle stops beating 心脏骤停; **cardiac asthma** = difficulty in breathing caused by heart failure 心源性哮喘; **cardiac catheterization** = passing a catheter into the heart to take samples of tissue *or* to check blood pressure 心导管检查; **cardiac cirrhosis** = cirrhosis of the liver caused by heart disease 心源性肝硬化; **cardiac compression** = compression of the heart by fluid in the pericardium 心脏受压; **cardiac conducting system** = nerve system in the heart which links an atrium to a ventricle, so that the two beat at the same rate 心脏传导系统; **cardiac cycle** = repeated beating of the heart, formed of the diastole and systole 心动周期; **cardiac decompression** = removal of a haematoma or constriction of the heart 心脏减压; **cardiac failure** *or* **heart failure** = situation where the heart cannot function in a satisfactory way and is unable to circulate blood normally 心力衰竭; **cardiac impression** = (i) concave area near the centre of the upper surface of the liver under the heart (肝脏上的)心切迹 (ii) depression on the mediastinal part of the lungs where they touch the pericardium (肺上的)心脏切迹; **external cardiac massage** = method of making a patient's heart start beating again by rhythmic pressing on the breastbone 心外按摩，体外心脏按摩; **internal cardiac massage** = method of making a patient's heart start beating again by pressing on the heart itself 心内

按压,开胸按摩; **cardiac monitor** = electrocardiograph, an apparatus for measuring and recording the electrical impulses of the muscles of the heart as it beats 心电监测; **cardiac murmur** = abnormal sound made by the heart, heard through a stethoscope 心脏杂音; **cardiac muscle** = special muscle which forms the heart 心肌; **cardiac neurosis** = da Costa's syndrome, condition where the patient suffers palpitations, breathlessness and dizziness, caused by effort or worry 心脏神经官能症,神经性循环衰弱; **cardiac notch** = (i) point in the left lung, where the right inside wall is bent 心脏切迹 (ii) notch at the point where the oesophagus joins the greater curvature of the stomach *or* cardiac orifice = opening where the oesophagus joins the stomach 贲门; **cardiac pacemaker** = electronic device implanted on a patient's heart, or which a patient wears attached to his chest, which stimulates and regulates the heartbeat 心脏起搏器 *see also* PACEMAKER; **cardiac patient** = patient suffering from heart disorder 心脏病患者; **cardiac reflex** = reflex which controls the heartbeat automatically 心跳反射; **cardiac surgery** = surgery to the heart 心脏手术,心脏外科; **cardiac tamponade** = pressure on the heart when the pericardial cavity fills with blood 心包填塞; **cardiac veins** = veins which lead from the myocardium to the right atrium 冠状静脉

◊ **cardialgia** *noun* heartburn, pain in the chest from indigestion 灼痛,烧心

◊ **cardiogram** *noun* graph showing the heartbeat, produced by a cardiograph 心电图

◊ **cardiograph** *noun* instrument which records the heartbeat 心电图机

◊ **cardiographer** *noun* technician who operates a cardiograph 心电图员,心电图师

◊ **cardiologist** *noun* heart specialist, a doctor who specializes in the study of the heart 心脏病专家

◊ **cardiology** *noun* study of the heart, its diseases and functions 心脏病学

◊ **cardiomegaly** *noun* enlarged heart 心脏肥大

◊ **cardiomyopathy** *noun* disorder of the heart muscle 心肌病

◊ **cardiomyotomy** *noun* Heller's operation, an operation to treat cardiac achalasia by splitting the ring of muscles where the oesophagus joins the stomach 贲门肌切开术

◊ **cardiopathy** *noun* any kind of heart disease 心脏病

◊ **cardiophone** *noun* microphone attached to a patient to record sounds (used to record the heart of an unborn baby) 心音描记器

◊ **cardiopulmonary bypass** *noun* machine or method for artificially circulating the patient's blood during open-heart surgery, where the heart and lungs are cut off from the circulation and replaced by a pump 心肺分流术

◊ **cardiopulmonary resuscitation** (**CPR**) *noun* method of resuscitation which stimulates both heart and lungs, consisting of a combination of external chest compression which serves to get the heart going again, and mouth-to-mouth ventilation to get the breathing going again 心肺复苏

◊ **cardioscope** *noun* instrument formed of a tube with a light at the end, used to inspect the inside of the heart 心脏镜

◊ **cardiospasm** *noun* = CARDIAC ACHALASIA 贲门痉挛

◊ **cardiothoracic** *adjective* referring to the heart and the chest region 心胸的; ***a cardiothoracic surgeon*** 心胸外科医师

◊ **cardiotocography** *noun* recording of the heartbeat of a fetus 胎心记录

◊ **cardiovascular** *adjective* referring to the heart and the blood circulation system 心血管的; **cardiovascular disease** = any disease (such as hypertension) which affects the circulatory system 心血管疾病; **cardiovascular system** = system of blood circulation 心血管系统

◇ **cardioversion** *noun* defibrillation, correcting an irregular heartbeat by using an electric impulse 心脏电复律,心脏除颤

◇ **carditis** *noun* inflammation of the connective tissue of the heart 心炎

> QUOTE: Cardiovascular diseases remain the leading cause of death in the United States.
> 引文:在美国,心血管疾病仍是死亡的首位原因。
>
> **Journal of American Medical Association** 美国医学会杂志

care *noun* attention *or* general treatment (of a patient) 关心,治疗: ***The patient is under the care of a cancer specialist.*** 这患者由肿瘤专家负责治疗。***She is responsible for the care of patients in the outpatients' department.*** 她负责医治门诊病人。**coronary care unit** = section of a hospital reserved to treat patients suffering from heart attacks 冠心病病房: ***A coronary care unit has been opened at a London hospital.*** 伦敦医院开设了冠心病病房。**intensive care** = continual supervision and treatment of a patient in a special section of a hospital 重症监护; **intensive care unit** (**ICU**) = special section of a hospital which supervises seriously ill patients who need constant supervision 重症监护病房: ***She is in intensive care*** *or* ***in the intensive care unit.*** 她在重症监护病房。***The patient was put in intensive care.*** 患者被送进了重症监护病房。***He came out of intensive care and was moved to the general ward.*** 他出了重症监护病房,被送往普通病房。

◇ **care for** *verb* to look after 照顾: ***Nurses were caring for the injured people at the scene of the accident.*** 护士在现场照顾受伤的群众。***Severely handicapped children are cared for in special clinics.*** 严重残障儿童由专科诊所负责照管。

◇ **care plan** *noun* plan drawn up by the nursing staff for the treatment of an individual patient 护理计划

◇ **carer** *or* **caregiver** *noun* someone who looks after a sick person 护理人员

> QUOTE: The experience of the ward sister is the most important factor in the standard of care.
> 引文:病房护士长的经验是护理标准中最重要的。
>
> **Nursing Times** 护理时代

> QUOTE: All relevant sections of the nurses' care plan and nursing process had been left blank.
> 引文:所有有关护理计划和护理进程的章节均为空白。
>
> **Nursing Times** 护理时代

> QUOTE: Most research has focused on those caring for older people or for adults with disability and chronic illness. Most studied are the carers of those who might otherwise have to stay in hospital for a long time.
> 引文:大多数研究着眼于照顾老年人或有功能障碍及慢性疾病病人的护理。大部分的研究对象是长期住院患者的看护人。
>
> **British Medical Journal** 英国医学杂志

caries *noun* decay in a tooth or bone 龋齿,骨疽; **dental caries** = decay in a tooth 龋齿

carina *noun* structure shaped like the bottom of a boat, such as the cartilage at the point where the trachea branches into the bronchi 隆凸

cariogenic *adjective* (substance) which causes caries 致龋的

carminative *adjective & noun* (substance) which relieves colic or indigestion 排气的,排气剂

carotenaemia *noun* xanthaemia, excessive amount of carotene in the blood as a result of eating mainly too many carrots or tomatoes, which gives the skin a yellow colour 胡萝卜素血症

◇ **carotene** *noun* orange or red pigment in carrots, egg yolk and some natural oils, which is converted by the liver into vitamin A,胡萝卜素

carotid *noun* artery in the neck 颈动脉; **common carotid artery** *or* **carotid** = main artery running up each side of the lower part of the neck 颈总动脉; **carotid body** = tissue in the carotid sinus which is concerned with cardiovascular reflexes 颈动脉球; **carotid pulse** = pulse in the carotid artery at the side of the neck 颈动脉搏动; **carotid sinus** = expanded part attached to the carotid artery, which monitors blood pressure in the skull 颈动脉窦

COMMENT: The common carotid artery is in the lower part of the neck and branches upwards into the external and internal carotids. The carotid body is situated at the point where the carotid divides.
注释:颈总动脉位于颈下部,向上分为颈内、颈外动脉。颈动脉球即位于分叉处。

carp- *or* **carpo-** *prefix* referring to the wrist 腕

◇ **carpal** *adjective* & *noun* referring to the wrist 腕的,腕; **carpal bones** *or* **carpals** = the eight bones which make up the carpus or wrist 腕骨 ◊ 见图 HAND; **carpal tunnel syndrome** = condition (usually in women) where the fingers tingle and hurt at night, caused by compression of the median nerve 腕管综合症; **carpal tunnel release** = operation to relieve the compression of the median nerve 腕管松解术

◇ **carpometacarpal joints (CM joints)** *plural noun* joints between the carpals and metacarpals 腕掌关节

◇ **carpopedal spasm** *noun* spasm in the hands and feet caused by lack of calcium 腕足痉挛

◇ **carpus** *noun* wrist, the bones by which the lower arm is connected to the hand 腕

COMMENT: The carpus is formed of eight small bones (the carpals): these are the capitate, hamate, lunate, pisiform, scaphoid, trapezium, trapezoid and triquetral.
注释:腕部由 8 块小骨构成,它们是头状骨、钩骨、月骨、豌豆骨、舟状骨、大多角骨、小多角骨和三角骨。

carphology *or* **floccitation** *noun* pulling at the bedclothes (a sign of delirium in typhoid and other fevers) 摸空,捉空摸床

carrier *noun* (**a**) person who carries bacteria of a disease in his body and who can transmit the disease to others without showing any sign of it himself 带菌者: ***Ten percent of the population are believed to be unwitting carriers of the bacteria***. 现认为大约 10% 的人口是此种细菌的无症状携带者。(**b**) insect which carries disease and infects humans 虫媒 (**c**) healthy person who carries the chromosome defect of a hereditary disease (such as haemophilia or Duchenne muscular dystrophy) 染色体异常的携带者

carry out *verb* to perform (an operation) 进行,实施

carsick *adjective* feeling sick because of the movement of a car 晕车的

◇ **carsickness** *noun* sickness caused by the movement of a car 晕车

cart *US* = TROLLEY 电车,小车

cartilage *noun* gristle, thick connective tissue which lines the joints and acts as a cushion and which forms part of the structure of an organ 软骨; **articular cartilage** = layer of cartilage at the end of a bone where it forms a joint with another bone 关节软骨; **costal cartilage** = cartilage which forms the end of each rib and either joins the rib to the breastbone or to the rib above 肋软骨; **cricoid cartilage** = ring-shaped cartilage in the lower part of the larynx 环状软骨; **elastic cartilage** = flexible cartilage such as that in the ear and epiglottis 弹性软骨; **epiphyseal cartilage** = type of cartilage in the bones of children and adolescents which expands and hardens as the bones grow to full size 骺软骨; **hyaline cartilage** = type of cartilage found in the nose, larynx and joints 透明软骨; **thyroid cartilage** = large cartilage in the larynx, part of which forms the Adam's apple 甲状软骨

◇ **cartilaginous** *adjective* made of cartilage 软骨的; (**primary**) **cartilaginous joint** *or* **synchondrosis** = joint, as in children, where the bones are linked by cartilage, before the cartilage has changed to bone (原发性)软骨性关节; (**secondary**) **cartilaginous joint** *or* **symphysis** = point (such as the pubic symphysis) where two bones are joined by cartilage which makes the joint rigid 继发性软骨结合 (NOTE: for other terms referring to cartilage, see words beginning with **chondr-**) ◇ 见图 BONE STRUCTURE, JOINTS

> COMMENT: Cartilage in small children is the first stage in the formation of bones.
> 注释：幼儿的软骨是骨形成的第一阶段。

caruncle *noun* small swelling 肉阜; **lacrimal caruncle** = small red point at the inner corner of each eye 泪阜

cascara (**sagrada**) *noun* laxative made from the bark of a tropical tree 美鼠李皮

case *noun* (i) single occurrence of a disease 病例(ii) person who has adisease or who is undergoing treatment 患者: ***There were two hundred cases of cholera in the recent outbreak.*** 最近的霍乱暴发中共有200个病例。The hospital is only admitting urgent cases. 这医院仅收急诊病例。There is an appendicectomy case waiting for the operating theatre. 有一例阑尾切除术等待手术室。**case history** = details of what has happened to a patient undergoing treatment 病历,病史

casein *noun* protein found in milk 酪蛋白

> COMMENT: Casein is precipitated when milk comes into contact with an acid and so makes milk form cheese.
> 注释：当牛奶与酸作用时酪蛋白会发生沉淀,据此可制乳酪。

cast *noun* (**a**) **plaster cast** = hard support made of bandage soaked in liquid plaster of Paris, which is allowed to harden after being wrapped round a broken limb and which prevents the limb moving while the bone heals 管形石膏夹 (**b**) mass of material formed in a hollow organ *or* tube and excreted in fluid 管型; **blood casts** = pieces of blood cells which are secreted by the kidneys in kidney disease 血细胞管型

castor oil *noun* vegetable oil which acts as a laxative 蓖麻油

castrate *verb* to remove the testicles 阉割

◇ **castration** *noun* surgical removal of the testicles 阉割术

casualty *noun* (**a**) person who has suffered an accident *or* who is suddenly ill 伤患人员: ***The fire caused several casualties.*** 火灾造成了几人受伤。***The casualties were taken by ambulance to the nearest hospital.*** 伤员被救护车送往最近的医院。**casualty department** *or* **hospital** *or* **ward** = department *or* hospital *or* ward which deals with accident victims 创伤科、创伤医院、创伤病房 (**b**) casualty department 创伤科: ***The accident victim was rushed to casualty.*** 事故受害者被推进急救科。

CAT = COMPUTERIZED AXIAL TOMOGRAPHY 计算机轴向体层扫描; **CAT scan** = scan where a narrow X-ray beam, guided by a computer, photographs a thin section of the body or an organ from different angles; the results are fed into the computer which analyses them and produces a picture of a slice of the body or organ 计算机轴向体层扫描

cata- *prefix* meaning downwards 向下

catabolism *noun* breaking down of complex chemicals into simple chemicals

分解代谢

◇ **catabolic** *adjective* referring to catabolism 分解代谢的

catalase *noun* enzyme present in the blood and liver which catalyses the breakdown of hydrogen peroxide into water and oxygen 过氧化氢酶

catalepsy *noun* condition often associated with schizophrenia, where a patient becomes incapable of sensation, his body is rigid and he does not move for long periods 强直症,木僵

catalysis *noun* process where a chemical reaction is helped by a substance (the catalyst) which does not change during the process 催化作用

◇ **catalyse** *or US* **catalyze** *verb* to act as a catalyst, to help make a chemical reaction take place 催化

◇ **catalyst** *noun* substance which produces or helps a chemical reaction without itself changing 催化剂; ***an enzyme which acts as a catalyst in the digestive process*** 在消化过程中起催化剂作用的酶

◇ **catalytic** *adjective* referring to catalysis 催化的; **catalytic reaction** = chemical reaction which is caused by a catalyst which does not change during the reaction 催化反应

catamenia *noun* menstruation 月经

cataplexy *noun* condition where the patient's muscles become suddenly rigid and he falls without losing consciousness, possibly caused by a shock 猝倒

cataract *noun* condition where the lens of the eye gradually becomes hard and opaque 白内障; **congenital cataract** = cataract which is present from birth 先天性白内障; **diabetic cataract** = cataract which develops in people suffering from diabetes 糖尿病性白内障; **senile cataract** = cataract which occurs in an elderly person 老年性白内障; **cataract extraction** = surgical removal of a cataract from the eye 白内障摘除术

COMMENT: Cataracts form most often in people after the age of 50. They are sometimes caused by a blow or an electric shock. Cataractscan easily and safely be removed by surgery.
注释:白内障多发生于50岁后,有时可因打击或电击引起,白内障可经手术方便、安全地摘除。

catarrh *noun* inflammation of mucous membranes in the nose and throat, creating an excessive amount of mucus 卡他,粘膜炎: ***He suffers from catarrh in the winter.*** 冬天他患了粘膜炎。***Is there anything I can take to relieve my catarrh?*** 有什么方法减轻我的卡他症状吗?

◇ **catarrhal** *adjective* referring to catarrh 卡他性的; ***a catarrhal cough*** 卡他性咳嗽

catatonia *noun* condition where a psychiatric patient is either motionless or shows violent reactions to stimulation 紧张症

◇ **catatonic** *adjective* (behaviour) where the patient is either motionless or extremely violent 紧张症的; **catatonic schizophrenia** = type of schizophrenia where the patient is alternately apathetic or very active and disturbed 紧张型精神分裂症

catch *verb* to get a disease 患: ***He caught a cold after standing in the rain.*** 他淋雨后得了感冒。***She caught mumps.*** 她患了流行性腮腺炎。(NOTE: **catches-catching-caught-has caught**)

◇ **catching** *adjective* infectious 传染的: ***Is the disease catching?*** 这病会传染吗?

◇ **catchment area** *noun* area around a hospital which is served by that hospital 医院的服务区

catecholamines *plural noun* the hormones adrenaline and noradrenaline which are released by the adrenal glands 儿茶酚胺

category *noun* classification, the way in which things can be classified 分类,类别: ***His condition is of a non-urgent category.*** 他的病不属于急诊范围。

catgut *noun* thread made from part of the intestines of sheep, now usually artificially hardened, used to sew up incisions made during surgery 肠线

> COMMENT: Catgut is slowly dissolved by fluids in the body after the wound has healed and therefore does not need to be removed. Ordinary catgut will dissolve in 5 to 10 days; hardened catgut takes up to three or four weeks.
> 注释:伤口愈合后肠线会被体液溶解,所以不需要拆线。吸收时间一般是 5 - 10 天,加强肠线会延至 3 - 4 周。

catharsis *noun* purgation of the bowels 导泻,通便

◊ **cathartic** *adjective* laxative *or* purgative 导泻的

catheter *noun* tube passed into the body along one of the passages in the body 导管; **cardiac catheter** = catheter passed through a vein into the heart, to take blood samples *or* to record pressure *or* to examine the interior of the heart before surgery 心导管; **ureteric catheter** = catheter passed through the ureter to the kidney, to inject an opaque solution into the kidney before taking an X-ray 输尿管插管; **urinary** *or* **urethral catheter** = catheter passed up the urethra to allow urine to flow out of the bladder, used to empty the bladder before an abdominal operation 导尿管

◊ **catheterization** *noun* putting a catheter into a patient's body 导管插入术; **cardiac catheterization** = passing a catheter into the heart to take samples of tissue or to check blood pressure 心导管插入术

◊ **catheterize** *verb* to insert a catheter into a patient 插入导管

> QUOTE: High rates of disconnection of closed urine drainage systems, lack of hand washing and incorrect positioning of urine drainage bags have been highlighted in a new report on urethral catheterization.
> 引文:一个新报告突出提到了导尿管插入术时存在的封闭排尿系统断开的发生率高、人工冲洗缺乏和导尿袋位置放置不当等问题。
>
> **Nursing Times** 护理时代

> QUOTE: The technique used to treat aortic stenosis is similar to that for any cardiac catheterization. A catheter introduced through the femoral vein is placed across the aortic valve and into the left ventricle.
> 引文:治疗主动脉狭窄术与其他心导管插入术相似。经股静脉插入导管,过主动脉瓣进入左心室。
>
> **Journal of the American Medical Association** 美国医学会杂志

cat scratch fever *noun* viral fever with inflammation of the lymph glands, caught from being scratched by a cat's claws or by other sharp points 猫抓热

cauda equina *noun* group of nerves which go from the spinal cord to the lumbar region and the coccyx 马尾

◊ **caudal** *adjective* (*in animals*) referring to the tail; (*in humans*) referring to the cauda equina 尾的,马尾的; **caudal analgesia** = technique often used in childbirth, where an analgesic is injected into the extradural space at the base of the spine to remove feeling in the lower part of the trunk 骨氐茇止痛法; **caudal block** = local analgesia of the cauda equina nerves 马尾阻滞

◊ **caudate** *adjective* like a tail 尾样的

caul *noun* (**a**) membrane which sometimes covers a baby's head at birth 胎头羊膜 (**b**) = OMENTUM 大网膜

cauliflower ear *noun* permanently swollen ear, caused by blows (in boxing) 菜花耳

causalgia *noun* burning pain in a limb, caused by a damaged nerve 灼痛

cauterize *verb* to use burning *or* radiation *or* laser beams to remove tissue *or* to stop bleeding 烧灼

◊ **cauterization** *noun* act of cauterizing 烧灼术: ***The growth was removed by cauterization.*** 新生物被烧灼掉了。

◇ **cautery** *noun* surgical instrument used to cauterize a wound 灼器; **cold cautery** = removal of a skin growth using carbon dioxide snow 冷灼术 *see also* 参见 ELECTROCAUTERY, GALVANOCAUTERY

cava 腔 *see* 见 VENA CAVA

cavernosa 阴茎海绵体 *see* 见 CORPUS

cavernous *adjective* hollow 空洞的; **cavernous breathing** *or* **breath sounds** = hollow sounds made by the lungs and heard through a stethoscope placed on a patient's chest, used in diagnosis 呼吸音; **cavernous haemangioma** = tumour in connective tissue with wide spaces which contain blood 海绵状血管瘤; **cavernous sinus** 海绵窦 *see* 见 SINUS

cavity *noun* (i) hole *or* space inside the body 体腔 (ii) hole in a tooth 牙洞; **abdominal cavity** = space in the body below the chest 腹腔; **buccal cavity** = the mouth 口腔; **cerebral cavity** = ventricles in the brain 脑室; **chest cavity** = space in the body containing the heart, lungs and diaphragm 胸腔; **cranial cavity** = space inside the bones of the cranium, in which the brain is situated 颅腔; **glenoid cavity** = socket in the shoulder joint into which the head of the humerus fits 肩盂 ◊ 见图 SHOULDER; **medullary cavity** = hollow centre of a long bone, containing bone marrow 骨髓腔 ◊ 见图 BONE STRUCTURE; **nasal cavity** = cavity behind the nose between the cribriform plates above and the hard palate below, divided in two by the nasal septum and leading to the nasopharynx 鼻腔 ◊ 见图 THROAT; **oral cavity** = the mouth 口腔; **pelvic cavity** = space below the abdominal cavity, above the pelvis 盆腔; **peritoneal cavity** = space between the layers of the peritoneum, containing the major organs of the abdomen 腹膜腔; **pleural cavity** = space between the inner and outer pleura of the chest 胸膜腔; **pulp cavity** = centre of a tooth containing soft tissue 牙髓腔 ◊ 见图 TOOTH; **synovial cavity** = space inside a synovial joint 滑膜腔; **thoracic cavity** = space in the body containing the heart, lungs and diaphragm 胸腔

◇ **cavitation** *noun* forming of a cavity 成洞,成腔

cavus 弓形足 *see* 见 PES

CBC = COMPLETE BLOOD COUNT 全血细胞计数

cc = CUBIC CENTIMETRE 立方厘米

CCU = CORONARY CARE UNIT 冠心病监护病房

Cd *chemical symbol for* cadmium 镉的化学元素符号

CDH = CONGENITAL DISLOCATION OF THE HIP 先天性髋关节脱位

cecum *noun US* = CAECUM 盲肠

-cele *suffix* referring to a hollow 腔的

celiac *US* = COELIAC 腹的

cell *noun* tiny unit of matter which is the base of all plant and animal tissue 细胞; **alpha cell** = one of the types of cells in glands (such as the pancreas) which have more than one type of cell α细胞; **beta cell** = cell which produces insulin β细胞; **blood cell** = corpuscle, any type of cell found in the blood 血细胞; **daughter cell** = one of the cells which develop by mitosis from a single parent cell 子细胞; **goblet cell** = tube-shaped cell in the epithelium which secretes mucus 杯状细胞; **mast cell** = large cell in connective tissue, which carries histamine and reacts to allergens 肥大细胞; **mother cell** *or* **parent cell** = original cell which splits into daughter cells by mitosis 母细胞; **mucous cell** = cell which contains mucinogen which secretes mucin 粘液细胞; **oxyntic cell** *or* **parietal cell** = cell in the gastric gland which secretes hydrochloric acid 泌酸细胞,壁细胞; **receptor cell** = cell which senses a change (such as cold or heat) in the surrounding environment or in the body and reacts to it by sending an impulse to the central nervous system 受体细胞; **cell body** = part of a nerve cell which surrounds the nucleus and from which the axon and dendrites begin 细胞体; **cell division** = way in which a cell reproduces itself by mitosis 细胞分裂; **cell membrane** = membrane enclosing the cytoplasm of a cell 细胞膜

◇ **cellular** *adjective* (**a**) referring to cells; formed of cells 细胞的 (**b**) made of many similar parts connected together 许多相似的部分聚集在一起; **cellular tissue** = form of connective tissue with large spaces 蜂窝组织 (NOTE: for other terms referring to cells, see words beginning with **cyt-**, **cyto-**)

> COMMENT: The cell is a unit which can reproduce itself. It is made up of a jelly-like substance (cytoplasm) which surrounds a nucleus and contains many other small organisms which are different according to the type of cell. Cells reproduce by division (mitosis) and their process of feeding and removing waste products is metabolism. The division and reproduction of cells is how the human body is formed.
> 注释:细胞是可自我复制的单位,由细胞核及其周围凝胶状的细胞质组成,不同类型的细胞的细胞质中含有很多不同的小的细胞器。细胞经分裂繁殖,其摄食、排泄的过程称为代谢。细胞的分裂和繁殖形成了人体。

cellulite *noun* lumpy deposits of subcutaneous fat, especially in the thighs and buttocks 蜂窝组织

cellulitis *noun* usually bacterial inflammation of connective tissue or of the subcutaneous tissue 蜂窝织炎

cellulose *noun* carbohydrate which makes up a large percentage of plant matter 纤维素

> COMMENT: Cellulose is not digestible and is passed through the digestive system as roughage.
> 注释:纤维素不能被消化,以粗糙食物形式通过胃肠道。

Celsius *noun* scale of temperature where the freezing and boiling points of water are 0° and 100° 摄氏度 (NOTE: used in many countries, except in the USA, where the Fahrenheit system is still preferred. Normally written as a **C** after the degree sign: **52°C** (say: 'fifty-two degrees Celsius'). Also called **centigrade**)

> COMMENT: To convert Celsius temperatures to Fahrenheit, multiply by 1.8 and add 32. So 20°C is equal to 68°F.
> 注释:摄氏度换算为华氏度是乘 1.8 再加 32,如 20°C 等于 68°F。

cement *noun* (**a**) adhesive used in dentistry to attach a crown to the base of a tooth 粘固粉 (**b**) = CEMENTUM 牙骨质

cementum *noun* layer of thick hard material which covers the roots of teeth 牙骨质 ◇ 见图 TOOTH

centi- *prefix* meaning one hundredth (10^{-2}) 百分之一 (NOTE: symbol is **c**)

centigrade *noun* scale of temperature where the freezing and boiling points of water are 0° and 100° 摄氏度 *see* 见 *note at* CELSIUS

centilitre *or US* **centiliter** *noun* unit of measurement of liquid (= one hundredth of a litre) 厘升 (NOTE: with figures usually written **cl**)

centimetre *or US* **centimeter** *noun* unit of measurement of length (= one hundredth of a metre) 厘米 (NOTE: with figures usually written **cm**: **10cm**: **'the appendix is about 6cm (six centimetres) in length'**)

central *adjective* referring to the centre 中心的; **central canal** = thin tube in the centre of the spinal cord containing cerebrospinal fluid 中央管; **central nervous system (CNS)** = the brain and spinal cord which link together all the nerves 中枢神经系统; **central sulcus** = one of the grooves which divide a cerebral hemisphere into lobes 中央沟; **central vein** = vein in the liver 中央静脉;

central venous pressure = blood pressure in the right atrium, which can be measured by means of a catheter 中心静脉压

◇ **centre** *or US* **center** *noun* (**a**) middle point *or* main part 中央点,主要部分: ***The aim of the examination is to locate the centre of infection.*** 检查的目的是确定感染的中心部位。(**b**) large building 中心,大的建筑物; **medical centre** = place where several different doctors and specialists practise 医疗中心 (**c**) point where a group of nerves come together 神经的交汇部; **vision centre** = point in the brain where the nerves relating to the eye come together 视中心

centralis 中央凹 *see* 见 FOVEA

centrifugal *adjective* which goes away from the centre 远心的,离心的

◇ **centrifugation** *or* **centrifuging** *noun* separating the components of a liquid in a centrifuge 离心

◇ **centrifuge** *noun* device to separate the components of a liquid by rapid spinning 离心机

centriole *noun* small structure found in the cytoplasm of a cell, which forms asters during cell division 中心粒

centripetal *adjective* which goes towards the centre 向心的

centromere *noun* kinetochore, constricted part of a cell, seen as the cell divides 着丝粒

centrosome *noun* structure of the cytoplasm in a cell, near the nucleus, and containing the centrioles 中心体

centrum *noun* centre *or* central part of an organ 器官的中央部 (NOTE: plural is **centra**)

cephal- *prefix* referring to the head 头的

◇ **cephalalgia** *noun* headache, a pain in the head 头痛

◇ **cephalhaematoma** *noun* swelling found mainly on the head of babies delivered with forceps 头部血肿

◇ **cephalic** *adjective* referring to the head 头的; **cephalic index** = measurement of the shape of the skull 头颅指数; **cephalic presentation** = normal position of a baby in the womb, where the baby's head will appear first 头先露; **cephalic version** = turning a wrongly positioned fetus round in the uterus, so that the head will appear first at birth 胎头倒转术

◇ **cephalocele** *noun* swelling caused by part of the brain passing through a weak point in the bones of the skull 脑膨出

◇ **cephalogram** *noun* X-ray photograph of the bones of the skull 头颅X线片

◇ **cephalometry** *noun* measurement of the head 头颅测量法

◇ **cephalopelvic** *adjective* referring to the head of the fetus and the pelvis of the mother 头盆的; **cephalopelvic disproportion** = condition where the pelvic opening of the mother is not large enough for the head of the fetus 头盆不称

cerea 蜡样屈曲 *see* 见 FLEXIBILITAS CEREA

cereal *noun* (**a**) plant whose seeds are used for food, especially to make flour 谷类: ***The Common Market grows large quantities of cereals or of cereal crops.*** 共同市场生产了大量的谷物。(**b**) food made of seeds of corn, etc. which is usually eaten at breakfast 麦片: ***He ate a bowl of cereal.*** 他吃了一碗麦片。***Put milk and sugar on your cereal.*** 在你的麦片里放些牛奶和糖。

cerebellar *adjective* referring to the cerebellum 小脑的; **cerebellar ataxia** = disorder where the patient staggers and cannot speak clearly, due to a disease of the cerebellum 小脑共济失调; **cerebellar gait** = way of walking where the patient staggers along, caused by a disease of the cerebellum 小脑步态; **cerebellar peduncle** = band of nerve tissue connecting parts of the cerebellum 小脑脚;

cerebellar syndrome = disease affecting the cerebellum, the symptoms of which are lack of muscle coordination, spasms in the eyeball and impaired speech 小脑综合症

◊ **cerebellum** *noun* section of the hindbrain, located at the back of the head beneath the back part of the cerebrum 小脑 ◊ 见图 BRAIN; **tentorium cerebelli** = part of the dura mater which separates the cerebellum from the cerebral hemispheres 小脑幕

> COMMENT: The cerebellum is formed of two hemispheres with the vermis in the centre. Fibres go into or out of the cerebellum through the peduncles. The cerebellum is the part of the brain where voluntary movements are coordinated and is associated with the sense of balance.
> 注释:小脑由两个半球组成,中间为小脑蚓部。神经纤维从小脑脚进出协调自主运动及平衡感觉的中枢。

cerebr- *or* **cerebro-** *prefix* referring to the cerebrum 大脑的

◊ **cerebral** *adjective* referring to the cerebrum or to the brain in general 大脑的或脑的; **cerebral aqueduct** *or* **aqueduct of Sylvius** = canal connecting the third and fourth ventricles in the brain 中脑导水管; **cerebral arteries** = main arteries which take blood into the brain 大脑动脉; **cerebral cavity** = ventricles in the brain 脑室; **cerebral cortex** = outer layer of grey matter which covers the cerebrum 大脑皮质; **cerebral decompression** = removal of part of the skull to relieve pressure on the brain 脑减压; **cerebral haemorrhage** = bleeding inside the brain from a cerebral artery 脑出血; **cerebral hemisphere** = one of the two halves of the cerebrum 大脑半球; **cerebral peduncle** = mass of nerve fibres connecting the cerebral hemispheres to the midbrain 大脑脚; **cerebral thrombosis** = stroke, condition where a blood clot enters and blocks a brain artery 脑栓塞

◊ **cerebral palsy** *noun* disorder of the brain, mainly due to brain damage occurring before birth, or due to lack of oxygen during birth 脑瘫,大脑性麻痹

> COMMENT: Cerebral palsy is the disorder affecting spastics. The patient may have bad coordination of muscular movements, impaired speech, hearing and sight, and sometimes mental retardation.
> 注释:脑瘫是一严重的大脑麻痹症,患者表现为肌肉运动失调,言语、听力、视力受损,有时可伴智力障碍。

cerebration *noun* working of the brain 脑活动

cerebrospinal *adjective* referring to the brain and the spinal cord 脑脊髓的; **cerebrospinal fever** *or* **cerebrospinal meningitis** = meningococcal meningitis *or* spotted fever, the commonest epidemic form of meningitis, caused by a bacterium *Neisseria meningitidis*, where the meninges become inflamed causing headaches and fever 脑脊髓膜炎; **cerebrospinal fluid** (**CSF**) = fluid which surrounds the brain and the spinal cord 脑脊液; **cerebrospinal tracts** = main motor pathways in the anterior and lateral white columns of the spinal cord 脑脊束

> COMMENT: CSF is found in the space between the arachnoid mater and pia mater of the brain, between the ventricles of the brain and in the central canal of the spinal cord. CSF consists mainly of water, with some sugar and sodium chloride. Its function is to cushion the brain and spinal cord and it is continually formed and absorbed to maintain the correct pressure.
> 注释:脑脊液位于蛛网膜和软脑膜的间隙、脑室间隙和脊髓中央管中。主要成分为水份,水中含有一些糖和氯化钠,对脑和脊髓起缓冲作用,并在不断的形成和吸收过程中保持适宜的压力。

cerebrovascular *adjective* referring to the blood vessels in the brain 脑血管

的；**cerebrovascular accident** (**CVA**) = stroke, a sudden blocking of or bleeding from a blood vessel in the brain resulting in temporary or permanent paralysis or death 脑血管意外；**cerebrovascular disease** = disease of the blood vessels in the brain 脑血管病

cerebrum *noun* main part of the brain 大脑；**falx cerebri** = fold of the dura mater between the two hemispheres of the cerebrum 大脑镰 ◊ 见图 BRAIN

> COMMENT: The cerebrum is the largest part of the brain, formed of two sections (the cerebral hemispheres) which run along the length of the head. The cerebrum controls the main mental processes, including the memory.
> 注释:大脑是脑的最大组成部分,由两半球组成,控制主要的智力活动,包括记忆。

certificate *noun* official paper which states something 证书；**birth certificate** = official document giving details of a person's date and place of birth and parents 出生证；**death certificate** = official document signed by a doctor, stating that a person has died and giving details of the person and the cause of death 死亡证明；**medical certificate** = official document signed by a doctor, giving a patient permission to be away from work or not to do certain types of work 医疗证明

◊ **certify** *verb* to make an official statement in writing 证明：***He was certified dead on arrival at hospital.*** 他被证明到达医院时已死亡。(NOTE: formerly used to refer to patients sent to a mental hospital)

cerumen *noun* wax which forms inside the ear 耵聍

◊ **ceruminous glands** *noun* glands which secrete earwax 耵聍腺 ◊ 见图 EAR

cervic- *or* **cervico-** *prefix* (i) referring to a neck 颈的 (ii) referring to the cervix of the uterus 子宫颈

◊ **cervical** *adjective* (i) referring to any neck 颈的 (ii) referring to the cervix of the uterus 宫颈的；**cervical canal** = tube running through the cervix from the point where the uterus joins the vagina to the entrance of the uterine cavity 宫颈管；**cervical cancer** = cancer of the cervix of the uterus 宫颈癌；**cervical cap** = DUTCH CAP 宫颈帽；**cervical collar** = special strong orthopaedic collar to support the head of a patient with neck injuries or a condition such as cervical spondylosis 颈圈；**cervical ganglion** = one of the bundles of nerves in the neck 颈神经节；**cervical (lymph) node** = lymph node in the neck 颈淋巴结；**cervical nerves** = spinal nerves in the neck 颈神经；**cervical rib** = extra rib sometimes found attached to the vertebrae above the other ribs and which may cause thoracic inlet syndrome 颈肋；**cervical smear** = test for cervical cancer, where cells taken from the mucus in the cervix of the uterus are examined 宫颈涂片；**cervical spondylosis** = degenerative change in the neck bones 颈椎关节强直 *see also* 参见 SPONDYLOS；**deep cervical vein** = vein in the neck, which drains into the vertebral vein 颈深静脉；**cervical vertebrae** = the seven bones which form the neck 颈椎 ◊ 见图 VERTEBRAL COLUMN

◊ **cervicectomy** *noun* surgical removal of the cervix uteri 子宫颈切除术

◊ **cervicitis** *noun* inflammation of the cervix uteri 宫颈炎

◊ **cervicography** *noun* photographing the cervix uteri: used as a method of screening for cervical cancer 宫颈造影术

◊ **cervicouterine canal** = CERVICAL CANAL 宫颈管

◊ **cervix** *noun* (i) any narrow neck of an organ 颈部 (ii) neck of the womb, the narrow lower part of the uterus leading into the vagina 宫颈 (NOTE: cervix means 'neck' and can refer to any neck; it is most usually used to refer to the narrow part of the uterus and is then referred to as the **cervix uteri**)

cestode *noun* type of tapeworm 绦虫

CFT = COMPLEMENT FIXATION TEST 补体结合试验

chafe *verb* to rub, especially to rub against the skin 刺激,尤其针对皮肤: ***The rough cloth of the collar chafed the patient's neck.*** 衣领处的粗糙布料刺激了患者的颈部皮肤。***She was experiencing chafing of the thighs.*** 她感觉到大腿处有刺激感。

Chagas' disease *noun* type of sleeping sickness found in South America, transmitted by insect bites which pass trypanosomes into the bloodstream 恰加斯氏病,南美洲锥虫病

> COMMENT: The first symptom is an inflamed spot at the place of the insect bite, followed later by fever, swelling of the liver and spleen and swelling of tissues in the face. Children are mainly affected and if untreated the disease can cause fatal heart block in early adult life.
> 注释:它的首发症状是虫咬处的炎性斑点,随后是发热、肝脾肿大和面部肿胀。儿童是主要的受累对象,如果不治疗步入成年时可出现致命的心脏传导阻滞。

chain *noun* (i) number of metal rings attached together to make a line 链条(ii) number of components linked together or number of connected events 一连串,一系列; **chain reaction** = reaction where each stage is started by the one before it 连锁反应

chair *noun* piece of furniture for sitting on 椅子: ***A badly made chair can affect the posture.*** 制作不良的椅子可影响坐姿。**dentist's chair** = special chair which can be made to tip backwards, used by dentists when operating on patients' teeth 牙科椅 *see also* 参见 BIRTHING

chalazion *or* **meibomian cyst** *noun* swelling of a sebaceous gland in the eyelid 睑板腺囊肿

chalone *noun* hormone which stops a secretion, as opposed to those hormones which stimulate secretion 抑素

chamber *noun* hollow space (atrium *or* ventricle) in the heart where blood is collected 房室腔; **anterior** *or* **posterior chambers of the eye** = parts of the aqueous chamber of the eye which are in front of or behind the iris 前或后房; **collection chambers** = sections of the heart where blood collects before being pumped out 收集腔; **pumping chambers** = sections of the heart where blood is pumped 泵出腔

chancre *noun* sore on the lip *or* penis *or* eyelid which is the first symptom of syphilis 下疳

◇ **chancroid** *noun* soft chancre, venereal sore with a soft base, situated in the groin or on the genitals and caused by the bacterium *Haemophilus ducreyi* 软下疳

change 1 *noun* being different 变化; ***We will try a change of treatment.*** 我们会尝试改变治疗方案。***This patient needs a change of bedclothes.*** 这患者需要更换被褥。**change of life** = MENOPAUSE 停经 **2** *verb* **(a)** to make something different; to become different 改变: ***Treatment of tuberculosis has changed a lot in the past few years.*** 在过去的几年里结核病的治疗有了很大的改变。***He's changed so much since his illness that I hardly recognized him.*** 他生病后变化很大,我差点儿认不出来了。***The doctor decided to change the dosage.*** 医生决定改变药物剂量。**(b)** to put on different clothes *or* bedclothes *or* bandages 更换(衣服,被褥,绷带): ***She changed into her uniform before going into the ward.*** 进病房前她换上了制服。***The nurses change the bedclothes every day.*** 护士每天更换被褥。***Make sure the dressing on the wound is changed every morning.*** 确保伤口上的敷料每早都更换。

channel *noun* tube *or* passage through which fluid flows 管道,沟

chaplain *noun* **hospital chaplain** =

religious minister attached to a hospital, who visits and comforts patients and their families and gives them the sacraments when necessary 医院的牧师

chapped *adjective* (skin) which is cracked due to cold 皲裂的：***Put some cream on your chapped lips.*** 在你干裂的唇上抹点儿油膏。

◇ **chapping** *noun* cracking of the skin due to cold 干裂：***Cream will prevent your hands chapping.*** 雪花膏可防止你的手干裂。

character *noun* way in which a person thinks and behaves 性格

◇ **characteristic** **1** *adjective* typical *or* special 特有的：***The inflammation is characteristic of shingles.*** 炎症是带状疱疹的特点。***symptoms characteristic of anaemia*** 贫血特有的症状 **2** *noun* difference which makes something special 特性：***Cancer destroys the cell's characteristics.*** 癌症破坏了细胞的特性。

◇ **characterize** *verb* to make something typical *or* special 成为…的特性：***The disease is characterized by the development of coarse features.*** 本病以逐渐发生面容粗陋为特点。

charcoal *noun* black substance, an impure form of carbon, formed when wood is burnt in the absence of oxygen 活性炭

> COMMENT: Charcoal tablets can be used to relieve diarrhoea *or* flatulence.
> 注释：活性炭可用来缓解腹泻或腹胀。

Charcot's joint *noun* joint which becomes deformed because the patient cannot feel pain in it when the nerves have been damaged by syphilis *or* diabetes *or* leprosy 夏科氏关节，神经源性关节病

charge nurse *noun* nurse in charge of a group of patients 主管护士

chart *noun* diagram *or* record of information shown as a series of lines *or* points on graph paper：***A chart showing the rise in cases of whooping cough during the first five months of 1993.*** 图示显示 1993 年头 5 月百日咳发病率增长了。temperature chart = chart showing changes in a patient's temperature over a period of time 体温图

ChB = BACHELOR OF SURGERY 外科学士

CHC = CHILD HEALTH CLINIC 儿童保健门诊

CHD = CORONARY HEART DISEASE 冠心病

checkup *noun* test to see if someone is fit; general examination by a doctor or dentist 体检，检查：***He had a heart checkup last week.*** 他上周做了心脏检查。***She has entered hospital for a checkup.*** 她去医院做体检。***He made an appointment with the dentist for a checkup.*** 他预约了牙科医生做检查。

cheek *noun* one of two fleshy parts of the face on each side of the nose 面颊；***A little girl with red cheeks*** 面颊红润的小女孩

◇ **cheekbone** *noun* zygomatic bone *or* malar bone *or* bone which forms the prominent part of the cheek and the lower part of the eye socket 颧骨

cheil- *prefix* referring to lips 唇的

◇ **cheilitis** *noun* inflammation of the lips 唇炎

◇ **cheilosis** *noun* swelling and cracks on the lips and corners of the mouth caused by lack of vitamin B 唇干裂

chelating agent *noun* chemical compound which can combine with certain metals, used as a treatment for metal poisoning 螯合剂

cheloid = KELOID 瘢痕瘤

chem- *prefix* referring to chemistry or to chemicals 化学的

◇ **chemical** **1** *adjective* referring to chemistry 化学的 **2** *noun* substance produced by a chemical process or formed of chemical elements 化合物

◇ **chemist** *noun* (**a**) scientist who specializes in the study of chemistry 化学家 (**b**) dispensing chemist = pharmacist who prepares and sells drugs according to doctors' prescriptions 药剂师,发药师; **a chemist's** = shop where you can buy medicine, toothpaste, soap, etc. 药店: ***Go to the chemist's to get some cough medicine.*** 去药店买些咳嗽药。***The tablets are sold at all chemists'.*** 这药在所有的药店都有售。***There's a chemist's on the corner.*** 在街角有家药店。

◊ **chemistry** *noun* study of substances, elements and compounds and their reactions with each other 化学; **blood chemistry** *or* **chemistry of the blood** = (i) substances which make up blood, which can be analysed in blood tests, the results of which are useful in diagnosing disease 血液的化学成分 (ii) record of changes which take place in blood during disease and treatment 血液化学检查成分变化的记录

> QUOTE: The MRI body scanner is able to provide a chemical analysis of tissues without investigative surgery.
> 引文:磁共振成像扫描不经手术探查就能对组织的化学成分进行分析。
> **Health Services Journal** 健康服务杂志

chemo- *prefix* referring to chemistry 化学的

◊ **chemoreceptor** *noun* cell which responds to the presence of a chemical compound by activating a sensory nerve (such as a taste bud reacting to food) 化学感受器 *see also* 参见 EXTEROCEPTOR, INTEROCEPTOR, RECEPTOR

◊ **chemosis** *noun* swelling of the conjunctiva 球结膜水肿

◊ **chemotaxis** *noun* movement of a cell which is attracted to or repelled by a chemical substance 趋化性

◊ **chemotherapeutic agent** *noun* chemical substance used to treat a disease 化疗剂

◊ **chemotherapy** *noun* using chemical drugs (such as antibiotics *or* painkillers *or* antiseptic lotions) to fight a disease, especially using toxic chemicals to destroy rapidly developing cancer cells 化疗

chest *noun* thorax, the cavity in the top part of the front of the body above the abdomen, containing the diaphragm, heart and lungs and surrounded by the rib cage 胸部: ***He placed the stethoscope on the patient's chest*** *or* ***he listened to the patient's chest.*** 他把听诊器放在患者的胸部,对患者的胸部进行听诊。***She is suffering from chest pains.*** 她胸痛。***After the fight he was rushed to hospital with chest wounds.*** 战斗后他因胸伤被送往医院。***a day unit set up for disabled chest patients*** 为胸部有残疾的病人开设的日间病房; **She has a cold in the chest.** = She coughs badly. 她咳嗽得厉害。**chest cavity** = space in the body containing the heart, lungs and diaphragm 胸腔; **chest examination** = examination of the patient's chest by percussion, stethoscopeor X-rays 胸部检查; **chest muscle** *or* **pectoral muscle** = one of two muscles which lie across the chest and control movements of the shoulder and arm 胸肌 (NOTE: for other terms referring to the chest, see words beginning with **pecto-**, **steth-**, **thorac-**)

chew *verb* to masticate, to crush food with the teeth 咀嚼: ***He was chewing a piece of meat.*** 他在嚼一块肉。***Food should be chewed slowly.*** 应慢慢咀嚼食物。

◊ **chewing gum** *noun* sweet substance which you can chew for a long time but not swallow 口香糖

> COMMENT: The action of chewing grinds the food into small pieces and mixes it with saliva to start the process of breaking down the food to extract nutrients from it.
> 注释:咀嚼可将食物磨成碎粒并与唾液混合,由此开始消化食物吸收养分的过程。

Cheyne-Stokes respiration *or* **breathing** *noun* condition (usually of unconscious patients) where breathing is irregular, with short breaths gradually increasing to deep breaths, then reducing again, until breathing appears to stop; caused by a disorder of the brain centre which controls breathing 陈-施呼吸

chiasm *or* **chiasma** *noun* cross-shaped crossing of fibres 交叉; **optic chiasma** = structure where some of the optic nerves from each eye partially cross each other in the hypothalamus 视交叉

chickenpox *noun* varicella, infectious disease of children, with fever and red spots which turn into itchy blisters 水痘

> COMMENT: Chickenpox is caused by a herpesvirus. In later life, shingles is usually a re-emergence of a dormant chickenpox virus and an adult with shingles can infect a child with chickenpox.
> 注释:水痘由疱疹病毒引起,成年后发生的带状疱疹通常是潜伏的水痘病毒的复发,患有带状疱疹的成人可使儿童感染水痘。

chigger *noun* harvest mite, a tiny insect which bites and causes irritation; its larva also can enter the skin near a hair follicle and travel under the skin causing intense irritation 恙螨

chilblain *noun* erythema pernio, condition where the skin of the fingers, toes, nose or ears becomes red, swollen and itchy because of exposure to cold 冻疮: ***He has chilblains on his toes.*** 他的脚趾上有冻疮。

child *noun* young boy or girl 儿童: ***Here is a photograph of my father as a child.*** 这是我父亲儿时的照片。 ***All the children were playing out in the field.*** 所有的儿童都在田里玩耍。 ***When do the children come out of school?*** 孩子们什么时候放学? **They have six children.** = They have six sons or daughters. 他们有6个孩子。**child abuse** = bad treatment of children, including sexual interference 虐待儿童; **children's hospital** = hospital which specializes in treating children 儿童医院 (NOTE: plural is **children.** Note also that **child** is the legal term for a person under 14 years of age)

◇ **childbearing** *noun* giving birth 分娩: ***45 is the upper age limit for childbearing.*** 45岁是分娩的年龄上限。

◇ **childbirth** *noun* parturition, the act of giving birth 出生; **natural childbirth** = childbirth where the mother is not given any pain-killing drugs or anaesthetic but is encouraged to give birth after having prepared herself through relaxation and breathing exercises and a new psychological outlook 自然分娩

◇ **child care** *noun* care of young children and study of their special needs 儿童护理

◇ **child health clinic (CHC)** *or* **child development clinic** *noun* special clinic for checking the health and development of small children under school age 儿童保健所

◇ **childhood** *noun* time when a person is a child 儿童期: ***He had a happy childhood in the country.*** 在乡村他度过了快乐的童年。 ***She spent her childhood in Canada.*** 他在加拿大度过了童年。**childhood illnesses** *or* **disorders** = disorders which mainly affect children and not adults 儿科病

◇ **child-proof** *adjective* which a child cannot use 防止儿童误用的: ***The pills are sold in bottles with child-proof lids.*** 药片放在有防止儿童误用瓶盖的药瓶中出售。(NOTE: for other terms referring to children, see words beginning with **paed-** *or* **ped-**)

chill *noun* feeling cold and shivering, usually the sign of the beginning of a fever, of flu or a cold 寒战,受凉: ***He caught a chill on the train.*** 他在火车上着凉了。

chin *noun* bottom part of the face, beneath the mouth 颏: ***She hit him on the chin.*** 她打了他下巴颏。 ***He rested his chin on his hand while he was thinking.*** 他思考时把下巴颏支在手上。

Chinese restaurant syndrome

noun allergic condition which gives people violent headaches after eating food flavoured with monosodium glutamate 中国餐馆综合症

chiropody *noun* study and treatment of minor diseases and disorders of the feet 足医术

◇ **chiropodist** *noun* person who specializes in treatment of minor disorders of the feet 足医 *see also* 参见 PODIATRIST, PODIATRY

chiropractic *noun* treatment of disorders by manipulating the bones of the spine 脊柱按摩疗法

◇ **chiropractor** *noun* person who treats disorders by manipulating the bones of the spine 脊柱按摩士

Chlamydia *noun* type of parasite, which is transmitted to humans by insects, causing psittacosis and trachoma 衣原体

chloasma *noun* presence of brown spots on the skin from various causes 褐黄斑

chlor(o)- *prefix* (i) referring to chlorine 氯的 (ii) referring to the colour green 绿色的

◇ **chloride** *noun* a salt of hydrochloric acid 氯化物; **sodium chloride** (**NaCl**) = common salt 氯化钠

◇ **chlorination** *noun* sterilizing by adding chlorine 加氯消毒

◇ **chlorinator** *noun* apparatus for adding chlorine to water 加氯器

◇ **chlorine** *noun* powerful greenish gas, used to sterilize water 氯气 (NOTE: chemical symbol is **Cl**)

> COMMENT: Chlorination is used to kill bacteria in drinking water, in swimming pools and sewage farms, and has many industrial applications such as sterilization in food processing.
> 注释:加氯消毒可用来杀灭饮用水、游泳池及污水中的细菌,并有许多工业用途如食品加工过程中的消毒。

chloroform (**$CHCl_3$**) *noun* powerful drug formerly used as an anaesthetic 氯仿

chloroma *noun* bone tumour associated with acute leukaemia 绿色瘤

chlorophyll *noun* green pigment in plants, also used in deodorants and toothpaste 叶绿素

chloroquine *noun* drug used to treat and prevent malaria 氯喹

chlorosis *noun* type of severe anaemia due to iron deficiency, affecting mainly young girls 萎黄病,绿色贫血

chlorothiazide *noun* drug which acts as a diuretic and also helps reduce high blood pressure 氯噻嗪

chlorpromazine *noun* tranquillizing drug 氯丙嗪

ChM = MASTER OF SURGERY 外科硕士

choana *noun* any opening shaped like a funnel, especially that leading from the nasal cavity to the pharynx 漏斗,后鼻孔 (NOTE: plural is **choanae**)

choke *verb* to stop breathing because the windpipe becomes blocked by a foreign body or by inhalation of water 哽噎; **to choke on something** = to take something into the windpipe instead of the gullet, so that the breathing is interrupted 被…呛了,被噎住了: ***He choked on a piece of bread** or **a piece of bread made him choke**.* 他被一片面包噎住了。

◇ **choking 1** *noun* asphyxia, a condition where someone is prevented from breathing 窒息 **2** *adjective* (smoke) which makes you choke 使人窒息的: ***The room filled with choking black smoke**.* 屋里弥漫着使人窒息的黑烟。

chol- *prefix* referring to bile 胆汁的

◇ **cholaemia** *noun* presence of abnormal amount of bile in the blood 胆汁血症

◇ **cholagogue** *noun* drug which encourages the production of bile 利胆药

◇ **cholangiography** *noun* X-ray examination of the bile ducts and gall bladder 胆管造影术

◇ **cholangiolitis** *noun* inflammation

of the small bile ducts 胆小管炎

◇ **cholangitis** *noun* inflammation of the bile ducts 胆管炎

◇ **chole-** *prefix* referring to bile 胆汁的

◇ **cholecystectomy** *noun* surgical removal of the gall bladder 胆囊切除术

◇ **cholecystitis** *noun* inflammation of the gall bladder 胆囊炎

◇ **cholecystoduodenostomy** *noun* surgical operation to join the gall bladder to the duodenum to allow bile to pass into the intestine when the main bile ductis blocked 胆囊十二指肠吻合术

◇ **cholecystogram** *noun* X-ray photograph of the gall bladder 胆囊片

◇ **cholecystography** *noun* X-ray examination of the gall bladder 胆囊造影术

◇ **cholecystotomy** *noun* surgical operation to make a cut in the gall bladder, usually to remove gallstones 胆囊切开术

◇ **choledoch-** *prefix* referring to the common bile duct 胆总管的

◇ **choledochotomy** *noun* surgical operation to make a cut in the common bile duct to remove stones 胆总管切开术

◇ **cholelithiasis** *or* **choledocholithiasis** *noun* condition where gallstones form in the gall bladder *or* bile ducts 胆石病

◇ **cholelithotomy** *noun* surgical removal of gallstones by cutting into the gall bladder 胆石切除术

cholera *noun* serious bacterial disease spread through food *or* water which has been infected by *Vibrio cholerae* 霍乱: ***He caught cholera while on holiday.*** 他度假时感染了霍乱。***A cholera epidemic broke out after the flood.*** 洪水后有霍乱暴发。

COMMENT: The infected person suffers diarrhoea, cramp in the intestines and dehydration. The disease is often fatal and vaccination is only effective for a relatively short period.
注释:患者有腹泻、肠痉挛及脱水症状。本病常是致命性的,接种疫苗的持效期很短。

choleresis *noun* production of bile by the liver 胆汁分泌

◇ **choleretic** *adjective* (substance) which increases the production and flow of bile 促胆汁分泌的

◇ **cholestasis** *noun* condition where all bile does not pass into the intestine but some remains in the liver and causes jaundice 胆汁淤积

cholesteatoma *noun* cyst containing some cholesterol found in the middle ear and also in the brain 胆脂瘤

cholesterol *noun* fatty substance found in fats and oils, also produced by the liver and forming an essential part of all cells 胆固醇

◇ **cholesterosis** *noun* inflammation of the gall bladder with deposits of cholesterol 胆固醇沉着病

COMMENT: Cholesterol is found in brain cells, the adrenal glands, liver and bile acids. High levels of cholesterol in the blood are found in diabetes. Cholesterol is formed by the body, and high blood cholesterol levels are associated with diets rich in animal fat (such as butter and fat meat). Excess cholesterol can be deposited in the walls of arteries, causing atherosclerosis.
注释:脑细胞、肾上腺、肝及胆汁酸中都有胆固醇。患糖尿病时血中胆固醇水平升高。胆固醇由机体产生,高胆固醇血症与饮食中富含动物脂肪(如黄油、肥肉)有关。过量的胆固醇在动脉壁沉着可引起动脉粥样硬化。

cholic acid *noun* one of the bile acids 胆汁酸

◇ **choline** *noun* essential basic compound which synthesizes acetylcholine 胆碱

◇ **cholinesterase** *noun* enzyme which breaks down a choline ester 胆碱酯酶

choluria *noun* bile in the urine 胆汁尿

chondr- *prefix* referring to cartilage 软骨的

◊ **chondritis** *noun* inflammation of a cartilage 软骨炎

◊ **chondroblast** *noun* cell from which cartilage develops in an embryo 成软骨细胞

◊ **chondrocalcinosis** *noun* condition where deposits of calcium phosphate are found in articular cartilage 软骨钙质沉着

◊ **chondrocyte** *noun* mature cartilage cell 软骨细胞

◊ **chondrodysplasia** *noun* hereditary disorder of cartilage which is linked to dwarfism 软骨发育异常

◊ **chondrodystrophy** *noun* general term for disorders of the cartilage 软骨营养障碍

◊ **chondroma** *noun* tumour formed of cartilaginous tissue 软骨瘤

◊ **chondromalacia** *noun* degeneration of the cartilage of a joint 软骨软化

◊ **chondrosarcoma** *noun* malignant, rapidly growing tumour involving cartilage cells 软骨肉瘤

chorda *noun* cord or tendon 索，腱；**chordae tendineae** = tiny fibrous ligaments in the heart which attach the edges of some of the valves to the walls of the ventricles 腱索（NOTE: plural is **chordae**）

◊ **chordee** *noun* painful condition where the erect penis is curved; a complication of gonorrhoea 痛性阴茎勃起

◊ **chorditis** *noun* inflammation of the vocal cords 声带炎

◊ **chordotomy** *noun* surgical operation to cut any cord, such as a nerve pathway in the spinal cord, to relieve intractable pain 脊髓切断术

chorea *noun* sudden severe twitching (usually of the face and shoulders), symptom of disease of the nervous system 舞蹈病；**Huntington's chorea** = progressive hereditary disease which affects adults, where the outer layer of the brain degenerates and the patient makes involuntary jerky movements and develops progressive dementia 杭廷顿氏舞蹈病，慢性舞蹈病，一种进行性遗传疾病，发生于成年人，因大脑皮质退化导致非自主性滑稽动作，进而痴呆；**Sydenham's chorea** = temporary chorea affecting children, frequently associated with endocarditis and rheumatism 西登哈姆氏舞蹈病，发生于儿童的暂时性舞蹈病，常伴随心内膜炎、风湿病发作

chorion *noun* membrane covering the fertilized ovum 绒毛膜

◊ **chorionic** *adjective* referring to the chorion 绒毛膜的；(**human**) **chorionic gonadotrophin** (**hCG**) = hormone produced by the placenta, which suppresses the mother's normal menstrual cycle during pregnancy; it is found in the urine during pregnancy; it can be given by injection to encourage ovulation and help a woman to become pregnant 人绒毛膜促性腺激素

◊ **chorionic villi** *noun* tiny finger-like folds in the chorion 绒毛

choroid *noun* middle layer of tissue which forms the eyeball, between the sclera and the retina 脉络膜；**choroid plexus** = part of the pia mater, a network of small blood vessels in the ventricles of the brain which produce cerebrospinal fluid 脉络丛 ⇨见图 EYE

◊ **choroiditis** *noun* inflammation of the choroid in the eyeball 脉络膜炎

Christmas disease *noun* haemophilia B, clotting disorder of the blood, similar to haemophilia A, but in which the blood coagulates badly due to deficiency of Factor IX 克里斯马斯病，B型血友病

◊ **Christmas factor** *noun* Factor IX, one of the coagulating factors in the blood 凝血因子 IX

> COMMENT: Haemophilia A is caused by deficiency of Factor VIII. 注释：A型血友病因缺乏凝血因子 VIII 引起。

chrom- *prefix* referring to colour 颜色的

chromatid *noun* one of two parallel filaments making up a chromosome 染色

单体

◇ **chromatin** *noun* network which forms the nucleus of a cell and can be stained with basic dyes 染色质; **sex chromatin** = Barr body, chromatin found only in female cells, which can be used to identify the sex of a baby before birth 性染色质

chromatography *noun* method of separating chemicals through a porous medium and analysing compounds 色谱法; **gas chromatography** = chromatography where chemicals are passed through a gas before being analysed 气相色谱法

chromatophore *noun* any pigment-bearing cell in the eyes, hair and skin 色素细胞

chromicized catgut *noun* catgut which is hardened with chromium to make it slower to dissolve in the body 加铬肠线

chromium *noun* metallic trace element 铬 (NOTE: chemical symbol is **Cr**)

chromosome *noun* rod-shaped structure in the nucleus of a cell, formed of DNA which carries the genes 染色体; **chromosome aberration** = abnormality in the number, arrangement, etc. of chromosomes 染色体异常

◇ **chromosomal** *adjective* referring to chromosomes 染色体的; **chromosomal aberration** = CHROMOSOME ABERRATION 染色体异常; **chromosomal deletion** = abnormality in which a part of the chromosome is lost or removed 染色体缺失

> COMMENT: Each human cell has 46 chromosomes, 23 inherited from each parent. The female has one pair of X chromosomes, and the male one pair of XY chromosomes, which are responsible for the sexual difference. Sperm from a male have either an X or aY chromosome; if a Y chromosome sperm fertilizes the female's ovum the child will be male.
> 注释：每一个人体细胞有46条染色体，从父母那儿各继承23条染色体。女性是一对X染色体，男性是XY，由此区分性别。精子有X或Y染色体，如果含Y染色体的精子与卵子结合生男孩。

chronic *adjective* (disease or condition) which lasts for a long time 慢性的: ***He has a chronic chest complaint.*** 他患有慢性胸部不适。***She is a chronic asthma sufferer.*** 她是慢性哮喘病患者。**chronic fatigue syndrome** = MYALGIC ENCEPHALOMYELITIS 慢性疲劳综合症 (NOTE: the opposite is **acute**)

chyle *noun* fluid in the lymph vessels in the intestine which contains fat, especially after a meal 乳糜

◇ **chylomicron** *noun* particle of chyle present in the blood 乳糜微粒

◇ **chyluria** *noun* presence of chyle in the urine 乳糜尿

chyme *noun* semi-liquid mass of food and gastric juices which passes from the stomach to the intestine 食糜

chymotrypsin *noun* enzyme which digests protein 糜蛋白酶

Ci *abbreviation for* (缩写) curie 居里的简写

cicatrix *noun* scar, a mark on the skin, left when a wound *or* surgical incision has healed 瘢痕

-cide *suffix* referring to killing 杀

cilia 睫 *see* 见 CILIUM

◇ **ciliary** *adjective* (i) referring to cilia 睫状的(ii) referring to the eyelid *or* eyelashes 眼睑的; **ciliary body** = part of the eye which connects the iris to the choroid 睫状体; **ciliary muscle** = muscle which makes the lens of the eye change its shape to focus on objects at different distances 睫状肌 ◊ 见图 EYE; **ciliary processes** = series of ridges behind the iris to which the lens of the eye is attached 睫状突

◇ **ciliated epithelium** *noun* simple epithelium where the cells have tiny hairs *or* cilia 纤毛上皮

◇ **cilium** *noun* (**a**) eyelash 睫毛 (**b**) one of many tiny hair-like processes which line cells in passages in the body and by moving backwards and forwards drive particles or fluid along the passage 纤毛 (NOTE: plural is **cilia**)

cinematics *noun* science of movement, especially of body movements 运动学

◇ **cineplasty** *noun* amputation where the muscles of the stump of the amputated limb are used to operate an artificial limb 运动成形切断术

◇ **cineradiography** *noun* taking a series of X-ray photographs for diagnosis *or* to show how something moves *or* develops in the body X线电影照相术

◇ **cinesiology** *noun* study of muscle movements, particularly in relation to treatment 运动学

cingulectomy *noun* surgical operation to remove the cingulum 扣带回切除术

◇ **cingulum** *noun* long curved bundle of nerve fibres in the cerebrum 扣带 (NOTE: plural is **cingula**)

circadian rhythm *noun* rhythm of daily activities and bodily processes (eating *or* defecating *or* sleeping, etc.) frequently controlled by hormones, which repeats every twenty-four hours 昼夜节律

circle of Willis *noun* circle of branching arteries at the base of the brain formed by the basilar, anterior and posterior cerebral, anterior and posterior communicating, and internal carotid arteries 韦利斯氏环,大脑动脉环

circular *adjective* in the form of a circle 环状的; **circular fold** = large transverse fold of mucous membrane in the small intestine 环状褶

circulate *verb* (of fluid) to move around 循环: ***Blood circulates around the body.*** 血液循环全身。***Bile circulates from the liver to the intestine through the bile ducts.*** 胆汁从肝经胆管进小肠。

◇ **circulation (of the blood)** *noun* movement of blood around the body from the heart through the arteries to the capillaries and back to the heart through the veins 血液循环: ***She has poor circulation in her legs.*** 她腿部血循环不好。***Rub your hands to get the circulation going.*** 摩擦你的手使血液流动。**collateral circulation** = enlargement of certain secondary blood vessels, as a response when the main vessels become slowly blocked 侧支循环; **pulmonary circulation** *or* **lesser circulation** = circulation of blood from the heart through the pulmonary arteries to the lungs for oxygenation and back to the heart through the pulmonary veins 肺循环,小循环; **systemic circulation** *or* **greater circulation** = circulation of blood around the whole body (except the lungs) starting with the aorta and returning through the venae cavae 体循环,大循环

◇ **circulatory** *adjective* referring to the circulation of the blood 血液循环的; **circulatory system** = system of arteries and veins, together with the heart, which makes the blood circulate around the body(血液)循环系统

COMMENT: Blood circulates around the body, carrying oxygen from the lungs and nutrients from the liver through the arteries and capillaries to the tissues; the capillaries exchange the oxygen for waste matter such as carbon dioxide which is taken back to the lungs to be expelled. At the same time the blood obtains more oxygen in the lungs to be taken to the tissues. The circulation pattern is as follows: blood returns through the veins to the right atrium of the heart; from there it is pumped through the right ventricle into the pulmonary artery, and then into the lungs. From the lungs it returns through the pulmonary veins to the

left atrium of the heart and is pumped from there through the left ventricle into the aorta and from the aorta into the other arteries.
注释：血液在全身循环，将肺脏的氧、肝的养分通过动脉和毛细血管输送到组织。在毛细血管，氧气同废料如二氧化碳进行交换，后者被带回肺脏排出体外。同时血液从肺脏摄取更多的氧送到组织。循环模式如下：血液从静脉回到右心房，再经右心室泵入肺动脉，然后入肺。从肺静脉回到左心房，经左心室，主动脉到其它动脉。

circumcise *verb* to remove the foreskin of the penis 包皮环切
◇ **circumcision** *noun* surgical removal of the foreskin of the penis 包皮环切术

circumduction *noun* moving a part in a circular motion 环行运动

circumflex *adjective* bent or curved 卷曲的；**circumflex arteries** = branches of the femoral artery in the upper thigh 旋动脉；**circumflex nerve** = sensory and motor nerve in the upper arm 旋（前或后）神经，伴旋动脉而行的神经

circumvallate papillae *noun* large papillae at the base of the tongue, which have taste buds 轮状乳头

cirrhosis of the liver *noun* hepatocirrhosis, condition where some cells of the liver die and are replaced by hard fibrous tissue 肝硬化
◇ **cirrhotic** *adjective* referring to cirrhosis 硬化的：***The patient had a cirrhotic liver.*** 患者患有肝硬化。

COMMENT: Cirrhosis can have many causes: the commonest cause is alcoholism (alcoholic cirrhosis or Laennec's cirrhosis); it can also be caused by heart disease (cardiac cirrhosis), by viral hepatitis (postnecrotic cirrhosis), by autoimmune disease(primary biliary cirrhosis), or by obstruction or infection of the bile ducts (biliary cirrhosis).
注释：硬化可由多种原因引起，最常见的是酒精中毒（酒精性硬化或 Laennec 硬化）。它还可因心脏疾病（心源性硬化）、病毒性肝炎（坏死后硬化）、自身免疫性疾病（原发性胆汁性肝硬化）或胆管阻塞、感染（胆汁性硬化）引起。

cirsoid *adjective* dilated (as of a varicose vein) 曲张的；**cirsoid aneurysm** = condition where arteries become swollen and twisted 曲张状动脉瘤

cistern *or* **cisterna** *noun* space containing fluid 池；**cisterna magna** = large space containing cerebrospinal fluid, situated underneath the cerebellum and behind the medulla oblongata 小脑延髓池；**lumbar cistern** = subarachnoid space in the spinal cord, where the dura mater ends, filled with cerebrospinal fluid 腰池

citric acid *noun* acid found in fruit such as oranges, lemons and grapefruit 柠檬酸
◇ **citric acid cycle** *noun* Krebs cycle, an important series of events concerning amino acid metabolism, taking place in the mitochondria 三羧酸循环，枸橼酸循环

citrulline *noun* an amino acid 瓜氨酸
◇ **citrullinaemia** *noun* deficiency of an enzyme which helps break down proteins 瓜氨酸血症，因缺乏代谢瓜氨酸的酶而致

CJD = CREUTZFELDT-JACOB DISEASE 克罗茨费尔特—雅各布综合征

Cl *chemical symbol for* chlorine 氯的化学元素符号

cl = CENTILITRE 立升

clamp 1 *noun* surgical instrument to hold something tightly (such as a blood vessel during an operation) 夹子 **2** *verb* to hold something tightly 夹紧

clap *noun* = GONORRHOEA（俚语）淋病

classic *adjective* typically well-known (symptom) 典型的：***She showed classic heroin withdrawal symptoms: sweating, fever, sleeplessness and anxiety.*** 她出现了典型的海洛因戒断症状：出汗、发热、失眠和焦虑。

classify *verb* **(a)** to put references or components into order so as to be able to refer to them again and identify them easily 分类: ***The medical records are classified under the surname of the patient.*** 病历根据患者的姓氏分类。***Blood groups are classified according to the ABO system.*** 血型根据ABO系统分类。(**b**) to make information secret 保密: ***Doctors' reports on patients are classified and may not be shown to the patients themselves.*** 患者的病情记录是保密的,不能被患者看到。

◇ **classification** *noun* putting references or components into order so as to be able to refer to them again and identify them easily 分类; ***the ABO classification of blood*** ABO血型分类

claudication *noun* limping or being lame 跛; **intermittent claudication** = condition caused by impairment of the arteries 间歇性跛行

> COMMENT: At first, the patient limps after having walked a short distance, then finds walking progressively more difficult and finally impossible. The condition improves after rest.
> 注释:初期,患者在短距离行走后出现跛行,行走困难逐渐加剧,最终不能行走。症状在休息后缓解。

claustrophobia *noun* being afraid of enclosed spaces or crowded rooms 幽闭恐惧

◇ **claustrophobic** *adjective* (room) which causes claustrophobia; (person) suffering from claustrophobia 引起幽闭恐惧的,患幽闭恐惧的 (NOTE: opposite is **agoraphobia**)

clavicle *noun* collarbone, one of two long thin bones which join the shoulder blades to the breastbone 锁骨 ◊ 见图 SHOULDER

◇ **clavicular** *adjective* referring to the clavicle 锁骨的

clavus *noun* (**a**) corn (on the foot) 鸡眼 (**b**) severe pain in the head, like a nail being driven in 头部刺痛

claw foot *noun* pes cavus, deformed foot with the toes curved towards the instep and with a very high arch 爪形足

◇ **claw hand** *noun* deformed hand with the fingers (especially the ring finger and little finger) bent towards the palm, caused by paralysis of the muscles 爪形手

clean 1 *adjective* not dirty 干净的: ***The beds have clean sheets every morning.*** 每天早晨床上都铺干净的床单。***These plates aren't clean.*** 这些盘子不干净。***The report suggested the hospital kitchens were not as clean as they should have been.*** 报告认为医院的厨房不够干净。(NOTE: **clean - cleaner - cleanest**) 2 *verb* to make clean by taking away dirt 使干净: ***The nurses have to make sure the wards are clean before the inspection.*** 护士在查房前必须使病房保持清洁。***Have you cleaned your teeth today?***; 你今天刷牙了吗? ***She was cleaning the patients' bathroom.*** 她在清洗患者的浴室。

◇ **cleanliness** *noun* state of being clean 清洁: ***The report criticized the cleanliness of the hospital kitchen.*** 报告对医院厨房的卫生情况提出了批评。

◇ **cleanse** *verb* to make very clean 使干净

◇ **cleanser** *noun* powder *or* liquid which cleanses 清洁剂

clear 1 *adjective* (**a**) easily understood 清晰的: ***The doctor made it clear that he wanted the patient to have a home help.*** 医生明确地表示他希望患者得到家庭的帮助。***The words on the medicine bottle are not very clear.*** 药瓶上的说明不太清楚。(**b**) which is not cloudy and which you can easily see through 清澈的: ***a clear glass bottle*** 明净的玻璃杯; ***The urine sample was clear, not cloudy.*** 尿样很清澈,不浑浊。(**c**) **clear of** = free from 无,没有: ***The area is now clear of infection.*** 这部位没有感染。(NOTE: **clear - clearer - clearest**) 2 *verb* to take away a blockage 清除: ***The inhalant will clear your blocked nose.*** 吸入剂可以解除你的鼻塞症状。***He is on antibiotics to try to clear the congestion in his lungs.*** 他服用

抗生素以解除肺充血。

◇ **clearance** *noun* 清除; **renal clearance** = measurement of the rate at which kidneys filter impurities from blood 肾清除率

◇ **clearly** *adverb* plainly *or* obviously 清楚地: ***The swelling is clearly visible on the patient's neck.*** 患者颈上的肿块清晰可见。

◇ **clear up** *verb* to get better 痊愈: ***His infection should clear up within a few days.*** 他的感染在几天内会痊愈。***I hope your cold clears up before the holiday.*** 我希望你的感冒在假期前痊愈。

cleavage *noun* repeated division of cells in an embryo 分裂,卵裂

cleft palate *noun* congenital defect, where there is a fissure in the hard palate allowing the mouth and nasal cavities to be linked 腭裂

> COMMENT: A cleft palate is usually associated with a harelip. Both are due to incomplete fusion of the maxillary processes. Both can be successfully corrected by surgery.
> 注释:腭裂常同时伴有兔唇。两者均由上颌突融合不全引起,可经手术矫正。

clerking *noun* (*informal* 非正式) writing down the details of a patient on admission to a hospital 入院病情记录

client *noun* person visited by a health visitor *or* social worker 病人,当事人

climacteric *noun* (**a**) = MENOPAUSE 绝经期、更年期 (**b**) period of diminished sexual activity in a man who reaches middle age (男性)性欲减退期

clinic *noun* (**a**) small hospital or department in a large hospital which deals only with walking patients or which specializes in the treatment of certain conditions 诊所,门诊部: ***He is being treated in a private clinic.*** 他在私人诊所治疗。***She was referred to an antenatal clinic.*** 她去产前门诊咨询。**antenatal clinic** *or* **maternity clinic** = clinic where expectant mothers are taught how to look after babies, do exercises and have medical checkups 产前门诊; **physiotherapy clinic** = clinic where patients can have physiotherapy 理疗门诊 (**b**) group of students under a doctor or surgeon who examine patients and discuss their treatment 病例示教

◇ **clinical** *adjective* (**a**) (i) referring to a clinic 门诊的 (ii) referring to a physical examination of patients by doctors (as opposed to a surgical operation *or* a laboratory test *or* experiment) 体检的; **clinical medicine** = treatment of patients in a hospital ward *or* in the doctor's surgery (as opposed to the operating theatre *or* laboratory) 临床医学; **clinical nurse specialist** = nurse who specializes in a particular branch of clinical care 专科临床护士; **clinical thermometer** = thermometer for taking a patient's body temperature 体温计 (**b**) referring to instruction given to students at the bedside of patients as opposed to class instruction with no patient present 病例示教; **clinical trial** = trial carried out in a medical laboratory on a patient or on tissue from a patient 临床试验

◇ **clinically** *adverb* using information gathered from the treatment of patients in a hospital ward *or* in the doctor's surgery 临床上地: ***Smallpox is now clinically extinct.*** 天花已临床绝迹。

◇ **clinician** *noun* doctor, usually not a surgeon, who has considerable experience in treating patients 临床医师

> QUOTE: We studied 69 patients who met the clinical and laboratory criteria of definite MS.
> 引文:我们研究了69例符合多发性硬化病临床和试验室诊断标准的病例。
> **Lancet** 柳叶刀

> QUOTE: The allocation of students to clinical areas is for their educational needs and not for service requirements.
> 引文:将学生分到临床是出于教育需要而不

是出于服务需要。

Nursing Times 护理时代

clip 1 *noun* piece of metal with a spring, used to attach things together 小夹; **Michel's clips** = clips used to suture a wound 密歇尔氏夹 2 *verb* to attach together 夹住: ***The case notes are clipped together with the patient's record card.*** 病历记录同患者的病历卡夹在一起。

clitoris *noun* small erectile female sex organ, a structure in females, situated at the anterior angle of the vulva, which can be excited by sexual activity 阴蒂 ◊ 见图 UROGENITAL SYSTEM (FEMALE)

cloaca *noun* end part of the hindgut in an embryo 泄殖腔

clone 1 *noun* group of cells derived from a single cell by a sexual reproduction and so identical to the first cell 纯系 2 *verb* to reproduce an individual organism by a sexual means 克隆

◊ **cloning** *noun* reproduction of an individual organism by asexual means 克隆化

clonic *adjective* (i) referring to clonus 阵挛的 (ii) having spasmodic contractions 挛缩的

◊ **clonus** *noun* rhythmic contraction and relaxation of a muscle (usually a sign of upper motor neurone lesions) 痉挛,阵挛

clonorchiasis *noun* liver condition, common in the Far East, caused by the fluke *Clonorchis sinensis* 支睾吸虫病

close *verb* (*of wound*) to be covered with new tissue 覆盖

Clostridium *noun* type of bacteria 梭状芽胞杆菌属

> COMMENT: Species of Clostridium cause botulism, tetanus and gas gangrene.
> 注释:梭状芽胞杆菌属的细菌引起肉毒中毒、破伤风及气性坏疽。

clot 1 *noun* soft mass of coagulated blood in a vein or an artery 血栓,栓子: ***The doctor diagnosed a blood clot in the brain.*** 医生诊断脑栓塞。***Blood clots occur in embolism and thrombosis.*** 在栓塞及血栓形成时有栓子存在。2 *verb* to coagulate, to change from liquid to semi-solid 凝血: ***His blood does not clot easily.*** 他的血不易凝固。(NOTE: **clotting-clotted**)

◊ **clotting** *noun* action of coagulating 凝血; **clotting factors** = coagulation factors *or* substances (called Factor I, Factor II, and so on) in plasma which act one after the other to make the blood coagulate when a blood vessel is damaged 凝血因子; **clotting time** = coagulation time, the time taken for blood to coagulate under normal conditions 凝血时间

> COMMENT: Deficiency in one or more of the clotting factors results in haemophilia.
> 注释:一种或多种凝血因子缺乏可导致血友病。

clothes *noun* things worn to cover the body and keep a person warm 衣服: ***All his clothes had to be destroyed.*** 他所有的衣服都得被销毁。***You ought to put some clean clothes on.*** 你应该穿些干净的衣服。**bedclothes** = sheets and blankets which cover a bed 被褥

cloud *noun* (**a**) (i) light white *or* grey mass of water vapour *or* ice particles in the sky which can produce rain 云 (ii) mass of particles suspended in the air 云状物: ***I think it is going to rain — look at those grey clouds.*** 我觉得要下雨了——看这些乌云。***Clouds of smoke were pouring out of the house.*** 烟雾从房子里冒了出来。(**b**) disturbed sediment in a liquid 混浊液

◊ **cloudy** *adjective* (i) (sky) which is covered with clouds 阴天的 (ii) (liquid) which is not transparent but which has an opaque substance in it 浑浊的: ***The patient is passing cloudy urine.*** 患者尿液浑浊。

clubbing *noun* thickening of the ends of the fingers and toes, a sign of many different diseases 杵状指

club foot *noun* talipes, a congenitally deformed foot 畸形足

COMMENT: The most usual form (talipes equinovarus) is where the person walks on the toes, because the foot is permanently bent forward; in other forms, the foot either turns towards the inside (talipes varus), towards the outside (talipes valgus) or upwards (talipes calcaneus) at the ankle so that the patient cannot walk on the sole of the foot.
注释:最常见的形式是因足持续前屈走路时脚尖着地。其他形式为足向外、向内、或向上使患者不能用脚底走路。

cluster *noun* group of small items which cling together 簇,丛; **cluster headache** = headache which occurs behind one eye for a short period 偏头痛

Clutton's joint *noun* swollen knee joint occurring in congenital syphilis 克莱顿关节

cm = CENTIMETRE 厘米

CMV = CYTOMEGALOVIRUS 巨细胞病毒

C/N = CHARGE NURSE 主管护士

CNS = CENTRAL NERVOUS SYSTEM 中枢神经系统

Co *chemical symbol for* cobalt 钴的化学元素符号

coagulate *verb* to clot, to change from liquid to semi-solid 凝固: ***His blood does not coagulate easily.*** 他的血不易凝固。

◇ **coagulant** *noun* substance which can make blood clot 促凝剂

◇ **coagulase** *noun* enzyme produced by Staphylococci which makes blood plasma clot 凝血酶

◇ **coagulation** *noun* action of clotting 凝血; **coagulation factors** = CLOTTING FACTORS 凝血因子; **coagulation time** = CLOTTING TIME 凝血时间

◇ **coagulum** *noun* blood clot *or* mass of clotted blood 血凝块

COMMENT: Blood coagulates with the conversion into fibrin of fibrinogen, a protein in the blood, under the influence of the enzyme thromboplastin.
注释:血凝是指血液中的纤维蛋白原在凝血激酶的作用下变为纤维蛋白。

coarctation *noun* narrowing 缩窄; **coarctation of the aorta** = congenital narrowing of the aorta which results in high blood pressure in the upper part of the body and low blood pressure in the lower part 主动脉狭窄

coarse *adjective* rough *or* not fine 粗糙的: ***Coarse hair grows on parts of the body at puberty.*** 青春期身体的某些部位会长出粗的体毛。***disease characterized by coarse features*** 以面容粗陋为特征的疾病

coat 1 *noun* layer of material covering an organ *or* a cavity 层,膜; **muscle coats** = two layers of muscle forming part of the lining of the intestine 肌层 **2** *verb* to cover 覆盖

◇ **coating** *noun* covering 包衣; ***pill with a sugar coating*** 糖衣片

cobalt *noun* metallic element 钴; **cobalt 60** = radioactive isotope which is used in radiotherapy to treat cancer 钴60 (NOTE: symbol is **Co**)

cocaine *noun* alkaloid from the coca plant, sometimes used as a local anaesthetic but not generally used because its use leads to addiction 可卡因

coccidioidomycosis *noun* lung disease, caused by inhaling spores of the fungus *Coccidioides immitis* 球孢子菌病

coccus *noun* bacterium shaped like a ball 球菌属 (NOTE: plural is **cocci**)

COMMENT: Cocci grow together in groups: either in groups (staphylococci) or in long chains (streptococci).
注释:球菌成群生长,可为团状(如葡萄球菌)或长链状(如链球菌)。

coccy- *prefix* referring to the coccyx 尾骨的

◇ **coccydynia** *or* **coccygodynia** *noun* sharp pain in the coccyx, usually caused by a blow 尾骨痛

◇ **coccygeal vertebrae** *noun* fused

bones in the coccyx 尾椎

◇ **coccyx** *noun* lowest bones in the backbone 尾骨 (NOTE: plural is **coccyges**) ◇ 见图 VERTEBRAL COLUMN

COMMENT: The coccyx is a rudimentary tail made of four bones which have fused together into a bone in the shape of a triangle.
注释:尾骨是由四块骨融合成三角形的退化了的尾部。

cochlea *noun* spiral tube, shaped like a snail shell, inside the inner ear, which is the essential organ of hearing 耳蜗 ◇ 见图 EAR

◇ **cochlear** *adjective* referring to the cochlea 耳蜗的; **cochlear duct** = spiral channel in the cochlea 耳蜗管; **cochlear nerve** = division of the auditory nerve 耳蜗神经

COMMENT: Sounds are transmitted as vibrations to the cochlea from the ossicles through the oval window. The lymph fluid in the cochlea passes the vibrations to the organ of Corti which in turn is connected to the auditory nerve.
注释:声音以振动的形式从听骨经卵圆窗传到耳蜗。耳蜗内的淋巴液再将振动传到与听神经相连的科蒂器。

code 1 *noun* signs which have a hidden meaning 密码; **genetic code** = characteristics which exist in the DNA of a cell and are passed on when the cell divides and so are inherited by a child from a parent 遗传密码 **2** *verb* to give a meaning 编码: ***Genes are sequences of DNA that code for specific proteins*.** 基因是编码特定蛋白的 DNA 序列。**coding gene** = gene which carries a particular genetic code 编码基因

codeine *noun* alkaloid made from opium, used as a painkiller and to reduce coughing 可待因(碱),以鸦片为原料制成的止痛药、镇静剂用于止痛和止咳

cod liver oil *noun* oil from the liver of codfish, which is rich in calories and vitamins A and D 鱼肝油(由鳕鱼肝脏提炼而成的药用脂肪油)

codon *noun* group of three of the four basic elements in DNA (adenine, cytosine, guanine and thymine) which governs the formation of enzymes 密码子

-coele *suffix* referring to a hollow 空的

coeli- *prefix* referring to a hollow, usually the abdomen 空的,多指腹的 (NOTE: words beginning **coeli-** are spelled **celi-** in US English)

◇ **coeliac** *adjective* referring to the abdomen 腹的; **coeliac artery** *or* **coeliac axis** *or* **coeliac trunk** = main artery in the abdomen leading from the abdominal aorta and dividing into the left gastric, hepatic and splenic arteries 腹主动脉; **coeliac disease** = gluten enteropathy *or* malabsorption syndrome, an allergic disease (mainly affecting children) in which the lining of the intestine is sensitive to gluten, preventing the small intestine from digesting fat 乳糜泻; **adult coeliac disease** = condition in adults where the villi in the intestine become smaller and so reduce the surface which can absorb nutrients 成人乳糜泻; **coeliac plexus** = network of nerves in the abdomen, behind the stomach 腹腔神经丛

COMMENT: Symptoms of coeliac disease include a swollen abdomen, pale diarrhoea, abdominal pains and anaemia.
注释:乳糜泻症状包括腹胀、腹泻、腹痛和贫血。

◇ **coelioscopy** *noun* examining the peritoneal cavity by inflating the abdomen with sterile air and passing an endoscope through the abdominal wall 腹腔镜检查

coelom *noun* body cavity in an embryo, which divides to form the thorax and abdomen 体腔

coffee ground vomit *noun* vomit containing dark pieces of blood, indicating that the patient is bleeding from the stomach or upper intestine 呕吐咖啡样物

cognitive *adjective* referring to the

mental processes of perception, memory, judgement and reasoning 认识的，认知的；***a cognitive disorder*** *or* **impairment** 认知障碍

coil *noun* spiral metal wire fitted into a woman's uterus as a contraceptive 子宫节育环

◇ **coiled** *adjective* spiral *or* twisted round and round 卷曲的；***a coiled tube at the end of a nephron*** 肾曲小管

coitus *noun* sexual intercourse 性交；**coitus interruptus** = form of contraception where the penis is removed from the vagina before ejaculation 体外射精避孕法，终止性交避孕法

> COMMENT: This is not a safe method of contraception.
> 注释：这不是安全的避孕方法。

◇ **coital** *adjective* referring to coitus 性交的

◇ **coition** *noun* sexual intercourse 性交

cold 1 *adjective* not warm *or* not hot 凉的：***He always has a cold shower in the morning.*** 他早晨总是要冲个冷水澡。***The weather is colder than last week and they say it will be even colder tomorrow.*** 天气比上周冷，他们说明天会更冷。***Many old people suffer from hypothermia in cold weather.*** 很多老人在冬天体温会降低。***Cold drinks give him colic pains.*** 冷饮使他肠绞痛。**cold burn** = injury to the skin caused by exposure to extreme cold *or* by touching a very cold surface 冷灼伤；**cold compress** = wad of cloth soaked in cold water, used to relieve a headache or bruise 冷敷料；**cold sore** = herpes simplex, a burning sore, usually on the lips 单纯疱疹 **2** *noun* **common cold** *or* **cold in the head** = coryza, an illness, with inflammation of the nasal passages, in which the patient sneezes and coughs and has a blocked and running nose 感冒，头伤风：***He caught a cold by standing in the rain.*** 他被雨淋后感冒了。***She's got a cold so she can't go out.*** 她感冒了不能出去。***Mother's in bed with a cold.*** 母亲感冒了躺在床上。***Don't come near me — I've got a cold and you may catch it.*** 不要靠近我——我感冒了，会传染你的。

> COMMENT: A cold usually starts with a virus infection which causes inflammation of the mucous membrane in the nose and throat. Symptoms include running nose, cough and loss of taste and smell; there is no cure for a cold at present, though the coronavirus which causes a cold has been identified.
> 注释：感冒早期多因病毒感染引起鼻、咽部粘膜炎，症状包括流涕、咳嗽、味觉及嗅觉的丧失。尽管引起感冒的冠状病毒已经被发现，但目前仍无治疗的方法。

colectomy *noun* surgical removal of the whole *or* part of the colon 结肠切除术

coli 结肠 *see* 见 TAENIA

colic *or* **enteralgia** *noun* (**a**) pain in any part of the intestinal tract 绞痛；**biliary colic** = pain in the abdomen caused by gallstones in the bile duct *or* by inflammation of the gall bladder 胆绞痛；**mucous colic** = inflammation of the colon, with painful spasms in the muscles of the walls of the colon 粘液性绞痛；**renal colic** = sudden pain caused by kidney stone or stones in the ureter 肾绞痛 (**b**) **right colic** *or* **middle colic** = arteries which lead from the superior mesenteric artery 右或中结肠动脉

◇ **colicky** *adjective* referring to colic 绞痛的：***He had colicky pains in his abdomen.*** 他感到腹部绞痛。

> COMMENT: Although colic can refer to pain caused by indigestion, it can also be caused by stones in the gall bladder or kidney.
> 注释：尽管绞痛可因消化不良引起，也可因胆囊或肾结石导致。

coliform bacteria *plural noun* bacteria which are similar to *Bacterium coli* 类大肠杆菌属

colitis *noun* inflammation of the colon 结肠炎；**mucous colitis** = irritable bowel syndrome, inflammation of the mucous membrane in the intestine, where the patient suffers pain caused by spasms in the muscles of the walls of the colon 粘液性结肠炎; **ulcerative colitis** = severe pain in the colon, with diarrhoea and ulcers in the rectum, often with a psychosomatic cause 溃疡性结肠炎

collagen *noun* bundles of protein fibres, which form the connective tissue, bone and cartilage 胶原; **collagen disease** = any of several diseases of the connective tissue 胶原病; **collagen fibre** = fibre which is the main component of fasciae, tendons and ligaments, and is essential in bone and cartilage 胶原纤维

◇ **collagenous** *adjective* (i) containing collagen 有胶原的 (ii) referring to collagen disease 胶原病的

> COMMENT: Collagen diseases include rheumatic fever, rheumatoid arthritis, periarteritis nodosa, scleroderma and dermatomyositis. Collagen diseases can be treated with cortisone.
> 注释:胶原病包括风湿热、类风湿性关节炎、结节性动脉外膜炎、硬皮病和皮肌炎。胶原病可用可的松治疗。

collapse 1 *noun* condition where a patient is extremely exhausted or semi-conscious 虚脱,耗竭或意识不清: ***He was found in a state of collapse.*** 他处于一种虚脱状态。**2** *verb* (**a**) to fall down in a semi-conscious state 进入半清醒状态,虚脱: ***After running to catch his train he collapsed.*** 他因为跑着赶火车,人都虚脱了。(**b**) to become flat *or* to lose air 塌陷,无空气; **collapsed lung** 肺萎陷 *see* 见 PNEUMOTHORAX

collar *noun* part of a coat, shirt, etc. which goes round the neck 颈圈,领圈: ***My shirt collar's too tight.*** 我衬衣的领子太紧了。***She turned up her coat collar because of the wind.*** 起风了,她竖起了衣领。**cervical collar** *or* **neck collar** *or* **orthopaedic collar** *or* **surgical collar** = special strong collar to support the head of a patient with neck injuries or a condition such as cervical spondylosis 颈圈(用于支持颈部受伤或颈椎关节强直患者的头部)

◇**collarbone** *noun* clavicle, one of two long thin bones which join the shoulderblades to the breastbone 锁骨; **collarbone fracture** = fracture of the collarbone (one of the most frequent fractures in the body) 锁骨骨折

collateral *adjective* secondary or less important 次要的; **collateral circulation** = enlargement of certain secondary blood vessels, as a response when the main vessels become slowly blocked 侧支循环

> QUOTE: Embolization of the coeliac axis is an effective treatment for severe bleeding in the stomach or duodenum, localized by endoscopic examination. A good collateral blood supply makes occlusion of a single branch of the coeliac axis safe.
> 引文:对严重的胃、十二指肠出血,经内镜定位后,进行腹腔动脉栓塞是有效的治疗手段。良好的侧支循环可保证单支腹腔动脉栓塞的安全性。
> **British Medical Journal** 英国医学杂志

collect *verb* to bring various things together; to come together 收集,聚集: ***Fluid collects in the tissues of patients suffering from dropsy.*** 水肿患者的体液聚积在组织内。

◇ **collecting duct** *noun* part of the system by which urine is filtered in the kidney 集合管

◇ **collection** *noun* bringing together of various things 收集: ***The hospital has a collection of historical surgical instruments.*** 这医院收集了一些以前的手术器械。

college *noun* place of further education where people study after they have left secondary school 学院,大学: ***I'm going to college to study pharmacy.*** 我将上大学学习药学。

Colles' fracture 科勒斯氏骨折,桡骨远端骨折 *see* 见 FRACTURE

colliculus *noun* one of four small

projections (the superior and inferior colliculi) in the midbrain 丘脑 ◊ 见图 BRAIN (NOTE: the plural is **colliculi**)

collodion *noun* liquid used to paint on a clean wound, where it dries to form a flexible covering 火棉胶

collyrium *noun* solution used to bathe the eyes 洗眼剂

coloboma *noun* condition where part of the eye, especially part of the iris, is missing 缺损,尤指虹膜

colon *noun* the main part of the large intestine (running from the caecum at the end of the small intestine to the rectum) 结肠; **ascending colon** = first part of the colon which goes up the right side of the body from the caecum 升结肠; **descending colon** = third section of the colon which goes down the left side of the body 降结肠; **sigmoid colon** = fourth section of the colon which continues as the rectum 乙状结肠; **transverse colon** = second section of the colon which crosses the body below the stomach 横结肠; **irritable** *or* **spastic colon** = MUCOUS COLITIS 结肠痉挛,粘液性结肠炎 ◊ 见图 DIGESTIVE SYSTEM

◊ **colonic** *adjective* referring to the colon 结肠的; **colonic irrigation** = washing out of the large intestine 结肠灌洗

◊ **colonoscope** *noun* surgical instrument for examining the interior of the colon 结肠镜

◊ **colonoscopy** *noun* examination of the inside of the colon, using a colonoscope passed through the rectum 结肠镜检查

> COMMENT: The colon is about 1.35 metres in length, and rises from the end of the small intestine up the right side of the body, then crosses beneath the stomach and drops down the left side of the body to end as the rectum. In the colon, water is extracted from the waste material which has passed through the small intestine, leaving only the faeces which are pushed forward by peristaltic movements and passed out of the body through the rectum.
> 注释:结肠长约1.35米,起自小肠末端,沿右侧上升,横过胃下部,从左侧下降,终于直肠。结肠主要吸收小肠排泄物中的水分,将粪质经蠕动通过直肠排出体外。

colony *noun* group *or* culture of microorganisms 集落

colostomy *noun* surgical operation to make an opening (stoma) between the colon and the abdominal wall to allow faeces to be passed out without going through the rectum 结肠造口术

◊ **colostomy bag** *noun* bag attached to the opening made by a colostomy, to collect faeces as they are passed out of the body 结肠袋

> COMMENT: A colostomy is carried out when the colon or rectum is blocked, or where part of the colon or rectum has had to be removed.
> 注释:当结肠、直肠阻塞,或必须切除部分结肠、直肠时实施结肠造口术。

colostrum *noun* fluid secreted by the breasts at the birth of a baby, but before the true milk starts to flow 初乳

colour *or US* **color 1** *noun* differing wavelengths of light (red, blue, yellow, etc.) which are reflected from objects and sensed by the eyes 颜色,色彩: ***What is the colour of a healthy liver?*** 正常肝脏是什么颜色? ***The diseased parts are shown by the colour red on the chart.*** 病变部位在图上显示为红色。 ***He looks unwell, and his face has no colour.*** 他好像生病了,气色很不好。 **2** *verb* to give colour to 着色: ***The arteries are coloured red on the diagram.*** 图谱上动脉被染为红色。 ***Bile colours the urine yellow.*** 尿液被胆汁染为黄色。

◊ **colour-blind** *adjective* not able to tell the difference between certain colours 色盲的: ***Several of the students are colour-blind.*** 有几个学生是色盲。

◊ **colour blindness** *noun* being unable to tell the difference between certain colours 色盲

> COMMENT: Colour blindness is a condition which almost never occurs in women. The commonest form is the inability to tell the difference between red and green. The Ishihara test is used to test for colour blindness.
> 注释:妇女几乎不患有色盲。色盲的最常见类型是不能区分红色和绿色。通常使用石原氏试验来检查色盲。

colouring (matter) *noun* substance which colours an organ 染料

◇ **colourless** *adjective* with no colour 无色的: ***A colourless fluid was discharged from the sore.*** 伤口分泌一种无色液体。

colp- *prefix* referring to the vagina 阴道的

◇ **colpocystopexy** *noun* surgical operation to lift and stitch the vagina and bladder to the abdominal wall 阴道膀胱固定术

◇ **colpopexy** *noun* surgical operation to fix a prolapsed vagina to the abdominal wall 阴道固定术

◇ **colpoplasty** *noun* surgical operation to repair a damaged vagina 阴道成形术

◇ **colpoptosis** *noun* prolapse of the walls of the vagina 阴道脱垂

◇ **colporrhaphy** *noun* surgical operation to suture a prolapsed vagina 阴道缝合术

◇ **colposcope** *noun* surgical instrument used to examine the inside of the vagina 阴道镜

◇ **colposcopy** *noun* examination of the inside of the vagina 阴道镜检查

◇ **colpotomy** *noun* any surgical operation to make a cut in the vagina 阴道切开术

column *noun* usually circular mass standing upright like a tree 柱; **spinal column** *or* **vertebral column** = backbone, the series of bones and discs which forms a flexible column running from the pelvis to the skull 脊柱

◇ **columnar** *adjective* shaped like a column 柱状的; **columnar cell** = type of epithelial cell 柱状细胞

coma *noun* state of unconsciousness from which a person cannot be awakened by external stimuli 昏迷: ***He went into a coma and never regained consciousness.*** 他昏迷了,再也没有恢复意识。***She has been in a coma for four days.*** 她已经昏迷了4天。**diabetic coma** = unconsciousness caused by untreated diabetes 糖尿病性昏迷

◇ **comatose** *adjective* (i) unconscious *or* in a coma 昏迷的 (ii) like a coma 像昏迷的

> COMMENT: A coma can have many causes: head injuries, diabetes, stroke, drug overdose. A coma is often fatal, but a patient may continue to live in a coma for a long time, even several months, before dying or regaining consciousness.
> 注释:昏迷可因多种原因引起:头部受伤、糖尿病、中风、药物过量等。昏迷常是致命性的,但昏迷患者在死亡或苏醒前可持续很长时间,甚至几个月。

combat *verb* to fight against 作战,斗争: ***The medical team is combating an outbreak of diphtheria.*** 医疗队正在同白喉的爆发进行斗争。***What can we do to combat the spread of the disease?*** 我们能做些什么来阻止疾病的传播?

combine *verb* to join together 联合

◇ **combination** *noun* act of joining together 联合,结合: ***Actomyosin is a combination of actin and myosin.*** 肌纤凝蛋白是肌动蛋白和肌球蛋白的复合物。

comedo *noun* blackhead, a small point of dark, hard matter in a sebaceous follicle, often found associated with acne on the skin of adolescents 粉刺 (NOTE: plural is **comedones**)

comfort *verb* to make relaxed *or* to help make a patient less miserable 安慰,抚慰: ***The paramedics comforted the injured until the ambulance arrived.*** 在救护车来到前,一直由医辅人员安慰受伤者。

commensal *noun* & *adjective* (plant

or animal) which lives on another plant or animal, but does not harm it in any way and both may benefit from the association 共生体(的): ***Candida is a normal commensal in the mouths of 50% of healthy adults.*** 念珠菌是大约50%的健康人口腔中正常的共生菌。(NOTE: if it causes harm it is a **parasite**)

comminuted fracture *noun* fracture where the bone is broken in several places 粉碎性骨折

commissure *noun* structure which joins two tissues of similar material, such as a group of nerves which crosses from one part of the central nervous system to another 连合; **grey commissure** *or* **white commissure** = parts of grey and white matter in the spinal cord nearest the central canal 灰质或白质连合 *see also* 参见 CORPUS CALLOSUM

common *adjective* (**a**) ordinary or not exceptional; which happens very frequently 平常的,普通的: ***Accidents are quite common on this part of the motorway.*** 这段快速路经常发生车祸。***It's a common mistake to believe that cancer is always fatal.*** 认为癌症总是致命的观点是一常见错误。**common cold** = coryza, a virus infection which causes inflammation of the mucous membrane in the nose and throat 普通型感冒(**b**) (**in**) **common** = belonging to more than one thing *or* person 共有的: ***Haemophilia and Christmas disease have several symptoms in common.*** 血友病甲和血友病乙有一些共同的症状。**common bile duct** = duct leading to the duodenum, formed of the hepatic and cystic ducts 胆总管; **common carotid artery** = large artery in the lower part of the neck 颈总动脉; **common hepatic duct** = duct from the liver formed when the right and left hepatic ducts join 肝总管; **common iliac arteries** = arteries which branch from the aorta and divide into the internal and external iliac arteries 髂总动脉; **common iliac veins** = veins draining the legs, pelvis and abdomen, which unite to form the inferior vena cava 髂总静脉; **final common pathway** = linked neurones which take all impulses from the central nervous system to a muscle 最终共同通路

◇ **commonly** *adverb* which happens often 经常地: ***A cold winter commonly brings a flu epidemic.*** 寒冷的冬季经常会暴发流感。

communicable disease *noun* disease which can be passed from one person to another *or* from an animal to a person 传染性疾病 *see also* 参见 CONTAGIOUS, INFECTIOUS

communicate *verb* to pass a message to someone *or* something 交流: ***Autistic children do not communicate, even with their parents.*** 孤独症患儿不与人交流,即使是他们的父母。**communicating arteries** = arteries which connect the blood supply from each side of the brain, forming part of the circle of Willis 交通动脉

community *noun* group of people who live and work in a district 社区,社团: ***The health services serve the local community.*** 健康服务部门为当地社区服务。***Community care is an important part of primary health care.*** 社区服务是初级卫生保健的重要内容。**community medicine** = study of medical practice which examines groups of people and the health of the community, including housing, pollution and other environmental factors 社区医学; **community physician** = doctor who specializes in community medicine 社区医生; **Community Psychiatric Nurse** (**CPN**) = psychiatric nurse who works in a district, visiting various patients in the area 社区心理护士; **community services** = nursing services which are available to the community 社区护理服务

compact bone *noun* type of bone tissue which forms the hard outer layer of a bone 密质骨 ◊见图 BONE STRUC-

TURE

compatibility *noun* (i) ability of two drugs not to interfere with each other when administered together 可配伍性 (ii) ability of a body to accept organs *or* tissue *or* blood from another person and not to reject them 相容性

◇ **compatible** *adjective* able to work together without being rejected 相容的: ***The surgeons are trying to find a compatible donor or a donor with a compatible blood group.*** 术者在设法寻找组织相容性或血型相合的供者。

compensate *verb* (*of an organ*) to make good the failure of another organ 代偿: ***The heart has to beat more strongly to compensate for the narrowing of the arteries.*** 心脏必须增强收缩来代偿动脉狭窄。

complain *verb* to say that something is not good 主诉,抱怨: ***The patients have complained about the food.*** 患者抱怨食物不好。 ***He is complaining of pains in his legs.*** 他主诉腿疼。

◇ **complaint** *noun* (**a**) illness 疾病: ***He is suffering from a nervous complaint.*** 他患有神经系统疾病。(**b**) saying that something is wrong. 抱怨: ***The hospital administrator wouldn't listen to the complaints of the consultants.*** 医院管理者不会倾听顾问们的抱怨。

complement *noun* substance which forms part of blood plasma and is essential to the work of antibodies and antigens 补体; **complement fixation test (CFT)** = test to measure the amount of complement in antibodies and antigens 补体结合试验

complete blood count (CBC) *noun* test to find the exact numbers of each type of blood cell in a certain amount of blood 全血细胞计数

complex 1 *noun* (**a**) (*in psychiatry*) group of ideas which are based on the experience a person has had in the past, and which influence the way he behaves 情结; **Electra complex** = condition where a woman feels sexually attracted to her father and sees her mother as an obstacle 恋父情结; **inferiority complex** = condition where the person feels he is inferior to others 自卑情结; **Oedipus complex** = condition where a man feels sexually attracted to his mother and sees his father as an obstacle 恋母情结; **superiority complex** = condition where the person feels he is superior to others and pays little attention to them 自尊情结 (**b**) group of items *or* buildings *or* organs 复合体: ***He works in the new laboratory complex.*** 他在新的综合试验室工作。**primary complex** = first lymph node to be infected by TB 初期复合体; **Vitamin B complex** = group of vitamins such as folic acid, riboflavine and thiamine 复合维生素 B (**c**) syndrome, a group of signs and symptoms due to a particular cause 综合症 **2** *adjective* complicated 复杂的: ***A gastrointestinal fistula can cause many complex problems, including fluid depletion.*** 胃肠瘘可导致许多复杂的问题,包括体液丢失。

complexion *noun* general colour of the skin on the face 气色: ***He has a red complexion.*** 他面色红润。 ***She has a fine pink complexion.*** 她的肤色是粉红的。 ***People with fair complexions burn easily in the sun.*** 浅色皮肤的人易被阳光灼伤。

complicated fracture *noun* fracture with an associated injury of tissue, as where the bone has punctured an artery 复杂性骨折

◇**complication** *noun* (**a**) condition where two or more diseases exist in a patient, and are not always connected 并发病,两种或多种不一定相关联的疾病同时存在 (**b**) situation where a patient develops a second disease which changes the course of treatment for the first 并发症: ***He was admitted to hospital suffering from pneumonia with complications.*** 他因患肺炎及并发症而入院。 ***She appeared to be improving, but complications set in***

***and she died in a few hours*.** 她看上去病情有所好转,但因出现并发症在几个小时内死亡。

QUOTE: Sickle cell chest syndrome disease, is a common complication of sickle cell presenting with chest pain, fever and leucocytosis. 引文:镰状细胞胸部综合征是镰状细胞病的常见并发症,包括胸疼、发热和白细胞增多。
British Medical Journal 英国医学杂志

QUTOE: Venous air embolism is a potentially fatal complication of percutaneous venous catheterization.
引文:静脉空气栓塞是经皮静脉导管插入术的致命并发症。
Southern Medical Journal 南方医学杂志

component *noun* substance or element which forms part of a complete item 成分

compos mentis *Latin phrase meaning* of sound mind *or* sane 精神健全: ***The patient was non compos mentis when he attacked the doctor*.** 患者在攻击医生时精神是不健全的。

compose *verb* to make up 组成: ***The lotion is composed of oil, calamine and camphor*.** 洗剂由油、炉甘石和樟脑组成的。

◇ **composition** *noun* way in which a compound is formed 组成; **chemical composition** = the chemicals which make up a substance 化学成分: ***They analysed the blood samples to find out their chemical composition*.** 他们分析血样找出血中的化学成分。

compound *noun* chemical substance made up of two or more components 化合物

◇ **compound fracture** *noun* fracture where the skin surface is damaged *or* where the broken bone penetrates the surface of the skin 开放性骨折

compress 1 *noun* wad of cloth soaked in hot or cold liquid and applied to the skin to relieve pain or to force pus out of an infected wound 敷布 **2** *verb* to squeeze *or* to press 按压; **compressed air sickness** = CAISSON DISEASE 减压病

◇ **compression** *noun* (**a**) squeezing *or* pressing 按压: ***The first aider applied compression to the chest of the casualty*.** 紧急救护者按压伤者的胸部。**compression stockings** = strong elastic stockings worn to support a weak joint in the knee or to hold varicose veins tightly 加压袜; **compression syndrome** = pain in muscles after strenuous exercise 压迫综合征 (**b**) serious condition where the brain is compressed by blood or cerebrospinal fluid accumulating in it or by a fractured skull 脑受压

compulsive *adjective* (feeling) which cannot be stopped 强迫的,被迫的: ***She has a compulsive desire to steal*.** 她患有偷窃癖。**compulsive eating** = psychological condition where the patient has a continual desire to eat 强迫进食 *see also* 参见 BULIMIA

computer *noun* electronic machine for calculating 计算机

◇ **computerized axial tomography** (**CAT**) *noun* system of scanning a patient's body, where a narrow X-ray beam, guided by a computer, can photograph a thin section of the body or of an organ from several angles, using the computer to build up an image of the section 计算机轴向体层扫描

concave *adjective* which curves towards the inside 凹的; ***a concave lens*** 凹透镜

conceive *verb* (**a**) (*of woman*) to become pregnant 受孕 *see* 见 CONCEPTION (**b**) (*of child*) **to be conceived** = to start existence 产生: ***Our son was conceived during our holiday in Italy*.** 我们的儿子是我们在意大利度假期间孕育的。

concentrate 1 *noun* (**a**) strength of a solution 浓度 (**b**) way of showing amounts of a substance in body tissues and fluids 浓缩 (**c**) strong solution which is to be diluted 浓缩物 **2** *verb* (**a**) **to concentrate on** = to examine something in particular 注意力集中于 (**b**) to reduce a solution and increase its strength by evaporation 浓缩

conception *noun* point at which a woman becomes pregnant and the development of a baby starts 受精，妊娠

◇ **conceptus** *noun* result of the fertilized ovum which will develop into an embryo and fetus 受精卵

> COMMENT: Conception is usually taken to be the moment when the sperm cell fertilizes the ovum, or a few days later, when the fertilized ovum attaches itself to the wall of the womb.
> 注释：受精是指精子与卵子结合的一刹那，或指几天后受精卵着床的时刻。

concha *noun* part of the body shaped like a shell 甲；**concha auriculae** = part of the outer ear 耳甲；**nasal conchae** = little projections of bone which form the sides of the nasal cavity 鼻甲（NOTE: the plural is **conchae**）

concretion *noun* mass of hard material which forms in the body (such as a gallstone *or* deposits on bone in arthritis) 凝结物，结石

concussion *noun* (**a**) applying force to any part of the body 打击，震荡 (**b**) disturbance of the brain, loss of consciousness for a short period, caused by a blow to the head 脑震荡

◇ **concussed** *adjective* (person) who has been hit on the head and has lost and then regained consciousness 脑震荡的：***He was walking around in a concussed state.*** 他在脑震荡状态下走来走去。

◇ **concussive** *adjective* which causes concussion 致脑震荡的

condensed *adjective* made compact *or* more dense 压缩的，浓缩的

condition *noun* (**a**) state (of health *or* of cleanliness) 状态：***The arteries are in very good condition.*** 动脉状况良好。***He is ill, and his condition is getting worse.*** 他病了，情况一天天恶化。***Conditions in the hospital are very bad.*** 医院的情况很糟。(**b**) illness *or* injury *or* disorder 疾病：***He is being treated for a heart condition.*** 他在接受心脏病治疗。

◇ **conditioned reflex** *noun* automatic reaction by a person to a stimulus, a normal reaction to a normal stimulus which comes from past experience 条件反射

condom *noun* rubber sheath worn on the penis during intercourse as a contraceptive and also as a protection against sexually transmitted disease 避孕套，阴茎套（通常为橡皮制，用于避孕或预防性病的器具）；**female condom** = rubber sheath inserted into the vagina before intercourse, covering the walls of the vagina and the cervix 阴道隔

conduction *noun* passing of heat *or* sound *or* nervous impulses from one part of the body to another 传导；**conduction fibres** = fibres (as in the bundle of His) which transmit impulses 传导纤维；**air conduction** = conduction of sounds from the outside to the inner ear through the auditory meatus 空气传导；**bone conduction** = osteophony, conduction of sound waves to the inner ear through the bones of the skull 骨传导 *see also* 参见 RINNE'S TEST

◇ **conducting system** *noun* nerve system in the heart which links an atrium to aventricle, so that the two beat at the same rate 传导系统

◇ **conductive** *adjective* referring to conduction 传导的；**conductive deafness** = deafness caused by a disorder in the conduction of sound into the inner ear, rather than a disorder of the hearing nerves 传导性耳聋

conduit *noun* channel *or* passage along which a fluid flows 管道；**ileal conduit** = using a loop of the ileum to which one or both ureters are anastomosed, in order to drain urine from the body 回肠导管（用一段回肠与一侧或两侧输尿管吻合，将尿液排出体外）

condyle *noun* rounded end of a bone which articulates with another 髁；**occipital condyle** = round part of the oc-

cipital bone which joins it to the atlas 枕骨髁
◇ **condyloid process** *noun* projecting part at each end of the lower jaw which forms the head of the jaw, joining the jaw to the skull 下颌髁突
◇ **condyloma** *noun* growth usually found on the vulva 湿疣
cone *noun* one of two types of cell in the retina of the eye which is sensitive to light 视锥细胞 *see also* 参见 ROD

> COMMENT: Cones are sensitive to bright light and colours and do not function in bad light.
> 注释:视锥细胞对亮光和颜色敏感,在暗光下不起作用。

confined *adjective* kept in a place 限制,监禁: ***She was confined to bed with pneumonia.*** 她因肺炎必须卧床。***Since his accident he has been confined to a wheelchair.*** 事故后,他只能坐在轮椅里。
confirm *verb* to agree officially that something is true 证实: ***X-rays confirmed the presence of a tumour.*** X线证实了肿瘤的存在。The number of confirmed cases of the disease has doubled. 患此病的确诊病例数增加了一倍。
confuse *verb* to make someone think wrongly; to make things difficult for someone to understand 使混乱: ***The patient was confused by the physiotherapist's instructions.*** 患者被理疗者的指示弄糊涂了。
◇ **confused** *adjective* (*of patient*) not clearly aware of where one is or what one is doing 糊涂的,迷惑的: ***Old people can easily become confused if they are moved from their homes.*** 老年人离家后容易迷路。***Many severely confused patients do not respond to spoken communication.*** 许多严重精神错乱的患者对口头交流无反应。
◇ **confusion** *noun* being confused 迷惑,错乱: ***He has attacks of mental confusion.*** 他精神错乱了。***the absence of any effective treatment for confusion*** 对精神错乱没有任何有效的治疗方法
congeal *verb* (*of fat or blood*) to become solid 凝固
congenita 先天 *see* 见 AMYOTONIA
congenital *adjective* which exists at or before birth 先天的; **congenital defect** = birth defect, a malformation which exists in a person's body from birth 先天性缺陷; **congenital dislocation of the hip** = condition where a baby is born with weak ligaments in the hip, so that the femur does not stay in position in the pelvis 先天性髋关节脱位; **congenital heart disease** = heart trouble caused by defects present in the heart at birth 先天性心脏病

> COMMENT: A congenital condition is not always inherited from a parent through the genes, as it may be due to abnormalities which develop in the fetus because of factors such as a disease which the mother has (as in the case of German measles) or a drug which she has taken.
> 注释:先天性疾病并不总是通过基因从父母那儿遗传的,也可以在胎儿发育中,因为母亲患病(如风疹)或服用药物等因素造成的异常而引起。

◇ **congenitally** *adverb* at *or* before birth 先天地: ***The baby is congenitally incapable of absorbing gluten.*** 这婴儿先天性不能吸收谷胶。
congestion *noun* accumulation of blood in an organ 充血; **nasal congestion** = blocking of the nose by inflammation as a response to a cold other infection 鼻充血
◇ **congested** *adjective* with blood *or* fluid inside 充血的; **congested face** = red face, caused by blood rushing to the face 充血面容
congestive *adjective* (heart failure) caused by congestion 充血的
conization *noun* surgical removal of a cone-shaped piece of tissue 锥形切除术
conjoined twins 连体双胞胎 *see* SIAMESE TWINS
conjugate *or* **true conjugate** *or* **conjugate diameter** *noun* measurements of space in the pelvis, used to

calculate if normal childbirth is possible 骨盆直径，真直径

conjunctiva *noun* membrane which covers the front of the eyeball and the inside of the eyelids 结膜

◇ **conjunctival** *adjective* referring to the conjunctiva 结膜的

◇ **conjunctivitis** *noun* inflammation of the conjunctiva 结膜炎 *see also* 参见 PINK EYE

connect *verb* to join 连接：***The lungs are connected to the mouth by the trachea.*** 肺通过气管与口腔相接。***The pulmonary artery connects the heart to the lungs.*** 肺动脉连接心肺。***The biceps is connected to both the radius and the scapula.*** 肱二头肌连接桡骨和肩胛骨。

◇ **connection** *noun* something which joins 连接体

◇ **connective tissue** *noun* tissue which forms the main part of bones and cartilage, ligaments and tendons, in which a large proportion of fibrous material surrounds the tissue cells 结缔组织

Conn's syndrome *noun* condition caused by excessive production of aldosterone 康恩氏综合症，原发性醛固酮增多症

consanguinity *noun* blood relationship between people 血缘关系

conscious *adjective* awake and knowing what is happening 苏醒的，清醒的：***He became conscious in the recovery room two hours after the operation.*** 手术后两个小时他在恢复室苏醒了。***It was two days after the accident before she became conscious.*** 出事两天后她才清醒过来。

◇ **consciously** *adverb* in a conscious way 清醒地

◇ **consciousness** *noun* being mentally awake and knowing what is happening 知觉；**to lose consciousness** = to become unconscious *or* to become unable to respond to stimulation by the senses 丧失知觉；**to regain consciousness** = to become conscious after being unconscious 恢复知觉

consent *noun* agreement 同意：***The parents gave their consent for their son's heart to be used in the transplant operation.*** 父母同意将儿子的心脏用于移植手术。***The nurses checked the patient's identity bracelet and that his consent had been given.*** 护士已核查患者的身份标签及同意书。**consent form** = form which a patient signs to show he agrees to have the operation 手术同意书

conserve *verb* to keep *or* not to waste 保存：***The body needs to conserve heat in cold weather.*** 天气寒冷时机体需要储存热量。

consolidation *noun* (i) stage in mending a broken bone, where the callus formed at the break changes into bone 骨化 (ii) condition where part of the lung becomes solid (as in pneumonia) 实变

constant *adjective* (**a**) continuous *or* not stopping 持续的，不间断的：***Patients with Alzheimer's disease need constant supervision.*** 阿耳茨默氏病患者需要连续监护。(**b**) level *or* not varying 不变的：***His blood pressure remained constant during the operation.*** 术中，他的血压平稳。

constipated *adjective* unable to pass faeces often enough 便秘的

◇ **constipation** *noun* difficulty in passing faeces often enough 便秘

> COMMENT: Constipated bowel movements are hard, and may cause pain in the anus. One bowel movement per day is the normal frequency. Constipation may be caused by worry or by a diet which does not contain enough roughage or by lack of exercise, as well as more serious diseases of the intestine.
> 注释：便秘时肠蠕动加剧可引起肛门疼痛。每天排便一次是正常的频率。便秘可因焦虑、饮食中缺少粗糙食物、缺乏运动以及严重的肠道疾病等引起。

constituent *noun* substance which forms part of something 组分，成分；***the chemical constituents of nerve cells*** 神经

细胞的化学成分

constitution *noun* general health and strength of a person 体质: ***She has a strong constitution** or **a healthy constitution**.* 她体质很强壮。***He has a weak constitution and is often ill*** 他体质虚弱，经常生病。

◊ **constitutional** *adjective* referring to a person's constitution 体质的

◊ **constitutionally** *adverb* in a person's constitution 体质上: ***He is constitutionally incapable of feeling tired.*** 从体质上讲，他不能劳累。

constrict *verb* to squeeze *or* to make a passage narrower 收缩，使狭窄

◊ **constriction** *noun* stenosis, becoming narrow 收缩，狭窄

◊ **constrictor** *noun* muscle which squeezes an organ or which makes an organ contract 收缩肌

◊ **constrictive** *adjective* which constricts 收缩的; **constrictive pericarditis** = condition where the pericardium becomes thickened and prevents the heart from functioning normally 缩窄性心包炎

consult *verb* to ask someone for his opinion 求教: ***He consulted an eye specialist.*** 他向眼科专家请教。

◊ **consultancy** *noun* post of consultant 顾问的职位: ***She was appointed to a consultancy with a London hospital.*** 她被委任为伦敦医院的顾问。

◊ **consultant** *noun* (i) doctor who is a senior specialist in a particular branch of medicine and who is consulted by a GP 顾问医生(ii) senior specialized doctor in a hospital 医院的高级专科医师: ***She was referred to the consultant orthopaedist*** 她被介绍给矫形科的高级医师

◊ **consultation** *noun* (i) discussion between two doctors about a case 会诊 (ii) meeting with a doctor who examines the patient, discusses his condition with him, and prescribes treatment 就诊

◊ **consulting room** *noun* room where a doctor sees his patients 诊室

consumption *noun* (**a**) taking food *or* liquid into the body 消耗: ***The patient's increased consumption of alcohol.*** 患者酒精的消耗量增加。(**b**) former name for pulmonary tuberculosis 痨病结核病的旧称

◊ **consumptive** *adjective* referring to consumption (patient) suffering from consumption 肺结核的；患肺结核的

contact 1 *noun* (**a**) touching someone *or* something 接触; **to have (physical) contact with someone** *or* **something** = to actually touch someone *or* something (身体)直接接触人; **to be in contact with someone** = to be near someone *or* to touch someone 接近或接触某人: ***The hospital is anxious to trace anyone who may have come into contact with the patient.*** 医院正在紧急追踪与此患者有过接触的人。**direct contact** = actually touching an infected person *or* object 直接接触; **indirect contact** = catching a disease by inhaling germs *or* being in contact with a vector 间接接触; **contact dermatitis** = inflammation of the skin, caused by touch (as in the case of some types of plant *or* soap, etc.) 接触性皮炎 (**b**) person who has been in contact with a person suffering from an infectious disease 接触者: ***Now that Lassa fever has been diagnosed, the authorities are anxious to trace all contacts which the patient may have met.*** 患者被确诊为 Lassa 热后，有关部分正在紧急跟踪与此患者有接触的所有人。**2** *verb* to meet *or* to get in touch with (someone) 接触，会见

◊ **contact lens** *noun* tiny plastic or glass lens which fits over the eyeball (worn instead of spectacles) 隐形眼镜

contagion *noun* spreading of a disease by touching an infected person or objects which an infected person has touched 接触传染: ***The contagion spread through the whole school.*** 接触传染遍及整个学校。

◊ **contagious** *adjective* (disease) which can be transmitted by touching an infected person or objects which an infected person has touched 有传染性的

contaminate *verb* to make something impure by touching it *or* by adding something to it 污染：***Supplies of drinking water were contaminated by refuse from the factories.*** 饮用水源被工厂的排泄废物污染了。***The whole group of tourists fell ill after eating contaminated food.*** 全队的旅游者在食用了污染的食物后都病倒了。

◇ **contaminant** *noun* substance which contaminates 污染物

◇ **contamination** *noun* action of contaminating 污染：***The contamination resulted from polluted water.*** 污染来源于污水。

content *noun* proportion of a substance in something 含量：***These foods have a high starch content.*** 这些食物含有大量淀粉。***Dried fruit has a higher sugar content than fresh fruit.*** 干果比新鲜水果含有更高的糖分。

continue *verb* to go on doing something; to do something which was being done before 继续做：***The fever continued for three days.*** 发热持续了3天。They continued eating as if nothing had happened. 他们继续吃饭，就像什么都没发生一样。The doctor recommended that the treatment should be continued for a further period. 医生建议治疗再继续一段时间。

◇ **continual** *adjective* which goes on all the time without stopping; which happens again and again 不停的，经常的：***He suffered continual recurrence of the disease.*** 他的疾病经常复发。

◇ **continually** *adverb* all the time 总是：***The intestine is continually infected.*** 肠道总是受到感染。

◇ **continuation** *noun* part which continues 连续的部分：***The radial artery is a continuation of the brachial artery.*** 桡动脉是臂动脉的继续。

◇ **continuous** *adjective* which continues without breaks or stops 连续不断的

contraception *noun* prevention of pregnancy by using devices (such as a condom *or* an IUD) or drugs (such as the contraceptive pill) or by other means 避孕 *see also* 参见 BIRTH CONTROL

◇ **contraceptive 1** *adjective* which prevents conception 避孕的；***a contraceptive device or contraceptive drug*** 避孕设备，避孕药；**oral contraceptive** = contraceptive pill which is taken through the mouth 口服避孕药 **2** *noun* drug *or* condom which prevents pregnancy 避孕剂

contract *verb* **(a)** (*of muscle*) to become smaller and tighter 收缩：***As the muscle contracts the limb moves.*** 肌肉收缩使肢体运动。***The diaphragm acts to contract the chest.*** 膈肌使胸廓收缩。**(b)** **to contract a disease** = to catch a disease 感染：***He contracted Lassa fever.*** 他感染了Lassa热。

◇ **contractile tissue** *noun* tissue in muscle which makes the muscle contract 收缩组织

◇ **contraction** *noun* (i) tightening movement which makes a muscle shorter *or* which makes the pupil of the eye smaller *or* which makes the skin wrinkle 收缩(ii) movement of the muscles of the uterus, marking the beginning of labour 宫缩

◇ **contracture** *noun* permanent tightening of a muscle caused by fibrosis 挛缩；**Dupuytren's contracture** = condition where the palmar fascia becomes thicker, causing the fingers to bend forwards 掌挛缩病；**Volkmann's contracture** = tightening and fibrosis of the muscles of the forearm because blood supply has been restricted, leading to deformity of the fingers 手挛缩(因为血运不足引起前臂肌肉僵硬、纤维化，最终导致手畸形)

contraindication *noun* something which suggests that a patient should not be treated with a certain drug *or* not continue to be treated in the same way as at present, because circumstances make that treatment unsuitable 禁忌症

contralateral *adjective* affecting the side of the body opposite the one referred to 对侧的

contrast medium *noun* radio-opaque dye or sometimes gas, put into an organ *or* part of the body so that it will show clearly in an X-ray photograph 造影剂(注入器官或体内的使 X 线片更清晰的不透光染料或气体)

> QUOTE: Comparing the MRI scan and the CT scan: in the first no contrast medium is required; in the second iodine-based contrast media are often required.
> 引文:比较磁共振成像和 CT 图像,前者不需造影剂,后者常需碘基造影剂。
> **Nursing 87 护理 87**

contrecoup *noun* injury to one point of an organ (for example, the brain) caused by a blow received on an opposite point of the organ 对冲伤

control 1 *noun* power *or* keeping in order 权力: ***The manager has no control over the consultants working in the hospital.*** 管理者对医院的顾问没有控制权。***The specialists brought the epidemic under control.*** = They stopped it from spreading. 专家控制住了流行病的传播。***The epidemic rapidly got out of control.*** = It spread quickly. 流行病很快传播开了。(*in experiments*) **control group** = group of people who are not being treated, but whose test data are used as a comparison 对照组 **2** *verb* to keep in order 控制: ***The medical authorities are trying to control the epidemic.*** 医疗当局在设法控制流行病的传播。***Certain drugs help to control the convulsions.*** 某些药物可控制惊厥的发作。***He controls his asthma with a bronchodilator.*** 他用支气管扩张剂控制哮喘发作。**controlled drugs** *or* **dangerous drugs** = drugs which are on the official list of drugs which are harmful and are not available to the general public 监控药品,危险药品; **controlled respiration** = control of a patient's breathing by an anaesthetist during an operation, when normal breathing has stopped 人工控制呼吸

contusion *noun* bruise, a dark painful area on the skin, where blood has escaped into the tissues but not through the skin, following a blow 挫伤,青肿

◊ **contused wound** *noun* wound caused by a blow where the skin is bruised as well as torn and bleeding 挫伤

conus *noun* structure shaped like a cone 圆锥

convalesce *verb* to get back to good health gradually after an illness *or* operation 康复

◊ **convalescence** *noun* period of time when a patient is convalescing 恢复期

◊ **convalescent** *adjective & noun* referring to convalescence 恢复期的; **convalescent patients** *or* **convalescents** = people who are convalescing 恢复期患者; **convalescent home** = type of hospital where patients can recover from illness *or* surgery 接纳疾病或手术恢复期患者的医院,康复医院

converge *verb* (*of rays*) to come together at a point 汇和,集合

◊ **convergent strabismus** *or* **squint** *noun* condition where a person's eyes look towards the nose 内斜视

conversion *noun* change 转化; ***the conversion of nutrients into tissue*** 将营养转化为组织

◊ **convert** *verb* to change something into something else 转化: ***Keratinization is the process of converting cells into horny tissue.*** 角质化是细胞转化为角质组织的过程。

convex *adjective* which curves towards the outside 凸的; ***a convex lens*** 凸透镜

convoluted *adjective* folded and twisted 卷曲的; **convoluted tubules** = coiled parts of a nephron 肾曲小管

◊ **convolution** *noun* twisted shape 卷曲; ***the convolutions of the surface of the cerebrum*** 大脑表面的沟回

convulsion *noun* fit, the rapid involuntary contracting and relaxing of the muscles in several parts of the body 惊厥 (NOTE: often used in the plural : **'the child had convulsions'**)

◇**convulsive** *adjective* referring to convulsions 惊厥的: ***He had a convulsive seizure.*** 他患有惊厥。*see also* 参见 ELECTROCONVULSIVE THERAPY

COMMENT: Convulsions in children may be caused by brain disease, such as meningitis, but can often be found at the beginning of a disease (such as pneumonia) which is marked by a sudden rise in body temperature. In adults, convulsions are usually associated with epilepsy. 注释:儿童惊厥可因脑部疾病如脑膜炎引起,但更多的是在某些疾病(如:肺炎)的早期出现,常伴体温的突然升高。成人惊厥多与癫痫有关。

cool 1 *adjective* not very warm *or* quite cold 凉的: ***The patient should be kept cool.*** 患者应保持凉爽。***Keep this bottle in a cool place.*** 把瓶子放在阴凉处。(NOTE : **cool - cooler - coolest**) **2** *verb* to become cool 使变凉

Cooley's anaemia = THALASSAEMIA 库利贫血,地中海贫血

Coombs' test *noun* test for antibodies in red blood cells, used as a test for erythroblastosis fetalis and other haemolytic syndromes 库姆斯试验,检查红细胞中抗体以诊断胎儿成红细胞增多症和其他溶血综合症的试验

coordinate *verb* to make things work together 协调: ***He was unable to coordinate the movements of his arms and legs.*** 他不能协调手脚的运动。

◇ **coordination** *noun* ability to work together 协调性: ***The patient showed lack of coordination between eyes and hands.*** 患者缺乏手眼的协调性。

QUOTE: There are four recti muscles and two oblique muscles in each eye, which coordinate the movement of the eyes and enable them to work as a pair.
引文:每只眼有四条直肌和两条斜肌来控制眼睛的协调运动,使两支眼睛成双运动。
Nursing Times 护理时代

QUOTE: Alzheimer's disease is a progressive disorder which sees a gradual decline in intellectual functioning and deterioration of physical coordination.
阿尔茨海默氏病是一渐进性疾病,表现为智力的逐渐减低和机体协调力的下降。
Nursing Times 护理时代

cope with *verb* to deal with *or* to manage 处理,对付: ***A hospital administrator has to cope with a lot of forms.*** 医院的管理者必须处理很多表格。***He walks with crutches and has difficulty in coping with the stairs.*** 他拄拐杖走路,上下楼梯有困难。

copper *noun* metallic trace element 铜 (NOTE: the chemical symbol is **Cu**)

coprolith *noun* hard faeces in the bowel 粪石

coproporphyrin *noun* porphyrin excreted by the liver 粪卟啉

copulate *verb* to have sexual intercourse 交配

◇ **copulation** *noun* coitus *or* sexual intercourse 交配

cor *noun* the heart 心脏; **cor pulmonale** = pulmonary heart disease where the right ventricle is enlarged 肺心病

coraco-acromial *adjective* referring to the coracoid process and the acromion 喙肩的,喙突肩峰的

◇ **coracobrachialis** *noun* muscle on the medial side of the upper arm, below the armpit 喙肱肌

◇ **coracoid process** *noun* projecting part on the shoulder blade 喙突

cord *noun* long flexible structure in the body like a thread 索条; **spermatic cord** = cord formed of the vas deferens, the blood vessels, nerves and lymphatics of the testis, running from the testis to the abdomen 精索; **spinal cord** = part of the central nervous system, running from the medulla oblongata to the filum terminale, in the vertebral canal of the spine 脊髓; **umbilical cord** = cord containing two arteries and one vein which links the fetus inside the womb to the placenta 脐带; **vocal cords** = cords in the larynx which can be brought together to make sounds as air passes between them 声带

◇ **cordectomy** *noun* surgical removal of a vocal cord 声带切除术

◇ **cordotomy** = CHORDOTOMY 脊髓切断术

core *noun* central part 核心

corectopia *noun* ectopia of the pupil 瞳孔异位

corium *noun* dermis, layer of living tissue beneath the epidermis 真皮

corn *noun* heloma, a hard painful lump of skin usually on the foot or hand, where something (such as tight shoe) has rubbed or pressed on the skin 鸡眼

cornea *noun* transparent part of the front of the eyeball 角膜(NOTE: plural is **corneae**)

◇ **corneal** *adjective* referring to a cornea 角膜的: ***Corneal tissue from donors is used in grafting to replace a damaged cornea.*** 供者的角膜组织被用来移植替代受损的角膜。**corneal abrasion** = scratch on the cornea, caused by something sharp getting into the eye 角膜擦伤; **corneal bank** = place where eyes of dead donors can be kept ready for use in corneal grafts 角膜库

◇ **corneal graft** *noun* keratoplasty, corneal tissue from a donor or from a dead person, grafted in place of diseased tissue 角膜移植 (NOTE: for terms referring to the cornea, see words beginning with **kerat-**)

corneum 角质层 *see* 见 STRATUM

cornification *noun* keratinization, process of converting cells into horny tissue 角质化

cornu *noun* structure in the body which is shaped like a horn 角形结构; **cornua of the thyroid** = four processes of the thyroid cartilage 甲状软骨角 (NOTE: the plural is **cornua**)

corona *noun* structure in the body which is shaped like a crown 冠状结构; **corona capitis** = the crown of the head *or* the top part of the skull 颅顶

◇ **coronal** *adjective* (i) referring to a corona 冠的(ii) referring to the crown of a tooth 牙冠; **coronal plane** = plane at right angles to the median plane, dividing the body into dorsal and ventral halves 冠状平面; **coronal suture** = horizontal joint across the top of the skull between the parietal and frontal bones 冠状缝 ◊ 见图 SKULL

coronary 1 *noun* (*non-medical term*) coronary thrombosis, a blood clot in the coronary arteries which leads to a heart attack 冠脉血栓,冠心病: ***He had a coronary and was rushed to hospital.*** 他得了冠心病被急送入医院。2 *adjective*. referring to any structure shaped like a crown, but especially to the arteries which supply blood to the heart muscles 冠状组织的,冠状动脉的; **coronary arteries** = arteries which supply blood to the heart muscles 冠状动脉; **coronary artery bypass graft** *or* **surgery** = surgical operation to treat angina by grafting pieces of vein to go around the diseased part of a coronary artery 冠状动脉旁路手术; **coronary care unit** (**CCU**) = section of a hospital caring for patients with heart disorders *or* who have had heart surgery 冠心病监护病房; **coronary circulation** = blood circulation through the arteries and veins of the heart muscles 冠脉循环; **coronary heart disease** (**CHD**) = any disease affecting the coronary arteries, which can lead to strain on the heart *or* a heart attack 冠心病; **coronary ligament** = folds of peritoneum connecting the back of the liver to the diaphragm 冠状韧带; **coronary obstruction** *or* **coronary occlusion** = thickening of the walls of the coronary arteries *or* a blood clot in the coronary arteries, which prevents blood reaching the heart muscles and leads to heart failure 冠脉阻塞; **coronary sinus** = vein which takes most of the venous blood from the heart muscles to the right atrium 冠脉窦; **coronary thrombosis** = blood clot which blocks the coronary arteries, leading to a heart attack 冠脉血栓形成

> QUOTE: Coronary heart disease (CHD) patients spend an average of 11.9 days in hospital. Among primary health care services, 1.5% of all GP consultations are due to CHD.
> 引文:冠心病患者的平均住院日为11.9天。在初级卫生保健服务中,有1.5%的人因冠心病就诊于开业医生。
> **Health Services Journal** 健康服务杂志

> QUOTE: Apart from death, coronary heart disease causes considerable morbidity in the form of heart attack, angina and a number of related diseases.
> 引文:除死亡外,冠心病可引起许多心脏病发生,如心脏骤停、心绞痛和其他相关疾病。
> **Health Education Journal** 健康教育杂志

coronavirus *noun* virus which causes the common cold 冠状病毒

coroner *noun* public official (either a doctor or a lawyer) who investigates sudden *or* violent deaths 验尸官,法医; **coroner's court** = court where a coroner is the chairman 法医法庭; **coroner's inquest** = inquest carried out by a coroner into a death 验尸

> COMMENT: Coroners investigate deaths which are violent or not expected, deaths which may be murder or manslaughter, deaths of prisoners and deaths involving the police.
> 注释:验尸官调查因暴力或意外导致的死亡,它可为谋杀、屠杀、罪犯或警察的死亡。

coronoid process *noun* (i) projecting piece of bone on the ulna 尺骨喙突 (ii) projecting piece on each of the lower jaw 下颌髁突

corpse *noun* body of a dead person 尸体

corpus *noun* any mass of tissue 任何组织; **corpus albicans** = scar tissue which replaces the corpus luteum in the ovary 白体; **corpus callosum** = tissue which connects the two cerebral hemispheres 胼胝体 ◊ 见图 BRAIN; **corpus cavernosum** = part of the erectile tissue in the penis and clitoris 海绵体 ◊ 见图 UROGENITAL SYSTEM (MALE); **corpus haemorrhagicum** = blood clot formed in the ovary where a Graafian follicle has ruptured 红体,出血体孵泡; **corpus luteum** = body which forms in the ovary after a Graafian follicle has ruptured (the corpora lutea secrete the hormone progesterone to prepare the uterus for implantation of the fertilized ovum) 黄体; **corpus spongiosum** = part of the penis round the urethra, forming the glans 尿道海绵体; **corpus striatum** = part of a cerebral hemisphere 纹状体 (NOTE: the plural is **corpora**)

corpuscle *noun* any small round mass 球形小体; **red corpuscle** *or* **erythrocyte** = red blood cell which contains haemoglobin and carries oxygen to the tissues and takes carbon dioxide from them 红血球,红细胞; **white corpuscle** *or* **leucocyte** = white blood cell, a colourless cell which contains a nucleus but has no haemoglobin 白血球,白细胞; **Krause corpuscles** = encapsulated nerve endings in mucous membrane of mouth, nose, eyes and genitals 克劳泽氏小体(口、鼻、眼及生殖器粘膜的神经末梢); **Meissner's corpuscle** = sensory nerve ending in the skin which is sensitive to touch 麦斯纳氏小体,触觉小体; **Pacinian corpuscle** = sensory nerve ending in the skin which is sensitive to touch and vibrations 帕西尼氏小体(位于皮肤的感觉神经末梢,感知触觉和震动) ◊ 见图 SKIN & SENSORY RECEPTORS; **renal cor-**

puscle *or* **Malpighian corpuscle** *or* **Malpighian body** = part of a nephron in the cortex of a kidney 马耳皮基氏小体,肾小体; **Ruffini corpuscles** *or* **Ruffini nerve endings** = branching nerve endings in the skin, which are thought to be sensitive to heat 鲁非尼氏小体,皮下神经终末端 ◊ 见图 SKIN & SENSORY RECEPTORS

correct *verb* to put faults right *or* to make something work properly 矫正: ***She wears a brace to correct the growth of her teeth.*** 她戴了牙箍矫形。***Doctors are trying to correct his speech defect.*** 医生在设法纠正他的语言缺陷。

◊ **correction** *noun* showing the mistake in something; making something correct 矫正

◊ **corrective** *noun* drug which changes the harmful effect of another drug 矫正药,缓解副作用的药物

Corrigan's pulse *noun* type of pulse, where there is a visible rise in pressure followed by a sudden collapse, of the arterial pulse in the neck, caused by aortic regurgitation 水冲脉

corrosive *adjective* & *noun* (substance, such as acid *or* alkali) which destroys tissue 有腐蚀性的,腐蚀剂(如酸或碱)

corrugator muscles *noun* muscles which produce vertical wrinkles on the forehead when frowning 皱眉肌

corset *noun* piece of stiff clothing, worn on the chest *or* over the trunk to support the body as after a back injury 围腰,胸衣

cortex *noun* outer layer of an organ, as opposed to the soft inner medulla 皮质; **adrenal cortex** = firm outside layer of the adrenal or suprarenal glands, which secretes various hormones, including cortisone 肾上腺皮质; **cerebellar cortex** = outer covering of grey matter which covers the cerebellum 小脑皮质; **cerebral cortex** = outer layer of grey matter which covers the cerebrum 大脑皮质; **olfactory cortex**, **visual cortex** = parts of the cerebral cortex which receive information about smell *or* sight 纹状区; **renal cortex** = outer covering of a kidney, immediately beneath the capsule, containing glomeruli 肾皮质 ◊ 见图 KIDNEY; **sensory cortex** = area of the cerebral cortex which receives information from nerves in all parts of the body 感觉区 (NOTE: the plural is **cortices**)

Corti 科蒂器 *see* 见 ORGAN

cortical *adjective* referring to a cortex 皮质的; (**suprarenal**) **cortical hormones** = hormones (such as cortisone) secreted by the cortex of the adrenal glands 肾上腺皮质激素; **subcortical** = beneath the cortex 皮质下

corticospinal *adjective* referring to both the cerebral cortex and the spinal cord 皮质脊髓的

corticosteroid *noun* any steroid hormone produced by the cortex of the adrenal glands 皮质类固醇

◊ **corticosterone** *noun* hormone secreted by the cortex of the adrenal glands 皮质酮

corticotrophin *or* **adrenocorticotrophic hormone** (**ACTH**) *noun* hormone produced by the anterior pituitary gland, which causes the cortex of the adrenal glands to release corticosteroids 促肾上腺皮质激素

cortisol *noun* hydrocortisone, steroid hormone produced by the cortex of the adrenal glands 氢化可的松,皮质醇

◊ **cortisone** *noun* hormone secreted in small quantities by the adrenal cortex 可的松: ***The doctor gave her a cortisone injection in the ankle.*** 医生给她踝关节内注射可的松。**cortisone treatment** = treatment of conditions by injections of cortisone 可的松治疗

> COMMENT: Cortisol is used by the body to maintain blood pressure, connective tissue and break down carbohydrates. It also reduces the body's immune response to infec-

tion. Synthetic cortisone is used in the treatment of arthritis, asthma and skin disorders, but can have powerful side-effects on some patients andis less often used.
注释:可的松可维持机体的血压、结缔组织并分解碳水化合物。它还可降低机体对感染的免疫力。人工合成的可的松可治疗关节炎、哮喘和皮肤疾病,但对某些患者可产生严重的副作用,因此很少应用。

Corynebacterium *noun* genus of bacteria which includes the bacterium which causes diphtheria 棒状杆菌属

coryza *noun* nasal catarrh *or* common cold *or* cold in the head, an illness, with inflammation of the nasal passages, in which the patients neezes and coughs and has a blocked and running nose 鼻伤风,鼻炎

cosmetic surgery *noun* surgical operation carried out to improve the appearance of the patient 美容手术

COMMENT: Whereas plastic surgery may be prescribed by a doctor to correct skin or bone defects or the effect of burns or after a disfiguring operation, cosmetic surgery is carried out on the instructions of the patient to remove wrinkles, enlarge breasts,etc..
注释:整形手术是由医生决定用来矫正皮肤或骨骼畸形、烧伤或毁容手术后的整容,而美容手术是根据患者的需要去除皱纹,使乳房丰满等。

cost- *prefix* referring to the ribs 肋的

◇ **costal** *adjective* referring to the ribs 肋骨的; **costal cartilage** = cartilage which forms the end of each rib and either joins the rib to the breastbone or to the rib above 肋软骨; **costal pleura** = part of the pleura lining the walls of the chest 肋胸膜

costive 1 *adjective* constipated, suffering from difficulty in passing bowel movements 便秘的 **2** *noun* drug which causes constipation 便秘药

costocervical trunk *noun* large artery in the chest 颈肋干

◇ **costodiaphragmatic** *adjective* referring to the ribs and the diaphragm 膈肋膜的

◇ **costovertebral joints** *noun* joints between the ribs and the vertebral column 肋椎关节

cot death *or US* **crib death** *noun* sudden infant death syndrome, the sudden death of a baby in bed, without any identifiable cause 婴儿猝死综合症

COMMENT: Occurs in very young children, up to the age of about 12 months; the causes are still being investigated, but may be related to the position of the baby, in particular whether it is lying on its back or front.
注释:发生于 12 月内的婴儿,病因待查,但可能与体位有关,尤其是仰卧或俯卧时。

co-trimoxazole *noun* drug used to combat bacteria in the urinary tract 增效磺胺甲基异噁唑

cottage hospital *noun* small local hospital sometimes set in pleasant gardens in the country 乡村医院

cotton *noun* fibres from a tropical plant; cloth made from cotton thread 棉花,棉布: ***She wore a cotton shirt.*** 她穿了件棉布衬衣。

◇ **cotton wool** *or* **absorbent cotton** *noun* purified fibres from the cotton plant used as a dressing on wounds, etc. 纱布,棉球: ***She dabbed the cut with cotton wool soaked in antiseptic.*** 她用消毒棉球轻拭伤口。***The nurse put a pad of cotton wool over the sore.*** 护士在伤处敷了层纱布。

cotyledon *noun* one of the divisions of a placenta 绒毛叶

cotyloid cavity *noun* acetabulum, part of the pelvic bone shaped like a cup, into which the head of the femur fits to form the hip joint 髋臼

couch *noun* long bed on which a patient lies when being examined by a doctor in a surgery 诊床

◇ **couching** *noun* in treatment of cataract, surgical operation to displace the opaque lens of an eye 白内障摘除术

cough 1 *noun* reflex action, caused by irritation in the throat, when the glottis is opened and air is sent out of the lungs suddenly 咳嗽: ***He gave a little cough to attract the nurse's attention.*** 他清了清喉咙以引起护士的注意。***She has a bad cough and cannot make the speech.*** 她咳嗽得厉害,不能说话。**cough medicine** *or* **cough linctus** = liquid taken to soothe the irritation which causes a cough 止咳剂; **barking cough** = loud noisy dry cough 犬吠样咳嗽; **dry cough** = cough where no phlegm is produced 干咳; **hacking cough** = continuous short dry cough 频咳; **productive cough** = cough where phlegm is produced 咳痰 2 *verb* to send air out of the lungs suddenly because the throat is irritated 咳嗽: ***The smoke made him cough.*** 烟使他咳嗽。***He has a cold and keeps on coughing and sneezing.*** 他感冒了,不停的咳嗽打喷嚏。**coughing fit** = sudden attack of coughing 咳嗽发作

◇ **cough up** *verb* to cough hard to produce a substance from the trachea. 咳出: ***He coughed up phlegm.*** 他咳出痰来。***She became worried when the girl started coughing up blood.*** 当女孩咳血时她很担心。

council *noun* group of people elected to manage something 议会; **town council** = elected committee which manages a town 镇议会; **General Medical Council** = body which registers all practising doctors (without such registration, a doctor cannot practise) 医师总会(英国)

counselling *noun* method of treating especially psychiatric disorders, where a specialist advises and talks with a patient about his condition and how to deal with it 交谈疗法,言语治疗

◇ **counsellor** *noun* person who advises and talks with someone about his problems 顾问

count 1 *verb* (**a**) to say numbers in order 按顺序数数: ***The little girl can count up to ten.*** 小女孩可以数到10。***Hold your breath and count to twenty to try to stop a hiccup.*** 可用屏住呼吸数到20的方法来治疗呃逆。(**b**) to add up to see how many things there are 计数: ***Count the number of tablets left in the bottle.*** 数一下瓶子里剩余多少药片。(**c**) to include 包括: ***There were thirty people in the ward if you count the visitors.*** 如果算上探视者,病房里有30个人。2 *noun* act of adding things to see how many there are 计数; **blood count** = test to count the number and types of different blood cells in a certain tiny sample of blood, to give an indication of the condition of the patient's blood as a whole 血细胞计数; **platelet count** = test to see the quantity of platelets in a patient's blood 血小板计数

> QUOTE: The normal platelet count during pregnancy is described as 150,000 to 400,000 per cu mm.
> 引文:妊娠时正常血小板计数是15－40万/立方毫米。
> **Southern Medical Journal** 南方医学杂志

counteract *verb* to act against something *or* to reduce the effect of something 抵消: ***The lotion should counteract the irritant effect of the spray on the skin.*** 这种擦剂可以减轻喷雾对皮肤引起的刺激反应。

◇ **counteraction** *noun* (*in pharmacy*) action of one drug which acts against another drug 拮抗

counterextension *noun* orthopaedic treatment, where the upper part of a limb is kept fixed and traction is applied to the lower part of it 对抗牵引术

counterirritant *noun* substance which alleviates the pain in an internal organ, by irritating an area of skin whose sensory nerves are close to those of the organ in the spinal cord 抗刺激物,来缓解内脏疼痛的一种物质,通过刺激与脊髓中感觉神经相近的皮肤感觉神经来起作用。

◇ **counterirritation** *noun* skin

irritation, applied artificially to alleviate the pain in another part of the body 抗刺激法

counterstain 1 *noun* stain used to identify tissue samples, such as red dye used to identify Gram-negative bacteria 复染剂 2 *verb* to stain specimens with a counterstain, as bacteria with a red stain after having first stained them with violet dye 复染 *see also* 参见 GRAM

course *noun* (**a**) passing of time 时间的流逝：***His condition has deteriorated in the course of the last few weeks.*** 在过去的几周内他的病情恶化了。(**b**) series of lessons 课程：***I'm taking a course in physiotherapy.*** 我正上理疗课。***She's taking a hospital administration course.*** 她在上医院管理课。(**c**) series of drugs to be taken *or* of sessions of treatment 疗程：***We'll put you on a course of antibiotics.*** 我们会给你进行一疗程的抗生素治疗。**course of treatment** = series of applications of a treatment (such as a series of injections *or* physiotherapy) 疗程；**to put someone on a course of drugs** *or* **of antibiotics** *or* **of injections** = to decide that a patient should take a drug *or* an antibiotic *or* should have a number of injections regularly over a certain period of time. 定期给予药物治疗。

court *noun* place where a trial is heard *or* where a legal judgement is reached 法庭；**court order** = order made by a court telling someone to do *or* not to do something 法庭判决：***He was sent to a mental institution by court order.*** 他被判决送往精神病院。

cover 1 *noun* (**a**) thing put over something to keep it clean, etc. 遮盖物：***Keep a cover on the petri dish.*** 在培养皿上盖上盖子。**cover test** = test for a squint, where an eye is covered and its movements are checked when the cover is taken off 遮盖试验 (**b**) doing work for someone who is absent 替班：***Out-of-hours cover is provided by the other GPs in the practice.*** 业余时间由诊室的其他医师替班。2 *verb* (**a**) to put something over something to keep it clean, etc. 加盖以保持干净：***You should cover the table with a plastic sheet before you start to mix the mouthwash.*** 在开始混合漱口水前，应该在桌子上铺块塑料布。***The fetus is covered with a membrane.*** 胎儿被膜覆盖。(**b**) to be available to work in place of someone who is absent 替班：***The other GPs will cover for him while he is on holiday.*** 他休假期间由其他医师替班。

◇ **covering** *noun* layer which covers *or* protects something 覆盖物；**brain covering** = the meninges 脑膜

Cowper's glands *noun* bulbourethral glands, two glands at the base of the penis which secrete into the urethra 库珀腺，尿道球腺

cowpox *or* **vaccinia** *noun* infectious viral disease of cattle 牛痘

> COMMENT: The virus can be transmitted to man, and is used as a constituent of the vaccine for smallpox.
> 注释：这病毒可以传播给人，也可用来制作天花疫苗。

coxa *noun* the hip joint 髋

◇ **coxalgia** *noun* pain in the hip joint 髋痛

Coxsackie virus *noun* one of a group of enteroviruses which enter the cells of the intestines but can cause diseases such as aseptic meningitis and Bornholm disease 柯萨奇病毒(侵入肠细胞的病毒，可导致带菌性脑膜炎和流行性胸肌痛)

CPR = CARDIOPULMONARY RESUSCITATION 心肺复苏

Cr *chemical symbol for* chromium 铬的化学符号

crab (louse) *or* **pubic louse** *noun* louse *Phthirius pubis* which infests the pubic region and other parts of the body with coarse hair 阴虱，毛虱

crack 1 *noun* thin break 裂隙：***There's***

a crack in one of the bones in the skull. 一块颅骨上有裂缝。**2** *verb* to make a thin break in something; to split 使破裂: ***She cracked a bone in her leg.*** 她腿骨折了。**cracked lips** = lips where the skin has split because of cold *or* dryness 唇裂

cradle *noun* (**a**) metal frame put over a patient in bed to keep the weight of the bedclothes off the body 支架 (**b**) carrying an injured child by holding him with one arm under the thigh and the other above the waist 搬运受伤患儿的一种姿势,一手在大腿下侧,另一手在腰上; **cradle cap** = yellow deposit on the scalp of babies, caused by seborrhoea 乳痂

cramp *noun* painful involuntary spasm in the muscles, where the muscle may stay contracted for some time 痛性痉挛: ***He went swimming and got cramp in the cold water.*** 他去游泳,因冷水刺激抽筋了。**menstrual cramps** = cramp in the muscles around the uterus during menstruation 痛经; **stomach cramp** = sharp spasm of the stomach muscles 胃痉挛; **swimmer's cramp** = spasms in arteries and muscles caused by cold water, or swimming soon after a meal 游泳痉挛; **writer's cramp** = spasms and pain in the muscles of the wrist and hand, caused by holding a pen for long periods 书写痉挛

crani- *or* **cranio-** *prefix* referring to the skull 颅

◇ **cranial** *adjective* referring to the skull 颅的; **cranial bone** = one of the bones in the skull 颅骨; **cranial cavity** = space inside the bones of the cranium, in which the brain is situated 颅腔; **cranial nerve** = one of the nerves, twelve on each side, which are connected directly to the brain, governing mainly the structures of the head and neck 颅神经 *see* 见 NERVE

◇ **craniometry** *noun* measuring skulls to find differences in size and shape 颅测量法

◇ **craniopharyngioma** *noun* tumour in the brain originating in hypophyseal duct 颅咽管瘤

◇ **craniostenosis** *or* **craniosynostosis** *noun* early closing of the bones in a baby's skull, so making the skull contract 颅狭小

◇ **craniotabes** *noun* thinness of the bones in the occipital region of a child's skull, caused by rickets, marasmus or syphilis 颅骨软化

◇ **craniotomy** *noun* any surgical operation on the skull, especially cutting away part of the skull 颅骨切开术

◇ **cranium** *or* **skull** *noun* the group of eight bones which surround the brain 头颅

> COMMENT: The cranium consists of the occipital bone, two parietal bones, two temporal bones and the frontal, ethmoid and sphenoid bones. See also SUTURE. The cranial nerves are: I: olfactory. II: optic. III: oculomotor. IV: trochlear. V: trigeminal (ophthalmic, maxillary, mandibular). VI: abducent. VII: facial. VIII: auditory (vestibular, cochlear). IX: glossopharyngeal. X: vagus. XI: accessory. XII: hypoglossal.
> 注释:头颅由枕骨、两块顶骨、两块颞骨和额骨、筛骨、蝶骨组成,参见 SUTURE。颅神经是 I: 嗅神经、II: 视神经、III: 动眼神经、IV: 滑车神经、V: 三叉神经、VI: 外展神经、VII: 面神经、VIII: 听神经、IX: 舌咽神经、X: 迷走神经、XI: 副神经、XII: 舌下神经。

cranky *adjective US* (*informal* 非正式) bad-tempered *or* difficult (child) 任性的

crash 1 *noun* accident where cars, planes, etc. are damaged 交通事故: ***He was killed in a car crash.*** 他在车祸中身亡。***None of the passengers was hurt in the crash.*** 在车祸中没有一位乘客受伤。**crash helmet** = hard hat worn by motorcyclists, etc. 头盔 **2** *verb* (*of vehicles*) to hit something and be damaged 撞坏: ***The car crashed into the wall.*** 车撞到墙上。**The plane crashed** = The plane hit the ground and was damaged. 飞机坠毁了。**3** *adjective*. rapid 急速的,速成的: ***She took a crash course in physiotherapy.*** = a course to learn physiotherapy very quickly 她上了个理疗速成班。

cream *noun* medicinal oily substance, used to rub on the skin 膏; **cold cream** = mixture of almond oil and borax 冷膏

create *verb* to make 制造

creatine *noun* compound of nitrogen found in the muscles and produced by protein metabolism, and excreted as creatinine 肌酸; **creatine phosphate** = store of energy-giving phosphate in muscles 磷酸肌酸

◊ **creatinase** *noun* enzyme which helps break down creatine into creatinine 肌酸酶

◊ **creatinine** *noun* substance which is the form in which creatine is excreted 肌酐; **creatinine clearance** = removal of creatinine from the blood by the kidneys 肌酐清除率

◊ **creatinuria** *noun* excess creatine in the urine 肌酸尿

◊ **creatorrhoea** *noun* presence of undigested muscle fibre in the faeces, occurring in some pancreatic diseases 肉质下泄(粪便中有未消化的肌肉纤维,见于胰岛病变)

Credé's method *noun* (**a**) method of extracting a placenta, by massaging the uterus through the abdomen 克勒德氏法,腹外用手压出胎盘法 (**b**) putting silver nitrate solution into the eyes of a baby born to a mother suffering from gonorrhoea, in order to prevent gonococcal conjunctivitis 新生儿硝酸银滴眼法

creeping eruption *noun* itching skin complaint, caused by larvae of various parasites which creep under the skin 匍行疹(因皮下寄生虫的蚴虫引起)

crepitation *noun* rale, abnormal soft crackling sound heard in the lungs through a stethoscope 捻发音

crepitus *noun* (i) harsh crackling sound heard through a stethoscope in a patient with inflammation of the lungs 捻发音(ii) scratching sound made by a broken bone *or* rough joint 咿轧音

crest *noun* long raised part on a bone 嵴; **crest of ilium** *or* **iliac crest** = curved top edge of the ilium 髂嵴

cretin *noun* patient suffering from congenital hypothyroidism 克汀病人,患先天性甲状腺机能减退的病人

◊ **cretinism** *noun* condition of being a cretin 克汀病

> COMMENT: The condition is due to a defective thyroid gland and affected children, if not treated, develop more slowly than normal, are mentally retarded and have coarse facial features.
> 注释:本病因甲状腺功能缺陷引起,见于儿童,如不治疗,将会发育迟缓、智力减退、面容粗陋。

Creutzfeldt-Jacob disease *noun* disease of the nervous system, caused by a slow-acting virus, which eventually affects the brain; it may be linked to BSE in cows 雅各布氏病, 痉挛性假硬化

crib death *noun US* = COT DEATH 婴儿猝死综合症

cribriform plate *noun* top part of the ethmoid bone which forms the roof of the nasal cavity, and part of the roof of the eye sockets(鼻腔、眼窝的)筛板

cricoid cartilage *noun* ring-shaped cartilage in the lower part of the larynx 环状软骨 ◊见图 LUNGS

cripple 1 *verb* to make someone physically handicapped 使残废: ***She was crippled by arthritis.*** 她因关节炎而残废。***He was crippled in a car crash.*** 他因车祸而残废。**2** *noun* person who is physically disabled 残疾人; **cardiac cripple** = person who has a cardiac disease which makes him unable to work normally 因心脏病而残

◇ **crippling** *adjective* (disease) which makes someone physically handicapped 致残的: ***Arthritis is a crippling disease.*** 关节炎是一种可致残的疾病。

crisis *noun* (**a**) turning point in a disease, after which the patient may start to become better or very much worse 转折点 (**b**) important point *or* time 紧要关头; **mid-life crisis** = MENOPAUSE 绝经(NOTE: plural is **crises**)

> COMMENT: Many diseases progress to a crisis and then the patient rapidly gets better; the opposite situation where the patient gets better very slowly is called lysis.
> 注释:很多疾病发展到转折点后患者会很快康复;相反,一些疾病进展慢恢复也慢,医学上称之为渐退。

crista *noun* crest 嵴; **crista galli** = projection from the ethmoid bone 鸡冠

critical *adjective* (**a**) referring to crisis 转折点的 (**b**) extremely serious 危重的: ***He was taken to hospital in a critical condition.*** 他病情危重被送入医院。***The hospital spokesman said that three of the accident victims were still on the critical list.*** 院方发言人说事故受害者中有3人仍处于危险中。(**c**) which criticizes 批评的: ***The report was critical of the state of aftercare provision.*** 报告对术后护理状况提出了批评。

◇ **critically** *adverb* in a way which criticizes 危重地; **critically ill** = very seriously ill, where it is not known if the patient will get better 危重病

criticize *verb* to say what is wrong with something 批评: ***The report criticized the state of the hospital kitchens.*** 报告批评了医院的厨房状况。

CRNA = CERTIFIED REGISTERED NURSE ANAESTHETIST 注册护理麻醉师

Crohn's disease 克隆氏病 *see* ILEITIS

cross *noun* (**a**) shape made with an upright line with another going across it, used as a sign of the Christian church; (*in anatomy*) any cross-shaped structure 十字形; **the Red Cross** = international organization which provides emergency medical help 红十字 (**b**) mixture of two different breeds 杂交

◇ **cross eye** *or* **convergent strabismus** *noun* condition where a person's eyes both look towards the nose 对眼

◇ **cross-eyed** *adjective* strabismal, with eyes looking towards the nose 对眼的

◇ **cross-infection** *noun* infection passed from one patient to another in hospital, either directly or from nurses, visitors or equipment 交叉感染

◇ **cross-match** *verb* (*in transplant surgery*) matching a donor to a recipient as closely as possible to avoid tissue rejection 交叉配型 *see* 见 BLOOD GROUP

◇ **cross-section** *noun* (**a**) sample cut across a specimen for examination under a microscope 切片: ***He examined a cross-section of the lung tissue.*** 他在检查肺组织切片。(**b**) small part of something, taken to be representative of the whole 样本: ***The team consulted a cross-section of hospital ancillary staff.*** 小组对医院的辅助人员进行抽样调查。

crotamiton *noun* drug used to treat scabies or pruritus 克罗米通(抗疥癣药)

crotch *noun* point where the legs meet the body, where the genitals are 会阴部

croup *noun* Children's disease, acute infection of the upper respiratory passages which blocks the larynx 格鲁布,哮吼(一种喉头炎,尤指儿童喉咙与气管的疾病,常有激烈咳嗽、呼吸困难现象)

> COMMENT: The patient's larynx swells, and he breathes with difficulty and has a barking cough. Attacks usually occur at night. They can be fatal if the larynx becomes completely blocked.
> 注释:患者的喉水肿、呼吸困难、有犬吠样咳嗽,经常夜间发作。如果喉头完全阻塞会引起死亡。

crown *noun* (i) top part of a tooth

(above the level of the gums) 牙冠(ii) artificial top attached to a tooth 牙套 (iii) top part of the head 头顶 ◊ 见图 TOOTH

◊ **crowning** *noun* (i) putting an artificial crown on a tooth 装牙套(ii) stage in childbirth, where the top of the baby's head becomes visible 儿头先露

cruciate ligament *noun* any ligament shaped like a cross, especially the ligaments behind the knee, which prevent the knee from bending forwards 十字韧带

crus *noun* long projecting part 脚,长形突起; **crus cerebri** = one of the nerve tracts between the cerebrum and the medulla oblongata 大脑脚底; **crus of penis** = part of corpus cavernosum attached to the pubic arch 阴茎海绵脚; **crura cerebri** = CEREBRAL PEDUNCLES 大脑脚; **crura of the diaphragm** = long muscle fibres joining the diaphragm to the lumbar vertebrae 膈角 (NOTE: plural is **crura**)

◊ **crural** *adjective* referring to the thigh, leg or shin 腿的

crush *verb* to squash *or* to injure with a heavy weight 压碎: ***He was crushed by falling stones.*** 他被掉下的石头压伤了。

◊ **crush syndrome** *noun* condition where the limb of a patient has been crushed, as in an accident 挤压综合症

> COMMENT: The condition causes kidney failure and shock.
> 注释:可引起肾衰竭和休克。

crutch *noun* strong support for a patient with an injured leg, formed of a stick with either a holding bar and elbow clasp or with a T-bar which fits under the armpit 拐杖; **human crutch** = method of helping an injured person to walk, where the patient puts his arm round the shoulders of a first aider 人体支撑,用肩膀作为支柱帮助患者行走 (**b**) = CROTCH 会阴部

cry 1 *noun* sudden vocal sound 叫喊 **2** *verb* to produce tears because of pain *or* shock *or* fear, etc. 哭: ***She cried when she heard her mother had been killed.*** 当她听说母亲被杀后哭了起来。***The pain made him cry.*** 他疼得哭了起来。***The baby started crying when it was time for its feed.*** 喂奶时间到了,婴儿开始哭了。

cry- *or* **cryo-** *prefix* referring to cold 冷的

◊ **cryaesthesia** *noun* being sensitive to cold 对冷过敏

◊ **cryoprecipitate** *noun* precipitate (such as that from blood plasma) which separates out on freezing and thawing 冷沉淀(物)

> COMMENT: Cryoprecipitate from plasma contains Factor VIII and is used to treat haemophiliacs.
> 注释:血浆的冷沉淀物含有 VIII 因子,可用来治疗血友病。

◊ **cryoprobe** *noun* instrument used in cryosurgery, where the tip is kept very cold to destroy tissue 冷探头,(用极低温度破坏身体某部组织的)冷冻探针

cryosurgery *noun* surgery which uses extremely cold instrument to destroy tissue 低温手术(用很冷的器械破坏组织)

cryotherapy *noun* treatment using extreme cold (as in removing a wart with dry ice) 冷冻治疗

crypt *noun* small cavity in the body 隐窝; **crypts of Lieberkuhn** *or* **Lieberkuhn's glands** = tubular glands found in the mucous membrane of the small and large intestine, especially those between the bases of the villi in the small intestine 利贝昆氏腺,肠腺

crypto- *prefix* hidden 隐藏

◊ **cryptococcal meningitis** *noun* form of meningitis caused by infection with a Cryptococcus fungus, occurring in persons who are immunodeficient 隐球菌脑膜炎

◊ **Cryptococcus** *noun* one of several single-celled yeasts, which exist in the soil and can cause disease 隐球菌(NOTE: plural is **Cryptococci**)

◊ **cryptomenorrhoea** *noun* retention

of menstrual flow probably caused by an obstruction 隐经

◇ **cryptorchidism** *or* **cryptorchism** *noun* condition in a male, where the testicles do not move down into the scrotum 隐睾病

crystal *noun* chemical formation of hard regular-shaped solids 晶体

◇ **crystal violet** *noun* gentian violet, blue antiseptic dye used to paint on skin infections 龙胆紫

◇ **crystalline** *adjective* clear like pure crystal 晶状的

Cs *chemical symbol for* caesium 铯的化学元素符号

CSF = CEREBROSPINAL FLUID 脑脊液

CT *or* **CAT** = COMPUTERIZED (AXIAL) TOMOGRAPHY 计算机轴向体层扫描; **CT scanner** = device which directs a narrow X-ray beam at a thin section of the body from various angles, using a computer to build up a complete picture of the cross-section CT 扫描仪

Cu *chemical symbol for* copper 铜的化学元素符号

cubital *adjective* referring to the ulna 肘的; **cubital fossa** = depression in the front of the elbow joint 肘窝

cuboid bone *noun* one of the tarsal bones in the foot 骰骨 ◊ 见图 FOOT

◇ **cuboidal** *adjective* **cuboidal cell** = cube-shaped epithelial cell 杯状细胞

cuff *noun* (i) inflatable ring put round a patient's arm and inflated when blood pressure is being measured 袖带(ii) inflatable ring put round an endotracheal tube to close the passage 气管插管上的可膨胀环用以封闭气道

cuirass respirator *noun* type of artificial respirator, which surrounds only the patient's chest 胸甲式呼吸器

culdoscope *noun* instrument used to inspect the interior of the female pelvis, introduced through the vagina 后穹窿镜

◇ **culdoscopy** *noun* examination of the interior of a woman's pelvis, using a culdoscope 后穹窿镜检查

cultivate *verb* to make something grow 培养: ***Agar is used as a culture medium to cultivate bacteria in a laboratory.*** 在实验室琼脂被用作培养细菌的培养基。

◇ **culture 1** *noun* bacteria or tissues grown in a laboratory 培养物; **culture medium** *or* **agar** = liquid *or* gel used to grow bacteria *or* tissue 培养基; **stock culture** = basic culture of bacteria from which other cultures can be taken 存储培养基 **2** *verb* to grow bacteria in a culture medium 培养 *see also* 参见 SUBCULTURE

cumulative *adjective* which grows by adding 加的,累积的; **cumulative action** = effect of a drug which is given more often than it can be excreted, and so accumulates in the tissues 积累作用

cuneiform bones *or* **cuneiforms** *noun* three of the tarsal bones in the foot 楔状骨 ◊ 见图 FOOT

cupola *noun* (i) cap 盖(ii) piece of cartilage in a semicircular canal which is moved by the fluid in the canal and connects with the vestibular nerve 钟形感器

curare *noun* drug derived from South American plants, used surgically to paralyse muscles during operations 箭毒

> COMMENT: Curare is the poison used to make poison arrows.
> 注释:箭毒可用来制备毒箭。

curdle *verb* (*of milk*) to coagulate 结成凝乳

cure 1 *noun* particular way of making a patient well *or* of stopping an illness 治疗: ***Scientists are trying to develop a cure for the common cold.*** 科学家正设法寻找治疗普通感冒的方法。**2** *verb* to make a patient healthy 治愈: ***He was completely cured.*** 他彻底治愈了。***Can the doctors cure his bad circulation?*** 医生能治好他的循环不良吗? ***Some forms of cancer can't be cured.*** 有些肿瘤不能治愈。

◇ **curable** *adjective* which can be cured 可治愈的; ***a curable form of*** *cancer* 可治愈的肿瘤 *see also* 参见 INCURABLE

◇ **curative** *adjective* which can cure 能治病的

curettage *or* **curettement** *noun* scraping the inside of a hollow organ to remove a growth or tissue for examination (often used in connection with the uterus) 刮除术 *see also* 参见 D AND C, DILATATION AND CURETTAGE

◇ **curette** *US* 刮匙

◇ **curet** 1 *noun* surgical instrument like a long thin spoon, used for scraping the inside of an organ 刮匙 2 *verb* to scrape with a curette 用刮匙刮

curie *noun* unit of measurement of radioactivity 居里 (NOTE: with figures usually written as **Ci**)

curvature *noun* way in which something bends from a straight line 弯曲; **curvature of the spine** = abnormal bending of the spine forwards or sideways 脊柱弯曲; **greater** *or* **lesser curvature of the stomach** = longer outside convex line of the stomach *or* shorter inside concave line of the stomach 胃大弯或小弯

◇ **curve** 1 *noun* line which bends round 曲线 2 *verb* to make a round shape; to bend something round 使弯曲

◇ **curved** *adjective* with a shape which is not straight or flat 弯的; ***a curved line*** 曲线; ***a curved scalpel*** 弯曲手术刀

Cushing's disease *or* **Cushing's syndrome** *noun* condition where the adrenal cortex produces too many corticosteroids 柯兴氏(病)综合症,肾上腺皮质功能亢进

◇ **cushingoid** *adjective* showing symptoms of Cushing's syndrome 类库兴氏病的

> COMMENT: The syndrome is caused either by a tumour in the adrenal gland, by excessive stimulation of the adrenals by the basophil cells of the pituitary gland, or by a corticosteroidsecreting tumour. The syndrome causes swelling of the face and trunk, the muscles weaken, the blood pressure rises and the body retains salt and water.
> 注释:本病既可因肾上腺肿瘤、垂体中嗜碱性细胞过度刺激肾上腺而致,也可由分泌皮质类固醇的肿瘤引起。症状有面部、躯干肿胀,肌无力,血压升高和水钠储留。

cusp *noun* (**a**) pointed tip of a tooth 牙尖 (**b**) flap of membrane forming a valve in the heart 心瓣膜

◇ **cuspid** *noun* a canine tooth, one of the four pointed teeth next to the incisors (two in the top jaw and two in the lower jaw) 尖牙,犬牙

cut 1 *noun* place where the skin has been penetrated by a sharp instrument 切口: ***She had a bad cut on her left leg.*** 她左腿上有一大切口。***The nurse will put a bandage on your cut.*** 护士会用绷带包扎你的伤口。2 *verb* (**a**) to make an opening using a knife, scissors, etc. 切开: ***The surgeon cut the diseased tissue away with a scalpel.*** 术者用手术刀切除病变组织。***She got tetanus after cutting her finger on the broken glass.*** 她手被碎玻璃划破后得了破伤风。(**b**) to reduce the number of something 减少: ***Accidents have been cut by 10%.*** 事故减少了10%。(NOTE: **cuts - cutting - has cut**)

cutaneous *adjective* referring to the skin 皮肤的; **cutaneous leishmaniasis** = form of skin disease caused by the tropical parasite *Leishmania* 利什曼皮肤病

cuticle *noun* (i) epidermis, the outer layer of skin 表皮 (ii) strip of epidermis attached at the base of a nail 护膜(附于甲床的表皮)

◇ **cutis** *noun* skin 皮肤; **cutis anserina** = goose flesh *or* goose pimples *or* reaction of the skin to being cold *or* frightened, where the skin is raised into many little bumps by the action of the arrector pili muscles 鸡皮疙瘩

CVA = CEREBROVASCULAR ACCIDENT 脑血管意外

cyanide *noun* prussic acid, salt of hydrocyanic acid, a poison which kills very rapidly when drunk or inhaled 氰化物

cyano- *prefix* blue 青,蓝

◇ **cyanocobalamin** = VITAMIN B_{12} 氰钴胺,维生素 B_{12}

◇ **cyanosis** *noun* blue colour of the peripheral skin and mucous membranes, symptom of lack of oxygen in the blood (as in a blue baby) 紫绀

◇ **cyanosed** *adjective* with blue skin 发绀的: ***The patient was cyanosed round the lips.*** 患者口唇发绀。

◇ **cyanotic** *adjective* suffering from cyanosis 患紫绀的; **cyanotic congenital heart disease** = cyanosis 紫绀性先心病

cyclandelate *noun* drug used to treat cerebrovascular disease 环扁桃酯

cycle *noun* (**a**) series of events which recur regularly 周期; **menstrual cycle** = period (usually 28 days) during which the endometrium develops, a woman ovulates, and menstruation takes place 月经周期; **ovarian cycle** = regular changes in the ovary during reproductive life 排卵周期 (**b**) bicycle, a vehicle with two wheels 自行车; **exercise cycle** = type of cycle which is fixed to the floor, so that someone can pedal on it for exercise 健身车

◇ **cyclical** *adjective* referring to cycles 周期性的; **cyclical vomiting** = repeated attacks of vomiting 周期性呕吐

cyclitis *noun* inflammation of the ciliary body in the eye 睫状体炎

cyclizine *noun* antihistamine drug used in the treatment of travel sickness, pregnancy sickness *or* inner ear disorders 赛克利嗪(抗组胺药,用于晕车、妊娠反应或耳内疾病)

cyclo- *prefix* meaning cyclical *or* referring to cycles 环

◇ **cyclodialysis** *noun* surgical operation to connect the anterior chamber of the eye and the choroid, as treatment of glaucoma 睫状体分离术

◇ **cycloplegia** *noun* paralysis of the ciliary muscle which makes it impossible for the eye to focus properly 睫状肌麻痹

◇ **cyclothymia** *noun* mild form of manic depression, where the patient suffers from alternating depression and excitement 躁狂抑郁性精神障碍

◇ **cyclotomy** *noun* surgical operation to make a cut in the ciliary body 睫状肌切开术

cyesis *noun* pregnancy, condition where a woman is carrying an unborn child in her womb 妊娠

cylinder 量筒,圆柱 *see* 见 OXYGEN

cyst *noun* abnormal growth in the body shaped like a pouch, containing liquid *or* semi-liquid substances 囊肿; **branchial cyst** = cyst on the side of the neck of an embryo 鳃裂囊肿; **dental cyst** = cyst near the root of a tooth 牙囊肿; **dermoid cyst** = cyst found under the skin, usually in the midline, containing hair, sweat glands and sebaceous glands 皮样囊肿; **ovarian cyst** = cyst which develops in the ovaries 卵巢囊肿; **parasitic cyst** = cyst produced by a parasite, usually in the liver 寄生虫囊肿; **pilonidal cyst** = cyst at the bottom of the spine near the buttocks 毛窝瘘,藏毛囊肿;**sebaceous cyst** *or* **wen** = cyst which forms in a sebaceous gland 皮脂囊肿

◇ **cyst-** *prefix* referring to the bladder 膀胱的

◇ **cystadenoma** *noun* adenoma in which fluid-filled cysts form 囊腺瘤

◇ **cystalgia** *noun* pain in the urinary bladder 膀胱痛

◇ **cystectomy** *noun* surgical operation to remove all *or* part of the urinary bladder 膀胱切除术

◇ **cystic** *adjective* (**a**) referring to cysts 胆囊的 (**b**) referring to a bladder 膀胱的; **cystic artery** = artery leading from the hepatic artery to the gall bladder 胆囊动脉; **cystic duct** = duct which takes bile from the gall bladder to the common bile duct 胆囊管; **cystic vein** = vein which drains the gall bladder 胆囊静脉

◇ **cystica** 囊肿 *see* 见 SPINA BIFIDA

◇ **cysticercosis** *noun* disease caused by infestation of tapeworm larvae from pork 囊尾蚴病(囊虫病)

◇ **cysticercus** *noun* bladder worm, the larva of a tapeworm found in pork, which is enclosed in a cyst, typical of *Taenia* 囊尾蚴

◇ **cystic fibrosis** *noun* fibrocystic disease of the pancreas *or* mucoviscidosis, hereditary disease in which there is malfunction of the exocrine glands, such as the pancreas, in particular those which secrete mucus 纤维性囊肿病或粘稠物阻塞症(遗传性疾病,胰腺等外分泌腺,尤其是分泌粘液的腺体功能不全)

> COMMENT: The thick mucous secretions cause blockage of ducts and many serious secondary effects in the intestines and lungs. Symptoms include loss of weight, abnormal faeces and bronchitis. If diagnosed early, cystic fibrosis can be controlled with vitamins, physiotherapy and pancreatic enzymes.
> 注释:分泌的粘稠粘液堵塞导管,并在肠道、肺导致许多严重的后果。症状有体重下降,粪便异常和支气管炎。如果早期诊断,可以用维生素、理疗和胰酶进行治疗。

◇ **cystine** *noun* amino acid found in protein: it can cause stones to form in the urinary system of patients suffering from a rare inherited metabolic disorder 胱氨酸

◇ **cystinosis** *noun* defective absorption of amino acids, which results in excessive amounts of cystine accumulating in the kidneys 胱氨酸病

◇ **cystinuria** *noun* cystine in the urine 胱氨酸尿

◇ **cystitis** *noun* inflammation of the urinary bladder, which makes a patient pass water often and giving a burning sensation 膀胱炎

◇ **cystocele** *noun* hernia of the urinary bladder into the vagina 膀胱突出

◇ **cystogram** *noun* X-ray photograph of the urinary bladder 膀胱造影

◇ **cystography** *noun* examination of the urinary bladder by X-rays after radio-opaque dye has been introduced 膀胱造影术

◇ **cystolithiasis** *noun* condition where stones are formed in the urinary bladder 膀胱结石

◇ **cystometer** *noun* apparatus which measures the pressure in the bladder 膀胱内压测量器

◇ **cystometry** *noun* measurement of the pressure in the bladder 膀胱内压测量

◇ **cystopexy** *noun* vesicofixation, surgical operation to fix the bladder in a different position 膀胱固定术

◇ **cystoscope** *noun* instrument made of a long tube with a light at the end, used to inspect the inside of the bladder 膀胱镜

◇ **cystoscopy** *noun* examination of the bladder using a cystoscope 膀胱镜检查

◇ **cystostomy** *noun* vesicostomy, surgical operation to make an opening between the bladder and the abdominal wall to allow urine to pass without going through the urethra 膀胱造口术

◇ **cystotomy** *noun* vesicotomy, surgical operation to make a cut in a bladder 膀胱切开术

cyt- *or* **cyto-** *prefix* referring to cells 细胞的

◇ **cytarabine** *noun* antiviral drug 阿糖胞苷

◇ **cytochemistry** *noun* study of the chemical activity of living cells 细胞化学

◇ **cytogenetics** *noun* branch of genetics, which studies the structure and function of cells, especially the chromosomes 细胞遗传学

◇ **cytokinesis** *noun* changes in the cytoplasm of a cell during division 胞质分裂

◇ **cytological smear** *noun* sample of tissue taken for examination under a microscope 细胞涂片

◇ **cytology** *noun* study of the structure and function of cells 细胞学

◇ **cytolysis** *noun* breaking down of

cells 细胞溶解

◇ **cytomegalovirus** (**CMV**) *noun* virus (one of the herpesviruses) which can cause serious congenital disorders in a fetus if it infects the pregnant mother 巨细胞病毒

◇ **cytometer** *noun* instrument attached to a microscope, used for measuring and counting the number of cells in a specimen 细胞计数器

◇ **cytopenia** *noun* deficiency of cellular elements in blood *or* tissue 细胞减少

◇ **cytoplasm** *noun* substance inside the cell membrane, which surrounds the nucleus of a cell 细胞质

◇ **cytoplasmic** *adjective* referring to the cytoplasm of a cell 细胞质的

◇ **cytosine** *noun* one of the four basic elements of DNA 胞嘧啶

◇ **cytosome** *noun* body of a cell, not including the nucleus 胞质体

◇ **cytotoxic drug** *noun* drug which reduces the reproduction of cells, and is used to treat cancer 细胞毒药物

◇ **cytotoxin** *noun* substance which has a toxic effect on cells of certain organs 细胞毒素

Dd

Vitamin D *noun* vitamin which is soluble in fat, and is found in butter, eggs and fish; it is also produced by the skin when exposed to sunlight 维生素 D

COMMENT: Vitamin D helps in the formation of bones, and lack of it causes rickets in children
注释:维生素 D 有助于骨的形成,缺乏维生素 D 可导致佝偻病。

d *symbol for* deci- 十分之一

da *symbol for* deca- 十

dab *verb* to touch lightly 轻触: ***He dabbed the cut with a piece of absorbent cotton.*** 他用吸水棉球轻拭伤口。

da Costa's syndrome *noun* disordered action of the heart, a condition where the patient suffers palpitations, breathlessness and dizziness, caused by effort or worry 达科斯塔氏综和症,神经性循环衰弱

dacryo- *prefix* referring to tears 泪的

◇ **dacryoadenitis** *noun* inflammation of the lacrimal gland 泪腺炎

◇ **dacryocystitis** *noun* inflammation of the lacrimal sac when the tear duct, which drains into the nose, becomes blocked 泪囊炎

◇ **dacryocystography** *noun* contrast radiography to determine the site of an obstruction in the tear ducts 泪囊造影术

◇ **dacryocystorhinostomy** (**DCR**) *noun* surgical operation to bypass a blockage from the tear duct which takes tears into the nose 泪囊鼻腔造口术

◇ **dacryolith** *noun* stone in the lacrimal sac 泪石

◇ **dacryoma** *noun* benign swelling in one of the tear ducts 泪囊肿大

dactyl 1 *noun* finger or toe 指,趾 **2** prefix **dactyl-** = referring to fingers or toes 指(趾)的

◇ **dactylitis** *noun* inflammation of the fingers or toes, caused by bone infection or rheumatic disease 指(趾)炎

◇ **dactylology** *noun* deaf and dumb language, signs made with the fingers, used in place of words when talking to a deaf and dumb person, or when a deaf and dumb person wants to communicate 手语

DAH = DISORDERED ACTION OF THE HEART 神经性循环衰弱

daily 1 *adjective* which happens every day 每天的: ***You should do daily exercises to keep fit.*** 你应该每天锻炼以保持身体健康。**2** *adverb* every day 每天地: ***Take the medicine twice daily.*** 每天吃两次药。

Daltonism *noun* protanopia, the commonest form of colour blindness, where the patient can not see red 红色盲 *compare* 比较 DEUTERANOPIA, TRITANOPIA

damage 1 *noun* harm done to things 损害: ***The disease caused damage to the brain cells.*** 这疾病可损害脑细胞。**bone damage** *or* **tissue damage** = damage caused to a bone *or* to tissue 骨损伤或组织损伤 **2** *verb* to harm something 损害: ***His hearing or his sense of balance was damaged in the accident.*** 他的听力或平衡感在事故中受了损害。***a surgical operation to remove damaged tissue*** 祛除损伤组织的手术

damp *adjective* slightly wet 潮湿的: ***You should put a damp compress on the bruise.*** 你应该拿块湿敷布放在瘀伤处。

D and C = DILATATION AND CURETTAGE 刮除术

D and V = DIARRHOEA AND VOMITING 腹泻和呕吐

dandruff *noun* scurf *or* pityriasis capitis, pieces of dead skin which form on the scalp and fall out when the hair is combed 头皮屑

danger *noun* possibility of harm *or* death 危险: ***Unless the glaucoma is treated quickly, there's a danger that the patient will lose his eyesight*** *or* ***a danger of the patient losing his***

eyesight*.**除非尽快治疗青光眼,否则患者有失明的危险。The doctors say she's out of danger*.** = She is not likely to die.医生说她已经度过了危险期。

◇ **dangerous** *adjective* which can cause harm or death 有危险的: ***Don't touch the electric wires - they're dangerous*.** 不要触电线,有危险。***Cigarettes are dangerous to health*.** 抽烟对身体有害。**dangerous drugs** = drugs (such as morphine or heroin) which are harmful and are not available to the general public, and also poisons which can only be sold to certain persons 危险药品

dark 1 *adjective* (**a**) with very little light 暗的: ***Switch the lights on — it's getting too dark to read*.** 把灯打开,天太黑得看不清字。***In the winter it gets dark early*.** 冬天天黑得早。**dark adaptation** = change in the retina and pupil of the eye to adapt to dim light after being in normal light 暗适应 (**b**) with black or brown hair 黑色或棕色头发的: ***He's dark, but his sister is fair*.** 他是黑发,但他姐姐是金发。(NOTE: **dark - darker - darkest**) **2** *noun* lack of light 黑暗: ***She is afraid of the dark*.** 她害怕黑暗。***Cats can see in the dark*.** 猫可以在黑暗中看见东西。

◇ **darkening** *noun* becoming darker in colour 色变深: ***Darkening of the tissue takes place after bruising*.** 挫伤后组织变青了。

◇ **darkroom** *noun* room with no light, in which photographic film can be developed 暗室: ***The X-rays are in the darkroom, so they should be ready soon*.** X线片在暗室里,很快就可以阅片了。He hopes to get a job as a darkroom technician. 他希望做个暗室技术员。

data *noun* any information (in words or figures) about a certain subject, especially information which is available on computer 数据; **data bank** *or* **bank of data** = *store of information in a computer* 数据库: ***The hospital keeps a data bank of information about possible kidney donors*.** 医院有个肾供者情况的数据库。

date *noun* number of a day or year, name of a month (when something happened) 日期: ***What's the date today?*** 今天是几号? ***What is the date of your next appointment*.** 你下一次约会是什么时候? ***Do you remember the date of your last checkup*** ?你还记得你上一次检查的时间吗? **up-to-date** = very modern *or* using very recent information *or* equipment 最新的,现代的: ***The new hospital is provided with the most up-to-date equipment*.** 这家医院配有最新的设备。**out-of-date** = not modern 过时的: ***The surgeons have to work with out-of-date equipment*.** 外科医师不得不用过时的设备进行工作。

daughter *noun* girl child of a parent 女儿: ***They have two sons and one daughter*.** 他们有 *2* 个儿子和 *1* 个女儿。**daughter cell** = one of the cells which develop by mitosis from a single parent cell 子细胞

day *noun* (i) period of 24 hours 天 (ii) period from morning until night, when it is light 白天: ***He works all day in the office, and then visits patients in the hospital in the evening*.** 他白天在办公室工作,晚上到医院探望患者。***Take two tablets three times a day*.** 每天3次,每次2片药。***She's attending a day unit for disabled patients*.** 她白天护理残疾病人。**day hospital** = hospital where patients are treated during the day and go home in the evenings 日间医院; **day nursery** = place where small children can be looked after during the daytime, while their parents are at work 日托幼儿园; **day patient** *or* **day case** = patient who is in hospital for treatment for a day (i.e. one who does not stay overnight) 日间病人,日间病例; **day recovery ward** = ward where day patients who have had minor operations can recover before going home 日间康复病房; **day surgery** = surgical operation which does not require the patient to stay overnight in hospital 日间手术

> QUOTE: Paediatric day-surgery patients spend on average between 2 and 8 hours in hospital.
> 引文：儿科的日间手术病人平均留院时间为2～8 小时。
> **British Journal of Nursing** 英国护理杂志

◊ **day blindness** = HEMERALOPIA 昼盲症

◊ **daylight** *noun* light during the day 日光

◊ **daytime** *noun* period of light between morning and night 白天: ***He works at night and sleeps during the daytime.*** 他晚上工作,白天睡觉。

dazed *adjective* confused in the mind 茫然的,迷乱的: ***She was found walking about in a dazed condition.*** 她被发现在恍惚状态下四处乱走。***He was dazed after the accident.*** 事故后他就处于茫然状态。

dB = DECIBEL 分贝

DCR = DACRYOCYSTORHINOSTOMY 泪囊鼻腔造口术

DDS *US* = DOCTOR OF DENTAL SURGERY 口腔外科医师

DDT = DICHLORODIPHENYLTRICHLOROETHANE 滴滴涕

de- *prefix* meaning removal *or* loss 除去

dead *adjective* (**a**) not alive 死的: ***My grandparents are both dead.*** 我的祖父母都去世了。***When the injured man arrived at hospital he was found to be dead.*** 当伤者被送到医院时他已经死了。***The woman was rescued from the crash, but was certified dead on arrival at the hospital.*** 这名妇女被从车祸中救了出来,但送到医院时被确认已经死亡。(**b**) not sensitive 麻木: ***The nerve endings are dead.*** 神经末梢麻木了。***His fingers went dead.*** 他的手指麻木了。(**c**) **dead space** = breath in the last part of the inspiration which does not get further than the bronchial tubes 死腔

◊ **deaden** *verb* to make (pain or noise) less strong 减轻(疼痛,噪音): ***The doctor gave him an injection to deaden the pain.*** 医生给他打了一针以减轻疼痛。

◊ **deadly** *adjective* likely to kill 致命的: ***Cyanide is a deadly poison.*** 氰化物是一种可致命的毒物。**deadly nightshade** = BELLADONNA 颠茄

◊ **dead (man's) fingers** = RAYNAUD'S DISEASE 雷诺氏病

deaf 1 *adjective* not able to hear 聋的: ***You have to shout when you speak to Mr Jones because he's quite deaf.*** 你跟约翰先生说话时必须大声嚷嚷,他相当耳背。**totally deaf** *or* **completely deaf** *or* **stone deaf** = unable to hear any sound at all 完全耳聋的; **partially deaf** = able to hear some sounds but not all 部分耳聋的; **deaf and dumb** = not able to hear or to speak 聋哑的; **deaf and dumb language** *or* **sign language** *or* **dactylology** = signs made with the fingers, used instead of words when talking to a trained deaf and dumb person, or when a deaf and dumb person wants to communicate 手语 **2** *noun* **the deaf** = people who are deaf 聋人: ***Hearing aids can be of great use to the partially deaf.*** 助听器对不完全耳聋的患者有很大帮助。

◊ **deafen** *verb* to make (someone) deaf for a time 使聋: ***He was deafened by the explosion.*** 他被爆炸声震聋了。

◊ **deafness** *noun* loss of hearing; being unable to hear 耳聋; **conductive deafness** = deafness caused by defective conduction of sound into the inner ear 传导性耳聋; **partial deafness** = (i) being able to hear some tones, but not all 不完全耳聋,不能听见某些音调的声音 (ii) general dulling of the whole range of hearing 不完全耳聋,对各种声调普遍的听力迟钝; **perceptive deafness** *or* **sensorineural deafness** = deafness caused by a disorder in the auditory nerves *or* the cochlea *or* the brain centres which receive impulses from the nerves 感受性耳聋; **progressive deafness** = condition, common in people as they get older, where a person gradually becomes more and more deaf 进行性耳聋；**total deafness** = being unable to hear any sound at all 完全耳聋

COMMENT：Deafness has many degrees and many causes：old age, viruses, exposure to continuous loud noise or intermittent loud explosions, and diseases such as German measles.
注释：耳聋分为很多级，病因也很多，如：老年、病毒、暴露于持续的高噪声或间断的爆炸声以及风疹等疾病。

deaminate *verb* to remove an amino group from an amino acid, forming ammonia 脱氨基

◊ **deamination** *noun* removal of an amino group from an amino acid, forming ammonia 脱氨基作用

COMMENT：After deamination, the ammonia which is formed is converted to urea by the liver, while the remaining carbon and hydrogen from the amino acid provide the body with heat and energy.
注释：脱氨基后产生的氨被肝脏转化为尿素，剩余的碳和氢为机体提供热能。

death *noun* dying; end of life 死亡：***His sudden death shocked his friends.*** 他的突然死亡使他的朋友很震惊。***He met his death in a car crash.*** 他在一场车祸中丧生。**death certificate** = official document signed by a doctor, stating that a person has died and giving details of the person and the cause of death 死亡证明；**death rate** = number of deaths per year per thousand of population 死亡率：***The death rate from cancer of the liver has remained stable.*** 肝癌的死亡率保持恒定。**brain death** = condition where the nerves in the brain stem have died, and the patient can be certified as dead, although the heart may not have stopped beating 脑死亡；**cot death** *US* **crib death** = sudden death of a baby in bed, with no identifiable cause 婴儿猝死（NOTE：for terms referring to death see words beginning with **necro-**）

debilitate *verb* to make weak 使虚弱：***He was debilitated by a long illness.*** 久病后他很虚弱。**debilitating disease** = disease which makes the patient weak 消耗性疾病

◊ **debility** *noun* general weakness 虚弱

debridement *noun* removal of dirt or dead tissue from a wound to help healing 清创术

deca- *prefix meaning* ten 十（NOTE：symbol is **da**）

decaffeinated *adjective* （coffee）with the caffeine removed 不含咖啡因的（咖啡）

decalcification *noun* loss of calcium salts from teeth and bones 脱钙

decapsulation *noun* surgical operation to remove a capsule from an organ, especially from a kidney 被膜剥除术

decay **1** *noun* process by which tissues become rotten, caused by the action of microbes and oxygen 腐蚀 **2** *verb*（*of tissue*）to rot 腐蚀：***The surgeon removed decayed matter from the wound.*** 术者从伤口清除掉腐败物。

deci- *prefix* meaning one tenth (10^{-1}) 十分之一（NOTE：symbol is **d**）

decibel *noun* unit of measurement of the loudness of sound, used to compare different levels of sound 分贝（NOTE：usually written **dB** with figures：**20dB**：say ‘twenty decibels’）

COMMENT：Normal conversation is at about 50dB. Very loud noise with a value of over 120dB（such as aircraft engines）can cause pain.
注释：一般谈话的声强是 50 分贝，大于 120 分贝以上的噪声（如飞机发动机）可引起疼痛。

decidua *noun* membrane which lines the uterus after fertilization 蜕膜

COMMENT：The decidua is divided into several parts：the decidua basalis, where the embryo is attached, the decidua capsularis, which covers the embryo and the decidua vera which is the rest of the decidua not touching the embryo；it is expelled

after the birth of the baby.
注释：蜕膜可分为几个部分：基底蜕膜，是胚胎附着部；蜕膜囊包绕胚胎；而壁蜕膜是不接触胚胎的蜕膜，在婴儿出生后被排出。

◇ **deciduous** *adjective* **deciduous teeth** *or* **milk teeth** = a child's first twenty teeth, which are gradually replaced by the permanent teeth 乳牙

decilitre *or US* **deciliter** *noun* unit of measurement of liquid (= one tenth of a litre) 分升（NOTE: with figures usually written **dl**）

decimetre *or US* **decimeter** *noun* unit of measurement of length (= one tenth of a metre) 分米（NOTE: with figures usually written **dm**）

decompensation *noun* condition where an organ such as the heart cannot cope with extra stress placed on it (and so is unable to circulate the blood properly) 失代偿

decompose *verb* to rot *or* to become putrefied 分解

◇ **decomposition** *noun* process where dead matter is rotted by the action of bacteria *or* fungi 分解作用

decompression *noun* (**a**) reduction of pressure 减压；**cardiac decompression** = removal of a haematoma *or* constriction of the heart 心脏减压；**cerebral decompression** = removal of part of the skull to relieve pressure on the brain 脑减压 (**b**) controlled reduction of atmospheric pressure which occurs as a diver returns to the surface 控制下减压；**decompression sickness** = CAISSON DISEASE 减压病

decongestant *adjective* & *noun* (drug) which reduces congestion and swelling, sometimes used to unblock the nasal passages 减轻充血剂、消肿剂

decortication *noun* surgical removal of the cortex of an organ 去皮质术；**decortication of a lung** = pleurectomy, a surgical operation to remove part of the pleura which has been thickened or made stiff by chronic empyema 胸膜外纤维层剥除术，胸膜切除术

decrease 1 *noun* lowering in numbers *or* becoming less 减少 ***a decrease in the numbers of new cases being notified*** 注意到了新发病例数的减少 **2** *verb* to become less *or* to make something less 使减少：***His blood pressure has decreased to a more normal level.*** 他的血压降到了正常水平。***The pressure in the vessel is gradually decreased.*** 血管内的压力逐渐下降。

decubitus *noun* position of a patient who is lying down 卧床；**decubitus ulcer** = BEDSORE 褥疮

decussation *noun* chiasma, crossing of nerve fibres in the central nervous system 交叉

deep *adjective* (**a**) which goes a long way down 深的：***Be careful — the water is very deep here.*** 当心，这儿水很深。***The wound is several millimetres deep.*** 伤口有几毫米深。**take a deep breath** = to inhale a large amount of air 深呼吸 (**b**) inside the body, further from the skin 深部的：***The internal intercostal muscle is deep to the external.*** 肋间内肌在肋间外肌的深面。**deep vein** = vein which is inside the body near a bone, as opposed to a superficial vein near the skin 深静脉；**deep vein thrombosis (DVT)** *or* **phlebothrombosis** = thrombus in the deep veins of a leg or the pelvis 深静脉血栓形成，深静脉血栓；**deep facial vein** = small vein which drains from the pterygoid process behind the cheek into the facial vein 面深静脉（NOTE: the opposite is **superficial.** Note also that a part is **deep to** another part）

◇ **deeply** *adverb* (breathing) which takes in a large amount of air 深吸气地：***He was breathing deeply.*** 他在深吸气。

defaecate *verb* to pass faeces from the bowels 排便

◇ **defaecation** *noun* passing out faeces from the bowels 排便

defect *noun* (i) wrong formation *or* something which is badly formed 畸形

(ii)lack of something which is necessary 缺陷; **birth defect** *or* **congenital defect** = malformation which exists in a person's body from birth 先天性缺陷

◇ **defective 1** *adjective* which works badly *or* which is wrongly formed 缺陷的,畸形的: ***The surgeons operated to repair a defective heart valve.*** 外科医师修补了有缺陷的心瓣膜。**2** *noun* person suffering from severe mental subnormality 智残

defence *noun* (i) resistance against an attack of a disease 抵抗力(ii) behaviour of a person which is aimed at protecting him from harm 防卫; **muscular defence** = rigidity of muscles associated with inflammation such as peritonitis 肌卫; **defence mechanism** = subconscious reflex by which a person prevents himself from showing emotion 防御机制

deferent *adjective* (i) which goes away from the centre 远离的,输出的(ii) referring to the vas deferens 输精管的

◇ **deferens** 输精管 *see* 见 VAS DEFERENS

defervescence *noun* period during which a fever is subsiding 退热期

defibrillation *noun* cardioversion, correcting an irregular heartbeat by using an electric impulse 除颤

◇ **defibrillator** *noun* apparatus used to apply an electric impluse to the heart to make it beat regularly 除颤器

defibrination *noun* removal of fibrin from a blood sample to prevent clotting 脱纤维蛋白

deficiency *noun* lack *or* not having enough of something 缺乏; **deficiency disease** = disease caused by lack of an essential element in the diet(such as vitamins, essential amino and fatty acids, etc.)营养缺乏性疾病; **iron-deficiency anaemia** = anaemia caused by lack of iron in red blood cells 缺铁性贫血; **vitamin deficiency** = lack of vitamins 维生素缺乏; **immunodeficiency** = lack of immunity to a disease 免疫缺陷

◇ **deficient** *adjective* **deficient in something** = not containing the necessary amount of something 缺少…: ***His diet is deficient in calcium*** *or* ***he has a calcium-deficient diet.*** 他的膳食缺少钙。

defloration *noun* breaking the hymen of a virgin usually at the first sexual intercourse 处女膜破裂,破膜

deflorescence *noun* disappearance of a rash 皮疹消退

deformed *adjective* not shaped or formed in a normal way 畸形的

◇ **deformans** 畸形的 *see* 见 OSTEITIS

◇ **deformation** *noun* becoming deformed 畸形: ***The later stages of the disease are marked by bone deformation.*** 疾病的晚期表现为骨骼变形。

◇ **deformity** *noun* abnormal shape of part of the body 畸形

degenerate *verb* to change so as not to be able to function 退化, 变性: ***His brain degenerated so much that he was incapable of looking after himself.*** 他的大脑严重退化,已不能自己照顾自己。

◇ **degeneration** *noun* change in the structure of a cell *or* organ so that it no longer works properly 变性; **adipose degeneration** *or* **fatty degeneration** = accumulation of fat in the cells of an organ (such as the heart *or* liver), making the organ less able to perform 脂肪变性; **calcareous degeneration** = deposits of calcium which form at joints in old age 石灰变性; **fibroid degeneration** = change of normal tissue to fibrous tissue (as in cirrhosis of the liver) 纤维样变性

◇ **degenerative** *adjective* (disease) where a part of the body stops functioning *or* functions abnormally 退化的

> QUOTE: The weight-bearing joints, such as the spine, hip and knees, are the most frequent sites of degenerative disease.
> 引文:承重关节如:脊柱、髋关节和膝关节是变性性疾病最常侵及的部位。
> **British Journal of Nursing**
> 英国护理杂志

deglutition *noun* swallowing, the action of passing food *or* liquid (sometimes also air) from the mouth into the oesophagus 吞咽

degree *noun* (**a**) (*in science*) unit of measurement 度: ***A circle has 360°.*** 圆是360度。***The temperature is only 20°Celsius.*** 温度只有20摄氏度。(NOTE: the word **degree** is written ° after figures: **40°C**: say: 'forty degrees Celsius') (**b**) title given by a university or college to a person who has successfully completed a course of studies 学位: ***He has a medical degree from London University.*** 他在伦敦大学获得了医学学位。***She was awarded a first-class degree in pharmacy.*** 她被授予药学一级学位。(**c**) level of how important *or* serious something is 等级; **to a minor degree** = in a small way 低等级、低水平; **degree of burn** = the amount of damage done to the skin and tissue by light *or* heat *or* radiation *or* electricity *or* chemicals 烧伤度; **first-degree burn** = burn where the skin turns red because the epidermis has been affected 一度烧伤; **second-degree burn** = burn where the skin becomes very red and blisters 二度烧伤 *see also* 参见 BURN

COMMENT: Burns were formerly classified by degrees and are still often referred to in this way. The modern classification is into two categories: deep and superficial.
注释:烧伤以前是按度分级,现在也经常应用。最新分法将其分为两类:深部烧伤和浅表烧伤。

dehisced *adjective* (wound) which has split open again 裂开的

◇ **dehiscence** *noun* opening wide 裂开; **wound dehiscence** = splitting open of a surgical incision 手术切口裂开

dehydrate *verb* to lose water 脱水: ***After two days without food or drink, he became dehydrated.*** 两天没吃没喝,他开始脱水。

◇ **dehydration** *noun* loss of water 脱水

COMMENT: Water is more essential than food for a human being's survival. If someone drinks during the day less liquid than is passed out of the body in urine and sweat, he begins to dehydrate.
注释:对人生存来说,水比食物更重要。如果有人一天的饮水少于从尿和汗中排泄的水分,他就会脱水。

QUOTE: An estimated 60 – 70% of diarrhoeal deaths are caused by dehydration.
引文:腹泻引起的死亡中60%~70%是因脱水造成的。

Indian Journal of Medical Sciences 印度医学科学杂志

déjà vu *noun* illusion that a new situation is a previous one being repeated, usually caused by a disease of the brain 似曾相识症

deletion *noun* 缺失; **chromosomal deletion** = chromosomal aberration in which a part of the chromosome is lost or removed 染色体缺失

Delhi boil *noun* cutaneous Leishmaniasis, a tropical skin disease caused by the parasite Leishmania 皮肤利什曼病

delicate *adjective* (i) easily broken or harmed 柔弱的(ii) easily falling ill 易患病的: ***The bones of a baby's skull are very delicate.*** 婴儿的头盖骨很稚嫩。***The eye is covered by a delicate membrane.*** 眼球覆有一层柔软的薄膜。***The surgeons carried out a delicate operation to join the severed nerves.*** 外科医师做了精细的手术来连接切断的神经。***His delicate state of health means that he is not able to work long hours.*** 他虚弱的身体状况意味着他不能长时间的工作。

delirium *noun* mental state where the patient is confused, excited, restless and has hallucinations 谵妄; **delirium tremens (DTs)** *or* **delirium alcoholicum** = state of mental disturbance, especially including hallucinations about insects, trembling and excitement, usually found in chronic alcoholics who attempt to give up alcohol consumption 震颤性谵妄

◇ **delirious** *adjective* suffering from delirium 谵妄的

> COMMENT: A person can become delirious because of shock, fear, drugs or fever.
> 注释:人会因为休克、恐惧、药物和发热而出现谵妄。

deliver *verb* to bring something to someone 送; **to deliver a baby** = to help a mother in childbirth 助产: ***The twins were delivered by the midwife.*** 这对双胞胎是由助产士帮助分娩的。

◇ **delivery** *noun* birth of a child 分娩: ***The delivery went very smoothly.*** 分娩很顺利。**breech delivery** = birth where the baby's buttocks appear first 臀先露; **face delivery** = birth where the baby's face appears first 面先露; **forceps delivery** *or* **instrumental delivery** = childbirth where the doctor uses forceps to help the baby out of the mother's womb 产钳分娩; **spontaneous delivery** = delivery which takes places naturally, without any medical or surgical help 自然分娩,顺产; **vertex delivery** = normal birth, where the baby's head appears first 头位分娩; **delivery bed** = special bed on which a mother lies to give birth 产床

delta *noun* fourth letter of the Greek alphabet 希腊字母表的第4个字母; **hepatitis** *or* **hepatitis delta** = severe form of hepatitis caused by the delta virus in conjunction with HBV 丁型肝炎; **delta virus** = virus which causes hepatitis delta 丁型肝炎病毒

deltoid (muscle) *noun* big triangular muscle covering the shoulder joint and attached to the humerus, which lifts the arm sideways 三角肌; **deltoid tuberosity** = raised part of the humerus to which the deltoid muscle is attached 三角肌粗隆

delusion *noun* false belief which a person holds which cannot be changed by reason 妄想: ***He suffered from the delusion that he was wanted by the police.*** 他有被警察追捕的妄想。

dementia *noun* loss of mental ability and memory, causing disorientation and personality changes, due to organic disease of the brain 痴呆; **AIDS dementia** = form of mental degeneration resulting from infection with HIV 艾滋病性痴呆; **presenile dementia** = form of mental degeneration affecting adults 早老性痴呆; **senile dementia** = form of mental degeneration affecting old people 老年性痴呆; **dementia paralytica** = general paralysis of the insane, a serious condition marking the final stages of syphilis 麻痹性痴呆; **dementia praecox** = formerly the name given to schizophrenia 早发性痴呆

◇ **dementing** *adjective* (patient) suffering from dementia 痴呆的

> QUOTE: AIDS dementia is a major complication of HIV infection, occurring in 70 - 90% of patients.
> 引文:艾滋病性痴呆是HIV病毒感染的主要并发症,发生率为70%~90%。
> **British Journal of Nursing** 英国护理杂志

demography *noun* study of populations and environments *or* changes affecting populations 人口学

◇ **demographic** *adjective* referring to demography 人口学的; **demographic forecasts** = forecasts of the numbers of people of different ages and sexes in an area at some time in the future 人口预测

demonstrate *verb* to show how something is done *or* is used 示教: ***The surgeon demonstrated how to make the incision or demonstrated the incision.*** 术者演示怎样做切口。

◇ **demonstrator** *noun* person who demonstrates, especially in a laboratory *or* surgical department 示教者

demulcent *noun* soothing substance which relieves irritation in the stomach 缓和药,和胃药。

demyelination *or* **demyelinating** *noun* destruction of the myelin sheath round nerve fibres 脱髓鞘作用

COMMENT: Can be caused by injury to the head, or is the main result of multiple sclerosis.
注释:可因头部创伤引起或是多发性硬化的主要后果。

denatured alcohol 变性酒精 *see* 见 ALCOHOL

dendrite *noun* branched process of a nerve cell, which receives impulses from nerve endings of axons of other neurones at synapses 树突 ◊ 见图 NEURONE

◊ **dendritic** *adjective* referring to a dendrite 树突的; **dendritic ulcer** = branching ulcer on the cornea, caused by herpesvirus 树状(角膜)溃疡 *see also* 参见 AXODENDRITE

denervation *noun* stopping or cutting of the nerve supply to a part of the body 去神经

dengue *noun* breakbone fever, tropical disease caused by an arbovirus, transmitted by mosquitoes, where the patient suffers a high fever, pains in the joints, headache and rash 登革热

Denis Browne splint *noun* metal splint used to correct a club foot 丹尼斯-布朗支架

dens *noun* tooth; something shaped like a tooth 齿,齿样物

dense *adjective* compact *or* tightly pressed together 紧的,密的; **dense bone** = type of bone tissue which forms the hard outer layer of a bone 密质骨

dental *adjective* referring to teeth *or* to a dentist 牙的; **dental auxiliary** = person who helps a dentist 牙科助手; **dental care** = looking after teeth 牙齿保健; **dental caries** *or* **dental decay** = rotting of a tooth 龋齿; **dental cyst** = cyst near the root of a tooth 牙囊肿; **dental floss** = soft thread used to clean between the teeth 牙线; **dental hygienist** = qualified assistant who cleans teeth and gums 牙科洁治师,洁牙师; **dental plaque** = hard smooth bacterial deposit on teeth, which is the probable cause of caries 牙菌斑; **dental practice** = office and patients of a dentist 牙科诊所; **dental pulp** = soft tissue inside a tooth 牙髓; **dental surgeon** = dentist, qualified doctor who practises surgery on teeth 牙外科医师; **dental surgery** = (i) office and operating room of a dentist 牙科手术室 (ii) surgery carried out on teeth 牙科手术; **dental technician** = person who makes dentures 牙科技师

◊ **dentifrice** *noun* paste or powder used with a toothbrush to clean teeth 牙粉,牙膏

◊ **dentine** *noun* hard substance which surrounds the pulp of teeth, beneath the enamel 牙本质 ◊ 见图 TOOTH

◊ **dentist** *noun* trained doctor who looks after teeth and gums 牙医: ***I must go to the dentist — I've got toothache.*** 我必须去看牙医,我的牙痛。***She had to wait for an hour at the dentist's.*** 她在牙科诊室不得不呆1小时。***I hate going to see the dentist.*** 我讨厌去看牙医。

◊ **dentistry** *noun* profession of a dentist; branch of medicine dealing with teeth and gums 牙科技术,牙科学

◊ **dentition** *noun* number, arrangement and special characteristics of all the teeth in a person's jaws 牙列; **adult** *or* ***permanent*** **dentition** = the thirty-two teeth which an adult has 恒牙; **milk** *or* ***deciduous*** **dentition** = the twenty teeth which a child has, and which are gradually replaced by the permanent teeth 乳牙

◊ **denture** *noun* set of false teeth, fixed to a plate which fits inside the mouth 牙托; **partial denture** = part of a set of false teeth, replacing only a few teeth 部分牙托

COMMENT: Children have incisors, canines and molars. These are replaced over a period of years by the permanent teeth, which are eight incisors, four canines, eight premolars and twelve molars (the last four molars being called the wisdom teeth).

注释:儿童有切牙、犬牙和磨牙,经过几年后将被恒牙代替,恒牙有 8 颗切牙,4 颗犬牙,8 颗双尖牙和 12 颗磨牙(最后 4 颗磨牙被称为智齿)。

deodorant *adjective & noun* (substance) which hides *or* prevents unpleasant smells 除臭的,除臭剂

deoxygenate *verb* to remove oxygen 去氧; **deoxygenated blood** = venous blood, blood from which most of the oxygen has been removed by the tissues and is darker than arterial oxygenated blood 静脉血

deoxyribonuclease *noun* enzyme which breaks down DNA 脱氧核糖核酸酶

◇ **deoxyribonucleic acid** (**DNA**) *noun* one of the nucleic acids, the basic genetic material present in the nucleus of each cell 脱氧核糖核酸 *see also* 参见 RNA

department *noun* (**a**) part of a large organization (such as a hospital) 部门,科室: ***If you want treatment for that cut, you must go to the outpatients department.*** 如果你想处理那个切口,应该去门诊部。***She is in charge of the physiotherapy department.*** 她负责理疗科。(**b**) section of the British government 英国政府部门; *GB* **Department of Social Security (DSS)** = section of British government which is in charge of national insurance, sickness and unemployment benefits, pensions, etc. 社会保险部

depend on *verb* to be sure that something will happen *or* that someone will do something; to rely on something 相信,信赖,依靠: ***We depend on the nursing staff in the running of the hospital.*** 医院运转有赖于护理人员。***He depends on drugs to relieve the pain.*** 他靠药物来缓解疼痛。***The blood transfusion service depends on a large number of donors.*** 输血服务需依靠大量的献血者。

◇ **dependence** *noun* being dependent on *or* addicted to (a drug) 依赖; **drug dependence** = being addicted to a drug and unable to exist without taking it regularly 药物依赖; **physical drug dependence** = state where a person is addicted to a drug (such as heroin) and suffers physical effects if he stops or reduces the drug 躯体性药物依赖; **psychological drug dependence** = state where a person is addicted to a drug (such as cannabis *or* alcohol) but suffers only mental effects if he stops taking it 心理性药物依赖

◇ **dependant** *noun* person who is looked after *or* supported by someone else 被抚养者,领养儿,受照顾者: ***He has to support a family of six children and several dependants.*** 他得抚养一家6个孩子和几个领养儿。

◇ **dependent** *adjective* (**a**) relying on (a person) 依赖的; **dependent relative** = person who is looked after by another member of the family 抚养关系 (**b**) addicted to (a drug) 成瘾的: ***He is physically dependent on amphetamines.*** 他对苯异丙胺躯体性成瘾。(**c**) (part of the body) which is hanging down 下垂的

depersonalization *noun* psychiatric state where the patient does not believe he is real 人格解体

depilatory *adjective & noun* (substance) which removes hair 脱发的,脱发剂

◇ **depilation** *noun* removal of hair 脱发术

deplete *verb* (i) to exhaust the strength *or* the numbers of something 耗竭,减少 (ii) to remove a component from a substance 排除,减去: ***Venous blood is depleted of oxygen by the tissues and returns to the lungs for oxygenation.*** 被组织脱氧的静脉血回到肺进行氧和。***Our nursing staff has been depleted by illness, and the outpatients' unit has had to be closed.*** 我们的护理人员因疾病人数减少,门诊部不得不停诊。

◇ **depletion** *noun* being depleted *or* lacking something 排除,缺失; **salt depletion** = loss of salt from the body, by sweating or vomiting, which causes cramp 脱盐

depolarization *noun* electrochemical reaction which takes place when an impulse travels along a nerve 去极化

deposit 1 *noun* substance which is attached to part of the body 沉积物: ***Some foods leave a hard deposit on teeth*** . 一些食物会在牙上留下些坚硬的沉积物。***A deposit of fat forms on the walls of the arteries*** . 脂肪沉积在动脉壁上。2 *verb* to attach a substance to part of the body 沉积: ***Fat is deposited on the walls of the arteries*** . 脂肪沉积在动脉壁上。

depressant *noun* drug (such as a tranquillizer) which reduces the activity of part of the body 阻滞的,阻滞剂; **thyroid depressant** = drug which reduces the activity of the thyroid gland 甲状腺阻滞剂

◇ **depressed** *adjective* (**a**) feeling miserable and worried 沮丧的: ***He was depressed after his exam results*** . 他知道考试结果后很沮丧。***She was depressed for some weeks after the death of her husband*** . 她丈夫死后几周她情绪抑郁。(**b**) (metabolic rate, freezing point, etc.) which is operating below the normal level 低于正常水平的

◇ **depressed fracture** *noun* fracture of a flat bone, such as those in the skull, where part of the bone has been pushed down lower than the surrounding parts 压缩性骨折,凹陷性骨折

◇ **depression** *noun* (**a**) mental state where the patient feels miserable and hopeless 抑郁; **pathological depression** = abnormally severe state of depression, possibly leading to suicide 病理性抑郁 (**b**) hollow on the surface of a part of the body 凹陷

◇ **depressive** *adjective & noun* (substance) which causes mental depression 抑郁的,致抑郁物; (state of) depression 抑郁状态: ***He is in a depressive state*** . 他处于抑郁状态。**manic-depressive** = person suffering from a psychological condition where he moves from mania to depression 躁狂抑郁患者

◇ **depressor** *noun* (i) muscle which pulls part of the body downwards 降肌 (ii) nerve which inhibits the activity of an organ such as the heart and lowers the blood pressure 减压神经; **tongue depressor** = instrument, usually a thin piece of wood, used by a doctor to hold the patient's tongue down while his throat is being examined 压舌板

deprivation *noun* (i) needing something 匮乏 (ii) loss of something which is needed 剥夺; **maternal deprivation** = psychological condition caused when a child does not have a proper relationship with a mother 母爱剥夺

deradenitis *noun* inflammation of the lymph nodes in the neck 颈部淋巴结炎

deranged *adjective* **mentally deranged** = suffering from a mental illness 精神紊乱

◇ **derangement** *noun* disorder 紊乱; **internal derangement of the knee (IDK)** = condition where the knee cannot function properly because of a torn meniscus 膝关节内错位

Derbyshire neck *noun* endemic goitre, a form of goitre which was once widespread in Derbyshire 地方性甲状腺肿

Dercum's disease = ADIPOSIS DOLOROSA 德尔肯氏病,痛性肥胖症

derealization *noun* psychological state where the patient feels the world around him is not real 失实症

derive *verb* to start from *or* to come into existence from 衍生,衍化; ***compounds which derive from or are derived from sugar*** 从糖中提取的化合物; ***The sublingual region has a rich supply of blood derived from the carotid artery*** . 舌下区有由颈动脉分支提供的丰富血供。

◇ **derivative** *noun* substance which is derived from another substance 衍生的: ***What are the derivatives of petroleum*** ? 汽油的衍生物是什么? *see also* 参见 PURIFIED

derm- *prefix* referring to skin 皮肤的

◇ **dermal** *adjective* referring to the skin 皮肤的

◇ **dermatitis** *noun* inflammation of the skin 皮炎; **contact dermatitis** = dermatitis caused by touching something (such as certain types of plant *or* soap) 接触性皮炎; **eczematous dermatitis** = itchy inflammation *or* irritation of the skin due to an allergic reaction to a substance which a person has touched or absorbed 湿疹性皮炎; **exfoliative dermatitis** = typical form of dermatitis where the skin becomes red and comes off in flakes 剥脱性皮炎; **occupational dermatitis** = dermatitis caused by materials touched at work 职业性皮炎; **dermatitis artefacta** = injuries to the skin caused by the patient himself 人为性皮炎; **dermatitis herpetiformis** = type of dermatitis where large itchy blisters form on the skin 疱疹样皮炎

QUOTE: Various types of dermal reaction to nail varnish have been noted. Also contact dermatitis caused by cosmetics such as toothpaste, soap, shaving creams.
引文:已经注意到了指甲油可引起多种皮炎。一些卫生用品如牙膏、肥皂和剃须膏等也可引起接触性皮炎。
Indian Journal of Medical Sciences 印度医学科学杂志

◇ **dermatoglyphics** *noun* study of the patterns of lines and ridges on the palms of the hands and the soles of the feet 皮纹学

◇ **dermatographia** *noun* swelling on the skin produced by pressing with a blunt instrument, usually an allergic reaction 皮肤划痕症

◇ **dermatological** *adjective* referring to dermatology 皮肤病学的

◇ **dermatologist** *noun* doctor who specializes in the study and treatment of the skin 皮肤病学家

◇ **dermatology** *noun* study and treatment of the skin and diseases of the skin 皮肤病学

◇ **dermatome** *noun* (**a**) special knife used for cutting thin sections of skin for grafting 取皮刀 (**b**) area of skin supplied by one spinal nerve 皮区

◇ **dermatomycosis** *noun* skin infections caused by a fungus 皮肤真菌病,癣

◇ **dermatomyositis** *noun* collagen disease with a wasting inflammation of the skin and muscles 皮肌炎

◇ **dermatophyte** *noun* fungus which affects the skin 皮霉菌

◇ **dermatophytosis** *noun* fungus infection of the skin 皮肤真菌病

◇ **dermatoplasty** *noun* skin graft, replacing damaged skin by skin taken from another part of the body *or* from a donor 植皮术

◇ **dermatosis** *noun* any skin disease 皮肤病

◇ **dermis** *or* **corium** *noun* thick layer of living skin beneath the epidermis 真皮 ➪见图 SKIN & SENSORY RECEPTORS

◇ **dermographia** = DERMATOGRAPHIA 皮肤划痕症

◇ **dermoid** *adjective* referring to the skin *or* like skin 皮样的; **dermoid cyst** = cyst found under the skin, usually in the midline, containing hair, sweat glands and sebaceous glands 皮样囊肿

Descemet's membrane *noun* one of the deep layers of the cornea 德斯密氏膜,后弹性层

descend *verb* to go down 下降; **descending aorta** = second part of the aorta as it goes downwards after the aortic arch 降主动脉; **descending colon** = third section of the colon which goes down the left side of the body 降结肠 ➪见图 DIGESTIVE SYSTEM; **descending tract** = tract of nerves which take impulses away from the head 降支

describe *verb* to say or write what something *or* someone is like 描述: ***Can you describe the symptoms?*** 你可以描述一下症状吗? ***She described how her right leg suddenly became inflamed.*** 她

描述了她的右腿是如何突然发炎的。

◇ **description** *noun* saying or writing what something *or* someone is like 描写; ***the patient's description of the symptoms*** 患者对症状的描绘

desensitize *verb* (i) to deaden a nerve *or* to remove sensitivity 减感,失敏 (ii) to treat a patient suffering from an allergy by giving graduated injections of the substance to which he is allergic over a period of time until he becomes immune to it 脱敏治疗: ***The patient was prescribed a course of desensitizing injections.*** 患者给予一疗程的脱敏治疗。

◇ **desensitization** *noun* (i) removal of sensitivity 减感,去感觉 (ii) treatment of an allergy by giving the patient injections of small quantities of the substance to which he is allergic over a period of time until he becomes immune to it 脱敏治疗

desire *noun* wanting greatly to do something 愿望,期望: ***He has a compulsive desire to steal.*** 他有一种强迫偷窃的欲望。

desquamate *verb* (*of skin*) to peel off 脱皮

◇ **desquamation** *noun* (i) continual process of losing the outer layer of dead skin 脱皮(ii) peeling off of the epithelial part of a structure 脱屑

destroy *verb* to ruin *or* kill completely 破坏: ***The nerve cells were destroyed by the infection.*** 神经细胞因感染受损了。

◇ **destruction** *noun* ruining *or* killing of something completely 破坏; ***the destruction of the tissue*** *or* ***the cells by infection.*** 感染对组织(细胞)的破坏; ***the destruction of bacteria by phagocytes.*** 吞噬细胞对细菌的破坏

detach *verb* to separate one thing from another 剥离; ***an operation to detach the cusps of the mitral valve*** 剥离二尖瓣的手术; **detached retina** *or* **retinal detachment** = condition where the retina is partially detached from the choroid 视网膜脱离

◇ **retinal detachment** = DETACHED RETINA 视网膜脱离

> COMMENT: A detached retina can be caused by a blow to the eye, or simply is a condition occurring in old age; if left untreated the eye will become blind. A detached retina can sometimes be attached to the choroid again using lasers.
> 注释:视网膜脱离可因眼部受打击造成或仅为老年的表现,如不经治疗会致盲。有时脱离的视网膜可用激光与脉络膜相贴。

detect *verb* to sense *or* to notice (usually something which is very small or difficult to see) 察觉,检测; ***an instrument to detect microscopic changes in cell structure*** 检测细胞镜下结构变化的仪器; ***The nurses detected a slight improvement in the patient's condition.*** 护士察觉患者状况有轻微的改善。

◇ **detection** *noun* action of detecting something 检测,发现; ***the detection of sounds by nerves in the ears*** 耳朵通过神经察觉声音; ***The detection of a cyst using an endoscope*** 用内镜检测囊肿

detergent *noun* cleaning substance which removes grease and bacteria 去污剂

> COMMENT: Most detergents are not allergenic but some biological detergents which contain enzymes to remove protein stains can cause dermatitis.
> 注释:大多数去污剂是没有致敏性的,但有些生物去污剂含有可祛除蛋白污渍的酶,会引起皮炎。

deteriorate *verb* to become worse 恶化: ***The patient's condition deteriorated rapidly.*** 患者的病情迅速恶化。

◇ **deterioration** *noun* becoming worse 恶化: ***The nurses were worried by the deterioration in the patient's mental state.*** 护士对患者精神状态恶化担忧。

determine *verb* to find out something correctly 明确: ***Health inspectors are trying to determine the cause of the outbreak of Salmonella poisoning.*** 卫生检查员在设法弄清沙门氏菌中毒的原因。

detoxication *or* **detoxification** *noun* removal of toxic substances to make a poisonous substance harmless 解毒

detrition *noun* wearing away by rubbing or use 磨耗

◊ **detritus** *noun* rubbish produced when something disintegrates 碎屑

detrusor muscle *noun* muscular coat of the urinary bladder 逼尿肌

detumescence *noun* (of penis *or* clitoris after an erection *or* orgasm) becoming limp; (of a swelling) going down 勃起消退;消肿

deuteranopia *noun* form of colour blindness, a defect in vision, where the patient cannot see green 绿色盲 *compare* 比较 DALTONISM, TRITANOPIA

develop *verb* (**a**) to grow *or* make grow; to mature 生长,发育: ***The embryo developed quite normally, in spite of the mother's illness.*** 尽管母亲有病,胎儿发育仍相当正常。***A swelling developed under the armpit.*** 腋下有肿块。***The sore throat developed into an attack of meningitis.*** 咽痛进展为脑膜炎。(**b**) to start to get 发生: ***She developed a cold*** 她得了感冒。***He developed complications and was rushed to hospital.*** 他产生了并发症,被送到医院。

◊ **development** *noun* thing which develops *or* is being developed; action of becoming mature 发育: ***The development of the embryo takes place in the uterus.*** 胚胎在子宫内发育。

◊ **developmental** *adjective* referring to the development of an embryo 发育的

> QUOTE: Rheumatoid arthritis is a chronic inflammatory disease which can affect many systems in the body, but mainly the joints. 70% of sufferers develop the condition in the metacarpophalangeal joints.
> 引文:类风湿性关节炎是一慢性炎症性疾病,可以影响机体的许多器官,主要是关节。70%的患者掌指关节受累。
> **Nursing Times** 护理时代

deviation *noun* variation from normal; abnormal position of a joint or of the eye (such as strabismus) 偏离;偏斜

◊ **deviance** *noun* abnormal sexual behaviour 性欲不正常

Devic's disease = NEUROMYELITIS OPTICA 德维克氏病,视神经脊髓病

device *noun* instrument *or* piece of equipment 设备; ***a device for weighing very small quantities of powder*** 用来称量极少量粉末的设备; ***He used a device for examining the interior of the ear.*** 他用一种仪器来检查内耳。

dextro- *prefix* referring to the right side of the body *or* to the right hand 右侧的

◊ **dextrocardia** *noun* congenital condition where the apex of the heart is towards the right of the body instead of the left 右位心 *compare* 比较 LAEVOCARDIA

dextrose *or* **glucose** *noun* simple sugar found in fruit, also broken down in the body from white sugar or carbohydrate and absorbed into the body or excreted by the kidneys 葡萄糖

DHA = DISTRICT HEALTH AUTHORITY 区卫生当局

dhobie itch *noun* contact dermatitis (believed to be caused by an allergy to the marking ink used by laundries) 接触性皮炎

diabetes *noun* one of a group of diseases, but most commonly used to refer to diabetes mellitus 糖尿病; **diabetes insipidus** = rare disease caused by a disorder of the pituitary gland, making the patient pass large quantities of urine and want to drink more than normal 尿崩症; **diabetes mellitus** = disease where the body cannot control sugar absorption because the pancreas does not secrete enough insulin 糖尿病; **bronze diabetes** = haemochromatosis, hereditary disease where the body absorbs and stores too much iron, giving a dark colour to the skin 血色素沉着症; **gestational**

diabetes = diabetes which develops in a pregnant woman 妊娠糖尿病；**insulin-dependent diabetes** = diabetes caused by inadequate production or utilization of insulin 胰岛素依赖性糖尿病

◇ **diabetic** *adjective* (**a**) referring to diabetes mellitus 糖尿病的；**diabetic coma** = state of unconsciousness caused by untreated diabetes 糖尿病性昏迷；**diabetic diet** = diet which is low in carbohydrates and sugar 糖尿病饮食；**diabetic retinopathy** = defect in vision caused by diabetes 糖尿病性视网膜病变（**b**）(food) which contains few carbohydrates and sugar 无糖的（食物）：***He bought some diabetic chocolate.*** 他买了些无糖巧克力。***She lives on diabetic soups.*** 她靠无糖汤食过活。**2** *noun* person suffering from diabetes 糖尿病患者

◇ **diabetologist** *noun* physician specializing in the treatment of diabetes mellitus 糖尿病学家

> COMMENT：Diabetes mellitus has two forms：Type I is caused by an infection which affects the cells in the pancreas which produce insulin；Type II is common in older people and is caused by a lower sensitivity to insulin or by obesity. Symptoms of diabetes mellitus are tiredness, abnormal thirst, frequent passing of water and sweet-smelling urine. Blood and urine tests will reveal high levels of sugar. Treatment for Type II diabetes involves keeping to a strict diet and reducing weight. Type I diabetes must be treated with regular injections of insulin.
> 注释：糖尿病有两种类型，I 型糖尿病是因产生胰岛素的胰腺细胞受感染所致，II 型糖尿病在老年人中较普遍，是因对胰岛素的敏感性降低或肥胖所致。糖尿病的症状表现为乏力、易渴、尿频及尿中有甜味儿。对 II 型糖尿病的治疗包括严格控制饮食和减轻体重，而 I 型糖尿病必须定期注射胰岛素。

diaclasia *noun* fracture made by a surgeon to repair a earlier fracture which has set badly *or* to correct a deformity 折骨术

diadochokinesis *noun* normal ability to make muscles move limbs in opposite directions 轮替运动

diagnose *verb* to identify a patient's condition *or* illness, by examining the patient and noting symptoms 诊断：***The doctor diagnosed appendicitis.*** 医生的诊断是患阑尾炎。

◇ **diagnosis** *noun* act of diagnosing a patient's condition *or* illness 诊断：***The doctor's diagnosis was cancer, but the patient asked for a second opinion.*** 医生的诊断是癌症，但患者仍寻求其他诊断。**differential diagnosis** = identification of one particular disease from other similar diseases by comparing the range of symptoms of each 鉴别诊断；**antenatal** *or* **prenatal diagnosis** = medical examination of a pregnant woman to see if the fetus is developing normally 产前诊断 (NOTE：plural is **diagnoses**)

◇ **diagnostic** *adjective* referring to diagnosis 诊断的；**diagnostic imaging** = scanning for the purpose of diagnosis, as of a pregnant woman to see if the fetus is healthy 影像诊断；**diagnostic process** = method of making a diagnosis 诊断过程；**diagnostic test** = test which helps a doctor diagnose an illness 诊断性试验 *compare* 比较 PROGNOSIS

diagonal *adjective* going across at an angle 对角线的

◇ **diagonally** *adverb* crossing at an angle 对角线地

diagram *noun* chart *or* drawing which records information as lines or points：***The book gives a diagram of the circulation of blood.*** 书上有血液循环的图谱。***The diagram shows the occurrence of cancer in the southern part of the town.*** 图例显示了城南癌症的发生情况。

dialyse *verb* to treat (a patient) using a kidney machine 透析

◇ **dialyser** *noun* apparatus which uses a membrane to separate solids from liquids, especially a kidney machine 透析器

◊ **dialysis** *noun* using a membrane as a filter to separate soluble waste substances from the blood 透析; **kidney dialysis** *or* **haemodialysis** = removing waste matter from a patient's blood by passing it through a kidney machine *or* dialyser 肾透析,血液透析; **peritoneal dialysis** = removing waste matter from the blood by introducing fluid into the peritoneum which then acts as the filter membrane 腹膜透析

diameter *noun* distance across a circle (such as a tube *or* blood vessel) 直径: ***They measured the diameter of the pelvic girdle.*** 他们在测量骨盆带的直径。

diapedesis *noun* movement of white blood cells through the walls of the capillaries into tissues in inflammation 伪足运动,白细胞渗出

diaper *noun US* cloth used to wrap round a baby's bottom and groin, to keep clothing clean and dry 尿布; **diaper rash** = sore red skin on a baby's buttocks and groin, caused by long contact with ammonia in a wet diaper 尿布疹 (NOTE: GB English is **nappy**)

diaphoresis *noun* excessive perspiration 大量出汗

◊ **diaphoretic** *adjective* (drug) which causes sweating 发汗的

diaphragm *noun* (**a**) thin layer of tissue stretched across an opening, especially the flexible sheet of muscle and fibre which separates the chest from the abdomen, and moves to pull air into the lungs in respiration 膈,横膈; **pelvic diaphragm** = sheet of muscle between the pelvic cavity and the peritoneum 盆膈; **urogenital diaphragm** = fibrous layer beneath the prostate gland through which the urethra passes 泌尿生殖膈 (**b**) **vaginal diaphragm** = circular contraceptive device for women, which is inserted into the vagina and placed over the neck of the uterus before sexual intercourse 阴道膈

◊ **diaphragmatic** *adjective* referring to a diaphragm; like a diaphragm 膈的;像膈的; **diaphragmatic hernia** = condition where a membrane and organ in the abdomen pass through an opening in the diaphragm into the chest 膈疝; **diaphragmatic pleura** = part of the pleura which covers the diaphragm 膈胸膜; **diaphragmatic pleurisy** = inflammation of the pleura which covers the diaphragm 膈胸膜炎; **diaphragmatic surface of pleura** = surface of the pleura which is in direct contact with the diaphragm 胸膜的膈面

> COMMENT: The diaphragm is a muscle which in breathing expands and contracts with the walls of the chest. The normal rate of respiration is about 16 times a minute.
> 注释:横膈是一肌性组织,随呼吸时胸廓的运动而扩张、收缩。正常的呼吸频率是每分钟16次。

diaphyseal *adjective* referring to a diaphysis 骨干的

◊ **diaphysis** *noun* shaft, the long central part of a long bone 骨干 *compare* 比较 EPIPHYSIS, METAPHYSIS ◊ 见图 BONE STRUCTURE

◊ **diaphysitis** *noun* inflammation of the diaphysis, often associated with rheumatic disease 骨干炎

diarrhoea *or US* **diarrhea** *noun* condition where a patient frequently passes liquid faeces 腹泻: ***He had an attack of diarrhoea after going to the restaurant.*** 他从饭馆回来后就开始腹泻。***She complained of mild diarrhoea.*** 她主诉轻微腹泻。

◊ **diarrhoeal** *adjective* referring to *or* caused by diarrhoea 腹泻的,腹泻引起的

> COMMENT: Diarrhoea can have many causes: types of food or allergy to food; contaminated or poisoned food; infectious diseases, such as dysentery; sometimes worry or other emotions.
> 注释:腹泻由多种原因引起:某种特殊的食物或对食物过敏;污染的食物或有毒的

食物；感染性疾病，如痢疾；有时焦虑或其他情绪波动也可导致腹泻。

diarthrosis *noun* synovial joint, a joint which moves freely 滑动关节

diastase *noun* enzyme which breaks down starch and converts it into sugar 淀粉酶

diastasis *noun* (i) condition where a bone separates into parts 分离(ii) dislocation of bones at an immovable joint (不动关节的)脱位

diastole *noun* phase in the beating of the heart between two contractions, where the heart dilates and fills with blood 舒张：***The period of diastole lasts about 0.4 seconds in a normal heart rate.*** 在正常的心率下舒张期持续约0.4秒。

◇ **diastolic pressure** *noun* blood pressure taken at the diastole 舒张压 *compare* 比较 SYSTOLE, SYSTOLIC

COMMENT: Diastolic pressure is always lower than systolic.
注释：舒张压总是比收缩压低。

diathermy *noun* using high frequency electric current to produce heat in body tissue 透热法；**medical diathermy** = using heat produced by electricity for treatment of muscle and joint disorders (such as rheumatism) 医用透热法；**surgical diathermy** = using a knife or electrode which is heated by a strong electric current until it coagulates tissue 手术电凝法；**diathermy knife** *or* **diathermy needle** = instrument used in surgical diathermy 电凝刀，电凝针

COMMENT: The difference between medical and surgical uses of diathermy is in the size of the electrodes used. Two large electrodes will give a warming effect over a large area (medical diathermy); if one of the electrodes is small, the heat will be concentrated enough to coagulate tissue (surgical diathermy).
注释：医用透热法和手术电凝法的区别在于所用电极的大小不同。两个大的电极将在大范围内产生热效应(医用透热法)，如果一个电极很小，热将会被集中使组织凝(固手术电凝法)。

diathesis *noun* general inherited constitution of a person, with his susceptibility to certain diseases *or* allergies 体质(易于患某种疾病的先天性因素)

dichlorodiphenyltrichloroethane (DDT) *noun* higly toxic insecticide, formerly commonly used, but now banned in many countries 滴滴涕(一种杀虫剂)

dichromatic *adjective* seeing only two of the three primary colours 二色视的 *compare* 比较 TRICHROMATIC

Dick test *noun* test to show if a patient is immune to scarlet fever 狄克试验，用来检测对猩红热的免疫性

dicrotism *noun* condition where the pulse dilates twice with each heartbeat 二波脉，重波脉

◇ **dicrotic pulse** *or* **dicrotic wave** *noun* pulse which beats twice 二波脉

didelphys *noun* **uterus didelphys** = double uterus, a condition where the uterus is divided in two by a membrane 双子宫

die 1 *noun* cast of the patient's mouth taken by a dentist before making a denture 齿模 **2** *verb* to stop living 死亡：***His father died last year.*** 他父亲去年去世了。***She died in a car crash.*** 她在车祸中丧生。(NOTE: **dies - dying - died - has died**)

diencephalon *noun* central part of the forebrain, formed of the thalamus, hypothalamus, pineal gland and third ventricle 间脑

diet 1 *noun* (i) amount and type of food eaten 饮食(ii) measured amount of food eaten, usually to try to lose weight 节食：***He lives on a diet of bread and beer.*** 他以面包和啤酒为食。***The doctor asked her to follow a strict diet.*** 医生让她严格节食。***He has been on a diet for some weeks, but still hasn't lost enough weight.*** 他已经节食几个星期了，但体重仍没有明显的减轻。**diet sheet** = list of suggestions for quantities and types of food given to a patient to follow 食谱；

balanced diet = diet which contains the right quantities of basic nutrients 平衡膳食; **bland diet** = diet in which the patient eats mainly milk-based foods, boiled vegetables and white meat, as a treatment for peptic ulcers 软食; **diabetic diet** = diet which is low in carbohydrates and sugar 糖尿病饮食; **low-calorie diet** = diet which provides less than the normal number of calories 低热量饮食; **salt-free diet** = diet which does not contain salt 无盐饮食 **2** *verb* to reduce the quantity of food eaten *or* to change the type of food eaten in order to become thinner *or* healthier 节食: ***She dieted for two weeks before going on holiday.*** 在假期前她已经节食两周。***He is dieting to try to lose weight.*** 他在节食减肥。

◇ **dietary 1** *noun* system of nutrition and energy 食谱: ***The nutritionist supervised the dietaries for the patients.*** 营养学家监督患者的食谱。**2** *adjective* referring to a diet. 饮食的; **dietary fibre** = roughage, fibrous matter in food, which cannot be digested 食用纤维素

> COMMENT: Dietary fibre is found in cereals, nuts, fruit and some green vegetables. It is believed to be necessary to help digestion and avoid developing constipation, obesity and appendicitis.
> 注释:食用纤维素在谷类、坚果、水果及一些绿色蔬菜中含量丰富。它被认为有助于消化,避免便秘、肥胖和阑尾炎。

◇ **dietetic** *adjective* referring to diet 饮食的; **dietetic principles** = rules concerning the body's needs in food *or* vitamins *or* trace elements 营养法则

◇ **dietetics** *noun* study of food, nutrition and health, especially when applied to the food intake 饮食学,营养学

◇ **dieting** *noun* attempting to reduce weight by reducing the amount of food eaten 节食

◇ **dietitian** *noun* person who specializes in the study of diet, especially an officer in a hospital who supervises dietaries as part of the medical treatment of patients 营养学家

Dietl's crisis *noun* painful blockage of the ureter, causing back pressure on the kidney which fills with urine, and swells 迪特耳危象,因尿路阻塞,肾脏内尿液淤积、肿胀,游动肾危象

difference *noun* way in which two things are not the same 差异,不同: ***Can you tell the difference between butter and margarine?*** 你能说出黄油和人造黄油的差别吗?

◇ **different** *adjective* not the same 不同的: ***Living in the country is very different from living in the town.*** 在乡村生活和在城镇生活截然不同。***He looks quite different since he had the operation.*** 他手术后完全变样了。

◇ **differential** *adjective* referring to a difference 鉴别的; **differential diagnosis** = identification of one particular disease from other similar diseases by comparing the range of symptoms of each 鉴别诊断; **differential blood count** *or* **differential white cell count** = showing the amounts of different types of (white) blood cell in a blood sample 血细胞或白细胞分类

◇ **differentiate** *verb* to tell the difference between; to be different from 区分; 不同于…: **The tumour is clearly differentiated.** = The tumour can be easily identified from the surrounding tissue. 肿瘤的界限很清楚。

◇ **differentiation** *noun* development of specialized cells during the early embryo stage 分化

difficult *adjective* hard to do *or* not easy 困难的: ***The practical examination was very difficult - half the students failed.*** 实习考试很难,一半学生不及格。***The heart-lung transplant is a particularly difficult operation.*** 心肺移植是很困难的手术。***The doctor had to use forceps because the childbirth was difficult.*** 因为难产,医生不得不用产钳。

◇ **difficulty** *noun* problem *or* thing which is not easy 困难: ***She has***

***difficulty in breathing** or **in getting enough vitamins*.她呼吸困难或她很难获得足够的维生素。

diffuse 1 *verb* to spread through tissue 扩散,弥散: ***Some substances easily diffuse through the walls of capillaries*.**一些物质很容易经毛细血管壁弥散。**2** *adjective* (disease) which is widespread in the body *or* which affects many organs *or* cells(疾病)播散的

◇ **diffusion** *noun* (i) mixing a liquid with another liquid, or a gas with another gas 扩散(ii) passing of a liquid *or* gas through a membrane 弥散

digest *verb* to break down food in the alimentary tract and convert it into elements which are absorbed into the body 消化

◇ **digestible** *adjective* which can be digested 可消化的: ***Glucose is an easily digestible form of sugar*.**葡萄糖是一种易消化的糖类。

◇ **digestion** *noun* process by which food is broken down in the alimentary tract into elements which can be absorbed by the body 消化

◇ **digestive** *adjective* referring to digestion 消化的; **digestive enzymes** = enzymes which encourage digestion 消化酶; **digestive system** = all the organs in the body (such as the liver and pancreas) which are associated with the digestion of food 消化系统; **digestive tract** *or* **alimentary tract** = passage from the mouth to the rectum, down which food passes and is digested 消化道

COMMENT: The digestive tract is formed of the mouth, throat, oesophagus, stomach and small and large intestines. Food is broken down by digestive juices in the mouth, stomach and small intestine, water is removed in the large intestine, and the remaining matter is passed out of the body as faeces.
注释:消化道由口腔、咽、食管、胃和大小肠组成。食物被口腔、胃和小肠内的消化液降解,水分在大肠吸收,剩余的物质以粪便的形式排出体外。

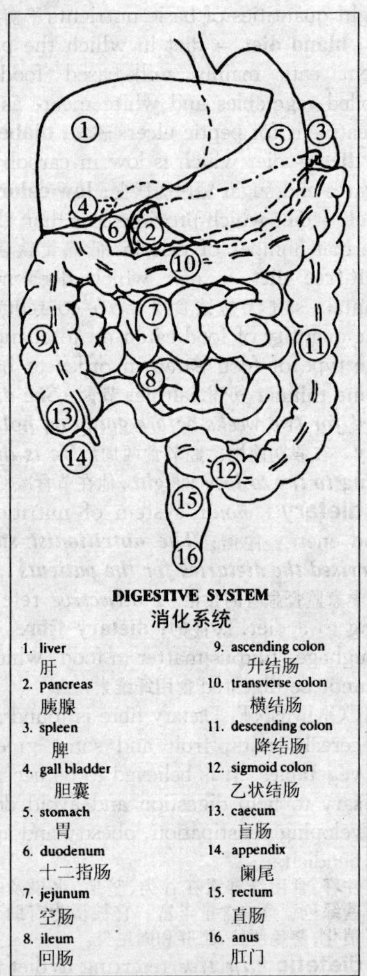

DIGESTIVE SYSTEM
消化系统

1. liver 肝	9. ascending colon 升结肠
2. pancreas 胰腺	10. transverse colon 横结肠
3. spleen 脾	11. descending colon 降结肠
4. gall bladder 胆囊	12. sigmoid colon 乙状结肠
5. stomach 胃	13. caecum 盲肠
6. duodenum 十二指肠	14. appendix 阑尾
7. jejunum 空肠	15. rectum 直肠
8. ileum 回肠	16. anus 肛门

digit *noun* (**a**) a finger *or* a toe 指(趾) (**b**) a number 数字

◇ **digital** *adjective* (**a**) referring to fingers *or* toes 指(趾)的; **digital veins** = veins draining the fingers *or* toes 指(趾)静脉 (**b**) **digital computer** = computer which calculates on the basis of numbers 数字计算机

◇ **digitalis** *noun* poisonous drug extracted from the foxglove plant, used in small doses to treat heart conditions 洋

地黄,洋地黄制剂

dilate *verb* to swell 扩张: ***The veins in the left leg have become dilated.*** 左腿的静脉开始扩张。***The drug is used to dilate the pupil of the eye.*** 这药用来扩张瞳孔。

◇ **dilatation** *or* **dilation** *noun* (i) expansion of a hollow space *or* a passage in the body 扩张 (ii) expansion of the pupil of the eye as a reaction to bad light *or* to drugs 瞳孔扩张; **dilatation and curettage (D & C)** = surgical operation to scrape the interior of the uterus to obtain a tissue sample *or* to remove a cyst 刮除术

◇ **dilator** *noun* (i) instrument used to widen the entrance to a cavity 扩张器 (ii) drug used to make part of the body expand 扩张药; **dilator pupillae muscle** = muscle in the iris which pulls the iris back and so dilates the pupil 瞳孔开大肌

dilute 1 *adjective* with water added 稀释的: ***Bathe the wound in a solution of dilute antiseptic.*** 用稀释的消毒液清洗伤口。**2** *verb* to add water to a liquid to make it weaker 稀释: ***The disinfectant must be diluted in four parts of water before it can be used on the skin.*** 消毒液在用于皮肤前必须用4倍体积的水稀释。

◇ **diluent** *noun* substance (such as water) which is used to dilute a liquid 稀释剂

◇ **dilution** *noun* (i) action of diluting 稀释 (ii) liquid which has been diluted 稀释液

dimetria *noun* condition where a woman has a double uterus 双子宫 *see also* 参见 DIDELPHYS

dioptre *or US* **diopter** *noun* unit of measurement of refraction of a lens 屈光度

> COMMENT: A one dioptre lens has a focal length of one metre; the greater the dioptre, the shorter the focal length.
> 注释:一个屈光度的镜片焦距是1米,屈光度越大,焦距越小。

dioxide 二氧化物 *see* 见 CARBON

DIP = DISTAL INTERPHALANGEAL JOINT 远端指关节

diphtheria *noun* serious infectious disease of children, caused by the bacillus *Corynebacterium diphtheriae*, with fever and the formation of a fibrous growth like a membrane in the throat which restricts breathing 白喉

◇ **diphtheroid** *adjective* (bacterium) like the diphtheria bacterium 类白喉杆菌的

> COMMENT: Symptoms of diphtheria begin usually with a sore throat, followed by a slight fever, rapid pulse and swelling of glands in the neck. The 'membrane' which forms can close the air passages, and the disease is often fatal, either because the patient is asphyxiated or because the heart becomes fatally weakened. The disease is also highly infectious, and all contacts of the patient must be tested. The Schick test is used to test if a person is immune or susceptible to diphtheria.
> 注释:白喉开始的症状是咽痛,随后是低热、脉速、颈部腺体肿大。形成的"假膜"可阻塞呼吸道,常因窒息或心衰而致死。本病有很高的传染性,所有接触过患者的人都应接受检查。锡克试验可用来检测机体对白喉是否有免疫力或易受感染。

dipl- *or* **diplo-** *prefix* meaning double 双的

◇ **diplacusis** *noun* (i) condition where a patient hears double sounds 复听 (ii) condition where a patient hears the same sound in a different way in each ear 双耳复听

◇ **diplegia** *noun* paralysis of a similar part on both sides of the body (such as both arms) 双侧瘫

◇ **diplegic** *adjective* referring to diplegia 双侧瘫的 *compare* 比较 HEMIPLEGIA

◇ **diplococcus** *noun* bacterium which occurs in pairs 双球菌 (NOTE: plural is **diplococci**)

diploe *noun* layer of spongy bone tissue filled with red bone marrow, between the inner and outer layers of the skull 板障

diploid *adjective* (cell) where each chromosome (except the sex chromosome) occurs twice 二倍体的 *compare* 比较 HAPLOID, POLYPLOID

diploma *noun* certificate showing that a person has successfully finished a course of specialized training 文凭,毕业证书: ***He has a diploma from a College of Nursing.*** 他有护士学院的文凭。***She is taking her diploma exams next week.*** 她下周进行毕业考试。

diplopia *noun* double vision, a condition where a patient sees single objects as double 复视 *compare* 比较 POLYOPIA

dipsomania *noun* uncontrollable desire to drink alcohol 嗜酒狂

direct 1 *adjective & adverb* straight *or* with nothing intervening 直接的(地): ***His dermatitis is due to direct contact with irritants.*** 他的皮炎是因直接接触刺激剂引起。**2** *verb* to tell someone what to do *or* how to go somewhere 指导: ***The police directed the ambulances to the scene of the accident.*** 警察指挥救护车来到事故现场。***Can you direct me to the outpatients' unit?*** 你能告诉我如何去门诊部吗? ***She spent two years directing the work of the research team.*** 她花了2年的时间指导研究小组的工作。

◇ **directly** *adverb* straight *or* with nothing in between 直接地: ***The endocrine or ductless glands secrete hormones directly into the bloodstream.*** 内分泌腺或无导管腺体直接将激素分泌入血。***The dressing should not be placed directly on the burn.*** 衣服不能直接放在阳光直射的地方。

◇ **director** *noun* (**a**) person in charge of a department 主管: ***He is the director of the burns unit.*** 他是烧伤病区的主任。(**b**) instrument used to limit the incision made with a surgical knife 导子

dirt *noun* material which is not clean, like mud, dust, earth, etc. 赃物,灰尘: ***He allowed dirt to get into the wound which became infected.*** 他允许脏东西进入感染伤口。

◇ **dirty** *adjective* not clean 脏的: ***Dirty sheets are taken off the beds every morning.*** 每天早晨脏床单都被拿走。***Every one concerned with patient care has to make sure that the wards are not dirty.*** 每一个关心患者的人都应注意不要弄脏病房。(NOTE: **dirty - dirtier - dirtiest**)

disable *verb* to make someone unable to do some normal activity 致残: ***He was disabled by the lung disease.*** 他因肺部疾病而致残。***a hospital for disabled soldiers*** 为伤残士兵服务的医院; **disabling disease** = disease which makes it impossible for a person to do some normal activity 致残疾病; **the disabled** = people suffering from a physical *or* mental handicaps which prevent them from doing some normal activity 残疾人

◇ **disablement** *noun* condition where a person has a physical *or* mental handicap 残疾

◇ **disability** *noun* condition where part of the body does not function normally 残障: ***Deafness is a disability which affects old people.*** 耳聋是老年人常患的一种残障。***People with severe disabilities can claim grants from the government.*** 严重残疾者可向政府申请补助。

disarticulation *noun* amputation of a limb at a joint, which does not involve dividing a bone 关节切断术,关节断离术

disc *or especially US* **disk** *noun* flat round structure like a plate 盘; **intervertebral disc** = round plate of cartilage which separates two vertebrae in the spinal column 椎间盘; **displaced intervertebral disc** *or* **prolapsed intervertebral disc or slipped disc** = condition where an intervertebral disc becomes displaced *or* where the soft centre of a disc passes through the hard cartilage outside and presses on a nerve 椎间盘脱出 ⇨ 见图 JOINTS, VERTEBRAL COLUMN; **Merkel's discs** = receptor cells in the lower part of the epidermis 美克耳氏体(表皮下层的感受细胞)◊见图 SKIN AND SENSORY RECEPTORS

discharge 1 *noun* (**a**) (i) secretion of liquid from an opening 分泌(ii) release of nervous energy 释放; **vaginal discharge** = flow of liquid from the vagina 阴道分泌物 (**b**) sending a patient away from a hospital because the treatment has ended 出院; **discharge rate** = number of patients with a certain type of disorder who are sent away from hospitals in a certain area (shown as a number per 10,000 of population) 出院率 2 *verb* (**a**) to secrete liquid out of an opening 分泌: ***The wound discharged a thin stream of pus.*** 伤口分泌稀薄的脓液。(**b**) to send a patient away from hospital because the treatment has ended 使…出院: ***He was discharged from hospital last week.*** 他上周出院了。**She discharged herself.** = She decided to leave hospital and stop taking the treatment provided. 她自己决定出院。

discolour *or US* **discolor** *verb* to change the colour of something 使变色: ***His teeth were discoloured from smoking cigarettes.*** 他的牙齿因抽烟而变色了。

◊ **discoloration** *noun* change in colour 变色

> COMMENT: Teeth can be discoloured in fluorosis; if the skin on the lips is discoloured it may indicate that the patient has swallowed a poison.
> 注释:在氟中毒时牙齿会变色;口唇变色提示患者服用了毒物。

discomfort *noun* feeling of not being comfortable *or* not being completely well 不舒服,不适: ***She experienced some discomfort after the operation.*** 手术后她感觉有些不适。

discontinue *verb* to stop doing something 停止,中断: ***The doctors decided to discontinue the treatment.*** 医生决定停止治疗。

◊ **discontinued** *adjective* no longer done 中断的: ***The use of the drug has been discontinued because of the possibility of side-effects.*** 因为可能的副作用此药已停止使用。

discover *verb* to find something which was hidden *or* not known before 发现: ***Scientists are trying to discover a cure for this disease.*** 科学家在设法寻找治愈此病的方法。

◊ **discoverer** *noun* person who discovers something 发明者: ***Who was the discoverer of penicillin?*** 谁是青霉素的发明者?

◊ **discovery** *noun* finding something which was not known before 发现: ***The discovery of penicillin completely changed hospital treatment.*** 青霉素的发现彻底改变了医院的治疗方案。***New medical discoveries are reported each week.*** 每周都报道医疗的新发现。

discrete *adjective* separate *or* not joined together 分散的; **discrete rash** = rash which is formed of many separate spots, which do not join together into one large red patch 稀疏皮疹

disease *noun* illness (of people *or* animals *or* plants, etc.) where the body functions abnormally 疾病: ***He caught a disease in the tropics.*** 他在热带得了病。***She is suffering from a very serious disease of the kidneys*** *or* ***from a serious kidney disease.*** 她患有严重的肾脏疾病。***He is a specialist in occupational diseases*** *or* ***in diseases which affect workers.*** 他是研究职业病的专家。

◊ **diseased** *adjective* (person *or* part of the body) affected by an illness *or* not whole or normal 有病的: ***The doctor cut away the diseased tissue.*** 医生切除了病变组织。(NOTE: although a particular disease may have few visible characteristic symptoms, the term 'disease' is applied to all physical and mental reactions which make a person ill. Diseases with distinct characteristics have names. For terms referring to disease, see words beginning with **path-** or **patho-**)

disfigure *verb* to change someone's appearance so as to make it less pleasant 变形: ***Her legs were disfigured by scars.***

她的腿因伤疤变形了。

disinfect *verb* to make a place free from germs *or* bacteria 消毒：***She disinfected the skin with surgical spirit*.** 她用外科酒精消毒皮肤。***All the patient's clothes have to be disinfected*.** 所有患者的衣服都应消毒。

◇ **disinfectant** *noun* substance used to kill germs *or* bacteria 消毒剂

◇ **disinfection** *noun* removal of infection caused by germs *or* bacteria 消毒 (NOTE: the words **disinfect** and **disinfectant** are used for substances which destroy germs on instruments, objects or the skin; substances used to kill germs inside infected people are **antibiotics, drugs, etc.**)

disintegrate *verb* to come to pieces 分裂,分解：***In holocrine glands the cells disintegrate as they secrete*.** 全泌腺中细胞分泌后就裂解了。

◇ **disintegration** *noun* act of disintegrating 分裂,分解

disk 盘 *see* 见 DISC

dislike 1 *noun* not liking something 不喜欢,讨厌：***He has a strong dislike of cats*.** 他很厌恶猫。2 *verb* not to like something 讨厌：***She dislikes going to the dentist*.** 她不喜欢去看牙医。

dislocate *verb* to displace a bone from its normal position at a joint 脱位：***He fell and dislocated his elbow*.** 他摔倒了,肘关节脱位了。***The shoulder joint dislocates easily* or *is easily dislocated*.** 肩关节很容易脱位。

◇ **dislocation** *noun* luxation, condition where a bone is displaced from its normal position at a joint 脱位；**pathological dislocation** = dislocation of a diseased joint 病理性脱位

dislodge *verb* to move something which is stuck 清除：***By coughing he managed to dislodge the bone stuck in his throat*.** 他通过咳嗽尽力清除卡在喉咙的骨头。

disorder *noun* (i) illness *or* sickness 疾病(ii) state where part of the body is not functioning correctly 障碍：***The doctor specializes in disorders of the kidneys* or *in kidney disorders*.** 这位医生是肾病专家。***The family has a history of mental disorder*.** 这家有精神病家族史。**cognitive disorder** = impairment of any of the mental processes of perception, memory, judgement and reasoning 认知障碍；**motor disorder** = impairment of the nerves *or* neurons that cause muscles to contract to produce movement 运动障碍

◇ **disordered** *adjective* (i) not functioning correctly 有障碍的 (ii) (organ) affected by adisease 有病的；**disordered action of the heart (DAH)** = da Costa's syndrome, condition where the patient suffers palpitations, breathlessness and dizziness, caused by effort or worry 神经性循环衰竭

disorientation *noun* condition where the patient is not completely conscious of space *or* time *or* place 定向障碍

◇ **disorientated** *adjective* (patient) who is confused and does not know where he is 定向障碍的

dispensary *noun* place (part of a chemist's shop *or* department of a hospital) where drugs are prepared *or* mixed and given out according to a doctor's prescription 药房

◇ **dispensing chemist** *noun* pharmacist who prepares and provides drugs according to a doctor's prescription 发药师

> COMMENT: In the UK, prescriptions can only be dispensed by qualified and registered pharmacists who must keep accurate records.
> 注释:在英国,处方只能由合格的、经注册的并保持良好记录的药剂师来拿药。

displace *verb* to put out of the usual place 移位；**displaced intervertebral disc** = disc which has moved slightly, so that the soft interior passes through the tougher exterior and causes pressure on a nerve 椎间盘脱出

◇ **displacement** *noun* movement out

of the normal position 错位; ***fracture of the radius together with displacement of the wrist*** 桡骨骨折合并腕错位

disposable *adjective* (item) which can be thrown away after use 可丢弃的,一次性的; ***disposable syringes*** 可丢弃的注射器,一次性注射器; ***disposable petri dishes*** 可丢弃的培养皿,一次性培养皿

disproportion *noun* lack of proper relationships between two things 不相称; **cephalopelvic disproportion** = condition where the pelvic opening of the mother is not large enough for the head of the fetus 头盆不称

dissecans 分离的 *see* 见 OSTEOCHONDRITIS

dissect *verb* to cut and separate tissues in a body to examine them 解剖,切开; **dissecting aneurysm** = aneurysm which occurs when the inside wall of the aorta is torn, and blood enters the membrane 壁间动脉瘤

◇ **dissection** *noun* cutting and separating parts of a body *or* an organ as part of a surgical operation *or* as part of an autopsy *or* as part of a course of study 解剖

> QUOTE: Renal dissection usually takes from 40 - 60 minutes, while liver and pancreas dissections take from one to three hours. Cardiac dissection takes about 20 minutes and lung dissection takes 60 to 90 minutes.
> 引文:肾脏解剖大约需要 40～60 分钟,而肝、胰腺解剖需 1～3 小时,心脏解剖需 20 分钟,肺解剖需 60～90 分钟。
> **Nursing Times** 护理时代

disseminated *adjective* occurring in every part of an organ *or* in the whole body 播散性的; **disseminated sclerosis** = MULTIPLE SCLEROSIS 多发性硬化; **disseminated lupus erythematosus** (**DLE**) = inflammatory disease where the skin rash is associated with widespread changes in the central nervous system, the cardiovascular system and many organs 播散性红斑狼疮

◇ **dissemination** *noun* being widespread throughout the body 播散

dissociate *verb* (i) to separate parts *or* functions 分离(ii) to separate part of the conscious mind from the rest 分裂; **dissociated anaesthesia** = loss of sensitivity to heat *or* pain *or* cold 分离性麻醉

◇ **dissociation** *noun* (**a**) separating of parts *or* functions 分离 (**b**) (*in psychiatry*) condition where part of the consciousness becomes separated from the rest and becomes independent 分裂

> COMMENT: Patients will dissociate their delusion from the real world around them as a way of escaping from the facts of the real world.
> 注释:患者通过妄想游离于自己所处的现实世界,以此作为逃避现实的一种手段。

dissolve *verb* to absorb *or* disperse something in liquid 溶解: ***The gut used in sutures slowly dissolves in the body fluids.*** 缝合用的肠线将被体液缓慢溶解。

distal *adjective* further away from the centre of a body 远端的; **distal interphalangeal joint** (**DIP**) = joint nearest the end of the finger *or* toe 远端指(趾)间关节; **distal phalanges** = bones nearest the ends of the fingers and toes 远端指(趾)骨; **distal convoluted tubule** = part of the kidney filtering system before the collecting ducts 远端肾曲小管

◇ **distally** *adverb* placed further away from the centre *or* point of attachment 远端地 (NOTE: the opposite is **proximal.** Note also that you say that a part is distal **to** another part)

distend *verb* to swell by pressure 膨胀,扩张 **distended bladder** = bladder which is full of urine 膀胱膨胀

◇ **distension** *noun* condition where something is swollen 膨胀,扩张: ***Distension of the veins in the abdomen is a sign of blocking of the portal vein.*** 腹壁静脉扩张是门静脉阻塞的体征。**abdominal distension** = swelling of the abdomen (because of gas *or* fluid) 腹膨隆

distil *verb* to separate the component

parts of a liquid by boiling and collecting the condensed vapour 蒸馏; **distilled water** *or* **purified water** = water which has been made pure by distillation 蒸馏水,纯净水

◇ **distillation** *noun* action of distilling a liquid 蒸馏

distinct *adjective* separate *or* not to be confused 明显的: ***The colon is divided into four distinct sections.*** 结肠分为界限明显的四部分。

◇ **distinctive** *adjective* easily noticed *or* characteristic 特征性的,与众不同的: ***Mumps is easily diagnosed by distinctive swellings on the side of the face.*** 流行性腮腺炎根据脸一侧的特征性肿胀很容易诊断。

distort *verb* to twist something into an abnormal shape 扭曲,变形: ***His lower limbs were distorted by the disease.*** 他的下肢因疾病而变形。

◇ **distortion** *noun* twisting of part of the body out of its normal shape 扭曲

distress *noun* suffering caused by pain *or* worry 痛苦,沮丧: ***Attempted suicide is often a sign of the person's mental distress.*** 企图自杀往往是精神痛苦的表现。**infant respiratory distress syndrome** = condition of newborn babies where the lungs do not function properly 婴儿呼吸窘迫综合征

district *noun* area *or* part of the country *or* town 地区; **district general hospital** = hospital which serves the needs of the population of a district 地区性综合医院; **District Health Authority (DHA)** = administrative unit in the National Health Service which is responsible for all health services provided in a district 地区卫生当局; **district nurse** = nurse who visits patients in their homes in a certain area 地段护士

disturb *verb* to worry someone *or* to stop someone working by talking, etc. 打扰: ***Don't disturb him when he's working.*** 他工作时不要打扰他。***His sleep was disturbed by the other patients in the ward.*** 病房里的其他患者干扰了他的睡眠。

◇ **disturbance** *noun* being disturbed 紊乱,失调,障碍: ***The blow to the head caused disturbance to the brain.*** 头部受击使大脑的活动紊乱。

diuresis *noun* increase in the production of urine 多尿,利尿

◇ **diuretic** *adjective* & *noun* (substance) which makes the kidneys produce more urine 利尿的,利尿剂

diurnal *adjective* happening in the daytime *or* happening every day 昼现的

divalent *adjectine* having a valency of two 二价的

divergent strabismus *noun* condition where a person's eyes both look away from the nose 散开性斜视

diverticulum *noun* little sac *or* pouch which develops in the wall of the intestine or other organ 憩室; **Meckel's diverticulum** = congenital formation of a diverticulum in the ileum 梅克尔憩室 (NOTE: the plural is **diverticula**)

◇ **diverticular disease** *noun* disease of the large intestine, where the colon thickens and diverticula form in the walls, causing the patient pain in the lower abdomen 大肠憩室

◇ **diverticulitis** *noun* inflammation of diverticula formed in the wall of the colon 憩室炎

◇ **diverticulosis** *noun* condition where diverticula form in the intestine but are not inflamed (in the small intestine, this can lead to blind loop syndrome) 憩室病

divide *verb* to separate into parts 分开: ***The common carotid divides into two smaller arteries.*** 颈总动脉分为两条较小的动脉。

◇ **division** *noun* cutting into parts *or* splitting into parts 分开,分裂; **cell division** = way in which a cell reproduces itself by mitosis 细胞分裂

divulsor *noun* surgical instrument used to expand a passage 扩张器

dizygotic twins = FRATERNAL

TWINS 异卵双胞胎

dizzy *adjective* having the sense of balance affected *or* feeling that everything is going round 眩晕: ***After standing in the sun, she became dizzy and had to lie down.*** 站在太阳下她感到眩晕,不得不躺下。***He suffers from dizzy spells.*** 他眩晕发作。

◇ **dizziness** *noun* feeling that everything is going round because the sense of balance has been affected 眩晕

dl = DECILITRE 分升

DLE = DISSEMINATED LUPUS ERYTHEMATOSUS 播散性红斑狼疮

dm = DECIMETRE 分米

DMD *US* = DOCTOR OF DENTAL MEDICINE 牙科医生

DNA = DEOXYRIBONUCLEIC ACID 脱氧核糖核酸

DOA = DEAD ON ARRIVAL 到达时已死亡

doctor *noun* (**a**) person who has trained in medicine and is qualified to examine people when they are ill to find out what is wrong with them and to prescribe a course of treatment 医生: ***His son is training to be a doctor.*** 他儿子在接受培训当医生。***If you have a pain in your chest, you ought to see a doctor.*** 如果胸疼,你应该去看医生。***He has gone to the doctor's.*** 他已经去医生那儿了。***Do you want to make an appointment with the doctor?*** 你要与医生预约吗? **family doctor** = general practitioner, a doctor who looks after the health of people in his area 家庭医生 (**b**) title given to a qualified person who is registered with the General Medical Council 医学博士: ***I have an appointment with Dr Jones.*** 我跟约翰博士有约会。(NOTE: **doctor** is shortened to **Dr** when written before a name. In the UK surgeons are traditionally not called 'Doctor', but are addressed as 'Mr', 'Mrs', etc. The title 'doctor' is also applied to persons who have a high degree from a university in a non-medical subject. So 'Dr Jones' may have a degree in music, or in any other subject without a connection with medicine)

Döderlein's bacillus *noun* bacterium usually found in the vagina 德得莱因氏杆菌,阴道中常见的杆菌

dolichocephaly *noun* condition of a person who has a skull which is longer than normal 长头者

◇ **dolichocephalic** *adjective* (person) with a long skull 长头的

> COMMENT: In dolichocephaly, the measurement across the skull is less than 75% of the length of the head from front to back.
> 注释:长头患者的头颅横径小于头前后距的75%。

dolor *noun* pain 痛

◇ **dolorimetry** *noun* measuring of pain 疼痛测量

◇ **dolorosa** 痛性的 *see* 见 ADIPOSIS

domicile *noun* (*in official use*) home *or* place where someone lives 家庭的

◇ **domiciliary** *adjective* at home *or* in the home 在家的: ***The doctor made a domiciliary visit.*** = He visited the patient at home. 医生进行家庭出诊。**domiciliary midwife** = nurse with special qualification in midwifery, who can assist in childbirth at home 家庭助产士; **domiciliary services** = nursing services which are available to patients in their homes 家庭护理

dominance *noun* being more powerful 优势; **cerebral dominance** = normal condition where the centres for various functions are located in one cerebral hemisphere 大脑半球优势; **ocular dominance** = condition where a person uses one eye more than the other 眼优势

◇ **dominant** *adjective & noun* (genetic trait) which is more powerful than other recessive genes 显性的,显性基因

> COMMENT: Since each physical trait is governed by two genes, if one is recessive and the other dominant, the resulting trait will be that of the dominant gene.

注释：每个生理表型都由两个基因控制，如果一个是隐性的，另一个是显性的，那么最终表型由显性基因控制。

donor *noun* person who gives his own tissue *or* organs for use in transplants 供体，捐献者；**blood donor** = person who gives blood which is then used in transfusions to other patients 献血者；**kidney donor** = person who gives one of his kidneys as a transplant 肾脏供体；**donor card** = card carried by a person stating that he approves of his organs being used for transplanting after he has died 供体卡

dopamine *noun* substance found in the medulla of the adrenal glands, which also acts as a neurotransmitter, lack of which is associated with Parkinson's disease 多巴胺

dormant *adjective* inactive for a time 休眠的，不活动的：***The virus lies dormant in the body for several years.*** 病毒可在体内潜伏几年。

dorsal *adjective* (i) referring to the back 背的 (ii) referring to the back of the body 背面的；**dorsal vertebrae** = twelve vertebrae in the back, between the cervical vertebrae and the lumbar vertebrae 胸椎 (NOTE: the opposite is **ventral**)

◇ **dorsi-** *or* **dorso-** *prefix* referring to the back 背

◇ **dorsiflexion** *noun* flexion towards the back of part of the body (such as raising the foot at the ankle, as opposed to plantar flexion) 背屈

◇ **dorsoventral** *adjective* (i) referring to the back of the body and the front 背腹侧的 (ii) extending from the back of the body to the front 后前位

◇ **dorsum** *noun* back of any part of the body 背面

dose 1 *noun* measured quantity of a drug *or* radiation which is to be administered to a patient at a time 剂量：***It is dangerous to exceed the prescribed dose.*** 超过处方剂量是危险的。**2** *verb* **to dose with** = to give a patient a drug 开药：***She dosed her son with aspirin and cough medicine before he went to his examination.*** 她在儿子考试前给他开了些阿司匹林和咳嗽药。***The patient has been dosing herself with laxatives.*** 患者自己开了些泻药。

◇ **dosage** *noun* correct amounts of a drug calculated by a doctor to be necessary for a patient 剂量：***The doctor decided to increase the dosage of antibiotics.*** 医生决定增加抗生素的剂量。***The dosage for children is half that for adults.*** 儿童的剂量是成人的一半。

◇ **dosimeter** *noun* instrument which measures the amount of X-rays or other radiation received 放射量计

◇ **dosimetry** *noun* measuring the amount of X-rays or radiation received, using a dosimeter X线放射量测定法

double *adjective* with two similar parts 双的；**double figures** = numbers from 10 to 99 两位数；**double pneumonia** = pneumonia in both lungs 双肺；**double uterus** = DIDELPHYS 双子宫；**bent double** = bent over completely so that the face is towards the ground 驼背：***He was bent double with arthritis.*** 他的关节炎使他驼背。

◇ **double-blind** *noun* way of testing a new drug, where neither the people taking the test, nor the people administering it know which patients have had the real drug and which have had the placebo 双盲

◇ **double-jointed** *adjective* able to bend joints to an abnormal degree 关节过伸

◇ **double vision** = DIPLOPIA 复视

douche *noun* (i) liquid forced into the body to wash out a cavity 冲洗，灌洗；(ii) device used for washing out a cavity 冲洗器；**vaginal douche** = device *or* liquid for washing out the vagina 阴道冲洗器，阴道冲洗液

Douglas Douglas bag = bag used for measuring the volume of air breathed out of the lungs 道格拉斯袋，用来测量肺呼

出气量的集气袋；**Douglas' pouch** = the rectouterine peritoneal recess 道格拉斯陷凹，直肠子宫陷凹

douloureux 三叉神经的 *see* TIC

Down's syndrome *noun* trisomy 21, a congenital defect, due to existence of an extra third chromosome at number 21; in which the patient has slanting eyes, a wide face, speech difficulties and is usually mentally retarded to some extent 道恩综合征，一种遗传性疾病，染色体21核型为三体，患儿表现为斜视、宽面、说话困难，常有一定程度的智力发育障碍 (NOTE: sometimes called 'mongolism' because of the shape of the eyes)

doze *verb* to sleep a little *or* to sleep lightly 打盹：***She dozed off for a while after lunch.*** 她午饭后打了会儿盹儿。

◇ **dozy** *adjective* sleepy 发困的：***These antihistamines can make you feel dozy.*** 抗组胺药会使你发困。

DPT = DIPHTHERIA, WHOOPING COUGH, TETANUS 白(喉)百(日咳)破(伤风)；**DPT vaccine** *or* **DPT immunization** = combined vaccine *or* immunization against the three diseases 白百破疫苗

drachm *noun* measure used in pharmacy (dry weight equals 3.8g, liquid measure equals 3.7ml) 打兰，英钱(重量单位；一打兰相当于1.771克常衡，或3.88克药衡)

dracontiasis *or* **dracunculiasis** *noun* tropical disease caused by the guinea worm *Dracunculus medinensis* which enters the body from infected drinking water and forms blisters on the skin, frequently leading to secondary arthritis, fibrosis and cellulitis 麦地那龙线虫病

◇ **Dracunculus** *noun* the guinea worm, a parasitic worm which enters the body and rises to the skin to form a blister 龙线虫属

dragee *noun* sugar-coated drug tablet *or* pill 糖衣片

drain 1 *noun* (**a**) pipe for carrying waste water from a house 下水道：***The report of the health inspectors was critical of the drains.*** 卫生监察员的报告中批评了下水管道的状况。(**b**) tube to remove liquid from the body 引流管 **2** *verb* to remove liquid from something 引流；***an operation to drain the sinus*** 窦的引流手术；***They drained the pus from the abscess.*** 他们引流了脓液。

◇ **drainage** *noun* removal of liquid from the site of an operation *or* pus from an abscess by means of a tube or wick left in the body for a time 引流

drape *noun* thin material used to place over a patient about to undergo surgery, leaving the operation site uncovered 被单，手术单

draw-sheet *noun* sheet under a patient in bed, folded so that it can be pulled out as it becomes soiled 垫单

dream 1 *noun* images which a person sees when asleep 梦：***I had a bad dream about spiders.*** 我做了个有关蜘蛛的恶梦。**2** *verb* to think you see something happening while you are asleep 做梦：***He dreamt he was attacked by spiders.*** 他做梦被蜘蛛攻击。(NOTE: **dreams- dreaming- dreamed** *or* **dreamt**)

drepanocyte = SICKLE CELL 镰状细胞

◇ **drepanocytosis** = SICKLE-CELL ANAEMIA 镰状细胞贫血

dress *verb* (**a**) to put on clothes 穿衣：***He (got) dressed and then had breakfast.*** 他穿好衣服后吃早餐。***The surgeon was dressed in a green gown.*** 外科医师穿了件绿色的手术衣。***You can get dressed again now.*** 你现在可以重新穿上衣服。(**b**) to clean a wound and put a covering over it 清洗包扎伤口：***Nurses dressed the wounds of the accident victims.*** 护士为事故中的伤者清洗包扎伤口。

◇ **dressing** *noun* covering *or* bandage applied to a wound to protect it 敷料：***The patient's dressings need to be changed every two hours.*** 患者的敷料需要每两小时更换一次。**gauze dressing** = dressing of thin light material 纱布敷料；

sterile dressing = dressing which is sold in a sterile pack, ready for use 消毒敷料; **adhesive dressing** 橡皮膏 *see* 见 ADHESIVE

dribble *verb* to let liquid flow slowly out of an opening, especially saliva out of the mouth 滴落: ***The baby dribbled over her dress.*** 婴儿的口水滴在了衣服上。

◇ **dribbling** *noun* (i) letting saliva flow out of the mouth 流涎 (ii) incontinence, being unable to keep back the flow of urine 尿失禁

drill 1 *noun* tool which rotates very rapidly to make a hole; surgical instrument used in dentistry to remove caries 钻,牙钻 **2** *verb* to make a hole with a drill 钻洞: ***A small hole is drilled in the skull.*** 在颅骨上钻了个小洞。***The dentist drilled one of her molars.*** 牙医在她的一颗磨牙上钻了个洞。

drink 1 *noun* (**a**) liquid which is swallowed 饮料: ***Have a drink of water.*** 喝口水。***Always have a hot drink before you go to bed.*** 就寝前喝杯热饮。**soft drinks** = drinks (like orange juice) with no alcohol in them 软饮料 (**b**) alcoholic drink 酒 **2** *verb* (**a**) to swallow liquid 喝: ***He drinks two cups of coffee for breakfast.*** 他早餐喝了两杯咖啡。***You need to drink at least five pints of liquid a day.*** 你每天至少需要喝 5 品脱的液体。(**b**) to drink alcoholic drinks 喝酒: ***Do you drink a lot?*** 你喝酒多吗? (NOTE: **drinks- drinking - drank - has drunk**)

Drinker respirator *noun* iron lung, a machine which encloses the whole of a patient's body except the head, and in which air pressure is increased and decreased, so forcing the patient to breathe in and out 人工呼吸器,铁肺

drip *noun* method of introducing liquid slowly and continuously into the body, where a bottle of liquid is held above the patient and the fluid flows slowly down a tube into a needle in a vein *or* into the stomach 滴注法; **intravenous drip** = drip which goes into a vein 静脉点滴; **saline drip** = drip containing salt solution 盐水滴注; **drip feed** = drip containing nutrients 滴注营养液,鼻饲

drop 1 *noun* (**a**) small quantity of liquid 滴: ***A drop of water fell on the floor.*** 一滴水掉在了地板上。***The optician prescribed her some drops for the eyes.*** 眼科医师给她开了些滴眼药。(**b**) reduction *or* fall in quantity of something 下降; **drop in pressure** = sudden reduction in pressure 血压下降 **2** *verb* to fall *or* to let something fall 下落: ***Pressure in the artery dropped suddenly.*** 血压突然下降。

◇ **drop attack** *noun* condition where a person suddenly falls down, though he is not unconscious, caused by sudden weakness of the spine 猝倒

◇ **drop foot** *or* **drop wrist** *noun* conditions, caused by muscular disorder, where the ankle *or* wrist is not strong, and the foot *or* hand hangs limp 垂腕,腕下垂,足下垂

◇ **droplet** *noun* very small drop of liquid 小滴

◇ **drop off** *verb* to fall asleep 入睡: ***She dropped off in front of the TV.*** 她在电视前睡着了。

◇ **dropper** *noun* small glass *or* plastic tube with a rubber bulb at one end, used to suck up and expel liquid in drops 滴管

dropsy *noun* swelling of part of the body because of accumulation of fluid in the tissues 积水

> COMMENT: Dropsy is usually caused by kidney failure or heart failure, leading to bad circulation. The legs (especially the ankles) and the arms become very swollen.
> 注释:积水多因肾衰竭或心力衰竭引起循环不良所致。腿(尤其是踝部)和胳膊会严重肿胀。

drown *verb* to die by inhaling liquid 溺死: ***He fell into the sea and (was) drowned.*** 他掉到海里淹死了。***Six people drowned when the boat sank.*** 船沉时有 6 人溺水身亡。

◇ **drowning** *noun* act of dying by inhaling liquid 淹死: ***The autopsy showed***

***that death was due to drowning*.**尸检显示死亡是溺水造成的。**dry drowning** = death where the patient's air passage has been constricted because he is under water, though he does not inhale any water 溺水窒息死亡

drowsy *adjective* sleepy 瞌睡的：***The injection will make you feel drowsy*.**这针将会使你瞌睡。

drug *noun* (**a**) chemical substance (either natural or synthetic) which is used in medicine and affects the way in which organs *or* tissues function 药：***The doctors are trying to cure him with a new drug*.** 医生在尝试用新药为他治疗。***She was prescribed a course of pain-killing drugs*.** 给她开了一疗程的止痛药。***The drug is being monitored for possible side-effects*.**正在监测这药可能的副作用。**drug dependence** = being addicted to a drug and unable to exist without taking it regularly (can also apply to habit-forming substances not used in medicine) 药物依赖 (**b**) habit-forming substance 毒品：***He has been taking drugs for several months*.**他吸毒已经几个月了。***The government is trying to stamp out drug pushing*.**政府力图消灭贩毒。**drug abuse** = taking habit-forming drugs药物滥用；**a high rate of drug-related deaths** = of deaths associated with the taking of drugs 吸毒高死亡率；**controlled drugs**, *US* **controlled substances** = drugs which are not freely available, which are restricted by law, and which are classified (Class A, B, C), and of which possession may be an offence 管制药物；**dangerous drugs** = drugs which may be harmful to people who take them, and so can be prohibited from import and general sale 危险药物 *see also* 参见 ADDICT, ADDICTION

◇ **drugstore** *noun US* shop where medicines and drugs can be bought (as well as many other goods) 杂货店

COMMENT: There are three classes of controlled drugs: *Class 'A'drugs*: (cocaine, heroin, crack, LSD, etc.); *Class 'B'drugs*: (amphetamines, cannabis, codeine, etc.); and Class 'C'drugs : (drugs which are related to the amphetamines, such as benzphetamine). The drugs are covered by five schedules under the Misuse of Drugs Regulations : Schedule 1: drugs which are not used medicinally, such as cannabis and LSD, for which possession and supply are prohibited ; Schedule 2: drugs which can be used medicinally, such as heroin, morphine, cocaine, and amphetamines: these are fully controlled as regards prescriptions by doctors, safe custody in pharmacies, registering of sales, etc. Schedule 3: barbiturates, which are controlled as regards prescriptions, but need not be kept in safe custody; Schedule 4: benzodiazepines, which are controlled as regards registers of purchasers ; Schedule 5: other substances for which invoices showing purchase must be kept.

注释：管制药物有3类：A类(可卡因、海洛因、麦角副酸二乙酰胺等)；B类(苯丙胺、大麻、可待因等)；C类(跟苯丙胺有关的药物，如苄甲苯丙胺)。药品由药物滥用管制委员会分为5类：1类是不能作为医用的药物，如大麻和麴乙二胺，无论是拥有还是提供都是被禁止的；2类是可用于医疗的，如海洛因、吗啡、可卡因和苯丙胺，但必须有医生处方，由药房负责安全监管，还必须有销售许可；3类是巴比妥类必须有医生处方但不必安全监管；4类是苯二氮草，购买者需登记；5类是其他需保存购买发票的药物。

drum 鼓，鼓膜 *see* 见 EARDRUM

drunk *adjective* intoxicated with too much alcohol 醉酒的，酒精中毒

◇ **drunken** *adjective* intoxicated 中毒的：***The doctors had to get help to control the drunken patient*.**医生不得不帮助处理酒精中毒患者。(NOTE: drunken is only used in front of a noun, and drunk is usually used after the verb to be **a drunken patient**; **that patient is drunk**)

dry 1 *adjective* not wet *or* with the smallest amount of moisture 干燥的: ***The surface of the wound should be kept dry.*** 伤口应保持干燥。***She uses a cream to soften her dry skin.*** 她用雪花膏滋润干燥的皮肤。**dry burn** = burn caused by touching a very hot dry surface 烫伤; **dry gangrene** = condition where the blood supply has been cut off and the tissue becomes black 干性坏疽; **dry ice** = CARBON DIOXIDE 干冰（NOTE: **dry - drier - driest**）**2** *verb* to remove moisture from something 使干燥; to wipe something untilitis dry 擦干

◊ **dryness** *noun* state of being dry 干: ***She complained of dryness in her mouth.*** 她主诉口干。***Dryness in the eyes, accompanied by rheumatoid arthritis.*** 眼干，伴类风湿性关节炎。

◊ **dry out** *verb* (i) to dry completely 使彻底干燥 (ii) (*informal* 非正式) to treat someone for alcoholism 戒酒

DSS = DEPARTMENT OF SOCIAL SECURITY 社会保险部

DTs = DELIRIUM TREMENS 震颤性谵妄

Duchenne muscular dystrophy *noun* hereditary disease of the muscles where some muscles (starting with the legs) swell and become weak 杜兴氏肌营养不良，一种遗传性肌病，表现为部分肌肉肿胀，虚弱（从腿部开始）

> COMMENT: Usually found in young boys. It is carried in the mother's genes.
> 注释：男孩儿中常见，由母系遗传。

Ducrey's bacillus *noun* type of bacterium found in the lungs, causing chancroid 杜克雷氏杆菌，杜克雷嗜血杆菌

duct *noun* tube which carries liquids, especially one which carries secretions 管; **bile duct** = tube which links the cystic duct and the hepatic duct to the duodenum 胆管; **common bile duct** = duct leading to the duodenum, formed of the hepatic and cystic ducts together 胆总管; **cystic duct** = duct which takes bile from the gall bladder to the common bile duct 胆囊管; **hepatic duct** = duct which links the liver to the bile duct leading to the duodenum 肝管; **common hepatic duct** = duct from the liver formed when the right and left hepatic ducts join 肝总管; **cochlear duct** = spiral channel in the cochlea 耳蜗管; **collecting duct** = part of the kidney filtering system 集合管; **efferent duct** = duct which carries liquid away from an organ 输出管; **ejaculatory ducts** = two ducts formed by the seminal vesicles and vas deferens, which go through the prostate and end in the urethra 射精管 ◊ 见图 UROGENITAL SYSTEM (MALE); **nasolacrimal duct** *or* **tear duct** = canal which takes tears from the lacrimal sac into the nose 鼻泪管; **right lymphatic duct** = one of the main terminal channels for carrying lymph, draining the right side of the head and neck and entering the junction of the right subclavian and internal jugular veins. It is the smaller of the two main discharge points of the lymphatic system into the venous system, the larger being the thoracic duct 右淋巴导管; **pancreatic ducts** = ducts leading through the pancreas to the duodenum 胰管; **semicircular ducts** = ducts in the semicircular canals in the ear 半规管 ◊ 见图 EAR; **thoracic duct** = one of the main terminal ducts carrying lymph, on the left side of the neck 胸导管

◊ **ductless gland** *or* **endocrine gland** *noun* gland without a duct which produces hormones which are introduced directly into the bloodstream (such as the pituitary gland, thyroid gland, the adrenals, and the gonads) 内分泌腺 ◊ 见图 GLAND

◊ **ductule** *noun* very small duct 小管

◊ **ductus** *noun* duct 管; **ductus arteriosus** = in a fetus, the blood vessel connecting the left pulmonary artery to the aorta so that blood does not pass through the lungs 动脉导管; **ductus deferens** *or* **vas deferens** = one of two tubes along which sperm passes from the epididymis to the prostate gland 输精管 ◊ 见图 UROGENITAL SYSTEM (MALE); **ductus venosus** = in a fetus, the blood vessel connecting the portal sinus to the inferior vena cava 静脉导管

ductile *adjective* soft *or* which can bend 延伸性的,易变形的 (NOTE: the opposite is **brittle**)

dull 1 *adjective* (pain) which is not sharp, but continuously painful 钝的: ***She complained of a dull throbbing pain in her head.*** 她主诉头部搏动性钝痛。***He felt a dull pain in the chest.*** 他感觉胸部钝痛。**2** *verb* to make less sharp 使迟钝: ***His senses were dulled by the drug.*** 药物使他的感觉变迟钝。

dumb *adjective* not able to speak 哑的
◊ **dumbness** *noun* being unable to speak 哑

dummy *noun* rubber teat given to a baby to suck, to prevent it crying 橡皮奶嘴 (NOTE: US English is **pacifier**)

dumping syndrome *noun* rapid passing of the contents of the stomach and duodenum into the jejunum, causing fainting, diarrhoea and sweating in patients who have had a gastrectomy 倾倒综合征

duoden- *prefix* referring to the duodenum 十二指肠的
◊ **duodenal** *adjective* referring to the duodenum 十二指肠的; **duodenal papillae** = small projecting parts in the duodenum where the bile duct and pancreatic duct open 十二指肠乳突; **duodenal ulcer** = ulcer in the duodenum 十二指肠溃疡
◊ **duodenoscope** *noun* instrument used to examine the inside of the duodenum 十二指肠镜
◊ **duodenostomy** *noun* permanent opening made between the duodenum and the abdominal wall 十二指肠造口术
◊ **duodenum** *noun* first part of the small intestine, going from the stomach to the jejunum 十二指肠 ◊ 见图 DIGESTIVE SYSTEM, STOMACH

> COMMENT: The duodenum is the shortest part of the small intestine, about 250 mm long. It takes bile from the gall bladder and pancreatic juice from the pancreas and continues the digestive processes started in the mouth and stomach.
> 注释:十二指肠是小肠最短的部分,大约250毫米长。接纳胆囊的胆汁和胰的胰液进行消化,继续从口腔和胃开始的消化过程。

Dupuytren's contracture *noun* condition where the palmar fascia becomes thicker, causing the fingers (usually the middle and ring fingers) to bend forwards 杜普依特伦氏挛缩,掌挛缩病

dura mater *noun* thicker outer meninx covering the brain and spinal cord 硬脑脊膜
◊ **dural** *adjective* referring to the dura mater 硬脑[脊]膜的

Dutch cap *noun* vaginal diaphragm, a contraceptive device for women, which is placed over the cervix uteri before sexual intercourse 子宫帽,阴道膈

duty *noun* requirement for a particular job *or* something which has to be done (especially in a particular job) *or* work which a person has to do 责任: ***What are the duties of a night sister?*** 夜班护士的责任是什么? **to be on duty** = to be doing official work at a special time 在岗,值班; **night duty** = work done at night 夜班: ***Nurse Smith is on night duty this week.*** 思密斯护士这周上夜班。**duty nurse** = nurse who is on duty 值班护士; ***A doctor owes a duty of care to his patient.*** = The doctor has to treat a patient in a proper way, as this is part of the work of being a doctor. 医生必须关心病人,这是他作为医生工作中的一部分。

d. v. t. *or* **DVT** = DEEP VEIN THROMBOSIS 深静脉血栓

dwarf *noun* person who is much smaller than normal 侏儒

◇ **dwarfism** *noun* condition where the growth of a person has stopped leaving him much smaller than normal 侏儒症

COMMENT: May be caused by achondroplasia, where the long bones in the arms and legs do not develop fully but the trunk and head are of normal size. Dwarfism can have other causes, such as rickets or deficiency in the pituitary gland.
注释:可能由软骨发育不全引起,躯干及头部骨发育正常,而手腿的长骨发育不全。侏儒症也可有其他原因如:佝偻病、垂体缺陷。

dynamometer *noun* instrument for measuring the force of muscular contraction 肌力计

-dynia *suffix* meaning pain 疼

dys- *prefix* meaning difficult *or* defective 困难,不良

◇ **dysaesthesia** *noun* (i) impairment of a sense, in particular the sense of touch 感觉迟钝(ii) unpleasant feeling of pain experienced when the skin is touched lightly 触物痛

◇ **dysarthria** *noun* difficulty in speaking words clearly, caused by damage to the central nervous system 发音障碍

◇ **dysbarism** *noun* any disorder caused by differences between the atmospheric pressure outside the body and the pressure inside 气压病

◇ **dysbasia** *noun* difficulty in walking, especially when caused by a lesion to a nerve 步行困难

◇ **dyschezia** *noun* difficulty in passing faeces 大便困难

◇ **dyschondroplasia** *noun* abnormal shortness of the long bones 软骨发育异常

◇ **dyscoria** *noun* (i) abnormally shaped pupil of the eye 瞳孔变形(ii) abnormal reaction of the pupil 瞳孔反应异常

◇ **dyscrasia** *noun* old term for any abnormal body condition 恶液质,体液不调

◇ **dysdiadochokinesia** *noun* inability to carry out rapid movements, caused by a disorder *or* lesion of the cerebellum 轮替运动障碍

dysentery *noun* infection and inflammation of the colon, causing bleeding and diarrhoea 痢疾

◇ **dysenteric** *adjective* referring to dysentery 痢疾的

COMMENT: Dysentery occurs mainly in tropical countries. The symptoms include diarrhoea, discharge of blood and pain in the intestines. There are two main types of dysentery: bacillary dysentery, caused by the bacterium Shigella in contaminated food; and amoebic dysentery or amoebiasis, caused by a parasitic amoeba Entamoeba histolytica spread through contaminated drinking water.
注释:痢疾主要发生在热带国家,症状包括腹泻、血便和腹痛。痢疾主要有两种:杆菌性痢疾,因志贺杆菌污染了食物引起;阿米巴痢疾或阿米巴病,因饮水中污染了溶组织内阿米巴引起。

dysfunction *noun* abnormal functioning of an organ 功能障碍

◇ **dysfunctional uterine bleeding** *noun* bleeding in the uterus, not caused by a menstrual period 功能性子宫出血

◇ **dysgenesis** *noun* abnormal development 发育不全

◇ **dysgerminoma** *noun* malignant tumour of the ovary *or* testicle 无性细胞瘤

◇ **dysgraphia** *noun* (i) difficulty in writing caused by a brain lesion 书写困难 (ii) writer's cramp 书写痉挛

◇ **dyskinesia** *noun* inability to control voluntary movements 运动障碍

◇ **dyslalia** *noun* disorder of speech, caused by abnormal formation of the tongue 发音困难

dyslexia *noun* disorder of development, where a person is unable to read or write properly and confuses letters 诵读困难

◇ **dyslexic** **1** *adjective* referring to dyslexia 诵读困难的 **2** *noun* person suffering from dyslexia 诵读困难患者

COMMENT : Caused either by an

inherited disability or by a brain lesion; dyslexia does not suggest any lack of normal intelligence.
注释:由于遗传性疾病或脑损伤引起,诵读困难并不意味着智力障碍。

dyslogia *noun* difficulty in putting ideas in words 精神性难语病
◇ **dysmenorrhoea** *noun* pain experienced at menstruation 痛经; **primary** *or* **essential dysmenorrhoea** = dysmenorrhoea which occurs at the first menstrual period 原发性痛经; **secondary dysmenorrhoea** = dysmenorrhoea which starts at some time after the first menstruation 继发性痛经
◇ **dysostosis** *noun* defective formation of bones 骨发育不全
◇ **dyspareunia** *noun* difficult *or* painful sexual intercourse in a woman 性交困难(指女性),性交痛
◇ **dyspepsia** *or* **indigestion** *noun* condition where a person feels pains *or* discomfort in the stomach, caused by indigestion 消化不良
◇ **dyspeptic** *adjective* referring to dyspepsia 消化不良的
◇ **dysphagia** *noun* difficulty in swallowing 咽下困难
◇ **dysphasia** *noun* difficulty in speaking and putting words into the correct order 言语困难
◇ **dysphemia** = STAMMERING 口吃
◇ **dysphonia** *noun* difficulty in speaking caused by impairment of the voice *or* vocal cords *or* by laryngitis 发声困难
◇ **dysplasia** *noun* abnormal development of tissue 发育异常
◇ **dyspnoea** *noun* difficulty or pain in breathing 呼吸困难; **paroxysmal dyspnoea** = attack of breathlessness at night, caused by heart failure 阵发性呼吸困难
◇ **dyspnoeic** *adjective* where breathing is difficult or painful 呼吸困难的
◇ **dyspraxia** *noun* difficulty in carrying out coordinated movements 运用障碍
◇ **dysrhythmia** *noun* abnormal rhythm (either in speaking *or* in electrical impulses in the brain) 节律障碍
◇ **dyssynergia** = ASYNERGIA 协同失调
◇ **dystocia** *noun* difficult childbirth 难产; **fetal dystocia** = difficult childbirth caused by an abnormality *or* malpresentation of the fetus 胎原性难产; **maternal dystocia** = difficult childbirth caused by an abnormality in the mother 母原性难产
◇ **dystonia** *noun* disordered muscle tone, causing involuntary contractions which make the limbs deformed 张力障碍

dystrophia *or* **dystrophy** *noun* wasting of an organ *or* muscle *or* tissue due to lack of nutrients in that part of the body 营养不良; **dystrophia adiposogenitalis** = FRÖLICH'S SYNDROME 肥胖性生殖器退化; **dystrophia myotonica** = hereditary disease with muscle stiffness followed by atrophy of the face and neck muscles 强直性肌营养不良; **muscular dystrophy** = condition where the tissue of the muscles wastes away 肌营养不良

dysuria *noun* difficulty in passing urine 排尿困难

Ee

Vitamin E *noun* vitamin found in vegetables, vegetable oils, eggs and wholemeal bread 维生素 E

ear *noun* organ which is used for hearing 耳朵: ***If your ears are blocked, ask a doctor to syringe them.*** 如果你耳朵堵了,让医生冲洗一下。***He has gone to see an ear specialist about his deafness.*** 他已经去找耳科专家看过他的耳聋了。**inner ear** = part of the ear inside the head containing the vestibule, the cochlea and the semicircular canals 内耳; **middle ear** = part of the ear between the eardrum and the inner ear, containing the ossicles 中耳; **outer ear** *or* **external ear** *or* **pinna** = the ear on the outside of the head together with the passage leading to the eardrum 外耳; **ear canal** = one of several passages in or connected to the ear, especially the external auditory meatus, the passage from the outer ear to the eardrum 耳道; **ear ossicle** *or* **auditory ossicle** = one of three small bones (the malleus, the incus and the stapes) in the middle ear 听小骨 (NOTE: for terms referring to the ear, see words beginning with **auric-**, **ot** - or **oto-**)

◇ **earache** *or* **otalgia** *noun* pain in the ear 耳痛

◇ **eardrum** *or* **myringa** *or* **tympanum** *noun* membrane at the end of the external auditory meatus leading from the outer ear, which vibrates with sound and passes the vibrations on to the ossicles in the middle ear 鼓膜 (NOTE: for terms referring to the eardrum, see words beginning with **auric** - or **tympan-**)

◇ **earwax** *or* **cerumen** *noun* wax which forms inside the ear 耵聍

COMMENT: The outer ear is shaped in such a way that it collects sound and channels it to the eardrum. Behind the eardrum, the three ossicles in the middle ear vibrate with sound and transmit the vibrations to the cochlea in the inner ear. From the cochlea, the vibrations are passed by the auditory nerve to the brain.
注释:外耳的形状有利于收集声音传导至鼓膜。位于鼓膜后中耳内的三块听小骨随声音振动并将振动传到内耳的耳蜗,再从耳蜗经听神经到脑。

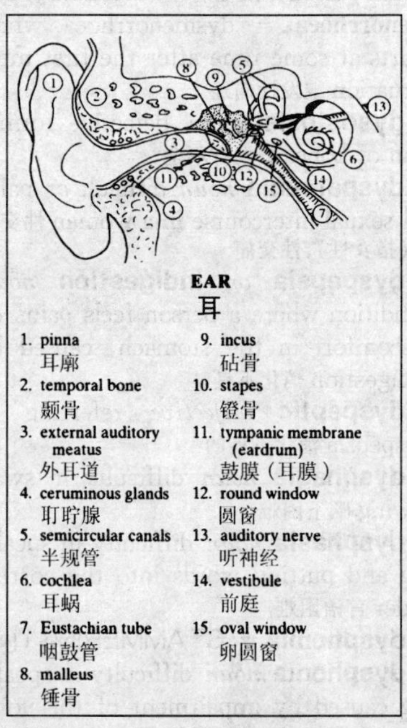

EAR
耳

1. pinna 耳廓
2. temporal bone 颞骨
3. external auditory meatus 外耳道
4. ceruminous glands 耵聍腺
5. semicircular canals 半规管
6. cochlea 耳蜗
7. Eustachian tube 咽鼓管
8. malleus 锤骨
9. incus 砧骨
10. stapes 镫骨
11. tympanic membrane (eardrum) 鼓膜(耳膜)
12. round window 圆窗
13. auditory nerve 听神经
14. vestibule 前庭
15. oval window 卵圆窗

ease *verb* to make (pain *or* worry) less 减轻: ***She had an injection to ease the pain in her leg.*** 她打了一针以减轻腿部的疼痛。***The surgeon tried to ease the patient's fears about the results of the scan.*** 外科医师设法缓解患者对扫描结果的恐惧。

eat *verb* to chew and swallow food 吃: ***I haven't eaten anything since breakfast.*** 早餐后我就再也没吃任何东西。***The patient must not eat anything for twelve hours before the operation.*** 患者术前 12

小时不能吃任何东西。**eating disorders** = illnesses (such as anorexia or bulimia) which are associated with eating 进食障碍; **eating habits** = types of food and quantities of food regularly eaten by a person 饮食习惯: ***The dietitian advised her to change her eating habits*** . 营养学家劝她改变饮食习惯。(NOTE: **eats - eating - ate - has eaten**)

EB virus = EPSTEIN-BARR VIRUS EB病毒

eburnation *noun* conversion of cartilage into a hard mass with a shiny surface like bone 软骨象牙化

ecbolic *adjective* & *noun* (substance) which produces contraction of the uterus and so induces childbirth or abortion 催产的,催产剂

ecchondroma *noun* benign tumour on the surface of cartilage or bone 外生软骨瘤

ecchymosis *or* **bruise** *or* **contusion** *noun* dark area on the skin, made by blood which has escaped into the tissues after a blow 瘀斑

eccrine *adjective* merocrine, (gland, especially a sweat gland) which does not disintegrate and remains intact during secretion 外分泌的

eccyesis = ECTOPIC PREGNANCY 异位妊娠,宫外孕

ecdysis *or* **desquamation** *noun* continuous process of losing the outer layer of dead skin 蜕皮

ECG = ELECTROCARDIOGRAM 心电图

echinococciasis *noun* disorder caused by a tapeworm *Echinococcus* which forms hydatid cysts in the lungs, liver, kidney or brain 棘球蚴病

◇ **Echinococcus granulosus** *noun* type of tapeworm, usually found in animals, but sometimes transmitted to humans, causing hydatid cysts 细粒棘球绦虫

echo- *prefix* referring to sound 回声

◇ **echocardiogram** *noun* recording of heart movements using ultrasound 超声心动图

◇ **echocardiography** *noun* ultrasonography of the heart 超声心动检查

◇ **echoencephalography** *noun* ultrasonography of the brain 脑回声波检查

◇ **echography** *noun* ultrasonography, passing ultrasound waves through the body and recording echoes to show details of internal organs 超声描计术

◇ **echokinesis** *noun* meaningless imitating of another person's actions 模仿运动

◇ **echolalia** *noun* repeating words spoken by another person 模仿语言

◇ **echopraxia** *noun* imitating another person's actions 模仿行动

◇ **echovirus** *noun* one of a group of viruses which can be isolated from the intestine and which can cause serious illnesses such as aseptic meningitis, gastroenteritis and respiratory infection in small children 埃柯病毒 *compare* 比较 REOVIRUS

eclabium *noun* turning the lips outwards, eversion of the lips 唇外翻

eclampsia *noun* serious condition of pregnant women at the end of pregnancy, where the patient has convulsions and high blood pressure and may go into a coma, caused by toxaemia of pregnancy 妊娠惊厥;子痫

ecmnesia *noun* not being able to remember recent events, while remembering clearly events which happened some time ago 近事遗忘

ecology *noun* study of the environment and the relationship of living organisms to it 生态学; **human ecology** = study of man's place in the natural world 人类生态学

◇ **ecological** *adjective* referring to ecology 生态学的

◇ **ecologist** *noun* scientist who studies ecology 生态学家

écraseur *noun* surgical instrument (usually with a wire loop) used to cut a part *or* a growth off at its base 绞勒器

ecstasy *noun* feeling of extreme happiness 狂喜

ECT = ELECTROCONVULSIVE THERAPY (electroshock treatment) 电惊厥疗法

ect- *or* **ecto-** *prefix* meaning outside 外面的

◇ **ectasia** *noun* dilatation of a passage 扩张,膨胀

◇ **ecthyma** *noun* skin disorder, a serious form of impetigo which penetrates deep under the skin and leaves scars 深脓疮

◇ **ectoderm** *or* **embryonic ectoderm** *noun* outer layer of an early embryo 外胚层

◇ **ectodermal** *adjective* referring to the ectoderm 外胚层的

◇ **ectomorph** *noun* type of person who tends to be quite thin 外胚层体型者

◇ **ectomorphic** *adjective* referring to an ectomorph 外胚层体型的 *compare* 比较 ENDOMORPH, MESOMORPH

-ectomy *suffix* referring to the removal of a part by surgical operation 切除术; **appendicectomy** = operation to remove the appendix 阑尾切除术

ectoparasite *noun* parasite which lives on the skin 外寄生虫 *compare* 比较 ENDOPARASITE

◇ **ectopia** *noun* condition where an organ *or* part of the body is not in its normal position 异位,出位

◇ **ectopic** *adjective* abnormal *or* not in the normal position 异位的; **ectopic heart beat** = abnormal extra beat of the heart which originates from a point other than the sinoatrial node 异位心跳; **ectopic pregnancy** *or* **extrauterine pregnancy** *or* **eccyesis** = pregnancy where the fetus develops outside the womb, often in one of the Fallopian tubes (tubal pregnancy) 异位妊娠 (NOTE: the opposite is **entopic**)

◇ **ectoplasm** *noun* (*in cells*) outer layer of cytoplasm which is the densest part of the cytoplasm 外胞浆;外胚层质;外质

ectro- *prefix* meaning absence *or* lack of something (usually congenital) 缺,少(常是先天的)

◇ **ectrodactyly** *noun* congenital absence of all *or* part of a finger 缺指(趾)

◇ **ectrogeny** *noun* congenital absence of a part at birth 先天性缺损

◇ **ectromelia** *noun* congenital absence of one or more limbs 缺肢畸形

ectropion *noun* eversion, turning of the edge of an eyelid outwards 睑外翻

eczema *noun* non-contagious inflammation of the skin, with itchy rash and blisters 湿疹; **atopic eczema** = type of eczema often caused by hereditary allergy 特应性湿疹; **endogenous eczema** = eczema which is caused internally 内源性湿疹; **seborrhoeic eczema** = type of eczema where scales form on the skin, usually on the scalp, and then move down the body 脂溢性湿疹; **varicose eczema** *or* **hypostatic eczema** = eczema which develops on the legs, caused by bad circulation 静脉曲张性湿疹

◇ **eczematous** *adjective* referring to eczema 湿疹的; **eczematous dermatitis** = itchy inflammation *or* irritation of the skin due an allergic reaction to a substance which a person has touched or absorbed 湿疹性皮炎

EDD = EXPECTED DATE OF DELIVERY 预产期

edema *US* = OEDEMA 水肿

edentulous *adjective* having lost all teeth 无牙的

edible *adjective* which can be eaten 可食的; **edible fungi** = fungi which can be eaten and are not poisonous 可食蕈

EEG = ELECTROENCEPHALOGRAM 脑电图

effect 1 *noun* result of a drug *or* a treatment *or* an action 药效,疗效,作用: ***The effect of the disease is to make the patient blind.*** 这疾病可使患者失明。***The antiseptic cream has had no effect on***

the rash. 抗菌软膏对皮疹无效。***Radiotherapy has a positive effect on cancer cells.*** 放疗对肿瘤细胞有肯定的疗效。**2** *verb* to make something happen 使…生效: ***The doctors effected a cure.*** 医生治疗有效。

◇ **effective** *adjective* which has an effect 有效的: ***His way of making the children keep quiet is very effective.*** 他使儿童保持安静的方法很有效。***Embolization is an effective treatment for severe haemoptysis.*** 栓塞法是治疗严重咯血的有效方法。

◇ **effector** *noun* special nerve ending in muscles *or* glands which is activated to produce contraction *or* secretion 效应器

efferens 输出的 *see* 见 VAS EFFERENS

efferent *adjective* carrying away from part of the body *or* from the centre 输出的; **efferent duct** = duct which carries a secretion away from a gland 输出管; **efferent vessel** = vessel which drains lymph from a gland 输出淋巴管 (NOTE: the opposite is **afferent**)

efficient *adjective* which works well *or* which functions correctly 有效的: ***The new product is an efficient antiseptic.*** 新产品是一种有效的抗菌剂。***The ward sister is extremely efficient.*** 病房护士长效率极高。

◇ **efficiently** *adverb* in an efficient way 有效地: ***She manages all her patients very efficiently.*** 她管理患者很有效。

effleurage *noun* form of massage where the skin is stroked in one direction to increase blood flow 轻抚法

effort *noun* using power, either mental or physical 努力,尝试: ***He made an effort and lifted his hands above his head.*** 他努力尝试将手举过头顶。***It took a lot of effort to walk even this short distance.*** 即使走这么短的路也需要很大的努力。***If he made an effort he would be able to get out of bed.*** 如果他努力的话,他可以下床。**effort syndrome** = da Costa's syndrome *or* disordered action of the heart, condition where the patient suffers palpitations caused by worry 神经性循环衰弱

effusion *noun* (i) discharge of blood *or* fluid *or* pus into or out of an internal cavity 渗,漏 (ii) fluid *or* blood *or* pus which is discharged 渗漏液; **pericardial effusion** = excess of fluid which forms in the pericardial sac 心包渗出; **pleural effusion** = excess of fluid formed in the pleural sac 胸膜渗出

egg *noun* (**a**) reproductive cell produced in the female body by the ovary, and which, if fertilized by the male sperm, becomes an embryo 卵,卵细胞; **egg cell** = immature ovum or female cell 卵细胞 (**b**) hen's egg = egg with a hard shell, laid by a hen, which is used for food 鸡蛋: ***He is allergic to eggs.*** 他对鸡蛋过敏。

ego *noun* (*in psychology*) part of the mind which is consciously in contact with the outside world and is influenced by experiences of the world 自我 *compare* 比较 ID, SUBCONSCIOUS, SUPEREGO

Egyptian ophthalmia 埃及眼炎 *see* 见 TRACHOMA

EHO = ENVIRONMENTAL HEALTH OFFICER 环境卫生官员

EIA = EXERCISE-INDUCED ASTHMA 运动诱发性哮喘

eidetic imagery *noun* recalling extremely clear pictures in the mind 逼真的表象

Eisenmenger syndrome *noun* heart disease caused by a septal defect between the ventricles, with pulmonary hypertension 艾森门格氏综合症(室间隔缺损引起肺动脉高压导致的心脏病)

ejaculation *noun* sending out of semen from the penis 射精; **premature ejaculation** = situation where the man ejaculates too early during sexual intercourse 早泄

◇ **ejaculate** *verb* to send out semen

from the penis 射精

◇ **ejaculatio praecox** *noun* situation where the man ejaculates too early during sexual intercourse 早泄

◇ **ejaculatory** *adjective* referring to ejaculation 射精的; **ejaculatory ducts** = two ducts, leading from the seminal vesicles and vas deferens, which go through the prostate and end in the urethra 射精管 ◊ 见图 UROGENITAL SYSTEM (MALE)

eject *verb* to send out something with force 排出,射出: ***Blood is ejected from the ventricle during systole.*** 血液在收缩期由心室射出。

◇ **ejection** *noun* sending out something with force 射出

EKG *US* = ELECTROCARDIOGRAM 心电图 (NOTE: GB English is **ECG**)

elastic *adjective* which can be stretched and compressed and return to its former shape 有弹性的; **elastic bandage** = stretch bandage used to support a weak joint or for treatment of a varicose vein 弹力绷带; **elastic cartilage** *or* **yellow elastic fibrocartilage** = flexible cartilage such as that in the ear and epiglottis 弹性软骨; **elastic fibres** *or* **yellow fibres** = basic components of elastic cartilage, also found in the skin and the walls of arteries or the lungs 弹力纤维,黄色纤维; **elastic tissue** = connective tissue, as in the walls of arteries or of the alveoli in the lungs, which contains elastic fibres 弹性组织

◇ **elasticity** *noun* being able to expand and be compressed and to return to the former shape 弹性

◇ **elastin** *noun* protein which occurs in elastic fibres 弹性硬蛋白

elation *noun* being stimulated and excited 激动,兴奋,欣快

elbow *noun* hinged joint where the arm bone (humerus) joins the forearm bones (radius and ulna) 肘; **tennis elbow** *or* **golf elbow** *US* **pitcher's elbow** = inflammation of the tendons of the extensor muscles in the hand which are attached to the bone near the elbow 网球肘,高尔夫球肘,投手肘 (NOTE: for other terms referring to the elbow, see **cubital**)

elderly *adjective* & *noun* old (person), (person) aged over 65 老年的,老年人: ***She looks after her two elderly parents.*** 她照顾她年迈的父母。***home for elderly single women*** 单身老年妇女之家; **the elderly** = old people 老年人

elective *adjective* (i) (chemical substance) which tends to combine with one particular substance rather than another 有选择性的(化学物质) (ii) (part of a course in a college or university) which a student can choose to take rather than another 选修课程; **elective surgery** *or* **elective treatment** = surgery *or* treatment which a patient can choose to have but is not urgently necessary to save his life 择期手术,选择性治疗

Electra complex *noun* (*in psychology*) condition where a girl feels sexually attracted to her father and sees her mother as an obstacle 恋父(厌母)情结

electricity *noun* electron energy which can be converted to light *or* heat *or* power 电: ***The motor is run by electricity.*** 这摩托靠电力驱动。***Electricity is used to administer shocks to a patient.*** 电可用来使患者休克。

◇ **electric** *adjective* worked by electricity 用电的; used for carrying electricity 带电的; **electric shock** = sudden passage of electricity into the body, causing a nervous spasm or, in severe cases, death 电击; **electric shock treatment** = treatment of a disorder by giving the patient light electric shocks 电击疗法

◇ **electro-** *prefix* referring to electricity 电的

◇ **electrocardiogram** (**ECG**) *noun* chart which records the electrical impulses in the heart muscle 心电图

◇ **electrocardiograph** *noun* apparatus for measuring and recording the electrical impulses of the muscles of the heart as it beats 心电图机

◇ **electrocardiography** *noun* process of recording the electrical impulses of the heart 心电描记法

◇ **electrocardiophonography** *noun* process of electrically recording the sounds of the heartbeats 心音描计法

◇ **electrocautery** = GALVANOCAUTERY 电烙术(器)

◇ **electrochemical** *adjective* referring to electricity and chemicals and their interaction 电化学的

◇ **electrocoagulation** *noun* control of haemorrhage in surgery by coagulation of divided blood vessels by passing a high-frequency electric current through them 电凝法

◇ **electroconvulsive therapy** (**ECT**) *or* **electroplexy** *noun* treatment of severe depression and some mental disorders by giving the patient small electric shocks in the brain to make him have convulsions 电惊厥疗法

◇ **electrode** *noun* conductor of an electrical apparatus which touches the body and carries an electric shock 电极

◇ **electrodesiccation** *or* **fulguration** *noun* destruction of tissue (such as the removal of a wart) by burning with an electric needle 电灼疗法

◇ **electroencephalogram** (**EEG**) *noun* chart on which are recorded the electrical impulses in the brain 脑电图

◇ **electroencephalograph** *noun* apparatus which records the electrical impulses in the brain 脑电图机

◇ **electroencephalography** *noun* process of recording the electrical impulses in the brain 脑电描记法,脑电图记录

◇ **electrolysis** *noun* destruction of tissue (such as removing unwanted hair) by applying an electric current 电解(作用)

◇ **electrolyte** *noun* chemical solution of a substance which can conduct electricity 电解质,电解液

◇ **electrolytic** *adjective* referring to electrolytes *or* to electrolysis 电解质的,电解的

◇ **electromyogram** (**EMG**) *noun* chart showing the electric currents in muscles in action 肌电图

◇ **electromyography** *noun* study of electric currents in active muscles 肌电学

◇ **electron** *noun* negative particle in an atom 电 子; **electron microscope** (**EM**) = microscope which uses a beam of electrons instead of light 电子显微镜

◇ **electronic** *adjective* referring to electrons *or* working with electrons 电子的,用电子的; **electronic stethoscope** = stethoscope fitted with an amplifier 电子听诊器

◇ **electro-oculogram** *noun* a record of the electric currents round the eye, induced by eye movements 眼电图

◇ **electro-oculography** *noun* recording the electric currents round the eye, induced by eye movements 电子眼动图,眼电图

◇ **electrophoresis** *noun* analysis of a substance by the movement of charged particles towards an electrode in a solution 电泳现象

◇ **electroplexy** *noun* 电惊厥疗法 *see* 见 ELECTROCONVULSIVE THERAPY

◇ **electroretinography** *noun* process of recording electrical changes in the retina when stimulated by light 视网膜电描记法

◇ **electroshock therapy** *or* **electroshock treatment** *or* **electroplexy** *noun* electroconvulsive therapy, the treatment of some mental disorders by giving the patient electric shocks in the brain to make him have convulsions(治疗精神的)电击疗法

◇ **electrotherapy** *noun* treatment of a disorder, such as some forms of paralysis, using low-frequency electric current to try to revive the muscles 电疗法

element *noun* basic simple chemical substance which cannot be broken down to a simpler substance 化学元素; **trace**

element = substance which is essential to the human body, but only in very small quantities 微量元素

elephantiasis *noun* oedematous condition where parts of the body swell and the skin becomes hardened, frequently caused by filariasis(infestation with various species of the parasitic worm *Filaria*) 象皮病

elevate *verb* to raise *or* to lift up 上升

◇ **elevation** *noun* raised part 上升; **elevation sling** = sling tied round the neck, used to hold the arm in a high position to prevent bleeding 高位吊带

◇ **elevator** *noun* (**a**) muscle which raises part of the body 提肌 (**b**) (i) surgical instrument used to lift part of a broken bone 起子(ii) instrument used by a dentist to remove a tooth *or* part of a tooth 牙铤; **periosteum elevator** = surgical instrument used to remove the periosteum from a bone 骨膜起子

elicit *verb* to make happen *or* to provoke 使发生: ***Muscle tenderness was elicited in the lower limbs*.** 引起了下肢肌触痛。

eliminate *verb* to get rid of waste matter from the body 清除,排除: ***The excess salts are eliminated through the kidneys*.** 多余的盐份由肾脏排除。

◇ **elimination** *noun* removal of waste matter from the body 清除

elixir *noun* sweet liquid which hides the unpleasant taste of a drug 酏剂

elliptocytosis *noun* condition where abnormal oval-shaped red cells appear in the blood 椭圆型红细胞增多症

EM = ELECTRON MICROSCOPE 电子显微镜

emaciated *adjective* very thin *or* extremely underweight 极度消瘦: ***Anorexic patients become emaciated and may need hospitalization*.** 厌食患者变得极度消瘦,需要住院治疗。

◇ **emaciation** *noun* being extremely thin; wasting away of body tissue 极度消瘦,憔悴

emaculation *noun* removing spots from the skin 除斑术

emasculation *noun* (i) removal of the penis 阴茎切除(ii) loss of male characteristics 阉

embalm *verb* to preserve a dead body by using special antiseptic chemicals to prevent decay 防腐

embolectomy *noun* surgical operation to remove a blood clot 栓子切除术

◇ **embolism** *noun* blocking of an artery by a mass of material (usually a bloodclot), preventing the flow of blood 栓塞; **air embolism** = interference with the flow of blood in vessels by bubbles of air 空气栓塞; **pulmonary embolism** = blockage of the pulmonary artery 肺梗塞

◇ **embolization** *noun* using emboli inserted down a catheter into a blood vessel to treat internal bleeding 栓塞术

◇ **embolus** *noun* mass of material (such as a blood clot *or* air bubble *or* fat globule) which blocks a blood vessel 栓子 (NOTE: plural is **emboli**)

> QUOTE: Once a bleeding site has been located, a catheter is manipulated as near as possible to it, so that embolization can be carried out. Many different materials are used as the embolus.
> 引文:一旦确定了出血部位,将导管尽量靠近出血处,进行栓塞。许多材料可用来制作栓子。
> **British Medical Journal** 英国医学杂志

embrocation *noun* liniment, oily liquid rubbed on the skin, which eases the pain *or* stiffness of a sprain *or* bruise by acting as a vasodilator *or* counterirritant 搽剂

embryo *noun* unborn baby during the first eight weeks after conception 胚胎 (NOTE: after eight weeks, the unborn baby is called a **fetus**)

◇ **embryological** *adjective* referring to embryology 胚胎学的

◇ **embryology** *noun* study of the early stages of the development of the embryo 胚胎学

◇ **embryonic** *adjective* (i) referring to an embryo 胚胎的(ii) in an early stage of development 发育早期的; **embryonic membranes** = skins around an embryo providing protection and food supply (the amnion and chorion) 胎膜

emergency *noun* situation where immediate action has to be taken 紧急; *US* **emergency medical technician (EMT)** = trained paramedic who gives care to victims at the scene of an accident or in an ambulance 急救医辅人员; **emergency ward** = hospital ward which deals with urgent cases (such as accident victims) 急诊室

emesis *noun* vomiting 呕吐

◇ **emetic** *adjective & noun* (substance) which causes vomiting 催吐的,催吐剂: ***The doctor administered an emetic.*** 医生开了催吐剂。

EMG = ELECTROMYOGRAM 肌电图

eminence *noun* something which protrudes from a surface, such as a lump on a bone *or* swelling on the skin 隆起 *see also* 参见 HYPOTHENAR, THENAR

emissary veins *noun* veins through the skull which connect the venous sinuses with the scalp veins 导静脉

emission *noun* discharge *or* release of fluid 排泄; **nocturnal emission** = production of semen from the penis while a man is asleep 遗精

emmenagogue *noun* drug which will help increase menstrual flow 通经药

emmetropia *noun* normal vision, the correct focusing of light rays by the eye onto the retina 屈光正常 *compare* 比较 AMETROPIA

emollient *adjective & noun* (substance) which smooths the skin 润肤的,润滑剂

emotion *noun* strong feeling 情感,情绪

◇ **emotional** *adjective* showing strong feeling 激动的; **emotional disorder** = disorder due to worry *or* stress, etc. 情感障碍

empathy *noun* being able to understand the problems and feelings of another person 投情,神入

emphysema *or* **pulmonary emphysema** *noun* condition where the alveoli of the lungs become enlarged *or* rupture *or* break down, with the result that the surface available for gas exchange is reduced, so reducing the oxygen level in the blood and making it difficult for the patient to breathe 肺气肿

> COMMENT: Emphysema can be caused by smoking or by living in a polluted environment, by old age, asthma or whooping cough.
> 注释:肺气肿可因抽烟、空气污染、年老、哮喘或百日咳引起。

employ *verb* (**a**) to use 使用: ***The dentist usually has to employ force to extract a tooth.*** 牙科医生拔牙时常要用力。(**b**) to pay a person for regular work 雇佣: ***The local health authority employs a staff of two thousand.*** 当地卫生部门雇佣了两千名员工。***She is employed by the dentist as a hygienist.*** 她被牙医雇为洁治师。***A practice nurse is employed by the practice, not by the health authority.*** 执业护士是由开业医生而不是由卫生行政机构雇佣的。

empty 1 *adjective* with nothing inside 空的: ***The medicine bottle is empty.*** 药瓶空了。***Take this empty bottle and provide a urine sample.*** 拿这个空瓶留取尿样。***The children's ward is never empty.*** 儿科房从来没有空过。**2** *verb* to take everything out of something 使空,倒空: ***She emptied the water out of the bottle.*** 她把瓶子里的水倒空。

empyema *noun* pyothorax, collection of pus in a cavity, especially in the pleural cavity 积脓,脓胸

EMT *US* = EMERGENCY MEDICAL TECHNICIAN 急救医辅人员

emulsion *noun* mixture of liquids which do not normally mix (such as oil and water) 乳剂

EN = ENROLLED NURSE 注册护士 (NOTE: enrolled nurses are classified according to their area of specialization; **EN(G)** = **Enrolled Nurse (General)**; **EN(M)** = **Enrolled Nurse (Mental)** **EN(MH)** = **Enrolled Nurse (Mental Handicap)**

enamel *noun* hard white shiny outer covering of the crown of a tooth 釉质◊见图 TOOTH

enanthema *noun* rash on a mucous membrane, as in the mouth or vagina, produced by the action of toxic substances on small blood vessels 粘膜疹

enarthrosis *noun* ball and socket joint, such as the hip joint 杵臼关节

ENB = ENGLISH NATIONAL BOARD 英国国家护理委员会

encapsulated *adjective* enclosed in a capsule *or* in a sheath of tissue 包在荚膜内的

encephal- *or* **encephalo-** *prefix* referring to the brain 脑的

◊ **encephalin** *noun* peptide produced in the brain 脑啡肽 *see also* 参见 ENDORPHIN

◊ **encephalitis** *noun* inflammation of the brain 脑炎; **encephalitis lethargica** *or* **lethargic encephalitis** = common type of encephalitis occurring in epidemics in the 1920s 嗜睡性脑炎

> COMMENT: Encephalitis is caused by any of several viruses (viral encephalitis) and is also associated with infectious viral diseases such as measles or mumps.
> 注释:脑炎(病毒性脑炎)可由几种病毒中的任一种引起,并与病毒感染性疾病如麻疹或流行性腮腺炎有关。

◊ **encephalocele** *noun* condition where the brain protrudes through a congenital *or* traumatic gap in the skull bones 脑膨出

◊ **encephalogram** *or* **encephalograph** *noun* X-ray photograph of the ventricles and spaces of the brain taken after air has been injected into the cerebrospinal fluid by lumbar puncture 气脑造影片

◊ **encephalography** *or* **pneumoencephalography** *noun* X-ray examination of the ventricles and spaces of the brain taken after air has been injected into the cerebrospinal fluid by lumbar puncture 气脑造影术

> COMMENT: The air takes the place of the cerebrospinal fluid and makes it easier to photograph the ventricles clearly. This technique has been superseded by CAT and MRI.
> 注释:空气占据脑脊液的位置使脑室造影清晰。此项技术现已被计算机轴向体层扫描和核磁共振成像替代。

◊ **encephaloid** **1** *adjective* which looks like brain tissue 脑样的 **2** *noun* large carcinoma of the breast 髓样瘤

◊ **encephaloma** *noun* tumour of the brain 脑瘤

◊ **encephalomalacia** *noun* softening of the brain 脑软化

◊ **encephalomyelitis** *noun* group of diseases which cause inflammation of the brain and the spinal cord 脑脊髓炎; **acute disseminated encephalomyelitis** = late reaction to a vaccination *or* disease 急性播散性脑脊髓炎; **myalgic encephalomyelitis (ME)** = postviral fatigue syndrome, a long-term condition affecting the nervous system, where the patient feels tired and depressed and has pain and weakness in the muscles 肌痛性脑脊髓炎(病毒后疲劳综合征,长期影响神经系统,患者感觉劳累、压抑和肌肉疼痛无力)

◊ **encephalomyelopathy** *noun* any condition where the brain and spinal cord are diseased 脑脊髓病

◊ **encephalon** *noun* the brain *or* the contents of the head 脑

◊ **encephalopathy** *noun* any disease of the brain 脑病 *see also* 参见 WERNICKE'S ENCEPHALOPATHY

enchondroma *noun* tumour formed of cartilage growing inside a bone 内生软骨瘤

enclose *verb* to surround *or* to keep something inside 包绕: ***The membrane enclosing the cytoplasm.*** 细胞膜包绕着胞浆。

encopresis *noun* faecal incontinence, being unable to control the faeces 大便失禁

encounter group *noun* form of treatment of psychological disorders, where people meet and talk about their problems in a group 邂逅小组,"交朋友小组"(现代美国的一种所谓精神治疗方式,受治疗者在组内自由与其他成员交流内心感情)

encourage *verb* to persuade someone that he should do something 鼓励: ***The surgeon encouraged her to get out of bed and start trying to walk.*** 外科医师鼓励她下床练习行走。***Children should not be encouraged to take medicines by themselves.*** 不应鼓励儿童自己服用药物。

encysted *adjective* enclosed in a capsule like a cyst 包绕的,被囊的

end 1 *noun* last part of something 末端,终结; **end artery** = last section of an artery which does not divide into smaller arteries and does not anastomose with other arteries 终动脉; **end organ** = nerve ending with encapsulated nerve filaments 终器(感觉神经); **end piece** = last part of the tail of a spermatazoon 精子尾的末端 **2** *verb* to finish; to come to an end 结束: ***He ended his talk by showing a series of slides of diseased parts.*** 他以展示一系列病变部位的幻灯结束了他的讲话。

◇ **ending** *noun* last part of something 终端; **nerve ending** = last part of a nerve, especially of a peripheral nerve 神经末梢 ◇ 见图 SKIN & SENSORY RECEPTORS

◇ **end plate** *noun* end of a motor nerve, where it joins muscle fibre 终板

endanger *verb* to put at risk 使危险: ***The operation may endanger the life of the patient.*** 手术有可能危及患者的生命。

end- *or* **endo-** *prefix* meaning inside 内的

◇ **endarterectomy** *noun* surgical removal of the lining of a blocked artery 动脉内膜切除术(NOTE: also called a **rebore**)

◇ **endarteritis** *noun* inflammation of the inner lining of an artery 动脉内膜炎; **endarteritis obliterans** = condition where inflammation in an artery is so severe that it blocks the artery 闭塞性动脉内膜炎

endemic *adjective* (any disease) which is very common in certain places 地方性流行的: ***This disease is endemic to Mediterranean countries.*** 这种病在地中海国家流行。**endemic syphilis** = BEJEL 地方性梅毒 *see also* 参见 EPIDEMIC, PANDEMIC

◇ **endemiology** *noun* study of endemic diseases 地方病学

end-expiratory 呼气末 *see* 见 POSITIVE

endo- *prefix* meaning inside 里面的

◇ **endocardial** *adjective* referring to the endocardium 心内膜的; **endocardial pacemaker** = pacemaker attached to the lining of the heart muscle 心内膜起搏器;

◇ **endocarditis** *noun* inflammation of the endocardium, the membrane lining of the heart 心内膜炎; (**subacute**) **infective endocarditis** *or* (**subacute**) **bacterial endocarditis** = infection of the endocardium (the membrane covering the inner surfaces of the heart) by bacteria (亚急性)感染性心内膜炎

◇ **endocardium** *noun* membrane which lines the heart 心内膜 ◇ 见图 HEART

endocervicitis *noun* inflammation of the membrane in the neck of the uterus 子宫颈内膜炎

◇ **endocervix** *noun* membrane which lines the neck of the uterus 子宫颈内膜

◇ **endochondral** *adjective* inside a cartilage 软骨内的

endocrine gland *noun* ductless gland, gland without a duct which produces hormones which are introduced directly into the bloodstream (such as the pituitary gland, thyroid gland, the adrenals, and the gonads) 内分泌腺; **endocrine system** = system of related ductless glands 内分泌系统

◇ **endocrinologist** *noun* doctor who specializes in the study of endocrinology 内分泌学家

◇ **endocrinology** *noun* study of the endocrine system, its function and effects 内分泌学

QUOTE: The endocrine system releases hormones in response to a change in concentration of trigger substances in the blood or other body fluids.
引文:内分泌系统根据血液或其他体液内激发物质浓度的变化释放激素。
Nursing 87 护理 87

endoderm *or* **entoderm** *noun* inner of three layers surrounding an embryo 内胚层

COMMENT: The endoderm gives rise to most of the epithelium of the respiratory system, the alimentary tract, some of the ductless glands, the bladder and part of the urethra.
注释:内胚层生成呼吸系统、消化道、一些无管腺体、膀胱和部分尿道的大部分上皮。

◇ **endodermal** *or* **entodermal** *adjective* referring to the endoderm 内胚层的

◇ **endodontia** *noun* treatment of chronic toothache by removing the roots of a tooth 牙根管治疗术,牙髓病学

◇ **endogenous** *adjective* developing *or* being caused by something inside an organism 内生的,内源的; **endogenous depression** = depression caused by something inside the body 内源性抑郁; **endogenous eczema** = eczema which is caused by no obvious external factor 内源性湿疹 *compare* 比较 EXOGENOUS

◇ **endolymph** *noun* fluid inside the membranous labyrinth in the inner ear 内淋巴

◇ **endolymphatic duct** *noun* duct which carries the endolymph inside the membranous labyrinth 内淋巴管

◇ **endolysin** *noun* substance present in cells, which kills bacteria 内溶素

◇ **endometrial** *adjective* referring to the endometrium 子宫内膜的

◇ **endometriosis** *noun* condition affecting women, where tissue similar to the tissue of the womb is found in other parts of the body 子宫内膜异位

◇ **endometritis** *noun* inflammation of the lining of the uterus 子宫内膜炎

◇ **endometrium** *noun* mucous membrane lining the uterus part of which is shed at each menstruation 子宫内膜

◇ **endomorph** *noun* type of person who tends to be quite fat with large intestines and small muscles 内胚层体型者

◇ **endomorphic** *adjective* referring to an endomorph 内胚层体型的 *see also* 参见 ECTOMORPH, MESOMORPH

◇ **endomyocarditis** *noun* inflammation of the muscle and inner membrane of the heart 心肌(心)内膜炎

◇ **endomysium** *noun* connective tissue around and between muscle fibres 肌内膜

◇ **endoneurium** *noun* fibrous tissue between the nerve fibres in a nerve trunk 神经内膜

◇ **endoparasite** *noun* parasite which lives inside its host (as in the intestines) 内寄生物 *compare* 比较 ECTOPARASITE

◇ **endophthalmitis** *noun* inflammation of the interior of the eyeball 眼内炎

◇ **endoplasm** *noun* inner layer of the cytoplasm, which is less dense than the rest 内浆,内质

◇ **endoplasmic reticulum(ER)** *noun* network of vessels forming a membrane in a cytoplasm 内质网

◇ **endorphin** *noun* peptide produced by the brain which acts as a natural pain killer 内啡肽 *see also* 参见 ENCEPHALIN

◇ **endoscope** *noun* instrument used to examine the inside of the body, made of a thin tube which is passed into the body down a passage (the tube has a fibre optic light, and may have small surgical instruments attached) 内镜

◇ **endoscopic retrograde cholangiopancreatography** (**ERCP**) *noun* method used to examine the pancreatic duct and bile duct for possible obstructions 逆行性胰胆管内镜检查

◇ **endoscopy** *noun* examination of the inside of the body using an endoscope 内镜检查

◇ **endoskeleton** *noun* inner structure of bones and cartilage in an animal 内骨骼 *compare* 比较 EXOSKELETON

◇ **endospore** *noun* spore formed inside a special spore case 内孢子

◇ **endosteum** *noun* membrane lining the bone marrow cavity inside a long bone 骨内膜

◇ **endothelial** *adjective* referring to the endothelium 内皮的

◇ **endothelioma** *noun* malignant tumour originating inside the endothelium 内皮瘤

◇ **endothelium** *noun* membrane of special cells which lines the heart, the lymph vessels, the blood vessels and various body cavities 内皮 *compare* 比较 EPITHELIUM

◇ **endotoxin** *noun* toxic substance released after the death of certain bacterial cells 内毒素

◇ **endotracheal** *adjective* inside the trachea 气管内的; **endotracheal tube** = tube passed down the trachea (through either the nose or mouth) in anaesthesia or to help the patient breathe 气管插管

enema *noun* liquid substance put into the rectum to introduce a drug into the body *or* to wash out the colon before an operation *or* for diagnosis 灌肠剂; **enema bag** = bag containing the liquid, attached to a tube into the rectum 灌肠袋; **barium enema** = enema made of barium sulphate, injected into the rectum so as to show up the bowel in X-rays 钡灌肠 (NOTE: plural is **enemas**, **enemata**)

energy *noun* force *or* strength to carry out activities 能量: ***You need to eat certain types of food to give you energy.*** 你需要吃某些种类的食物提供能量。**energy value** *or* **calorific value** = heat value of food, the number of Calories which a certain amount of a certain food contains 热量价: ***The tin of beans has an energy value of 250 calories.*** 一听豆罐头的热能是250卡。

> COMMENT: Energy is measured in calories, one calorie being the amount of heat needed to raise the temperature of one gram of water by one degree Celsius. The kilocalorie or Calorie is also used as a measurement of the energy content of food, and to show the amount of energy needed by an average person.
> 注释:热能用卡来衡量,一卡的热量是使1克水升温1摄氏度所需要的热能。千卡也被用来衡量食物中蕴含的能量,以及人均所需的热能。

◇ **energetic** *adjective* full of energy *or* using energy 有能量的,用能的: ***The patient should not do anything energetic.*** 患者不能做任何费力的活动。

enervate *verb* to deprive someone of nervous energy 使神经衰弱,削瘦

◇ **enervation** *noun* (i) general nervous weakness 神经无力 (ii) surgical operation to resect a nerve 神经切除

engagement *noun* (in obstetrics) moment where the presenting part of the fetus (usually the head) enters the pelvis at the beginning of labour 衔接

English National Board (**ENB**) *noun* official body responsible for training nurses, for setting nursing examinations and for approving nursing schools 英国国家护理委员会

engorged *adjective* filled with liquid (usually blood) 充盈的

◇ **engorgement** *noun* congestion, the excessive filling of a vessel with blood 充血

enlarge *verb* to make larger *or* wider 扩充,扩大; ***operation to enlarge a defec-***

tive vessel 血管扩张

◇ **enlargement** *noun* (i) widening 扩大(ii) point where something becomes wider 膨大部; **lumbar enlargement** = point where the spinal cord widens in the lower part of the spine 腰膨大

enophthalmos *noun* condition where the eyes are very deep in their sockets 眼球内陷

enostosis *noun* benign growth inside a bone (usually in the skull *or* in a long bone) 内生骨疣

enrolled *adjective* registered on an official list 注册的; (**State**) **Enrolled Nurse** (**SEN**) = nurse who has passed examinations successfully in one of the special courses of study 国家注册护士

COMMENT: Enrolled Nurses follow a two year course to qualify in general nursing (ENG), mental nursing (ENM) or nursing mentally handicapped patients (ENMH).
注释:注册护士需要两年的时间取得全科护士、精神科护士或护理精神障碍患者的资格。

ensiform *adjective* shaped like a sword 剑形的; **ensiform cartilage** *or* **xiphoid process** = bottom part of the breastbone, which in young people is formed of cartilage, but becomes bone by middle age 剑突

ensure *verb* to make sure of something 保证: ***Please ensure that the patient takes his medicine.*** 请确保患者服用药物。

ENT = EAR, NOSE AND THROAT 耳鼻喉: ***She was sent to see an ENT specialist.*** 她去看耳鼻喉专家。

Entamoeba *noun* genus of amoeba which lives in the intestine 内阿米巴属; **Entamoeba coli** = harmless intestinal parasite 结肠内阿米巴; **Entamoeba gingivalis** = amoeba living in the gums and tonsils, and causing gingivitis 龈内阿米巴; **Entamoeba histolytica** = intestinal amoeba which causes amoebic dysentery 溶组织内阿米巴

enter- *or* **entero-** *prefix* referring to the intestine 肠的

◇ **enteral** *adjective* (i) referring to the intestine 肠的 (ii) (drug *or* food) which is taken through the intestine 经肠的(药物,食物); **enteral nutrition** *or* **feeding** = feeding of a patient by a nasogastric tube or directly into the intestine 经肠道营养 *compare* 比较 PARENTERAL

◇ **enteralgia** = COLIC 肠痛

◇ **enterally** *adverb* (to feed a patient) by nasogastric tube or directly into the intestine 经胃肠道地

QUOTE: Standard nasogastric tubes are usually sufficient for enteral feeding in critically ill patients.
引文:标准鼻胃管可为危重病人提供足够的肠内营养。
British Journal of Nursing 英国护理杂志

QUOTE: All patients requiring nutrition are fed enterally, whether nasogastrically or directly into the small intestine.
引文:无论是通过鼻胃管还是直接进入小肠,所有患者所需的营养均经肠道提供。
British Journal of Nursing 英国护理杂志

enterectomy *noun* surgical removal of part of the intestine 肠切除术

◇ **enteric** *adjective* referring to the intestine 肠的; **enteric fever** = (i) any one of three fevers (typhoid, paratyphoid A and paratyphoid B) 伤寒 (ii) *US* any febrile disease of the intestines 因肠道病变引起的发热性疾病

◇ **enteric-coated** *adjective* (pill) with a coating which prevents it from being digested in the stomach, so that it goes through whole into the intestine and can release the drug there 包有肠溶衣的(药丸)

◇ **enteritis** *noun* inflammation of the mucous membrane of the intestine 肠炎; **infective enteritis** = enteritis caused by bacteria 细菌性肠炎; **post-irradiation enteritis** = enteritis caused by X-rays 放射后肠炎 *see also* 参见 GASTROENTERITIS

◇ **Enterobacteria** *noun* important family of bacteria, including Salmonella, Shigella, Escherichia and Klebsiella 肠杆菌
◇ **enterobiasis** *noun* oxyuriasis, infection with *Enterobius vermicularis*, a common children's disease, caused by threadworms in the large intestine which give itching round the anus 蛲虫病
◇ **Enterobius** *noun* threadworm, a small thin nematode which infests the large intestine and causes itching round the anus 蛲虫属
◇ **enterocele** *noun* hernia of the intestine 肠疝
◇ **enterocentesis** *noun* surgical puncturing of the intestines where a hollow needle is pushed through the abdominal wall into the intestine to remove gas *or* fluid 肠穿刺
◇ **enterococcus** *noun* streptococcus in the intestine 肠球菌
◇ **enterocoele** *noun* the abdominal cavity 腹腔
◇ **enterocolitis** *noun* inflammation of the colon and small intestine 小肠结肠炎
◇ **enterogastrone** *noun* hormone released in the duodenum, which controls secretions of the stomach 肠抑胃素
◇ **enterogenous** *adjective* originating in the intestine 肠生的
◇ **enterolith** *noun* calculus, stone in the intestine 肠石
◇ **enteron** *noun* the whole intestinal tract 肠道
◇ **enteropathy** *noun* any disorder of the intestine 肠病; **gluten-induced enteropathy** (**coeliac disease**) = (i) allergic disease (mainly affecting children) in which the lining of the intestine is sensitive to gluten, preventing the small intestine from digesting fat 谷胶性肠病(乳糜泻) (ii) condition in adults where the villi in the intestine become smaller and so reduce the surface which can absorb nutrients 小肠绒毛萎缩症
◇ **enteropeptidase** *noun* enzyme produced by glands in the small intestine 肠肽酶
◇ **enteroptosis** *noun* condition where the intestine is lower than normal in the abdominal cavity 肠下垂
◇ **enterorrhaphy** *noun* surgical operation to stitch up a perforated intestine 肠缝合术
◇ **enterospasm** *noun* irregular painful contractions of the intestine 肠痉挛
◇ **enterostomy** *noun* surgical operation to make an opening between the small intestine and the abdominal wall 大肠造口术
◇ **enterotomy** *noun* surgical incision of the intestine 肠切开术
◇ **enterotoxin** *noun* bacterial exotoxin which particularly affects the intestine 肠毒素
◇ **enterovirus** *noun* virus which prefers to live in the intestine 肠病毒

> COMMENT: The enteroviruses are an important group of viruses, and include poliomyelitis virus, Coxsackie viruses and the echoviruses.
> 注释：肠病毒是一类重要的病毒，包括脊髓灰质炎病毒、柯萨奇病毒和埃可病毒。

◇ **enterozoon** *noun* parasite which infests the intestine 肠寄生虫 (NOTE: plural is **enterozoa**)
entoderm *or* **endoderm** *noun* inner of three layers surrounding an embryo 内胚层
◇ **entodermal** *adjective* referring to the entoderm 内胚层的 *see* 见 *comment at* ENDODERM
entopic *adjective* in the normal place 正位的 (NOTE: the opposite is **ectopic**)
entropion *noun* turning of the edge of the eyelid towards the inside 睑内翻
enucleate *verb* to remove an eyeball 剜除
◇ **enucleation** *noun* (i) surgical removal of all of a tumour (肿瘤)摘除术 (ii) surgical removal of the whole eyeball(眼球)剜除术
enuresis *noun* involuntary passing of

urine 遗尿; **nocturnal enuresis** = bed-wetting, passing urine when asleep in bed at night(especially used of children) 夜尿症

◇ **enuretic** *adjective* referring to enuresis *or* causing enuresis 遗尿的

envenomation *noun* using snake venom as part of a therapeutic treatment 螯刺毒作用

environment *noun* conditions and influences under which an organism lives 环境

> COMMENT: Man's environment can be the country or town, house or room where he lives; a parasite's environment can be the intestine or the scalp and different parasites have different environments.
> 注释:人类的环境可以是乡村或城镇,或居住的房屋;寄生虫的环境可以是小肠或头皮,不同的寄生虫有不同的环境。

◇ **environmental** *adjective* referring to the environment 环境的; **Environmental Health Officer** (**EHO**) = official of a local authority who examines the environment and tests for air pollution *or* bad sanitation *or* noise pollution,etc. 环境卫生官员

enzyme *noun* protein substance produced by living cells which catalyses a biochemical reaction in the body 酶

◇ **enzymatic** *adjective* referring to enzymes 酶的 (NOTE: the names of enzymes mostly end with the suffix **-ase**)

> COMMENT: Many different enzymes exist in the body, working in the digestive system, in the metabolic processes and helping the synthesis of certain compounds.
> 注释:体内有很多种酶,在消化、新陈代谢及某些物质的合成等过程中发挥作用。

eosin *noun* red dye used in staining tissue samples 伊红

◇ **eosinopenia** *noun* reduction in the number of eosinophils in the blood 嗜酸性细胞减少症

◇ **eosinophil** *noun* type of cell which can be stained with eosin 嗜酸性细胞

◇ **eosinophilia** *noun* having an excess of eosinophils in the blood 嗜酸细胞增多

eparterial *adjective* situated over *or* on an artery 动脉上的

ependyma *noun* thin membrane which lines the ventricles of the brain and the central canal of the spinal cord 室管膜

◇ **ependymal** *adjective* referring to the ependyma 室管膜的; **ependymal cell** = one of the cells which form the ependyma 室管膜细胞

◇ **ependymoma** *noun* tumour in the brain originating in the ependyma 室管膜瘤

epi- *prefix* meaning on *or* over 上

◇ **epiblepharon** *noun* abnormal fold of skin over the eyelid, which may press the eyelashes against the eyeball 睑赘皮

◇ **epicanthus** *or* **epicanthic fold** *noun* large fold of skin in the inner corner of the eye, common in babies, and Mongoloid races 内眦赘皮

◇ **epicardial** *adjective* referring to the epicardium 心外膜的; **epicardial pacemaker** = pacemaker attached to the surface of the ventricle 心外膜起搏器

◇ **epicardium** *noun* inner layer of the pericardium which lines the walls of the heart,outside the myocardium 心外膜

◇ **epicondyle** *noun* projecting part of the round end of a bone above the condyle 上髁; **lateral epicondyle** (**of the humerus**) = lateral projection on the condyle of the humerus 肱骨外上髁; **medial epicondyle** (**of the humerus**) = medial projection on the condyle of the humerus 肱骨内侧髁

◇ **epicranium** *noun* the five layers of the scalp, the skin and hair on the head covering the skull 头被,头皮

◇ **epicranius** *noun* a scalp muscle 颅顶肌

◇ **epicritic** *adjective* referring to the nerves which govern the fine senses of touch and temperature 细觉的 *see also* 参

见 PROTOPATHIC

epidemic *adjective & noun* (infectious disease) which spreads quickly through a large part of the population 流行的,流行病: ***The disease rapidly reached epidemic proportions.*** 疾病迅速达到流行程度。***The health authorities are taking steps to prevent an epidemic of cholera*** *or* ***a cholera epidemic.*** 卫生部门在采取措施预防霍乱的流行。**epidemic pleurodynia** *or* **Bornholm disease** 流行性胸肌病 *see* 见 PLEURODYNIA *see also* 参见 ENDEMIC, PANDEMIC

◇ **epidemiological** *adjective* concerning epidemiology 流行病学的

◇ **epidemiologist** *noun* person who specializes in the study of diseases in groups of people 流行病学家

◇ **epidemiology** *noun* study of diseases in the community, in particular how they spread and how they can be controlled 流行病学

epidermis *noun* outer layer of skin, including the dead skin on the surface 表皮 ◊ 见图 SKIN & SENSORY RECEPTORS

◇ **epidermal** *adjective* referring to the epidermis 表皮的

◇ **epidermolysis** *noun* loose condition of the epidermis 表皮松解

◇ **Epidermophyton** *noun* fungus which grows on the skin and causes athlete's foot among other disorders 表皮癣菌属

◇ **epidermophytosis** *noun* fungus infection of the skin, such as athlete's foot 表皮癣

epididymis *noun* long twisting thin tube at the back of the testis, which forms part of the efferent duct of the testis, and in which spermatozoa are stored before ejaculation 附睾 ◊ 见图 UROGENITAL SYSTEM (MALE)

◇ **epididymal** *adjective* referring to the epididymis 附睾的

◇ **epididymitis** *noun* inflammation of the epididymis 附睾炎

◇ **epididymo-orchitis** *noun* inflammation of the epididymis and the testes 睾丸附睾炎

epidural *or* **extradural** *adjective* on the outside of the dura mater 硬膜外的; **epidural anaesthesia** = local anaesthesia (used in childbirth) in which anaesthetic is injected into the space between the vertebral canal and the dura mater 硬膜外麻醉; **epidural block** = analgesia produced by injecting an analgesic solution into the space between the vertebral canal and the dura mater 硬膜外阻滞; **epidural space** = space in the spinal cord between the vertebral canal and the dura mater 硬膜外腔

epigastric *adjective* referring to the upper abdomen 上腹部的: ***The patient complained of pains in the epigastric area.*** 患者诉上腹部疼痛。

◇ **epigastrium** *noun* pit of the stomach, the part of the upper abdomen between the ribcage and the navel 上腹部

◇ **epigastrocele** *noun* hernia in the upper abdomen 上腹疝

epiglottis *noun* cartilage at the root of the tongue which moves to block the windpipe when food is swallowed, so that the food does not go down the trachea 会厌软骨 ◊ 见图 THROAT

◇ **epiglottitis** *noun* inflammation and swelling of the epiglottis 会厌炎

epilation *noun* removing hair by destroying the hair follicles 脱发

epilepsy *noun* disorder of the nervous system in which there are convulsions and loss of consciousness due to disordered discharge of cerebral neurones 癫痫; **focal epilepsy** = epilepsy arising from a localized area of the brain 局病灶性癫痫; **Jacksonian epilepsy** = form of epilepsy where the jerking movements start in one part of the body before spreading to others 杰克逊氏癫痫(皮质性癫痫); **idiopathic epilepsy** = epilepsy not caused by lesions of the brain 特发性癫痫; **psychomotor epilepsy**

or **temporal lobe epilepsy** = epilepsy caused by abnormal discharges from the temporal lobe 颞叶性癫痫(精神运动性癫痫) *see also* 参见 TEMPORAL

◇ **epileptic** *adjective* & *noun* referring to epilepsy *or* (person) suffering from epilepsy 癫痫的,癫痫病患者; **epileptic fit** = attack of convulsions (and sometimes unconsciousness) due to epilepsy 癫痫发作

◇ **epileptiform** *adjective* similar to epilepsy 癫痫样的

◇ **epileptogenic** *adjective* which causes epilepsy 引起癫痫的

> COMMENT: The commonest form of epilepsy is major epilepsy or 'grand mal', where the patient loses consciousness and falls to the ground with convulsions. A less severe form is minor epilepsy or 'petit mal', where attacks last only a few seconds, and the patient appears simply to be hesitating or thinking deeply.
> 注释:癫痫最常见的形式是癫痫大发作,表现为意识丧失,惊厥倒地。癫痫小发作是较温和的形式,仅持续几秒钟,患者多表现为踌躇或沉思状态。

epiloia *noun* hereditary disease of the brain, where the child is mentally retarded, suffers from epilepsy and has tumours on the kidney and heart(脑)结节性硬化

epimenorrhagia *noun* very heavy bleeding during menstruation occurring at very short intervals 月经过多过频

◇ **epimenorrhoea** *noun* menstruation at shorter intervals than twenty-eight days 月经过频

◇ **epimysium** *noun* connective tissue binding striated muscle fibres 肌外膜

◇ **epinephrine** *noun US* adrenaline, hormone secreted by the medulla of the adrenal glands which has an effect similar to stimulation of the sympathetic nervous system 肾上腺素

◇ **epineurium** *noun* sheath of connective tissue round a nerve 神经外膜

◇ **epiphenomenon** *noun* strange symptom which may not be caused by a disease 副现象,表面现象

◇ **epiphora** *noun* condition where the eye fills with tears either because the lacrimal duct is blocked or because excessive tears are being secreted 泪溢

epiphysis *noun* centre of bone growth separated from the main part of the bone by cartilage 骺; **epiphysis cerebri** = pineal gland 松果体 ◊ 见图 BONE STRUCTURE

◇ **epiphyseal** *adjective* referring to an epiphysis 骺的; **epiphyseal cartilage** = type of cartilage in the bones of children and adolescents, which expands and hardens as the bone grows to full size 骺软骨; **epiphyseal line** = plate of epiphyseal cartilage separating the epiphysis and the diaphysis of a long bone 骺线

◇ **epiphysitis** *noun* inflammation of an epiphysis 骺炎 *compare* 比较 DIAPHYSIS, METAPHYSIS

epiplo- *prefix* referring to the omentum 网膜的

◇ **epiplocele** *noun* hernia containing part of the omentum 网膜疝

◇ **epiploic** *adjective* referring to the omentum 网膜的

◇ **epiploon** = OMENTUM 网膜

episcleritis *noun* inflammation of the outer surface of the sclera in the eyeball 巩膜外层炎

episio- *adjective* referring to the vulva 外阴的

◇ **episiorrhaphy** *noun* stitching of torn labia majora 外阴缝合术

◇ **episiotomy** *noun* surgical incision of the perineum near the vagina to prevent tearing during childbirth 外阴切开术

episode *noun* separate occurrence of an illness 发作

◇ **episodic** *adjective* (asthma) which occurs in separate attacks 发作的

epispadias *noun* congenital defect where the urethra opens on the top of the penis and not at the end 尿道上裂

compare 比较 HYPOSPADIAS
◇ **epispastic** = VESICANT 起疱剂
◇ **epistaxis** *noun* nosebleed 鼻衄
epithalamus *noun* part of the forebrain containing the pineal body 上丘脑
epithelium *noun* layer(s) of cells covering an organ, including the skin and the lining of all hollow cavities except blood vessels, lymphatics and serous cavities 上皮 *see also* 参见 ENDOTHELIUM, MESOTHELIUM
◇ **epithelial** *adjective* referring to the epithelium 上皮的; **epithelial layer** = the epithelium 上皮层; **epithelial tissue** = epithelial cells arranged as a continuous sheet consisting of one or several layers 上皮组织
◇ **epithelialization** *noun* growth of skin over a wound 上皮形成
◇ **epithelioma** *noun* tumour arising from epithelial cells 上皮瘤(癌)

COMMENT: Epithelium is classified according to the shape of the cells and the number of layers of cells which form it. The types of epithelium according to the number of layers are: simple epithelium (epithelium formed of a single layer of cells) and stratified epithelium (epithelium formed of several layers of cells). The main types of epithelial cells are: columnar epithelium (simple epithelium with long narrow cells, forming the lining of the intestines); ciliated epithelium (simple epithelium where the cells have little hairs, forming the lining of air passages); cuboidal epithelium (with cube-shaped cells, forming the lining of glands and intestines); squamous epithelium or pavement epithelium (with flat cells like scales, which forms the lining of pericardium, peritoneum and pleura).
注释:上皮组织根据组成细胞的形态及层数分类。根据组成细胞的层数分为:简单上皮(只由一层细胞组成)和复层上皮(由几层上皮组成)。根据上皮细胞形态主要分为:柱状上皮(由狭长细胞组成的简单上皮,构成肠上皮)、纤毛上皮(具有纤毛的细胞组成的简单上皮,构成呼吸道内皮)、杯状上皮(由杯形细胞组成,构成腺体和肠上皮)、扁平上皮或鳞状上皮(由鳞状的扁平细胞组成,构成心包、腹膜和胸膜上皮)。

epituberculosis *noun* swelling of the lymph node in the thorax, due to tuberculosis 浸润型肺结核
eponym *noun* procedure *or* disease *or* part of the body which is named after a person 以人名命名的词
◇ **eponymous** *adjective* named after a person 以人名命名词的

COMMENT: An eponym can refer to a disease or condition (Dupuytren's contracture, Guillain-Barré syndrome), a part of the body (circle of Willis), an organism (Leishmania), a surgical procedure (Trendelenburg's operation) or an appliance (Kirschner wire).
注释:以人名命名的词包括疾病或症状(Dupuytren's 挛缩, Guillain- Barré 综合征)、机体的某一部分(Willis 环)、微生物(利什曼原虫)、手术(Trendelenburg's 手术)或器械(Kirschner 钢丝)。

Epsom salts *noun* magnesium sulphate ($MgSO_4 \cdot 7H_2O$), white powder which when diluted in water is used as a laxative 泻盐(指硫酸镁)
Epstein-Barr virus *or* **EB virus** *noun* virus which probably causes glandular fever and is associated with tension headaches E-B 病毒
epulis *noun* small fibrous swelling on a gum 龈瘤
equal 1 *adjective* exactly the same in quantity, size, etc. as something else 同样的: ***The twins are of equal size and weight.*** 双胞胎具有同样的身高和体重。2 *verb* to be exactly the same as something 相同
equilibrium *noun* state of balance 平衡
equina 马的 *see* 见 CAUDA EQUINA
equinovarus 马蹄内翻足 *see* 见 TAL-

IPES

equip *verb* to provide the necessary apparatus 配备：***The operating theatre is equipped with the latest scanning devices.*** 手术室配有最先进的扫描设备。

◇ **equipment** *noun* apparatus *or* tools which are required to do something 装备：***The centre urgently needs surgical equipment.*** 中心急需手术器械。***The surgeons complained about the out-of-date equipment in the hospital.*** 外科医师抱怨医院的装备过时。(NOTE：no plural：for one item say '**a piece of equipment**')

ER = ENDOPLASMIC RETICULUM 内质网

eradicate *verb* to wipe out *or* to remove completely 根除；***international action to eradicate tuberculosis*** 根除结核病的国际行动

◇ **eradication** *noun* removing completely 根除

Erb's palsy *or* **Erb's paralysis** 欧勃氏麻痹,假肥大性肌营养不良 *see* 见 PALSY

ERCP = ENDOSCOPIC RETROGRADE CHOLANGIOPANCREATOGRAPHY 逆行胰胆管内镜检查

erect *adjective* stiff and straight 勃起,竖立

◇ **erectile** *adjective* which can become erect 可勃起的；**erectile tissue** = vascular tissue which can become erect and stiff when engorged with blood (as the corpus cavernosa in the penis) 勃起组织

◇ **erection** *noun* state where a part, such as the penis, becomes swollen because of engorgement with blood 勃起

◇ **erector spinae** *noun* large muscle starting at the base of the spine, and dividing as it runs up the spine 骶棘肌

erepsin *noun* mixture of enzymes produced by the glands in the intestine, used in the production of amino ac-ids 肠肽酶

erethism *noun* abnormal irritability 兴奋增盛

erg *noun* unit of measurement of work *or* energy 尔格(功的单位)

◇ **ergograph** *noun* apparatus which records the work of one or several muscles 测力器

◇ **ergonomics** *noun* study of man at work 人体功率学

ergometrine *noun* drug derived from ergot, used in obstetrics to reduce bleeding and to produce contractions of the uterus 麦角新碱

ergot *noun* fungus which grows on rye 麦角

◇ **ergotism** *noun* poisoning by eating rye which has been contaminated with ergot 麦角中毒

> COMMENT：The symptoms are muscle cramps and dry gangrene in the fingers and toes.
> 注释：症状是肌肉痉挛和指趾干性坏疽。

erode *verb* to wear away *or* to break down 侵蚀,腐蚀

◇ **erosion** *noun* wearing away of tissue *or* breaking down of tissue 侵蚀,腐蚀；**cervical erosion** = condition where the epithelium of the mucous membrane lining the cervix uteri extends outside the cervix 宫颈糜烂

erogenous *noun* which produces sexual excitement 使发生性欲的,产生性欲的；**erogenous zone** = part of the body which, if stimulated, produces sexual excitement (such as penis *or* clitoris *or* nipples, etc.) 性欲发生区

ERPC = EVACUATION OF RETAINED PRODUCTS OF CONCEPTION 不全娩出后清宫术

eructation *noun* belching, allowing air in the stomach to come up through the mouth 嗳气,打嗝

erupt *verb* to break through the skin 长出,萌出：***The permanent incisors erupt before the premolars.*** 恒切牙在前磨牙前出牙。

◇ **eruption** *noun* (i) something which breaks through the skin (such as a rash *or* pimple) 皮疹 (ii) appearance of a new tooth in a gum 出牙

ery- *prefix* meaning red 红的

◇ **erysipelas** *noun* contagious skin disease, where the skin on the face becomes hot and red and painful, caused by *Streptococcus pyogenes* 丹毒

◇ **erysipeloid** *noun* bacterial skin infection caused by touching infected fish *or* meat 类丹毒

◇ **erythema** *noun* redness on the skin, caused by hyperaemia of the blood vessels near the surface 红斑; **erythema ab igne** = pattern of red lines on the skin caused by exposure to heat 火激红斑; **erythema induratum** *or* **Bazin's disease** = tubercular disease where ulcerating nodules appear on the legs of young women 硬红斑,白塞氏病; **erythema multiforme** = sudden appearance of inflammatory red patches and sometimes blisters on the skin 多形性红斑; **erythema nodosum** = inflammatory disease where red swellings appear on the front of the legs 结节性红斑; **erythema pernio** = CHILBLAIN 冻疮; **erythema serpens** = bacterial skin infection caused by touching infected fish *or* meat 匐行性红斑

◇ **erythraemia** *or* **polycythaemia vera** *noun* blood disorder where the number of red blood cells increases sharply, together with an increase in the number of white cells, making the blood thicker and slower to flow 真性红细胞增多症

◇ **erythematosus** 红斑的 *see* 见 DISSEMINATED, LUPUS

erythrasma *noun* chronic bacterial skin condition in a fold in the skin *or* where two skin surfaces touch (such as between the toes), caused by a Corynebacterium 红癣

◇ **erythroblast** *noun* cell which forms an erythrocyte or red blood cell 成红细胞

◇ **erythroblastosis** *noun* presence of erythroblasts in the blood, usually found in haemolytic anaemia 成红细胞增多症; **erythroblastosis fetalis** = blood disease affecting newborn babies, caused by a reaction between the rhesus factor of the mother and the fetus 胎儿成红细胞增多症

> COMMENT: Usually this occurs where the mother is rhesus negative and has developed rhesus positive antibodies, which are passed into the blood of a rhesus positive fetus.
> 注释:本病常发生于 Rh 阴性的母亲,产生了 Rh 抗体,并进入 Rh 阳性的胎儿血内。

◇ **erythrocyanosis** *noun* red and purple patches on the skin of the thighs, often accompanied by chilblains and made worse by cold 绀红皮病

erythrocyte *noun* mature non-nucleated red blood cell, a blood cell which contains haemoglobin and carries oxygen 红细胞; **erythrocyte sedimentation rate** (**ESR**) = diagnostic test to see how fast erythrocytes settle in a sample of blood plasma 红细胞沉降率

◇ **erythrocytosis** *noun* increase in the number of red blood cells in the blood 红细胞增多症

> QUOTE: Anemia may be due to insufficient erythrocyte production, in which case the corrected reticulocyte count will be low, or it may be due to hemorrhage or hemolysis, in which cases there should be reticulocyte response.
> 引文:贫血可因红细胞生成不足引起,此时矫正的网织红细胞数是较低的;出血或溶血也可导致贫血,但网织红细胞是升高的。
> **Southern Medical Journal** 南部医学杂志

erythroderma *noun* condition where the skin becomes red and flakes off 红皮病

◇ **erythroedema** *or* **pink disease** *noun* disease of infants where the child's hands and feet swell and become pink, with a fever and loss of appetite, probably formerly caused by allergic reaction to mercury in lotions 红皮病

◇ **erythrogenesis** *or* **erythropoiesis** *noun* formation of red blood cells in red bone marrow 红细胞生成

◊ **erythromelalgia** *noun* painful swelling of blood vessels in the extremities 红斑性肢痛病

◊ **erythromycin** *noun* antibiotic used to combat bacterial infections 红霉素

◊ **erythropenia** *noun* condition where a patient has a low number of erythrocytes in his blood 红细胞减少

◊ **erythropoiesis** = ERYTHROGENESIS 红细胞生成

◊ **erythropoietin** *noun* hormone which regulates the production of red blood cells 红细胞生成素

> COMMENT: Erythropoietin can now be produced by genetic techniques and is being used to increase the production of red blood cells in anaemia.
> 注释:红细胞生成素现已可通过基因技术生产,被用于刺激贫血时红细胞的生成。

◊ **erythropsia** *noun* condition where the patient sees things as if coloured red 红视病

Esbach's albuminometer *noun* glass for measuring albumin in urine, using Esbach's method 埃斯巴赫氏尿蛋白检测仪

eschar *noun* dry scab, such as one on a burn 焦痂

◊ **escharotic** *noun* substance which produces an eschar 腐蚀药

Escherichia *noun* one of the Enterobacteria commonly found in faeces 大肠杆菌; **Escherichia coli** = Gram-negative bacillus associated with acute gastroenteritis in infants 埃希杆菌属

escort *verb* to go with someone, especially to go with a patient to make sure he arrives at the right place 陪伴,护送; **escort nurse** = nurse who goes with patients to the operating theatre and back again to the ward 护送护士

Esmarch's bandage *noun* rubber band wrapped round a limb as a tourniquet before a surgical operation and left in place during the operation so as to keep the site free of blood 埃斯马赫氏绷带,止血带

eso- *US* = OESO- 在内,向内

esophagus *US* = OESOPHAGUS 食管

esotropia *noun* convergent strabismus, a type of squint, where the eyes both look towards the nose 内斜视

espundia 利什曼病 *see* 见 LEISHMANIASIS

ESR = ERYTHROCYTE SEDIMENTATION RATE 红细胞沉降率

essence *noun* concentrated oil from a plant, used in cosmetics, and sometimes as analgesics or antiseptics 露,香精剂

◊ **essential** *adjective* (**a**) idiopathic, (disease) with no obvious cause 原发的; **essential hypertension** = high blood pressure without any obvious cause 原发性高血压; **essential uterine haemorrhage** = heavy uterine bleeding for which there is no obvious cause 原发性子宫出血 (**b**) extremely important *or* necessary 必需的,必要的; **essential amino acid** = amino acid which is necessary for growth but which cannot be synthesized and has to be obtained from the food supply 必需氨基酸; **essential elements** = chemical elements (such as carbon, oxygen, hydrogen, nitrogen and many others) which are necessary to the body's growth or function 必要元素; **essential fatty acid** (**EFA**) = unsaturated fatty acid which is necessary for growth and health 必需脂肪酸; **essential oils** *or* **volatile oils** = concentrated oils from a scented plant used in cosmetics or as antiseptics 挥发油

> COMMENT: The essential amino acids are: isoleucine, leucine, lysine, methionine, phenylalanine, threonine, tryptophan and valine. The essential fatty acids are linoleic acid, linolenic acid and arachidonic acid.
> 注释:必需氨基酸是:异亮氨酸、亮氨酸、赖氨酸、甲氨酸、苯丙氨酸、苏氨酸、酪氨酸、缬氨酸。必需脂肪酸是亚麻酸、亚油酸和花生四烯酸。

estrogen *US* = OESTROGEN 雌激

素

ethanol *noun* ethyl alcohol, a colourless liquid, present in drinking alcohols (whisky *or* gin *or* vodka, etc.) and also used in medicines and as a disinfectant 乙醇

ether *noun* anaesthetic substance, now rarely used 乙醚

ethical *adjective* (i) concerning ethics 伦理的,传统的 (ii) *US* (drug) available to prescription only 只凭处方出售的(药品); **ethical committee** = group of specialists who monitor experiments involving human beings *or* who regulate the way in which members of the medical profession conduct themselves 伦理委员会

◇ **ethically** *adverb* concerning ethics 伦理地

◇ **ethics** *noun* code of working which shows how a professional group (such as doctors and nurses) should work, and in particular what type of relationship they should have with their patients 伦理学,(某种职业的)规范

ethmoid bone *noun* bone which forms the top of the nasal cavity and part of the orbits 筛骨

◇ **ethmoidal** *adjective* referring to the ethmoid bone *or* near to the ethmoid bone 筛骨的; **ethmoidal sinuses** = air cells inside the ethmoid bone 筛窦

◇ **ethmoiditis** *noun* inflammation of the ethmoid bone *or* of the ethmoidal sinuses 筛窦炎,筛骨炎

ethyl alcohol 乙醇 *see* 见 ALCOHOL

ethylene *noun* gas used as an anaesthetic 乙烯

etiology, etiological *US* = AETIOLOGY, AETIOLOGICAL 病因学

eu- *prefix* meaning good 好,佳

◇ **eubacteria** *noun* true bacteria with rigid cell walls 真菌

eucalyptus *noun* genus of tree growing mainly in Australia, from which a strongly smelling oil is distilled 桉树

◇ **eucalyptol** *noun* substance obtained from eucalyptus oil 桉油醇

> COMMENT: Eucalyptus oil is used in pharmaceutical products especially to relieve congestion in the respiratory passages.
> 注释:桉油醇被用来制药,尤其是缓解呼吸道充血。

eugenics *noun* study of how to improve the human race by genetic selection 优生学

eunuch *noun* castrated male 阉人

eupepsia *noun* good digestion 消化良好

euphoria *noun* feeling of extreme happiness 欣快,安乐症

euplastic *adjective* (tissue) which heals well 易于愈合的(组织)

Eustachian tube *or* **syrinx** *or* **pharyngotympanic tube** *noun* tube which connects the pharynx to the middle ear 咽鼓管 ◇ 见图 EAR

> COMMENT: The Eustachian tubes balance the air pressure on either side of the eardrum. When a person swallows or yawns, air is allowed into the Eustachian tubes and equalizes the pressure with the normal atmospheric pressure outside the body. The tubes can be blocked by an infection (as in a cold) or by pressure differences (as inside an aircraft) and if they are blocked, the hearing is impaired.
> 注释:咽鼓管平衡鼓膜两侧的气压。吞咽或哈欠时,空气进入咽鼓管使鼓膜内气压等于外界正常大气压。咽鼓管可因炎症(感冒时)、气压差(在飞机上)堵塞,而损伤听力。

euthanasia *noun* mercy killing, the killing of a sick person to put an end to his suffering 安乐死

euthyroidism *or* **euthyroid state** *noun* having a normal thyroid gland 甲状腺功能正常

eutocia *noun* normal childbirth 顺产

evacuate *verb* to discharge faeces from the bowel *or* to have a bowel movement 排泄

◇ **evacuant** *noun* medicine which makes a person have a bowel movement 泻药

◇ **evacuation** *noun* removing the contents of something, especially discharging faeces from the bowel 排泄; **evacuation of retained products of conception (ERPC)** = D & C operation performed after an abortion 不全娩出后清宫术

◇ **evacuator** *noun* instrument used to empty a cavity such as the bladder *or* bowel 排出器

evaluate *verb* (i) to examine and calculate the quantity *or* level of something 评估;(ii) to examine a patient and calculate the treatment required 检查病人并核计所需的治疗: ***The laboratory is still evaluating the results of the tests.*** 试验室仍在对试验结果进行评估。

◇ **evaluation** *noun* examining and calculating 评价: ***In further evaluation of these patients no side-effects of the treatment were noted.*** 对患者的进一步评估未发现此治疗的副作用。

> QUOTE: All patients were evaluated and followed up at the hypertension unit.
> 引文:对所有的患者均进行了评估,并在高血压门诊随访。
> **British Medical Journal** 英国医学杂志

> QUOTE: Evaluation of fetal age and weight has proved to be of value in the clinical management of pregnancy, particularly in high-risk gestations.
> 引文:胎儿胎龄、体重的评估,在妊娠的临床处理尤其是高危妊娠中非常重要。
> **Southern Medical Journal** 南部医学杂志

evaporate *verb* to convert liquid into vapour 蒸发

◇ **evaporation** *noun* converting liquid into vapour 蒸发

eversion *noun* turning towards the outside *or* turning inside out 外翻; **eversion of the cervix** = condition after laceration during childbirth, where the edges of the cervix sometimes turn outwards 子宫颈外翻

◇ **evertor** *noun* muscle which makes a limb turn outwards 外翻肌

evisceration *noun* (i) surgical removal of the abdominal viscera 去脏术 (ii) removal of the contents of an organ 掏空内容物; **evisceration of the eye** = surgical removal of the contents of an eyeball 剜除术

evolution *noun* changes in organisms which take place over a long period involving many generations 进化

Ewing's tumour *or* **Ewing's sarcoma** *noun* malignant tumour in the marrow of a long bone 尤文氏瘤,长骨骨髓中的恶性肿瘤

ex- *or* **exo-** *prefix* meaning out of 出,离

exacerbate *verb* to make a condition more severe 使加重: ***The cold damp weather will only exacerbate his chest condition.*** 寒冷潮湿的天气只会加重他的肺病

◇ **exacerbation** *noun* (i) making a condition worse 使加重;(ii) period when a condition becomes worse 加重期,恶化期

> QUOTE: Patients were re-examined regularly or when they felt they might be having an exacerbation. Exacerbation rates were calculated from the number of exacerbations during the study.
> 引文:患者定期或自觉症状加重时复查,计算研究期间病情恶化的例数求出恶化率。
> **Lancet** 柳叶刀

exact *adjective* correct *or* precise 精确的

exaltation *noun* sense of being extremely cheerful and excited(异常)兴奋,激越

examine *verb* (i) to look at *or* to investigate someone *or* something carefully 检查(ii) to look at and test a patient to find what is wrong with him 体检,查体: ***The doctor examined the patient's heart.*** 医生检查患者的心脏。***The tissue***

samples were examined in the laboratory. 组织样本在试验室进行检查。

◇ **examination** *noun* (**a**) (i) looking at someone *or* something carefully 仔细检查(ii) looking at a patient to find out what is wrong with him 对患者进行体检: ***From the examination of the X-ray photographs, it seems that the tumour has not spread.*** X线检查未发现肿瘤扩散。***The surgeon carried out a medical examination before operating.*** 外科医师在手术前进行身体检查。(**b**) written or oral test to see if a student is progressing satisfactorily 考试,测验: ***There will be a written and an oral examination in German.*** 德语将有笔试和口试。(NOTE: in this sense often abbreviated to **exam**)

exanthem *noun* skin rash found with infectious diseases like measles *or* chickenpox 皮疹; **exanthem subitum** = ROSEOLA INFANTUM 幼儿急诊(玫瑰疹)

◇ **exanthematous** *adjective* referring to an exanthem *or* like an exanthem 发疹的,疹的

excavator *noun* surgical instrument shaped like a spoon 挖器

◇ **excavatum**漏斗状 *see* 见 PECTUS

exceed *verb* to do more than *or* to be more than 超过: ***His pulse rate exceeded 100.*** 他的心率超过100次。Do not exceed the stated dose. = Do not take more than the stated dose. 不要超过规定剂量。

exceptional *adjective* strange *or* not common 例外的,特别的: ***In exceptional cases, treatment can be carried out in the patient's home.*** 某些特殊病例,可在家中进行治疗。

excess *noun* too much of a substance 过量: ***The gland was producing an excess of hormones.*** 腺体分泌了过量的激素。***The body could not cope with an excess of blood sugar.*** 机体无法消耗过量的血糖。**in excess of** = more than 超过: ***Short men who weigh in excess of 100 kilos are very overweight.*** 体重超过100公斤的矮个男人属于严重超重。

◇ **excessive** *adjective* more than normal 过多的,极端的: ***The patient was passing excessive quantities of urine.*** 患者多尿。***The doctor noted an excessive amount of bile in the patient's blood.*** 医生发现患者血胆红素水平过高。

◇ **excessively** *adverb* too much 过多地: ***He has an excessively high blood pressure.*** 他血压过高。***If the patient sweats excessively, it may be necessary to cool his body with cold compresses.*** 如果患者大量出汗,应用冷敷降低体温。

exchange 1 *noun* giving one thing and taking another 交换; **gas exchange** = process where oxygen in air is exchanged in the lungs for waste carbon dioxide from the blood 气体交换; **exchange transfusion** = method of treating leukaemia *or* erythroblastosis in newborn babies, where almost all the abnormal blood is removed from the body and replaced by normal blood 换血 **2** *verb* to take something away and give something in its place 交换: ***In the lungs, carbon dioxide in the blood is exchanged for oxygen from the air.*** 血液中的二氧化碳在肺脏与空气中的氧气交换。

excipient *noun* substance added to a drug so that it can be made into a pill 赋形剂

excise *verb* to cut out 切除

◇ **excision** *noun* operation by a surgeon to cut and remove part of the body (such as a growth) 切除术 *compare* 比较 INCISION

excite *verb* to stimulate *or* to give an impulse to a nerve *or* muscle 使兴奋

◇ **excited** *adjective* (i) very lively and happy 高兴的,幸福的 (ii) aroused 兴奋的

◇ **excitation** *noun* state of being mentally *or* nervously aroused 兴奋

◇ **excitatory** *adjective* which tends to excite 易兴奋的

◇ **excitement** *noun* (i) being excited; 兴奋(ii) second stage of anaesthesia 兴奋期

excoriation *noun* raw skin surface

or mucous membrane after rubbing *or* burning 表皮脱落

excrement *noun* faeces 粪便

excrescence *noun* growth on the skin 赘生物,赘疣

excrete *verb* to pass waste matter out of the body, especially to discharge faeces 排泄: ***The urinary system separates waste liquids from the blood and excretes them as urine.*** 泌尿系统从血液中分离出废液,以尿的形式排出体外。

◇ **excreta** *plural noun* waste material from the body (such as faeces) 排泄物

◇ **excretion** *noun* passing waste matter (faeces *or* urine *or* sweat) out of the body 排泄

excruciating *adjective* (pain) which is extremely painful 剧痛的: ***He had excruciating pains in his head.*** 他感觉头部剧烈疼痛。

exenteration = EVISCERATION 去脏术

exercise 1 *noun* physical or mental activity *or* active use of the muscles as a way of keeping fit *or* to correct a deformity *or* to strengthen apart 锻炼: ***Regular exercise is good for your heart.*** 经常锻炼对你的心脏有好处。***You should do five minutes' exercise every morning.*** 你应该每天早上进行5分钟的锻炼。***He doesn't do or take enough exercise — that's why he's too fat.*** 锻炼不够,这是他发胖的原因。**exercise cycle** = cycle which is fixed to the floor so that you can pedal on it to get exercise 健身车; **exercise-induced asthma** (**EIA**) = asthma which is caused by exercise such as running or cycling 运动诱发性哮喘 **2** *verb* to take exercise 锻炼,运动: ***He exercises twice a day to keep fit.*** 他每天运动两次以保持健康。

exert *verb* to use (force *or* pressure) 用力,使劲

◇ **exertion** *noun* physical activity 用劲

exfoliation *noun* losing layers of tissue (such as sun burnt skin) 表皮脱落

◇ **exfoliative** *adjective* referring to exfoliation 脱落的; **exfoliative dermatitis** = condition where the skin becomes red and flakes off 剥脱性皮炎

exhale *verb* to breathe out 呼出

◇ **exhalation** *noun* (i) expiration *or* breathing out 呼出 (ii) air which is breathed out 呼气 (NOTE: the opposite is **inhale**, **inhalation**)

exhaust *verb* to tire someone out; to drain energy 竭尽全力,耗尽: ***He was exhausted by his long walk.*** 长途跋涉后他已经精疲力尽了。***The patient was exhausted after the second operation.*** 经历第二次手术后患者已经完全衰竭了。

◇ **exhaustion** *noun* extreme tiredness *or* fatigue 衰竭,虚脱; **heat exhaustion** = collapse caused by physical exertion in hot conditions 热虚脱

exhibit *verb* to show signs of 展示,显示: ***The patient exhibited significant mental and psychological impairment.*** 病人表现出明显的精神和心理上的缺陷。

exhibitionism *noun* sexual aberration in which there is a desire to show the genitals to a person of the opposite sex 暴露癖,露阴症

exo- *prefix* meaning outside 外的

◇ **exocrine gland** *noun* gland (such as the liver, the sweat glands, the pancreas and the salivary glands) with ducts which channel secretions to particular parts of the body 外分泌腺; **exocrine secretions of the pancreas** = enzymes carried from the pancreas to the second part of the duodenum 胰腺的外分泌

exogenous *adjective* developing *or* caused by something outside the organism 外源的 *compare* 比较 ENDOGENOUS

exomphalos = UMBILICAL HERNIA 脐疝

exophthalmic goitre *or* **Graves' disease** 突眼性甲状腺肿 *see* 见 THYROTOXICOSIS

◇ **exophthalmos** *noun* protruding eyeballs 突眼

exoskeleton *noun* outer skeleton of some animals such as insects 外骨骼 *compare* 比较 ENDOSKELETON

exostosis *noun* benign growth on the surface of a bone 外生骨疣

exotic *adjective* (disease) which is not native *or* which comes from a foreign country 外来的

exotoxin *noun* poison produced by bacteria, which affects parts of the body away from the place of infection (such as the toxins which cause botulism or tetanus) 外毒素

> COMMENT: Diphtheria is caused by a bacillus; the exotoxin released causes the generalized symptoms of the disease (such as fever and rapid pulse) while the bacillus itself is responsible for the local symptoms in the patient's upper throat.
> 注释:白喉由白喉杆菌引起,分泌的外毒素引起全身症状(如发热,速脉),杆菌本身导致上咽部的局部症状。

exotropia *noun* divergent strabismus, a form of squint where both eyes look away from the nose 散开性斜视,外斜视

expand *verb* to spread out 扩张: ***The chest expands as the person breathes in.*** 人吸气时胸廓扩张。

◇ **expansion** *noun* growing larger *or* becoming swollen 扩大,肿胀

expect *verb* to think *or* to hope that something is going to happen 期待: ***She's expecting a baby in June.*** = She is pregnant and the baby is due to be born in June. 她的预产期是6月。**expected date of delivery** = day on which a doctor calculates that the birth will take place 预产期

◇ **expectant mother** *noun* pregnant woman 待产妇

expectorate *verb* to cough up phlegm *or* sputum from the respiratory passages 咳出

◇ **expectorant** *noun* drug which helps the patient to expectorate *or* to cough up phlegm 祛痰药

◇ **expectoration** *noun* coughing up fluid *or* phlegm from the respiratory tract 咳出

expel *verb* to send out of the body 排出: ***Air is expelled from the lungs when a person breathes out.*** 患者呼气时空气从肺排出。

experiment *noun* scientific test conducted under set conditions 试验: ***The scientists did some experiments to try the new drug on a small sample of people.*** 科学家选用小样本对新药进行了试验。

experience 1 *noun* (**a**) having worked in many types of situation, and so knowing how to cope with different problems 经验: ***He has had six years' experience in tropical medicine.*** 他在热带病学方面有6年的经验。His research is based on his experience as a nurse in a teaching hospital. 他的研究基于他在教学医院当护士时的经验。(**b**) thing which has happened to someone 经历: ***He told the complaints board about his experiences as an outpatient.*** 他对投诉委员会诉说了他门诊的经历。**2** *verb* to live through a situation 经过,经历: ***She experienced acute mental disturbance.*** 她经历了急性精神紊乱。***He is experiencing pains in his right upper leg.*** 他的右大腿疼痛。

◇ **experienced** *adjective* (person) who has lived through many situations and has learnt how to deal with problems 有经验的: ***She is the most experienced member of our nursing staff.*** 她是我们护理人员中最有经验的。***We require an experienced nurse to take charge of a geriatric ward.*** 我们需要有经验的护士负责管理老年病区。

expert 1 *noun* person who is trained *or* who has experience in a certain field 专家: ***He was referred to an expert in tropical diseases.*** 他被转诊到热带病专家那里。***She is an expert in the field of optics.*** 她是眼科领域的专家。***They asked for a second expert opinion.*** 他们询问第二位专家的意见。**2** *adjective* done well *or* showing experience 熟练的: ***The***

clinic offers expert treatment of sexually transmitted diseases. 门诊部对性传播疾病提供专业治疗。

expire *verb* (i) to breathe out 呼出(ii) to die 死亡

◇ **expiration** *noun* (i) breathing out *or* pushing air out of the lungs 呼出(ii) dying 死亡: ***Expiration takes place when the chest muscles relax and the lungs become smaller.*** 呼气时,胸肌舒张,肺脏缩小。(NOTE: the opposite is **inspiration**)

explain *verb* to give reasons for something; to make something clear 解释: ***The doctors cannot explain why he suddenly got better.*** 医生不能解释他突然好转的原因。***She tried to explain her symptoms to the doctor.*** 她尽力向医生解释她的症状。

◇ **explanation** *noun* reason for something 原因,解释: ***The staff of the hospital could not offer any explanation for the strange behaviour of the consultant.*** 医护人员不能解释会诊医师的奇怪举止。

explant 1 *noun* tissue taken from a body and grown in a culture in a laboratory 移出物 **2** *verb* (**a**) to take tissue from a body and grow it in a culture in a laboratory 体外培养 (**b**) to remove an implant 植入物移出

◇ **explantation** *noun* (**a**) taking tissue from a body and growing it in a culture in a laboratory 体外培养 (**b**) removal of an implant 移出

exploration *noun* procedure *or* surgical operation where the aim is to discover the cause of the symptoms *or* the nature and extent of the illness 探查

◇ **exploratory** *adjective* referring to an exploration 探查的; **exploratory surgery** = surgical operations in which the aim is to discover the cause of the patient's symptoms *or* the nature and extent of the illness 探查手术

expose *verb* (**a**) to show something which was hidden 暴露,披露: ***The operation exposed a generalized cancer.*** 手术中发现了一个扩散的癌肿。***The report exposed a lack of medical care on the part of some of the hospital staff.*** 报告披露部分医院职工缺乏医疗保健。(**b**) to place something *or* someone under the influence of something 使暴露于,遭受: ***He was exposed to the disease for two days.*** 他患此病已经两天了。***She was exposed to a lethal dose of radiation.*** 她接受了致死剂量的放射线。

◇ **exposure** *noun* (**a**) being exposed 暴露; ***his exposure to radiation*** 他接触放射线 (**b**) being damp, cold and with no protection from the weather 露天: ***The survivors of the crash were all suffering from exposure after spending a night in the snow.*** 事故的幸存者都经受了一夜风雪,领受了霜寒之苦。

express *verb* to squeeze out 压出; ***to express pus*** 挤脓

expression *noun* (**a**) look on a person's face which shows his emotions *or* what he thinks and feels 表情: ***His expression showed that he was annoyed.*** 他的表情显示他很生气。(**b**) pushing something out of the body 压出; ***the expression of the fetus and placenta during childbirth*** 分娩时压出胎儿和胎盘

exsanguinate *verb* to drain blood from the body 放血

◇ **exsanguination** *noun* removal of blood from the body 放血

exsufflation *noun* forcing breath out of the body 排气

extend *verb* to stretch out 伸展: ***The patient is unable to extend his arms fully.*** 患者不能充分伸展他的胳膊。

◇ **extension** *noun* (**a**) (i) stretching *or* straightening out of a joint 伸展(ii) stretching of a joint by traction 牵伸 (**b**) something built on afterwards 增建部分: ***The hospital has had an extension built to house its new X-ray equipment.*** 医院增建了房屋放置新的 X 线设备。

◇**extensor** (**muscle**) *noun* muscle which makes a joint become straight 伸肌 *compare* 比较 FLEXOR

exterior *noun* the outside 外的：***The interior of the disc has passed through the tough exterior and is pressing on a nerve.*** 椎间盘的内环穿过了坚硬的外环，压迫了神经。
◇ **exteriorization** *noun* surgical operation to bring an internal organ to the outside surface of the body 外置术
externa 外的 *see* 见 OTITIS
external *adjective* which is outside, especially outside the surface of the body 外的，外在的：***The lotion is for external use only.*** = It should only be used on the outside of the body. 仅供外用的洗剂。**external auditory meatus** = tube in the skull leading from the outer ear to the eardrum 外耳道；**external cardiac massage** *or* **external chest** *or* **cardiac compression** = method of making a patient's heart start beating again by rhythmic pressing on the breastbone 心外按摩，体外心脏按压；**external jugular** = main jugular vein in the neck, leading from the temporal vein 颈外静脉；**external oblique** = outer muscle covering the abdomen 外斜肌
◇ **externally** *adverb* on the outside of the body 在外部，外表上：***The ointment should only be used externally.*** 药膏仅供外用。*compare* 比较 INTERNAL, INTERNALLY
exteroceptor *noun* sensory nerve such as those in the eye *or* ear, which is affected by stimuli from outside the body 外感受器 *see also* 参见 CHEMORECEPTOR, INTEROCEPTOR, RECEPTOR
extirpate *verb* to remove by surgery 摘除
◇ **extirpation** *noun* total removal of a structure *or* an organ *or* growth by surgery 摘除术
extra- *prefix* meaning outside 外面的
◇ **extracapsular** *adjective* outside a capsule 囊外的；**extracapsular fracture** = fracture of the upper part of the femur, but which does not involve the capsule round the hip joint 关节囊外骨折
◇ **extracellular** *adjective* outside cells 细胞外的；**extracellular fluid** = fluid which surrounds cells 细胞外液
extract 1 *noun* preparation made by removing water *or* alcohol from a substance, leaving only the essence 浸膏，提取；**liver extract** = concentrated essence of liver 肝浸膏 **2** *verb* (i) to take out 提取(ii) to remove the essence from a liquid 提取溶质(iii) to pull out a tooth 拔牙：***Adrenaline extracted from the animal's adrenal glands is used in the treatment of asthma.*** 从动物肾上腺提取的肾上腺素可用来治疗哮喘。
◇ **extraction** *noun* (i) removal of part of the body, especially a tooth 拔除，拔牙 (ii) in obstetrics, delivery, usually a breech presentation, which needs medical assistance 取胎术；**cataract extraction** = surgical removal of a cataract from the eye 白内障摘除术；**vacuum extraction** = pulling on the head of the baby with a suction instrument to aid birth 吸出术

> QUOTE: All the staff are RGNs, partly because they do venesection, partly because they work in plasmapheresis units which extract plasma and return red blood cells to the donor.
> 引文：所有工作人员都是注册全科护士，一方面是因为她们做静脉切开术，另一方面因为他们在血浆置换病房工作，抽取供者的血浆后回输红细胞。
> **Nursing Times** 护理时代

extradural *or* **epidural** *adjective* lying on the outside of the dura mater 硬膜外的；**extradural haematoma** = blood clot which forms in the head outside the dura mater, caused by a blow 硬膜外血肿；**extradural haemorrhage** = serious condition where bleeding occurs between the dura mater and the skull 硬膜外出血
◇ **extraembryonic** *adjective* (part of a fertilized ovum, such as the amnion,

allantois and chorion) which is not part of the embryo 胚外的

◇ **extrapleural** *adjective* outside the pleural cavity 胸膜外的

◇ **extrapyramidal** *adjective* outside the pyramidal tracts 椎体束外的；**extrapyramidal system** *or* **tracts** = motor system which carries motor nerves outside the pyramidal system 椎体外系统

◇ **extrasystole** *or* **ectopic beat** *noun* abnormal extra heartbeat which originates from a point other than the sinoatrial node 期外收缩

◇ **extrauterine pregnancy** *or* **ectopic pregnancy** *noun* pregnancy where the embryo develops outside the uterus, often in one of the Fallopian tubes 宫外孕，异位妊娠

◇ **extravasation** *noun* escaping of bodily fluid (such as blood *or* secretions) into tissue 外渗

◇ **extravert, extraversion** *noun* = EXTROVERT, EXTROVERSION 外向性格，外翻

extreme *adjective* very severe 严重的：***Extreme forms of the disease can cause blindness.*** 疾病严重时可致盲。

◇ **extremities** *noun* parts of the body at the ends of limbs, such as the fingers, toes, nose and ears 肢体末端

extrinsic *adjective* external *or* which originates outside a structure 外部的；**extrinsic allergic alveolitis** = condition where the lungs are allergic to fungus and other allergens 外源性过敏性肺泡炎；**extrinsic factor** = former term for vitamin B_{12}, which is necessary for the production of red blood cells 外因子，维生素$_{12}$的旧称；**extrinsic ligament** = ligament between the bones in a joint which is separate from the joint capsule 外韧带；**extrinsic muscle** = muscle which is some way away from the part of the body (such as the eye) which it operates 外附肌

extroversion *noun* (**a**) (in psychology) condition where a person is mainly interested in people and things other than himself 外向性格 (**b**) congenital turning of an organ inside out 外翻

◇ **extrovert** *noun* person who is interested in people and things apart from himself 外向性格者

◇ **extroverted** *adjective* (**a**) (*person*) interested in people and things apart from himself 外倾性格的 (**b**) (*organ*) turned inside out 外翻的 *compare* 比较 INTROVERSION, INTROVERT

exudate *noun* fluid which is deposited on the surface of tissue as the result of a condition *or* disease 渗出物

◇ **exudation** *noun* escape of exudate into tissue as a defence mechanism 渗出

eye *noun* part of the body with which a person sees 眼：***She has blue eyes.*** 她有一双蓝色的眼睛。***Shut your eyes while the doctor gives you an injection.*** 医生给你注射时请闭上眼睛。***He has got a speck***

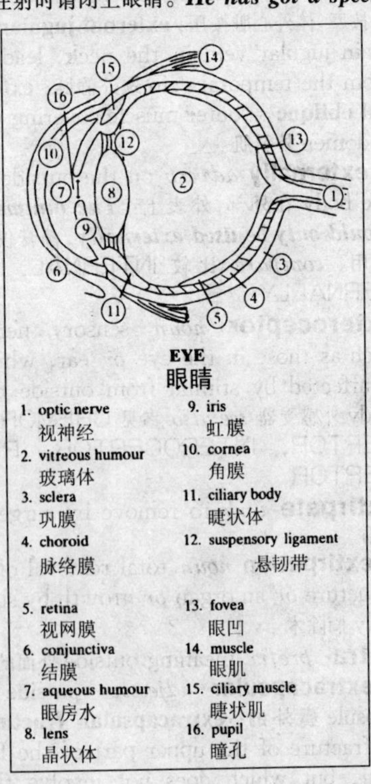

EYE
眼睛

1. optic nerve 视神经
2. vitreous humour 玻璃体
3. sclera 巩膜
4. choroid 脉络膜
5. retina 视网膜
6. conjunctiva 结膜
7. aqueous humour 眼房水
8. lens 晶状体
9. iris 虹膜
10. cornea 角膜
11. ciliary body 睫状体
12. suspensory ligament 悬韧带
13. fovea 眼凹
14. muscle 眼肌
15. ciliary muscle 睫状肌
16. pupil 瞳孔

of dust in his eye. 他眼睛里进了灰尘。*She has been having trouble with her eyes* or *she has been having eye trouble*. 她的眼睛一直有毛病。*He is an outpatient at the local eye hospital*. 他是当地眼科医院的门诊病人。**black eye** = darkening and swelling of the tissues round an eye, caused by a blow 眼圈青肿: *He got two black eyes in the fight*. 打斗中他双眼给打成乌眼青。**glass eye** = artificial eye made of glass 眼镜; **pink eye** *or* **red eye** = epidemic conjunctivitis, common in schools, and caused by the Koch-Weeks bacillus 急性结膜炎; **eye bath** = small dish into which a solution can be placed for bathing the eye 洗眼杯; **eye drops** = medicine in liquid form which is put into the eye in small amounts 眼药水; **eye ointment** = smooth oily medicinal preparation which is put into *or* around the eye 眼药膏: *The doctor prescribed some eye drops or eye ointment*. 医生开了些眼药水或膏。

◊ **eyeball** *noun* the receptor part of the eye, a round ball of tissue through which light passes and which is controlled by various muscles 眼球

COMMENT: Light rays enter the eye through the cornea, pass through the pupil and are refracted through the aqueous humour onto the lens, which then focuses the rays through the vitreous humour onto the retina at the back of the eyeball. Impulses from the retina pass along the optic nerve to the brain.
注释:光线经角膜进入眼内,通过瞳孔,经房水折射到晶体,后者将光线经玻璃体液聚焦于眼球后部的视网膜。视网膜产生的冲动通过视神经传到大脑。

◊ **eye bank** *noun* place where parts of eyes given by donors can be kept for use in grafts 眼库

◊ **eyebath** *noun* small dish into which a solution can be put for bathing the eye 洗眼杯

◊ **eyebrow** *noun* arch of skin with a line of hair above the eye 眉毛: *He raised his eyebrows*. = He looked surprised. 他扬起了眉毛,表示吃惊

◊ **eyeglasses** *noun US* glasses *or* spectacles 眼镜

◊ **eyelash** *noun* small hair which grows out from the edge of the eyelid 睫毛

◊ **eyelid** *or* **blepharon** *or* **palpebra** *noun* piece of skin which covers the eye 眼睑 (NOTE: for terms referring to the eyelids, see words beginning with **blepharo-**)

◊ **eyesight** *noun* being able to see 视力: *He has got very good eyesight*. 他视力良好。*Failing eyesight is common in old people*. 老年人常视力下降。

◊ **eyestrain** *or* **asthenopia** *noun* tiredness in the muscles of the eye, with a headache, caused by reading in bad light, watching television, working on a computer screen, etc. 眼疲劳

◊ **eyetooth** *noun* canine tooth, one of two pairs of pointed teeth next to the incisors 上尖牙 (NOTE: plural is **eyeteeth**. For other terms referring to the eye, see words beginning with **oculo-**, **ophth- and opt-**)

Ff

F **1** *abbreviation for* (缩写) Fahrenheit 华氏温度的简称 **2** *chemical symbol for* fluorine 氟的化学元素符号

face **1** *noun* front part of the head, where the eyes, nose and mouth are placed 面,脸: ***Don't forget to wash the patient's face.*** 不要忘了给患者洗脸。**face delivery** = birth where the baby's face appears first 面先露;(in cosmetic surgery) **face lift** *or* **face-lifting operation** = surgical operation to remove wrinkles on the face and neck 除去面部皱纹的整形手术: ***She's gone into hospital for a face lift.*** 她去医院做面部整容手术。**face mask** = (i) rubber mask that fits over the patient's nose and mouth and is used to administer an anaesthetic 面罩(ii) piece of gauze which fits over the mouth and nose to prevent droplet infection 口罩; **face presentation** = position of a baby in the womb where the face will appear first at birth 面先露 **2** verb to have your face towards *or* to look towards 面对: ***Please face the screen.*** 请面对荧光屏。***The hospital faces east.*** 医院朝向东。

> COMMENT: The fourteen bones which make up the face are: two maxillae forming the upper jaw; two nasal bones forming the top part of the nose; two lacrimal bones on the inside of the orbit near the nose; two zygomatic or malar bones forming the sides of the cheeks; two palatine bones forming the back part of the top of the mouth; two nasal conchae or turbinate bones which form the sides of the nasal cavity; the mandible or lower jaw; and the vomer in the centre of the nasal septum. 构成颜面的 14 块骨头是:2 块上颌骨形成上腭;2 块鼻骨构成鼻梁;2 块泪骨位于眶内侧;2 块颧骨形成面颊;2块腭骨形成口盖;2块鼻甲骨构成鼻腔;还有下颌骨和鼻中隔。

facet *noun* flat surface on a bone 骨平面; **facet syndrome** = condition where a joint in the vertebrae becomes dislocated 椎关节脱位综合征

facial *adjective* referring to the face 面的: ***The psychiatrist examined the patient's facial expression.*** 心理医生研究患者的面部表情。**facial bones** = the fourteen bones which form the face 面骨; **facial artery** = artery which branches off the external carotid into the face and mouth 面动脉; **facial nerve** = seventh cranial nerve, which governs the muscles of the face, the taste buds on the front of the tongue, and the salivary and lacrimal glands 面神经; **facial paralysis** *or* **facial palsy** = BELL'S PALSY 面瘫; **facial vein** = vein which drains down the side of the face into the internal jugular vein 面静脉; **deep facial vein** = small vein which drains from behind the cheek into the facial vein 面深静脉

-facient *suffix* which makes 做; **abortifacient** = drug or instrument which produces an abortion 堕胎药(设备)

facies *noun* facial appearance of a patient, used as a guide to diagnosis 气色,面色

facilitate *verb* to help *or* to make something easy 使容易

◊ **facilitation** *noun* act where several slight stimuli help a neurone to be activated 助长,接通,刺激

◊ **facilities** *plural noun* equipment *or* counselling *or* rooms which can be used to do something 设备,装置; ***provision of aftercare facilities*** 提供术后护理设备

fact *noun* something which is real and true 事实,真实: ***It is a fact that the disease is rarely fatal.*** 事实上,此病很少有生命危险。***Tell me all the facts of your son's illness so that I can decide what to do.*** 告诉我所有有关你儿子疾病的情况以便我决定如何做。**the facts of life** = description of how sexual intercourse is performed and how conception takes place, given to children 性教育

factor *noun* (**a**) something which has an influence, which makes something else take place 因素,因子,原动力; **extrinsic factor** = form of vitamin B_{12} 外因子; **growth factor** = chemical substance produced in one part of the body which encourages the growth of a type of cell (such as red blood cells) 生长因子; **intrinsic factor** = protein produced in the gastric glands which controls the absorption of extrinsic factor, and the lack of which causes pernicious anaemia 内因子 (**b**) substance (called Factor I, Factor II, etc.) in the plasma which makes the blood coagulate when a blood vessel is injured 凝血因子; **Factor VIII** = substance in plasma which is lacking in haemophiliacs VIII 因子; **Christmas factor** *or* **Factor IX** = substance in plasma, the lack of which causes Christmas disease IX 因子

faculty *noun* ability to do something 能力; **mental faculties** = power of the mind to think or decide 脑力活动: ***A reduction in blood supply to the brain can have a lasting effect on the mental faculties.*** 脑供血不足对智力有持久的影响。

faeces *plural noun* stools *or* bowel movements, solid waste matter passed from the bowels through the anus 粪便

◊ **faecal** *adjective* referring to faeces 粪便的; **faecal matter** = solid waste matter from the bowels 渣滓,粪质 (NOTE: spelt feces, fecal especially in the USA. For other terms referring to faeces, see words beginning with **sterco-**)

Fahrenheit *noun* scale of temperatures where the freezing and boiling points of water are 32° and 212° 华氏温度 *compare* 比较 CELSIUS, CENTIGRADE (NOTE: used in the USA, but less common in the UK. Normally written with an **F** after the degree sign: **32°F** (say: 'thirty-two degrees Fahrenheit').)

fail *verb* not to be successful in doing something *or* not to succeed *or* not to do something which you are trying to do 失败,不成功,不及格: ***The doctor failed to see the symptoms.*** 医生没有发现症状。***She has failed her pharmacy exams.*** 她没有通过药学考试。***He failed his medical and was rejected by the police force.*** 他没有通过体检,未被警局录取。

◊ **failing** *adjective* weakening, becoming closer to death 虚弱的,濒死的

◊ **failure** *noun* not a success 失败: ***The operation to correct the bone defect was a failure.*** 矫正骨畸形的手术失败了。**heart failure** = situation where the heart cannot function in a satisfactory way and is unable to circulate blood normally 心力衰竭; **kidney failure** = situation where a kidney does not function properly 肾衰竭; **failure to thrive** = wasting disease of small children who have difficulty in absorbing nutrients or who are suffering from malnutrition 消瘦病

faint 1 *verb* to lose consciousness *or* to stop being conscious for a short time 昏厥: ***She fainted when she saw the blood.*** 她看见血后晕倒了。***It was so hot standing in the sun that he fainted.*** 站在烈日下他热的晕倒了。**2** *noun* loss of consciousness for a short period, caused by a temporary reduction in the flow of blood to the brain 晕厥: ***He collapsed in a faint.*** 他虚脱了。**3** *adjective* not very clear *or* difficult to see or hear 模糊的,不清楚的: ***He could detect a faint improvement in the patient's condition.*** 他发现患者的病情有了轻微的改善。***There's a faint smell of apples in the urine.*** 尿有一股淡淡的苹果味儿。(NOTE: **faint - fainter - faintest**)

◊ **fainting** *noun* syncope, becoming unconscious for a short time 昏倒; **fainting fit** *or* **fainting spell** = becoming unconscious for a short time 昏厥: ***She often had fainting fits when she was dieting.*** 她节食时经常昏厥。

COMMENT: A fainting spell happens when the supply of blood to the brain is reduced for a short time, and this can be due to many causes, including lack of food, heat exhaustion, standing upright for a long time, and fear.
注释:昏厥因短时间内脑供血不足引起,原因很多,包括进食不足、热虚脱、长期站立以及恐惧。

fair *adjective* light-coloured (hair *or* skin) 浅色的: ***She's got fair hair.*** 她有一头金色的头发。***He's dark, but his sister is fair.*** 他肤色发暗,但他姐姐的皮肤很白嫩。

◇ **fair-haired** *adjective* (person) with light-coloured hair 金发的

◇ **fairly** *adverb* quite 很: ***I'm fairly certain I have met him before.*** 我肯定以前见过他。***He has been working as a doctor only for a fairly short time.*** 他只当过很短时间的大夫。

Fairbanks' splint *noun* special splint used for correcting Erb's palsy 法尔奔克氏夹板

falciform ligament *noun* tissue which separates the two lobes of the liver and attaches it to the diaphragm 镰状韧带

fall 1 *noun* losing balance and going onto the ground 失去平衡而落下: ***She had a fall and hurt her back.*** 她摔了下去,摔伤了后背。***He broke a bone in his hip after a fall.*** 他摔下后,摔断了髋骨。**2** *verb* (**a**) to drop down onto the ground 落下,降落: ***He fell down the stairs.*** 他从楼梯上摔了下来。***She fell off the wall.*** 她从墙上掉了下来。***Don't put the baby's bottle on the cushion - it will fall over.*** 不要把奶瓶放在垫子上,它会翻倒的。(NOTE: **falls - falling - fell - has fallen**)

◇ **fall asleep** *verb* to go to sleep 入睡: ***He fell asleep in front of the TV.*** 他在电视机前睡着了。

◇ **fall ill** *verb* to get ill *or* to start to have an illness 生病: ***He fell ill while on holiday and had to be flown home.*** 他在旅途中病倒了,不得不飞回家。

◇ **fall off** *verb* to become less 减少: ***The number of admissions has fallen off this month.*** 这个月住院人数有所减少。

Fallopian tube *noun* one of two tubes which connect the ovaries to the uterus 输卵管 (NOTE: also called **oviduct** *or* **salpinx** *or* **uterine tube**) ◊ 见图 UROGENITAL SYSTEM(female) (NOTE: for other terms referring to Fallopian tubes, see words beginning with **salping-**)

COMMENT: Once a month, ova (unfertilized eggs) leave the ovaries and move down the Fallopian tubes to the uterus; at the point where the Fallopian tubes join the uterus an ovum may be fertilized by a sperm cell. Sometimes fertilization and development of the embryo take place in the Fallopian tube itself.
注释:每一个月有一个卵细胞离开卵巢,通过输卵管进入子宫,在输卵管与子宫交界处可与精子结合。有时卵细胞在输卵管受精发育成胚胎。

Fallot's tetralogy 法乐氏四联症 *see* 见 TETRALOGY, WATERSTON'S OPERATION

false *adjective* not true *or* not real 假的; **false pains** = pains which appear to be labour pains but are not 假性疼痛; **false ribs** = ribs which are not attached to the breastbone 假肋,浮肋; **false teeth** *or* **dentures** = artificial teeth made of plastic, which fit in the mouth and take the place of teeth which have been extracted 义齿,假牙

falx (cerebri) *noun* fold of the dura mater between the two hemispheres of the cerebrum 大脑镰

family *noun* group of people who are related to each other, especially mother, father and children 家,家人: ***John is the youngest in our family.*** 约翰是我们家最小的。***They have a very big family — two sons and three daughters.*** 他们是一个大家庭,有两个儿子和三个女儿。**family doctor** = general practitioner, especially one who looks after all the members of a family 家庭医生; **family planning** = using contraception to control the number of children in a family 计划生育; **family planning clinic** = clinic which gives advice on contraception 计划生育门诊; **Family Practitioner Committee** = committee which organizes the management of GPs, dentists, opticians and pharmacists offering their services in an area 家庭医生协会: ***Drugs account for the largest element of expenditure in the Family Practitioner Service.*** 药费是家庭医生协会开支中最大的一项。

◇ **familial** *adjective* referring to a family 家的; **familial adenomatous polyposis (FAP)** = hereditary disorder where polyps develop in the small intestine 家族性腺瘤样息肉病; **familial disorder** = hereditary disorder which affects several members of the same family 家族性疾病

Fanconi syndrome *noun* kidney disorder where amino acids are present in the urine 范康尼氏综合症，一种肾脏疾病伴氨基酸尿

fantasy *noun* series of imaginary events which a patient believes really took place 幻觉

◇ **fantasize** *verb* to imagine that things have happened 幻想

FAP = FAMILIAL ADENOMATOUS POLYPOSIS 家族性腺瘤样息肉病

farcy *noun* form of glanders which affects the lymph nodes 慢性鼻疽

farinaceous *adjective* referring to flour *or* containing starch 含淀粉的; **farinaceous foods** = foods (such as bread) which are made of flour and have a high starch content 含淀粉的食物

farm *noun* land used for growing crops and keeping animals 农场: ***He's going to work on the farm during the holidays.*** 他假期要去农场工作。***You can buy eggs and vegetables at the farm.*** 你可以在农场买鸡蛋和蔬菜。

◇ **farmer** *noun* man who looks after or owns a farm 农场主; **farmer's lung** = type of asthma caused by an allergy to rotting hay 农民肺

farsightedness *noun* longsightedness *or* hypermetropia *or US* hypertropia, condition where the patient sees clearly objects which are a long way away but cannot see objects which are close 远视 (NOTE: the opposite is **shortsightedness** *or* **myopia**)

fascia *noun* fibrous tissue covering a muscle or an organ 筋膜; **fascia lata** = wide sheet of tissue covering the thigh muscles 阔筋膜 (NOTE: plural is **fasciae**)

fasciculus *noun* bundle of nerve fibres 神经束(NOTE: plural is **fasciculi**)

◇ **fasciculation** *noun* small muscle movements which appear as trembling skin 肌纤颤

Fasciolopsis *noun* type of liver fluke, often found in the Far East, which is transmitted to humans through contaminated waterplants 姜片虫属

fast 1 *adjective* quick, not slow 快的: ***This is a very fast-acting drug.*** 此药起效很快。2 *noun* going without food (either to lose weight *or* for religious reasons) 禁食: ***He went on a fast to lose some weight.*** 他为了减肥禁食。3 *verb* to go without food 禁食: ***The patient should fast from midnight of the night before an operation.*** 患者从手术前一夜的午夜开始禁食。

fastigium *noun* highest temperature during a bout of fever 最高温度

fat 1 *adjective* big and round in the body 胖的: ***You ought to eat less — you're getting too fat.*** 应该少吃些，你太胖了。***That fat man has a very thin wife.*** 这个胖男人有个很瘦的妻子。***He's the fattest boy in the class.*** 他是班里最胖的男孩。(NOTE : **fat - fatter - fattest**) 2 *noun* (**a**) white oily substance in the body, which stores energy and protects the body against cold 脂肪; **body fat** *or* **adipose tissue** = tissue where the cells contain fat, which replaces the normal fibrous tissue when too much food is eaten 脂肪组织; **brown fat** = animal fat which can easily be converted to energy, and is believed to offset the effects of ordinary white fat 棕色脂肪; **saturated fat** = fat which has the largest amount of hydrogen possible 饱和脂肪; **unsaturated fat** = fat which does not have a large amount of hydrogen, and so can be broken down more easily 不饱和脂肪 (**b**) type of food which supplies protein and Vitamins A and D, especially that part of meat which is white *or* solid substances(like lard *or* butter) produced from animals and used for cooking *or* liquid substances like oil 肥肉,油: ***If you don't like the fat on the meat, cut it off.*** 如果你不喜欢肥肉,把它切掉。***Fry the eggs in some fat.*** 放一些油煎鸡蛋。

◇ **fat-soluble** *adjective* which can dissolve in fat 脂溶的: ***Vitamin D is fat-soluble.*** 维生素 D 是脂溶性的。(NOTE: **fat** has no plural when it means the substance; the plural **fats** is used to mean different types of fat. For other terms referring to fats, see also **lipid** and words beginning with **steato-**)

COMMENT: Fat is a necessary part of diet because of the vitamins and energy-giving calories which it contains. Fat in the diet comes from either animal fats or vegetable fats. Animal fats such as butter, fat meat or cream, are saturated fatty acids. It is believed that the intake of unsaturated and polyunsaturated fats (mainly vegetable fats and oils, and fish oil) in the diet, rather than animal fats, helps keep down the level of cholesterol in the blood and so lessens the risk of atherosclerosis. A low-fat diet does not always help to reduce weight.

注释:脂肪是饮食中的必需成分,它含有维生素,并提供能量。食物中的脂肪来于动物或植物。动物脂肪如黄油、肥肉或奶酪是饱和脂肪酸。现认为摄入不饱和或多不饱和脂肪(主要是植物脂肪、植物油和鱼油)更有利于降低血胆固醇水平,减少发生动脉硬化的危险。低脂肪饮食并不总能帮助减轻体重。

fatal *adjective* which causes *or* results in death 致死的: ***He had a fatal accident.*** 他发生了致命性意外。***Cases of bee stings are rarely fatal.*** 被蜜蜂蜇伤一般不会致死。

◇ **fatality** *noun* case of death 死亡: ***There were three fatalities during the flooding.*** 有三人死于洪水。

◇ **fatally** *adverb* in a way which causes death 死地: ***His heart was fatally weakened by the lung disease.*** 他的心脏因为肺病而衰竭。

father *noun* man who has a son or daughter 父亲: ***Ask your father if you can borrow his car.*** 问问你父亲能否借他的汽车。***She is coming to tea with her father and mother.*** 她要和父母一起喝茶。

fatigue 1 *noun* very great tiredness 疲劳; **muscle fatigue** *or* **muscular fatigue** = tiredness in the muscles after strenuous exercise 肌肉疲劳; **chronic fatigue syndrome** = MYALGIC ENCEPHALOMYELITIS 慢性疲劳综合征,慢性肌痛性脑脊髓炎 **2** *verb* to tire someone out 使疲劳: ***He was fatigued by the hard work.*** 他被艰巨的工作弄得很疲劳。

fatty *adjective* containing fat 含脂的; **fatty acid** = acid (such as stearic acid) which is an important substance in the body 脂肪酸; **essential fatty acid** = unsaturated fatty acid which is essential for growth but which cannot be synthesized by the body and has to be obtained from the food supply 必需脂肪酸; **fatty degeneration** = accumulation of fat in the cells of an organ (such as the liver or heart), making the organ less able to perform 脂肪变性

fauces *noun* opening between the tonsils at the back of the throat, leading to the pharynx 咽门

favism *noun* type of inherited anaemia caused by an allergy to beans 蚕豆病,由蚕豆过敏导致的遗传性贫血

favus *noun* highly contagious type of

ringworm caused by a fungus which attacks the scalp 毛囊癣

Fe *chemical symbol for* iron 铁的化学元素符号

fear *noun* state where a person is afraid of something happening 害怕: ***He has a morbid fear of flying or of spiders.*** 他对苍蝇或蜘蛛有一种病态的恐惧。

features *noun* appearance of a person's face 面色: ***He has heavy features.*** 他面色阴沉。

febricula *noun* low fever 低热

◇ **febrifuge** *adjective & noun* (drug such as aspirin) which prevents *or* lowers a fever 退热的,退热剂

◇ **febrile** *adjective* referring to a fever *or* caused by a fever 热的,发热的; **febrile disease** = disease which is accompanied by fever 发热性疾病

feces *or* **fecal** *US* = FAECES, FAECAL 粪便

feeble *adjective* very weak 虚弱的: ***She is old and feeble.*** 她又老又弱。***Some of the patients in the geriatric ward are very feeble.*** 老年病房的一些患者很虚弱。

◇ **feebleminded** *adjective* being less than normally intelligent 低能的

◇ **feeblemindedness** *noun* state of less than normal intelligence 低能

feed *verb* to give food (to someone *or* an animal) 喂养: ***He has to be fed with a spoon.*** 他必须用匙喂。***The baby has reached the stage when she can feed herself.*** 这个婴儿已经到了可以搬自己吃饭的时候。(NOTE: **feeds - feeding - fed - has fed**)

◇ **feedback** *noun* linking of the result of an action back to the action itself 反馈; **negative feedback** = situation where the result represses the process which caused it 负反馈; **positive feedback** = situation where the result stimulates the process again 正反馈

◇ **feeding** *noun* action of giving someone something to eat 喂; **feeding cup** = special cup with a spout, used for feeding patients who cannot feed themselves 带喷嘴的杯子,用来给不能自己进食的患者喂水 *see also* 参见 BREAST FEEDING, BOTTLE FEEDING, INTRAVENOUS FEEDING

feel *verb* (**a**) to touch (usually with your finger) 触摸: ***Feel how soft the cushion is.*** 摸摸垫子有多软。***When the lights went out we had to feel our way to the door.*** 灯灭了,我们不得不摸索着找到门。(**b**) to give a sensation when touched 给人…感觉: ***The knife felt cold.*** 刀很凉。***The floor feels hard.*** 地板很硬。(**c**) to have a sensation 感觉: ***I felt the table move.*** 我觉得桌子在动。***Did you feel the lift go down suddenly?*** 你感到电梯在突然下降吗? ***He felt ill after eating the fish.*** 吃了鱼后他感觉不舒服。***When she saw the report she felt better.*** 看了报告后,她感觉好多了。(**d**) to believe *or* to think; to have an opinion 认为,相信: ***He feels it would be wrong to leave the children alone in the house.*** 她认为把孩子独自留在家中是不对的。***The police felt that the accident was the fault of the driver of the car.*** 警察认为事故的责任在汽车司机。***The doctor feels the patient is well enough to be moved out of intensive care.*** 医生认为患者的情况在好转,可以搬出监护病房。(NOTE: **feels - feeling - felt - felt**)

◇ **feeling** *noun* sensation *or* something which you feel 感觉: ***I had a feeling that someone was watching me.*** 我感觉有人在看我。***She had an itchy feeling inside her stomach.*** 她胃里有种痒的感觉。

Fehling's solution *noun* solution used to detect sugar in urine 费林氏溶液,检测尿糖用

felon = WHITLOW 瘭疽,化脓性指头炎

Felty's syndrome *noun* condition where the spleen is enlarged, and the number of white blood cells increases, associated with rheumatoid arthritis 费耳提氏综合征,表现为脾大,白细胞增多,伴有类风湿性关节炎

female *adjective & noun* (animal *or* plant) of the same sex as a woman or girl; animal which produces ova and bears young 母性的,女的,母性; ***a female cat*** 一只母猫;***a condition found more often in females aged 40～60*** 一种在40—60岁的女性中更常见的情况

◇ **feminization** *noun* development of female characteristics in a male 女性化

femoral *adjective* referring to the femur *or* to the thigh 股的,大腿的; **femoral artery** = continuation of the external iliac artery, which runs down the front of the thigh and then crosses to the back 股动脉; **femoral canal** = inner tube of the sheath surrounding the femoral artery and vein 股管; **femoral hernia** = hernia of the bowel at the top of the thigh 股疝; **femoral nerve** = nerve which governs the muscle at the front of the thigh 股神经; **femoral triangle** *or* **Scarpa's triangle** = slight hollow at the side of the thigh 股三角; **femoral vein** = vein running up the upper leg, a continuation of the popliteal vein 股静脉

◇ **femoris** *noun* 二头的 *see* 见 BICEPS, RECTUS

◇ **femur** *noun* thighbone, the bone in the top part of the leg which joins the acetabulum at the hip and the tibia at the knee 股骨 ◊ 见图 PELVIS (NOTE: plural is **femora**)

fenestra *noun* small opening in the ear 窗; **fenestra ovalis** *or* **fenestra vestibuli** *or* **oval window** = oval opening between the middle ear and the inner ear, closed by a membrane and covered by the stapes 前庭窗; **fenestra rotunda** *or* **fenestra cochleae** *or* **round window** = round opening between the middle ear and the cochlea, and closed by a membrane 蜗窗

◇ **fenestration** *noun* surgical operation to relieve deafness by making a small opening in the inner ear(耳科手术中的)开窗术

fennel *noun* herb which tastes of aniseed and is used to treat flatulence 茴香

fermentation *or* **zymosis** *noun* process where carbohydrates are broken down by enzymes from yeast and produce alcohol 发酵

fertile *adjective* able to bear fruit *or* to produce children 能生育的

◇ **fertility** *noun* being fertile 生育力; **fertility rate** = number of births per year, per thousand females aged between 15 and 44 生育率

◇ **fertilization** *noun* joining of an ovum and a sperm to form a zygote and so start the development of an embryo 受精

◇ **fertilize** *verb* (*of a sperm*) to join with an ovum 受精 (NOTE: the opposite is **sterile**, **sterility**, **sterilize**)

fester *verb* (*of an infected wound*) to become inflamed and produce pus 化脓: ***His legs were covered with festering sores.*** 他的腿有脓疮。

festination *noun* way of walking where the patient takes short steps, seen in patients suffering from Parkinson's disease 慌张步态,见于帕金森病患者

fetal 胎儿的 *see* 见 FETUS

◇ **fetalis** 胎儿的 *see* 见 ERYTHROBLASTOSIS

fetishism *or* **fetichism** *noun* psychological disorder where the patient gets sexual satisfaction from touching objects 恋物癖

◇ **fetishist** *or* **fetichist** *noun* person suffering from fetishism 恋物癖者

fetoprotein 胎蛋白 *see* 见 ALPHA

fetor *or* **foetor** *noun* bad smell 臭气

fetoscopy *noun* examination of a fetus inside the womb, taking blood samples to diagnose blood disorders 胎儿镜检查,取胎儿血检查宫内的胎儿有无血液疾病

fetus *or* **foetus** *noun* unborn baby in the womb 胎儿

◇ **fetal** *or* **foetal** *adjective* referring to a fetus 胎儿的: ***A sample of fetal blood was examined.*** 检查胎儿的血样。**fetal position** = position where a person lies curled up on his side, like a fetus in the womb 胎儿姿式，蜷曲侧卧位如同宫内的胎儿（NOTE：**fetus** is used to refer to unborn babies from two months after conception until birth. Before then, the baby is an **embryo**）

fever *or* **pyrexia** *noun* (i) rise in the body temperature 发热（ii）sickness when the temperature of the body is higher than normal 发热性疾病：***She is running a slight fever.*** 她有些发热。***You must stay in bed until the fever has gone down.*** 你必须卧床直至热退。**intermittent fever** = fever which rises and falls regularly, as in malaria 间歇热；**relapsing fever** = disease caused by a bacterium, where attacks of fever recur from time to time 回归热；**remittent fever** = fever which goes down for a period each day, as in typhoid fever 弛张热；**fever sore** *or* **fever blister** = cold sore *or* burning sore, usually on the lips 急性天疱疮

◇ **feverfew** *noun* herb, formerly used to reduce fevers, but now used to relieve migraine 小白菊，龙牙草

◇ **feverish** *adjective* with a fever 热的：***He felt feverish and took an aspirin.*** 他感觉发烧，吃了片阿司匹林。***She is in bed with a feverish chill.*** 她发烧寒战躺在床上。

> COMMENT：Normal oral body temperature is about 98.6°F or 37℃ and rectal temperature is about 99°F or 37.2℃. A fever often makes the patient feel cold, and is accompanied by pains in the joints. Most fevers are caused by infections; infections which result in fever include cat scratch fever, dengue, malaria, meningitis, psittacosis, Q fever, rheumatic fever, Rocky mountain spotted fever, scarlet fever, septicaemia, typhoid fever, typhus, and yellow fever.
> 注释：正常的口表温度是 98.6°F 或 37℃，直肠温度是 99°F 或 37.2℃。发热时患者感觉到冷，关节痛。发热常因感染引起，常见的有猫抓热、登革热、疟疾、脑脊髓膜炎、鹦鹉热、Q 热、风湿热、落基山斑疹热、腥红热、败血症、伤寒、斑疹伤寒和黄热病。

fibr- *prefix* referring to fibres *or* fibrous 纤维的

fibre *or* US **fiber** *noun* (**a**) structure in the body shaped like a thread 纤维；**collagen fibre** = fibre which is the main component of fasciae, tendons and ligaments and is essential in bones and cartilage 胶原纤维；**elastic fibres** *or* **yellow fibres** = fibres which can expand easily and are found in elastic cartilage, the skin and the walls of arteries and the lungs 弹性纤维；**nerve fibre** = thread-like structure (axon *or* dendron) leading from a nerve cell and carrying nerve impulses 神经纤维（**b**）**optical fibres** = artificial fibres which carry light *or* images 光导纤维（**c**）**dietary fibre** = fibrous matter in food, which cannot be digested 纤维素，不能被消化的食物纤维；**high fibre diet** = diet which contains a high percentage of cereals, nuts, fruit and vegetables 高纤维素膳食

> COMMENT：Dietary fibre is found in cereals, nuts, fruit and some green vegetables. There are two types of fibre in food：insoluble fibre (in bread and cereals) which is not digested and soluble fibre (in vegetables and pulses). Foods with the highest proportion of fibre are bread, beans and dried apricots. Fibre is thought to be necessary to help digestion and avoid developing constipation, obesity and appendicitis.
> 注释：纤维素在谷物、坚果、水果和绿色蔬菜中含量丰富。食物中的纤维有两种：不能被消化的不溶性纤维(面包和谷物)以及可溶性纤维(蔬菜和豆类)。食物中纤维含量最高的是面包、豆类和干杏。纤维可以帮助消化，避免便秘、肥胖和阑尾炎。

◇ **fibre optics** *or* **fibreoptics** *noun* examining internal organs using thin fibres which conduct light and images 纤维镜检查

◇ **fibrescope** *noun* device made of bundles of optical fibres which is passed into the body, used for examining internal organs 纤维镜

fibril *noun* very small fibre 原纤维,纤丝

◇ **fibrillating** *adjective* with fluttering of a muscle 纤颤的: ***They applied a defibrillator to correct a fibrillating heartbeat.*** 他们用除颤器治疗心脏纤颤。

◇ **fibrillation** *noun* fluttering of a muscle 肌纤颤; **atrial fibrillation** = rapid uncoordinated fluttering of the atria of the heart, causing an irregular heartbeat 心房颤动; **ventricular fibrillation** = serious heart condition where the ventricular muscles flutter and the heart no longer beats to pump blood 心室颤动

> QUOTE: Cardiovascular effects may include atrial arrhythmias but at 30℃ there is the possibility of spontaneous ventricular fibrillation.
> 引文:它的心血管作用是引起房性心律失常,但在30℃时可能发生自发性室颤。
> **British Journal of Nursing** 英国护理杂志

fibrin *noun* protein produced by fibrinogen, which helps make blood coagulate 纤维蛋白; **fibrin foam** = white material made artificially from fibrinogen, used to prevent bleeding 纤维蛋白泡沫

> COMMENT: Removal of fibrin from a blood sample is called defibrination.
> 注释:去除血中的纤维蛋白叫脱纤维。

◇ **fibrinogen** *noun* substance in blood plasma which produces fibrin when activated by thrombin 纤维蛋白原

◇ **fibrinolysin** *noun* plasmin, an enzyme which digests fibrin 纤维蛋白溶酶,纤溶酶

◇ **fibrinolysis** *noun* removal of blood clots from the system by the action of plasmin on fibrin 纤维蛋白溶解

fibro- *prefix* referring to fibres 纤维的

◇ **fibroadenoma** *noun* benign tumour formed of fibrous and glandular tissue 纤维腺瘤

◇ **fibroblast** *noun* long flat cell found in connective tissue, which develops into collagen 成纤维细胞

◇ **fibrocartilage** *noun* cartilage and fibrous tissue combined 纤维软骨

> COMMENT: Fibrocartilage is found in the discs of the spine. It is elastic like cartilage and pliable like fibre.
> 注释:纤维软骨位于椎盘上,它具软骨的弹性和纤维的柔韧性。

◇ **fibrochondritis** *noun* inflammation of the fibrocartilage 纤维软骨炎

◇ **fibrocyst** *noun* benign tumour of fibrous tissue 囊性纤维瘤

◇ **fibrocystic** *adjective* referring to a fibrocyst 纤维囊性的; **fibrocystic disease** *or* **cystic fibrosis** = hereditary disease in which there is malfunction of the exocrine glands such as the pancreas, and in particular those which secrete mucus 纤维囊性疾病,遗传性外分泌腺如胰腺,尤其是分泌粘液的腺体功能不全

◇ **fibrocyte** *noun* cell which derives from a fibroblast and is found in connective tissue 纤维细胞

◇ **fibroelastosis** *noun* deformed growth of the elastic fibres, especially in the ventricles of the heart 纤维弹性组织增生

◇ **fibroid** *adjective* & *noun* like fibre 纤维样的,类纤维; **fibroid degeneration** = changing of normal tissue into fibrous tissue (as in cirrhosis of the liver) 纤维样变性; **a fibroid** *or* **fibroid tumour** *or* **fibromyoma** *or* **uterine fibroma** = benign tumour in the muscle fibres of the uterus 纤维肌瘤(一种良性瘤)

◇ **fibroma** *noun* small benign tumour formed in connective tissue 纤维瘤

◇ **fibromuscular** *adjective* referring to fibrous tissue and muscular tissue 纤维肌性的

◇ **fibromyoma** *noun* benign tumour in the muscle fibres of the uterus 纤维肌瘤

◇ **fibroplasia** 纤维组织形成 *see* 见 RETROLENTAL

◇ **fibrosa** 纤维性 *see* 见 OSTEITIS

◇ **fibrosarcoma** *noun* malignant tumour of the connective tissue, common in the legs 纤维肉瘤

◇ **fibrosis** *noun* replacing damaged tissue by scar tissue 纤维化; **cystic fibro-**

sis = FIBROCYSTIC DISEASE 囊性纤维化

◇ **fibrositis** *noun* painful inflammation of the fibrous tissue which surrounds muscles and joints, especially the muscles of the back 纤维肌炎

◇ **fibrous** *adjective* made of fibres or like fibre 纤维性的；**fibrous capsule** = fibrous tissue surrounding a kidney 纤维囊；**fibrous joint** = joint where fibrous tissue holds two bones together so that they cannot move (as in the bones of the skull) 纤维关节；**fibrous pericardium** = outer part of the pericardium which surrounds the heart, and is attached to the main blood vessels 纤维性心包；**fibrous tissue** = tissue made of collagen fibres 纤维组织：***Muscles are attached to bones by bands of strong fibrous tissue called tendons.*** 肌肉通过由纤维组织形成的肌腱附着于骨上。

> COMMENT: Fibrous tissue is the strong white tissue which makes tendons and ligaments; also forms scar tissue.
> 注释：纤维组织是一种白色坚硬的组织，形成肌腱、韧带以及瘢痕。

fibula *noun* long thin bone running between the ankle and the knee, the other thicker bone in the lower leg is the tibia 腓骨 (NOTE: plural is **fibulae**)

◇ **fibular** *adjective* referring to the fibula 腓骨的

field *noun* (**a**) area of interest 领域：***He specializes in the field of community medicine.*** 他的专业是社区医学。***Don't see that specialist with your breathing problems — his field is obstetrics.*** 不要找那位医生看你的呼吸系统疾病，他是产科大夫。(**b**) **field of vision** = area which can be seen without moving the eye 视野

fil- *prefix* like a thread 丝状的

◇ **filament** *noun* long thin structure like a thread 丝

◇ **filamentous** *adjective* like a thread 丝状的

◇ **Filaria** *noun* thin parasitic worm which is found especially in the lymph system, and is passed to humans by mosquitoes 丝虫属 (NOTE: plural is **Filariae**)

> COMMENT: Infestation with Filariae in the lymph system causes elephantiasis.
> 注释：淋巴系统感染了丝虫会导致象皮病。

◇ **filariasis** *noun* tropical disease caused by parasitic threadworms in the lymph system, transmitted by mosquito bites 丝虫病

◇ **filiform** *adjective* shaped like a thread 丝状的；**filiform papillae** = papillae on the tongue which are shaped like threads, and have no taste buds 丝状乳头 ◊ 见图 TONGUE

◇ **filipuncture** *noun* putting a wire into an aneurysm to cause blood clotting 线刺法

fill *verb* (**a**) to make something full 填满：***She was filling the bottle with water.*** 她把瓶子灌满了水。(**b**) **to fill a tooth** = to put metal into a hole in a tooth after it has been drilled 牙充填

◇ **filling** *noun* (i) surgical operation carried out by a dentist to fill a hole in a tooth with amalgam 补牙 (ii) amalgam, metallic mixture put into a hole in a tooth by a dentist 填料：***I had to have two fillings when I went to the dentist's.*** 我去看了牙科大夫，填充了两颗牙。

film *noun* (**a**) roll of material which is put into a camera for taking photographs 胶卷：***I must buy a film before I go on holiday.*** 旅行前我必须买卷胶卷。***Do you want a colour film or a black and white one?*** 你是想要彩卷还是黑白卷？(**b**) very thin layer of a substance, especially on the surface of a liquid 薄膜；***a film of oil on the surface of water*** 水上的一层油膜

filter 1 *noun* piece of paper or cloth through which a liquid is passed to remove solid substances in it 滤纸 **2** *verb* to pass a liquid through a piece of paper or cloth to remove solid substances 过滤：***Impurities are filtered from the blood***

***by the kidneys*.** 血中的杂质通过肾过滤。

◇ **filtrate** *noun* substance which has passed through a filter 滤液

◇ **filtration** *noun* passing a liquid through a filter 过滤

filum *noun* structure which is shaped like a thread 丝状的; **filum terminale** = thin end section of the pia mater in the spinal cord 终丝

fimbria *noun* fringe, especially the fringe of hair-like processes at the end of a Fallopian tube near the ovaries 输卵管伞(NOTE: plural is **fimbriae**)

final *adjective* last 最后的: ***This is your final injection*.** 这是你最后的一针。 **final common pathway** = lower motor neurones, linked neurones which take all motor impulses from the spinal cord to a muscle 最后共同通道

fine *adjective* (**a**) healthy 健康的: ***He was ill last week, but he's feeling fine now*.** 他上周生病了,但现在感觉好多了。(**b**) (hair, thread, etc.) which is very thin 细的: ***There is a growth of fine hair on the back of her neck*.** 她的颈后有一些细小的汗毛。***Fine sutures are used for delicate operations*.** 精细的手术用细线。

finger *noun* one of the five parts at the end of the hand, but usually not including the thumb 手指: ***He touched the switch with his finger*.** 他用手指触开关。 **finger-nose test** = test of coordination, where the patients is asked to close his eyes, stretch out his arm and then touch his nose with his index finger 指鼻试验(NOTE: the names of the fingers are **little finger**, **third finger** *or* **ring finger**, **middle finger**, **forefinger** or **index finger and the thumb**)

> COMMENT: Each finger is formed of three finger bones (the phalanges), but the thumb has only two.
> 注释:每根手指由三块指骨组成,但拇指只有两块。

◇ **fingernail** *noun* hard thin growth covering the end of a finger 指甲: ***She painted her fingernails red*.** 她将指甲染成红色。

◇ **fingerprint** *noun* mark left by a finger when you touch something 指纹: ***The police found fingerprints near the broken window*.** 警察在破碎的窗户旁发现了指纹。

◇ **fingerstall** *noun* cover for an infected finger, attached to the hand with strings 指套

fireman's lift *noun* way of carrying an injured person by putting him over one's shoulder 消防员抬法

firm *noun* (*informal* 非正式) group of doctors and consultants in a hospital (especially one to which a trainee doctor is attached during clinical studies) 医务人员

first *adjective* coming before everything else 首先的; **first-ever stroke** = stroke which a patient has for the first time in his life 初发卒中; **first intention** = healing of a clean wound where the tissue forms again rapidly and no prominent scar is left 一期愈合

◇ **first aid** *noun* help given by an ordinary person to someone who is suddenly ill *or* hurt, given until full-scale medical treatment can be given 急救: ***She ran to the man who had been knocked down and gave him first aid until the ambulance arrived*.** 她跑到摔倒的人身旁进行急救直到救护车赶到。**first-aid kit** = box with bandages and dressings kept ready to be used in an emergency 急救箱; **first-aid post** *or* **station** = special place where injured people can be taken for immediate attention 急救站

◇ **first-aider** *noun* person who gives first aid to someone who is suddenly ill *or* injured 急救者

> QUOTE: Cerebral infarction (embolic or thrombolic) accounts for about 80% of first-ever strokes.
> 引文:脑血栓或脑栓塞占初发卒中的80%。
> **British Journal of Hospital Medicine** 英国医院医学杂志

fish *noun* cold-blooded animal which swims in water, eaten for food 鱼: ***They***

***live on a diet of fish and rice*.**他们以鱼和米饭为主食。(NOTE: no plural when referring to the food: **you should eat some fish every week**)

COMMENT: Fish are high in protein, phosphorus, iodine and vitamins A and D. White fish has very little fat. Certain constituents of fish oil are thought to help prevent the accumulation of cholesterol on artery walls.
注释:鱼富含蛋白、磷酸盐、碘、维生素 A 和 D。白鱼的脂肪含量很低。鱼油中的某些物质可阻止胆固醇在动脉壁的沉积。

fissile *adjective* which can split *or* can be split 可裂的

◇ **fission** *noun* splitting (as of the cells of bacteria) 分裂

fissure *noun* crack or groove in the skin *or* tissue *or* an organ 裂纹; **anal fissure** *or* **rectal fissure** *or* **fissure in ano** = crack in the mucous membrane wall of the anal canal 肛裂; **horizontal and oblique fissures** = grooves between the lobes of the lungs 水平裂和斜裂◊见图 LUNGS; **lateral fissure** = groove along the side of each cerebral hemisphere 侧裂; **longitudinal fissure** = groove separating the two cerebral hemispheres 大脑纵裂

fist *noun* hand which is tightly closed 拳头: ***The baby held the spoon in its fist*.** 婴儿把匙攥在拳头中。***He hit the nurse with his fist*.**他用拳头打护士。

fistula *noun* passage *or* opening which has been made abnormally between two organs, often near the rectum *or* anus 瘘管; **anal fistula** *or* **fistula in ano** = fistula which develops between the rectum and the outside of the body after an abscess near the anus 肛瘘; **biliary fistula** = opening which discharges bile on to the surface of the skin from the gall bladder, bile duct or liver 胆瘘; **branchial fistula** = cyst on the side of the neck of an embryo 支气管瘘; **vesicovaginal fistula** = abnormal opening between the bladder and the vagina 膀胱阴道瘘

fit 1 *adjective* strong and physically healthy 强壮的: ***The manager is not a fit man*.** 经理不是个强壮的男人。***You'll have to get fit before the football match*.** 你必须在足球赛前使自己进入状态。***She exercises every day to keep fit*.** 她每天都锻炼使自己保持健康。***The doctors decided the patient was not fit for surgery*.**医生认为患者的身体状况不适于手术。***He isn't fit enough to work*.** = He is still too ill to work.他的身体没有复原,不能工作。(NOTE : **fit - fitter - fittest**)**2** *noun* sudden attack of a disorder, especially convulsions and epilepsy 发作: ***She had a fit of coughing*.** 她突然咳嗽。***He had an epileptic fit*.** 他癫痫发作。***The baby had a series of fits*.**婴儿惊厥发作。**3** *verb* (**a**) to be the right size *or* shape 适合: ***He's grown so tall that his trousers don't fit him any more*.** 他长得太高了,裤子已经不合适了。***These shoes don't fit me - they're too tight*.**这双鞋不适合我,太紧了。(**b**) to attach an appliance correctly 安装: ***The surgeons fitted the artificial hand to the patient's arm*** *or* ***fitted the patient with an artificial hand*.**外科医师给患者安上假肢。(NOTE: you fit someone **with** an appliance)

◇ **fitness** *noun* being healthy 健康: ***He had to pass a fitness test to join the police force*.** 在做警察之前他必须通过体格检查。***Being in the football team demands a high level of physical fitness*.**加入橄榄球队需要有高水平的身体素质。

fix *verb* (**a**) (i) to fasten *or* to attach; 固定,安装(ii) to treat a specimen which is permanently attached to a slide 固化: ***The slide is fixed with an alcohol solution*.**玻片用酒精固定。**fixed oils** = liquid fats, especially those used as food 不挥发油 (**b**) to arrange 安排: ***The meeting has been fixed for next week*.**此会定在下周召开。

◇ **fixated** *adjective* (person) with a fixation on a parent 固恋父(母)的

◇ **fixation** *noun* (i) psychological disorder where a person does not develop beyond a certain stage 发育停滞(ii) way of preserving a specimen on a slide 固定; **mother-fixation** = condition where a person's development has been stopped at a stage where he remains like a child, dependent on his mother 恋母情结

◇ **fixative** *noun* chemical used in the preparation of samples on slides 固定液

flab *noun* (*informal* 非正式) soft fat flesh 赘肉: ***He's doing exercises to try to fight the flab.*** 他在进行锻炼去除赘肉。

◇ **flabby** *adjective* with soft flesh 松弛的: ***She has got flabby from sitting at her desk all day.*** 她整天坐在桌前,肌肉都松弛了。

flaccid *adjective* soft or flabby 不结实的,松软的

flagellate *noun* type of parasitic protozoan which uses whip-like hairs to swim (such as Leishmania) 鞭毛虫

◇ **flagellum** *noun* tiny growth on a microorganism, shaped like a whip 鞭毛 (NOTE: plural is **flagella**)

flail chest *noun* condition where the chest is not stable, because several ribs have been broken 连枷胸

flake 1 *noun* thin piece of tissue 絮片,碎片: ***Dandruff is formed of flakes of dead skin on the scalp.*** 头皮屑是死去皮肤的碎片。**flake fracture** = fracture where thin pieces of bone come off 碎片样骨折 2 *verb* **to flake off** = to fall off as flakes 碎片样剥脱

flap *noun* flat piece, especially a piece of skin *or* tissue still attached to the body at one side and used in grafts 瓣,皮瓣

flare *noun* red colouring of the skin at an infected spot *or* in urticaria 潮红

flat *adjective* & *adverb* level *or* not curved 平的,平地: ***Spread the paper out flat on the table.*** 把纸在桌上铺平。**flat foot** *or* **flat feet** *or* **pes planus** = condition where the soles of the feet lie flat on the ground instead of being arched as normal 扁平足

◇ **flatworm** *noun* any of several types of parasitic worm with a flat body (such as a tapeworm) 扁虫,扁平无环节的寄生虫(如绦虫)

flatulence *noun* gas *or* air which collects in the stomach *or* intestines causing discomfort 胀气

◇ **flatulent** *adjective* caused by flatulence 胀气的

◇ **flatus** *noun* air and gas which collects in the intestines and is painful 肠胃胀气

> COMMENT: Flatulence is generally caused by indigestion, but can be made worse if the patient swallows air (aerophagy).
> 注释:胃肠积气常由消化不良引起,患者吞气时加重。

flea *noun* tiny insect which sucks blood and is a parasite on animals and humans 蚤

> COMMENT: Fleas can transmit disease, most especially bubonic plague which is transmitted by infected rat fleas.
> 注释:蚤可以传播疾病,尤其是由鼠蚤传播的腺鼠疫。

flesh *noun* tissue containing blood, forming the part of the body which is not skin, bone or organs 肉; **flesh wound** = wound which only affects the fleshy part of the body 轻伤: ***She had a flesh wound in her leg.*** 她腿受了轻伤。

◇ **fleshy** *adjective* (i) made of flesh 血肉的(ii) fat 脂肪

flex *verb* to bend 弯,曲; **to flex a joint** = to use a muscle to make a joint bend 屈曲关节

◇ **flexible** *adjective* which bends easily 可弯曲的

◇ **flexibilitas cerea** *noun* condition where if a patient's arms or legs are moved, they remain in that set position for some time 蜡样屈曲

◇ **flexion** *noun* bending of a joint 曲; **plantar flexion** = bending of the toes downwards 跖曲

Flexner's bacillus *noun* bacterium

which causes bacillary dysentery 弗氏痢疾杆菌

flexor *noun* muscle which makes a joint bend 曲肌 *compare* 比较 EXTENSOR

◇ **flexure** *noun* bend in an organ; fold in the skin 曲; **hepatic flexure** = bend in the colon, where the ascending and transverse colons join 肝曲; **splenic flexure** = bend in the colon where the transverse colon joins the descending colon 脾曲

float *verb* to lie on top of a liquid *or* not to sink 漂浮: ***The unborn baby floats in amniotic fluid***. 胎儿浮在羊水中。**floating kidney** = NEPHROPTOSIS 肾下垂; **floating ribs** = the two lowest ribs on each side, which are not attached to the breastbone 浮肋

floccitation = CARPHOLOGY 摸空

flooding *or* **menorrhagia** *noun* very heavy bleeding during menstruation 血崩

floppy baby syndrome = AMYOTONIA CONGENITA 先天性肌弛缓

flora *noun* bacteria which exist in a certain part of the body 菌丛

floss 1 *noun* **dental floss** = soft thread which can be pulled between the teeth to help keep them clean 牙线 **2** *verb* to clean the teeth with floss 用牙线清牙

flow 1 *noun* (**a**) movement of liquid *or* gas 气流,水流: ***They used a tourniquet to try to stop the flow of blood***. 他们用止血带止血。(**b**) amount of liquid *or* gas which is moving 流量: ***The meter measures the flow of water through the pipe***. 水表测定水管中的水流。**2** *verb* (*of liquid*) to move past 流: ***The water flowed down the pipe***. 水从水管流出。***Blood was flowing from the wound***. 血从伤口流出来。

◇ **flowmeter** *noun* meter attached to a pipe (as in anaesthetic equipment) to measure the speed at which a liquid *or* gas moves in the pipe 流量计,水表

flu *or* **influenza** *noun* common illness like a bad cold, but with a fever 流感: ***He's in bed with flu***. 他患了流感,躺在床上。***She caught flu and had to stay at home***. 她得了流感不得不呆在家里。***There is a lot of flu about this winter***. 这个冬季有很多人患流感。**Asian flu** = type of flu which originated in Asia 亚洲型流感; **gastric flu** = general term for any mild stomach disorder 胃肠型流感; **twenty-four hour flu** = type of flu which lasts for a short period 轻型流感 (NOTE: sometimes written **'flu** to show it is a short form of **influenza**)

fluctuation *noun* feeling of movement of liquid inside part of the body *or* inside a cyst when pressed by the fingers 波动感

fluid *noun* liquid substance 液体; **amniotic fluid** = fluid in the amnion in which an unborn baby floats 羊水; **cerebrospinal fluid** (**CSF**) = fluid which surrounds the brain and the spinal cord 脑脊液; **pleural fluid** = fluid which forms between the layers of pleura in pleurisy 胸膜液

fluke *noun* parasitic flatworm which settles inside the liver (liver flukes), in the blood stream (Schistosoma), and other parts of the body 吸虫

fluorescence *noun* sending out of light from a substance which is receiving radiation 荧光

◇ **fluorescent** *adjective* (substance) which sends out light 发荧光的

fluoride *noun* chemical compound of fluorine and sodium *or* potassium *or* tin 氟化物

◇ **fluoridate** *verb* to add fluoride to a substance, usually to drinking water, in order to help prevent tooth decay 加氟,氟化

◇ **fluoridation** *noun* adding fluoride to a substance, usually to drinking water, in order to help prevent tooth decay 加氟,氟化作用

COMMENT: Fluoride will reduce decay in teeth and is often added to

drinking water or to toothpaste. Some people object to fluoridation and it is thought that too high a concentration (such as that achieved by highly fluoridated water and the use of a highly fluoridated toothpaste) may damage the teeth of children.
注释：氟化物可防止龋齿，经常被加入饮用水或牙膏中。一些人反对加氟，认为高浓度的氟（如高浓度氟化水或用高氟牙膏）会损害儿童的牙齿。

◇ **fluorine** *noun* chemical element found in bones and teeth 氟（NOTE：chemical symbol is **F**）

◇ **fluoroscope** *noun* apparatus which projects an X-ray image of a part of the body on to a screen, so that the part of the body can be examined as it moves 荧光屏，荧光镜

◇ **fluoroscopy** *noun* examination of the body using X-rays projected onto a screen X线透视检查

◇ **fluorosis** *noun* condition caused by excessive fluoride in drinking water 氟中毒

COMMENT：At a low level, fluorosis causes discoloration of the teeth, and as the level of fluoride rises, ligaments can become calcified.
注释：轻度氟中毒可使牙齿变色，随着氟化物浓度的增高可引起韧带钙化。

flush 1 *noun* red colour in the skin 潮红；**hot flush** = condition in menopausal women, where the patient becomes hot, and sweats, often accompanied by redness of the skin 热潮红，多见于更年期的妇女，表现为发热，出汗伴皮肤发红 2 *verb* (**a**) to wash a wound with liquid 冲洗伤口 (**b**) (*of person*) to turn red 变红

◇ **flushed** *adjective* with red skin (due to heat *or* emotion *or* overeating) 发红的：***His face was flushed and he was breathing heavily.*** 他面色发红，呼吸沉重。

flutter *or* **fluttering** *noun* rapid movement, especially of the atria of the heart, which is not controlled by impulses from the SA node 脉博、心脏快速跳动，扑动

flux *noun* excessive production of liquid from the body 溢出，流出

fly *noun* small insect with two wings, often living in houses 苍蝇：***Flies can walk on the ceiling; flies can carry infection onto food.*** 苍蝇可在天花板上行走，可污染食物。

focus 1 *noun* (**a**) point where light rays converge through a lens 焦点 (**b**) centre of an infection 病灶（NOTE：plural is **foci**）2 *verb* to change the lens of an eye so that you see clearly at different distances 聚焦：***He has difficulty in focusing on the object.*** 他聚焦有困难。

◇ **focal** *adjective* referring to a focus 焦点的；**focal distance** *or* **focal length** = distance between the lens of the eye and the point behind the lens where light is focused 焦距；**focal epilepsy** = form of epilepsy arising from a localized area of the brain 局灶性癫痫；**focal myopathy** = destruction of muscle tissue caused by the substance injected in an intramuscular injection 局灶性肌病，由肌肉注射引起

foetor = FETOR 臭气

foetus, **foetal** = FETUS, FETAL 胎儿

folacin = FOLIC ACID 叶酸

fold 1 *noun* part of the body which is bent so that it lies on top of another part 褶皱；**circular fold** = large transverse fold of mucous membrane in the small intestine 环状褶；**vestibular folds** = folds in the larynx above the vocal fold, which are not used for speech (sometimes called 'false vocal cords') 室襞，假声带；**vocal folds** = VOCAL CORDS 声带 2 *verb see* 见 CORD, to bend something so that part of it is on top of the rest 折叠：***He folded the letter and put it in an envelope.*** 他把信折好，放入信封。**to fold your arms** = to rest one arm on the other across your chest 把手放在对侧胸上

folic acid *noun* vitamin in the Vitamin B complex found in milk, liver, yeast and green vegetables like spinach, which is essential for creating new blood cells 叶酸

COMMENT: Lack of folic acid can cause anaemia, and it can be caused by alcoholism.
注释：缺乏叶酸可导致贫血，酒精中毒可引起叶酸缺乏。

folieà deux *noun* rare condition where a psychological disorder is communicated between two people who live together 感应性精神病

follicle *noun* tiny hole *or* sac in the body 小囊，滤泡；**atretic follicle** = scarred remains of an ovarian follicle 闭锁卵泡；**Graafian follicle** *or* **ovarian follicle** = cell which contains the ovum 囊状卵泡；**hair follicle** = tiny hole in the skin with a gland from which a hair grows 毛囊

COMMENT: An ovarian follicle goes through several stages in its development. The first stage is called a primordial follicle, which then develops into a primary follicle and becomes a mature follicle by the sixth day of the period. This follicle secretes oestrogen until the ovum has developed to the point when it can break out, leaving the corpus luteum behind.
注释：卵泡的发育经过几个阶段：首先是原始卵泡，然后为初级卵泡，在第 6 天时变为成熟卵泡，释放卵子，形成黄体。

◇ **follicle-stimulating hormone (FSH)** *noun* hormone produced by the pituitary gland which stimulates ova in the ovaries and sperm in the testes 促卵泡激素

◇ **follicular** *or* **folliculate** *adjective* referring to follicles 小囊的，小泡的；**follicular tumour** = tumour in a follicle 卵泡瘤

◇ **folliculin** *noun* oestrone, a type of oestrogen 雌酮：***She is undergoing folliculin treatment.*** 她在接受雌酮治疗。

◇ **folliculitis** *noun* inflammation of the hair follicles, especially where hair has been shaved 毛囊炎

follow (up) *verb* to check on a patient who has been examined before in order to assess the progress of the disease or the results of treatment 随访

◇ **follow-up** *noun* check on a patient who has been examined before 随访

QUOTE: Length of follow-ups varied from three to 108 months. Thirteen patients were followed for less than one year, but the remainder were seen regularly for periods from one to nine years.
引文：随访期持续 3 个月到 9 年不等。其中 13 例随访期短于 1 年，其余的病例都定期随访 1－9 年。
New Zealand Medical Journal
新西兰医学杂志

fomentation = POULTICE 热敷

fomites *plural noun* objects (such as bed clothes) touched by a patient with a communicable disease which can therefore pass on the disease to others 污染物

fontanelle *noun* soft cartilage between the bony sections of a baby's skull 囟门；**anterior fontanelle** = cartilage at the top of the head where the frontal bone joins the two parietals 前囟；**posterior fontanelle** = cartilage at the back of the head where the parietal bones join the occipital 后囟 *see also* 参见 BREGMA

COMMENT: The fontanelles gradually harden over a period of months and by the age of 18 months the bones of the baby's skull are usually solid.
注释：囟门在随后的几个月中逐渐变硬，18 个月时完全闭合。

food *noun* things which are eaten 食物：***This restaurant is famous for its food.*** 这个餐馆的饭菜很出名。***Do you like Chinese food?*** 你喜欢中餐吗？***This food tastes funny.*** 这个菜的味道很怪。**health food** = food with no additives *or* food consisting of natural cereals, dried fruit and nuts 健康食品；**food allergies** =

allergies which are caused by food (the commonest are oranges, eggs, tomatoes, strawberries) 食物过敏; **food canal** *or* **alimentary canal** = passage from the mouth to the rectum through which food passes and is digested 消化道; **food poisoning** = illness caused by eating food which is contaminated with bacteria 食物中毒: ***The hospital had to deal with six cases of food poisoning.*** 医院有6名食物中毒病例。***All the people at the party went down with food poisoning.*** 所有参加宴会的人都因食物中毒病倒了。(NOTE: **food** is usually used in the singular, but can sometimes be used in the plural)

foot *noun* end part of the leg on which a person stands 脚, 足: ***He has got big feet.*** 他有一双大脚。***You stepped on my foot.*** 你踩了我的脚。**athlete's foot** = infectious skin disorder between the toes, caused by a fungus 脚癣; **drop foot** *or* **foot drop** = being unable to keep the foot at right angles to the leg 足下垂; **flat foot** *or* **feet** 扁平足 *see* 见 FLAT; **Madura foot** 足分支菌病 *see* 见 MADUROMYCOSIS; **trench foot** *or* **immersion foot** = condition, caused by exposure to cold and damp, where the skin of the foot becomes red and blistered and in severe cases turns black when gangrene sets in. (The condition was common among soldiers serving in the trenches during the First World War) 战壕足或浸泡足 (NOTE: plural is **feet**)

> COMMENT: The foot is formed of 26 bones: 14 phalanges in the toes, five metatarsals in the main part of the foot and seven tarsals in the heel.
> 注释: 足有 26 块骨头组成: 趾有 14 块趾骨, 足背有 5 块跖骨, 足跟有 7 块跗骨。

foramen *noun* natural opening inside the body, such as the opening in a bone through which veins or nerves pass 孔, 窗; **foramen magnum** = the hole at the bottom of the skull where the brain is joined to the spinal cord 枕骨大孔; **intervertebral foramen** = space between two vertebrae 椎间孔; **vertebral foramen** = hole in the centre of a vertebra which links with others to form the vertebral canal through which the spinal cord passes 椎孔; **foramen ovale** = opening between the two parts of the heart in a fetus 卵圆孔 (NOTE: plural is **foramina**)

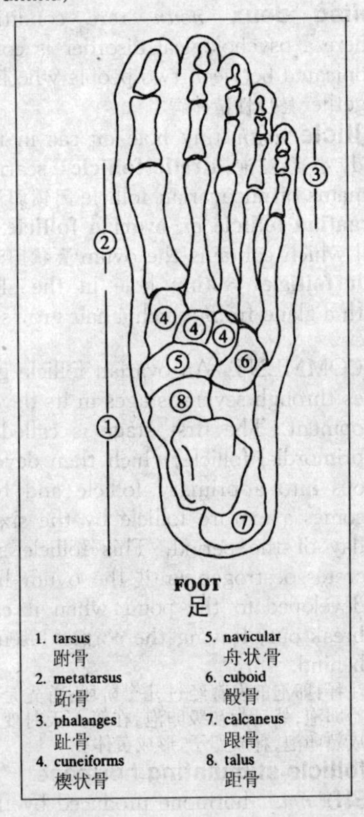

FOOT
足

1. tarsus 跗骨
2. metatarsus 跖骨
3. phalanges 趾骨
4. cuneiforms 楔状骨
5. navicular 舟状骨
6. cuboid 骰骨
7. calcaneus 跟骨
8. talus 距骨

> COMMENT: The foramen ovalex normally closes at birth, but if it stays open the blood from the veins can mix with the blood going to the arteries, causing cyanosis (blue baby disease).
> 注释: 卵圆孔一般在出生时关闭, 如果未闭, 动静脉血会混合, 引起紫绀。

forbid *verb* to tell someone not to do something 禁止: ***Smoking is forbidden in the cinema.*** 戏院禁止吸烟。***The health***

committee has forbidden any contact with the press. 健康委员会禁止与新闻界联系。***She has been forbidden all starchy food.*** 她被禁止食用含淀粉食物。***The doctor forbade him to go back to work.*** 医生禁止他恢复工作。(NOTE: **forbids - forbidding - forbade - has forbidden**)

force 1 *noun* strength 力量: ***The tree was blown down by the force of the wind.*** 树被大风吹倒了。***He has no force in his right hand.*** 他的右手没有一点力气。**2** *verb* to make someone do something 强迫,迫使: ***They forced him to lie down on the floor.*** 他们强迫他躺在地板上。***She was forced to do whatever they wanted.*** 她被迫作他们吩咐的任何事。

forceps *noun* surgical instrument like a pair of scissors, made in different sizes and with differently shaped ends, used for holding and pulling 钳; **obstetrical forceps** = type of large forceps used to hold a baby's head during childbirth 产钳

fore- *prefix* in front 前

◇ **forearm** *noun* lower part of the arm from the elbow to the wrist 前臂; **forearm bones** = the ulna and the radius 前臂骨

◇ **forebrain** *noun* cerebrum, the front part of the brain in an embryo 前脑

◇ **forefinger** *noun* first finger on the hand, next to the thumb 食指

◇ **foregut** *noun* front part of the gut in an embryo 前肠

◇ **forehead** *noun* part of the face above the eyes 前额

foreign *adjective* not belonging to your own country 外国的: ***He speaks several foreign languages.*** 他说好几种外语。**foreign body** = piece of material which is not part of the surrounding tissue and should not be there (such as sand in a cut *or* dust in the eye *or* pin which has been swallowed) 异物: ***The X-ray showed the presence of a foreign body.*** X线显示有异物存在。**swallowed foreign bodies** = anything (a pin *or* coin *or* button) which should not have been swallowed 被吞食的异物

◇ **foreigner** *noun* person who comes from another country 外国人

forensic medicine *noun* medical science concerned with finding solutions to crimes against people (such as autopsies on murdered people *or* taking blood samples from clothes) 法医学

foreskin *or* **prepuce** *noun* skin covering the top of the penis, which can be removed by circumcision 包皮

forewaters *noun* fluid which comes out of the vagina at the beginning of childbirth when the amnion bursts 前羊水

forget *verb* not to remember to do something *or* not to remember a piece of information 忘记,遗忘: ***Old people start to forget names.*** 老人开始忘记名字。***She forgot to take the tablets.*** 她忘了吃药。***He forgot his appointment with the specialist.*** 他忘了跟大夫的约会。(NOTE: **forgetting - forgot - has forgotten**)

◇ **forgetful** *adjective* (person) who often forgets things 健忘的: ***She became very forgetful, and had to be looked after by her sister.*** 她变得很健忘,不得不由她妹妹照顾。

◇ **forgetfulness** *noun* condition where someone often forgets things 遗忘: ***Increasing forgetfulness is a sign of old age.*** 经常健忘是衰老的迹象。

form 1 *noun* (**a**) shape 形状: ***She has a ring in the form of the letter A.*** 她戴着一个A字形的戒指。(**b**) paper with blank spaces which you have to write in 表格: ***You have to fill in a form when you are admitted to hospital.*** 你住院时必须填表。(**c**) state *or* condition 状态: ***Our team was in good form and won easily.*** 我们的队伍状态良好,轻易就获胜了。***He's in good form today.*** = He is very amusing *or* is doing things well. 他今天的状态很好。**off form** = not very well *or* slightly ill 小恙 **2** *verb* to make *or* to be the main part of 形成: ***Calcium is one***

the elements which forms bones *or* ***bones are mainly formed of calcium.*** 钙是组成骨的重要成分。***an ulcer formed in his duodenum*** 他的十二指肠有一溃疡；***In diphtheria a membrane forms across the larynx.*** 患白喉时，喉部有一层薄膜形成。

◇ **formation** *noun* action of forming something 形成：***Drinking milk helps the formation of bones.*** 喝牛奶有助于骨的形成。

formaldehyde *noun* strong antiseptic derived from formic acid 甲醛

◇ **formalin** *noun* solution of formaldehyde in water used to preserve specimens 福尔马林

formication *noun* itching feeling where the skin feels as if it were covered with insects 蚁走感

formula *noun* (**a**) way of indicating a chemical compound using letters and numbers (such as H_2SO_4) 分子式(**b**) instructions on how to prepare a drug 处方 (**c**) *US* powdered milk for babies 婴儿奶粉 (NOTE: plural is **formulae**)

◇ **formulary** *noun* book containing formulae for making drugs 处方集

fornix *noun* arch 穹窿；**fornix cerebri** = section of white matter in the brain between the hippocampus and the hypothalamus 大脑穹窿 ◊ 见图 BRAIN；**fornix of the vagina** = space between the cervix of the uterus and the vagina 阴道穹窿 (NOTE: plural is **fornices**)

fortification figures *noun* patterns of coloured light, seen as part of the aura before a migraine attack occurs(偏头痛时)闪烁幻想

fossa *noun* shallow hollow in a bone *or* the skin 窝，凹；**cubital fossa** = depression in the front of the elbow joint 肘窝；**glenoid fossa** = socket in the shoulder joint into which the humerus fits 下颌窝；**iliac fossa** = depression on the inner side of the hip bone 髂窝；**pituitary fossa** = hollow in the upper surface of the sphenoid bone in which the pituitary gland sits 垂体窝；**temporal fossa** = depression in the side of the head, in the temporal bone above the zygomatic arch 颞窝 (NOTE: plural is **fossae**)

Fothergill's operation *noun* surgical operation to correct prolapse of the womb 法沙吉尔氏手术，治疗子宫脱垂

fourchette *noun* fold of skin at the back of the vulva 阴唇系带

fovea (centralis) *noun* depression in the retina which is the point where the eye sees most clearly 中央凹 ◊ 见图 EYE

FPC = FAMILY PRACTITIONER COMMITTEE 家庭医生委员会

fracture 1 *verb* to break a bone 骨折：***He fractured his wrist.*** 他腕骨骨折。(*of bone*) to break 断：***The tibia fractured in two places.*** 胫骨有两处骨折。**2** *noun* break in a bone 骨折：***facial fracture*** *or* ***nasal fracture*** *or* ***skull fracture*** 面骨或鼻骨或颅骨骨折；**rib fracture** *or* **fracture of a rib** 肋骨骨折；**breastbone fracture** *or* **fracture of the breastbone** 胸骨骨折；**simple** *or* **closed fracture** = fracture where the skin surface around the damaged bone has not been broken and the broken ends of the bone are close together 单纯性骨折；**Bennett's fracture** 贝奈特氏骨折(第一掌骨纵折) *see* 见 BENNETT'S；**Colles' fracture** = fracture of the lower end of the radius with displacement of the wrist backwards, usually when someone has stretched out his hand to try to break a fall 科勒斯氏骨折(桡骨远端骨折)；**comminuted fracture** = fracture where the bone is broken in several places 粉碎性骨折；**complicated fracture** = fracture with an associated injury of tissue, as where the bone has punctured an artery 复杂性骨折；**compound fracture** *or* **open fracture** = fracture where the skin surface is damaged *or* where the broken bone penetrates the surface of the skin 开放性骨折；**extracapsular fracture** = fracture of the upper part of the femur, but which does not involve the capsule round the hip joint 关节囊外骨折; **greenstick fracture** = fracture occurring in children, where a long bone bends but does not break completely 青枝骨折; **impacted fracture** = fracture where the broken parts of the bones are pushed into each other 嵌入性骨折; **march fracture** = fracture of one of the metatarsal bones in the foot, caused by too much exercise 行军性骨折; **multiple fracture** = condition where a bone is broken in several places 多发性骨折; **oblique fracture** = fracture where the bone is broken diagonally 斜骨折; **pathological fracture** = fracture of a diseased bone 病理性骨折; **Pott's fracture** = fracture of the end of the fibula together with the end of the malleolus 波特氏骨折,腓骨下端骨折; **stellate fracture** = fracture of the kneecap shaped like a star 星状骨折; **stress fracture** = fracture of a bone caused by excessive force, as in certain types of sport 应力性骨折; **transverse fracture** = fracture where the bone is broken straight across 横骨折 *see also* 参见 AVULSION, DEPRESSED, FLAKE

◇ **fractured** *adjective* broken (bone) 骨折的: ***He had a fractured skull.*** 他颅骨骨折。***She went to hospital to have her fractured leg reset.*** 她去医院将断腿重接。

fragile *adjective* easily broken 脆弱的: ***Old people's bones are more fragile than those of adolescents.*** 老年人的骨质比青少年脆弱。**fragile-X syndrome** = hereditary condition where part of an X chromosome is defective, causing mental defects 脆性 X 染色体综合征

◇ **fragilitas** *noun* being fragile *or* brittle 脆性; **fragilitas ossium** *or* **osteogenesis imperfecta** = hereditary condition where the bones are brittle and break easily 脆骨症

frail *adjective* weak *or* easily broken 脆弱的: ***Grandfather is getting frail, and we have to look after him all the time.*** 祖父越来越衰弱了,我们必须整天照顾他。***The baby's bones are still very frail.*** 婴儿的骨质还十分脆弱。

framboesia = YAWS 雅司病

frame *noun* (**a**) main part of a building *or* ship *or* bicycle, etc., which holds it together 构架: ***The bicycle has a very light frame.*** 自行车的骨架很轻。***I've broken the frame of my glasses.*** 我把镜架摔断了。(**b**) solid support 支架; **walking frame** *or* **Zimmer frame** = metal frame used by patients who have difficulty in walking 助行拐

◇ **framework** *noun* main bones which make up the structure of part of the body 骨架

fraternal twins *or* **dizygotic twins** *noun* twins who are not identical (and not always of the same sex) because they come from two different ova fertilized at the same time 异卵双胞胎 *compare* 比较 IDENTICAL, MONOZYGOTIC

freckles *plural noun* brown spots on the skin, often found in people with fair hair 雀斑

◇ **freckled** *adjective* with brown spots on the skin 雀斑的

freeze *verb* (**a**) to be so cold that water turns to ice 结冰: ***It is freezing outside.*** 外面结冰了。***They say it will freeze tomorrow.*** 他们说明天有冰冻。***I'm freezing.*** = I'm very cold. 我冻僵了。(**b**) to make something very cold *or* to become very cold 使冻,使结冰: ***The surgeon froze the tissue with dry ice.*** 外科医师用干冰冰冻组织。

◇ **freeze drying** *noun* method of preserving food *or* tissue specimens by freezing rapidly and drying in a vacuum 冻干法(NOTE: **freezes - freezing - froze - has frozen**)

Frei test *noun* test for the venereal disease lymphogranuloma inguinale 弗莱氏试验,检查腹股沟淋巴肉芽肿

Freiberg's disease *noun* osteochondritis of the head of the second metatarsus Freiberg 弗莱伯氏病，第二跖骨头骨软骨炎

fremitus *noun* trembling *or* vibrating (of part of a patient's body, felt by the doctor's hand or heard through a stethoscope) 震颤；**friction fremitus** = scratching felt when the hand is placed on the chest of a patient suffering from pericarditis 摩擦性震颤；**vocal fremitus** = vibration of the chest when a person speaks *or* coughs 语颤

French letter *noun* (*informal* 非正式) = CONDOM 阴茎套

Frenkel's exercises *plural noun* exercises for patients suffering from locomotor ataxia, to teach coordination of the muscles and limbs 弗兰克耳氏运动，治疗共济失调

frenulum *or* **frenum** *noun* fold of mucous membrane (under the tongue *or* by the clitoris) 系带

fresh *adjective* (**a**) not used *or* not dirty 新的：***I'll get some fresh towels.*** 我要些新的毛巾。***She put some fresh sheets on the bed.*** 她在床上铺了些新床单。**fresh air** = open air 新鲜空气：***They came out of the mine into the fresh air.*** 他们从矿井出来呼吸新鲜空气。(**b**) recently made 新鲜的；**fresh bread** 鲜面包；**fresh frozen plasma** = plasma made from freshly donated blood, and kept frozen 新鲜冰冻血浆 (**c**) not tinned *or* frozen 未冻的：**fresh fish** 鲜鱼；**fresh fruit salad** 新鲜水果沙拉；**Fresh vegetables are expensive in winter.** 冬季新鲜的蔬菜很贵。

fretful *adjective* (baby) which cries *or* cannot sleep *or* seems unhappy 烦躁的，烦人的

friars' balsam *noun* mixture of various plant oils, including benzoin and balsam, which can be inhaled as a vapour to relieve bronchitis *or* congestion 复方安息香酊

friction *noun* rubbing together of two surfaces 摩擦；**friction fremitus** = scratching felt when the hand is placed on the chest of a patient suffering from pericarditis 摩擦性震颤；**friction murmur** = scratching sound around the heart, heard with a stethoscope in patients suffering from pericarditis 摩擦音

Friedlder's bacillus *noun* bacterium *Klebsiella pneumoniae* which can cause pneumonia 弗里德兰德氏杆菌，可引起肺炎

Friedman's test *noun* test for pregnancy 弗里德曼氏试验，妊娠试验

Friedreich's ataxia *noun* inherited nervous disease which affects the spinal cord (ataxia is associated with club foot, and makes the patient walk unsteadily and speak with difficulty) 弗里德赖希氏共济失调，遗传性共济失调

frighten *verb* to make someone afraid 使害怕：***The noise frightened me.*** 那声响吓着了我。***She watched a frightening film about insects which eat people.*** 她看了部有关昆虫吃人的恐怖片。

◇ **frightened** *adjective* afraid 害怕的：***I'm frightened of spiders.*** 我怕蜘蛛。***Don't leave the patient alone — she's frightened of the dark.*** 别把患者独自留下，她怕黑。

frigid *adjective* (woman) who cannot experience orgasm *or* sexual pleasure 性冷淡的

◇ **frigidity** *noun* being unable to experience orgasm *or* sexual pleasure *or* who does not feel sexual desire 性感缺乏

fringe medicine *noun* types of medicine which are not part of normal treatment taught in medical schools (such as homeopathy, acupuncture, etc.) 边缘医学

frog *noun* small animal with no tail, which lives in water or on land and can jump 蛙；**frog plaster** = plaster cast made to keep the legs in a correct position after an operation to correct a dislocated hip 蛙形石膏架

Fröhlich's syndrome *or* **dystrophia adiposogenitalis** *noun* condition where the patient becomes obese and the genital system does not develop, caused by an adenoma of the pituitary gland 弗勒利氏综合征,肥胖性生殖器退化综合征

front *noun* part of something which faces forwards 前部: ***The front of the hospital faces south.*** 医院面朝南。***He spilt soup down the front of his shirt.*** 他把汤洒在了衬衣上。***The Adam's apple is visible in the front of the neck.*** 从颈前面可以看见喉结。

◊ **frontal** *adjective* referring to the forehead *or* to the front of the head 额的; **frontal bone** = bone forming the front of the upper part of the skull behind the forehead 额骨 ◊ 见图 SKULL; **frontal lobe** = front lobe of each cerebral hemisphere 额叶; **frontal lobotomy** = surgical operation on the brain to treat mental illness by removing part of the frontal lobe 额叶切除术; **frontal sinus** = one of two sinuses in the front of the face above the eyes and near the nose 额窦 (NOTE: the opposite is **occipital**)

frost *noun* freezing weather when the temperature is below the freezing point of water. (It may lead to a deposit of crystals of ice on surfaces) 霜: ***There was a frost last night.*** 昨晚有霜。

◊ **frostbite** *noun* injury caused by very severe cold which freezes tissue 冻疮

◊ **frostbitten** *adjective* suffering from frostbite 有冻疮的

> COMMENT: In very cold conditions, the outside tissue of the fingers, toes, ears and nose can freeze, becoming white and numb. Thawing of frostbitten tissue can be very painful and must be done very slowly. Severe cases of frostbite may require amputation because the tissue has died and gangrene has set in.
> 注释:在很冷的情况下,指、趾、耳、鼻的外部组织会冻伤、发白、进而麻木。冻伤的组织在复温时会很痛,复温必须缓慢。严重冻伤可引起组织坏死,坏疽形成,此时需截肢。

frozen shoulder *noun* stiffness and pain in the shoulder, caused by inflammation of the membranes of the shoulder joint after injury *or* after the shoulder has been immobile for a time, when deposits may be forming in the tendons 冻肩

fructose *noun* fruit sugar found in honey and some fruit, which together with glucose forms sucrose 果糖

◊ **fructosuria** *noun* presence of fructose in the urine 果糖尿

fruit *noun* usually sweet part of a plant which contains the seeds, and is eaten as food 水果; **a diet of fresh fruit and vegetables** 含新鲜水果和蔬菜的饮食 (NOTE: no plural when referring to the food: **you should eat a lot of fruit**)

> COMMENT: Fruit contains fructose and is a good source of vitamin C and some dietary fibre. Dried fruit have a higher sugar content but less vitamin C than fresh fruit.
> 注释:水果含有果糖和维生素 C 以及纤维素。干果比新鲜水果糖含量高,维生素 C 少。

FSH = FOLLICLE-STIMULATING HORMONE 促卵泡激素

fugax 一时的 *see* 见 AMAUROSIS

-fuge *suffix* which drives away 离开,去; **vermifuge** = substance which removes worms 驱虫剂

fugue *noun* condition where the patient loses his memory and leaves home 神游症

fulguration *or* **electrodesiccation** *noun* removal of a growth (such as a wart) by burning with an electric needle 电灼疗法

full *adjective* complete *or* with no empty space 满的: ***The hospital cannot take in any more patients — all the wards are full.*** 医院不能接纳更多的病人,所有的房都满了。***My appointments book is full for the next two weeks.*** 我下两周的约会都定满了。

◊ **full-scale** *adjective* complete *or* going into all details 全面的: ***The doctors***

put him through a full-scale medical examination. 医生给他做了全面体格检查。***The local health authority has ordered a full-scale inquiry into the case.*** 当地的卫生部门要求对此事件做详细的调查。

◇ **full term** *noun* complete pregnancy of forty weeks 足月的: ***She has had several pregnancies but none has reached full term.*** 她怀了几次孕,但没有一次足月。

◇ **fully** *adverb* completely 完全地: ***The fetus was not fully developed.*** 胎儿还没有发育完全。***Is the muscle fully relaxed?*** 肌肉完全放松了吗?

fulminant *or* **fulminating** *adjective* (dangerous disease) which develops very rapidly 暴发性的

> QUOTE: The major manifestations of pneumococcal infection in sickle-cell disease are septicaemia, meningitis and pneumonia. The illness is frequently fulminant.
> 引文:镰状细胞贫血患者感染肺炎球菌的主要症状为败血症、脑膜炎、肺炎。此病常呈暴发性。
> **The Lancet** 柳叶刀杂志

fumes *plural noun* gas *or* smoke 烟雾; **toxic fumes** = poisonous gases or smoke given off by a substance or a machine 有毒烟雾

fumigate *verb* to kill germs *or* insects by using gas 用熏烟消毒

◇ **fumigation** *noun* killing germs *or* insects by gas 熏烟消毒法

function 1 *noun* particular work done by an organ 功能: ***What is the function of the pancreas?*** 胰腺的功能是什么? ***The function of an ovary is to form ova.*** 卵巢的功能是产生卵子。**2** *verb* to work in a particular way 运行: ***The heart and lungs were functioning normally.*** 心肺功能良好。***His kidneys suddenly stopped functioning.*** 他的肾突然停止工作。

◇ **functional** *adjective* (disorder *or* illness) which does not have a physical cause and may have a psychological cause, as opposed to an organic disorder 功能性的; **functional enuresis** = bedwetting which has a psychological cause 功能性遗尿症

> QUOTE: Insulin's primary metabolic function is to transport glucose into muscle and fat cells, so that it can be used for energy.
> 引文:胰岛素的基本代谢功能是将葡萄糖转入肌肉和脂肪细胞,产生能量。
> **Nursing '87** 护理 '87

> QUOTE: The AIDS virus attacks a person's immune system and damages the ability to fight other disease. Without a functioning immune system to ward off other germs, the patient becomes vulnerable to becoming infected.
> 引文:艾滋病病毒攻击人的免疫系统,损害机体对其他疾病的抵抗力。免疫系统功能的丧失导致对外来病菌的易感性。
> **Journal of American Medical Association** 美国医学会杂志

fund 1 *noun* sum of money set aside for a special purpose 基金; **fund-holding GP** = doctor who manages himself the budget of money provided for his practice by the National Health Service, deciding how much money to allocate to such items as the purchase of hospital services, equipment and drugs, staff wages, maintenance of premises, etc. 自主支配基金的全科医师 **2** *verb* to pay for 支付: ***How will the new health centre be funded?*** = Who will provide the money to pay for it? 新的保健中心由谁支付?

◇ **fundholder** = FUNDHOLDING GP 自主支配基金的全科医师

fundus *noun* (i) bottom of a hollow organ (such as the uterus) 基底 (ii) top section of the stomach (above the body of the stomach) 胃底 ◊ 见图 STOMACH; **optic fundus** = back part of the inside of the eye, opposite the lens 眼底

fungus *noun* simple plant organism with thread-like cells (such as yeast, mushrooms, mould), and without green chlorophyll 真菌; **fungus disease** = disease caused by a fungus 真菌病; **fungus**

poisoning = poisoning by eating a poisonous fungus 真菌中毒 (NOTE: plural is **fungi**. For other terms referring to fungi, see words beginning with **myc-**)

◇ **fungal** *adjective* referring to fungi 真菌的: ***He had a case of fungal skin infection.*** 他患有皮肤真菌感染。

◇ **fungicide** *adjective* & *noun* (substance) used to kill fungi 杀真菌的,杀真菌剂

◇ **fungiform papillae** *noun* rounded papillae on the tip and sides of the tongue, which have taste buds 蕈状乳头 ◊见图 TONGUE

◇ **fungoid** *adjective* like a fungus 蕈样的

> COMMENT: Some fungi can become parasites of man, and cause diseases such as thrush. Other fungi, such as yeast, react with sugar to form alcohol. Some antibiotics (such as penicillin) are derived from fungi.
> 注释:一些真菌寄生于人体导致疾病如鹅口疮。其他真菌如酵母菌,与糖作用形成酒精。一些抗生素(如青霉素)由真菌产生。

funiculitis *noun* inflammation of the spermatic cord 精索炎

◇ **funiculus** *noun* one of the three parts (lateral *or* anterior *or* posterior funiculus) of the white matter in the spinal cord 脊髓前后侧三索中的一索

funis *noun* umbilical cord 脐带

funnel chest *or* **pectus excavatum** *noun* congenital deformity, where the chest is depressed in the centre because the lower part of the breastbone is curved backwards 漏斗胸

funny *adjective* (*informal* 非正式) unwell 不舒服: ***She felt funny after she had eaten the fish.*** 吃了鱼后她觉得不舒服。***He had a funny turn.*** = He had a dizzy spell. 他晕头转向。**funny bone** = part of the elbow where the ulnar nerve passes by the internal condyle of the humerus, which gives a painful tingling sensation when hit by accident 肱骨内髁

fur *verb* (*of the tongue*) to feel as if covered with soft hair 长舌苔

> COMMENT: The tongue is furred when a patient is feeling unwell, and the papillae on the tongue become covered with a whitish coating.
> 注释:当患者不适时,会感觉舌苔厚,舌乳头上覆有一层白膜。

furfuraceous *adjective* scaly (skin) 皮屑状的

Furley stretcher 弗耳利氏担架 *see* 见 STRETCHER FURly

furor *noun* attack of wild violence (especially when mentally deranged) 狂热

furuncle *noun* boil, a tender raised mass of infected tissue and skin, usually caused by infection of a hair follicle by the bacterium *Staphylococcus aureus* 疖

◇ **furunculosis** *noun* condition where several boils appear at the same time 疖病

fuse *verb* to join together to form a single structure 融合: ***The bones of the joint fused.*** 关节骨融合在一起。

fusiform *adjective* (muscles, etc.) shaped like a spindle, with a wider middle section which becomes narrower at each end 梭形的

fusion *noun* joining, especially a surgical operation to join the bones at a joint permanently so that they cannot move and so relieve pain in the joint 融合; **spinal fusion** = surgical operation to join two vertebrae together to make the spine more rigid 脊椎融合术

Gg

g = GRAM 克

GABA = GAMMA AMINOBUTYRIC ACID γ氨基丁酸

gag 1 *noun* instrument placed between a patient's teeth to stop him closing his mouth 开口器 **2** *verb* to choke, to try to vomit but be unable to do so 阻塞,干呕: ***He gagged on his food.*** 他被食物噎住了。***Every time the doctor tries to examine her throat, she gags.*** 每次医生要检查她的咽部她都想吐。***He started gagging on the endotracheal tube.*** 他因气管内插管的刺激开始干呕。

gain 1 *noun* act of adding *or* increasing 增加: ***The baby showed a gain in weight of 25g*** *or* ***showed a weight gain of 25g.*** 婴儿的体重增加了25克。**2** *verb* to add *or* to increase 增加; ***to gain in weight*** *or* ***to gain weight*** 增加体重

gait *noun* way of walking 步态; **ataxic gait** = way of walking where the patient walks unsteadily due to a disorder of the nervous system 共济失调步态; **cerebellar gait** = way of walking where the patient staggers along, caused by a disease of the cerebellum 小脑病步态; **spastic gait** = way of walking where the legs are stiff and the feet not lifted off the ground 痉挛步态 *see also* 参见 FESTINATION

galact- *prefix* referring to milk 乳,乳液

◊ **galactagogue** *noun* substance which stimulates the production of milk 催乳药

◊ **galactocele** *noun* breast tumour which contains milk 乳腺囊肿

◊ **galactorrhoea** *noun* excessive production of milk 乳溢

◊ **galactosaemia** *noun* congenital defect where the liver is incapable of converting galactose into glucose, with the result that a baby's development may be affected 半乳糖血症(遗传性疾病,肝脏不能将半乳糖转化为葡萄糖,可影响婴儿的发育)

> COMMENT: The treatment is to remove galactose from the diet.
> 注释:治疗方法是去除饮食中的半乳糖。

◊ **galactose** *noun* sugar which forms part of milk, and is converted into glucose by the liver 半乳糖

galea *noun* (i) any part of the body shaped like a helmet, especially the loose band of tissue in the scalp 帽 (ii) type of bandage wrapped round the head 帽状绷带

gall *or* **bile** *noun* thick bitter yellowish-brown fluid secreted by the liver and stored in the gall bladder or passed into the stomach, used to digest fatty substances and to neutralize acids 胆汁

◊ **gall bladder** *noun* sac situated underneath the liver, in which bile produced by the liver is stored 胆囊 ◊ 见图 DIGESTIVE SYSTEM

> COMMENT: Bile is stored in the gall bladder until required by the stomach. If fatty food is present in the stomach, bile moves from the gall bladder along the bile duct to the stomach. Since the liver also secretes bile directly into the duodenum, the gallbladder is not an essential organ and can be removed by surgery.
> 注释:胆汁在排入胃前存于胆囊,如胃内含有脂肪食物,胆汁会经胆管排入,因为肝脏也能直接分泌胆汁入十二指肠,所以胆囊不是主要器官,可以手术切除。

Gallie's operation *noun* surgical operation where tissues from the patient's thigh are used to hold a hernia in place 加利氏手术

gallipot *noun* little pot for ointment 药罐

gallon *noun* measurement of liquids which equals eight pints or 4.5 litres 加仑(1加仑等于8品脱或4.5升): ***The bucket can hold four gallons.*** 这桶的容积为4加仑。***The body contains about two gallons of blood.*** 机体有大约2加仑的血液。

gallop rhythm *noun* rhythm of heart sounds, three to each cycle, when a patient is experiencing tachycardia 奔马律

gallstone *or* **calculus** *noun* small stone formed from insoluble deposits from bile in the gall bladder 胆石

> COMMENT: Gallstones can be harmless, but some cause pain and inflammation and a serious condition can develop if a gallstone blocks the bile duct. Sudden pain going from the right side of the stomach towards the back indicates that a gallstone is passing through the bile duct.
> 注释:胆石可以是无害的,但有些会引起疼痛和炎症,如果阻塞胆管还可产生一系列严重的并发症。胃右侧突发疼痛向后背放射提示胆石通过胆管。

galvanism *noun* treatment using low voltage electricity 流电疗法

◇ **galvanocautery** *or* **electrocautery** *noun* removal of diseased tissue using an electrically heated needle *or* loop of wire 电烙器

gamete *noun* sex cell, either a spermatozoon or an ovum 配子

◇ **gametocide** *noun* drug which kills gametocytes 杀配子剂

◇ **gametocyte** *noun* cell which is developing into a gamete 配子体

◇ **gametogenesis** *noun* process by which a gamete is formed 配子形成

Gamgee tissue *noun* surgical dressing, formed of a layer of cotton wool between two pieces of gauze 加姆季敷料

gamma *noun* third letter of the Greek alphabet 希腊字母表的第三个字母

◇ **gamma aminobutyric acid** (**GABA**) *noun* amino acid found in the brain and many nerve terminals γ氨基丁酸

◇ **gamma camera** *noun* camera for taking photographs of parts of the body into which radioactive isotopes have been introduced γ相机

◇ **gamma globulin** *noun* protein found in plasma, forming antibodies as protection against infection 丙种球蛋白

> COMMENT: Gamma globulin injections are sometimes useful as a rapid source of protection against a wide range of diseases.
> 注释:丙种球蛋白针剂有时被用来作为快速预防多种疾病的一种手段。

◇ **gamma rays** *noun* rays which are shorter than X-rays and are given off by radioactive substances γ射线

ganglion *noun* (**a**) mass of nerve cell bodies and synapses usually covered in connective tissue, found along the peripheral nerves with the exception of the basal ganglia 神经节; **basal ganglia** = masses of grey matter at the base of each cerebral hemisphere which receive impulses from the thalamus and influence the motor impulses from the frontal cortex 基底神经节; **ciliary ganglion** = parasympathetic ganglion in the orbit of the eye, supplying the intrinsic eye muscles 睫状神经节; **coeliac ganglion** = ganglion on each side of the origins of the diaphragm, connected with the coeliac plexus 腹腔神经节; **mesenteric ganglion** = plexus of sympathetic nerve fibres and ganglion cells around the superior mesenteric artery 肠系膜神经节; **otic ganglion** = ganglion associated with the mandibular nerve where it leaves the skull 耳神经节; **pterygopalatine ganglion** *or* **sphenopalatine ganglion** = ganglion in the pterygopalatine fossa associated with the maxillary nerve (postganglionic fibres going to the nose, palate, pharynx and lacrimal glands) 蝶腭神经节; **spinal ganglion** = cone-shaped mass of cells on the posterior root, the main axons of which form the posterior root of the spinal nerve 脊神经节; **stellate ganglion** = group of nerve cells in the neck, shaped like a star 星状神经节; **submandibular ganglion** = ganglion associated with the lingual nerve, relaying impulses to the submandibular and sublingual salivary glands 下颌下神经节; **superior ganglion** = small collection of cells in the jugular foramen 舌咽神经上节; **trigeminal ganglion** *or* **Gasserian ganglion** = sensory ganglion containing the cells of origin of the sensory fibres in the fifth cranial nerve 三叉神经节; **vertebral ganglion** = ganglion in front of the origin of the vertebral artery 椎神经节 (**b**) cyst of a tendon sheath *or* joint capsule (usually at the wrist) which results in a painless swelling containing fluid 腱鞘囊肿 (NOTE: plural is **ganglia**)

◇ **ganglionic** *adjective* referring to a ganglion 神经节的; **postganglionic neurone** = neurone in a ganglion *or* plexus, the axon of which supplies muscle or glandular tissue directly 节后神经元

◇ **ganglionectomy** *noun* surgical removal of a ganglion 神经节切除术

gangrene *noun* condition where tissues die and decay, as a result of bacterial action, because the blood supply has been lost through injury or disease of the artery 坏疽: ***After he had frostbite, gangrene set in and his toes had to be amputated.*** 他的脚趾冻伤后发生了坏疽不得不被截除。**dry gangrene** = condition where the blood supply is cut off and the limb becomes black 干性坏疽; **gas gangrene** = complication of severe wounds in which the bacterium *Clostridium welchii* breeds in the wound and then spreads to healthy tissue which is rapidly decomposed with the formation of gas 气性坏疽; **hospital gangrene** = gangrene caused by insanitary hospital conditions 医院坏疽; **moist gangrene** = condition where dead tissue decays and swells with fluid because of infection and the tissues have an unpleasant smell 湿性坏疽

Ganser state = PSEUDODEMENTIA 甘塞氏状态,假性痴呆

gap *noun* space 空隙: ***There is a gap between his two front teeth.*** 他两前牙间有空隙。***The muscle has passed through a gap in the mucosa.*** 肌肉穿过粘膜的间隙。

gargle 1 *noun* mildly antiseptic solution used to clean the mouth. 漱口液: ***If diluted with water, the product makes a useful gargle.*** 这产品用水稀释后可成为有用的漱口液。**2** *verb* to put some antiseptic liquid solution into the back of the mouth and throat and then breathe out air through it 漱口: ***The doctor recommended gargling twice a day with a saline solution.*** 医生建议每天用盐水漱口两次。

gargoylism *or* **Hurler's syndrome** *noun* congenital defect of a patient's metabolism which causes polysaccharides and fat cells to accumulate in the body, resulting in mental defects, swollen liver and coarse features 脂肪软骨营养不良(遗传性代谢病)

gas *noun* (**a**) (i) state of matter in which particles occupy the whole space in which they occur 空气(ii) substance often produced from coal or found underground, and used to cook or heat 煤气; ***a gas cooker*** 煤气炉; ***We heat our house by gas.*** 我们用煤气取暖。**gas exchange** = process by which oxygen in air is exchanged in the lungs for waste carbon dioxide carried by the blood 气体交换; **gas gangrene** = complication of severe wounds in which the bacterium *Clostridium welchii* breeds in the wound and then spreads to healthy tissue which is rapidly decomposed with the formation of gas 气性坏疽; **gas poisoning** = poisoning by breathing in carbon monoxide or other toxic gas 煤气中毒 (**b**) gas which accumulates in the stomach or alimentary canal and causes pain 消化道积气; **gas pains** = flatus, excessive formation of gas in the stomach *or* intestine which is painful 肠胀气 (NOTE: plural **gases** is only used to mean different types of gas)

gash 1 *noun* long cut, as made with a

knife 长切口：***She had to have three stitches in the gash in her thigh.*** 她大腿上的伤口缝了3针。**2** *verb* to make a long cut. 做长切口：***She gashed her hand on the broken glass.*** 她的手被碎玻璃划了一道长切口。

gasp 1 *noun* trying to breathe *or* breath taken with difficulty 气喘：***His breath came in short gasps.*** 他的呼吸开始短促。**2** *verb* to try to breathe taking quick breaths 喘息：***She was gasping for breath.*** 她在喘息。

Gasserian ganglion *noun* trigeminal ganglion, sensory ganglion containing the cells of origin of the sensory fibres in the fifth cranial nerve 加塞神经节,半月神经节

gastr- *prefix* referring to the stomach 胃的

◇ **gastralgia** *noun* pain in the stomach 胃痛

◇ **gastrectomy** *noun* surgical removal of the stomach 胃切除术；**partial gastrectomy** = surgical removal of only the lower part of the stomach 部分胃切除术；**subtotal gastrectomy** = surgical removal of all but the top part of the stomach in contact with the diaphragm 胃大部切除术

◇ **gastric** *adjective* referring to the stomach 胃的；**gastric acid** = hydrochloric acid secreted into the stomach by acid-forming cells 胃酸；**gastric artery** = artery leading from the coeliac trunk to the stomach 胃动脉；**gastric flu** = general term for any mild stomach disorder 胃不适；**gastric juices** = mixture of hydrochloric acid, pepsin, intrinsic factor and mucus secreted by the cells of the lining membrane of the stomach to help the digestion of food 胃液：***The walls of the stomach secrete gastric juices.*** 胃壁分泌胃液。**gastric pit** = deep hollow in the mucous membrane forming the walls of the stomach 胃小凹；**gastric ulcer** = ulcer in the stomach 胃溃疡；**gastric vein** = vein which follows the gastric artery 胃静脉

◇ **gastrin** *noun* hormone which is released into the bloodstream from cells in the lower end of the stomach, stimulated by the presence of protein, and which in turn stimulates the flow of acid from the upper part of the stomach 胃泌素

◇ **gastritis** *noun* inflammation of the stomach 胃炎

◇ **gastrocele** *noun* stomach hernia, a condition where part of the stomach wall becomes weak and bulges out 胃膨出

◇ **gastrocnemius** *noun* large calf muscle 腓肠肌

◇ **gastrocolic reflex** *noun* sudden peristalsis of the colon produced when food is taken into an empty stomach 胃结肠反射

◇ **gastroduodenal** *adjective* referring to the stomach and duodenum 胃十二指肠的；**gastroduodenal artery** = artery leading from the gastric artery towards the pancreas 胃十二指肠动脉

◇ **gastroduodenostomy** *noun* surgical operation to join the duodenum to the stomach so as to bypass a blockage in the pylorus 胃十二指肠吻合术

◇ **gastroenteritis** *noun* inflammation of the membrane lining the intestines and the stomach, caused by a viral infection and resulting in diarrhoea and vomiting 胃肠炎

◇ **gastroenterologist** *noun* doctor who specializes in disorders of the stomach and intestine 胃肠病专家

◇ **gastroenterology** *noun* study of the stomach, intestine and other parts of the digestive system and their disorders 胃肠病学

◇ **gastroenterostomy** *noun* surgical operation to join the small intestine directly to the stomach so as to bypass a peptic ulcer 胃肠吻合术

◇ **gastroepiploic** *adjective* referring to the stomach and greater omentum 胃网膜的；**gastroepiploic artery** = artery linking the gastroduodenal artery to the splenic artery 胃网膜动脉

◇ **gastroileac reflex** *noun* automatic relaxing of the ileocaecal valve when food is present in the stomach 胃回肠反射

◇ **gastrointestinal**（**GI**）*adjective* referring to the stomach and intestine 胃肠道的：***He experienced some gastrointestinal（GI）bleeding.*** 他患过胃肠道出血。

◇ **gastrojejunostomy** *noun* surgical operation to join the jejunum to the stomach 胃空肠吻合术

◇ **gastrolith** *noun* stone in the stomach 胃石

◇ **gastro-oesophageal reflux** *noun* return of bitter-tasting, partly digested food from the stomach to the oesophagus when the patient has indigestion 胃食管返流

◇ **gastropexy** *noun* attaching the stomach to the wall of the abdomen 胃固定术

◇ **gastroplasty** *noun* surgery to correct a deformed stomach 胃成形术

◇ **gastroptosis** *noun* condition where the stomach hangs down 胃下垂

◇ **gastrorrhoea** *noun* excessive flow of gastric juices 胃液分泌过多

◇ **gastroscope** *noun* instrument formed of a tube *or* bundle of glass fibres with a lens attached, by which a doctor can examine the inside of the stomach（it is passed down into the stomach through the mouth）胃镜

◇ **gastroscopy** *noun* examination of the stomach using a gastroscope 胃镜检查

◇ **gastrostomy** *noun* surgical operation to create an opening into the stomach from the wall of the abdomen, so that food can be introduced without passing through the mouth and throat 胃造口术

◇ **gastrotomy** *noun* surgical operation to open up the stomach 胃切开术

gastrula *noun* second stage of the development of an embryo 原肠胚

gather *verb*（**a**）to bring together *or* to collect 收集：***She was gathering material for the study of children suffering from rickets.*** 她在收集佝偻病患儿的研究材料。***Pus had gathered round the wound.*** 脓液在伤口周围聚集。***The lecturer gathered up his papers.*** 演讲者将讲稿收起来。***A group of students gathered round the professor of surgery as he demonstrated the incision.*** 一群学生聚集在外科教授周围看他演示如何做切口。（**b**）to understand 明白，知道：***Did you gather who will be speaking at the ceremony?*** 你知道谁将会在典礼上讲话吗？

Gaucher's disease *noun* enzyme disease where fatty substances accumulate in the lymph glands, spleen and liver 戈谢氏病（酶缺陷病，脂质在淋巴结、脾和肝堆积）

> COMMENT：Symptoms are anaemia, a swollen spleen and darkening of the skin; the disease can be fatal in children.
> 注释：症状是贫血、脾肿大、皮肤发黑。在儿童可以是致命性的。

gauze *noun* thin light material used to make dressings 纱布：***She put a gauze dressing on the wound.*** 她在伤口上敷纱布垫。***The dressing used was a light paraffin gauze.*** 所用的敷料是淡的石蜡纱布。

gavage *noun* forced feeding of a patient who cannot eat *or* who refuses to eat 管饲法强迫进食

GC = GONORRHOEA 淋病

GDC = GENERAL DENTAL COUNCIL 牙科医师总会

Gehrig's disease = AMYOTROPHIC LATERAL SCLEROSIS 淀粉样侧索硬化

Geiger counter *noun* instrument for detection and measurement of radiation 盖格尔计数器

gel *noun* substance that has coagulated to form a jelly-like solid 凝胶

gelatin *noun* protein which is soluble

in water, made from collagen 明胶

> COMMENT: Gelatin is used in foodstuffs (such as desserts or meat jellies) and is also used to make capsules in which to put medicine.
> 注释:明胶可用于做食料(如餐后甜点和肉冻),也可用来做装药的胶囊。

◇ **gelatinous** *adjective* like jelly 胶状的

gemellus *noun* twin *or* double 双; **gemellus superior** *or* **inferior muscle** = two muscles arising from the ischium 坐骨上或下肌

gene *noun* unit of DNA on a chromosome which governs the synthesis of one protein, usually an enzyme, and determines a particular characteristic 基因 *see* 见 GENETIC

> COMMENT: Genes are either dominant, where the characteristicis always passed on to the child, or recessive, where the characteristic only appears if both parents have contributed the same gene.
> 注释:基因可以是显性基因,它的表型常传到子代;也可以是隐性基因,只有当父母双方的基因相同时表型才显现。

general *adjective* not particular; which concerns everything or everybody 普遍的,全面的; **general amnesia** = sudden and complete loss of memory *or* state where a person does not even remember who he is 完全性遗忘; **general anaesthesia** = loss of feeling and loss of sensation, after having been given an anaesthetic 全身麻醉; **general anaesthetic** = substance given to make a patient lose consciousness so that a major surgical operation can be carried out 全身麻醉剂; **general paralysis of the insane** (**GPI**) = widespread damage of the nervous system, marking the final stages of untreated syphilis 麻痹痴呆(四期梅毒); **general practice** = doctor's practice where patients from a district are treated for all types of illness 全科医疗: ***She qualified as a doctor and went into general practice.*** 她取得了医生资格,并可做全科医疗。

◇ **General Dental Council** (**GDC**) official body which registers and supervises dentists in the UK 牙科医师总会

◇ **generalized** *adjective* occurring throughout the body 泛发的,扩散的; ***The cancer became generalized.*** 肿瘤播散了。(NOTE: the opposite is **localized**)

◇ **generally** *adverb* normally 通常

◇ **General Medical Council** (**GMC**) official body which registers and supervises doctors in the UK 医师总会

◇ **General Optical Council** (**GOC**) official body which registers and supervises opticians in the UK 验光师总会

◇ **general practitioner** (**GP**) *noun* doctor who treats many patients in a district for all types of illness, though not specializing in any one branch of medicine 全科医师 (NOTE: plural is **Gps**)

> COMMENT: A GP usually has either a MB (bachelor of Medicine) or ChB (Bachelor of surgery) degree. He may also be a MRCS (Member of the Royal College of Surgeons) or LRCP (Licentiate of the Royal College of Physicians). GPs train in hospital as well in general practice, and often have specialist qualifications, such as in obstetrics or child care.
> 注释:GP 一般具有医学学士或外科学士学位,他可以是皇家外科学会会员或皇家内科学会领照者,GP 在医院除进行全科训练外还包括专科培训,如:产科或儿童护理。

generation *noun* all people born at about the same period 世代

generic *adjective* (i) referring to a genus 属的 (ii) (name) given to a drug generally, as opposed to a proprietary name used by the manufacturer 药品的通用名

genetic *adjective* referring to the genes 遗传的; **genetic code** = information which determines the synthesis of a cell, is held in the DNA of a cell and is passed on when the cell divides 遗传密码; **genetic engineering** = techniques

used to change the genetic composition of a cell so as to change certain characteristics which can be inherited 遗传工程
◇ **geneticist** *noun* person who specializes in the study of the way in which characteristics are inherited through the genes 遗传学家
◇ **genetics** *noun* study of genes, and of the way characteristics are inherited through the genes 遗传学

-genic *suffix* produced by *or* which produces 由…产生,生产; **photogenic** = produced by light *or* which produces light 由光产生的,发光的

genicular *adjective* referring to the knee 膝的

genital *adjective* referring to reproductive organs 生殖器的; **genital herpes** = venereal infection, caused by a herpesvirus, which forms blisters in the genital region and can have a serious effect on a fetus 生殖器疱疹; **genital organs** *or* **genitals** = external organs for reproduction (penis and testicles in male, vulva in female) 外生殖器
◇ **genitalia** *noun* genital organs 生殖器
◇ **genitourinary** *adjective* referring to both reproductive and urinary systems 泌尿生殖的; **genitourinary system** = organs of reproduction and urination, including the kidneys 泌尿生殖系统

genome *noun* (i) basic set of chromosomes in a person 染色体组 (ii) set of genes which are inherited from one parent 基因组

genotype *noun* genetic composition of an organism 基因型

gentian violet *noun* antiseptic blue dye used to paint on skin infections; dye used to stain specimens 龙胆紫

gentle *adjective* soft; kind 柔软的,温和的: ***The doctor has gentle hands.*** 医生有双轻柔的手。***You must be gentle when you are holding a little baby.*** 当你抱着婴儿时一定要非常温柔小心。***Use a gentle antiseptic on the rash.*** 在皮疹上用些温和的抗生素。(NOTE: **gentle - gentler - gentlest**)

genu *noun* the knee 膝盖
◇ **genual** *adjective* referring to the knee 膝的
◇ **genupectoral position** *noun* position of a patient when kneeling with the chest on the floor 膝胸位
◇ **genu valgum** *noun* knock knee, a state where the knees touch and the ankles are apart when a person is standing straight 膝外翻
◇ **genu varum** *noun* bow legs, a state where the ankles touch and the knees are apart when a person is standing straight 膝内翻

genus *noun* main group of related living organisms 属: ***A genus is divided into different species.*** 属可以分为不同的种。(NOTE: plural is **genera**)

geriatric *adjective* referring to old people 老年的; **geriatric unit** *or* **ward** *or* **hospital** = unit *or* ward *or* hospital which specializes in the treatment of old people 老年单位,老年病区,老年医院
◇ **geriatrician** *noun* doctor who specializes in the treatment *or* study of diseases of old people 老年病学家
◇ **geriatrics** *noun* study of the diseases and disorders of old people 老年医学 *compare* 比较 PAEDIATRICS

germ *noun* (**a**) microbe (such as a virus *or* bacterium) which causes a disease 病菌: ***Germs are not visible to the naked eye.*** 病菌用肉眼是看不见的。(NOTE: in this sense 'germ' is not a medical term) (**b**) part of an organism which develops into a new organism 胚; **germ cell** *or* **gonocyte** = cell which is capable of developing into a spermatozoon or ovum 生殖细胞; **germ layers** = two or three layers of cell in animal embryos which form the organs of the body 胚层
◇ **germicide** *adjective* & *noun* (substance) which can kill germs 杀菌的

German measles *or* **rubella** *noun* common infectious viral disease of children with mild fever, swollen lymph nodes and rash 风疹 *compare* 比较 MEASLES, RUBEOLA

COMMENT: German measles can cause stillbirth or malformation of an unborn baby if the mother catches the disease while pregnant. It is advisable that girls should catch the disease in childhood, or should be immunized against it.
注释:母亲在怀孕期间如果感染了风疹会引起死胎或发育畸形,因此建议若女孩在儿童时期未感染此病应当针对此病进行免疫。

germinal *adjective* (i) referring to a germ 病菌的(ii) referring to an embryo 胚胎的; **germinal epithelium** = outer layer of the ovary 胚层上皮

gerontology *noun* study of the process of ageing and the diseases of old people 老年医学

Gerstmann's syndrome *noun* condition where a patient no longer recognises his body image, cannot tell the difference between left and right, cannot recognise his different fingers and is unable to write 格斯特曼综合征(患者不能识别自身,分不清左右和不同的手指,也不能书写)

gestate *verb* to carry a baby in the womb from conception to birth 妊娠

◇ **gestation** *or* **pregnancy** *noun* period (usually 266 days) from conception to birth, during which the baby develops in the mother's womb 妊娠期

◇ **gestational diabetes** *noun* form of diabetes mellitus which develops in a pregnant woman 妊娠糖尿病

QUOTE: Evaluation of fetal age and weight has proved to be of value in the clinical management of pregnancy, particularly in high-risk gestations.
引文:对胎儿的年龄和体重进行评估被证明在妊娠尤其是高危妊娠的临床处理中有重要意义。
Southern Medical Journal 南部医学杂志

get *verb* (**a**) to become 变得: ***The muscles get flabby from lack of exercise.*** 因为缺少锻炼,肌肉变得松弛。***She got fat from eating too much.*** 她因为吃得太多而肥胖起来。***Waiting lists for operations are getting longer.*** 等待手术的名单越来越长。(**b**) (i) to make something happen 使…发生(ii) to pay someone to do something 付钱让人做某事 (iii) to persuade someone to do something 劝告某人做某事: ***He got the hospital to admit the patient as an emergency case.*** 他让医院以急诊收治这个患者。***Did you get the sister to fill in the form?*** 你让护士长填表了吗? ***He got the doctor to repeat the prescription.*** 他让医生重新开了处方。**to have got to** = must 必须: ***You have got to be at the surgery before 9.30.*** 你必须在9:30前到达手术室。***He is leaving early because he has got to drive a long way.*** 他很早就离开,因为他需要开很长的一段路。***Has she got to take the tablets every day?*** 她必须每天都吃这药吗? (**c**) to catch (a disease) 得病: ***I think I'm getting a cold.*** 我觉得我得了感冒。***She can't go to work because she's got flu.*** 因为患了流感她不能去上班了。

◇ **get along** *verb* to manage *or* to work 做,进行: ***We seem to get along quite well without any electricity.*** 没有电我们过得也很好。

◇ **get around** *verb* to move about 行走: ***Since she had the accident she gets around on two sticks.*** 出事故后她依靠两个拐杖行走。

◇ **get better** *verb* to become well again after being ill 好转: ***He was seriously ill, but seems to be getting better.*** 他曾病得很厉害,但现在似乎有所好转。***Her cold has got better.*** 她的感冒好多了。***His flu has not got any better, so he will have to stay in bed.*** 他的流感还没有见好,所以必须躺在床上。

◇ **get dressed** *verb* to put your clothes on 穿衣: ***He got dressed quickly because he didn't want to be late for work.*** 他很快穿好了衣服,因为他不想上班迟到。***She was getting dressed when the phone rang.*** 当来电话时她正在穿衣服。***The patient has to be helped to get***

dressed. 患者必须有人帮助穿衣。

◇ **get on** *verb* (**a**) to go into (a bus, etc.) 上(车): ***We got on the bus at the post office.*** 我们在邮局站上了车。***She got on her bike and rode away.*** 她骑上自行车走了。(**b**) to become old 衰老: ***He's getting on and is quite deaf.*** 他变老了,耳朵也背了。

◇ **get on with**(**a**) to be friendly with someone 相处融洽: ***He gets on very well with everyone.*** 他跟每个人都相处得很好。***I didn't get on with the boss.*** 我跟老板处得不好。(**b**) to continue to do some work 继续做某事: ***I must get on with the blood tests.*** 我必须再做血液检查。

◇ **get over** *verb* to become better after an illness *or* a shock 好转: ***He got over his cold.*** 他感冒好了。***She never got over her mother's death.*** 她还没有从她母亲死亡的打击中缓过来。

◇ **get up** *verb* to stand up;to get out of bed 站起;起床: ***He got up from his chair and walked out of the room.*** 他从椅子上站起来走出了房间。***At what time did you get up this morning?*** 今天早晨你几点起床的?

◇ **get well** *verb* to become healthy again after being ill 恢复: ***We hope your mother will get well soon.*** 我们希望你母亲尽快恢复。**get well card** = card sent to a person who is ill, with good wishes for a rapid recovery 慰问卡

GH = GROWTH HORMONE 生长激素

Ghon's focus *noun* spot on the lung produced by the tuberculosis bacillus 冈氏病灶,结核病灶

GI = GASTROINTESTINAL 消化道的: ***They diagnosed a GI disease.*** 他们诊断了一例消化道病人。***operation on a GI fistula*** 消化道瘘手术

giant *noun* very tall person 巨人; **giant cell** = very large cell such as an osteoclast *or* megakaryocyte 巨大细胞; **giant hives** = large flat white blisters caused by an allergic reaction 荨麻疹 *see also* 参见 ARTERITIS, GIGANTISM

Giardia *noun* microscopic protozoan parasite in the intestine which causes giardiasis 贾第虫属

◇ **giardiasis** *or* **lambliasis** *noun* disorder of the intestine caused by the parasite *Giardia lamblia* , usually with no symptoms, but in heavy infections the absorption of fat may be affected, causing diarrhoea 贾第虫病(肠道感染了贾第虫,通常无症状,严重感染时会影响脂肪吸收,引起腹泻)

gibbosity *or* **gibbus** *noun* sharp angle in the curvature of the spine caused by the weakening of a vertebra by tuberculosis of the backbone 驼背

giddiness *noun* condition in which someone feels that everything is turning around, and so cannot stand up 眩晕: ***He began to suffer attacks of giddiness.*** 他开始感到一阵眩晕。*see* 见 LABYRINTH

◇ **giddy** *adjective* feeling that everything is turning round 眩晕的: ***She has had a giddy spell.*** 她刚刚发作了一次眩晕。

gigantism *noun* condition in which the patient grows very tall, caused by excessive production of growth hormone by the pituitary gland 巨人症(垂体分泌生长激素过多引起)

Gilliam's operation *noun* surgical operation to correct retroversion of the womb 吉列姆氏手术,子宫后倾矫正术

gingiva *noun* gum, the soft tissue covering the part of the jaw which surrounds the teeth 龈◇见图 TOOTH

◇ **gingivalis** 龈的 *see* 见 ENTAMOEBA

◇ **gingivectomy** *noun* surgical removal of excess gum tissue 牙龈切除术

◇ **gingivitis** *noun* inflammation of the gums as a result of bacterial infection 牙龈炎; **ulcerative** *or* **ulceromembranous gingivitis** = ulceration of the gums which can also affect the membrane of the mouth 溃疡型牙龈炎

ginglymus *noun* hinge joint, a joint (like the knee or elbow) which allows movement in two directions only 屈戌关

节

gippy tummy *noun* (*informal* 非正式) diarrhoea which affects people travelling in foreign countries as a result of eating unwashed fruit or drinking water which has not been boiled(俚)热带腹泻(吃了未冲洗的水果或饮用未煮沸的水所致)

girdle *noun* set of bones making a ring or arch 带; **hip girdle** *or* **pelvic girdle** = the sacrum and the two hip bones to which the thigh bones are attached 骨盆带; **pectoral girdle** *or* **shoulder girdle** = the shoulder bones (scapulae and clavicles) to which the upper arm bones are attached 肩胛带

Girdlestone's operation *noun* surgical operation to relieve osteoarthritis of the hip 格德尔斯通手术(缓解髋骨关节炎)

girl *noun* female child 女孩: ***She's only got a little girl.*** 她只有一个小女孩。***They have three children — two boys and a girl.*** 他们有3个孩子,2个男孩1个女孩。

give *verb* (**a**) to pass something to someone 给: ***He was given a pain-killing injection.*** 给他打了止痛针。***The surgeons have given him a new pacemaker.*** 外科医师给他装了个新的起搏器。(**b**) to allow someone time 允许某人的时间: ***The doctors have only given her two weeks to live.*** = The doctors say she will die in two weeks' time. 医生宣告她只能活两周的时间。(NOTE: **gives - giving - gave - has given**)

◊ **give up** *verb* not to do something any more 放弃: ***He was advised to give up smoking.*** 他被劝告戒烟。***She has given up eating chocolate.*** 她已经不再吃巧克力了。

glabella *noun* flat area of bone in the forehead between the eyebrows 眉间

gladiolus *noun* middle section of the sternum 胸骨体

gland *noun* (**a**) organ in the body containing cells which secrete substances which act elsewhere (such as a hormone *or* sweat *or* saliva) 腺体; **endocrine gland** = gland without a duct which produces hormones which are introduced directly into the bloodstream (such as pituitary gland, thyroid gland, the pancreas, the adrenals, the gonads, the thymus) 内分泌腺; **exocrine gland** = gland with a duct down which its secretions pass to a particular part of the body (such as the liver, the sweat glands, the salivary glands) 外分泌腺; **adrenal glands** *or* **suprarenal glands** = two endocrine glands at the top of the kidneys which secrete cortisone, adrenaline and other hormones 肾上腺 ◊ 见图 KIDNEY; **bulbourethral glands** *or* **Cowper's glands** = two glands at the base of the penis which secrete into the urethra 尿道球腺; **ceruminous glands** = glands which secrete earwax 耵聍腺 ◊ 见图 EAR; **lacrimal gland** *or* **tear gland** = gland which secretes tears 泪腺; **Lieberkn's glands** = small glands between the bases of the villi in the small intestine 肠腺; **mammary gland** = gland in female mammals which produces milk 乳腺; **meibomian gland** = sebaceous gland on the edge of the eyelid which secretes the liquid which lubricates the eyelid 睑板腺; **parathyroid glands** = four glands in the neck near the thyroid gland, which secrete a hormone which regulates the level of calcium in blood plasma 甲状旁腺; **parotid gland** = one of the glands which produce saliva, situated in the neck behind the joint of the jaw 腮腺 ◊ 见图 THROAT; **pineal gland** *or* **pineal body** = small cone-shaped gland near the midbrain, which produces melatonin and is believed to be associated with Circadian rhythms 松果体 ◊ 见图 BRAIN; **pituitary gland** *or* **hypophysis cerebri** = main endocrine gland, about the size of a pea, situated in the sphenoid bone below the hypothalamus, which secretes hormones which stimulate other glands 垂体 ◊ 见图 BRAIN; **salivary gland** = gland which secretes saliva 涎腺；**sebaceous gland** = gland which secretes oil at the base of each hair follicle 皮脂腺；**sublingual gland** = salivary gland under the tongue 舌下腺 ◊ 见图 THROAT；**submandibular gland** = salivary gland in the lower jaw 下颌下腺 ◊ 见图 THROAT；**sweat gland** = gland which produces sweat, situated beneath the dermis and connected to the skin surface by a sweat duct 汗腺；**thymus gland** = endocrine gland in the front of the top of the thorax, behind the breastbone 胸腺；**thyroid gland** = endocrine gland in the neck, which secretes a hormone which regulates the body's metabolism 甲状腺；**greater vestibular glands** *or* **Bartholin's glands** = two glands at the side of the entrance to the vagina, which secrete a lubricating substance 前庭大腺 (**b**) **lymph** *or* **lymphatic glands** = glands situated in various points of the lymphatic system (especially under the armpits and in the groin) through which lymph passes 淋巴结

glanders *noun* bacterial disease of horses, which can be caught by humans, with symptoms of high fever and inflammation of the lymph nodes 鼻疽，马的细菌感染性疾病，可传染给人，表现为高热和淋巴结炎 *see also* 参见 FARCY

glandular *adjective* referring to glands 腺的

◊ **glandular fever** *or* **infectious mononucleosis** *noun* infectious disease where the body has an excessive number of white blood cells 腺热，传染性单核细胞增多症

> COMMENT: The symptoms include sore throat, fever and swelling of the lymph glands in the neck. Glandular fever is probably caused by the Epstein-Barr virus. The test for glandular fever is the Paul-Bunnell reaction. 注释：症状包括咽痛、发热、颈部淋巴结肿大，本病可能由 E-B 病毒感染引起，腺热的诊断试验是保－邦二氏反应。

glans *or* **glans penis** *noun* bulb at the end of the penis 阴茎球 ◊ 见图 URO-GENITAL SYSTEM (male)

glass *noun* (**a**) material which you can see through, used to make windows 玻璃：***The doors are made of glass.*** 门是玻璃的。***The specimen was kept in a glass jar.*** 样本保存在玻璃罐里。(NOTE: no plural **some glass, a piece of glass**) (**b**) thing to drink out of, usually made of glass 玻璃杯：***She poured the mixture into a glass.*** 她将混合物倒入玻璃杯内。(**c**) the contents of a glass 一杯的容量：***He drinks a glass of milk every evening.*** 他每天晚上喝一杯牛奶。***You may drink a small glass of wine with your evening meal.*** 晚餐你可以喝一小杯酒。(NOTE: plural is **glasses** for (b) and (c))

◊ **glasses** *plural noun* two pieces of glass or plastic, made into lenses, which are worn in front of the eyes to help the patient see better 眼镜：***She was wearing dark glasses.*** 她戴了副墨镜。***He has glasses with gold frames.*** 他戴着副金边儿眼镜。***She needs glasses to read.*** 她看书时需戴眼镜。

glaucoma *noun* condition of the eyes, caused by abnormally high pressure of fluid inside the eyeball, resulting in disturbances of vision and blindness 青光眼；**angle-closure glaucoma** *or* **acute glaucoma** = abnormally high pressure of fluid inside the eyeball caused by pressure of the iris against the lens, trapping the aqueous humour 闭角型青光眼，急性青光眼；**open-angle glaucoma** *or* **chronic glaucoma** = abnormally high pressure of fluid inside the eyeball caused by a blockage in the channel through which the aqueous humour drains 开角型青光眼，慢性青光眼

gleet *noun* thin discharge from the vagina, penis, a wound or an ulcer 慢性淋病性尿道炎，从阴道、阴茎、伤口或溃疡排出的粘薄液体

glenohumeral *adjective* referring to both the glenoid cavity and the humerus

盂肱的; **glenohumeral joint** = shoulder joint 盂肱关节

◇ **glenoid cavity** *or* **glenoid fossa** *noun* socket in the shoulder joint into which the head of the humerus fits 肩盂 ⇨见图 SHOULDER

glia *or* **neuroglia** *or* **glial tissue** *noun* connective tissue of the central nervous system, surrounding cell bodies, axons and dendrites 神经胶质

◇ **glial cells** *noun* cells in the glia 胶质细胞

◇ **glio-** *prefix* referring to brain tissue 胶质的

◇ **glioblastoma** *or* **spongioblastoma** *noun* rapidly developing malignant brain tumour in the glial cells 成胶质细胞瘤,恶性胶质瘤

◇ **glioma** *noun* any tumour of the glial tissue in the brain *or* spinal cord 神经胶质瘤

◇ **gliomyoma** *noun* tumour of both the nerve and muscle tissue 胶质肌瘤

globin *noun* protein which combines with other substances to form compounds such as haemoglobin and myoglobin 球蛋白

globule *noun* round drop (of fat) 球形

◇ **globulin** *noun* class of protein, present in blood, including antibodies 球蛋白; **gamma globulin** *or* **immunoglobulin** = protein found in plasma, and which forms antibodies as protection against infection 丙种球蛋白,免疫球蛋白

◇ **globulinuria** *noun* presence of globulins in the urine 球蛋白尿

globus *noun* any ball-shaped part of the body 球形的; **globus hystericus** = lump in the throat, feeling of not being able to swallow caused by worry *or* embarrassment 癔病球

glomangioma *noun* tumour of the skin at the ends of the fingers and toes 血管球瘤

glomerular *adjective* referring to a glomerulus 肾小球的; **glomerular capsule** = Bowman's capsule, the expanded end of a renal tubule, surrounding a glomerular tuft 肾小球囊; **glomerular tuft** = group of blood vessels in the kidney which filter the blood 肾小球丛

◇ **glomerulitis** *noun* inflammation causing lesions of glomeruli in the kidney 肾小球炎

◇ **glomerulonephritis** *noun* form of nephritis where the glomeruli in the kidneys are inflamed 肾小球肾炎

◇ **glomerulus** *noun* group of blood vessels which filter waste matter from the blood in a kidney 肾小球 *see also* 参见 MALPIGHIAN (NOTE: plural is **glomeruli**)

gloss- *prefix* referring to the tongue 舌的

◇ **glossa** *noun* the tongue 舌

◇ **glossectomy** *noun* surgical removal of the tongue 舌切除术

Glossina *noun* genus of African flies (such as the tsetse fly), which cause trypanosomiasis 舌蝇属

glossitis *noun* inflammation of the surface of the tongue 舌炎

◇ **glossodynia** *noun* pain in the tongue 舌痛

◇ **glossopharyngeal nerve** *noun* ninth cranial nerve which controls the pharynx, the salivary glands and part of the tongue 舌咽神经

◇ **glossoplegia** *noun* paralysis of the tongue 舌麻痹

glottis *noun* opening in the larynx between the vocal cords, which forms the entrance to the main airway from the pharynx 声门

glove *noun* piece of clothing which you wear on your hand 手套: ***The doctor was wearing rubber gloves*** *or* ***surgical gloves.*** 医生戴着橡胶手套。

gluc- *prefix* referring to glucose 葡萄糖的

◇ **glucagon** *noun* hormone secreted by the islets of Langerhans in the pancreas, which increases the level of blood sugar by stimulating the breakdown of glycogen 胰高血糖素

◇ **glucocorticoid** *noun* any corticosteroid which breaks down carbohydrates and fats for use by the body, produced by the adrenal cortex 糖(肾上腺)皮质激素

glucose *or* **dextrose** *noun* simple sugar found in some fruit, but also broken down from white sugar or carbohydrate and absorbed into the body or secreted by the kidneys 葡萄糖; **blood-glucose level** = amount of glucose present in the blood 血糖水平: ***The normal blood-glucose level stays at about 60 to 100 mg of glucose per 100 ml of blood.*** 正常的血糖水平是60—100mg/dl。**glucose tolerance test** = test for diabetes mellitus, where the patient eats glucose and his urine and blood are tested at regular intervals 葡萄糖耐量试验

◇ **glucuronic acid** *noun* acid formed by glucose and which acts on bilirubin 葡萄糖醛酸

> COMMENT: Combustion of glucose with oxygen to form carbondioxide and water is the body's main source of energy.
> 注释:消耗葡萄糖、氧形成二氧化碳和水是体内主要的能量来源。

glue 1 *noun* material which sticks things together 胶,胶水; **glue ear** *or* **secretory otitis media** = condition where fluid forms behind the eardrum and causes deafness 分泌性中耳炎(鼓膜后液体形成,引起耳聋); **glue-sniffing** = type of solvent abuse where a person is addicted to inhaling the toxic fumes given off by certain types of glue 吸胶毒,一种滥用溶剂的方法 **2** *verb* to stick things together with glue 胶合

glutamic acid *noun* amino acid in protein 谷氨酸

◇ **glutaminase** *noun* enzyme in the kidneys, which helps to break down glutamine 谷酰胺酶

◇ **glutamine** *noun* amino acid in protein 谷酰胺

gluteal *adjective* referring to the buttocks 臀的; **superior** *or* **inferior gluteal artery** = arteries supplying the buttocks 臀上、下动脉; **superior** *or* **inferior gluteal vein** = veins draining the buttocks 臀上、下静脉; **gluteal muscles** = muscles in the buttocks 臀肌 *see also* 参见 GLUTEUS

gluten *noun* protein found in certain cereals, which makes a sticky paste when water is added 谷胶; **gluten enteropathy** *or* **coeliac disease** = (i) allergic disease (mainly affecting children) in which the lining of the intestine is sensitive to gluten, preventing the small intestine from digesting fat 谷胶性肠病(主要见于儿童的过敏性疾病,因肠道粘膜对谷胶过敏影响小肠对脂肪的吸收)(ii) condition in adults where the villi in the intestine become smaller, and so reduce the surface which can absorb nutrients 乳糜泻(成人小肠绒毛变短,使吸收营养的面积减少)

gluteus *noun* one of three muscles in the buttocks, responsible for movements of the hip (the largest is the gluteus maximus, while gluteus medius and minimus are smaller) 臀肌

glyc- *prefix* referring to sugar 糖的

◇ **glycaemia** *noun* normal level of glucose found in the blood 血糖 *see also* 参见 HYPOGLYCAEMIA, HYPERGLYCAEMIA

◇ **glycerin(e)** *or* **glycerol** *noun* colourless viscous sweet-tasting liquid present in all fats 甘油

◇ **glycine** *noun* amino acid in protein 甘氨酸

> COMMENT: Synthetic glycerine is used in various medicinal preparations and also as a lubricant in toothpaste, cough medicines, etc. A mixture of glycerine and honey is useful to soothe a sore throat.
> 注释:合成甘油被广泛地应用于医药制剂,在牙膏、止咳药等中作为润滑剂,甘油和蜂蜜的混合物可用来缓解咽痛。

glycocholic acid *noun* one of the bile acids 甘氨胆汁酸

glycogen *noun* type of starch, converted from glucose by the action of insulin, and stored in the liver as a source of energy 糖原
◇ **glycogenesis** *noun* process by which glucose is converted into glycogen in the liver 糖异生
◇ **glycogenolysis** *noun* process by which glycogen is broken down to form glucose 糖原分解
◇ **glycosuria** *noun* high level of sugar in the urine, a symptom of diabetes mellitus 糖尿
GMC = GENERAL MEDICAL COUNCIL 医师总会
gnathoplasty *noun* plastic surgery to correct a defect in the jaw 颌成形术
goal *noun* that which is expected to be achieved by a certain treatment 目标,目的
goblet cell *noun* tube-shaped cell in the epithelium which secretes mucus 杯状细胞
GOC = GENERAL OPTICAL COUNCIL 眼科医师总会
go down *verb* to become smaller 减小: ***When the blood sugar level goes down, the swelling has started to go down.*** 当血糖水平下降时,肿胀开始消退。
goitre *or US* **goiter** *noun* excessive enlargement of the thyroid gland, seen as a swelling round the neck, caused by a lack of iodine 甲状腺肿; **exophthalmic goitre** *or* **Graves' disease** = form of goitre caused by hyperthyroidism, where the heart beats faster, the thyroid gland swells, the eyes protrude and the limbs tremble 突眼性甲状腺肿,格雷夫斯氏病
◇ **goitrogen** *noun* substance which causes goitre 致甲状腺肿物质
gold *noun* soft yellow-coloured precious metal, used as a compound in various drugs, and sometimes as a filling for teeth 金; **gold injections** = injections of a solution containing gold, used to relieve rheumatoid arthritis 注射金制剂,用于治疗类风湿性关节炎 (NOTE: the chemical symbol is **Au**)
◇ **golden** *adjective* coloured like gold 金色的; **golden eye ointment** = yellow ointment, made of an oxide of mercury, used to treat inflammation of the eyelids 金色眼药膏(黄色的氧化汞药膏,治疗眼睑炎症)
Golgi apparatus *noun* folded membranous structure inside the cell cytoplasm which stores and transports enzymes and hormones 高尔基体
◇ **Golgi cell** *noun* type of nerve cell in the central nervous system, either with long axons (Golgi type 1) or without axons (Golgi type 2) 高尔基细胞
gomphosis *noun* joint which cannot move, like a tooth in a jaw 嵌合,钉状关节
gonad *noun* sex gland which produces gametes (the testicles produce spermatozoa in males, and the ovaries produce ova in females) and also sex hormones 性腺
◇ **gonadotrophic hormones** *plural noun* hormones (the follicle-stimulating hormone (FSH) and the luteinizing hormone (LH)) produced by the anterior pituitary gland which have an effect on the ovaries in females and on the testes in males 促性腺激素
◇ **gonadotrophin** *noun* any of a group of hormones produced by the pituitary gland which stimulates the sex glands at puberty 促性腺激素 *see also* 参见 CHORIONIC
gonagra *noun* form of gout which occurs in the knees 膝关节痛风
goni- *prefix* meaning angle 角的
◇ **goniopuncture** *noun* surgical operation for draining fluid from the eyes of a patient who has glaucoma 前房角穿刺术
◇ **gonioscope** *noun* lens for measuring the angle of the front part of the eye 前房角镜
◇ **goniotomy** *noun* surgical operation to treat glaucoma by cutting Schlemm's

canal 前房角切开术

gonococcus *noun* type of bacterium, *Neisseria gonorrhoea*, which produces gonorrhoea 淋球菌（NOTE：plural is **gonococci**）

◇ **gonococcal** *adjective* referring to gonococcus 淋球菌的

◇ **gonocyte** *noun* germ cell, a cell which is able to develop into a spermatozoon or an ovum 生殖母细胞

◇ **gonorrhoea** *noun* sexually transmitted disease, which produces painful irritation of the mucous membrane and a watery discharge from the vagina or penis 淋病

◇ **gonorrhoeal** *adjective* referring to gonorrhoea 淋病的

Goodpasture's syndrome *noun* rare lung disease where the patient coughs up blood, is anaemic, and which may result in kidney failure 古德帕斯特氏综合征(一种少见的肺病，患者咯血、贫血、可导致肾衰竭)

goose flesh *or* **goose pimples** *or* **cutis anserina** *or US* **goose bumps** *noun* reaction of the skin to being cold *or* frightened, where the skin is raised into many little bumps by the action of the arrector pili muscles 鸡皮疙瘩

Gordh needle *noun* needle with a bag attached, so that several injections can be made one after the other 一种带有小囊的针，可以连续注射

gorget *noun* surgical instrument used to remove stones from the bladder 有槽导子

gouge *noun* surgical instrument like a chisel used to cut bone 圆凿

goundou *noun* condition caused by yaws, in which growths form on either side of the nose 鼻骨增殖性骨膜炎

gout *or* **podagra** *noun* disease in which abnormal quantities of uric acid are produced and precipitated as crystals in the cartilage round joints 痛风(机体产生过量的尿酸，并在关节周围的软骨内沉淀形成结晶)

COMMENT：Formerly associated with drinking strong wines such as port, but now believed to arise in three ways：excess uric acid in the diet, excess uric acid synthesized by the body and defective excretion of uric acid. It is likely that both overproduction and defective excretion are due to inherited biochemical abnormalities. Excess intake of alcohol can provoke an attack by interfering with the excretion of uric acid.
注释：以前认为由喝烈性酒如波尔图葡萄酒引起，现认为有3种原因：饮食中尿酸含量高、机体合成尿酸过剩和尿酸排泄减少。无论是合成增加还是排泄减少都与遗传性生化异常有关，过量饮酒可干扰尿酸排泄诱发痛风发作。

gown *noun* long robe worn over other clothes to protect them 罩衣：***The surgeons were wearing green gowns.*** 外科医师穿着绿色的罩衣。***The patient lay on his bed in a theatre gown, ready to go to the operating theatre.*** 患者穿着手术罩衣躺在床上，等待进入手术室。

GP *noun* general practitioner 全科医师：***Some GP practices will manage their own budget of NHS funds if they choose to do so.*** 一些全科医师如果愿意的话可以管理自己的国民保健事业基金预算。(NOTE：plural is **GPs**)

GPI = GENERAL PARALYSIS OF THE INSANE 麻痹性痴呆

gr = GRAIN 谷

Graafian follicle 囊状卵泡 *see* 见 FOLLICLE

gracilis *noun* thin muscle running down the inside of the leg from the top of the leg down to the top of the tibia 薄肌

graduate 1 *noun* person who has completed a university course and has a degree 大学毕业生：***She is a graduate from the School of Tropical Medicine.*** 她是从热带医学院毕业的。**2** *verb* to finish a course of study at a university and have a degree 毕业：***He graduated in Pharmacy last year.*** 他去年从药学院毕业。

◇ **graduated** *adjective* with marks showing various degrees *or* levels 分等级的；***a graduated measuring jar*** 量瓶

Graefe's knife *noun* sharp knife used in operations on cataracts 格雷费氏刀,白内障刀

graft 1 *noun* (i) act of transplanting an organ (heart *or* lung *or* kidney) or tissue (bone *or* skin) to replace an organ or tissue which is not functioning or which is diseased 移植(ii) organ *or* tissue which is transplanted 移植物：***She had to have a skin graft.*** 她必须进行皮肤移植。***The corneal graft was successful.*** 角膜移植很成功。***The patient was given drugs to prevent the graft being rejected.*** 患者服用药物预防移植物被排斥。**graft versus host disease** = condition which develops when cells from the grafted tissue react against the patient's own tissue, causing skin disorders 移植物抗宿主反应(移植物的细胞对抗患者自身组织,引起皮肤病变) *see also* 参见 AUTOGRAFT, HOMOGRAFT **2** *verb* to take a healthy organ *or* tissue and transplant it into a patient in place of diseased or defective organ or tissue 移植：***The surgeons grafted a new section of bone at the side of the skull.*** 外科医师在头颅的一侧移植了一段新骨。

grain *noun* measure of weight equal to 0.0648 grams 格令,重量单位,相当于0.0648克 (NOTE: when used with numbers, **grain** is usually written **gr**)

gram measure of weight 克：***A thousand grams make one kilogram.*** 1,000克等于1千克。***I need 5 g of morphine.*** 我需要5克的吗啡。(NOTE: when used with numbers, **gram** is usually written **g**)

-gram *suffix* meaning a record in the form of a picture 图,像；**cardiogram** = X-ray picture of the heart 心动图

Gram's stain *noun* method of staining bacteria so that they can be identified 革兰氏染色；**Gram-positive bacterium** = bacterium which retains the first dye and appears blue-black when viewed under the microscope 革兰氏阳性细菌；**Gram-negative bacterium** = bacterium which takes up the red counterstain, after the alcohol has washed out the first violet dye 革兰氏阴性细菌

> COMMENT: The tissue sample is first stained with a violet dye, treated with alcohol, and then counterstained with a red dye.
> 注释：组织样本先用紫色染料染色,然后用酒精处理,最后用红色染料复染。

grandchild *noun* child of a son or daughter(外)孙儿(女) (NOTE: plural is **grandchildren**)

◇ **granddaughter** *noun* daughter of a son or daughter(外)孙女

◇ **grandfather** *noun* father of a mother or father(外)祖父

◇ **grandmother** *noun* mother of a mother of father(外)祖母

◇ **grandparents** *plural noun* parents of a mother or father(外)祖父母

◇ **grandson** *noun* son of a son or daughter(外)孙子

grandes 经产妇 *see* 见 MULTIPARA

grand mal *or* **major epilepsy** *noun* type of epilepsy, in which the patient becomes unconscious and falls down, while the muscles become stiff and twitch violently 癫痫大发作

granular *adjective* like grains 颗粒状的；**granular cast** = cast composed of cells filled with protein and fatty granules 颗粒管型；**granular leucocytes** *or* **granulocytes** = leucocytes with granules (basophils, eosinophils, neutrophils) 粒细胞；**nongranular leucocytes** = leucocytes without granules (lymphocytes, monocytes) 非粒白细胞

◇ **granulation** *noun* formation of rough red tissue on the surface of a wound or site of infection, the first stage in the healing process 肉芽形成；**granulation tissue** *or* **granulations** = soft tissue, consisting mainly of tiny blood vessels and fibres, which forms over a wound 肉芽组织

◇ **granule** *noun* small particle *or* grain 颗粒; **Nissl granules** *or* **Nissl bodies** = coarse granules surrounding the nucleus in the cytoplasm of nerve cells 虎斑小体(神经细胞胞浆内环绕胞核的粗糙颗粒)

◇ **granulocyte** *noun* type of leucocyte *or* white blood cell which contains granules(such as basophils, eosinophils and neutrophils) 粒细胞

◇ **granulocytopenia** *noun* usually fatal disease caused by the lowering of the number of granulocytes in the blood due to a defect in the bone marrow 粒细胞减少症

granuloma *noun* mass of granulation tissue which forms at the site of bacterial infections 肉芽肿; **granuloma inguinale** = tropical venereal disease affecting the anus and genitals in which the skin becomes covered with ulcers 腹股沟肉芽肿 (NOTE: plural is **granulomata** or **granulomas**)

◇ **granulomatosis** *noun* chronic inflammation leading to the formation of nodules 肉芽肿病; **Wegener's granulomatosis** = disease of the connective tissue in which the nasal passages and lungs are inflamed and ulcerated 弗格内氏肉芽肿病(一种结缔组织病,表现为鼻道、肺的炎症及溃疡)

◇ **granulopoiesis** *noun* normal production of granulocytes in the bone marrow 粒细胞生成

graph *noun* diagram which shows the relationship between quantities as a line 图表; **temperature graph** = graph showing how a patient's temperature rises and falls over a period of time 体温图

-graph *suffix* meaning a machine which records as pictures 记录器的

◇ **-grapher** *suffix* meaning a technician who operates a machine which records 用记录器检查的技术员; **radiographer** = technician who operates an X-ray machine X线仪技术员

◇ **-graphy** *suffix* meaning the technique of study through pictures 通过图像检查的方法; **radiography** = X-ray examination of part of the body 放射线检查

grattage *noun* scraping the surface of an ulcer which is healing slowly, in order to make it heal more quickly 刷除术(刮搔愈合缓慢的溃疡表面,促使其尽快愈合)

grave *noun* place where a dead person is buried 坟墓: ***His grave is covered with flowers*.** 他的墓上覆盖着鲜花。

gravel *noun* small stones which pass from the kidney to the urinary system, causing pain in the ureter 尿砂

Graves' disease *or* **exophthalmic goitre** = THYROTOXICOSIS 格雷夫斯氏病,甲状腺毒症,突眼性甲状腺肿

gravid *adjective* pregnant 妊娠的; **hyperemesis gravidarum** = vomiting in pregnancy 妊娠剧吐; **gravides multiparae** = women who have given birth to at least four live babies 多产妇

Grawitz tumour *noun* malignant tumour in kidney cells 格腊维茨氏瘤,肾上腺样瘤

gray 1 *adjective US* = GREY 灰的 **2** *noun* SI unit of measurement of absorbed radiation equal to 100 rads 戈瑞,吸光度的单位 *see also* 参见 RAD (NOTE: **gray** is written **Gy** with figures)

graze 1 *noun* scrape on the skin surface, making some blood flow 擦伤 **2** *verb* to scrape the skin surface 抓破,擦伤

great *adjective* large 大的: **great cerebral vein** = median vein draining the choroid plexuses of the lateral and third ventricles 大脑大静脉; **great toe** = big toe, largest of the five toes, near the inside of the foot 大跗趾 (NOTE : **great - greater - greatest**)

◇ **greater** *adjective* larger 更大的; **greater curvature** = convex line of the stomach 胃大弯 *see also* 参见 OMENTUM, TROCHANTER

◇ **greatly** *adverb* very much 非常,很

greedy *adjective* always wanting to eat a lot of food 贪婪的,馋的 (NOTE : **greedy - greedier - greediest**)

green *adjective & noun* of a colour like the colour of leaves 绿色,绿色的: ***When he saw the blood he turned green.*** 他看见血后脸立刻变绿了。

◇ **green monkey disease** = MARBURG DISEASE 绿猴病

◇ **greenstick fracture** *noun* type of fracture occurring in children, where a long bone bends, but is not completely broken 青枝骨折

grey *or US* **gray** *adjective & noun* of a colour between black and white 灰色的,灰色: ***His hair is quite grey.*** 他的头发花白了。***a grey-haired man*** 一个花白老人; **grey commissure** = part of the grey matter nearest to the central canal of the spinal cord, where axons cross over each other 灰质连合; **grey matter** = nervous tissue of a dark grey colour, formed of cell bodies and occurring in the central nervous system 灰质

> COMMENT: In the brain, grey matter encloses the white matter, but in the spinal cord, white matter encloses grey matter.
> 注释:在大脑,灰质包绕在白质外层;但在脊髓,白质包绕着灰质。

grief *noun* feeling of great sadness felt when someone dies 悲伤,居丧; **grief counsellor** = person who helps someone to cope with the feelings they have when someone, such as a close relative, dies 抚慰居丧者的人

Griffith's types *noun* various types of haemolytic streptococci, classified according to the antigens present in them 格里菲思氏分类,根据抗原对溶血性链球菌进行分类的一种

gripe *noun* pains in the abdomen 肠绞痛; **gripe water** = solution of glucose and alcohol, used to relieve gripe in babies 止痛水(一种葡萄糖和酒精的溶液)缓解婴儿腹痛

grippe *noun* influenza 流感

gristle *noun* cartilage 软骨

grocer *noun* person who sells sugar, butter, tins of food, etc. 食品杂货商

◇ **grocer's itch** *noun* form of dermatitis on the hands caused by handling flour and sugar 食品商痒病(因接触面粉和糖引起的手部皮炎)

groin *noun* junction at each side of the body where the lower abdomen joins the top of the thighs 腹股沟: ***He had a dull pain in his groin.*** 他腹股沟感觉钝痛。(NOTE: for other terms referring to the groin, see **inguinal**)

grommet *noun* tube which can be passed from the external auditory meatus into the middle ear, usually to allow fluid to drain off, as in a patient suffering from secretory otitis media 中耳引流管(从外耳道插入中耳的管道,引流液体,如用于分泌性中耳炎的患者)

groove *noun* long shallow depression in a surface 沟; **atrioventricular groove** = groove round the outside of the heart, showing the division between the atria and the ventricles 房室沟

gross anatomy *noun* study of the structure of the body which can be seen without the use of a microscope 大体解剖

ground *noun* (**a**) soil *or* earth 土地 (**b**) surface of the earth 地面

◇ **ground substance** *or* **matrix** *noun* amorphous mass of cells forming the basis of connective tissue 基质

group 1 *noun* (**a**) several people *or* animals *or* things which are all close together 一群: ***A group of patients were waiting in the surgery.*** 一群患者等候在手术室。**group practice** = practice where several doctors *or* dentists share the same office building and support services 集体行医; **group therapy** = type of psychotherapy where a group of people with the same disorder meet together with a therapist to discuss their condition and try to help each other 群体治疗 (**b**) way of putting similar things together 分组; **age group** = all people of a certain age 年龄组; **blood group** 血型 *see* 见 BLOOD **2** *verb* to bring together in a group 分组,分群: ***The drugs are***

grouped under the heading 'antibiotics'. 药物归类为"抗生素"。**blood grouping** = classifying patients according to their blood groups 根据血型分组

grow *verb* (**a**) to become taller *or* bigger 生长：***Your son has grown since I last saw him.*** 你儿子比我上次看见他时长大了。***He grew three centimetres in one year.*** 他一年长高了3厘米。(**b**) to become 成为，变：***It's growing colder at night now.*** 现在夜间变冷了。***She grew weak with hunger.*** 她因为饥饿变得虚弱。(NOTE: **grows - growing - grew - grown**)

◊ **growing pains** *noun* pains associated with adolescence, which can be a form of rheumatic fever 生长痛(见于青少年的疼痛，可以是风湿热的一种)

◊ **grown-up** *noun* adult 成人：***There are three grown-ups and ten children.*** 那儿有3个成人和10个小孩。

◊ **growth** *noun* (**a**) increase in size 增长，生长：***The disease stunts children's growth.*** 这疾病阻碍儿童的生长。***the growth in the population since 1960*** 自1960年以来人口的增长；growth factor = chemical substance produced in the body which encourages a type of cell (such as a blood cell) to grow 生长因子；**growth hormone** (**GH**) *or* **somatotrophin** = hormone secreted by the pituitary gland during deep sleep, which stimulates growth of the long bones and protein synthesis 生长激素 (NOTE: no plural for this meaning) (**b**) lump of tissue which is not natural *or* a cyst *or* a tumour 赘生物：***The doctor found she had a cancerous growth on the left breast.*** 医生发现她左乳有一癌样赘生物。***He had an operation to remove a small growth from his chin.*** 他做了去除颏部小赘生物的手术。

grumbling appendix *noun* (*informal* 非正式) chronic appendicitis, condition where the vermiform appendixis always slightly inflamed 慢性阑尾炎

GU = GASTRIC ULCER, GENITOURINARY 胃溃疡，泌尿生殖的

guanine *noun* one of the nitrogen-containing bases in DNA 鸟嘌呤

gubernaculum *noun* fibrous tissue connecting the testes in a fetus (the gonads) to the groin 引带

guide 1 *noun* person *or* book which shows you how to do something *or* what to do 引导者，指南：***Read this guide to services offered by the local authority.*** 读读这本当地机关的服务指南。***The council has produced a guide for expectant mothers.*** 协会为待产妇准备了指南。**2** *verb* to show someone where to go *or* how to do something 向导

◊ **guide dog** *noun* dog which shows a blind person where to go 导盲犬

Guillain-Barré syndrome *noun* nervous disorder, in which after a non-specific infection, demyelination of the spinal roots and peripheral nerves takes place, leading to generalized weakness and sometimes respiratory paralysis 格林巴利综合征，急性感染性多神经炎(一种神经系统疾病，非特异性感染后脊髓根和周围神经脱髓鞘，导致全身乏力，有时会引起呼吸麻痹)

guillotine *noun* surgical instrument for cutting out tonsils 铡除刀(用于切除扁桃体)

guinea worm = DRACUNCULUS 麦地那龙线虫

gullet *or* **oesophagus** *noun* tube down which food and drink passes from the mouth to the stomach 食管，咽喉：***She had a piece of bread stuck in her gullet.*** 面包卡在了她咽喉部。

gum *or* **gingiva** *noun* part of the mouth, the soft epithelial tissue covering the part of the jaw which surrounds the teeth 龈：***His gums are red and inflamed.*** 他的牙龈发红，有炎症。***A build-up of tartar can lead to gum disease.*** 牙垢形成可导致牙龈疾病。

◊ **gumboil** *noun* abscess on the gum near a tooth 牙龈脓肿 (NOTE: for other terms referring to the gums, see words beginning with **gingiv-**, **ul(o)-**)

gumma *noun* abscess of dead tissue and overgrown scar tissue, which develops in the later stages of syphilis 梅毒瘤，树胶肿

gustation *noun* act of tasting 品尝

◇ **gustatory** *noun* referring to the sense of taste 味觉

gut *noun* (**a**) (*also informal* 非正式) **guts** = digestive tract *or* alimentary canal *or* the intestines, the tubular organ for the digestion and absorption of food 肠道，消化道：***He complained of having a pain in his gut*** *or* ***he said he had gut pain*.** 他主诉消化道疼痛。(**b**) type of thread, made from the intestines of sheep, used to sew up internal incisions; it dissolves slowly so does not need to be removed 肠线 *see also* 参见 CATGUT

Guthrie test *noun* test used on babies to detect the presence of phenylketonuria 加思里氏试验，用来检查婴儿苯丙酮尿症

gutta *noun* drop of liquid (as used in treatment of the eyes) 滴 (NOTE: plural is **guttae**)

gutter splint *noun* shaped container in which a broken limb can rest without being completely surrounded 沟形夹板，用于使断肢保持在休息位而不必整个用石膏包绕

Gy *abbreviation for* (缩写) gray 戈瑞的简写

gyn- *prefix* referring to (i) woman "妇女的" (ii) the female reproductive system "女性生殖系统的"

◇ **gynaecological** *adjective* referring to the treatment of diseases of women 妇科的

◇ **gynaecologist** *noun* doctor who specializes in the treatment of diseases of women 妇科学家

◇ **gynaecology** *noun* study of female sex organs and the treatment of diseases of women in general 妇科学

◇ **gynaecomastia** *noun* abnormal development of breasts in a male 男子女性型乳房 (NOTE: words beginning with **gynae-** are spelled **gyne-** in US English)

gyrus *noun* raised part of the cerebral cortex between the sulci 脑回；**postcentral gyrus** = sensory area of the cerebral cortex, which receives impulses from receptor cells and senses pain, heat, touch, etc. 中央后回；**precentral gyrus** = motor area of the cerebral cortex 中央前回 (NOTE: plural is **gyri**)

Hh

H *chemical symbol for* hydrogen 氢的化学元素符号

HA = HEALTH AUTHORITY 卫生行政部门

habit *noun* (**a**) action which is an automatic response to a stimulus 习惯 (**b**) regular way of doing something 习惯: ***He got into the habit of swimming every day before breakfast.*** 他养成了每天早饭前游泳的习惯。***She's got out of the habit of taking any exercise.*** 她丢掉了锻炼的习惯。**from force of habit** = because you do it regularly 出于习惯: ***I wake up at 6 o'clock from force of habit.*** 出于习惯我每天6点起床。

◇ **habit-forming** *adjective* which makes someone addicted *or* which makes someone get into the habit of taking something 易成瘾的,有习惯性的; **habit-forming drugs** = drugs which are addictive 成瘾药物

◇ **habitual** *adjective* which is done frequently *or* as a matter of habit 习惯的; **habitual abortion** = condition where a woman has abortions with successive pregnancies 习惯性流产

◇ **habituation** *noun* being psychologically but not physically addicted to *or* dependent on (a drug *or* alcohol, etc.) 成瘾(心理上的,非躯体性的); ***his habituation to nicotine*** 他对尼古丁成瘾

◇ **habitus** *noun* general physical appearance of the person (including build and posture) 体型

hacking cough *noun* continuous short dry cough 频咳

haem *noun* molecule containing iron which binds proteins to form haemoproteins such as haemoglobin and myoglobin 血红素

◇ **haem-** *prefix* referring to blood 血的 (NOTE: words beginning with the prefix **haem-** are written **hem-** in US English)

◇ **haemangioma** *noun* benign tumour which forms in blood vessels and appears on the skin as a birthmark 血管瘤; **cavernous haemangioma** = tumour in connective tissue with wide spaces which contain blood 海绵状血管瘤 (NOTE: plural is **haemangiomata**)

◇ **haemarthrosis** *noun* pain and swelling caused by blood getting into a joint 关节积血

◇ **haematemesis** *noun* vomiting of blood (usually because of internal bleeding) 咯血

◇ **haematin** *noun* substance which forms from haemoglobin when bleeding takes place 正铁血红素

◇ **haematinic** *noun* drug, such as an iron compound, which increases haemoglobin in blood, used to treat anaemia 补血药

◇ **haematocoele** *noun* swelling caused by blood getting into an internal cavity 腹腔积血

◇ **haematocolpos** *noun* condition where the vagina is filled with blood at menstruation because the hymen has no opening 阴道积血

◇ **haematocrit** *noun* (i) volume of red blood cells in a patient's blood, shown as a percentage of the total blood volume 红细胞压积 (ii) instrument for measuring haematocrit 红细胞比容管

◇ **haematocyst** *noun* cyst which contains blood 血囊肿,膀胱积血

◇ **haematogenous** *adjective* (i) which produces blood; 造血的(ii) which is produced by blood 血原性的

◇ **haematological** *adjective* referring to haematology 血液学的

◇ **haematologist** *noun* doctor who specializes in haematology 血液学家

◇ **haematology** *noun* scientific study of blood, its formation and its diseases 血液学

◇ **haematoma** *noun* mass of blood under the skin caused by a blow *or* by the effects of an operation 血肿; **extradural**

haematoma = haematoma in the head, between the dura mater and the skull 硬膜外血肿; **intracerebral haematoma** = haematoma inside the cerebrum 颅内血肿; **perianal haematoma** = haematoma in the anal region 肛周血肿; **subdural haematoma** = blood plasma, clot between the dura mater and the arachnoid, which displaces the brain, caused by a blow on the head 硬膜下血肿 (NOTE: plural is **haematomata**)

◇ **haematometra** *noun* (i) excessive bleeding in the womb 子宫出血过多 (ii) swollen womb, caused by haematocolpos 子宫积血

◇ **haematomyelia** *noun* condition where blood gets into the spinal cord 脊髓出血

◇ **haematopoiesis** = HAEMOPOIESIS 血细胞生成

◇ **haematoporphyrin** *noun* porphyrin produced from haemoglobin 血卟啉

◇ **haematosalpinx** = HAEMOSALPINX 输卵管积血

◇ **haematozoon** *noun* parasite living in the blood 血原虫 (NOTE: plural is **haematozoa**)

◇ **haematuria** *noun* abnormal presence of blood in the urine, as a result of injury *or* disease of the kidney or bladder 血尿

◇ **haemochromatosis** *or* **bronze diabetes** *noun* hereditary disease in which the body absorbs and stores too much iron, causing cirrhosis of the liver, and giving the skin a dark colour 血色素沉着症(遗传性疾病,机体吸收、储存过量的铁,导致肝硬化,皮肤发黑)

◇ **haemoconcentration** *noun* increase in the percentage of red blood cells because the volume of plasma is reduced 血液浓缩 (NOTE: *opposite is* **haemodilution**)

◇ **haemocytoblast** *noun* embryonic blood cell in the bone marrow from which red and white blood cells and platelets develop 成血细胞

◇ **haemocytometer** *noun* glass jar in which a sample of blood is diluted and the blood cells counted 血细胞计数器

◇ **haemodialysis** *noun* removing waste matter from blood using a dialyser (kidney machine) 血液透析(用透析器除去血中的废物)

◇ **haemodilution** *noun* decrease in the percentage of red blood cells because the volume of plasma has increased 血液稀释 (NOTE: *opposite is* **haemoconcentration**)

◇ **haemoglobin** (**Hb**) *noun* red respiratory pigment (formed of haem and globin) in red blood cells which gives blood its red colour 血红蛋白 *see also* 参见 OXYHAEMOGLOBIN

> COMMENT: Haemoglobin absorbs oxygen in the lungs and carries it in the blood to the tissues.
> 注释:血红蛋白在肺吸收氧,经血液输送至组织。

◇ **haemoglobinaemia** *noun* haemoglobin in the plasma 血红蛋白血症

◇ **haemoglobinopathy** *noun* inherited disease where production of haemoglobin is abnormal 血红蛋白病

◇ **haemoglobinuria** *noun* condition where haemoglobin is found in the urine 血红蛋白尿

◇ **haemogram** *noun* printed result of a blood test 血象

◇ **haemolysin** *noun* protein which destroys red blood cells 溶血素

◇ **haemolysis** *noun* destruction of red blood cells 溶血

◇ **haemolytic** *adjective* (substance, such as snake venom) which destroys red blood cells 溶血的; **haemolytic anaemia** = condition where the destruction of red blood cells is about six times the normal rate, and the supply of new cells from the bone marrow cannot meet the demand 溶血性贫血(红细胞的破坏率是正常的 6 倍,超过骨髓的代偿能力); **haemolytic disease of the newborn** = condition where the red blood cells of the fetus are destroyed because antibodies in the mother's blood react against the blood of the fetus in the womb 新生儿溶

血性贫血(母体血液内的抗体与宫内的胎儿发生反应,破坏其红细胞); **haemolytic jaundice** = jaundice caused by haemolysis of red blood cells 溶血性黄疸(红细胞破坏引起的黄疸); **haemolytic uraemic syndrome** = condition in which haemolytic anaemia damages the kidneys 溶血性血尿综合征(溶血性贫血导致肾损害)

◊ **haemopericardium** *noun* blood in the pericardium 心包积血

◊ **haemoperitoneum** *noun* blood in the peritoneal cavity 腹腔积血

haemophilia A *noun* familial disease, in which inability to synthesize Factor VIII (a clotting factor), means that patient's blood clots very slowly, prolonged bleeding occurs from the slightest wound and internal bleeding can occur without any cause 血友病 A(家族性疾病,合成 VIII 因子障碍,表现为小伤口的出血时间延长和自发性内出血); **haemophilia B** *or* **Christmas disease** = clotting disorder of the blood, similar to haemophilia A, but in which the blood coagulates badly due to deficiency of Factor IX 血友病 B(凝血障碍,同血友病 A 相似,IX 严重缺乏引起)

◊ **haemophiliac** *noun* person who suffers from haemophilia 血友病患者

◊ **haemophilic** *adjective* referring to haemophilia 血友病的

COMMENT: Because haemophilia A is a sex-linked recessive characteristic, it is found only in males, but females are carriers. It can be treated by injections of Factor VIII.
注释:因为血友病是性连锁隐性遗传病,故仅男性发病,但女性是携带者,可通过注射 VIII 因子进行治疗。

Haemophilus *noun* genus of bacteria, which need certain factors in the blood to grow 嗜血杆菌; **Haemophilus influenzae** = bacterium which lives in healthy throats, but if the patient's resistance is lowered by a bout of flu, then it can cause pneumonia 流感嗜血杆菌; **Haemophilus influenzae type b** (**Hib**) = bacterium which causes meningitis 乙型流感嗜血杆菌

QUOTE: The Haemophilus influenzae type b vaccine will be introduced into the programme of immunization for children in October.
引文:乙型流感嗜血杆菌疫苗将在 10 月份列入儿童计划免疫范围。
Guardian 卫报

haemophthalmia *noun* blood in the eye 眼球积血

◊ **haemopneumothorax** = PNEUMOHAEMOTHORAX 血气胸

◊ **haemopoiesis** *noun* continual production of blood cells and blood platelets by the bone marrow 血细胞生成,造血

◊ **haemopoietic** *adjective* referring to the formation of blood 造血的

◊ **haemoptysis** *noun* condition where the patient coughs blood from the lungs, caused by a serious illness such as anaemia, pneumonia, tuberculosis or cancer 咯血; **endemic haemoptysis** = PARAGONIMIASIS 寄生虫性咯血,肺吸虫病

haemorrhage 1 *noun* bleeding where a large quantity of blood is lost, especially bleeding from a burst blood vessel 出血: ***She had a haemorrhage and was rushed to hospital.*** 她因大出血被急送入医院。***He died of a brain haemorrhage.*** 他死于脑出血。**arterial haemorrhage** = haemorrhage of bright red blood from an artery 动脉出血; **brain haemorrhage** *or* **cerebral haemorrhage** = bleeding inside the brain from a cerebral artery 脑出血; **extradural haemorrhage** = serious condition where bleeding occurs between the duramater and the skull 硬膜外出血; **internal haemorrhage** = haemorrhage which takes place inside the body 内出血; **primary haemorrhage** = haemorrhage which occurs immediately after an injury is suffered 原发性出血; **secondary haemorrhage** = haemorrhage which occurs some time after the injury, due to infection of the wound 继

发性出血；**venous haemorrhage** = haemorrhage of dark blood from a vein 静脉出血 2 *verb* to bleed heavily 大出血：***The injured man was haemorrhaging from the mouth.*** 大量的鲜血从伤者的口腔涌出。

◊ **haemorrhagic** *adjective* referring to heavy bleeding 大出血的；**haemorrhagic disease of the newborn** = disease of babies, which makes them haemorrhage easily, caused by temporary lack of prothrombin 新生儿出血性疾病；**haemorrhagic disorders** = disorders (such as haemophilia) where haemorrhages occur 出血性疾病；**haemorrhagic stroke** = stroke caused by a burst blood vessel 出血性卒中

haemorrhoids *or* **piles** *plural noun* swollen veins in the anorectal passage 痔疮；**external haemorrhoids** = haemorrhoids in the skin just outside the anus 外痔；**internal haemorrhoids** = swollen veins inside the anus 内痔；**first-degree haemorrhoids** = haemorrhoids which remain in the rectum I 度痔疮(痔疮限于直肠内)；**second-degree haemorrhoids** = haemorrhoids which protrude into the anus but return into the rectum automatically II 度痔疮(痔疮脱入肛门,但可自动退回直肠)；**third-degree haemorrhoids** = haemorrhoids which protrude into the anus permanently III 度痔疮(痔疮永久性脱入肛门)

◊ **haemorrhoidectomy** *noun* surgical removal of haemorrhoids 痔疮切除术

haemosalpinx *noun* blood accumulating in the Fallopian tubes 输卵管积血

◊ **haemosiderosis** *noun* disorder in which iron forms large deposits in the tissue, causing haemorrhaging and destruction of red blood cells 含铁血黄素沉着症(铁大量沉积于组织,引起出血和红细胞破坏)

◊ **haemostasis** *noun* stopping bleeding *or* slowing the movement of blood 止血

◊ **haemostat** *noun* device, such as a clamp, which stops bleeding 止血器

◊ **haemostatic** *adjective* & *noun* (drug) which stops bleeding 止血的,止血药

◊ **haemothorax** *noun* blood in the pleural cavity 血胸

hair *noun* (**a**) long thread growing on the body of an animal, from a small pit in the skin called a follicle (hair is mainly made up of adense form of keratin) 毛发：***He's beginning to get a few grey hairs.*** 他的头发已经开始有些灰白了。***Hairs are growing on his chest.*** 他长有胸毛。**hair cell** = cell in the organ of Corti in the ear, which senses sound vibrations in the tectorial membrane 毛细胞；**hair follicle** = tube of epidermal cells containing the root of a hair 毛囊；**hair papilla** = part of the skin containing capillaries which feed blood to the hair 毛乳头 ◊ 见图 SKIN & SENSORY RECEPTORS (NOTE: plural in this meaning is **hairs**)
(**b**) mass of hairs growing on the head 头发：***She's got long black hair.*** 她有一头乌黑的长发。***You ought to wash your hair.*** 你该洗头了。***His hair is too long.*** 他的头发太长了。***He is going to have his hair cut.*** 他要去理发。**superfluous** *or* **unwanted hair** = hair which is growing in places where it is not thought to be beautiful 体毛过重有碍美观 (NOTE: no plural in this sense. For other terms referring to hair, see words beginning with **pilo-**, **tricho**)

◊ **hairline fracture** *noun* fracture with a very thin crack 劈裂骨折

◊ **hairy** *adjective* covered with hair 毛茸茸的,有毛发的：***He's got hairy arms.*** 他胳膊上有汗毛。**hairy cell leukaemia** = form of leukaemia with abnormal white blood cells with thread-like process on them 毛细胞白血病(有丝状突起的异常白细胞增多的白血病)

> COMMENT: Hair is dead tissue and grows out of hair follicles. The follicles are tubes leading into the skin and lined with sebaceous glands

which secrete the oil which covers the hair. Hair grows on almost all parts of the body, but is thicker and stronger on the head (the scalp, the eyebrows, inside the nose and ears). After puberty, hair becomes thicker on other parts of the body (the chin, chest and limbs in men, the pubic region and the armpits in both men and women). Hair on the head stops growing in many men in middle age, giving various degrees of baldness. Certain treatments, especially chemotherapy, can cause the hair to fall out. In later middle age, hair loses its natural pigmentation and becomes grey or white.
注释:毛发是长出毛囊的死亡组织。毛囊是穿过皮肤的管状结构,覆有皮脂腺分泌油脂覆盖于毛发。毛发遍布身体的所有部位,但在头部更密更硬(如头发、眉毛、鼻毛和耳毛)。青春期后,身体其他部位的毛发开始变密(如男性的下颏、胸部、四肢;女性的耻骨区以及男女两性的腋窝)。很多男人从中年开始头发就不再生长,形成不同程度的秃顶。某些治疗,尤其是化疗也可引起脱发。中年后期,头发的色素开始丢失,变成灰白或白色。

halitosis *noun* condition where a person has breath which smells unpleasant 口臭

COMMENT: Halitosis can have several causes: caries in the teeth, infection of the gums, and indigestion are the most usual. The breath can also have an unpleasant smell during menstruation, or in association with certain diseases such as diabetes mellitus and uraemia.
注释:口臭有多种原因:龋齿、牙龈炎及消化不良是最常见的。行经期或某些疾病如糖尿病、尿毒症也可使呼吸带有难闻的气味。

hallucination *noun* seeing an imaginary scene *or* hearing an imaginary sound as clearly as if it were really there 幻觉: ***He had hallucinations and went into a coma.*** 他产生了幻觉,并进入昏迷状态。

◇ **hallucinate** *verb* to have hallucinations 产生幻觉: ***The patient was hallucinating.*** 患者产生了幻觉。

◇ **hallucinatory** *adjective* (drug, such as cannabis *or* LSD) which causes hallucinations 致幻的

◇ **hallucinogen** *noun* drug which causes hallucinations (such as cannabis *or* LSD)致幻药

◇ **hallucinogenic** *adjective* (substance) which produces hallucinations 引起幻觉的; ***a hallucinogenic fungus*** 引起幻觉的蕈类

hallux *noun* big toe 踇趾; **hallux valgus** = deformity of the foot, where the big toe turns towards the other toes and a bunion is formed on the protruding joint 踇趾外翻 (NOTE: plural is **halluces**)

hamamelis 北美金缕梅 *see* 见 WITCH HAZEL

hamartoma *noun* benign tumour containing tissue from any organ 错构瘤

hamate (bone) *or* **unciform bone** *noun* one of the eight small carpal bones in the wrist, shaped like a hook 钩骨 ◊ 见图 HAND

hammer *noun* (**a**) heavy metal tool for knocking nails into wood, etc. 锤子: ***He hit his thumb with the hammer.*** 他的拇指被锤子砸了。**hammer toe** = toe where the middle joint is permanently bent downwards 锤状趾(趾的中间关节永久性向下弯曲) (**b**) malleus, one of the three ossicles in the middle ear 锤骨

hamstring *noun* group of tendons behind the knee, which link the thigh muscles to the bones in the lower leg 腘绳肌腱; **hamstring muscles** = group of muscles at the back of the thigh, which flex the knee and extend the gluteus maximus 腘绳肌

hand 1 *noun* terminal part of the arm, beyond the wrist, which is used for holding things 手: ***He injured his hand with a saw.*** 他的手被锯伤了。***The commonest hand injuries occur at work.***

手伤最常发生于工作时。**2** *verb* to pass 递 ***Can you hand me that book***？你能递给我那本书吗？ ***He handed me the key to the cupboard.*** 他给了我碗柜的钥匙。

COMMENT：The hand is formed of twenty-seven bones：fourteen phalanges (in the fingers), five metacarpals in the main part of the hand, and eight carpals in the wrist.
注释：手由27块骨组成：14块指骨(位于手指)，中部的5块掌骨和8块腕骨。

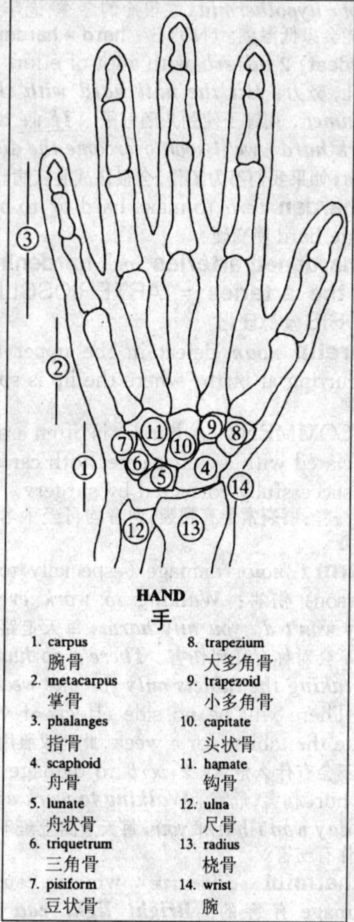

HAND
手
1. carpus 腕骨
2. metacarpus 掌骨
3. phalanges 指骨
4. scaphoid 舟骨
5. lunate 舟状骨
6. triquetrum 三角骨
7. pisiform 豆状骨
8. trapezium 大多角骨
9. trapezoid 小多角骨
10. capitate 头状骨
11. hamate 钩骨
12. ulna 尺骨
13. radius 桡骨
14. wrist 腕

handicap 1 *noun* physical or mental disability *or* condition which prevents someone from doing some normal activity 身体或智力障碍：***In spite of her handicaps, she tries to live as normal a life as possible.*** 尽管她有残疾，仍尽量设法过正常的生活。***After having both legs amputated, he fought to overcome the handicap.*** 双腿都截肢后，他努力克服身体上的障碍。**2** *verb* to prevent someone from doing a normal activity 妨碍，阻碍：***He is handicapped by only having one arm.*** 他因为只有一只胳膊而残疾。

◇ **handicapped** *adjective* (person) who suffers from a handicap 有残疾的，有障碍的；**the physically handicapped** = people with physical disabilities 躯体残疾；**the mentally handicapped** = people with impaired behavioural reactions 智力残疾

Hand-Schüller-Christian disease *noun* disturbance of cholesterol metabolism in young children which causes defects in membranous bone, mainly in the skull, exophthalmos, diabetes insipidus, and a yellow-brown colour of the skin 汉－许－克三氏病，慢性特发性黄瘤病(儿童的胆固醇代谢障碍，引起膜性骨主要是颅骨畸形、突眼、尿崩症和皮肤棕黄色)

hang *verb* to attach (something) above the ground (to a nail or hook, etc.); to be attached above the ground (to a nail or hook, etc.) 悬吊；被悬挂：***Hang your coat on the hook.*** 把你的外衣挂在钩上。***She hung the photograph over her bed.*** 她把照片挂在床头上。***His hand was almost severed, it was hanging by a band of flesh.*** 他的手几乎被切断了，仅由一小条肌肉组织相连。(NOTE：**hangs - hanging - hung - has hung**)

◇ **hangnail** *noun* piece of torn skin at the side of a nail 甲刺

◇ **hangover** *noun* condition after having drunk too much alcohol, with dehydration caused by inhibition of the antidiuretic hormone in the kidneys 宿醉(过量饮酒后，因肾脏抗利尿激素减少导致脱水)

COMMENT：The symptoms of a hangover are pain in the head, inability to stand noise and trembling of

the hands.
注释:宿醉的症状是头痛、不能耐受噪声和手颤。

Hansen's bacillus *noun Mycobacterium leprae*, the bacterium which causes leprosy 汉森氏杆菌,麻风分枝杆菌
◇ **Hansen's disease** = LEPROSY 麻风病

haploid *adjective* (cell, such as a gamete) with a single set of unpaired chromosomes 单倍体 *compare* 比较 DIPLOID, POLYPLOID

happen *verb* (**a**) to take place 发生: ***The accident happened at the corner of the street.*** 事故发生于街角。***How did it happen?*** 它是怎么发生的? ***What's happened to his brother?*** = What is his brother doing now? 他兄弟现在在干什么? (**b**) to be *or* to do something (by chance) 碰巧: ***She happened to be standing near the cooker when the fire started.*** 火着起来时她正站在炉子旁。***Luckily a doctor happened to be passing in the street when the baby fell out of the window.*** 幸运的是当婴儿从窗户上摔下来时碰巧有医生走过这条街。***Do you happen to have an antidote for snake bites?*** 你有蛇咬的解毒药吗?

hapten *noun* substance which causes an allergy, probably by changing a protein so that it becomes antigenic 半抗原(通过改变蛋白使其产生抗原性导致过敏的物质)

harbour *verb* to hold and protect 藏匿; **to harbour a disease** = to hold germs *or* bacteria and allow them to breed and spread disease *or* soiled clothing can harbour dysentery 病原隐藏处; ***Stagnant water harbours malaria mosquitoes.*** 停滞不动的水藏有可传播疟疾的蚊子。

hard 1 *adjective* (**a**) not soft 硬的: ***This bed is not too hard — a hard bed is good for someone suffering from back problems.*** 这床不太硬——硬床对患背部疾病的人有好处。***If you have a slipped disc, you will be made to lie on a hard surface for several weeks.*** 如果患有椎间盘突出,你应该在硬的平板上躺几周。**hard palate** = front part of the roof of the mouth between the upper teeth 硬腭; **hard water** = tap water which contains a high percentage of calcium 硬质水 (**b**) difficult 困难的: ***If the exam is too hard, nobody will pass.*** 如果考试很难的话,不会有人通过。***He's hard of hearing.*** = He's rather deaf. 他耳背。(**c**) **a hard winter** = a very cold winter 寒冷的冬季: ***In a hard winter, old people can suffer from hypothermia.*** 在很冷的冬季,老年人可能会患低温症。(NOTE: **hard - harder - hardest**) **2** *adverb* with a lot of effort 使劲儿,努力: ***Hit the nail hard with the hammer.*** 用锤子使劲儿砸钉子。***If we all work hard, we'll soon overcome the disease.*** 如果我们努力工作,会很快战胜疾病。
◇ **harden** *verb* to make hard *or* to become hard 使变硬
◇ **hardened arteries** *or* **hardening of the arteries** = ARTERIOSCLEROSIS 动脉硬化

harelip *noun* defect in the upper lip occurring at birth, where the lip is split 唇裂

COMMENT: A harelip is often associated with a cleft palate. Both can be successfully corrected by surgery.
注释:唇裂常伴有腭裂,两者均可经手术纠正。

harm 1 *noun* damage (especially to a person) 伤害: ***Walking to work every day won't do you any harm.*** 每天走路上班不会对你有任何伤害。***There's no harm in taking the tablets only for one week.*** = There will be no side effects if you take the tablets for a week. 此药仅服用一周不会有什么危害。**2** *verb* to damage *or* to hurt 伤害,危害: ***Walking to work every day won't harm you.*** 每天走路上班不会对你有伤害。
◇ **harmful** *adjective* which causes damage 有害的: ***Bright light can be harmful to your eyes.*** 明亮的光线对你的眼睛有害。***Sudden violent exercise can be harmful.*** 突然的剧烈运动是有害的。
◇ **harmless** *adjective* which causes no

damage 无害的: ***These herbal remedies are quite harmless.*** 这些草药完全无害。

Harrison's sulcus *noun* hollow on either side of the chest which develops in children who have rickets and breathe in with difficulty 郝氏沟

Harris's operation *noun* surgical removal of the prostate gland 哈里斯手术,前列腺切除术

Hartmann's solution *noun* chemical solution used in drips to replace body fluids lost in dehydration, particularly as a result of infantile gastroenteritis 哈特曼氏溶液(用来补充脱水尤其是婴儿患胃肠炎时丢失的体液)

Hartnup disease *noun* condition caused by a hereditary defect in amino acid metabolism, producing thick skin and retarded mental development 海特那普病(遗传性氨基酸代谢缺陷,引起肤色加深,智力发育停滞)

harvest *verb* to take a piece of skin for a graft 采集

◇ **harvest mite** *or* **harvest tick** = CHIGGER 恙螨

Hashimoto's disease *noun* type of goitre in middle-aged women, where the patient is sensitive to secretions from her own thyroid gland, and, in extreme cases, the face swells and the skin turns yellow 桥本氏病(中年妇女发生的一种甲状腺肿,表现为对自身甲状腺分泌的激素敏感,严重时面部肿胀,皮肤发黄)

hashish *or* **cannabis** *or* **marijuana** *noun* addictive drug made from the leaves *or* flowers of the Indian hemp plant 大麻(成瘾药物)

haustrum *noun* sac on the outside of the colon 结肠袋 (NOTE: plural is **haustra**)

HAV = HEPATITIS A VIRUS 甲型肝炎病毒

Haversian canal *noun* fine canal which runs vertically through the Haversian systems in compact bone, containing blood vessels and lymph ducts 哈佛管

◇ **Haversian system** *noun* osteon, unit of compact bone built around a Haversian canal, made of a series of bony layers which form a cylinder 哈佛系统

hay fever *or* **allergic rhinitis** *or* **pollinosis** *noun* inflammation in the nasal passage and eyes caused by an allergic reaction to flowers and their pollen and scent, also to dust 枯草热(因对花朵、花粉、花香或尘土过敏引起鼻道和眼的炎症反应): ***When he has hay fever, he has to stay indoors.*** 他患枯草热时不得不待在屋内。***The hay fever season starts in May.*** 枯草热季节开始于5月。

H band *noun* part of pattern in muscle tissue, a light band in the dark A band, seen through a microscope H带(显微镜下,肌肉组织暗带A中的亮带)

Hb = HAEMOGLOBIN 血红蛋白

HBV = HEPATITIS B VIRUS 乙型肝炎病毒

hCG = HUMAN CHORIONIC GONADOTROPHIN 人绒毛膜促性腺激素

HDL = HIGH DENSITY LIPOPROTEIN 高密度脂蛋白

He *chemical symbol for* helium 氦的化学元素符号

head 1 *noun* (**a**) top part of the body, which contains the eyes, nose, mouth, brain, etc. 头部: ***Can you stand on your head?*** 你能倒立吗? ***He hit his head on the lowbranch.*** 矮树枝碰了他的头。***He shook his head.*** = He moved his head from side to side to mean 'no'. 他摇了摇头。**head lice** = small insects of the *Pediculus* genus, which live on the scalp and suck the blood of the host 头虱 (NOTE: for other terms referring to the head, see words beginning with **cephal-**) (**b**) first place 首位: ***He stood at the head of the queue.*** 他站在队伍的第一位。***who's name is at the head of the list*** ? 谁的名字排在名单的首位? (**c**) (i) rounded top part of a bone which fits into a socket (骨)头 (ii) round main part of a spermatozoon 精子的头部; ***head of humerus*** 肱骨头; ***head of radius*** 桡骨头;

the head of a sperm 精子头; **head of femur** = rounded projecting end part of the thigh bone which joins the acetabulum at the hip 股骨头 (**d**) most important person 首脑,重要的人物: ***He's the head of the anatomy department.*** 他是解剖系的主任。***She was head of the research unit for some years.*** 她曾担任过几年研究组的领导。**2** *verb* (**a**) to be the first *or* to lead 站在前头,领导: ***His name heads the list.*** 他的名字在名单的第一位。(**b**) to go towards 向前: ***They are heading north.*** 他们向北走。***He headed for the administrator's office.*** 他向管理员办公室走去。

◇ **headache** *noun* pain in the head, caused by changes in pressure in the blood vessels feeding the brain which act on the nerves 头痛: ***I must lie down — I've got a headache.*** 我必须躺下——我头痛。***She can't come with us because she has got a headache.*** 因为头痛,她不能和我们在一起。**cluster headache** = headache which occurs behind one eye for a short period 阵发性头痛; **migraine headache** = very severe throbbing headache which can be accompanied by nausea, vomiting, visual disturbance and vertigo 偏头痛; **tension headache** *or* **muscular contraction headache** = headache over all the head, caused by worry *or* stress, and thought to result from chronic contraction of the muscles of the scalp and neck 紧张性头痛

> COMMENT: Headaches can be caused by a blow to the head, by lack of sleep or food, by eye strain, sinus infections and many other causes. Mild headaches can be treated with aspirin and rest. Severe headaches which recur may be caused by serious disorders in the head or nervous system.
> 注释:头痛可以因头部受到打击、睡眠或饮食缺乏、眼疲劳、鼻窦炎或其他原因引起。轻微头痛可服用阿司匹林或经休息治疗,头部或神经系统的严重疾病可导致反复发作的剧烈头痛。

heal *verb* (*of wound*) to mend *or* to become better 愈合: ***After six weeks, his wound had still not healed.*** 过去6周了他的伤口还没有愈合。***A minor cut will heal faster if it is left without a bandage.*** 小的伤口如果不用绷带包扎的话,会愈合得更快。

◇ **healing** *noun* process of getting better 痊愈: ***A substance which will accelerate the healing process.*** 可加速愈合的物质。

health *noun* being well *or* not being ill; state of being free from physical *or* mental disease 健康: ***He's in good health.*** 他很健康。***She had suffered from bad health for some years.*** 她身体不好已经有几年了。***The council said that fumes from the factory were a danger to public health.*** 委员会说工厂放出的烟雾对公众的健康有害。***All cigarette packets carry a government health warning.*** 所有的烟盒上都印有政府的健康警告。**Medical Officer of Health** (**MOH**) = formerly, a local government official in charge of the health services in an area 卫生官员; **Health and Safety at Work Act** = Act of Parliament which rules how the health of workers should be protected by the companies they work for 劳动法; **District Health Authority** (**DHA** *or* **HA**) = administrative unit in the National Health Service which is responsible for health services in a district 地区卫生部门; **Regional Health Authority** (**RHA**) = administrative unit in the National Health Service which is responsible for planning the health service in a region 地段卫生部门; **health care** = general treatment of patients, especially using preventive measures to stop a disease from occurring 卫生保健; **health centre** = public building in which a group of doctors practise, which contains a children's clinic, etc. 卫生中心; **health education** = teaching people (school children and adults) to do things to improve their health, such as taking more exercise, stopping smoking, etc. 健康教育; **health insurance** = insurance which pays the cost of treatment for illness, especially when travelling abroad 健康保险; *US* **Health Maintenance Organization** (**HMO**) = private doctors' practice offering health care to patients who pay a regular subscription 私立保健组织; **Environmental Health Officer** (**EHO**) *or* **Public Health Inspector** = official of a local authority who examines the environment and tests for air pollution *or* bad sanitation *or* noise pollution, etc. 环境卫生官员,公共卫生检查员; **health service** = organization in a district *or* country which is in charge of doctors, hospitals, etc. 卫生局; **National Health Service** (**NHS**) = British organization which provides medical services free of charge or at a low cost, to the whole population 国家保健事业; **Health Service Commissioner** *or* **Health Service Ombudsman** = official who investigates complaints from the public about the National Health Service 保健事业督察员; **health tax** = tax which will be used to help fund the health service 卫生保健税: ***They have proposed a health tax on tobacco.*** 他们提出了一项对烟草征收卫生保健税的提案。**health visitor** = registered nurse with qualifications in obstetrics, midwifery and preventive medicine, who visits babies and sick patients at home and advises on treatment 保健访视员

◇ **healthy** *adjective* (i) well *or* not ill 健康的 (ii) likely to make you well 有益健康的: ***Being a farmer is a healthy job.*** 做农场主是一项有益健康的工作。***People are healthier than they were fifty years ago.*** 人们比 50 年前要更加健康。***This town is the healthiest place in England.*** 这个小镇是英格兰最有益于健康的地方。***If you eat a healthy diet and take plenty of exercise there is no reason why you should fall ill.*** 如果吃有益健康的食物,并做大量的运动,你就不会生病。(NOTE: **healthy - healthier - healthiest**)

QUOTE: In the UK, the main screen is carried out by health visitors at 6–10 months.
引文:在英国,主要的筛查工作是由卫生访视员每隔 6–10 月开展一次。
Lancet 柳叶刀杂志

QUOTE: Large numbers of women are dying of cervical cancer in health authorities where the longest backlog of smear tests exists.
引文:在宫颈涂片积压时间最长的卫生局,大量妇女死于宫颈癌。
Nursing Times 护理时代

QUOTE: The HA told the Health Ombudsman that nursing staff and students now received full training in the use of the nursing process.
引文:区卫生局告知保健事业督察员:护理人员和学生们都已接受了应用护理过程的全部训练。
Nursing Times 护理时代

QUOTE: Occupational health nurses should be part of health care teams in local health centres.
引文:职业保健护士应当是当地保健中心卫生保健队伍的成员。
Nursing Times 护理时代

hear *verb* (**a**) to sense sounds with the ears 听: ***Can you hear footsteps?*** 你能听见脚步声吗? ***I can't hear what you're saying because of the noise of the aircraft.*** 因为飞机的噪声我听不见你说什么。***I heard her shut the front door.*** 我听见她关了前门。***He must be getting deaf, because often he doesn't hear the telephone.*** 他一定开始耳背了,因为他经常听不见电话铃响。(**b**) to get information 听说: ***Have you heard that the Prime Minister has died?*** 你听说总理去世了吗? ***Where did you hear about the new drug for treating AIDS?*** 你从哪儿听说这种可治疗艾滋病的新药的? (NOTE: **hears - hearing - heard - has heard**)

◇ **hearing** *noun* ability to hear; function performed by the ear of sensing sounds and sending sound impulses to the brain 听力: ***His hearing is failing.*** 他的听力下降了。***She suffers from bad hearing.*** 她的听力不好。**hearing aid** = tiny electronic device fitted into or near the ear, to improve the hearing of a deaf person by making sounds louder. 助听器 (NOTE: for other terms referring to hearing, see words beginning with **audi-**)

heart *noun* main organ in the body, which maintains the circulation of the blood around the body by its pumping action 心脏: ***The doctor listened to his heart.*** 医生对他的心脏进行听诊。***She has heart trouble.*** 她患有心脏病。**chambers of the heart** = the two sections (an atrium and a ventricle) of each side of the heart 心腔; **heart block** = slowing of the action of the heart because the impulses from the SA node to the ventricles are delayed or interrupted 传导阻滞; **heart disease** = any disease of the heart in general 心脏病: ***He has a long history of heart disease.*** 他有长期心脏病史。**heart failure** = failure of the heart to maintain the output of blood to meet the demands of the body 心力衰竭; **heart massage** = treatment to make a heart which has stopped beating start working again 心脏按摩; **heart murmur** = abnormal sound made by turbulent flow, usually the result of an abnormality in the structure of the heart 心脏杂音; **heart rate** = number of times the heart beats per minute 心率; **heart sounds** = two different sounds made by the heart as it beats 心音 *see* 见 LUBB-DUPP; **heart stoppage** = situation where the heart has stopped beating 心脏停搏; **heart surgeon** = surgeon who specializes in operations on the heart 心脏外科医生; **heart surgery** = surgical operation to remedy a condition of the heart 心脏外科; **heart transplant** = surgical operation to transplant a heart into a patient 心脏移植

◇ **heart attack** *noun* condition where the heart suffers from defective blood supply because one of the arteries becomes blocked by a blood clot (coronary thrombosis), causing myocardial ischaemia and myocardial infarction 心脏病急性发作

◇ **heartbeat** *noun* regular noise made by the heart as it pumps blood 心跳

◇ **heartburn** *or* **pyrosis** *noun* indigestion, causing a burning feeling in the abdomen and oesophagus, and a flow of acid saliva into the mouth 烧心,胃灼热

◇ **heart-lung** *noun* referring to both the heart and the lungs 心肺; **heart-lung machine** *or* **cardiopulmonary bypass** = machine used to pump blood round the body of a patient and maintain the supply of oxygen to the blood during heart surgery 心肺机,心肺转流机; **heart-lung transplant** = operation to transplant a new heart and lungs into a patient 心肺移植 (NOTE: for other terms referring to the heart, see also words beginning with **card-** or **cardi**)

> COMMENT: The heart is situated slightly to the left of the central part of the chest, between the lungs. It is divided into two parts by a vertical septum; each half is itself divided into an upper chamber (the atrium) and a lower chamber (the ventricle). The veins bring blood from the body into the right atrium; from there it passes into the right ventricle and is pumped into the pulmonary artery which takes it to the lungs. Oxygenated blood returns from the lungs to the left atrium, passes to the left ventricle and from there is pumped into the aorta for circulation round the arteries. The heart expands and contracts by the force of the heart muscle (the myocardium) under impulses from the sinoatrial node, and a normal heart beats about 70 times a minute; the contracting beat as it pumps blood out (the systole) is followed by a weaker diastole, where

the muscles relax to allow blood to flow back into the heart. In a heart attack, part of the myocardium is deprived of blood because of a clot in a coronary artery; this has an effect on the rhythm of the heartbeat and can be fatal. In heart block, impulses from the sinoatrial node fail to reach the ventricles properly; there are either longer impulses (first degree block) or missing impulses (second degree block) or no impulses at all (complete heartblock), in which case the ventricles continue to beat slowly and independently of the SA node.
注释：心脏位于胸腔略偏左处，两肺之间。由室间隔分为两部分，每一部分再分为上腔(心房)和下腔(心室)。静脉收集全身的血液进入右心房，经右心室泵入肺动脉到达肺脏。从肺脏来的氧合血回到左心房经左心室泵入主动脉，进入动脉循环。心脏在窦房结冲动的控制下由心肌的运动而扩张、收缩，正常的心率是每分钟 70 次。心脏收缩时泵出血液，舒张期心肌舒张，血液流回心脏。心脏卒中时因为冠脉堵塞，部分心肌缺血，这可影响心跳节律甚至是致命的。传导阻滞时，窦房结产生的冲动不能正常到达心室，表现为传导延长(I 度传导阻滞)，冲动丢失(II 度传导阻滞)或完全没有冲动传导(完全传导阻滞)，此时心室可不受窦房结控制，继续缓慢跳动。

heat 1 *noun* being hot 热：***The heat of the sun made the road melt.*** 太阳的热力使马路融化。**heat cramp** = cramp produced by loss of salt from the body in very hot conditions 中暑性痉挛；**heat exhaustion** = collapse due to overexertion in hot conditions 中暑衰竭；**heat rash** = MILIARIA 痱子；**heat spots** = little red spots which develop on the face in very hot weather 热疹；**heat treatment** *or* **heat therapy** = using heat (from hot lamps *or* hot water) to treat certain conditions, such as arthritis and bad circulation 热疗 **2** *verb* to make hot 加热：***The solution should be heated to 25℃.*** 溶液应加热至摄氏 25 度。

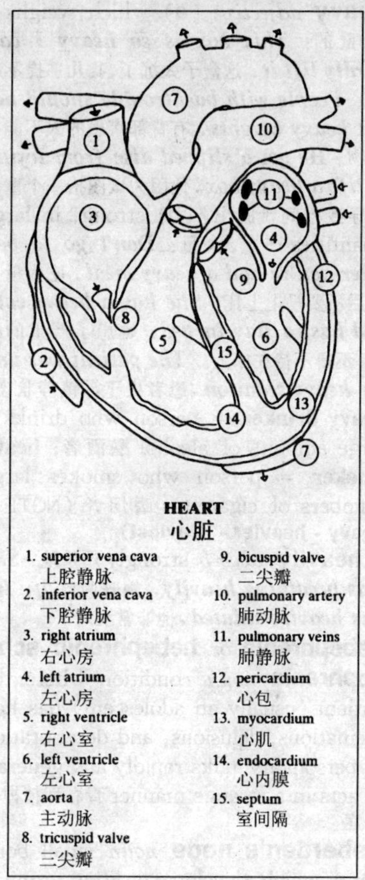

HEART
心脏

1. superior vena cava 上腔静脉
2. inferior vena cava 下腔静脉
3. right atrium 右心房
4. left atrium 左心房
5. right ventricle 右心室
6. left ventricle 左心室
7. aorta 主动脉
8. tricuspid valve 三尖瓣
9. bicuspid valve 二尖瓣
10. pulmonary artery 肺动脉
11. pulmonary veins 肺静脉
12. pericardium 心包
13. myocardium 心肌
14. endocardium 心内膜
15. septum 室间隔

◇ **heatstroke** *noun* condition where the patient becomes too hot and his body temperature rises abnormally 中暑

COMMENT: Heat exhaustion involves loss of salt and body fluids; heat stroke is also caused by high outside temperatures, but in this case the body is incapable of producing sweat and the body temperature rises, leading to headaches, stomach cramps and sometimes loss of consciousness.
注释：热衰竭伴有盐和体液的丢失；中暑也是由外界高温引起，但此时机体不能出汗散热，体温升高，导致头痛、胃痉挛，有时意识丧失。

heavy *adjective* (**a**) which weighs a lot 重的：***This box is so heavy I can hardly lift it.*** 这盒子太沉了，我几乎提不起来。***People with backtrouble should not lift heavy weights.*** 有背部疾患的人不能提重物。***He got a slipped disc from trying to lift a heavy box.*** 他因为试图抬一个重盒子导致椎间盘脱出。(**b**) strong; in large quantities 严重，大量：***Don't go to bed after you've had a heavy meal.*** 吃大量食物后不要马上上床。***She has a heavy cold and has to stay in bed.*** 她患了严重的感冒，不得不待在床上。***The patient was under heavy sedation.*** 患者处于深镇静状态。**heavy drinker** = person who drinks a large amount of alcohol 酗酒者；**heavy smoker** = person who smokes large numbers of cigarettes 嗜烟者（NOTE：**heavy - heavier - heaviest**）

◊ **heavily** *adverb* strongly 严重地：***She was breathing heavily.*** 她呼吸吃力。***He was heavily sedated.*** 他非常沉着。

hebephrenia *or* **hebephrenic schizophrenia** *noun* condition where the patient (usually an adolescent) has hallucinations, delusions, and deterioration of personality, talks rapidly and generally acts in a strange manner 青春型精神分裂症

Heberden's node *noun* small bony lump which develops on the terminal phalanges of fingers in osteoarthritis 希伯登氏结节，骨关节炎时指关节末端的骨性突起

hebetude *noun* stupidity *or* dullness of the senses during acute fever *or* being uninterested in one's surroundings and not responding to stimuli 精神迟钝

hectic *adjective* which recurs regularly 有规律发生的；**hectic fever** = attack of fever which occurs each day in patients suffering from tuberculosis 痨病热

heel *noun* (**a**) back part of the foot 脚后跟；**heel bone** *or* **calcaneus** = bone forming the heel, beneath the talus 跟骨 (**b**) block under the back part of a shoe 鞋跟：***She wore shoes with very high heels.*** 她穿了双后跟很高的鞋。

Hegar's sign *noun* way of detecting pregnancy, by inserting the fingers into the womb and pressing with the other hand on the pelvic cavity to feel if the neck of the uterus has become soft 黑加氏征，宫颈变软，为妊娠的指征

height *noun* (**a**) measurement of how tall *or* how high someone *or* something is 高度：***He is of above average height.*** 他高于平均身高。***The patient's height is 1.23m.*** 患者的身高是1.23米。(**b**) high place 高处：***He has a fear of heights.*** 他恐高。

helcoplasty *noun* skin graft to cover an ulcer to aid healing 溃疡成形术

heliotherapy *noun* treatment of patients by sunlight *or* sunbathing 日光疗法

helium *noun* very light gas used in combination with oxygen, especially to relieve asthma *or* sickness caused by decompression 氦（NOTE：chemical symbol is **He**）

helix *noun* curved outer edge of the ear 耳轮

Heller's operation = CARDIOMYOTOMY 海勒氏手术，贲门肌切开术

◊ **Heller's test** *noun* test for protein in the urine 海勒氏试验，用来检测尿蛋白

helminth *noun* general term for a parasitic worm (such as a tapeworm *or* fluke) 蠕虫

◊ **helminthiasis** *noun* infestation with parasitic worms 蠕虫病

heloma *noun* corn, hard lump of skin, usually on the foot or hand where something has pressed or rubbed against the skin 鸡眼

help 1 *noun* (**a**) something which makes it easier for you to do something 帮助：***He cut his nails with the help of a pair of scissors.*** 他用一把剪刀剪指甲。***Do you need any help with the patients?*** 需要帮助你照顾患者吗？**home help** = person who helps an invalid or handicapped person in their house by doing house work 家务帮手,保姆(**b**) making someone safe 救助: ***They went to his help.*** = They went to rescue him. 他们过去对他进行救助。***She was calling for help.*** 她寻求帮助。***They phoned the police for help.*** 他们给警察局打电话求助。**2** *verb* (**a**) to make it easier for someone to do something 帮助: ***She has a home help to help her with the housework.*** 她雇了保姆帮她做家务。***She got another nurse to help put the patients to bed.*** 她找另一护士帮忙将患者放在床上。***He helped the old lady across the street.*** 他帮助那位年老的女士过街。(**b**) (used with **cannot**) not to be able to stop doing something 禁不住做…: ***She can't help dribbling.*** 她忍不住流口水。***He can't help it if he's deaf.*** 如果他聋了就无能为力了。**3** *interjection* **help**! = call showing that someone is in difficulties 救命: ***Help! help! call a doctor quickly!*** 救命! 救命! 快叫大夫! ***Help, the patient is vomiting blood!*** 救命! 病人吐血了!

◇ **helper** *noun* person who helps 提供帮助者

◇ **helpful** *adjective* which helps 有帮助的,有益的

◇ **helping hand** *noun* handle *or* grip fitted to a wall, bath side, etc. to help a patient to stand up, etc. 把手

◇ **helpless** *adjective* not able to do anything 无助的

hem- 血 *US see* 见 HAEM-

hemeralopia *or* **day blindness** *noun* being able to see better in bad light than in ordinary daylight (usually a congenital condition) 昼盲症

hemi- *prefix* meaning half 半

◇ **hemianopia** *noun* state of partial blindness, where the patient has only half the normal field of vision in each eye 偏盲

◇ **hemiatrophy** *noun* condition where half of the body *or* half of an organ or part is atrophied 半侧萎缩

◇ **hemiballismus** *noun* sudden movement of the limbs on one side of the body, caused by a disease of the basal ganglia 抽搐

◇ **hemicolectomy** *noun* surgical removal of part of the colon 结肠部分切除术

◇ **hemicrania** *noun* headache *or* migraine in one side of the head 偏头痛

◇ **hemimelia** *noun* congenital condition where the patient has excessively short or defective arms and legs 半肢畸形

◇ **hemiparesis** *noun* slight paralysis of the muscles of one side of the body 轻偏瘫

◇ **hemiplegia** *noun* severe paralysis affecting one side of the body due to damage of the central nervous system 偏瘫 *compare* 比较 DIPLEGIA

◇ **hemiplegic** *adjective* referring to paralysis of one side of the body 偏瘫的

◇ **hemisphere** *noun* half of a sphere 半球; **cerebral hemisphere** = one of the two halves of the cerebrum 大脑半球

hemp 大麻 *see* 见 INDIAN HEMP

Henle's loop 享利袢,髓袢 *see* 见 LOOP

Henoch's purpura *noun* blood disorder of children, where the skin becomes dark blue and they suffer abdominal pains 神经性紫癜,儿童的血液疾病,皮肤青紫及腹痛

heparin *noun* anticoagulant substance found in the liver and lungs, and also produced artificially for use in the treatment of thrombosis 肝素

hepat- *or* **hepato-** *prefix* referring to the liver 肝的

◇ **hepatalgia** *noun* pain in the liver 肝痛

◇ **hepatectomy** *noun* surgical removal of part of the liver 肝切除术

◇ **hepatic** *adjective* referring to the liver 肝的; **hepatic artery** = artery which takes the blood to the liver 肝动脉; **hepatic cells** = epithelial cells of the liver acini 肝细胞; **hepatic duct** = duct which links the liver to the bile duct leading to the duodenum 肝管; **common hepatic duct** = duct from the liver formed when the right and left hepatic ducts join 总胆管; **hepatic flexure** = bend in the colon, where the ascending and transverse colons join 肝曲; **hepatic portal system** = group of veins linking to form the portal vein, which brings blood from the pancreas, spleen, gall bladder and the abdominal part of the alimentary canal to the liver 肝门静脉; **hepatic vein** = vein which takes blood from the liver to the inferior venacava 肝静脉

◇ **hepaticostomy** *noun* surgical operation to make an opening in the hepatic duct taking bile from the liver 肝管造口术

◇ **hepatis**肝 *see* 见 PORTA

hepatitis *noun* inflammation of the liver 肝炎; **infectious virus hepatitis** *or* **infective hepatitis** *or* **hepatitis A** = hepatitis transmitted by a carrier through food or drink 传染性病毒肝炎,甲型肝炎 **hepatitis A virus (HAV)** = virus which causes hepatitis A 甲型肝炎病毒; **serum hepatitis** *or* **hepatitis B** *or* **B viral hepatitis** = serious form of hepatitis transmitted by infected blood *or* unsterilized surgical instruments *or* shared needles *or* sexual intercourse 血清型肝炎,乙型肝炎; **hepatitis B virus (HBV)** = virus which causes hepatitis B 乙型肝炎病毒; **hepatitis delta** *or* **delta hepatitis** = severe form of hepatitis caused by the delta virus 丁型肝炎

> COMMENT: Infectious hepatitis and serum hepatitis are caused by different viruses (called A and B), and having had one does not give immunity against an attack of the other. Hepatitis B is more serious than the A form, and can vary in severity from a mild gastrointestinal upset to severe liver failure and death.
> 注释:传染性肝炎和血清型肝炎由不同的肝炎病毒(甲、乙)引起,感染其中一种不能对另一种产生免疫力。乙型肝炎比甲型更严重,其程度从轻度的胃肠道不适到严重的肝衰竭和死亡。

hepatoblastoma *noun* malignant tumour in the liver, made up of epithelial-type cells often with areas of immature cartilage and embryonic bone 肝母细胞瘤

◇ **hepatocele** *noun* hernia of the liver through the diaphragm or the abdominal wall 肝突出

◇ **hepatocellular** *adjective* referring to liver cells 肝细胞的; **hepatocellular jaundice** = jaundice caused by injury to *or* disease of the liver cells 肝细胞性黄疸

◇ **hepatocirrhosis** = CIRRHOSIS OF THE LIVER 肝硬化

◇ **hepatocolic ligament** *noun* ligament which links the gall bladder and the right flexure of the colon 肝结肠韧带

◇ **hepatocyte** *noun* liver cell which synthesizes and stores substances, and produces bile 肝细胞

◇ **hepatolenticular degeneration** = WILSON'S DISEASE 肝豆状核变性

◇ **hepatoma** *noun* malignant tumour of the liver formed of mature cells, especially found in patients with cirrhosis 肝细胞瘤

◇ **hepatomegaly** *noun* condition where the liver becomes very large 肝肿大

◇ **hepatotoxic** *adjective* which destroys the liver cells 肝细胞毒性的

herald patch *noun* small spot of a rash (such as pityriasis rosea) which appears some time before the main rash 前驱斑

herb *noun* plant which can be used as a medicine *or* to give a certain taste to food *or* to give a certain scent 草药

◇ **herbal** *adjective* referring to herbs 草药的; **herbal remedies** = remedies made from plants, such as infusions made from dried leaves or flowers in hot water 草药提取物

◇ **herbalism** *noun* science of treatment of illnesses *or* disorders by medicines extracted from plants 草药学

◇ **herbalist** *noun* person who treats

illnesses *or* disorders by medicine extracted from plants 草药郎中

hereditary *adjective* which is transmitted from parents to children 遗传的

◇ **heredity** *noun* occurrence of physical *or* mental characteristics in children which are inherited from their parents 遗传

COMMENT: The characteristics which are most commonly inherited are the pigmentation of skin and hair, eyes (including pigmentation, shortsightedness and other eye defects), blood grouping, and disorders which are caused by defects in blood composition, such as haemophilia.
注释:最常见的可遗传特征是皮肤和头发的颜色、眼睛(包括颜色、近视及其它眼部缺陷)、血型及其它因血液中成分的缺陷导致的疾病,如:血友病。

Hering-Breuer reflex *noun* reflex which regulates breathing 赫-布二氏反射,迷走神经反射

hermaphrodite *noun* person with both male and female characteristics 两性人

◇ **hermaphroditism** *noun* condition where a person has both male and female characteristics 两性畸形

hernia *noun* condition where an organ bulges through a hole *or* weakness in the wall which surrounds it 疝; **diaphragmatic hernia** = condition where the abdominal contents pass through an opening in the diaphragm into the chest 膈疝 (NOTE: also called in US English **upside-down stomach**); **femoral hernia** = hernia of the bowel at the top of the thigh 股疝; **hiatus hernia** = hernia where the stomach bulges through the opening in the diaphragm muscle through which the oesophagus passes 食管裂孔疝; **incisional hernia** = hernia which breaks through the abdominal wall at a place where a surgical incision was made during an operation 切口疝; **inguinal hernia** = hernia where the intestine bulges through the muscles in the groin 腹股沟疝; **irreducible hernia** = hernia where the organ cannot be returned to its normal position 难复性疝; **reducible hernia** = hernia where the organ can be pushed back into place without an operation 可复性疝; **strangulated hernia** = condition where part of the intestine is squeezed in a hernia and the supply of blood to it is cut off 绞窄性疝; **umbilical hernia** *or* **exomphalos** = hernia which bulges at the navel, usually in young children 脐疝

◇ **hernial** *adjective* referring to a hernia 疝的; **hernial sac** = sac formed where a membrane has pushed through a cavity in the body 疝囊

◇ **herniated** *adjective* (organ) which has developed a hernia 成疝的

◇ **herniation** *noun* development of a hernia 疝形成

◇ **hernioplasty** *noun* surgical operation to reduce a hernia 疝根治术

◇ **herniorrhaphy** *noun* radical surgical operation to repair a hernia 疝缝术

◇ **herniotomy** *noun* surgical operation to relieve a hernia which results in its reduction 疝切开术

heroin *noun* narcotic drug, a white powder derived from morphine 海洛因

herpangina *noun* infectious disease of children, where the tonsils and back of the throat become inflamed and ulcerated, caused by a Coxsackie virus 疱疹性咽峡炎

herpes *noun* inflammation of the skin or mucous membrane, caused by a virus, where small blisters are formed 疱疹; **herpes simplex (Type I)** *or* **cold sore** = burning sore, usually on the lips 单纯疱疹; **herpes simplex (Type II)** *or* **genital herpes** = sexually transmitted disease which forms blisters in the genital region 生殖器疱疹; **herpes zoster** *or* **shingles** *or* **zona** = inflammation of a sensory nerve, characterized by pain along the nerve causing a line of blisters to form on the skin, usually found mainly on the abdomen or back, or on the face 带状疱疹

◇ **herpesvirus** *noun* one of a group of viruses which cause herpes and chickenpox(herpesvirus Type I), and genital herpes (herpesvirus Type II) 疱疹病毒

◇ **herpetic** *adjective* referring to herpes 疱疹的; **post herpetic neuralgia** = pains felt after an attack of shingles 疱疹后神经痛

◇ **herpetiformis**疱疹样的 *see* 见 DERMATITIS

> COMMENT: Because the same virus causes herpes and chickenpox, anyone who has had chickenpox as a child carries the dormant herpesvirus in his bloodstream and can develop shingles in later life. It is not known what triggers the development of shingles, though it is known that an adult suffering from shingles can infect a child with chickenpox.
> 注释:疱疹和水痘由同一种病毒引起,童年患有水痘的人其血液中可带有潜伏的疱疹病毒,在成年后发作带状疱疹。尽管已知患有此病的成人可使儿童感染水痘,但带状疱疹发生的因素尚不清楚。

hetero- *prefix* meaning different 不同的

◇ **heterochromia** *noun* condition where the irises of the eyes are different colours 异色性,两眼虹膜的颜色不同

◇ **heterogametic** *adjective* (person) who produces gametes with different sex chromosomes(as a human male) 异型配子的 *see* 见 *note at* SEX

◇ **heterogeneous** *adjective* having different characteristics *or* qualities 异质的

◇ **heterogenous** *adjective* coming from a different source 异源的

◇ **heterograft** *noun* tissue taken from one species and grafted onto an individual of another species 异种移植物

◇ **heterophoria** *noun* condition where if an eye is covered it tends to squint 隐斜视

◇ **heteropsia** *noun* condition where the two eyes see differently 两眼不等视

◇ **heterosexual 1** *adjective* referring to the normal relation of the two sexes 异性的 **2** *noun* person who is sexually attracted to persons of the opposite sex 异性恋

◇ **heterosexuality** *noun* condition where a person has sexual attraction towards persons of the opposite sex 异性性欲 *compare* 比较 BISEXUAL, HOMOSEXUAL

◇ **heterosis** *or* **hybrid vigour** *noun* increase in size *or* rate of growth *or* fertility *or* resistance to disease found in offspring of a cross between two species 杂种优势

◇ **heterotopia** *noun* state where an organ is placed in a different position from normal or is malformed or deformed; development of tissue which is not natural to the part in which it is produced 异位

◇ **heterotropia** *noun* strabismus, a condition where the two eyes focus on different points 斜视

Hg *chemical symbol for* mercury 汞的化学元素符号

Hib *noun* haemophilus influenzae type B, bacterium which causes meningitis 乙型流感嗜血杆菌; **Hib vaccine** = vaccine used to inoculate against the Hib bacterium in order to prevent meningitis B 乙型流感嗜血杆菌疫苗

> QUOTE: Hib kills 65 people every year.
> 引文:每年有 65 人死于乙型流感嗜血杆菌感染。
> **Guardian** 卫报

hiatus *noun* opening *or* space 裂孔; **hiatus hernia** *US* **hiatal hernia** = hernia where the stomach bulges through the opening in the diaphragm muscle through which the oesophagus passes 食管裂孔疝; **oesophageal hiatus and aortic hiatus** = openings in the diaphragm through which the oesophagus and aorta pass 食管及主动脉裂孔疝

hiccup *or* **hiccough** *or* **singultus** **1** *noun* spasm in the diaphragm which causes a sudden inhalation of breath followed by sudden closure of the glottis which makes a characteristic sound 呃逆,打嗝: ***She had an attack of hiccups or a hiccuping attack.*** 她打嗝了。***He got the hiccups from laughing too much, and found he couldn't stop them.*** 他因为笑得太厉害而打嗝不止。**2** *verb* to make a hiccup 打嗝儿: ***She patted him on the back when he suddenly started to hiccup.*** 当他突然打嗝儿时,她轻拍他的后背。***Do you know how to stop someone hiccuping?*** 你知道怎样制止人打嗝儿吗? ***He hiccuped so loudly that everyone in the restaurant looked at him.*** 他打嗝儿那么大声,饭馆里所有的人都在看他。

COMMENT: Many cures have been suggested for hiccups, but the main treatment is to try to get the patient to think about something else. A drink of water, holding the breath and counting, breathing into a paper bag, are all recommended.
注释:有多种方法被提议用来治疗呃逆,但最主要的是设法使患者思考其他问题。喝水、屏住呼吸数数、用纸袋罩住呼吸均可尝试。

hidr- *prefix* meaning sweat(前缀)汗

◊ **hidradenitis** *noun* inflammation of the sweat glands 汗腺炎

◊ **hidrosis** *noun* (especially excessive) sweating 多汗

◊ **hidrotic** **1** *adjective* referring to sweating 出汗的 **2** *noun* substance which makes someone sweat 发汗药

Higginson's syringe *noun* syringe with a rubber bulb in the centre that allows flow in one direction only (used mainly to give enemas) 希京森氏注射器,一种灌肠器

high *adjective* (**a**) tall *or* reaching far from the ground level 高的: ***The hospital building is 60m high.*** 医院的建筑有60米高。The operating theatre has a high ceiling. 手术示教室的天花板很高。(**b**) (*referring to numbers*) big 数目大的: ***The patient has a very high temperature.*** 患者的体温很高。***There was a high level of glucose in the patient's blood.*** 患者的血糖水平高。**high blood pressure** *or* **hypertension** = condition where the pressure of blood in the arteries is too high, causing the heart to strain 高血压; **high-energy foods** = foods containing a large number of calories, such as fats or carbohydrates, which give a lot of energy when they are broken down 高能食物; **high temperature short time (HTST) method** = usual method of pasteurizing milk, where the milk is heated to 72℃ for 15 seconds and then rapidly cooled 短时高温法(用于消毒牛奶,72 ℃加热 15 秒后快速冷却)(NOTE: **high - higher - highest**)

◊ **highly strung** *adjective* very nervous and tense 紧张的: ***She is highly strung, so don't make comments about her appearance, or she will burst into tears.*** 她很紧张,不要对她的外表做什么评论,否则她会哭出来的。

◊ **high-risk** *adjective* (person) who is very likely to catch a disease *or* develop a cancer *or* suffer an accident 高危的(人群),易感的(人群); **High-risk categories of worker** 高危工种; **high-risk patient** = patient who has a high risk of catching an infection 易感染的患者

Highmore *noun* **antrum of Highmore** = MAXILLARY SINUS 海墨尔氏窦,上颌窦

hilar *adjective* referring to a hilum 门的

◊ **hilum** *noun* hollow where blood vessels *or* nerve fibres enter an organ such as a kidney *or* lung 门(如:肾门,肺门)(NOTE: the plural is **hila**)

hindbrain *noun* part of brain of an embryo, from which the medulla oblongata, the pons and the cerebellum eventually develop 后脑

◊ **hindgut** *noun* part of an embryo which develops into the colon and rectum 后肠

hinge joint *noun* synovial joint (like

the knee) which allows two bones to move in one direction only 屈戌关节 *compare* 比较 BALL AND SOCKET JOINT

hip *noun* ball and socket joint where the thigh bone *or* femur joins the acetabulum of the hip bone 髋部; **hip bath** = small low bath in which a person can sit but not lie down 坐浴; **hip bone** *or* **innominate bone** = bone made of the ilium, the ischium and the pubis which are fused together, forming part of the pelvic girdle 髋骨; **hip fracture** = fracture of the ball at the top of the femur 股骨头骨折; **hip girdle** *or* **pelvic girdle** = the sacrum and the two hip bones 骨盆带; **hip joint** = joint where the rounded end of the femur joins a socket in the acetabulum 髋关节 ◊ 见图 PELVIS; **hip replacement** = surgical operation to replace the whole ball and socket joint with an artificial one 髋关节置换

Hippel-Lindau 希佩尔-井道 *see* 见 VON HIPPEL-LINDAU

hippocampal formation *noun* curved pieces of cortex inside each part of the cerebrum 海马结构

◊ **hippocampus** *noun* long rounded elevation projecting into the lateral ventricle in the brain 海马

Hippocratic oath *noun* oath sworn by medical students when they become doctors, in which they swear not to do anything to harm their patients and not to tell anyone the details of each patient's case 希波克拉底誓言(医学生毕业时的誓言,宣誓不做任何对患者有害的事,不向任何人透露有关患者病情的细节)

hippus *noun* alternating rapid contraction and dilatation of the pupil of the eye 虹膜震颤(瞳孔的快速收缩和扩张)

Hirschsprung's disease *noun* congenital condition where parts of the lower colon lack nerve cells, making peristalsis impossible, so that food accumulates in the upper colon which becomes swollen 赫希施普龙氏病,巨结肠病(遗传性疾病,下部结肠缺乏神经元导致蠕动不能,食物聚集在上部结肠,使之肿胀)

hirsutism *noun* having excessive hair, especially condition where a woman grows hair on the body in the same way as a man 多毛症

hirudin *noun* anticoagulant substance produced by leeches, which is injected into the bloodstream while the leech is feeding 水蛭素(水蛭产生的抗凝物质)

His *noun* **bundle of His** *or* **atrioventricular bundle** = bundle of modified cardiac muscle which conducts impulses from the atrioventricular node to the septum and then divides to connect with the ventricles 希氏束,房室束(变异的心肌束,可将房室结的冲动传导至室间隔,然后分支与心室相连)

histamine *noun* substance released from mast cells throughout the body which stimulates tissues in various ways 组织胺(机体的肥大细胞产生,以多种形式刺激组织): ***Excess of histamine causes inflammation of the tissues.*** 组胺过量可导致组织炎症。***The presence of substances to which a patient is allergic releases large amounts of histamine into the blood.*** 患有接触过敏物质时可释放大量的组胺入血。**histamine test** = test to determine the acidity of gastric juice 组胺试验(测胃液的酸度)

> COMMENT: Histamines dilate the blood vessels (giving nettle rash) or constrict the muscles of the bronchi (giving asthmatic attacks).
> 注释:组胺可扩张血管(产生荨麻疹)或收缩支气管平滑肌(产生哮喘)。

◊ **histaminic** *adjective* referring to histamines 组胺的; **histaminic headache** *or* **Horton's disease** = headache affecting the region over the external carotid artery, caused by release of histamines (and associated with rise in temperature and lacrimation) 组胺性头痛(因为组胺释放导致的颈外动脉区的头痛)

◊ **histidine** *noun* amino acid which may be a precursor of histamine 组氨酸

histiocyte *noun* macrophage of the connective tissue, involved in tissue defence 组织细胞

◇ **histiocytoma** *noun* tumour containing histiocytes 组织细胞瘤

◇ **histiocytosis** *noun* condition where histiocytes are present in the blood 组织细胞增多症; **histiocytosis X** = any form of histiocytosis (such as Hand-Schler-Christian disease) where the cause is not known 组织细胞增多症 X

histo- *prefix* referring to tissue 组织的

◇ **histochemistry** *noun* study of the chemical constituents of cells and tissues and also their function and distribution, using a light or electron microscope to evaluate the stains 组织化学

◇ **histocompatibility** *noun* compatibility between antigens of donors and recipients of transplanted tissues 组织相容性

◇ **histocompatible** *adjective* (two organisms) which have tissues which are antigenically compatible 组织相容性的

◇ **histogenesis** *noun* formation and development of tissue from the embryological germ layer 组织发生

◇ **histoid** *adjective* made of *or* developed from a particular tissue; like normal tissue 某一种组织的;组织样的

◇ **histology** *noun* study of anatomy of tissue cells and minute cellular structure, done using a microscope after the cells have been stained 组织学

◇ **histological** *adjective* referring to histology 组织学的

◇ **histolysis** *noun* disintegration of tissue 组织溶解

◇ **histolytica** 溶组织的 *see* 见 ENTAMOEBA

◇ **histoplasmosis** *noun* lung disease caused by infection with a fungus *Histoplasma* 组织胞浆菌病(肺部的组织胞浆菌感染)

◇ **histotoxic** *adjective* (substance) which is poisonous to tissue 组织毒性的

history *noun* study of what happened in the past 历史,病史: ***He has a history of serious illness or a history of Parkinsonism.*** 他有严重疾病(帕金森病)的病史。**case history** = details of what has happened to a patient undergoing treatment 病史; **medical history** = details of a patient's medical records over a period of time 医疗史; **to take a patient's history** = to ask a patient to tell his case history in his own words on being admitted to hospital 问病史

> QUOTE: These children gave a typical history of exercise-induced asthma.
> 引文:这些儿童有典型的运动诱发型哮喘病史。
> **Lancet** 柳叶刀杂志

> QUOTE: The need for evaluation of patients with a history of severe heart disease.
> 引文:对有严重心脏病史的患者进行评估的必要性。
> **Southern Medical Journal** 南部医学杂志

HIV = HUMAN IMMUNODEFICIENCY VIRUS 人类免疫缺陷病毒; **HIV-negative** = (patient) who has been tested and shown not to have HIV HIV 阴性; **HIV-positive** = (patient) who has been tested and shown to have HIV HIV 阳性: ***Tests showed that he was HIV-positive.*** 试验显示他 HIV 阳性。The hospital is carrying out screening tests for HIV infection. 医院开展了 HIV 感染的筛查试验。HIV-infected patients need careful counselling. 感染 HIV 的患者需要仔细的检查。

> COMMENT: HIV is the virus which causes AIDS. Two strains of HIV virus have been identified: HIV-1 and HIV-2; a third, HIV-3, is claimed to exist but it is, as yet, unconfirmed.
> 注释:HIV 是引起艾滋病的病毒。已确定有两型:HIV-I 和 HIV-II;第三型 HIV-III被认为存在但尚未被证实。

> QUOTE: HIV-associated dementia is characterized by psychomotor slowing and inattentiveness.

引文:HIV相关性痴呆的特征是心理活动减慢和注意力不集中。
British Journal of Nursing 英国护理杂志

hives *or* **urticaria** *or* **nettlerash** *noun* affection of the skin where white, pink or red patches are formed which itch or sting 荨麻疹; **giant hives** = ANGIONEUROTIC OEDEMA 血管神经性水肿

HLA = HUMAN LEUCOCYTE ANTIGEN 人类白细胞抗原

◇ **HLA system** *noun* system of HLA antigens on the surface of cells which need to be histocompatible to allow transplants to take place HLA系统

COMMENT: HLA-A is the most important of the antigens responsible for rejection of transplants.
注释:HLA-A是移植排异反应中最重要的抗原。

HMO *US* = HEALTH MAINTENANCE ORGANIZATION 保健组织

hoarse *adjective* (voice) which is harsh and rough 声音嘶哑的: ***He became hoarse after shouting too much.*** 他大声叫喊得声音都嘶哑了。***She spoke in a hoarse whisper.*** 她说话的声音低哑。

◇ **hoarseness** *noun* harsh and rough sound of the voice, often caused by laryngitis 声嘶

hobnail liver *or* **atrophic cirrhosis** *noun* advanced portal cirrhosis in which the liver has become considerably smaller, where clumps of new cells are formed on the surface of the liver where fibrous tissue has replaced damaged liver cells 萎缩性肝硬化

Hodgkin's disease *noun* malignant disease in which the lymph glands are enlarged and there is an increase in the lymphoid tissues in the liver, spleen and other organs 何杰金氏病 *see also* 参见 PEL-EBSTEIN FEVER

COMMENT: The lymph glands swell to a very large size, and the disease can then attack the liver, spleen and bone marrow. It is frequently fatal if not treated early.
注释:淋巴结可极度肿大,进而侵犯肝脏、脾和骨髓,如果不及早治疗常会致死。

hoist *noun* device with pulleys and wires for raising a bed or a patient 升降机

hole *noun* opening *or* space in something 洞; **hole in the heart** = congenital defect where a hole exists in the wall between the two halves of the heart and allows blood to flow abnormally through the heart and lungs 室间隔(房间隔)缺损

Holger-Nielsen method *noun* method of giving artificial ventilation by hand, where the patient lies face down and the first-aider alternately presses on his back and pulls his arms outwards 霍耳格-尼耳森氏法,一种人工呼吸法,患有俯卧,救护人员交替压迫背部和外拉手臂

holistic *adjective* (method of treatment) involving all the patient's mental and family circumstances rather than just dealing with the condition from which he is suffering 机能整体性的

hollow 1 *adjective* (space) which is empty *or* with nothing inside 空的: ***The surgeon inserted a hollow tube into the lung.*** 术者将一段空管插入肺内。***The hollow cavity filled with pus.*** 空腔充满了脓液。**2** *noun* recess *or* place which is lower than the rest of the surface 穴,凹

holocrine *adjective* (gland) which is secretory only and where the secretion is made up of disintegrated cells of the gland itself 全浆分泌

Homans' sign *noun* pain in the calf when the foot is bent back, a sign of deep vein thrombosis 霍氏征,深静脉血栓的体征

home 1 *noun* (**a**) place where you live; house which you live in 家: ***Are you going to be at home tomorrow?*** 你明天在家吗? ***The doctor told her to stay at home instead of going to work.*** 医生让她待在家里不要去工作。**home help** = person who does housework for an invalid or handicapped person 家庭帮手,保姆;

home nurse *or* **district nurse** = nurse who visits patients in their homes 家庭护士 (**b**) house where people are looked after 疗养院; ***an old people's home*** 敬老院; **children's home** = house where children with no parents are looked after 儿童福利院, 孤儿院; **convalescent home** = type of hospital where patients can recover from illness surgery 疗养院, 休养所; **nursing home** = house where convalescents or old people can live under medical supervision by a qualified nurse 疗养院 **2** *adverb* towards the place where you usually live 回家: ***I'm going home.*** 我要回家了。***I'll take it home with me.*** 我要把它带回家。***I usually get home at 7 o'clock.*** = I reach the house where I live. 我通常7点到家。***She can take the bus home.*** = She can go to where she lives by bus. 她可以坐公交车回家。(NOTE: used without a preposition: **he went home, she's coming home.**)

homeo- *or* **homoeo-** *prefix* meaning like *or* similar 相同的,类似的

◇ **homeopathic** *or* **homoeopathic** *adjective* (**a**) referring to homeopathy 顺势疗法的: ***a homeopathic clinic*** 顺势疗法诊所: ***She is having a course of homeopathic treatment.*** 她在接受一疗程的顺势疗法治疗。(**b**) (drug) given in very small quantities 小剂量给药的

◇ **homeopathist** *or* **homoeopathist** *noun* person who practises homeopathy 顺势疗法医生

◇ **homeopathy** *or* **homoeopathy** *noun* treatment of a condition by giving the patient very small quantities of a substance which, when given to a healthy person, would cause symptoms like those of the condition being treated 顺势疗法 *compare* 比较 ALLOPATHY

homeostasis *noun* process by which the functions and chemistry of a cell *or* internal organ are kept stable, even when external conditions vary greatly 体内平衡,内稳态

homo- *prefix* meaning the same 相同的

◇ **homogenize** *verb* to make something all the same *or* to give something a uniform nature 匀化; **homogenized milk** = milk where the cream has been mixed up into the milk to give the same consistency throughout 匀化牛奶

◇ **homograft** *or* **allograft** *noun* graft of an organ *or* tissue from a donor to a recipient of the same species (as from one person to another) 同种移植物 *compare* 比较 AUTOGRAFT

homoiothermic *adjective* (animal) with warm blood *or* warm-blooded (animal) 温血的, 恒温的 *compare* 比较 POIKILOTHERMIC

> COMMENT: Warm-blooded animals are able to maintain a constant body temperature whatever the outside temperature.
> 注释:温血动物不管外界温度如何,仍能保持恒定的体温。

homologous *adjective* (chromosomes) which form a pair 同源的

homonymous *adjective* affecting the two eyes in the same way 同侧的; **homonymous hemianopia** = condition where the same half of the field of vision is lost in each eye 同侧偏盲

homophobia *noun* fear of and hostility towards homosexuals 对同性恋者的恐惧

homoplasty *noun* surgery to replace lost tissues by grafting similar tissues from another person 同种移植术,同种成形术

homosexual 1 *adjective* referring to homosexuality 同性恋的 **2** *noun* person who is sexually attracted to people of the same sex, especially a man who experiences sexual attraction for other males 同性恋者

◇ **homosexuality** *noun* condition where a person experiences sexual attraction for persons of the same sex *or* has sexual relations with persons of the same sex 同性恋 *compare* 比较 BISEXUAL,

HETEROSEXUAL, LESBIAN (NOTE: although **homosexual** can apply to both males and females, it is commonly used for males only, and **lesbian** is used for females)

hook 1 *noun* surgical instrument with a bent end used for holding structures apart in operations 钩 **2** *verb* to attach something with a hook 用钩钩

◇ **hookworm** = ANCYLOSTOMA 钩虫; **hookworm disease** = ANCYLOSTOMIASIS 钩虫病

hordeolum *or* **stye** *noun* infection of the gland at the base of an eyelash 睑腺炎

horizontal *adjective* which is lying flat *or* at a right angle to the vertical 水平的; **horizontal plane** = TRANSVERSE PLANE 水平面

hormone *noun* substance which is produced by one part of the body, especially the endocrine glands and is carried to another part of the body by the bloodstream where it has particular effects or functions 激素; **growth hormone** = hormone which stimulates the growth of long bones 生长激素; **sex hormones** = oestrogens and androgens which promote the growth of secondary sexual characteristics 性激素; **hormone replacement therapy** (**HRT**) *or* **hormone therapy** = (i) treatment for a patient whose endocrine glands have been removed 激素替代治疗 (ii) generally, treatment to relieve the symptoms of the menopause by supplying oestrogen and reducing the risk of osteoporosis 更年期激素补充治疗

◇ **hormonal** *adjective* referring to hormones 激素的

horn *noun* (**a**) (*in animals*) hard tissue which protrudes from the head 角, 犄角 (**b**) (*in humans*) (i) tissue which grows out of an organ 角 (ii) one of the H-shaped limbs of grey matter seen in a cross-section of the spinal cord 灰质脚 (iii) extension of the pulp chamber of a tooth towards the cusp 髓根

◇ **horny** *adjective* like horn *or* hard (skin) 角的,(皮肤)角化的 (NOTE: for terms referring to horny tissue, see words beginning with **kerat**)

Horner's syndrome *noun* condition caused by paralysis of the sympathetic nerve in one side of the neck, making the patient's eyelids hang down and the pupils contract 霍纳氏综合征,一侧颈部交感神经瘫痪引起眼睑下垂和瞳孔缩小

horseshoe kidney *noun* congenital defect of the kidney, where sometimes the upper but usually the lower parts of both kidneys are joined together 马蹄肾

Horton's disease *or* **Horton's headache** *noun* headache repeatedly affecting the region over the external carotid artery, caused by release of histamine in the body 霍顿氏头痛,组胺性头痛

hose *noun* (**a**) long rubber or plastic tube 长的橡皮管或塑料管 (**b**) stocking 长统袜; **surgical** *or* **elastic hose** = special stocking worn to support and relieve varicose veins 弹力袜

hospice *noun* hospital which cares for terminally ill patients 临终关怀医院

hospital *noun* place where sick or injured people are looked after 医院: ***She's so ill she has been sent to hospital.*** 她病得很厉害,被送往医院。***He's been in hospital for several days.*** 他已经住院好几天了。***The children's hospital is at the end of our street.*** 儿童医院位于我们这条街的尽头。**cottage hospital** = small local hospital set in pleasant gardens in the country 诊疗所; **day hospital** = hospital where the patients are treated during the day and go home in the evenings 日间医院; **general hospital** = hospital which cares for all types of patient 综合医院; **geriatric hospital** = hospital which specializes in the treatment of old people 老年医院; **isolation hospital** = hospital where patients suffering from dangerous infectious diseases can be isolated 传染病医院, 隔离医院; **mental**

hospital = hospital for the treatment of mentally ill patients 精神病院; **private hospital** = hospital which takes only paying patients 私人医院; **teaching hospital** = hospital attached to a medical school where student doctors work and study as part of their training 教学医院; **Hospital Activity Analysis** = regular detailed report on patients in hospitals, including information about treatment, length of stay, death rate. etc. 医院管理分析; **hospital bed** = (i) special type of bed used in hospitals 病床 (ii) place in a hospital which can be occupied by a patient 床位: ***A hospital bed is needed if the patient has to have traction.*** 如果患者不得不做牵引的话,必须有一张病床。***There will be no reduction in the number of hospital beds.*** 医院的床位不会减少。**hospital trust** = self-governing hospital, a hospital which earns its revenue from services provided to the District Health Authorities and family doctors 自我管理医院,所有权医院

◇ **hospitalize** *verb* to send someone to hospital 住院: ***He is so ill that he has had to be hospitalized.*** 他病得很厉害,不得不住院。

◇ **hospitalization** *noun* sending someone to hospital 住院: ***The doctor recommended immediate hospitalization.*** 医生建议马上住院。

host *noun* person *or* animal on which a parasite lives 宿主

hot *adjective* very warm; of a high temperature 热的: ***The water in my bath is too hot.*** 浴盆里的水太热了。***If you're hot, take your coat off.*** 如果你觉得热的话,把外衣脱了。***Affected skin will feel hot.*** 受影响的皮肤会觉得发热。**hot flush** = condition in menopausal women, where the patient becomes hot and sweats, often accompanied by redness of the skin 热疹 (NOTE: **hot - hotter - hottest**)

hour *noun* period of time lasting sixty minutes 小时: ***There are 24 hours in a day.*** 一天有24小时。***The hours of work are from 9 to 5.*** 工作时间是从9点到5点。***When is your lunch hour?*** = When do you stop work for lunch? 几点是你的午餐时间? ***I'll be ready in a quarter of an hour or in half an hour.*** = in 15 minutes *or* 30 minutes. 我15分钟(半个小时)内准备好。

◇ **hourglass contraction** *noun* condition where an organ (such as the stomach) is constricted in the centre 葫芦状收缩

◇ **hourly** *adjective* happening every hour 每小时

house *noun* building which someone lives in 家,房子: ***He has a flat in the town and a house in the country.*** 他在镇上有套公寓,在乡村有座房子。***All the houses in our street look the same.*** 我们街上所有的房子看上去都一样。***His house has six bedrooms.*** 他的房子里有6间卧室。**house mite** = small insect living in houses, which can cause an allergic reaction 尘螨; **house officer** = doctor who works in a hospital (as house surgeon *or* house physician) during the final year of training before registration by the GMC 住院医生

◇ **housemaid's knee** *or* **prepatellar bursitis** *noun* condition where the fluid sac in the knee becomes inflamed, caused by kneeling on hard surfaces 膑前粘液囊炎

◇ **houseman** *noun* house surgeon *or* house physician 实习医生 (NOTE: the US English is **intern**)

HRT = HORMONE REPLACEMENT THERAPY 激素替代治疗

HTST method = HIGH TEMPERATURE SHORT TIME METHOD 短时高温法

Huhner's test *noun* test carried out several hours after sexual intercourse to determine the number and motility of spermatozoa 胡讷氏试验,检测精子的数量和活性

human 1 *adjective* referring to any man, woman or child 人的; **a human being** = a person 人; **human chorionic go-**

nadotrophin (**hCG**) = hormone produced by the placenta, which suppresses the mother's normal menstrual cycle during pregnancy; it is found in the urine during pregnancy; it can be given by injection to encourage ovulation and help a woman to become pregnant 人绒毛膜促性腺激素; **human immunodeficiency virus** (**HIV**) = virus which causes AIDS 人类免疫缺陷病毒 *see* 见 AIDS, HIV; **human leucocyte antigen** (**HLA**) = any of the system of antigens on the surface of cells which need to be histocompatible to allow transplants to take place 人类白细胞抗原 *see* 见 HLA SYSTEM **2** *noun* person 人: ***Most animals are afraid of humans*.** 大多数动物都惧怕人类。

humeroulnar joint *noun* part of the elbow joint, where the trochlea of the humerus and the trochlear notch of the ulna articulate 肱尺关节

◇ **humerus** *noun* top bone in the arm, running from the shoulder to the elbow 肱骨 ◊ 见图 SHOULDER (NOTE: plural is **humeri**)

humid *adjective* which is damp *or* which contains moisture vapour 潮湿的

◇ **humidity** *noun* measurement of how much water vapour is contained in the air 湿度

humour *noun* fluid in the body 体液; **aqueous humour** = fluid in the eye between the lens and the cornea 房水; **vitreous humour** = jelly behind the lens in the eye 玻璃体液 ◊ 见图 EYE

hunchback *noun* (i) excessive curvature of the spine 驼背,脊柱后凸 (ii) person suffering from excessive curvature of the spine 驼背者

hunger *noun* feeling a need to eat 饥饿; **hunger pains** = pains in the abdomen when a person feels hungry (sometimes a sign of a duodenal ulcer) 饥饿痛; **air hunger** 呼吸困难 *see* 见 AIR

◇ **hungry** *adjective* wanting to eat 饥饿的: ***I'm hungry***; ***are you hungry***? 我饿了,你饿吗? ***You must be hungry after that long walk*.** 你走了那么长的路一定饿了。***The patient will not be hungry after the operation*.** 患者术后不会觉得饥饿。***I'm not very hungry — I had a big breakfast*.** 我不很饿,我早饭吃得很多。(NOTE: **hungry - hungrier - hungriest**)

Huntington's chorea 亨廷顿氏舞蹈病,遗传性慢性舞蹈病 *see* 见 CHOREA

Hurler's syndrome = GARGOYLISM 胡尔勒氏综合征,脂肪软骨营养不良

hurry 1 *noun* rush 匆忙,仓促: ***Get out of the way — we're in a hurry*!** 快让道,我们有急事。***He's always in a hurry*.** = He is always rushing about *or* doing things very fast. 他总是匆匆忙忙的 ***What's the hurry*?** = Why are you going so fast? 为什么那么着急? **2** *verb* to go or do something fast 赶紧做;to make someone go faster 使赶紧: ***She hurried along the passage*.** 她急急地走过走廊。***you'll have to hurry if you want to see the doctor, he's just leaving the hospital*.** 如果想见医生的话必须快点儿,他要离开医院。***Don't hurry - we've got plenty of time*.** 别着急,我们有充足的时间。***Don't hurry me, I'm working as fast as I can*.** 别催我,我正尽快干着呢。

hurt 1 *noun* (*used by children*) painful spot 疼痛点: ***She has a hurt on her knee*.** 她膝盖疼。**2** *verb* (i) to have pain; 疼痛,受伤 (ii) to give pain 使疼痛,伤害: ***He's hurt his hand*.** 他手疼。***Where does your foot hurt*?** 你脚哪儿疼? ***His arm is hurting so much he can't write*.** 他的胳膊疼得厉害,不能写字。***She fell down and hurt herself*.** 她摔了下来,伤了自己。***Are you hurt*?** 你疼吗? ***Is he badly hurt*?** 他伤得很厉害吗? ***My foot hurts*.** 我脚疼。***He was slightly hurt in the car crash*.** 他在车祸中受了轻伤。***Two players got hurt in the football game*.** 有两名队员在足球赛中受伤。(NOTE: **hurts - hurting - hurt - has hurt**)

husky *adjective* slightly hoarse 嘶哑的; ***husky voice*** 声音嘶哑

Hutchinson's tooth *noun* narrow upper incisor tooth, with notches along the cutting edge, a symptom of congenital syphilis but also occurring naturally 哈钦森牙(为先天性梅毒的体征,但不一定由先天梅毒引起)

◇ **Hutchinson-Gilford syndrome** *noun* progeria, premature senility 哈-吉综合征,早老症

hyal- *prefix* like glass 玻璃样的

◇ **hyalin** *noun* transparent substance produced from collagen and deposited around blood vessels and scars when certain tissues degenerate 透明蛋白

◇ **hyaline** *adjective* nearly transparent like glass 透明的; **hyaline cartilage** = type of cartilage found in the nose, larynx and joints 透明软骨 ◊ 见图 JOINTS; **hyaline membrane disease** *or* **respiratory distress syndrome** = condition of newborn babies, where the lungs do not expand properly 透明膜病(呼吸窘迫综合征)

◇ **hyalitis** *noun* inflammation of the vitreous humour or the hyaloid membrane in the eye 玻璃体炎

◇ **hyaloid membrane** *noun* transparent membrane round the vitreous humour in the eye 玻璃体膜

◇ **hyaluronic acid** *noun* substance which binds connective tissue and is found in the eyes 透明质酸

◇ **hyaluronidase** *noun* enzyme which destroys hyaluronic acid 透明质酸酶

hybrid *adjective* & *noun* cross between two species of plant *or* animal 杂种的,杂种; **hybrid vigour** = increase in size *or* rate of growth *or* fertility *or* resistance to disease found in offspring of a cross between two species 杂交优势

hydatid (cyst) *noun* cyst which covers the larvae of the tapeworm *Taenia solium* 棘球囊

◇ **hydatid disease** *or* **hydatidosis** *noun* disease caused by hydatid cysts in the lung *or* brain 棘球蚴病

◇ **hydatidiform mole** *noun* growth in the uterus, which looks like a hydatid cyst, and is formed of villous sacs swollen with fluid 葡萄胎

hydr- *prefix* referring to water 水

◇ **hydraemia** *noun* excess of water in the blood 稀血症

◇ **hydragogue** *noun* laxative *or* substance which produces watery faeces 水泻剂

◇ **hydrarthrosis** *noun* swelling caused by excess synovial liquid at a joint 关节积水

hydro- *prefix* referring to water 水

◇ **hydroa** *noun* eruption of small itchy blisters (as those caused by sunlight) 水疱

◇ **hydrocele** *noun* collection of watery liquid found in a cavity such as the scrotum 水囊肿

◇ **hydrocephalus** *noun* excessive quantity of cerebrospinal fluid in the brain 脑积水

◇ **hydrochloric acid(HCl)** *noun* acid found in the gastric juices which helps the maceration of food 盐酸

◇ **hydrocolpos** *noun* cyst in the vagina containing clear fluid 阴道积水

◇ **hydrocortisone** *noun* steroid hormone secreted by the adrenal cortex, used to treat rheumatism and inflammatory and allergic conditions 氢化可的松

◇ **hydrocyanic acid(HCN)** *noun* acid which forms cyanide 氢氰酸

◇ **hydrogen** *noun* chemical element, a gas which combines with oxygen to form water, and with other elements to form acids, and is present in all animal tissue 氢 (NOTE: chemical symbol is **H**)

◇ **hydrometer** *noun* instrument which measures the density of a liquid 比重计

◇ **hydromyelia** *noun* condition where fluid swells the central canal of the spinal cord 脊髓积水

◇ **hydronephrosis** *noun* swelling of the pelvis of a kidney caused by accumulation of water due to infection *or* a kidney stone blocking the ureter 肾盂积

水

◇ **hydropericarditis** *or* **hydropericardium** *noun* accumulation of liquid round the heart 心包积液,积水性心包炎

◇ **hydrophobia** *or* **rabies** *noun* frequently fatal virus disease transmitted by infected animals 恐水症,狂犬病

> COMMENT: Hydrophobia affects the mental balance, and the symptoms include difficulty in breathing or swallowing and a horror of water.
> 注释:狂犬病影响精神平衡,症状包括呼吸或吞咽困难及恐水。

◇ **hydrorrhoea** *noun* discharge of watery fluid 液溢

◇ **hydrotherapy** *noun* treatment of patients with water, where the patients are put in hot baths *or* are encouraged to swim 水疗法

◇ **hydrothorax** *noun* collection of liquid in the pleural cavity 胸膜(腔)积水

◇ **hydroxide** *noun* chemical compound containing a hydroxyl group 氢氧化物; **aluminium hydroxide** *US* **aluminum hydroxide** ($Al(OH)_3$ *or* $Al_2O_3.3H_2O$) = chemical substance used as an antacid 氢氧化铝

◇ **hydroxyproline** *noun* amino acid present in some proteins, especially in collagen 羟脯氨酸

hygiene *noun* (i) being clean and keeping healthy conditions 卫生(ii) science of health 卫生学: ***Nurses have to maintain a strict personal hygiene.*** 护士必须维持严格的个人卫生。**dental hygiene** = keeping the teeth clean and healthy 牙卫生; **oral hygiene** = keeping the mouth clean by gargling and mouthwashes 口腔卫生

◇ **hygienic** *adjective* (i) clean 干净的 (ii) which produces healthy conditions 有助于卫生的: ***Don't touch the food with dirty hands — it isn't hygienic.*** 不要用脏手碰食物,这不卫生。

◇ **hygienist** *noun* person who specializes in hygiene and its application 卫生学家; **dental hygienist** = person who helps a dentist by cleaning teeth and gums, removing plaque from teeth and giving fluoride treatment 牙科洁治师

hymen *noun* membrane which partially covers the vaginal passage in a virgin 处女膜

◇ **hymenectomy** *noun* surgical removal of the hymen *or* operation to increase the size of the opening of the hymen *or* surgical removal of any membrane 处女膜切除术,粘膜切除术

◇ **hymenotomy** *noun* incision of the hymen during surgery 处女膜切开术

hyoglossus *noun* muscle which is attached to the hyoid bone and depresses the tongue 舌骨舌肌

hyoid bone *noun* small U-shaped bone at the base of the tongue 舌骨

hyoscine *noun* drug used as a sedative, in particular for treatment of motion sickness 东莨菪碱

hyp- *or* **hypo-** *prefix* meaning less *or* too little *or* too small 少,小(NOTE: *opposite is* **HYPER-**)

◇ **hypaemia** *noun* insufficient amount of blood in the body 贫血

◇ **hypalgesia** *noun* low sensitivity to pain 痛觉减退

hyper- *prefix* meaning higher *or* too much 高,多(NOTE *opposite is* **HYP-, HYPO-**)

◇ **hyperacidity** *noun* increase in acid in the stomach 胃酸过多

◇ **hyperactive** *adjective* being very active 机能亢进的

◇ **hyperactivity** *noun* condition where something (a gland *or* a child) is too active 机能亢进; **hyperactivity syndrome** = condition where a child is extremely active, restless, breaks things for no reason and will not study 多动症

◇ **hyperacusis** *or* **hyperacousia** *noun* being very sensitive to sounds 听觉过敏

◇ **hyperaemia** *noun* excess blood in any part of the body 充血

◇ **hyperaesthesia** *noun* extremely high sensitivity in the skin 感觉过敏

◇ **hyperalgesia** *noun* increased sensitivity to pain 痛觉过敏

◇ **hyperbaric** *adjective* (treatment) where a patient is given oxygen at high pressure, used to treat carbon monoxide poisoning 高压氧治疗的

◇ **hypercalcaemia** *noun* excess of calcium in the blood 高钙血症

◇ **hyperchlorhydria** *noun* excess of hydrochloric acid in the stomach 胃酸过多

◇ **hyperdactylism** *or* **polydactylism** *noun* having more than the normal number of fingers or toes 多指(趾)

◇ **hyperemesis gravidarum** *noun* uncontrollable vomiting in pregnancy 妊娠剧吐

◇ **hyperglycaemia** *noun* excess of glucose in the blood 高血糖

◇ **hyperinsulinism** *noun* reaction of a diabetic to an excessive dose of insulin or to hypoglycaemia 胰岛素分泌过多

◇ **hyperkinesia** *noun* condition where there is abnormally great strength or movement 运动机能亢进; **essential hyperkinesia** = condition of children where their movements are excessive and repeated 特发性运动过度

◇ **hyperkinetic syndrome** *or* **effort syndrome** *noun* condition where the patient experiences fatigue, shortness of breath, pain under the heart and palpitation 运动过度综合征

◇ **hypermenorrhoea** *noun* menstruation in which the flow is excessive 月经过多

◇ **hypermetropia** *or* **longsightedness** *or US* **hypertropia** *noun* condition where the patient sees more clearly objects which are a long way away, but cannot see objects which are close 远视 *compare* 比较 MYOPIA

◇ **hypernephroma** = GRAWITZ TUMOUR 肾上腺样瘤

◇ **hyperostosis** *noun* excessive overgrowth on the outside surface of a bone, especially the frontal bone 骨肥厚

◇ **hyperpiesis** *noun* abnormally high pressure, especially of the blood 压力过高

◇ **hyperplasia** *noun* condition in which there is an increase in the number of cells in an organ 增生

◇ **hyperpyrexia** *noun* high body temperature (above 41.1℃) 高烧

◇ **hypersensitive** *adjective* (person) who reacts more strongly than normal to an antigen 过敏的

◇ **hypersensitivity** *noun* condition where the patient reacts very strongly to something (such as an allergic substance) 过敏: ***Her hypersensitivity to dust.*** 她对灰尘过敏。***Anaphylactic shock shows hypersensitivity to an injection.*** 过敏性休克提示对注射药过敏。

◇ **hypertension** *noun* high blood pressure, condition where the pressure of the blood in the arteries is too high 高血压; **portal hypertension** = high pressure in the portal vein, caused by cirrhosis of the liver *or* a clot in the vein and causing internal bleeding 门脉高压; **pulmonary hypertension** = high blood pressure in the blood vessels supplying the lungs 肺动脉高压

> COMMENT: High blood pressure can have many causes: the arteries are too narrow, causing the heart to strain; kidney disease; Cushing's syndrome, etc. High blood pressure is treated with drugs such as beta blockers.
> 注释:高血压可有多种原因:动脉狭窄并导致心脏受到压力、肾脏疾病、库兴氏综合征等等,高血压可用药物如β受体阻滞剂治疗。

◇ **hypertensive** *adjective* referring to high blood pressure 高血压的; **hypertensive headache** = headache caused by high blood pressure 高血压性头疼

◇ **hyperthermia** *noun* very high body temperature 高烧

◇ **hyperthyroidism** *noun* condition where the thyroid gland is too active and swells, as in Graves' disease 甲状腺功

能亢进

◇ **hypertonia** *noun* increased rigidity and spasticity of the muscles 肌张力增高

◇ **hypertrichosis** *noun* condition where the patient has excessive growth of hair on the body *or* on part of the body 多毛症

◇ **hypertrophic** *adjective* associated with hypertrophy 增生的,肥厚的; **hypertrophic rhinitis** = condition where the mucous membranes in the nose become thicker 肥厚性鼻炎

◇ **hypertrophy** *noun* increase in the number or size of cells in a tissue 肥大,增生

◇ **hypertropia** *noun US* = HYPERMETROPIA 上斜眼

◇ **hyperventilate** *verb* to breathe very fast 换气过度: ***We all hyperventilate as an expression of fear or excitement.*** 当恐惧或兴奋时我们都会换气过度。

◇ **hyperventilation** *noun* very fast breathing which can be accompanied by dizziness or tetany 过度换气

◇ **hypervitaminosis** *noun* condition caused by taking too many synthetic vitamins, especially Vitamins A and D 维生素过多症

hyphaema *noun* bleeding into the front chamber of the eye 眼前房出血

hypn- *prefix* referring to sleep 睡眠的

◇ **hypnosis** *noun* state like sleep, but caused artificially, where the patient can remember forgotten events in the past *or* will do whatever the hypnotist tells him to do 催眠状态

◇ **hypnotherapy** *noun* treatment by hypnosis, used in treating some addictions 催眠治疗

◇ **hypnotic** *adjective* referring to hypnotism 催眠术的(drug) which causes sleep 安眠药的; (state) which is like sleep but which is caused artificially 催眠的

◇ **hypnotism** *noun* inducing hypnosis 催眠术

◇ **hypnotist** *noun* person who hypnotizes other people 催眠术士: ***The hypnotist passed his hand in front of her eyes and she went immediately to sleep.*** 催眠术士将他的手放在她眼前,她很快就入睡了。

◇ **hypnotize** *verb* to make someone go into a state where he appears to be asleep, and will do whatever the hypnotist suggests 催眠: ***He hypnotizes his patients, and then persuades them to reveal their hidden problems.*** 他催眠了他的患者,然后诱导他们揭示隐藏的问题。

hypo (*informal* 非正式) = HYPODERMIC SYRINGE 皮下注射器

hypo- *prefix* meaning less *or* too little *or* beneath 少、小、下

◇ **hypoaesthesia** *noun* condition where the patient has a diminished sense of touch 感觉减退

◇ **hypocalcaemia** *noun* abnormally low amount of calcium in the blood, which can cause tetany 低钙血症

◇ **hypochondria** *noun* condition where a person is too worried about his health and believes he is ill 疑病症

◇ **hypochondriac 1** *noun* person who worries about his health too much 疑病症者 **2** *adjective* **hypochondriac regions** = two parts of the upper abdomen, on either side of the epigastrium below the floating ribs 季肋部

◇ **hypochondrium** *noun* one of the hypochondriac regions in the upper part of the abdomen 季肋部

◇ **hypochromic anaemia** *noun* anaemia where haemoglobin is reduced in proportion to the number of red blood cells, which then appear very pale 低色素性贫血

◇ **hypodermic** *adjective* beneath the skin 皮下的; **hypodermic syringe** *or* **a hypodermic** = syringe which injects liquid under the skin 皮下注射器; **hypodermic needle** = needle for injecting liquid under the skin 皮下针头

◇ **hypogastrium** *noun* part of the abdomen beneath the stomach 下腹,腹下部

◇ **hypoglossal nerve** *noun* twelfth cranial nerve which governs the muscles of the tongue 舌下神经

◇ **hypoglycaemia** *noun* low concentration of glucose in the blood 低血糖

◇ **hypoglycaemic** *adjective* suffering from hypoglycaemia 低血糖的; **hypoglycaemic coma** = state of unconsciousness affecting diabetics after taking an overdose of insulin 低血糖性昏迷

COMMENT: Hypoglycaemia affects diabetics who feel weak from lack of sugar. A hypoglycaemic attack can be prevented by eating glucose or a lump of sugar when feeling faint.
注释:糖尿病患者因低血糖而感觉虚弱时可吃一些葡萄糖或糖块预防发作。

◇ **hypohidrosis** *or* **hypoidrosis** *noun* producing too little sweat 少汗

◇ **hypokalaemia** *noun* deficiency of potassium in the blood 低血钾

◇ **hypomenorrhoea** *noun* production of too little blood at menstruation 月经过少

◇ **hyponatraemia** *noun* lack of sodium in the body 低血钠

◇ **hypophyseal** *adjective* referring to the hypophysis *or* pituitary gland 垂体的; **hypophyseal stalk** = stalk which attaches the pituitary gland to the hypothalamus 垂体柄

◇ **hypophysis cerebri** 大脑垂体 *see* 见 PITUITARY GLAND

◇ **hypoplasia** *noun* lack of development *or* defective formation of tissue or an organ 发育不全

◇ **hypopyon** *noun* pus in the aqueous humour in the front chamber of the eye 眼前房积脓

◇ **hyposensitive** *adjective* being less sensitive than normal 低敏的

◇ **hypospadias** *noun* congenital defect of the wall of the male urethra or the vagina, so that the opening occurs on the under side of the penisor in the vagina 尿道下裂 *compare* 比较 EPISPADIAS

◇ **hypostasis** *noun* condition where fluid accumulates in part of the body because of poor circulation 血液坠积

◇ **hypostatic** *adjective* referring to hypostasis 血液坠积的; **hypostatic eczema** = eczema which develops on the legs, caused by bad circulation 静脉曲张性湿疹; **hypostatic pneumonia** = pneumonia caused by fluid accumulating in the lungs of a bedridden patient with a weak heart 坠积性肺炎

◇ **hypotension** *noun* low blood pressure 低血压

◇ **hypotensive** *adjective* suffering from low blood pressure 低血压的

◇ **hypothalamic** *adjective* referring to the hypothalamus 下丘脑的; **hypothalamic hormones** *or* **releasing factors** = substances that cause the pituitary gland to release its hormones 下丘脑激素,释放激素

◇ **hypothalamus** *noun* part of the brain above the pituitary gland, which controls the production of hormones by the pituitary gland and regulates important bodily functions such as hunger, thirst and sleep 下丘脑 ◇ 见图 BRAIN

◇ **hypothenar** *adjective* referring to the soft fat part of the palm beneath the little finger 小鱼际的; **hypothenar eminence** = lump on the palm beneath the little finger 鱼际突起 *compare* 比较 THENAR

◇ **hypothermia** *noun* reduction in body temperature below normal, for official purposes taken to be below 35℃ 低温

QUOTE: Inadvertent hypothermia can readily occur in patients undergoing surgery when there is reduced heat production and a greater potential for heat loss to the environment.
引文:接受手术的患者因为产热减少,向环境中散热能潜力增加,会出现无伤害性低体温。
British Journal of Nursing 英国护理杂志

◇ **hypothermic** *adjective* suffering from hypothermia 低温的: ***Examination revealed that she was hypothermic, with a rectal temperature of only***

29.4℃. 检查表明她体温低,直肠温度仅有 29.4℃。

◇ **hypothyroidism** *noun* underactivity of the thyroid gland 甲状腺功能减退

◇ **hypotonia** *noun* reduced tension in any part of the body 张力减退

◇ **hypotonic** *adjective* with reduced tension 低张的;(solution) with lower osmotic pressure than plasma 低渗(液)

◇ **hypotropia** *noun* form of squint where one eye looks downwards 下斜视

◇ **hypoventilation** *noun* very slow breathing 肺换气不足

◇ **hypovitaminosis** *noun* lack of vitamins 维生素缺乏症

◇ **hypoxia** *noun* inadequate supply of oxygen to tissue or an organ 缺氧

hyster- *prefix* referring to the womb 子宫的

◇ **hysteralgia** *noun* pain in the womb 子宫痛

◇ **hysterectomy** *noun* surgical removal of the womb, either to treat cancer or because of the presence of fibroids 子宫切除术; **subtotal hysterectomy** = removal of the womb, but not the cervix 子宫次全切除术; **total hysterectomy** = removal of the whole womb 全子宫切除术

hysteria *noun* neurotic state, where the patient is unstable, and may scream and wave the arms about, but also is repressed, and may be slow to react to outside stimuli 癔病

◇ **hysterical** *adjective* (reaction) of hysteria 癔病的,歇斯底里的: ***He burst into hysterical crying.*** 他突然歇斯底里地哭起来。**hysterical personality** = mental condition of a person who is unstable, lacks normal feelings and is dependent on others 癔病人格

◇ **hysterically** *adverb* in a hysterical way 歇斯底里地: ***She was laughing hysterically.*** 她歇斯底里地大笑。

◇ **hysterics** *noun* attack of hysteria 癔病发作: ***She had an attack*** *or* ***a fit of hysterics*** *or* ***she went into hysterics.*** 她癔病发作。

◇ **hystericus**癔病的 *see* 见 GLOBUS

hystero- *prefix* referring to the womb 子宫

◇ **hysterocele** *noun* hernia of the womb 子宫疝

◇ **hysteroptosis** *noun* prolapse of the womb 子宫下垂

◇ **hysterosalpingography** *or* **uterosalpingography** *noun* X-ray examination of the womb and Fallopian tubes following injection of radio-opaque material 子宫输卵管造影术

◇ **hysteroscope** *noun* tube for inspecting the inside of the womb 宫腔镜

◇ **hysterotomy** *noun* surgical incision into the womb (as in Caesarean section *or* for some types of abortion) 子宫切开术

Ii

I *chemical symbol for* iodine 碘的化学元素符号

-iasis *suffix* meaning disease caused by something 病; **amoebiasis** = disease caused by an amoeba 阿米巴病

iatrogenic *adjective* condition which is caused by a doctor's treatment for another disease *or* condition 医源性的

> COMMENT: Can be caused by a drug (a side effect), by infection from the doctor, or simply by worry about possible treatment.
> 注释:可以因药物(副作用)、注射或仅仅因为对可能的治疗担心而引起。

I band *noun* part of the pattern in muscle tissue, seen through a microscope as a light-coloured band I 带(在显微镜下可见的肌肉组织的亮带)

ice *noun* (**a**) frozen water 冰 (**b**) **dry ice** = solid carbon dioxide 干冰(固态的二氧化碳)

◇ **ice cream** *noun* frozen sweet made from cream, water and flavouring 冰激凌: ***After a tonsillectomy, children can be allowed ice cream.*** 扁桃体切除术后,患儿被允许吃冰激凌。

◇ **icebag** *or* **ice pack** *noun* cold compress made of lumps of ice wrapped in a cloth or put in a special bag, applied to a bruise *or* swelling to reduce the pain 冰袋(装有冰的袋子,可减轻青紫或肿胀引起的疼痛)

ichor *noun* watery liquid which comes from a wound *or* suppurating sore 脓液

ICRC = INTERNATIONAL COMMITTEE OF THE RED CROSS 国际红十字委员会

ichthyosis *noun* hereditary condition where the skin is dry and covered with scales 鳞癣

ICSH = INTERSTITIAL CELL STIMULATING HORMONE 促间发细胞激素,促黄体生成激素

icterus = JAUNDICE 黄疸; **icterus gravis neonatorum** = jaundice associated with erythroblastosis fetalis 新生儿重黄疸

◇ **icteric** *adjective* (patient) with jaundice 患有黄疸的

ictus *noun* stroke *or* fit 暴发,发作

ICU = INTENSIVE CARE UNIT 重症监护病房

id *noun* (*in psychology*) basic unconscious drives which exist in hidden forms in a person 本我,私我

ideal *adjective* very suitable *or* perfect 理想的,适合的,完美的; referring to an idea 观念的,思想的: ***This is an ideal place for a new hospital.*** 这是建造新医院的理想地方。

identical *adjective* exactly the same 同一的; **identical twins** *or* **monozygotic twins** = two children born at the same time and from the same ovum, and therefore of the same sex and exactly the same in appearance 同卵双胞胎(由同一受精卵分裂而来,同时出生,具有相同的性别和外貌) *compare* 比较 FRATERNAL

identify *verb* to determine the identity of something *or* someone 认出,鉴定: ***The next of kin were asked to identify the body.*** 最近的亲属被叫去确认尸体。***Doctors have identified the cause of the outbreak of dysentery.*** 医生确定了痢疾暴发的原因。

◇ **identifiable** *adjective* which can be identified 可确认的: ***Cot deaths often have no identifiable cause.*** 婴儿猝死常无明确的原因。

◇ **identification** *noun* act of identifying 确定,鉴定; **identification with someone** = taking on some characteristics of an older person (such as a parent *or* teacher)具有某年长者(父母或老师)的特征

◇ **identity** *noun* who a person is 身份; **identity bracelet** *or* **label** = label attached to the wrist of a newborn baby *or* patient in hospital, so that he can be identified 身份标签(戴在新生儿和住院患者腕上的用以识别身份的标志)

idio- *prefix* referring to one particular person 个体,特异,自体

idiocy *noun* severe mental subnormality (IQ below 20) 白痴

idiopathic *adjective* (i) referring to idiopathy 自发病的(ii) (disease) with no obvious cause 特发的; **idiopathic epilepsy** = epilepsy not caused by a brain disorder, beginning during childhood or adolescence 特发性癫痫

◇ **idiopathy** *noun* condition which develops without any known cause 特发病, 自发病

◇ **idiosyncrasy** *noun* (i) way of behaving which is particular to one person 特应性 (ii) one person's strong reaction to treatment *or* to a drug 特异体质

◇ **idioventricular rhythm** *noun* slow natural rhythm in the ventricles of the heart, but not in the atria 心室自主节律

idiot *noun* person suffering from severe mental subnormality 白痴; **idiot savant** = person with mental subnormality who also possesses a single particular mental ability (such as the ability to play music by ear, to draw remembered objects, to do mental calculations) 白痴特才(拥有某一项特殊智能的白痴,如:仅凭耳朵听记即能重复音乐,画出记忆中物体的形状,心算) (NOTE: the term idiot is no longer used by the medical profession)

IDK = INTERNAL DERANGEMENT OF THE KNEE 膝关节内错位

Ig = IMMUNOGLOBULIN 免疫球蛋白

IHD = ISCHAEMIC HEART DISEASE 缺血性心脏病

IL-2 = INTERLEUKIN-2 白介素-2

ile- *prefix* referring to the ileum 回肠

◇ **ileal** *adjective* referring to the ileum 回肠的; **ileal bladder** *or* **ileal conduit** = artificial tube formed when the ureters are linked to part of the ileum, and that part is linked to an opening in the abdominal wall 回肠代膀胱,(人造的管道,将输尿管与回肠相连并开口于腹壁)

◇ **ileectomy** *noun* surgical removal of all *or* part of the ileum 回肠切除术

◇ **ileitis** *noun* inflammation of the ileum 回肠炎; **regional ileitis** *or* **regional enteritis** *or* **Crohn's disease** = inflammation of part of the intestine (usually the ileum) resulting in pain, diarrhoea and loss of weight 局限性回肠炎, 克隆氏病(小肠的一部分,通常为回肠的炎症,表现为疼痛、腹泻和体重下降)

> COMMENT: No certain cause has been found for Crohn's disease, where only one section of the intestine becomes inflamed and can be blocked.
> 注释:至今未发现克隆氏病的病因,本病仅一段小肠发生炎症,可引起梗阻。

◇ **ileocaecal** *adjective* referring to the ileum and the caecum 回盲肠的; **ileocaecal orifice** = point where the small intestine joins the large intestine 回盲孔

◇ **ileocolic** *adjective* referring to both the ileum and the colon 回结肠的; **ileocolic artery** = branch of the superior mesenteric artery 回结肠动脉

◇ **ileocolitis** *noun* inflammation of both the ileum and the colon 回结肠炎

◇ **ileocolostomy** *noun* surgical operation to make a link directly between the ileum and the colon 回结肠吻合术

◇ **ileoproctostomy** *noun* surgical operation to create a link between the ileum and the rectum 回肠直肠吻合术

◇ **ileorectal** *adjective* referring to both the ileum and the rectum 回肠直肠的

◇ **ileosigmoidostomy** *noun* surgical operation to create a link between the ileum and the sigmoid colon 回肠乙状结肠吻合术

◇ **ileostomy** *noun* surgical operation to make an opening between the ileum and the abdominal wall to act as an artificial opening for excretion of faeces 回肠造口术; **ileostomy bag** = bag attached to the opening made by an ileostomy, to collect faeces as they are passed out of the body 回肠造口袋(连接于回肠造口术后开口的袋子,用于收集排出体外的粪便)

◇ **ileum** *noun* lower part of the small intestine, between the jejunum and the caecum 回肠 *compare* 比较 ILIUM ◊ 见

图 DIGESTIVE SYSTEM

COMMENT: The ileum is the longest section of the small intestine, being about 2.5 metres long.
注释:回肠是最长的一段小肠,有2.5米长。

◇ **ileus** *noun* obstruction in the intestine, but usually distension caused by loss of muscular action in the bowel (paralytic *or* a dynamic ileus) 肠梗阻

ili- *prefix* referring to the ilium 髂

◇ **iliac** *adjective* referring to the ilium 髂的; **common iliac artery** = one of two arteries which branch from the aorta in the abdomen and in turn divide into the internal iliac artery (leading to the pelvis) and the external iliac artery (leading to the leg) 髂总动脉; **common iliac veins** = two veins draining the legs, pelvis and abdomen, which join to form the inferior vena cava 髂总静脉; **iliac crest** = curved top edge of the ilium 髂嵴 ◇ 见图 PELVIS; **iliac fossa** = depression on the inner side of the hip bone 髂窝; **iliac regions** = two regions of the lower abdomen, on either side of the hypogastrium 髂区; **iliac spine** = projection at the posterior end of the iliac crest 髂棘

◇ **iliacus** *noun* muscle in the groin which flexes the thigh 髂肌

◇ **iliococcygeal** *adjective* referring to both the ilium and the coccyx 髂尾骨的

◇ **iliolumbar** *adjective* referring to the iliac and lumbar regions 髂腰的

◇ **iliopectineal** *or* **iliopubic** *adjective* referring to both the ilium and the pubis 髂耻的; **iliopectineal** *or* **iliopubic eminence** = raised area on the inner surface of the innominate bone 髂耻突起

◇ **iliopsoas** *noun* muscle formed from the iliacus and psoas muscles 髂腰肌

◇ **iliotibial tract** *noun* thick fascia which runs from the ilium to the tibia 髂胫束

◇ **ilium** *noun* top part of each of the hip bones, which form the pelvis 髂骨 *compare* 比较 ILEUM ◇ 见图 PELVIS

ill *adjective* not well *or* sick 有病的: ***Eating green apples will make you ill.*** 吃青苹果会使你生病。***If you feel ill you ought to see a doctor.*** 如果你觉得有病,应该去看医生。***He's not as ill as he was last week.*** 他不像上周病得那样厉害。(NOTE: **ill - worse - worst**)

◇ **ill health** *noun* not being well 健康不佳: ***He has been in ill health for some time.*** 他身体不适已经有一段时间了。***She has a history of ill health.*** 她以前健康情况不佳。***He had to retire early for reasons of ill health.*** 他因为身体不佳不得不提前退休。

◇ **illness** *noun* (**a**) state of being ill *or* of not being well 疾病: ***His illness makes him very tired.*** 疾病使他很疲倦。***Most of the children stayed away from school because of illness.*** 很多儿童因为疾病离开学校。(**b**) type of disease 某种疾病: ***He is in hospital with an infectious tropical illness.*** 他因感染性热带疾病住院。***Scarlet fever is no longer considered to be a very serious illness.*** 猩红热已不再被认为是一种严重疾病。

illegal *adjective* not done according to the law 不合法的: ***She had an illegal abortion.*** 她非法堕胎。

illusion *noun* condition where a person has a wrong perception of external objects 错觉; **optical illusion** = something which is seen wrongly, usually when it is moving, so that it appears to be something else 视错觉

i.m. *or* **IM** = INTRAMUSCULAR 肌肉注射

image *noun* sensation (such as smell *or* sight *or* taste) which is remembered clearly 影像

◇ **imagery** *noun* producing visual sensations clearly in the mind 想像,意象

◇ **imaging** *noun* technique for creating pictures of sections of the body, using scanners attached to computers 影像术; **magnetic resonance imaging (MRI)** = scanning technique, using magnetic fields and radio waves, for examining soft tissue and cells 核磁共振成像; **X-ray imaging** = showing X-ray pictures of the inside of part of the body on a screen X 线成像

imagine *verb* to see *or* hear *or* feel something in your mind 想像,设想: ***Imagine yourself sitting on the beach in the sun.*** 设想你自己坐在阳光下的海滩上。***I thought I heard someone shout, but I must have imagined it because there is no one there.*** 我听见有人叫喊,但可能是我的幻觉,因为那儿没有一个人。**to imagine things** = to have delusions 妄想: ***She keeps imagining things.*** 她始终存有幻想。***Sometimes he imagines he is swimming in the sea.*** 他有时幻想自己在海里游泳。

◇ **imaginary** *adjective* which does not exist but which is imagined 想像中的; **imaginary playmates** = friends who do not exist but who are imagined by a small child to exist 虚构的玩伴

◇ **imagination** *noun* being able to see things in your mind 想像力,想像: ***In his imagination he saw himself sitting on a beach in the sun.*** 在想像中,他看见自己坐在阳光下的海滩上。

imbalance *noun* wrong proportions of substances as, for example, in the diet 不平衡

imbecile *noun* person who is mentally subnormal 痴愚者

◇ **imbecility** *noun* mental subnormality (where the IQ is below 50) 痴愚(智商值小于 50)(NOTE: these terms are no longer used by the medical profession)

imitate *verb* to do what someone else does 模仿: ***When he walks he imitates his father.*** 他走路时模仿他的父亲。***She is very good at imitating the English teacher.*** 她擅长模仿英语老师。***Children learn by imitating adults or older children.*** 儿童通过模仿成人或年长者进行学习。

immature *adjective* not mature 不成熟的; **an immature cell** = cell which is still developing 未成熟的细胞

immediate *adjective* which happens now *or* without waiting 立刻的,刻不容缓的: ***His condition needs immediate treatment.*** 他的疾病需要立即治疗。

◇ **immediately** *adverb* just after 马上,立刻: ***He became ill immediately after he came back from holiday.*** 他休假回来后就病了。***She will phone the doctor immediately (after) her father regains consciousness.*** 待父亲一恢复知觉,她就给医生打电话。***If the child's temperature rises, you must call the doctor immediately.*** 如果患儿的体温升高,你要立刻给医生打电话。

immersion foot *or* **trench foot** *noun* condition, caused by exposure to cold and damp, where the skin of the foot becomes red and blistered and in severe cases turns black when gangrene sets in. (The condition was common among soldiers serving in the trenches during the First World War) 浸泡足,战壕足(由于暴露于寒冷潮湿的环境中,足部皮肤发红,起泡,严重时坏疽发黑。第一次世界大战时,战壕中的士兵常发生)

Immiscible *adjective* (*of liquids*) which cannot be mixed (液体)不可混合的

immobile *adjective* not moving *or* which cannot move 不动的,不能动的

◇ **immobilization** *noun* being kept still, without moving 制动术

◇ **immobilize** *verb* to make someone keep still and not move *or* to attach a splint to a joint to prevent the bones moving 制动

◇ **immovable** *adjective* (joint) which cannot be moved 不能活动的

immune *adjective* protected against an infection *or* allergic disease 免疫: ***She seems to be immune to colds.*** 她似乎对感冒有免疫力。***The injection should make you immune to yellow fever.*** 这针可帮助你对黄热病产生免疫力。**immune deficiency** = lack of immunity to a disease 免疫缺陷 *see also* 参见 AIDS; **immune reaction** *or* **immune response** = reaction of a body to an antigen 免疫反应;

immune system = complex network of cells and cell products which protects the body from disease; it includes the thymus, spleen, lymph nodes, white blood cells and antibodies 免疫系统(细胞及其产物组成的复杂网络,帮助机体抵抗疾病,包括胸腺、脾、淋巴结、白细胞和抗体)

◇ **immunity** *noun* ability to resist attacks of a disease because antibodies are produced 免疫力: ***The vaccine gives immunity to tuberculosis.*** 疫苗可对结核产生免疫力。**acquired immunity** = immunity which a body acquires (from having caught a disease *or* from immunization), not one which is congenital 获得性免疫; **active immunity** = immunity which is acquired by catching and surviving an infectious disease or by vaccination with a weakened form of the disease which makes the body form antibodies 自动免疫; **natural immunity** = immunity which a body acquires in the womb or from the mother's milk 自然免疫; **passive immunity** = immunity which is acquired by the transfer of an immune mechanism from another animal 被动免疫

◇ **immunization** *noun* making a person immune to an infection, either by injecting an antiserum (passive immunization) or by giving the body the disease in such a small dose that the body does not develop the disease, but produces antibodies to counteract it 免疫

◇ **immunize** *verb* to give someone immunity from an infection 免疫 (NOTE: you immunize someone **against a disease**)

◇ **immunoassay** *noun* test for the presence and strength of antibodies 免疫检测

◇ **immunocompetent** *adjective* able to participate in the process of immunization 有免疫力的

◇ **immunocompromised** *adjective* not able to offer resistance to infection 免疫功能低下的

◇ **immunodeficiency** *noun* lack of immunity to a disease 免疫缺陷; **immunodeficieny virus** = retrovirus which attacks the immune system 免疫缺陷病毒 *see also* 参见 HIV

◇ **immunodeficient** *adjective* lacking immunity to a disease 免疫缺陷的: ***This form of meningitis occurs in persons who are immunodeficient.*** 这类脑膜炎发生于免疫功能低下者。

◇ **immunoelectrophoresis** *noun* method of identifying antigens in a laboratory, using electrophoresis 免疫电泳

◇ **immunoglobulin (Ig)** *noun* antibody, a protein produced in blood plasma as protection against infection (the commonest is gamma globulin) 免疫球蛋白

◇ **immunological** *adjective* referring to immunology 免疫学的; **immunological tolerance** = tolerance of the lymphoid tissues to an antigen 免疫耐受

◇ **immunology** *noun* study of immunity and immunization 免疫学

◇ **immunosuppression** *noun* suppressing the body's natural immune system so that it will not reject a transplanted organ 免疫抑制

◇ **immunosuppressive** *adjective* & *noun* (drug) used to counteract the response of the immune system to reject a transplanted organ 免疫抑制的,免疫抑制剂

◇ **immunotherapy** 免疫疗法 *see* 见 ADOPTIVE

◇ **immunotransfusion** *noun* transfusion of blood, serum or plasma containing immune bodies 免疫输血法

> QUOTE: The reason for this susceptibility is a profound abnormality of the immune system in children with sickle-cell disease.
> 引文:易感性的原因是镰状细胞病患儿的免疫系统有严重缺陷。
> **Lancet** 柳叶刀杂志

> QUOTE: The AIDS virus attacks a person's immune system and damages

his or her ability to fight other diseases. 引文：艾滋病病毒侵犯机体的免疫系统，损毁机体对其他疾病的抵抗力。

Journal of the American Medical Association 美国医学会杂志

QUOTE: Vaccination is the most effective way to prevent children getting the disease. Children up to 6 years old can be vaccinated if they missed earlier immunization.
引文：疫苗是预防儿童感染此病最有效的方法。错过早期免疫的儿童，在6岁前都可进行疫苗注射。

Health Visitor 保健访视员

impacted *adjective* tightly pressed *or* firmly lodged against something 嵌入的；**impacted fracture** = fracture where the broken parts of the bones are driven against each other 嵌入性骨折；**impacted tooth** = tooth which is held against another tooth and so cannot grow normally 阻生齿；**impacted ureteric calculus** = stone which is lodged in a ureter 输尿管结石嵌入

◇ **impaction** *noun* condition where two things are impacted 阻生，嵌塞；**dental impaction** = condition where a tooth is impacted in the jaw 牙阻生；**faecal impaction** = condition where a hardened mass of faeces stays in the rectum 粪便嵌塞

impair *verb* to harm (a sense *or* function) so that it does not work properly 损害；**impaired hearing** = hearing which is not acute 听力损伤；**impaired vision** = eyesight which is not fully clear 视力受损；**visually impaired person** = person whose eyesight is not clear 视力受损的人

◇ **impairment** *noun* condition where a sense *or* function is harmed so that it does not work properly 损伤：***His hearing impairment does not affect his work.*** 听力的损伤并没有影响他的工作。***The impairment was progressive, but she did not notice that her eyesight was getting worse.*** 损害在进行性加重，但她没有发觉视力在恶化。

impalpable *adjective* which cannot be felt when touched 不可触知的

impediment *noun* obstruction 障碍；**speech impediment** = condition where a person cannot speak properly because of a deformed mouth 言语障碍(因口腔畸形导致不能正常说话)

imperfecta 不全的 *see* 见 OSTEOGENESIS

imperforate *adjective* without an opening 无孔的；**imperforate anus** = condition where the anus does not have an opening 肛门闭锁；**imperforate hymen** = membrane in the vagina which has no opening for the menstrual fluid 处女膜闭锁

impetigo *noun* irritating and very contagious skin disease caused by staphylococci, which spreads rapidly and is easily passed from one child to another, but can be treated with antibiotics 脓疱病(葡萄球菌引起的皮肤病，极易传染，但可用抗生素治疗)

implant **1** *noun* tissue *or* drug *or* inert material *or* device (such as a pacemaker) grafted *or* inserted into a patient 植入物；**implant material** = substance grafted *or* inserted into a patient 植入物；**implant site** = place in *or* on the body where the implant is positioned 植入部位 **2** *verb* to become fixed; to graft *or* insert (tissue *or* drug *or* inert material *or* device) 固定，植入，种植：***The ovum implants in the wall of the uterus.*** 受精卵植入子宫壁。***The site was implanted with the biomaterial.*** 这部位植入了生物材料。

◇ **implantation** *noun* (**a**) grafting *or* inserting of a drug *or* tissue *or* inert material *or* device into a patient 移植，植入；introduction of one tissue into another surgically 手术移植 (**b**) place in *or* on the body where an implant is positioned 移植部位 (**c**) point in the development of an embryo when the fertilized ovum reaches the uterus and becomes fixed in the wall of the uterus 着床，植入 *see also* 参见 NIDATION

impotence *noun* inability in a male to have an erection *or* to ejaculate, and so have sexual intercourse 阳痿

◇ **impotent** *adjective* (*of a man*) unable to have sexual intercourse 阳痿的

impregnate *verb* (**a**) to make (a female) pregnant 受孕 (**b**) to soak (a cloth) with a liquid 浸渗：***A cloth impregnated with antiseptic*.** 浸有抗菌剂的敷料。

◇ **impregnation** *noun* action of impregnating 受孕

impression *noun* (**a**) mould of a patient's jaw made by a dentist before making a denture 印模 (**b**) depression on an organ *or* structure into which another organ *or* structure fits 压迹；**cardiac impression** = (i) concave area near the centre of the upper surface of the liver under the heart 肝的心压迹 (ii) depression on the mediastinal part of the lungs where they touch the pericardium 肺的心压迹

improve *verb* to get better 好转；to make better 改善：***He was very ill, but he is improving now*.** 他曾经病得很厉害，但他正在好转。

◇ **improvement** *noun* getting better 好转：***The patient's condition has shown a slight improvement*.** 患者的病情有轻微的好转。***Doctors have not detected any improvement in her asthma*.** 医生没有发现她的哮喘有任何好转的迹象。

impulse *noun* (i) message transmitted by a nerve 神经冲动 (ii) sudden feeling that you want to act in a certain way 冲动

impure *adjective* not pure 不纯的

◇ **impurities** *plural noun* substances which are not pure *or* clean 不纯物，杂质：***The kidneys filter impurities out of the blood*.** 肾脏过滤血液中的杂质。

inability *noun* being unable to do something 无能，无能为力：***He suffered from a temporary inability to pass water*.** 他患有暂时性尿潴留。

inactive *adjective* (**a**) not being active *or* not moving 不活动的：***Patients must not be allowed to become inactive*.** 患者无需制动。(**b**) which does not work 无用的：***The serum makes the poison inactive*.** 血清使毒物失去作用。

◇ **inactivity** *noun* lack of activity 无活力：***He has periods of complete inactivity*.** 他有一段时期完全丧失活力。

inadequate *adjective* not sufficient 不全的，不够的：***The hospital has inadequate staff to deal with a major accident*.** 医院缺乏处理重大事故的足够人力。

in articulo mortis *Latin phrase meaning* 'at the onset of death' 濒死(拉丁语)

inborn *adjective* which is in the body from birth 先天的：***A body has an inborn tendency to reject transplanted organs*.** 机体具有排斥植入器官的固有倾向。

inbreeding *noun* breeding between a closely related male and female, who have the same parents or grandparents, so making congenital defects spread 近亲繁殖

◇ **inbred** *adjective* suffering from inbreeding 近亲繁殖的

incapacitated *adjective* not able to act 不能动的：***He was incapacitated for three weeks by his accident*.** 因为事故，他有3个星期不能动。

incapable *adjective* not able to do something 不能的：***She was incapable of feeding herself*.** 她不能自己进食。

incarcerated *adjective* (hernia) which cannot be corrected by physical manipulation 箝闭的

inception rate *noun* number of new cases of a disease during a period of time, per thousand of population 发病率(每千人中某一时期新发病例数)

incest *noun* crime of having sexual intercourse with a close relative (daughter, son, mother, father) 乱伦

◇ **incestuous** *adjective* referring to incest 乱伦的：***They had an incestuous***

***relationship*.** 他们曾经乱伦。

incidence *noun* number of times something happens in a certain population over a period of time 发生率: ***The incidence of drug-related deaths*.** 药物引起死亡的发生率。***Men have a higher incidence of stroke than women*.** 男性比女性更易中风。**incidence rate** = number of new cases of a disease during a given period, per thousand of population 发病率

incipient *adjective* which is just beginning *or* which is in its early stages 初发的: ***He has an incipient appendicitis*.** 他患早期阑尾炎。***The tests detected incipient diabetes mellitus*.** 此试验检测初发糖尿病。

incise *verb* to cut 切; **incised wound** = wound with clean edges, caused by a sharp knife or razor 切伤

◇ **incision** *noun* cut in a patient's body made by a surgeon using a scalpel 手术切口; any cut made with a sharp knife *or* razor 切口: ***The first incision is made two millimetres below the second rib*.** 第一切口在第二肋骨下 2 毫米。*compare* 比较 EXCISION

◇ **incisional** *adjective* referring to an incision 切口的; **incisional hernia** = hernia which breaks through the abdominal wall at a place where a surgical incision was made during an operation 切口疝

incisor (**tooth**) *noun* one of the front teeth (four each in the upper and lower jaws) which are used to cut off pieces of food 切牙 ◊ 见图 TEETH

include *verb* to count something *or* someone with others 包括: ***Does the number of cases include the figures for outpatients?*** 病例数包括了门诊病人吗? ***The dentist will be on holiday up to and including next Tuesday*.** 牙医将休假到下周二(包括周二)。

◇ **inclusion** *noun* something enclosed inside something else 包括; **inclusion bodies** = very small particles found in cells infected by virus 包涵体

incoherent *adjective* not able to speak in a way which makes sense 不连贯的

incompatible *adjective* which does not go together with something else 不相容的; (drugs) which must not be used together because they undergo chemical change and the therapeutic effect is lost or changed to something undesirable 配伍禁忌的; (tissue) which is genetically different from other tissue, making it impossible to transplant into that tissue 配型不合的; **incompatible blood** = blood from a donor that does not match the blood of the patient receiving the transfusion 血型不合

◇ **incompatibility** *noun* being incompatible 不相容: ***The incompatibility of the donor's blood with that of the patient*.** 供者的血型与患者不合。

incompetence *noun* (i) not being able to do a certain act 功能不全(ii) (*of valves*) not closing properly 闭锁不全; **aortic incompetence** = condition where the aortic valve does not close properly, causing regurgitation 主动脉闭锁不全; **mitral incompetence** = situation where the mitral valve does not close completely so that blood flows back into the atrium 二尖瓣闭锁不全

◇ **incompetent** *adjective* (**a**) (part of the body) which is unable to function 功能不全的; ***an incompetent mitral valve*** 二尖瓣功能不全 (**b**) (person) who is mentally deficient 无能力的

incomplete *adjective* which is not complete 不全的; **incomplete abortion** 不全流产 *see* 见 ABORTION

incontinence *noun* inability to control the discharge of urine 尿失禁; **faecal incontinence** *or* **encopresis** = inability to control the bowel movements 便失禁; **stress incontinence** = condition in women where the sufferer is incapable of retaining urine when the intra-abdominal pressure is raised by coughing or laughing 压迫性尿失禁(妇女咳嗽或大笑时腹内压增高发生); **incontinence pad** = pad of material to absorb urine 尿垫

◇ **incontinent** *adjective* unable to control the discharge of urine *or* faeces 失禁的

incoordination *noun* situation where the muscles in various parts of the body do not act together, making it impossible to do certain actions 共济失调

incorrect *adjective* not correct 不正确的: ***The doctor made an incorrect diagnosis.*** 医生做出了错误诊断。***The dosage prescribed was incorrect.*** 处方的剂量不正确的。

increase **1** *noun* getting larger *or* higher 增长: ***an increase in heart rate*** 心率加快 **2** *verb* to get larger *or* higher 增长: ***His pulse rate increased by 10 per cent.*** 他的脉率增加10%。

incubation period *noun* (i) time during which a virus *or* bacterium develops in the body after contamination *or* infection, before the appearance of the symptoms of the disease 潜伏期 (ii) time during which a bacterial sample grows in a laboratory culture 孵育期

◇ **incubator** *noun* (**a**) apparatus for growing bacterial cultures 培养箱 (**b**) specially controlled container in which a premature baby can be kept in ideal conditions 保温箱,孵化器

incurable *noun* & *adjective* (patient) who will never be cured *or* (illness) which can not be cured 不治之症,不能治愈的: ***He is suffering from an incurable disease of the blood.*** 他患了不能治愈的血液病。***She has been admitted to a hospital for incurables.*** 她因患不治之症被送入院。

incus *noun* one of the three ossicles in the middle ear, shaped like an anvil 砧骨 ⇨见图 EAR

COMMENT: The incus is the central one of the three bones: the malleus articulates with it, and the incus articulates with the stapes.

注释:砧骨是三块骨中间的一块:锤骨与它连接,砧骨再与镫骨相连。

independent *adjective* free *or* not controlled by someone *or* something else 独立的

◇ **independently** *adverb* not being controlled by anyone *or* anything 自主地,不受控制地: ***The autonomic nervous system functions independently of the conscious will.*** 自主神经系统不受意识的控制。

index finger *noun* first finger next to the thumb 食指

Indian hemp *noun* tropical plant from whose leaves or flowers cannabis (*or* marijuana *or* hashish) is produced 大麻(一种热带植物,其叶和花可提取大麻)

indican *noun* potassium salt 钾盐

indicate *verb* (**a**) to show 指示,显示: ***The skin reaction indicates a highly allergenic state.*** 皮肤反应显示处于高敏状态。(**b**) to suggest that a certain type of treatment should be given 治疗指征: ***A course of antibiotics is indicated.*** 需要应用一疗程的抗生素。***Therapeutic intervention was indicated in nine of the patients tested.*** 被检验的患者中有9人需要治疗。

◇ **indication** *noun* situation *or* sign which suggests that a certain type of treatment should be given or that a condition has a particular cause 适应证: ***Sulpha drugs have been replaced by antibiotics in many indications.*** 在很多情况下,磺胺类药物被抗生素所取代。*see also* 参见 CONTRAINDICATION

◇ **indicator** *noun* substance which shows something, especially a substance secreted in body fluids which shows which blood group a person belongs to 指示剂

indigestion *or* **dyspepsia** *noun* disturbance of the normal process of digestion, where the patient experiences pain *or* discomfort in the stomach 消化不良: ***He is taking tablets to relieve his indigestion*** *or* ***he is taking indigestion tablets.*** 他吃药以减轻消化不良。

indirect *adjective* not direct 间接的; **indirect contact** = catching a disease by inhaling bacteria *or* by being in contact with a vector, but not in direct contact with an infected person 间接接触

indisposed *adjective* slightly ill 不适的,违和的: ***My mother is indisposed and cannot see any visitors.*** 我母亲身体不适,不能见任何客人。

◇ **indisposition** *noun* slight illness 不适,小恙

individual *noun* & *adjective* one particular person 个体,个别的

indolent *adjective* causing little pain 不痛的,微痛的;(ulcer) which develops slowly and does not heal 逐渐发生未愈合的(溃疡)

indrawing *noun* pulling towards the inside 吸入

◇ **indrawn** *adjective* which is pulled inside 吸入的

induce *verb* to make something happen 诱导; **to induce labour** = to make a woman go into labour 做引产; **induced abortion** = abortion which is produced by drugs *or* by surgery 引产

◇ **induction of labour** *noun* action of starting childbirth artificially 引产

induration *noun* hardening of tissue *or* of an artery because of pathological change 硬结

induratum 硬的 *see* 见 ERYTHEMA

industrial *adjective* referring to industries *or* factories 工业的,工厂的; **industrial disease** = disease which is caused by the type of work done by a worker (such as by dust produced *or* chemicals used in the factory) 工业病,职业病

indwelling catheter *noun* catheter left in place for a period of time after its introduction 留置导管

inebriation *noun* state where a person is habitually drunk 醉酒状

inertia *noun* complete lack of activity *or* condition of indolence of the body or mind 惰性

in extremis *Latin phrase meaning* 'at the moment of death' 濒死

infant *noun* small child under two years of age 婴幼儿; **infant mortality rate** = number of infants who die per thousand births 婴幼儿死亡率

◇ **infantile** *adjective* (i) referring to small children 婴幼儿的 (ii) (disease) which affects children 婴幼儿罹患的(疾病); **infantile convulsions** *or* **spasms** = convulsions, minor epileptic fits in small children 幼儿惊厥; **infantile paralysis** 脊髓灰质炎,小儿麻痹 *see* 见 POLIOMYELITIS

◇ **infantilism** *noun* condition where a person keeps some characteristics of an infant when he becomes an adult 幼稚型

infarct *noun* area of tissue which is killed when the blood supply is cut off by the blockage of an artery 梗死灶

◇ **infarction** *noun* killing of tissue by cutting off the blood supply 梗死; **cardiac** *or* **myocardial infarction** = death of part of the heart muscle after coronary thrombosis 心肌梗死; **cerebral infarction** = death of brain tissue as a result of reduction in the blood supply to the brain 脑梗死

> QUOTE: Cerebral infarction accounts for about 80% of first-ever strokes.
> 引文:脑梗死在初发卒中中占80%。
> **British Journal of Hospital Medicine** 英国医院医学杂志

infect *verb* to contaminate with disease-producing microorganisms *or* toxins; to transmit infection 感染,传染: ***The disease infected his liver.*** 疾病侵及了他的肝脏。***The whole arm soon became infected.*** 很快整条胳膊都感染了。**infected wound** = wound which has become poisoned by bacteria 感染伤口

◇ **infection** *noun* entry of microbes into the body, which then multiply in the body 感染: ***As a carrier he was spreading infection to other people in the office.*** 作为携带者他将疾病传染给了办公室里的其他人。***She is susceptible to***

minor infections. 她对轻微的感染易感。

◇ **infectious** *adjective* (disease) which is caused by microbes and can be transmitted to other persons by direct means 有传染性的: ***This strain of flu is highly infectious.*** 这型流感有很强的传染性。***Her measles is at the infectious stage.*** 她的风疹处于传染期。**infectious hepatitis** *or* **hepatitis A** = hepatitis transmitted by a carrier through food or drink 传染性肝炎,甲肝; **infectious mononucleosis** *or* **glandular fever** = infectious disease where the body has an excessive number of white blood cells 传染性单核细胞增多症

> COMMENT: The symptoms include sore throat, fever and swelling of the lymph glands in the neck. The disease is probably caused by the Epstein-Barr virus.
> 注释:症状包括咽痛、发热和颈部淋巴结肿大,本病可能由 EB 病毒引起。

◇ **infective** *adjective* (disease) caused by a microbe, which can be caught from another person but which cannot always be directly transmitted 感染的; (**subacute**) **infective endocarditis** = infection of the endocardium (the membrane covering the inner surfaces of the heart) by bacteria(亚急性)感染性心内膜炎; **infective enteritis** = enteritis caused by bacteria 感染性肠炎; **infective hepatitis** *or* **hepatitis A** = hepatitis transmitted by a carrier through food or drink 传染性肝炎,甲型肝炎

◇ **infectivity** *noun* being infective 传染性: ***The patient's infectivity can last about a week.*** 患者的传染性可持续一周。

inferior *adjective* lower (part of the body) 下的; **inferior aspect** = view of the body from below 仰视; **inferior vena cava** = main vein carrying blood from the lower part of the body to the heart 下腔静脉

◇ **inferiority** *noun* being lower *or* less important *or* less intelligent than others 自卑,低劣; **inferiority complex** = mental state where the patient feels very inferior to others and compensates for this by behaving violently towards them 自卑情结 (NOTE: the opposite is **superior, superiority**)

infertile *adjective* not fertile *or* not able to reproduce 不育的

◇ **infertility** *noun* not being fertile *or* able to reproduce 不育症

infest *verb* (*of parasites*) to be present in large numbers 大批出现,侵染,感染: ***The child's hair was infested with lice.*** 这孩子的头发上全是虱子。

◇ **infestation** *noun* having large numbers of parasites 有大批寄生虫; invasion of the body by parasites 感染寄生虫: ***The condition is caused by infestation of the hair with lice.*** 这病是因为头发上有大量的虱子引起的。

infiltrate 1 *verb* (*of liquid or waste*) to pass from one part of the body to another through a wall *or* membrane and be deposited in the other part 浸润 **2** *noun* substance which has infiltrated part of the body 浸润物

◇ **infiltration** *noun* passing of a liquid through the walls of one part of the body into another part 渗透,液体浸润; condition where waste is brought to and deposited round cells 浸润

> QUOTE: The chest roentgenogram often discloses interstitial pulmonary infiltrates, but may occasionally be normal.
> 引文:胸部 X 线片常可发现肺间质浸润,但偶尔表现正常。
> **Southern Medical Journal** 南部医学杂志

> QUOTE: The lacrimal and salivary glands become infiltrated with lymphocytes and plasma cells. The infiltration reduces lacrimal and salivary secretions which in turn leads to dry eyes and dry mouth.
> 引文:淋巴细胞和浆细胞浸润泪腺和涎腺,使两腺分泌减少,造成眼干和口干。
> **American Journal of Nursing**
> 美国护理杂志

infirm *adjective* old and weak 衰弱的:

My grandfather is quite infirm now. 我祖父现在很衰弱。

◇ **infirmity** *noun* (i) being old and weak 衰弱 (ii) illness 疾病: ***In spite of his infirmities he still reads all the newspapers.*** 尽管身体虚弱,他仍阅读所有的报纸。

◇ **infirmary** *noun* (**a**) room in a school *or* factory where people can go if they are ill 医务所 (**b**) old name for a hospital 医院的旧称 (NOTE: **infirmary** is still used in names of hospitals: **the Glasgow Royal Infirmary**)

inflame *verb* to make an organ *or* a tissue react to an infection *or* an irritation *or* a blow by becoming sore, red and swollen 发炎: ***The skin has become inflamed around the sore.*** 溃疡周围皮肤已经发炎。

◇ **inflammation** *noun* being inflamed *or* having become sore, red and swollen as a reaction to an infection *or* an irritation *or* a blow 炎症: ***She has an inflammation of the bladder or a bladder inflammation.*** 她膀胱发炎了。***The body's reaction to infection took the form of an inflammation of the eyelid.*** 机体对抗感染的反应表现为眼睑发炎。

◇ **inflammatory** *adjective* which makes an organ *or* a tissue become sore, red and swollen 炎症的; **inflammatory bowel disease** = any condition (such as Crohn's disease *or* colitis *or* ileitis) where the bowel becomes inflamed 炎症性肠病; **inflammatory response** *or* **reaction** = any condition where an organ *or* a tissue reacts to an external stimulus by becoming inflamed 炎症反应: ***She showed an inflammatory response to the ointment.*** 她对药膏出现了炎症反应。

inflate *verb* to fill with air 充气: ***The abdomen is inflated with air before a coelioscopy.*** 结肠镜检查前,腹腔要进行充气。***In valvuloplasty, a balloon is introduced into the valve and inflated.*** 在瓣膜成形术中,气囊引入瓣膜并充气。

◇ **inflatable** *adjective* which can be inflated 可充气的

influence 1 *noun* being able to have an effect on someone *or* something 影响 **2** *verb* to have an effect on someone *or* something 影响: ***The development of the serum has been influenced by research carried out in the USA.*** 血浆制品的发展受在美国开展的研究的影响。

influenza *noun* infectious disease of the upper respiratory tract with fever, malaise and muscular aches, transmitted by a virus, which occurs in epidemics 流感: ***She is in bed with influenza.*** 她因流感卧床。***Half the staff in the office are off work with influenza.*** 办公室一半的人员因为流感不能上班。***The influenza epidemic has killed several people.*** 流感的流行已经造成几名患者的死亡。

> COMMENT: Influenza virus is spread by droplets of moisture in the air, so the disease can be spread by coughing or sneezing. Influenza can be quite mild, but virulent strains occur from time to time (Spanish influenza, Hong Kong flu) and can weaken the patient so much that he becomes susceptible to pneumonia and other more serious infections.
> 注释:流感病毒由空气飞沫传播,所以本病可经咳嗽或喷嚏传染。流感可以很轻微,但有时会产生强毒性的病毒株(西班牙流感,香港流感),使患者体质虚弱,增加对肺炎及其他更严重感染的易感性。

inform *verb* to tell someone 通知: ***Have you informed the police that the drugs have been stolen?*** 你告诉警察药品被偷了吗?

◇ **information** *noun* facts about something 信息,消息: ***Have you any information about the treatment of sunburn?*** 你对治疗阳光灼伤有什么消息吗? ***The police won't give us any information about how the accident happened.*** 警察不会告诉我们有关事故发生的任何消息。***You haven't given me enough information about when your symptoms started.*** 你没有提供症状开始时的足够信息。***That's a very useful piece or bit of information.*** 这是一则很有价值的信息。(NOTE: no plural **some information; a piece of information**)

informal *adjective* not official 非正式的; **informal patient** = patient who has admitted himself to a hospital, without being referred by a doctor 未经医生介绍，主动去医院看病的患者。

infra- *prefix* meaning below 下

◇ **infraorbital nerve** *noun* continuation of the maxillary nerve below the orbit of the eye 眶下神经

◇**infraorbital vein** *noun* vessel draining the face through the infraorbital canal to the pterygoid plexus 眶下静脉

◇ **infrared rays** *or* **infrared radiation** *noun* long invisible rays, below the visible red end of the colour spectrum, used to produce heat in body tissues in the treatment of traumatic and inflammatory conditions 红外线: ***She was advised to take a course of infrared ray treatment.*** 她被建议接受一疗程的红外线治疗。

infundibulum *noun* any part of the body shaped like a funnel, especially the stem which attaches the pituitary gland to the hypothalamus 漏斗，圆锥（垂体柄）

infusion *noun* (i) drink made by pouring boiling water on a dry substance(such as herb tea *or* a powdered drug) 浸剂，冲剂(ii) putting liquid into a body, using a drip 输注 *see also* 参见 CAVAL

ingestion *noun* (i) taking in food *or* drink *or* medicine by the mouth 咽下，摄入(ii) process by which a foreign body (such as a bacillus) is surrounded by a cell 吞噬

ingredient *noun* substance which is used with others to make something (food to eat *or* lotion to put on the skin, etc.) 成分; **active ingredient** 活性成分 *see* 见 ACTIVE

ingrowing toenail *noun* condition where the nail cuts into the tissue at the side of it, and creates inflammation; sepsis and ulceration can also occur 内生趾甲，趾甲长入肌肉内，可引起炎症、败血症和溃疡: ***If the nail is slightly ingrown, it can be treated by cutting at the sides.*** 如果指甲略向肌肉内长入，可在侧面将其剪去。

inguinal *adjective* referring to the groin 腹股沟的; **inguinal canal** = passage in the lower abdominal wall, carrying the spermatic cord in the male and the round ligament of the uterus in the female 腹股沟管; **inguinal hernia** = hernia where the intestine bulges through the muscles in the groin, especially through the inguinal canal 腹股沟疝; **inguinal ligament** *or* **Poupart's ligament** = ligament in the groin, running from the spine to the pubis 腹股沟韧带; **inguinal region** = groin, the part of the body where the lower abdomen joins the top of the thigh 腹股沟区

◇ **inguinale** 腹股沟的 *see* 见 GRANULOMA

inhale *verb* to breathe in 吸入: ***He inhaled some toxic gas fumes and was rushed to hospital.*** 他吸入了些有毒气体，被急送入医院。***Even smoking cigars can be bad for you if you inhale the smoke.*** 即使是雪茄，如果吸入了烟雾也会对你有害。

◇ **inhalant** *noun* medicinal substance which is breathed in 吸入剂

◇ **inhalation** *noun* (**a**) action of breathing in 吸入; **smoke inhalation** = breathing in smoke (as in a fire) 吸入烟雾 (**b**) action of breathing in a medicinal substance as part of treatment 吸入疗法; medicinal substance which is breathed in 吸入剂; **steam inhalation** = treatment of respiratory disease by breathing in steam with medicinal substances in it 雾化吸入

◇ **inhaler** *noun* small device for administering medicinal substances into the mouth *or* nose so that they can be breathed in 吸入器 (NOTE: opposite is **exhale, exhalation**)

inherent *adjective* thing which is part of the essential character of a person *or* a permanent characteristic of an organism固有的

inherit *verb* to receive characteristics from a parent's genes 遗传: ***She inherited her father's red hair.*** 她遗传了父亲的红头发。***Haemophilia is a condition which is inherited through the mother's genes.*** 血友病是一种由母亲基因遗传的疾病。

inhibit *verb* to block *or* to prevent an action happening; to stop a functional process 抑制,阻止: ***Aspirin inhibits the clotting of blood.*** 阿司匹林抑制血液凝固。**to have an inhibiting effect on something** = to block something *or* to stop something happening 对…有抑制作用

◇ **inhibition** *noun* (**a**) action of blocking *or* preventing something happening, especially preventing a muscle *or* organ from functioning properly 抑制(尤其是抑制肌肉或器官的正常功能) (**b**) (*in psychology*) suppressing a thought which is associated to a sense of guilt 压制与罪恶感有关的思想; blocking of a normal spontaneous action by some mental influence 抑郁,因精神原因使正常的自发活动受抑

◇ **inhibitor** *noun* substance which inhibits 抑制剂

◇ **inhibitory nerve** *noun* nerve which stops a function taking place 抑制神经: ***The vagus nerve is an inhibitory nerve which slows down the action of the heart.*** 迷走神经是使心脏活动减弱的抑制神经。

inject *verb* to put a liquid into a patient's body under pressure, by using a hollow needle inserted into the tissues 注射: ***He was injected with morphine.*** 他被注射了吗啡。***She injected herself with a drug.*** 她给自己注射药物。

◇ **injection** *noun* (**a**) act of injecting a liquid into the body 注射; **intracutaneous injection** = injection of a liquid between the layers of skin (as for a test for an allergy) 皮内注射; **intramuscular injection** = injection of liquid into a muscle (as for a slow release of a drug) 肌肉注射; **intravenous injection** = injection of liquid into a vein (as for fast release of a drug) 静脉注射; **hypodermic injection** *or* **subcutaneous injection** = injection of a liquid beneath the skin (as for pain-killing drugs) 皮下注射 (**b**) liquid introduced into the body 注射剂: ***He had a penicillin injection.*** 给他用了青霉素注射剂。

injure *verb* to hurt 伤害,损伤: ***Six people were injured in the accident.*** 有6人在事故中受伤。

◇ **injured 1** *adjective* (person) who has been hurt 受伤的 **2** *noun* **the injured** = people who have been injured 伤员: ***All the injured were taken to the nearest hospital.*** 所有的伤员都被送到最近的医院。

◇ **injury** *noun* damage *or* wound caused to a person's body 损伤: ***His injuries required hospital treatment.*** 他的伤需要住院治疗。***She never recovered from her injuries.*** 她再也没有从损伤中恢复过来。***He received severe facial injuries in the accident.*** 事故中他的面部严重受伤。**accidental injury** = injury sustained in an accident 意外伤; **non-accidental injury** = injury which is not caused accidentally 非意外伤害

ink *noun* coloured liquid which is used for writing 墨水; **ink blot test** = RORSCHACH TEST 墨迹测验

inlay *noun* (*in dentistry*) type of filling for teeth 嵌体

inlet *noun* passage *or* opening through which a cavity can be entered 入口; **thoracic inlet** = upper bony margin of the thorax 胸廓上口

innate *adjective* inherited *or* which is present in a body from birth 天生的

inner *adjective* (part) which is inside 内部的; **inner ear** = part of the ear inside the head, behind the eardrum, containing the semicircular canals, the vestibule and the cochlea 内耳; **inner pleura** = membrane attached to the surface of a lung 内胸膜,脏层胸膜

(NOTE: the opposite is **outer**)

◇ **innermost** *adjective* furthest inside 最里面的

innervation *noun* nerve supply to an organ (both motor nerves and sensory nerves) 神经分布

innocent *adjective* (growth) which is benign *or* not malignant 良性的

innominate *adjective* with no name 无名的，匿名的；**innominate artery** *or* **brachiocephalic artery** = largest branch of the arch of the aorta, which continues as the right common carotid and right subclavian arteries 无名动脉；**innominate bone** = HIPBONE 髋骨；**innominate veins** *or* **brachiocephalic veins** = two veins which continue the subclavian and jugular veins to the superior vena cava 无名或头臂静脉

inoculate *verb* to introduce vaccine into a person's body in order to make the body create antibodies, so making the person immune to the disease 接种：***The baby was inoculated against diphtheria.*** 婴儿已经接种了白喉疫苗。(NOTE: you inoculate someone **with or against a disease**)

◇ **inoculation** *noun* action of inoculating someone 接种：***Has the baby had a diphtheria inoculation?*** 已经给孩子接种白喉疫苗了吗?

◇ **inoculum** *noun* substance (such as a vaccine) used for inoculation 接种物

inoperable *adjective* (condition) which cannot be operated on 不能手术的：***The surgeon decided that the cancer was inoperable.*** 外科医师认为肿瘤已经不能手术治疗了。

inorganic *adjective* (substance) which is not made from animal or vegetable sources 无机的

inotropic *adjective* which affects the way muscles contract, especially those of the heart 影响收缩力的

inpatient *noun* patient living in a hospital for treatment *or* observation 住院病人 *compare* 比较 OUTPATIENT

inquest *noun* inquiry (by a coroner) into the cause of a death 验尸

> COMMENT: An inquest has to take place where death is violent or not expected, where death could be murder, or where a prisoner dies and when police are involved.
> 注释：当因暴力或意外死亡、被谋杀、罪犯死亡或有警察介入者，都需进行验尸。

inquire *verb* to ask questions about something 询问：***He inquired if anything was wrong.*** 他问有什么不舒服。***She inquired about the success rate of that type of operation.*** 她询问此类手术的成功率。***The committee is inquiring into the administration of the District Health Authority.*** 委员会对地区卫生部门的管理提出质询。

◇ **inquiry** *noun* official investigation 调查：***There has been a government inquiry into the outbreak of legionnaires' disease.*** 政府已经在对军团菌病的暴发进行调查。

insane *adjective* mad *or* suffering from a mental disorder 精神错乱的

◇ **insanity** *noun* psychotic mental disorder *or* illness 精神病

> COMMENT: Insanity is the legal term used to describe patients whose mental condition is so unstable that they need to be placed in a hospital to prevent them doing actions which could harm themselves or other people, although some are cared for in the community.
> 注释：精神病是法律术语，用来指那些精神状态不稳定，需住院治疗以防止他们作出危害自身或他人举动的患者，部分患者可由社区照看。

insanitary *adjective* not sanitary *or* unhygienic 不卫生的：***Cholera spread rapidly because of the insanitary conditions in the town.*** 由于城镇恶劣的卫生状况，霍乱迅速传播。

insect *noun* small animal with six legs and a body in three parts 昆虫：***Insects were flying round the lamp.*** 昆虫在灯周围飞舞。***He was stung by an insect.*** 他被

昆虫螫了一下。**insect bites** = stings caused by insects which puncture the skin to suck blood, and in so doing introduce irritants 昆虫螫咬

◇ **insecticide** *noun* substance which kills insects 杀虫剂

> COMMENT: Most insect bites are simply irritating, but some patients can be extremely sensitive to certain types of insect(such as bee stings). Other insect bites can be more serious, as insects can carry the bacteria which produce typhus, sleeping sickness, malaria, filariasis, etc.
> 注释:大部分的虫咬仅引起刺激反应,但有些人对某类昆虫(如:蜜蜂)极其敏感。另一些虫咬因昆虫携带细菌可以传播伤寒、昏睡病、疟疾、丝虫病等而更危险。

insemination *noun* (i) fertilization of an ovum by a sperm 授精(ii) introduction of sperm into the vagina 授精,将精子植入阴道; **artificial insemination** = introduction of semen into a woman's womb by artificial means 人工授精 *see also* 参见 AID, AIH

insert *verb* to put something into something 插,植入: ***The catheter is inserted into the passage.*** 导管插入了管道。

◇ **insertion** *noun* (i) point of attachment of a muscle to a bone 肌肉附着点 (ii)point where an organ is attached to its support 附着点(iii) change in the structure of a chromosome, where a segment of the chromosome is introduced into another member of the complement 插入点

insides *plural noun* (*informal* 非正式) internal organs, especially the stomach and intestines 内脏器官: ***He says he has a pain in his insides.*** 他说内脏疼痛。***You ought to see the doctor if you think there is something wrong with your insides.*** 如果你觉得内脏有问题,应该去看医生。

insight *noun* ability of a patient to realise that he is ill 自知力;洞察力

insipidus 无助的 *see* 见 DIABETES

in situ *adjective* in place 原位

insoluble *adjective* which cannot be dissolved in liquid 不溶解的; **insoluble fibre** = fibre in bread and cereals, which is not digested, but which swells inside the intestine 不溶纤维

insomnia *noun* inability to sleep *or* sleeplessness 失眠: ***She suffers from insomnia.*** 她患有失眠。***What does the doctor give you for your insomnia?*** 对于你的失眠症,医生开了些什么药?

◇ **insomniac** *noun* person who suffers from insomnia 失眠患者

inspect *verb* to examine *or* to look at something carefully 检查: ***The doctor inspected the boy's throat.*** 医生检查了男孩的喉咙。***He used a bronchoscope to inspect the inside of the lungs.*** 他用支气管镜检查了肺。

◇ **inspection** *noun* act of examining something 检查: ***The officials have carried out an inspection of the hospital kitchens.*** 官员对医院的厨房进行了检查。

◇ **inspector** *noun* person who inspects 检查员; **Government Health Inspector** = government official who examines offices *or* factories to see if they are clean and healthy 政府卫生检查员

inspiration *noun* breathing in *or* taking air into the lungs 吸气 (NOTE: the opposite is **expiration**)

> COMMENT: Inspiration takes place when the muscles of the diaphragm contract, allowing the lungs to expand.
> 注释:吸气时膈肌收缩,肺扩张。

inspissated *adjective* (liquid) which is thickened by removing water from it 浓缩的

◇ **inspissation** *noun* removing water from a solution to make it thicker 浓缩

instep *noun* arched top part of the foot 足弓

instil *or* **instill** *verb* to put a liquid in drop by drop 滴注: ***Instil four drops in each nostril twice a day.*** 每个鼻孔滴 4 滴,一天两次。

◇ **instillation** *noun* (**a**) putting a liquid in drop by drop 滴注法 (**b**) liquid put in drop by drop 一滴滴的液体

instinct *noun* tendency *or* ability which the body has from birth, and does not need to learn 本能: ***The body has a natural instinct to protect itself from danger.*** 机体有保护自身逃离危险的本能。

◇ **instinctive** *adjective* referring to instinct 本能的: ***Everyone has an instinctive reaction to move away from fire.*** 每个人都有避开火焰的本能反应。

institution *noun* hospital *or* clinic, especially a psychiatric hospital *or* children's home 机构,医院(尤其是精神病院,育儿院): ***He has lived all his life in institutions.*** 他终身都住在医院里。

◇ **institutionalize** *verb* to put a person into an institution 入院

◇ **institutionalization** *or* **institutional neurosis** *noun* condition where a patient has become so adapted to life in an institution that it is impossible for him to live outside it 患者完全适应住院生活,以致不愿出院。

instruction *noun* teaching how to do something 指示,说明: ***The students are given instruction in dealing with emergency cases.*** 给学生演示如何处理紧急病例。 **instructions** = words which explain how something is used *or* how to do something 说明: ***The instructions are written on the medicine bottle.*** 说明写在药瓶上。 ***We can't use this machine because we have lost the book of instructions.*** 因为弄丢了说明书,我们没法使用这机器。 ***She gave the taxi driver instructions how to get to the hospital.*** 她告诉出租车司机怎么去医院。

instrument *noun* piece of equipment; tool 器械,仪器: ***The doctor had a box of surgical instruments.*** 医生有一盒子的手术器械。

◇ **instrumental** *adjective* (**a**) using an instrument 用器械的; **Instrumental delivery** = childbirth where the doctor uses forceps to help the baby out of the mother's womb 器械助产 (**b**) **instrumental in** = helping to do something 帮助: ***She was instrumental in developing the new technique.*** 她帮助发明了这项新技术。

insufficiency *noun* (i) not being enough to perform normal functions 功能不全(ii)incompetence of an organ 器官功能不全: ***The patient is suffering from a renal insufficiency.*** 患者肾功能不全。

insufflation *noun* blowing something, such as air *or* a powder, into a cavity in the body 吹入法

insula *noun* part of the cerebral cortex which is covered by the folds of the sulcus 岛

insulin *noun* hormone produced by the islets of Langerhans in the pancreas 胰岛素; **insulin-dependent** 胰岛素依赖 *see* 见 DIABETES

◇ **insulinase** *noun* enzyme which breaks down insulin 胰岛素酶

◇ **insulinoma** *or* **insuloma** *noun* tumour in the islets of Langerhans 胰岛瘤

> COMMENT: Insulin controls the way in which the body converts sugar into energy and regulates the level of sugar in the blood; a lack of insulin caused by diabetes mellitus makes the level of glucose in the blood rise. Insulin injections are regularly used to treat diabetes mellitus, but care has to be taken not to exceed the dose as this will cause hyperinsulinism.
> 注释:胰岛素调控机体将糖转化为能量,并维持血糖水平;糖尿病时胰岛素缺乏可使血糖升高,定期注射胰岛素可以治疗糖尿病,但必须注意不要过量,否则会造成高胰岛素症。

insure *verb* to agree with a company that they will pay you money if something is lost or damaged 保险: ***Is your car insured?*** 你的汽车上保险了吗?

◇ **insurance** *noun* agreement with a company that they will pay you money if something is lost or damaged 保险; **accident insurance** = insurance which pays out money when an accident happens 意外伤害保险; **life insurance** = insurance which pays out money when someone dies 人寿保险; **medical insurance** = insurance which pays for private medical treatment 医疗保险; **National Insurance** = weekly payment from a person's wages (with a supplement from the employer) which pays for state assistance, medical treatment, etc. 国民保险

intake *noun* amount of a substance taken in; taking in (of a substance) 摄入: ***a high intake of alcohol*** 摄入大量酒精; ***She was advised to reduce her intake of sugar.*** 她被建议减少糖的摄入。**suggested daily intake** = amount of a substance which it is recommended to take in each day 每日建议摄入量

integration *noun* process where a whole is made into a single unit by the functional combination of the parts 整合

> COMMENT: There are two modes of integration: nervous and hormonal.
> 注释:有两种形式的整合:神经性和体液性。

integument *noun* covering layer, such as the skin 包膜,体被

intelligent *adjective* clever *or* able to learn quickly 聪明的: ***He's the most intelligent boy in the class.*** 他是班上最聪明的男孩。

◇ **intelligence** *noun* ability to learn and understand quickly 智力: **intelligence quotient (IQ)** = ratio of the mental age as given by an intelligence test, to the actual age of the person 智商; **intelligence test** = test to see how intelligent someone is, giving a mental age, as opposed to the chronological age of the person 智力测验

> COMMENT: The average IQ is between 90 and 110.
> 注释:平均智商是 90—110。

intense *adjective* very strong (pain) 强烈的(疼痛): ***She is suffering from intense post herpetic neuralgia.*** 她患有严重的疱疹后神经痛。

◇ **intensity** *noun* strength (of pain) (疼痛)强度

intensive care *noun* continual supervision and treatment of a patient in a special section of a hospital 重症监护: ***The patient was put in intensive care.*** 患者处于重症监护中。***He came out of intensive care and was moved to the general ward.*** 他出了重症监护病房,移入普通病房。**intensive care unit (ICU)** = special section of a hospital which supervises seriously ill patients who need constant supervision 重症监护病房

intention *noun* **(a)** healing process 愈合; **healing by first intention** = healing of a clean wound where the tissue reforms quickly 一级愈合; **healing by second intention** = healing of an infected wound *or* ulcer, which takes place slowly and may leave a permanent scar 二级愈合 **(b)** aiming to do something 意向; **intention tremor** = trembling of the hands when a person makes a voluntary movement to try to touch something 意向性震颤

inter- *prefix* meaning between 之间的

◇ **interaction** *noun* effect which two *or* more substances (such as drugs) have on each other 相互作用

◇ **interatrial septum** *noun* membrane between the right and left atria in the heart 房间膈

◇ **interbreed** *verb* to reproduce with another member of the same species 种内杂交

◇ **intercalated** *adjective* inserted between other tissues 插入; **intercalated disc** = closely applied cell membranes at the end of adjacent cells in cardiac muscle, seen as transverse lines 闰盘

◇ **intercellular** *adjective* between the cells in tissue 细胞间的

◇ **intercostal** *adjective* between the ribs 肋间的; **intercostal muscles** *or* **the intercostals** = muscles between the ribs 肋间肌

> COMMENT: The intercostal muscles expand and contract the thorax, so

changing the pressure in the thorax and making the person breathe in or out. There are three layers of intercostal muscle: external, internal and innermost or intercostalis intimis.
注释:肋间肌通过使胸腔扩张和收缩改变其压力,从而使人呼吸。肋间肌有3层:外层、中层和内层或肋间内肌。

◊ **intercourse** *noun* (**sexual**) **intercourse** = action of inserting the man's penis into the woman's vagina, releasing spermatozoa from the penis by ejaculation, which may fertilize an ovum from the woman's ovaries 性交

◊ **intercurrent disease** *or* **infection** *noun* disease *or* infection which affects someone who is suffering from another disease 间发疾病

◊ **interdigital** *adjective* referring to the space between the fingers or toes 指间的

interest 1 *noun* (**a**) special attention 兴趣: ***The consultant takes a lot of interest in his students.*** 会诊医生对他的学生显示出浓厚的兴趣。***She has no interest in what goes on in the ward around her.*** 她对身边病房发生的事情一点儿也不感兴趣。***Why doesn't he take more interest in physiotherapy***? 为什么他对理疗不太感兴趣?(**b**) something which attracts you particularly 引起兴趣的事: ***Her main interest is the treatment of cardiac patients.*** 她的主要兴趣是治疗心脏病患者。***Do you have any special interests apart from your work***? 除了工作外你有什么特殊兴趣吗? **2** *verb* to attract someone's attention 吸引,有兴趣: ***He's specially interested in the work of the physiotherapy department.*** 他对理疗科的工作很有兴趣。***Nothing seems to interest her very much.*** 似乎没有什么可以吸引她的。

◊ **interesting** *adjective* which attracts your attention 有趣的: ***There's an interesting article on the treatment of drug addiction in the magazine.*** 杂志上有篇有关治疗药瘾的有趣文章。

interfere *verb* to get involved *or* to stop or hinder a function 干扰

◊ **interference** *noun* act of interfering 干扰,干涉

interferon *noun* protein produced by cells, usually in response to a virus and which then reduces the spread of viruses 干扰素

COMMENT: Although it is now possible to synthesize interferon outside the body, large-scale production is extremely expensive and the substance has not proved as successful at combating viruses as had been hoped.
注释:尽管目前已经可以体外合成干扰素,但大规模的生产仍很昂贵,而且在对抗病毒方面没有显示出预想的疗效。

interleukin *noun* protein produced by the body's immune system 白介素; **interleukin-1** (**IL-1**) = protein which causes high temperature 白介素-1; **interleukin-2** (**IL-2**) = protein which stimulates T-cell production, used in the treatment of cancer 白介素-2

interior *adjective* & *noun* (part) which is inside 内部的,内部: ***The interior of the intestine is lined with millions of villi.*** 小肠内部衬有大量的微绒毛。

interlobar *adjective* between lobes 叶间的; **interlobar artery** = artery running towards the cortex on each side of a renal pyramid 叶间动脉

◊ **interlobular** *adjective* between lobules 小叶间的; **interlobular arteries** = arteries running to the glomeruli of the kidneys 小叶间动脉

◊ **intermediate** *adjective* which is in the middle between two things 中间的

◊ **intermedius** 中间的 *see* 见 VASTUS

◊ **intermenstrual** *adjective* between the menstrual periods 经间期的

◊ **intermittent** *adjective* occurring at intervals 间歇性的; **intermittent claudication** = condition of the arteries causing severe pain in the legs which makes the patient limp after having walked a short distance (the symptoms increase with more walking, but stop after a short rest, and recur when the patient walks again) 间歇性跛行; **intermittent fever** = fever which rises and falls, like malaria 间歇热

intern *noun US* medical school graduate who is working in a hospital while at the same time continuing his studies 实习医师 (NOTE: the GB English is **houseman, house officer**)

◇ **internist** *noun* specialist who treats diseases of the internal organs by non-surgical means 内科医师

◇ **internship** *noun US* position of an intern in a hospital 实习医师职位

◇ **interna** 内的 *see* 见 OTITIS

internal *adjective* (**a**) inside the body 内部的: ***The drug is for internal use only.*** = It should not be used on the outside of the body. 此药仅供内服。**internal auditory meatus** = channel which takes the auditory nerve through the temporal bone 内听道; **internal bleeding** = loss of blood from an injury inside the body 内出血; **internal capsule** = broad band of fibres passing to and from the cerebral cortex 内囊; **internal carotid** = artery in the neck, behind the external carotid, which gives off the ophthalmic artery and ends by dividing into the anterior and middle cerebral arteries 颈内动脉; **internal derangement of the knee (IDK)** = condition where the knee cannot function properly because of a torn meniscus 膝关节内错位; **internal ear** = the part of the ear inside the head, behind the eardrum, containing the semicircular canals, the vestibule and the cochlea 内耳; **internal haemorrhage** = haemorrhage which takes place inside the body 内出血; **internal jugular** = largest jugular vein in the neck, leading to the brachiocephalic veins 颈内静脉; *US* **internal medicine** = treatment of diseases of the internal organs by specialists 内科学; **internal oblique** = middle layer of muscle covering the abdomen, beneath the external oblique 腹内斜肌; **internal organs** = organs situated inside the body 内脏器官 *compare* 比较 EXTERNAL (**b**) **internal market** = system within the NHS, where hospitals are considered as suppliers of health care services and health authorities and GPs are considered as purchasers of services, the aim being to improve the efficiency of the system by introducing a more commercial approach to its organization 内部交易,国家保健事业的一种体制,医院提供卫生保健服务,而卫生部门和全科医师作为服务的购买者,其目的在于引进更商业化的手段提高体制的效率

◇ **internally** *adverb* inside the body 内在地: ***He was bleeding internally.*** 他内出血了。

international unit (IU) *noun* internationally agreed standard used in pharmacy as a measure of a substance such as drug or hormone 国际单位

internodal *adjective* between two nodes 结间的

◇ **interneurone** *noun* neurone with short processes which is a link between two other neurones in sensory *or* motor pathways 中间神经元

◇ **internuncial neurone** *noun* neurone which links two other nerve cells 联络神经元

◇ **internus** *noun* medial rectus muscle in the orbit of the eye 眼内直肌

◇ **interoceptor** *noun* nerve cell which reacts to a change taking place inside the body 内感受器 *see also* 参见 CHEMORECEPTOR, EXTEROCEPTOR, PROPRIOCEPTOR, RECEPTOR, VISCEROCEPTOR

◇ **interosseous** *adjective* between bones 骨间的

◇ **interpeduncular cistern** *noun* subarachnoid space between the two cerebral hemispheres beneath the midbrain and the hypothalamus(脑)脚间池

◇ **interphalangeal joint** *or* **IP joint** *noun* joint between the phalanges 指(趾)间关节; **distal interphalangeal joint (DIP)** = joint nearest the end of the finger or toe 远端指(趾)间关节; **proximal**

interphalangeal joint (**PIP**) = joint nearest the point of attachment of a finger or toe 近端指(趾)间关节

◇ **interphase** *noun* stage of a cell between divisions 分裂间期

◇ **interpret** *verb* to examine and decide what something means 检查说明; ***to interpret an X-ray*** 阅 X 片

◇ **interpubic joint** *or* **pubic symphysis** *noun* piece of cartilage which joins the two sections of the pubic bone 耻骨间关节

◇ **interruptus** 中断的 *see* 见 COITUS

◇ **intersexuality** *noun* condition where a baby has both male and female characteristics, as in Klinefelter's syndrome and Turner's syndrome 两性,间性(同时具有两性特征)

◇ **interstices** *plural noun* small spaces between parts of the body *or* between cells 小间隙

◇ **interstitial** *adjective* (tissue, etc.) in the spaces between parts of something, especially the tissue between the active tissue in an organ 间质的; **interstitial cells** *or* **Leydig cells** = testosterone-producing cells between the tubules in the testes 间质细胞; **interstitial cell stimulating hormone** (**ICSH**) *or* **luteinizing hormone** (**LH**) = hormone produced by the pituitary gland which stimulates the formation of corpus luteum in females and testosterone in males 间质细胞刺激素,黄体生成激素

◇ **intertrigo** *noun* irritation which occurs when two skin surfaces rub against each other (as in the armpit *or* between the buttocks) 擦烂

◇ **intertubercular plane** *noun* imaginary horizontal line drawn across the lower abdomen at the level of the projecting parts of the iliac bones 结节间平面

intervention *noun* treatment 治疗,干预; **medical intervention** *or* **surgical intervention** = treatment of illness by drugs *or* by surgery 内科或外科治疗; **nursing intervention** = treatment of illness by nursing care, without surgery 护理治疗

interventricular *adjective* between ventricles (in the heart *or* brain) 室间的; **interventricular septum** = wall in the lower part of the heart, separating the ventricles 室间膈; **interventricular foramen** = opening in the brain between the lateral ventricle and the third ventricle, through which the cerebrospinal fluid passes 室间孔

intervertebral *adjective* between vertebrae 椎间的; **intervertebral disc** = thick piece of cartilage which lies between two vertebrae 锥间盘; **intervertebral foramen** = hole between two vertebrae 锥间孔 *see also* 参见 VERTEBRAL ◊见图 JOINTS, VERTEBRAL COLUMN

intestine *noun* **the intestines** = the bowel *or* gut, the tract which passes from the stomach to the anus in which food is digested as it passes through 肠道; **small intestine** = section of the intestine from the stomach to the caecum, consisting of the duodenum, the jejunum and the ileum 小肠; **large intestine** = the colon, the section of the intestine from the caecum to the rectum, consisting of the caecum, the ascending, transverse, descending and sigmoid colons and the rectum 大肠

◇ **intestinal** *adjective* referring to the intestine 肠的; **intestinal anastomosis** = surgical operation to join one part of the intestine to another (after a section has been removed) 肠吻合术; **intestinal flora** = bacteria which are always present in the intestine 肠道菌群; **intestinal glands** *or* **glands of Lieberkuhn** = tubular glands found in the mucous membrane of the small and large intestine, especially those between the bases of the villi in the small intestine 肠腺; **intestinal infection** = infection in the intestines 肠道感染; **intestinal juice**

= colourless fluid secreted by the small intestine which contains enzymes that help digestion 肠液; **intestinal obstruction** = blocking of the intestine 肠梗阻; **intestinal wall** = layers of tissue which form the intestine 肠壁 (NOTE: for other terms referring to the intestine, see words beginning with **entero-**)

> COMMENT: Absorption of substances in partly digested food is the main function of the small intestine. This is carried out by the little villi in the walls of the intestine which absorb nutrients into the bloodstream. The large intestine absorbs water from the food after it has passed through the small intestine, and the remaining material passes out of the body through the anus as faeces.
> 注释:吸收已部分消化的食物中的养分入血是小肠的主要功能,由肠壁上的微绒毛完成。大肠吸收由小肠来的食物中的水分,其余物质通过肛门以粪便的形式排出体外。

intima *noun* & *adjective* (**tunica**) **intima** = inner layer of the wall of an artery *or* vein 内膜(的)

intolerance *noun* (i) being unable to endure something, such as pain 不耐受 (ii) being unable to take certain drugs because of the body's reaction to them 对药物不耐受: ***He developed an intolerance to penicillin.*** 他对青霉素不耐受。

intoxicate *verb* to make a person drunk *or* to make a person incapable of controlling his actions, because of the influence of alcohol on his nervous system 使醉酒: ***He drank six glasses of whisky and became completely intoxicated.*** 他喝了6杯威士忌,完全醉了。

◇ **intoxicant** *noun* substance, such as an alcoholic drink, which induces a state of intoxication or poisoning 中毒药(如酒精)

◇ **intoxication** *noun* condition which results from the absorption and diffusion in the body of a poison, such as alcohol 醉酒: ***She was driving a bus in a state of intoxication.*** 她在醉酒状态下开车。

intra- *prefix* meaning inside 内,在内的

◇ **intra-abdominal** *adjective* inside the abdomen 腹内的

◇ **intra-articular** *adjective* inside a joint 关节内的

◇ **intracellular** *adjective* inside a cell 细胞内的

◇ **intracerebral haematoma** *noun* blood clot inside a cerebral hemisphere 颅内血肿

◇ **intracranial** *adjective* inside the skull 颅内的

intractable *adjective* which cannot be treated 难治的: **an operation to relieve intractable pain** 缓解难治性疼痛的手术

intracutaneous *or* **intradermal** *adjective* inside layers of skin tissue 皮内的

◇ **intradural** *adjective* inside the dura mater 硬膜内的

◇ **intramedullary** *adjective* inside the bone marrow *or* spinal cord 髓内的

◇ **intramural** *adjective* inside the wall of an organ 壁内的

◇ **intramuscular** *adjective* inside a muscle 肌肉内的; **intramuscular injection** = injection made into a muscle 肌肉注射

◇ **intraocular** *adjective* inside the eye 眼内的; **intraocular lens (IOL)** = artificial lens implanted inside the eye 眼内晶体(植入眼内的人工晶体); **intraocular pressure** = pressure inside the eyeball (if too high, it gives glaucoma) 眼内压

◇ **intrathecal** *adjective* inside a sheath *or* inside the intradural or subarachnoid space 鞘内的

◇ **intratubercular plane** *noun* plane at right angles to the sagittal plane, passing through the tubercles of the iliac crests 结节间平面

◇ **intrauterine** *adjective* inside the uterus 子宫内的; **intrauterine device (IUD)** = plastic coil placed inside the uterus to prevent conception 宫内节育器

◇ **intravenous (IV)** *adjective* into a vein 静脉内的; **intravenous feeding** = giving liquid food to a patient by means of a tube inserted into a vein 静脉营养 *see also* 参见 DRIP; **intravenous injection** = injection into a vein for fast release of a drug 静脉注射; **intravenous pyelogram (IVP)** = series of X-ray photographs of the kidneys using pyelography 静脉肾盂造影片; **intravenous pyelography** = X-ray examination of the kidneys after an opaque substance is injected intravenously into the body, and is carried by the blood into the kidneys 静脉肾盂造影术

◇ **intravenously** *adverb* into a vein 静脉内地; ***a fluid given intravenously*** 静脉用液体

◇ **intra vitam** *Latin phrase meaning* 'during life' 生活期间

intrinsic *adjective* referring to the essential nature of an organism *or* included inside an organ or part 本质的,内在的; **intrinsic factor** = protein produced in the gastric glands which reacts with the extrinsic factor, and which, if lacking, causes pernicious anaemia 内因子; **intrinsic ligament** = ligament which forms part of the capsule surrounding a joint 内韧带(构成关节囊的一部分); **intrinsic muscle** = muscle lying completely inside the part or segment, especially of a limb which it moves 内附肌

introduce *verb* **(a)** to put something into something 插入: ***He used a syringe to introduce a medicinal substance into the body.*** 他用注射器将药物注入体内。***The nurse introduced the catheter into the vein.*** 护士将导管插入静脉。**(b)** to present two people to one another when they have never met before 介绍: ***Can I introduce my new assistant?*** 介绍一下我的新助手? **(c)** to start a new way of doing something 采用,引进: ***The hospital has introduced a new screening process for cervical cancer.*** 医院对宫颈癌采用了新的筛查方法。

◇ **introduction** *noun* **(a)** putting something inside 放入: ***The introduction of semen into the woman's uterus.*** 将精子送入妇女的子宫。***The introduction of an endotracheal tube into the patient's mouth.*** 将气管内插管插入患者的口腔。**(b)** starting a new process 引进,采用

introitus *noun* opening into any hollow organ *or* canal 入口

introversion *noun* condition where a person is excessively interested in himself and his own mental state 内向

◇ **introvert** *noun* person who thinks only about himself and his own mental state 内向性格的人 *compare* 比较 EXTROVERT, EXTROVERSION

◇ **introverted** *adjective* (person) who thinks only about himself 内向的

intubate *verb* to catheterize, to insert a tube into any organ *or* part of the body 插管

◇ **intubation** *noun* catheterization, therapeutic insertion of a tube into the larynx through the glottis to allow passage of air 插管法

intumescence *noun* swelling of an organ 肿大

intussusception *noun* condition where part of the gastrointestinal tract telescopes into the part beneath it, causing an obstruction and strangulation of the part which has telescoped 套叠

invagination *noun* (i) intussusception 套叠 (ii) surgical treatment of hernia, in which a sheath of tissue is made to cover the opening 疝修补术的一种,以组织鞘覆盖疝口

invalid *noun* & *adjective* (person) who has had an illness and has not fully recovered from it 未完全恢复的(患者) (person) who is disabled 病残的(人): ***He has been an invalid since he had the accident six years ago.*** 自从6年前的事故后,他就病残了。***She is looking after her invalid parents.*** 她照顾她病残的双亲。**invalid carriage** = small car, specially made for use by an invalid 残障车; **invalid chair** *or* **wheelchair** = chair with wheels in which an invalid can sit and move about 轮椅: ***She manages to do all her shopping using her invalid chair.*** 她设法坐轮椅进行全部的购物。***Some buildings have special entrances for invalid chairs.*** 一些建筑物有特殊的入口供轮椅出入。

◇ **invalidity** *noun* being disabled 残疾; **invalidity benefit** = money paid by the government to someone who is permanently disabled 病残救济金

invasion *noun* entry of bacteria into a body *or* first attack of a disease 侵入

invasive *adjective* (**a**) (cancer) which tends to spread throughout the body 侵袭的 (**b**) (inspection *or* treatment) which involves entering the body by making an incision 介入性的,有创性 *see also* 参见 NON-INVASIVE

invent *verb* (**a**) to make something which has never been made before 发明: ***He invented a new type of catheter.*** 他发明了一种新型导管。(**b**) to make up, using your imagination 虚构: ***He invented the whole story.*** 他虚构了整个故事。***Small children often invent imaginary friends.*** 幼儿常会虚构玩伴。

◇ **invention** *noun* thing which someone has invented 发明物: ***We have seen his latest invention, a brain scanner.*** 我们见了他的最新发明——脑扫描仪

inversion *noun* being turned towards the inside *or* turning of part of the body (such as the foot) towards the inside 内翻; **inversion of the uterus** = condition where the top part of the uterus touches the cervix, as if it were inside out (which may happen after childbirth) 子宫内翻

invertase *noun* enzyme in the intestine which splits sucrose 转化酶,蔗糖酶

investigate *verb* to examine something to try to find out what caused it 调查研究: ***Health inspectors are investigating the outbreak of legionnaires' disease.*** 卫生视察员对军团菌病的暴发进行调查。

◇ **investigation** *noun* examination to find out the cause of something which has happened 调查: ***The Health Authority ordered an investigation into how the drugs were stolen.*** 卫生部门命令对药品的失窃进行调查。

◇ **investigative surgery** *noun* surgery to investigate the cause of a condition 探查手术

invisible *adjective* which cannot be seen 不可见的: ***The microbes are invisible to the naked eye, but can be clearly seen under a microscope.*** 微生物用肉眼看不见,但在显微镜下清晰可见。

in vitro *Latin phrase meaning* 'in a glass' 体外的; **in vitro activity** *or* **in vitro experiment** = experiment which takes place in the laboratory 体外实验; **in vitro fertilization** (**IVF**) = fertilization of an ovum in the laboratory 体外受精 *see also* 参见 TEST-TUBE BABY

in vivo *Latin phrase meaning* 'in living tissue': experiment which takes place on the living body 体内的; **in vivo experiment** = experiment on a living body (such as an animal) 体内实验

involucrum *noun* covering of new bone which forms over diseased bone 包壳

involuntary *adjective* independent of the will *or* done without any mental processes being involved 无意的,不随意的: ***Patients are advised not to eat or drink, to reduce the risk of involuntary vomiting while on the operating table.*** 建议患者不要进食,以减少在手术台上不自觉呕吐的危险性。**involuntary action** = action where a patient does not use his will power 不自主运动; **involuntary muscle** = muscle supplied by the autonomic nervous system, and therefore not under voluntary control (such as the muscle which activates a vital organ like the heart) 不随意肌

involution *noun* (**a**) return of an organ to normal size, such as the return of the uterus to normal size after childbirth 复旧（**b**）period of decline of organs which sets in after middle age 退化

◇ **involutional** *adjective* referring to involution 复旧的; **involutional melancholia** = depression which occurs in people (mainly women) after middle age, probably caused by a change of endocrine secretions 更年期忧郁症

involve *verb* to concern *or* to have to do with 卷入，涉及: ***The operation involves removing part of the duodenum and attaching the stomach directly to the jejunum.*** 手术包括切除部分十二指肠，将胃直接与空肠连接。

iodine *noun* chemical element which is essential to the body, especially to the functioning of the thyroid gland 碘; **tincture of iodine** = weak solution of iodine in alcohol, used as an antiseptic 碘酊（NOTE: chemical symbol is **I**）

> COMMENT: Lack of iodine in the diet can cause goitre.
> 注释：食物中缺乏碘可引起甲状腺肿。

IOL = INTRAOCULAR LENS 眼内晶体

ion *noun* atom which has an electric charge. (Ions with a positive charge are called cations and those with a negative charge are anions) 离子

◇ **ionize** *verb* to give an atom an electric charge 离子化

◇ **ionizer** *or* **negative ion generator** *noun* machine that increases the amount of negative ions in the atmosphere of a room, so counteracting the effect of positive ions 电离器，阴离子发生器

> COMMENT: It is believed that living organisms, including human beings, react to the presence of ionized particles in the atmosphere. Hot dry winds contain a higher proportion of positive ions than normal and these winds cause headaches and other illnesses. If negative ionized air is introduced into an air-conditioning system, the incidence of headaches and nausea among people working in the building may be reduced.
> 注释：现认为活的生物，包括人类，可以与大气中的电离颗粒相作用。干热风含有更多比例的阳离子，可以引起头疼和其他疾病。如果在空调系统内加入阴离子气体，就能减少屋内工作人员患头痛和恶心的发生率。

IP = INTERPHALANGEAL JOINT 指间关节

ipecacuanha *or US* **ipecac** *noun* drug made from the root of an American plant, used as treatment for coughs, and also as an emetic 吐根

ipsilateral *adjective* on the same side of the body 同侧的

IQ = INTELLIGENCE QUOTIENT 智商

irid- *prefix* referring to the iris 虹膜的

◇ **iridectomy** *noun* surgical removal of part of the iris 虹膜切除术

◇ **iridencleisis** *noun* operation to treat glaucoma, where part of the iris is used as a drainage channel through a hole in the conjunctiva 虹膜箝顿术

◇ **iridocyclitis** *noun* inflammation of the iris and the tissues which surround it 虹膜睫状体炎

◇ **iridodialysis** *noun* separation of the iris from its insertion 虹膜根部分离术

◇ **iridoplegia** *noun* paralysis of the iris 虹膜麻痹

◇ **iridotomy** *noun* surgical incision into the iris 虹膜切开术

◇ **iris** *noun* coloured ring in the eye, with the pupil at its centre 虹膜 ◇ 见图 EYE

◇ **iritis** *noun* inflammation of the iris 虹膜炎

> COMMENT: The iris acts like the aperture in a camera shutter, opening and closing to allow more or less light through the pupil into the eye.
> 注释：虹膜的作用相当于相机快门中的小孔，它的开、关控制通过瞳孔进入眼内光线的多少。

iron *noun* （**a**） chemical element

essential to the body, found in liver, eggs, etc. 铁元素 (NOTE: chemical symbol is **Fe**) (**b**) common grey metal 铁

> COMMENT: Iron is an essential part of the red pigment in red blood cells. Lack of iron in haemoglobin results in iron-deficiency anaemia. Storage of too much iron in the body results in haemochromatosis.
> 注释:铁是红细胞中红色色素的基本成分,缺铁会引起缺铁性贫血;体内铁储存过多会造成血色素沉着症。

◇ **iron lung** = DRINKER RESPIRATOR 铁肺

irradiation *noun* (**a**) spread from a centre, as nerve impulses 扩散 (**b**) use of rays to treat patients *or* to kill bacteria in food 放疗,光疗: **total body irradiation** = treating the whole body with radiation 全身放疗

irreducible *adjective* (hernia) where the organ cannot be returned to its original position without an operation 不能复位的

irregular *adjective* not regular *or* abnormal 不规则的: ***The patient's breathing was irregular.*** 患者的呼吸不规律。***The nurse noted that the patient had developed an irregular pulse.*** 护士注意到患者的脉搏不规律。***He has irregular bowel movements.*** 他的肠蠕动不规律。

irrigate *verb* to wash out a cavity in the body 冲洗

◇ **irrigation** *noun* washing out of a cavity in the body 冲洗; **colonic irrigation** = washing out the large intestine 结肠灌洗

irritate *verb* to make something painful *or* itchy *or* sore 刺激: ***Some types of wool can irritate the skin.*** 有些种类的羊毛对皮肤有刺激。

◇ **irritability** *noun* state of being irritable 过敏

◇ **irritable** *adjective* which can be easily excited 过敏的; **irritable colon** *or* **irritable bowel syndrome** = MUCOUS COLITIS 激惹性结肠,肠易激综合征

◇ **irritant** *noun* substance which can irritate 刺激剂; **irritant dermatitis** = contact dermatitis, a skin inflammation caused by touching 刺激性皮炎

◇ **irritation** *noun* action of irritating 刺激作用: ***An irritation caused by the ointment.*** 药膏引起的刺激作用。

isch- *prefix* meaning reduction *or* too little 减少

◇ **ischaemia** *noun* deficient blood supply to part of the body 缺血

◇ **ischaemic** *adjective* lacking in blood 缺血的; **ischaemic heart disease (IHD)** = disease of the heart caused by a failure in the blood supply (as in coronary thrombosis) 缺血性心脏病; **transient ischaemic attack (TIA)** = mild stroke caused by a brief stoppage of blood supply 短暂缺血发作

> QUOTE: Changes in life style factors have been related to the decline in total mortality from IHD. In many studies a sedentary life style has been reported as a risk factor for IHD.
> 引文:生活习惯的改变与缺血性心脏病总死亡率的减低有关。很多研究显示安静少动的生活习惯是缺血性心脏病的危险因素。
> **Journal of the American Medical Association** 美国医学会杂志

> QUOTE: The term stroke does not refer to a single pathological entity. Stroke may be haemorrhagic or ischaemic: the latter is usually caused by thrombosis or embolism.
> 引文:卒中这一术语并不指单一的病理改变,可以是出血性的或缺血性的,后者可以是血栓形成或栓塞。
> **British Journal of Hospital Medicine** 英国医院医学杂志

ischial *adjective* referring to the ischium *or* hip joint 坐骨的,髋关节的; **ischial tuberosity** = lump of bone forming the ring of the ischium 坐骨结节粗隆

◇ **ischiocavernosus muscle** *noun* muscle along one side of the perineum 坐骨海绵体肌

◇ **ischiorectal** *adjective* referring to both the ischium and the rectum 坐骨直

肠的; **ischiorectal abscess** = abscess which forms in fat cells between the anus and the ischium 坐骨直肠脓肿; **ischiorectal fossa** = space on either side of the lower end of the rectum and anal canal 坐骨直肠窝

◇ **ischium** *noun* lower part of the hip bone in the pelvis 坐骨 ◇ 见图 PELVIS

ischuria *noun* retention *or* suppression of urine 尿闭

Ishihara test *noun* test for colour blindness where the patient is asked to identify letters or numbers among a mass of coloured dots 石原试验(查色盲用)

islets of Langerhans *or* **islet cells** *plural noun* groups of cells in the pancreas which secrete the hormones glucagon and insulin 胰岛

iso- *prefix* meaning equal 相等的

◇ **isoantibody** *noun* antibody which forms in one person as a reaction to antigens from another person 同种抗体

◇ **isograft** *or* **syngraft** *noun* graft of tissue from an identical twin 同基因移植物

◇ **isoimmunization** *noun* immunization of a person with antigens derived from another person 同种免疫

isolate *verb* (**a**) to keep one patient apart from others (because he has a dangerous infectious disease) 隔离 (**b**) to identify a single virus *or* bacteria among many 病毒、细菌分离: ***Scientists have been able to isolate the virus which causes legionnaires' disease.*** 科学家已经可以分离出引起军团菌病的病原体。***Candida is easily isolated from the mouths of healthy adults.*** 念珠菌可以很容易地从健康成人的口腔内分离到。

◇ **isolation** *noun* separation of a patient, especially one with an infectious disease, from other patients 隔离; **isolation hospital** *or* **isolation ward** = special hospital *or* special ward in a hospital where patients suffering from infectious dangerous diseases can be isolated 隔离医院,隔离病房

isoleucine *noun* essential amino acid 异亮氨酸

isometric exercises *noun* exercises which strengthen the muscles, where the muscles contract but do not shorten 等长运动

isoniazid *noun* drug used to treat tuberculosis 异烟肼

◇ **isotonic** *adjective* (solution, such as a saline drip) which has the same osmotic pressure as blood and which can therefore be passed directly into the body 等张的

◇ **isotonicity** *noun* equal osmotic pressure of two or more solutions 等渗性

◇ **isotope** *noun* form of a chemical element which has the same chemical properties as other forms, but different atomic mass 同位素; **radioactive isotope** = isotope which sends out radiation, used in radiotherapy and scanning 放射性同位素

isthmus *noun* (i) short narrow canal *or* cavity 峡(ii) narrow band of tissue joining two larger masses of similar tissue (such as the section in the centre of the thyroid gland, which joins the two lobes)峡部,连接相似的两部分较大组织的狭窄组织,如甲状腺峡部

itch **1** *noun* any irritated place on the skin, which makes a person want to scratch 痒; **the itch** = scabies, an infection of the skin caused by a mite, producing violent irritation 疥疮 **2** *verb* to produce an irritating sensation, making a person want to scratch 发痒: ***The cream made his skin itch more.*** 雪花膏使他的皮肤更痒了。

◇ **itching** *or* **pruritus** *noun* irritation of the skin which makes a person want to scratch 瘙痒

◇ **itchy** *adjective* which makes a person want to scratch 发痒的: ***The main symptom of the disease is an itchy red rash.*** 疾病的主要症状是发痒性红色皮疹。

-itis *suffix* meaning inflammation 炎症 **otitis** = inflammation of the ear 耳炎

rhinitis = inflammation of the nasal passages 鼻炎

IU = INTERNATIONAL UNIT 国际单位

IUD = INTRAUTERINE DEVICE 宫内节育器

IV = INTRAVENOUS 静脉内

IVP = INTRAVENOUS PYELOGRAM 静脉肾盂造影片

IVF = IN VITRO FERTILIZATION 体外受精

Jj

J = JOULE 焦耳

jab *noun* (*informal* 非正式) injection *or* inoculation 注射,接种: ***He has had a tetanus jab.*** 他注射了破伤风疫苗。***Go to the doctor to get a cholera jab.*** 去医生那儿接种霍乱菌苗。

jacket *noun* short coat 短外衣: ***The dentist was wearing a white jacket.*** 牙医师穿了件白色短外衣。**bed jacket** = short warm jacket which a patient can wear when sitting in bed 睡衣

Jacksonian epilepsy 杰克逊癫痫 *see* 见 EPILEPSY

Jacquemier's sign *noun* sign of early pregnancy, when the vaginal mucosa becomes bluish in colour due to an increased amount of blood in the arteries 惹克米埃氏征,妊娠的早期指征,因动脉充血宫颈粘膜变蓝

jar 1 *noun* pot (usually glass) for keeping liquids *or* food in 瓶,罐子: ***Specimens of diseased organs can be kept in glass jars.*** 病变器官的标本可保存在玻璃瓶内。**2** *verb* to give a shock with a blow 震动: ***The patient fell awkwardly and jarred his spine.*** 患者踉跄地摔倒了,震伤了他的脊柱。

jaundice *or* **icterus** *noun* condition where there is an excess of bile pigment in the blood, and where the pigment is deposited in the skin and the whites of the eyes which have a yellow colour 黄疸,因血中胆色素过高使皮肤、巩膜发黄; **haemolytic jaundice** *or* **prehepatic jaundice** = jaundice caused by haemolysis of the red blood cells 溶血性黄疸或肝前性黄疸,因红细胞溶血引起; **hepatocellular jaundice** = jaundice caused by injury to *or* disease of the liver cells 肝细胞性黄疸,因肝细胞受损或病变引起; **infective jaundice** = jaundice caused by a viral disease such as hepatitis 传染性黄疸,病毒性疾病如肝炎引起; **obstructive jaundice** *or* **posthepatic jaundice** = jaundice caused by an obstruction of the bile ducts 阻塞性黄疸或肝后性黄疸,因胆管阻塞引起 *see also* 参见 ACHOLURIC

> COMMENT: Jaundice can have many causes, usually relating to the liver: the most common are blockage of the bile ducts by gallstones or by disease of the liver, infectious diseases such as the two forms of hepatitis and Weil's disease.
> 注释:黄疸有多种原因,常与肝脏有关:最常见的是结石阻塞胆管或肝病、感染性疾病如甲乙肝炎和钩端螺旋体病。

jaw *noun* bones in the face which hold the teeth and form the mouth 颌骨,面骨之一,附着牙齿,构成嘴部; **upper jaw and lower jaw** = the two parts of the jaw, the upper (the maxillae) being fixed parts of the skull, and the lower (the mandible) being attached to the skull with a hinge so that it can move up and down 上下颌骨,上颌骨(maxillae)是颅骨的固定部分,下颌骨(mandible)通过关节与颅骨相连,可以上下运动: ***Teeth are fixed in both the upper and lower jaw.*** 牙齿附着于上下颌骨。***He fell down and broke his jaw or the punch on his mouth broke his lower jaw.*** 他摔了下来或一拳打到了嘴上,摔折了下颌骨。

◇ **jawbone** *noun* one of the bones (the maxillae and the mandible) which form the jaw 颌骨之一(NOTE: **jawbone** usually refers to the lower jaw or mandible)

jejun- *prefix* referring to the jejunum 空肠

◇ **jejunal** *adjective* referring to the jejunum 空肠的; **jejunal ulcer** = ulcer in the jejunum 空肠溃疡

◇ **jejunectomy** *noun* surgical removal of all *or* part of the jejunum 空肠切除术

◇ **jejunoileostomy** *noun* surgical operation to make an artificial link between the jejunum and the ileum 空肠回肠吻合术

◇ **jejunostomy** *noun* surgical operation to make an artificial passage to the jejunum through the wall of the abdomen 空肠造口术

◇ **jejunotomy** *noun* surgical operation to cut into the jejunum 空肠切开术

◇ **jejunum** *noun* part of small intestine between the duodenum and the ileum 空肠，十二指肠和回肠之间的一段小肠 ◊ 见图 DIGESTIVE SYSTEM

COMMENT：The jejunum is about 2 metres long.
注释：空肠长约 2 米。

jelly *noun* semi-solid substance 凝胶；**lubricating jelly** = jelly used to make a surface slippery 润滑胶

jerk 1 *noun* sudden movement of part of the body which indicates that the local reflex arc is intact 反射；**ankle jerk** = jerk as a reflex action of the foot when the back of the ankle is tapped 踝反射；**knee jerk** = jerk made as a reflex action by the knee, when the legs are crossed and the patellar tendon is tapped sharply 膝反射 **2** *verb* to make sudden movements 抽动：***Some forms of epilepsy are accompanied by jerking of the limbs.*** 一些类型的癫痫伴有四肢的抽动。

◇ **jerky** *adjective* with sudden movement 颤抖：***The patient made jerky movements with his hand.*** 患者的手颤。

jet lag *noun* condition suffered by people who travel long distances in planes, caused by rapid changes in time zones which affect sleep patterns and meal times and thus interfere with the body's metabolism 时差反应，坐飞机长途旅行，因时差的改变影响了睡眠、进餐时间，干扰了机体的新陈代谢（NOTE：does not take **the** or **a**：**'she is suffering from jet lag'**；**'he took several days to get over his jet lag'**）

jigger = SANDFLEA 恙螨，沙蚤

join *verb* to put things together 使聚集；to come together 结合，聚集：***The bones are joined together by a cartilage.*** 骨由软骨连接。***The inflammation started at the point where the ileum joins the caecum.*** 炎症开始于回结肠连接部。

joint *noun* junction of two or more bones, especially one which allows movement of the bones 关节：***The elbow is a joint in the arm.*** 肘是上肢的关节。***Arthritis is accompanied by stiffness in the joints.*** 关节炎伴有关节强直。**hip joint** = place where the hip is joined to the upper leg 髋关节；**wrist joint** = place where the wrist joins the arm 腕关节；**ball and socket joint** = joint (like the shoulder) where the rounded end of a long bone fits into a socket on another bone 杵臼关节；**primary cartilaginous joint** = temporary joint where the intervening cartilage is converted into adult bone 初级软骨性关节，暂时性的关节中间的软骨、成人后转为骨；**secondary cartilaginous joint** = joint where the surfaces of the two bones are connected by a piece of cartilage so that they cannot move (such as the pubic symphysis) 次级软骨性关节，两骨的表面覆有一层软骨，不能运动，如耻骨联合；**fibrous joint** = joint where two bones are fixed together by fibrous tissue, so that they can move only slightly (as in the bones of the skull) 纤维关节，由纤维组织连接，可轻微活动，如颅骨；**hinge joint** = joint (like the knee) which allows the two bones to move in one plane only 屈戌关节，只能在一个平面上运动的关节；**locking joints** = joints (such as the knee *or* elbow) which can be locked in an extended position 绞锁关节，伸位时锁住的关节，如膝和肘关节；**pivot joint** *or* **trochoid joint** = joint where a bone can rotate easily 旋转关节或枢轴关节，可旋转的关节；**synovial joint** = joint where the two bones are separated by a space filled with synovial fluid which nourishes and lubricates the surfaces of the bones 滑膜关节，两关节骨间有充满滑液的间隙，起营养和润滑作用；**joint capsule** = white fibrous tissue which surrounds and holds a joint together 关节囊，包绕、固定关节的白色纤维组织；**joint mice** = loose pieces of bone *or* cartilage in the knee joint, making the joint lock 关节鼠,膝关节内游离的骨或软骨片,可使关节绞锁 *see also* 参见 CHARCOT'S JOINT (NOTE: for other terms referring to joints, see words beginning with **arthr-**, **articul-**)

◇ **jointed** *adjective* linked with joints 有关节连接的

◇ **joint-breaker fever** = O'NYONG-NYONG FEVER 关节断裂热

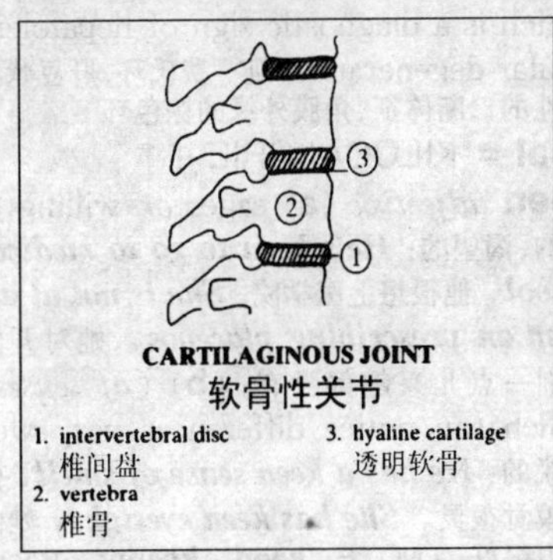

CARTILAGINOUS JOINT
软骨性关节

1. intervertebral disc 椎间盘
2. vertebra 椎骨
3. hyaline cartilage 透明软骨

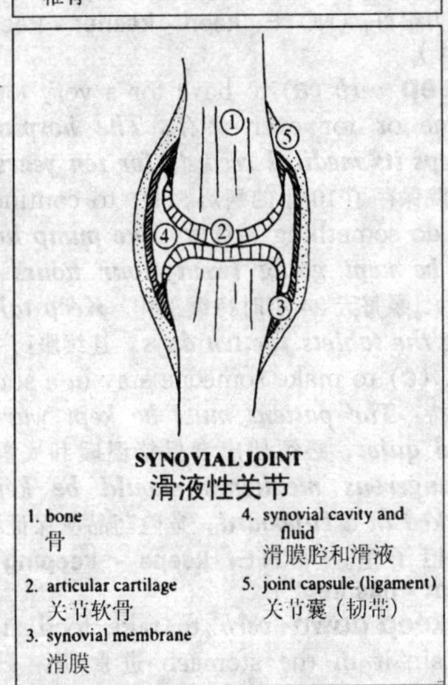

SYNOVIAL JOINT
滑液性关节

1. bone 骨
2. articular cartilage 关节软骨
3. synovial membrane 滑膜
4. synovial cavity and fluid 滑膜腔和滑液
5. joint capsule (ligament) 关节囊(韧带)

joule *noun* SI unit of measurement of energy 焦耳,能量的国际单位 (NOTE: usually written **J** with figures: **25J**)

COMMENT: One joule is the amount of energy used to move one kilogram the distance of one metre, using the force of one newton. 4.184 joules equals one calorie.
注释:1 焦耳的能量相当于用 1 牛顿的力使 1 千克的物体移动 1 米。4.184 焦耳等于 1 卡。

jugular *adjective* referring to the throat or neck 颈的; **jugular nerve** = one of the nerves in the neck 颈神经; **jugular trunk** = terminal lymph vessel in the neck, draining into the subclavian vein 颈干,颈部的终末淋巴管,进入锁骨下静脉; **jugular vein** *or* **jugular** = one of the veins which pass down either side of the neck 颈静脉

COMMENT: There are three jugular veins on each side: the internal jugular is large and leads to the brachiocephalic vein, the external jugular is smaller and leads to the subclavian vein and the anterior jugular is the smallest.
注释:每侧有 3 条颈静脉:颈内静脉是最大的,进入头臂静脉,其次是颈外静脉,进入锁骨下静脉,颈前静脉是最小的静脉。

juice *noun* fluid secretion of an animal or plant 汁,液: **a glass of orange juice** *or* **tomato juice** 一玻璃杯橘汁或番茄汁; **a tin of grapefruit juice** 一听葡萄汁; **gastric juice** = acid liquid secreted by the stomach which helps digest food 胃液,胃分泌的帮助消化的酸性液体; **intestinal juice** = alkaline liquid secreted by the small intestine which helps digest food 肠液,小肠分泌的帮助消化的碱性液体

junction *noun* joining point 接点

juvenile *adjective* referring to children *or* adolescents 青少年的: ***The area has six new cases of juvenile diabetes mellitus.*** 这地区新发现 6 例青少年型糖尿病。

juxta- *prefix* meaning beside *or* near 近,旁

Kk

K 1 *chemical symbol for* potassium 钾的化学元素符号 2 *noun* **Vitamin K** = vitamin found in green vegetables like spinach and cabbage, and which helps the clotting of blood and is needed to activate prothrombin 维生素K,菠菜和圆白菜等绿色蔬菜中含有的维生素,可促进凝血,为激活凝血酶原所需

k *symbol for* kilo- 千

Kahn test *noun* test of blood serum to diagnose syphilis 康瓦氏试验,诊断梅毒的血清学检查

kala-azar *noun* severe infection, occurring in tropical countries 黑热病

> COMMENT: Kala-azar is a form of leishmaniasis, caused by the infection of the intestines and internal organs by a parasite *Leishmania* spread by flies. Symptoms are fever, anaemia, general wasting of the body and swelling of the spleen and liver.
> 注释:利什曼病的一种,由苍蝇传播的小肠和内脏器官的利什曼原虫感染,症状有发热、贫血、体重下降和肝脾肿大。

kalium = POTASSIUM 钾

kaolin *noun* white powder, the natural form of aluminium silicate or china clay 白陶土

> COMMENT: Kaolin is used internally in liquid form to reduce diarrhoea and can also be used externally as a talc or as a poultice.
> 注释:作为液体内服可减轻腹泻,也可作为滑石粉或泥敷剂外用。

Kaposi's sarcoma *noun* cancer which takes the form of many haemorrhagic nodes affecting the skin, especially on the extremities 卡波西肉瘤,表现为皮肤尤其是指端的出血性结节

> COMMENT: Formerly a relatively rare disease, found mainly in tropical countries; now more common as it is one of the sequelae of AIDS.
> 注释:以前作为一种少见疾病主要见于热带地区,现今作为艾滋病的并发症较为常见。

karyotype *noun* the chromosome complement of a cell, shown as a diagram or as a set of letters and numbers 核型,以图或一组字母和数字的形式描述细胞的染色体组成

Kayser-Fleischer ring *noun* brown ring on the outer edge of the cornea, which is a diagnostic sign of hepatolenticular degeneration 凯-费氏环,肝豆状核变性的诊断体征,角膜外缘的棕色环

kcal = KILOCALORIE 千卡

keen *adjective* (**a**) eager *or* willing 热切的,渴望的: ***He's keen to go to medical school.*** 他很想上医学院。***She is not at all keen on prescribing placebos.*** 她对开安慰剂一点儿兴趣都没有。(**b**) (*of senses*) which can notice differences very well 敏锐的: ***He has a keen sense of smell.*** 他的嗅觉很灵。***She has keen eyesight.*** 她的视力很好。(NOTE: **keen - keener - keenest**)

keep *verb* (**a**) to have for a very long time or for ever 保存: ***The hospital keeps its medical records for ten years.*** 医院保存了10年的病历。(**b**) to continue to do something 持续做: ***The pump has to be kept going twenty-four hours a day.*** 泵每天24小时持续工作。***Keep taking the tablets for ten days.*** 连续服药10天。(**c**) to make someone stay in a state 保持: ***The patient must be kept warm and quiet.*** 必须使患者保持温暖和安静。***Dangerous medicines should be kept locked in a cupboard.*** 危险药品应保证锁在柜子里。(NOTE: **keeps - keeping - kept - has kept**)

◇ **keep down** *verb* to take food and retain it in the stomach 进食,吃: ***He managed to keep down some soup.*** 他尽力喝了些汤。***She could not even keep a glass of orange juice down.*** 她连一杯橘子汁都喝不下。

◇ **keep on** *verb* to continue to do something 继续做: ***The patient kept on calling out in his sleep.*** 患者在睡梦中不

停的叫喊。***You should keep on doing the exercises at home for several weeks.*** 你应该在家里坚持锻炼几周。

Keller's operation *noun* operation on the big toe, to remove a bunion *or* to correct an ankylosed joint 凯勒氏手术,祛除踇囊肿和纠正关节强直的手术

keloid *noun* excessive amount of scar tissue at the site of a skin injury 斑痕瘤

kerat- *prefix* referring to horn *or* horny tissue *or* the cornea 角的,角化组织的,角膜的

◇ **keratectasia** *noun* condition where the cornea bulges 角膜扩张

◇ **keratectomy** *noun* surgical removal of the whole *or* part of the cornea 角膜切除术

◇ **keratin** *noun* protein found in horny tissue (such as fingernails *or* hair *or* the outer surface of the skin) 角蛋白

◇ **keratinize** *verb* to convert into keratin *or* into horny tissue 角化: ***The cells are gradually keratinized.*** 细胞逐渐角化。

◇ **keratinization** *or* **cornification** *noun* appearance of horny characteristics in tissue 角质化

◇ **keratitis** *noun* inflammation of the cornea 角膜炎

◇ **keratoacanthoma** *noun* type of benign skin tumour, which disappears after a few months 角化棘皮病,一种皮肤的良性肿瘤,几个月后可消失

◇ **keratoconjunctivitis** *noun* inflammation of the cornea with conjunctivitis 角膜结膜炎

◇ **keratoconus** *noun* cone-shaped lump on the cornea 圆锥形角膜

◇ **keratoglobus** *noun* swelling of the eyeball 球形角膜

◇ **keratoma** *noun* hard thickened growth due to hypertrophy of the horny zone of the skin 角化病,皮肤角质层增生引起 (NOTE: plural is **keratomata**)

◇ **keratomalacia** *noun* (i) softening of the cornea frequently caused by Vitamin A deficiency 角膜软化,通常因缺乏维生素 A 引起 (ii) softening of the horny layer of the skin 皮肤角质层软化

◇ **keratome** *noun* surgical knife used for operations on the cornea 角膜刀

◇ **keratometer** *noun* instrument for measuring the curvature of the cornea 角膜散光计

◇ **keratometry** *noun* process of measuring the curvature of the cornea 角膜散光测量法

◇ **keratoplasty** *or* **corneal graft** *noun* grafting corneal tissue from a donor in place of diseased tissue 角膜成形术,角膜移植

◇ **keratoscope** *or* **Placido's disc** *noun* instrument for examining the cornea to see if it has an abnormal curvature 角膜镜

◇ **keratosis** *noun* lesion of the skin 角化病,一种皮肤病变

◇ **keratotomy** *noun* surgical operation to make a cut in the cornea, the first step in many intraocular operations 角膜切开术

kerion *noun* painful soft mass, usually on the scalp, caused by ringworm 脓癣,因癣引起的痛性软组织肿块,常位于头皮

kernicterus *noun* yellow pigmentation of the basal ganglia and other nerve cells in the spinal cord and brain, found in children with icterus 核黄疸,新生儿重症黄疸,患儿的基底神经节和脊索、脑内的神经细胞有色素沉着

> COMMENT: The symptoms are convulsions, anorexia and drowsiness. The disease can be fatal, and where it is not fatal, spasticity and mental defects appear.
> 注释:症状为抽搐、厌食和嗜睡。本病可是致命性的,即使不致命也会出现痉挛状态和智力损伤。

Kernig's sign *noun* symptom of meningitis, when the knee cannot be straightened if the patient is lying down with the thigh brought up against the abdomen 克氏征,脑膜炎的一种体征,平躺时向上抬腿,膝关节不能伸直

ketoacidosis *noun* accumulation of ketone bodies in tissue in diabetes, causing acidosis 酮症酸中毒,糖尿病患者体内酮体过多,引起酸中毒

◇ **ketogenesis** *noun* production of ketone bodies 酮生成

◇ **ketogenic diet** *noun* diet with a high fat content, producing ketosis 富含脂肪的饮食

◇ **ketonaemia** *noun* morbid state where ketone bodies exist in the blood 酮血症

◇ **ketone** *noun* chemical compound containing the group CO attached to two alkyl groups 酮; **ketone bodies** = ketone compounds formed from fatty acids 酮体

◇ **ketonuria** *noun* state where ketone bodies are excreted in the urine 酮尿

◇ **ketosis** *noun* state where ketone bodies (such as acetone and acetic acid) accumulate in the tissues, a late complication of juvenile diabetes mellitus 酮症,青少年糖尿病的晚期并发症,酮体在组织内沉积 *see also* 参见 ACETONE, ACETONURIA

key 1 *noun* (**a**) piece of shaped metal used to open a lock 钥匙: ***She has a set of keys to the laboratory.*** 她有试验室的一套钥匙。***He signed for the key to the medicine cupboard.*** 他做手势要药柜的钥匙。(**b**) part of a piano *or* a typewriter *or* a computer which you push down with your fingers 键盘 (**c**) answer to a problem *or* explanation 答案,关键: ***The key to successful treatment of arthritis is movement.*** 治疗关节炎成功的秘诀是运动。**2** *adjective* most important 关键的: ***He has the key position in the laboratory.*** 他是试验室的关键人物。***Penicillin is the key factor in the treatment of gangrene.*** 青霉素是治疗坏疽的关键药物。

◇ **keyhole surgery** *noun* (*informal* 非正式) laparoscopic surgery involving inserting tiny surgical instruments through an endoscope 腹腔镜手术

kg = KILOGRAM 千克

kick 1 *noun* hitting with your foot 踢: ***She could feel the baby give a kick.*** 她感觉到胎儿踢了一下。**2** *verb* to hit something with your foot 踢: ***She could feel the baby kicking.*** 她感觉到胎儿在踢。

kidney *noun* one of two organs situated in the lower part of the back on either side of the spine behind the abdomen, whose function is to maintain normal concentrations of the main constituents of blood, passing the waste matter into the urine 肾,位于腹后腰部脊柱两侧的器官,其功能是维持血液内主要成分的正常浓度,将废物排入尿中: ***He has a kidney infection.*** 他患肾脏感染。***The kidneys have begun to malfunction.*** 肾功能开始减退。***She is being treated for kidney trouble.*** 她接受肾病治疗。**kidney dialysis** = removing waste matter from the blood of a patient by passing it through a kidney machine 肾透析,用人工肾排泄废物; **kidney failure** = situation where a patient's kidneys do not function properly 肾衰竭; **kidney machine** = apparatus through which a patient's blood is passed to be cleaned by dialysis if the patient's kidneys have failed 人工肾; **kidney stone** = hard mass of calcium like a little piece of stone, which forms in the kidney 肾结石; **floating kidney** = NEPHROPTOSIS 游动肾; **horseshoe kidney** = congenital defect of the kidney, where sometimes the upper but usually the lower parts of both kidneys are joined together 马蹄肾,一种先天性疾病,两肾的上极通常与下极相连 (NOTE: for other terms referring to the kidney, see words beginning with **nephr-**, **ren-**, **reno-**)

> COMMENT: A kidney is formed of an outer cortex and an inner medulla. The nephrons which run from the cortex into the medulla filter the blood and form urine. The urine is passed through the ureters into the bladder. Sudden sharp pain in back of the abdomen, going downwards, is an indication of a kidney stone passing into the ureter.
> 注释:肾分为外部的皮质和内部的髓质,肾

小球从皮质进入髓质，过滤血液形成尿液，尿通过输尿管排入膀胱，腰部突然的锐痛，向下放射，提示有结石排入输尿管。

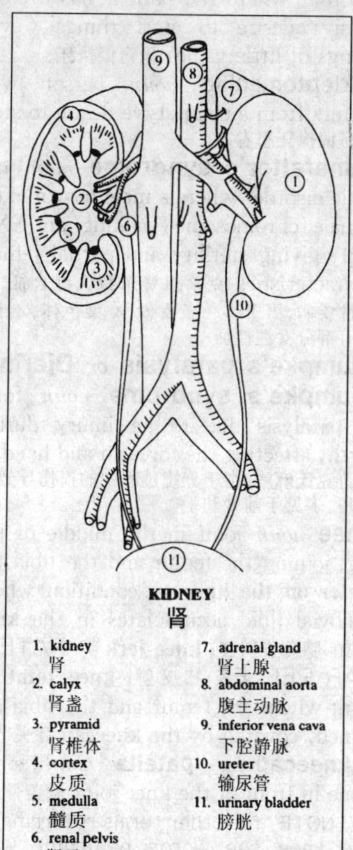

kill *verb* to make someone *or* something die 杀: ***She was given the kidney of a person killed in a car crash.*** 她接受了车祸中遇害者的肾脏。***Heart attacks kill more people every year.*** 每年有越来越多的人死于心脏疾病。***Antibodies are created to kill bacteria.*** 抗生素可杀死细菌。

◇ **killer** *noun* person *or* disease which kills 杀手: ***Virulent typhoid fever can be a killer disease.*** 毒性伤寒是种致命性疾病。***In the winter, bronchitis is the killer of hundreds of old people.*** 冬季，有成百上千的老人死于支气管炎。*see also* 参见 PAINKILLER

Killian's operation *noun* clearing of the frontal sinus by curetting 基利安氏手术，额窦术

COMMENT: In Killian's operation the incision is made in the eyebrow.
注释：额窦手术切口位于眉处。

kilo *abbreviation for* （缩写）KILOGRAM 千克

kilo- *prefix* meaning one thousand (10^3) 千 (NOTE: symbol is **k**)

◇ **kilocalorie** *noun* SI unit of measurement of heat (= 1000 calories) 千卡 (NOTE: with figures usually written **kcal.** Note also that it is now more usual to use the term **joule**)

◇ **kilogram** *or* **kilo** *noun* base SI unit of measurement of weight (= 1000 grams) 千克; ***two kilos of sugar*** 2 千克糖; ***He weighs 62 kilos (62 kg).*** 他重 62 千克。(NOTE: with figures usually written **kg**)

◇ **kilojoule** *noun* SI unit of measurement of energy *or* heat (= 1000 joules) 千焦 (NOTE: with figures usually written **kJ**)

◇ **kilopascal** *noun* SI unit of measurement of pressure (= 1000 pascals) 千帕 (NOTE: with figures usually written **kPa**)

Kimmelstiel-Wilson disease *or* **syndrome** *noun* form of nephrosclerosis found in diabetics 基－威二氏威病（综合症），糖尿病性肾小球硬化

kin *noun* relatives or close members of the family 亲戚; **next of kin** = person or persons who are most closely related to someone 至亲: ***The hospital has notified the next of kin of the death of the accident victim.*** 医院将事故遇害者死亡的消息通知了他的亲属。

kin- *or* **kine-** *prefix* meaning movement 运动

◇ **kinaesthesia** *noun* being aware of the movement and position of parts of the body 运动觉

COMMENT: Kinaesthesia is the result of information from muscles and ligaments which is passed to the brain and which allows the brain to recognize movements *or* touch *or* weight.
注释:运动觉是来自肌肉、韧带的信息传到脑,从而识别运动、触觉和重量。

◇ **kinanaesthesia** *noun* not being able to sense the movement and position of parts of the body 运动觉缺失

◇ **kinematics** *or* **cinematics** *noun* science of movement, especially of body movements 运动医学

◇ **kineplasty** *or* **cineplasty** *noun* amputation where the muscles of the stump of the amputated limb are used to operate an artificial limb 运动成形切断术

◇ **kinesiology** *or* **cinesiology** *noun* study of human movements, referring particularly to their use in treatment 运动医学

◇ **kinesitherapy** *noun* therapy involving movement of parts of the body 运动疗法

◇ **kinetochore** = CENTROMERE 着丝点

Kirschner wire *noun* wire attached to a bone and tightened to provide traction to a fracture 基施纳氏钢丝,固定骨折处进行牵引

kiss of life *noun* method of artificial respiration where the aider breathes into the patient's lungs (either through the mouth *or* through the nose) 人工呼吸(口对口或口对鼻): ***He was given the kiss of life.*** 对他进行人工呼吸。

kit *noun* equipment put together in a container 盒,用具; **first-aid kit** = box with bandages and dressings kept ready to be used in an emergency 急救箱

kJ = KILOJOULE 千焦

Klebsiella *noun* form of Gram negative bacteria, one of which, *Klebsiella pneumoniae*, can cause pneumonia 克雷白杆菌

Klebs-Loeffler bacillus *noun* diphtheria bacillus 克-吕氏杆菌,白喉杆菌

kleptomania *noun* form of mental disorder where the patient has a compulsive desire to steal things (even things of little value) 偷窃偏执狂

◇ **kleptomaniac** *noun* person who suffers from a compulsive desire to steal 偷窃偏执狂患者

Klinefelter's syndrome *noun* genetic disorder where a male has an extra female chromosome (making an XXY set), giving sterility and partial female characteristics 克莱恩费尔特氏综合征,遗传性疾病,男子多一条女性 X 染色体,不育,并有部分女性性征

Klumpke's paralysis *or* **Djerine-Klumpke's syndrome** *noun* form of paralysis due to an injury during birth, affecting the forearm and hand 克隆普克氏麻痹,由于分娩过程中的损伤导致的麻痹,多见于前臂和手

knee *noun* joint in the middle of the leg, joining the femur and the tibia 膝; **water on the knee** = condition where synovial fluid accumulates in the knee joint 膝关节积液; **knee jerk** = PATELLAR REFLEX 膝反射; **knee joint** = joint where the femur and the tibia are joined, covered by the kneecap 膝关节

◇ **kneecap** *or* **patella** *noun* small bone in front of the knee joint 膝盖骨,髌骨 (NOTE: for other terms referring to the knee see words beginning with **genu-**)

knit *verb* (**a**) to make something out of wool, using two long needles 编织 (**b**) (*of broken bones*) to join together again 愈合: ***Broken bones take longer to knit in old people than in children.*** 断骨愈合在老人要比儿童慢。(NOTE: **knits - knitting - has knitted** *or* **has knit**)

knock 1 *noun* (**a**) sound made by hitting something 敲击声,叩诊音 (**b**) hitting of something 碰撞: ***He was concussed after having had a knock on the head.*** 头受碰击后他得了脑震荡。**2** *verb* to hit something 敲,打: ***He knocked his***

head on the floor as he fell. 摔倒时,头碰在了地板上。

◊ **knock down** *verb* to make something fall down by hitting it hard 打倒: ***he was knocked down by a car.*** 他被汽车撞倒了。

◊ **knock knee** *noun* genu valgum, a state where the knees touch and the ankles are apart when a person is standing straight 膝外翻 *compare* 比较 BOW LEGS

◊ **knock-kneed** *adjective* (person) whose knees touch when he stands straight with feet slightly apart 膝外翻的

◊ **knock out** *verb* to hit someone so hard that he is no longer conscious 打晕,击昏: ***He was knocked out by a blow on the head.*** 他头上受了一击晕倒了。

knot 1 *noun* place where two pieces of string *or* gut are tied together 结: ***He tied a knot at the end of the piece of string.*** 他在绳的末端打了一个结。**2** *verb* to attach with a knot 打结: ***The nurse knotted the two bandages.*** 护士将绷带打结。(NOTE: **knotting - knotted**)

knuckles *plural noun* the backs of the joints on a person's hand 指节

Koch's bacillus *noun* bacillus, *Mycobacterium tuberculosis*, which causes tuberculosis 郭霍氏杆菌,结核杆菌

◊ **Koch-Weeks bacillus** *noun* bacillus which causes conjunctivitis 结膜炎嗜血杆菌

Köhler's disease *or* **scaphoiditis** *noun* degeneration of the navicular bone in children 科勒氏病,足舟骨炎,儿童足舟骨变性

koilonychia *or* **spoon nail** *noun* state where the fingernails are brittle and concave, caused by iron-deficiency anaemia 反甲,缺铁性贫血时指甲变脆、变凹

Koplik's spots *plural noun* small bluish-white spots surrounded by red areola, found in the mouth in the early stages of measles 科波力克氏斑,麻疹早期口腔内小的青白色的斑疹,有红晕

Korsakoff's syndrome *noun* condition where the patient's memory fails and he invents things which have not happened and is confused, caused usually by chronic alcoholism or disorders in which there is a deficiency of vitamin B 科罗特科夫氏综合征,因慢性酒精中毒或其他引起维生素 B 缺乏的疾病导致,表现为记忆力减退、幻想和精神错乱

kraurosis *noun* dryness and shrivelling of a part 干燥; **kraurosis penis** = state where the foreskin becomes dry and shrivelled 干燥性龟头炎; **kraurosis vulvae** = condition where the vulva becomes thin and dry due to lack of oestrogen (found usually in elderly women) 外阴干燥

Krause corpuscles 克劳泽氏小体,球状小体 *see* 见 CORPUSCLE ◊ 见图 SKIN AND SENSORY RECEPTORS

Krebs cycle = CITRIC ACID CYCLE 克雷布氏循环,三羧酸循环

Krukenberg tumour *noun* malignant tumour in the ovary secondary to a tumour in the stomach 克鲁肯伯格氏瘤,粘液细胞癌,胃癌转移至卵巢

Kuntscher nail *or* **Küntscher nail** *noun* long steel nail used to pin fractures of long bones through the bone marrow 金彻氏钉,骨髓腔内插钉

Kupffer's cells *noun* large specialized liver cells which break down haemoglobin into bile 枯否氏细胞,肝脏的特殊细胞,可将血红蛋白降解为胆汁

Kveim test *noun* skin test to confirm the presence of sarcoidosis 科维姆试验,检查结节病的皮肤试验

kwashiorkor *noun* malnutrition of small children, mostly in tropical countries, causing anaemia, wasting of the body and swollen liver 恶性营养不良病,最多见于热带国家,引起贫血、衰竭和肝大

kyphos *noun* lump on the back in kyphosis 驼背

◊ **kyphoscoliosis** *noun* condition where the patient has both backward and lateral curvature of the spine 脊柱后侧突

◊ **kyphosis** *noun* hunchback, excessive backward curvature of the top part of the spine 脊柱后突 *see also* 参见 LORDOSIS

◇ **kyphotic** *adjective* referring to kyphosis 驼背的

LI

l = LITRE 升

lab *noun* (*informal* 非正式) = LABORATORY 试验室: ***We'll send the specimens away for a lab test.*** 我们将把标本送往试验室进行检查。***The lab report is negative.*** 试验结果是阴性。***The samples have been returned by the lab.*** 标本已经被试验室退了回来。

lab- *prefix* referring to the lips *or* to labia 唇

label 1 *noun* piece of paper *or* card attached to an object *or* person to identify them 标签; **identity label** = label attached to the wrist of a newborn baby *or* a patient in hospital, so that he can be identified easily 身份标签,新生儿或患者腕上戴的标签,便于识别身份 **2** *verb* to write on a label *or* to attach a label to an object 做标签: ***The bottle is labelled 'poison'.*** 瓶上贴有标签"有毒"。

labia 唇 *see* 见 LABIUM

◇ **labial** *adjective* referring to the lips *or* to labia 口唇的,阴唇的

labile *adjective* (drug) which is unstable and likely to change if heated or cooled 不稳定的(药品)

labio- *prefix* referring to lips *or* to labia 口唇的,阴唇的

◇ **labioplasty** *noun* surgical operation to repair damaged *or* deformed lips 口唇成形术

◇ **labium** *noun* (i) lip 口唇 (ii) structure which looks like a lip 唇样组织; **labia majora** = two large fleshy folds at the outside edge of the vulva 大阴唇; **labia minora** *or* **nymphae** = two small fleshy folds on the inside edge of the vulva 小阴唇 ◊ 见图 UROEGNITAL SYSTEM (female) (NOTE: plural is **labia**)

laboratory *noun* special room(s) where scientists can do research *or* can test chemical substances *or* can grow tissues in culture, etc. 试验室: ***The new drug has passed its laboratory tests.*** 新药通过了试验室检查。***The samples of water from the hospital have been sent to the laboratory for testing.*** 从医院采集的水样被送往试验室进行检查。**laboratory officer** = qualified person in charge of a laboratory 试验室负责人; **laboratory techniques** = methods *or* skills needed to perform experiments in a laboratory 试验技术,技巧; **laboratory technician** = person who does practical work in a laboratory and has particular care of equipment 试验室技师

labour *or US* **labor** *noun* childbirth, especially the contractions in the womb which take place during childbirth 分娩; **woman in labour** = experiencing the physical changes, contractions in the womb, pains, etc. which precede the birth of a child 产妇; **to go into labour** = to start to experience the contractions which indicate the birth of a child is imminent 临产妇: ***She was in labour for 14 hours.*** 她分娩用了14个小时。***She went into labour at 6 o'clock.*** 她6点开始的临产。*see also* 参见 INDUCE, PREMATURE

> COMMENT: Labour usually starts about nine months (or 266 days) after conception. The cervix expands and the muscles in the uterus contract, causing the amnion to burst. The muscles continue to contract regularly, pushing the baby into, and then through, the vagina.
> 注释:分娩开始于妊娠9个月(266天)后。宫颈扩张,子宫肌收缩,羊膜破裂,子宫肌进一步的规律收缩,将胎儿经阴道推出体外。

labyrinth *noun* interconnecting tubes, especially those in the inside of the ear 迷路,相互连接的管道,常指耳内的迷路; **bony labyrinth** *or* **osseous labyrinth** = hard part of the temporal bone surrounding the membranous labyrinth in the inner ear 骨迷路,颞骨的硬部,环绕内耳的膜迷路; **membranous labyrinth** = series of ducts and canals formed of membrane inside the osseous labyrinth 膜迷路,骨迷路Z内的由膜组成的一系列管腔

◇ **labyrinthitis** *or* **otitis interna** *noun* inflammation of the labyrinth 迷路炎

> COMMENT: The labyrinth of the inner ear is in three parts: the three semicircular canals, the vestibule and the cochlea. The osseous labyrinth is filled with a fluid (perilymph) and the membranous labyrinth is a series of ducts and canals inside the osseous labyrinth. The membranous labyrinth contains a fluid (endolymph). As the endolymph moves about in the membranous labyrinth it stimulates the vestibular nerve which communicates the sense of movement of the head to the brain. If a person turns round and round and then stops, the endolymph continues to move and creates the sensation of giddiness.
> 注释:内耳的迷路分为3部分:3个半规管、前庭和耳蜗。骨迷路内充满了淋巴液(外淋巴),膜迷路是骨迷路内的由膜组成的一系列管腔,也含有淋巴液(内淋巴)。内淋巴在膜迷路内流动,刺激前庭神经将头部的运动感觉传到脑。如果不停地旋转,然后停下,内淋巴继续流动,就会产生眩晕。

lacerated *adjective* torn *or* with a rough edge 撕裂的; **lacerated wound** = wound where the skin is torn, as by a rough surface *or* barbed wire 撕裂伤

◇ **laceration** *noun* act of tearing tissue 撕裂; wound which has been cut *or* torn with rough edges, and not the result of stabbing *or* pricking 撕裂伤

lachrymal 泪的 *see* 见 LACRIMAL

lack 1 *noun* not having something 缺乏: ***The children are dying because of lack of food.*** 儿童因缺乏食物而死亡。***The hospital had to close two wards because of lack of money.*** 医院因为缺少资金不得不关闭两个病房。2 *verb* not to have enough of something 缺少,短缺: ***The children lack winter clothing.*** 儿童缺乏冬衣。***Their diet lacks essential proteins.*** 他们的饮食缺少必需的蛋白质。***He lacks the strength to feed himself.*** = He isn't strong enough to feed himself. 他连自己吃饭的力气都没有。

lacrimal *or* **lacrymal** *or* **lachrymal** *adjective* referring to tears *or* tear ducts *or* tear glands 泪的,泪管的,泪腺的; **lacrimal apparatus** *or* **system** = arrangement of glands and ducts which produce and drain tears 泪器; **lacrimal bones** = two little bones which join with others to form the orbits 泪骨; **lacrimal canaliculus** = small canal draining tears into the lacrimal sac 泪小管; **lacrimal caruncle** = small red point at the inner corner of each eye 泪阜; **lacrimal duct** *or* **tear duct** *or* **nasolacrimal duct** = canal which takes tears from the lacrimal sac to the nose 泪管,鼻泪管; **lacrimal gland** *or* **tear gland** = gland beneath the upper eyelid which secretes tears 泪腺; **lacrimal puncta** = small openings of the lacrimal canaliculus at the corners of the eyes through which tears drain into the nose 泪点; **lacrimal sac** = sac at the upper end of the nasolacrimal duct, linking it with the lacrimal canaliculus 泪囊

◇ **lacrimation** *noun* crying, the production of tears 流泪

◇ **lacrimator** *noun* substance which irritates the eyes and makes tears flow 催泪剂

lact- *prefix* referring to milk 奶的,乳汁的

◇ **lactase** *noun* enzyme, secreted in the small intestine, which converts milk sugar into glucose and galactose 乳糖酶,小肠分泌的酶,将乳糖转化为葡萄糖和半乳糖

◇ **lactate** *verb* to produce milk 产乳

◇ **lactation** *noun* (i) production of milk 泌乳 (ii) period during which a mother is breast feeding a baby 哺乳期

> COMMENT: Lactation is stimulated by the production of the hormone

prolactin by the pituitary gland. It starts about three days after childbirth, during which period the breasts secrete colostrum.
注释:垂体产生的泌乳素刺激泌乳,大约开始于产后3天,期间乳腺分泌初乳。

lacteal 1 *adjective* referring to milk 乳的 2 *noun* lymph vessel in a villus, which helps the digestive process in the small intestine by absorbing fat 乳糜管,肠绒毛内的淋巴管,帮助小肠消化,吸收脂肪

lactic acid *noun* sugar which forms in cells and tissue, also in sour milk, cheese and yoghurt 乳酸

COMMENT: Lactic acid is produced as the body uses up sugar during exercise. Excessive amounts of lactic acid in the body can produce muscle cramp.
注释:在机体运动时消耗糖产生乳酸,过量的乳酸堆积可引起肌肉痉挛。

◇ **lactiferous** *adjective* which produces *or* secretes *or* carries milk 泌乳的,输乳的; **lactiferous duct** = duct in the breast which carries milk 输乳管; **lactiferous sinus** = dilatation of the lactiferous duct at the base of the nipple 输乳窦

◇ **Lactobacillus** *noun* genus of Gram-positive bacteria which can produce lactic acid from glucose and may be found in the digestive tract and the vagina 乳酸杆菌,位于消化道和阴道,可将葡萄糖转化为乳酸的革兰氏阳性杆菌

◇ **lactogenic hormone** = PROLACTIN 催乳素

◇ **lactose** *or* **milk sugar** *noun* sugar found in milk 乳糖; **lactose intolerance** = condition where a person cannot digest lactose because lactase is absent in the intestine, or because of an allergy to milk, causing diarrhoea 乳糖不耐受,因为肠道内缺乏乳糖酶不能消化乳糖或对牛奶过敏,引起腹泻

◇ **lactosuria** *noun* excretion of lactose in the urine 乳糖尿

◇ **lactovegetarian** *noun & adjective* (person) who does not eat meat, but eats vegetables, fruit, dairy produce and eggs and sometimes fish 乳制品蔬菜食者(的),不吃肉,但吃蔬菜、水果、乳制品、鸡蛋,有时也吃鱼: ***He has been on a lactovegetarian diet for twenty years.*** 他是乳制品蔬菜食者已经20年了。*compare* 比较 VEGAN, VEGETARIAN

lacuna *noun* small hollow *or* cavity 腔隙,陷窝 (NOTE: plural is **lacunae**)

Laennec's cirrhosis *noun* commonest form of alcoholic cirrhosis of the liver 拉埃奈克氏肝硬化,酒精性肝硬化最常见的一种

laevocardia *noun* normal position of the apex of the heart towards the left side of the body 左位心 *compare* 比较 DEXTROCARDIA

lambda *noun* point at the back of the skull where the sagittal suture and lambdoidal suture meet 人字缝尖

◇ **lambdoid(al) suture** *noun* horizontal joint across the back of the skull between the parietal and occipital bones 人字缝,颅顶顶骨和枕骨之间的水平连接◊见图 SKULL

lamblia 贾弟虫属 *see* 见 GIARDIA

◇ **lambliasis** 贾弟虫病 *see* 见 GIARDIASIS

lame *adjective* not able to walk normally because of pain, stiffness or deformity in a leg or foot 跛的: ***He has been lame since his accident.*** 事故后他就跛了。

◇ **lameness** *noun* limping, the inability to walk normally because of pain, stiffness or deformity in a leg or foot 跛

lamella *noun* (i) thin sheet of tissue 板,薄的组织层 (ii) thin disc placed under the eyelid to apply a drug to the eye 眼用薄片 (NOTE: plural is **lamellae**)

lamina *noun* (i) thin membrane 板,层 (ii) side part of the posterior arch in a vertebra 椎弓板; **lamina propria** = connective tissue of mucous membrane containing blood vessels, lymphatics, etc. 粘膜的固有层 (NOTE: plural is **laminae**)

◇ **laminectomy** *or* **rachiotomy** *noun*

surgical operation to cut through the lamina of a vertebra in the spine to get to the spinal cord 椎板切除术

lamp *noun* electric device which makes light 灯：***an electric lamp*** 电灯；***An endoscope can have a small lamp at the end of it.*** 内镜末端可以有个小灯。***The ear specialist shone his lamp into the patient's ear.*** 耳科医生用他的灯照患者的耳内。***She lay for thirty minutes under an ultraviolet lamp.*** 她在紫外灯下躺了 30 分钟。

lance *verb* to make a cut in a boil *or* abscess to remove the pus 刀割

◇ **lancet** *noun* sharp two-edged pointed knife formerly used in surgery 柳叶刀

◇ **lancinate** *verb* to lacerate *or* cut 撕裂，刀割

◇ **lancinating** *adjective* (pain) which is sharp and cutting 刀割样(疼痛)

Landry's paralysis 兰德里氏麻痹，急性热病性多神经炎 *see* 见 Guillain-Barré syndrome

Lange test *noun* method of detecting globulin in the cerebrospinal fluid 郎格试验，检查脑脊液中的球蛋白

Langerhans *noun* **islets of Langerhans** = groups of cells in the pancreas which secrete the hormones glucagon, insulin and gastrin 郎格罕氏小岛，胰岛，胰腺中的一群细胞，分泌胰高血糖素、胰岛素和胃泌素；**Langerhans' cells** = cells on the outer layers of the skin 郎格罕氏小细胞，位于皮肤的外层

lanolin *noun* grease (from sheep's wool) which absorbs water, and is used to rub on dried skin, or in the preparation of cosmetics 羊毛脂，可吸收水分，用于涂在干燥的皮肤上，制备化妆品

lanugo *noun* soft hair on the body of a fetus *or* newborn baby 胎毛；soft hair on the body of an adult (except on the palms of the hands, the soles of the feet, and the parts where long hair grows) 体毛

laparo- *prefix* referring to the lower abdomen 下腹部，胁腹

◇ **laparoscope** *or* **peritoneoscope** *noun* surgical instrument which is inserted through a hole in the abdominal wall to allow a surgeon to examine the inside of the abdominal cavity 腹腔镜，通过腹壁的孔洞插入腹腔的手术器械，用于检查腹腔内器官

◇ **laparoscopic** *adjective* using a laparoscope 腹腔镜的；**laparoscopic surgery** = surgery involving inserting tiny surgical instruments through an endoscope 腹腔镜手术

◇ **laparoscopy** *or* **peritoneoscopy** *noun* using a laparoscope to examine the inside of the abdominal cavity 腹腔镜检查

◇ **laparotomy** *noun* surgical operation to cut open the abdominal cavity 剖腹术

large *adjective* very big 大的：***He has a large tumour on the right cerebrum.*** 他右脑长了个大肿瘤。(NOTE: **large - larger - largest**)

◇ **large intestine** *noun* section of the digestive system from the caecum to the rectum 大肠，包括结肠和直肠

larva *noun* stage in the development of an insect *or* tapeworm, after the egg has hatched but before the animal becomes adult 蚴虫期，昆虫或绦虫发育过程中卵孵出后至成虫的阶段 (NOTE: plural is **larvae**)

laryng- *or* **laryngo-** *prefix* referring to the larynx 喉的

◇ **laryngeal** *adjective* referring to the larynx 喉；**laryngeal inlet** = entrance from the laryngopharynx leading through the vocal cords to the trachea 喉入口；**laryngeal prominence** = Adam's apple 喉结；**laryngeal reflex** = cough 喉反射，咳嗽

◇ **laryngectomy** *noun* surgical removal of the larynx, usually as treatment for throat cancer 喉切除术

◇ **laryngismus** (**stridulus**) *noun* spasm of the throat muscles with a sharp intake of breath which occurs when the larynx is irritated, as in children suffering from croup 喉痉挛

◇ **laryngitis** *noun* inflammation of the larynx 喉炎

◇ **laryngofissure** *noun* surgical operation to make an opening into the larynx through the thyroid cartilage 喉裂开术

◇ **laryngologist** *noun* doctor who specializes in diseases of the larynx, throat and vocal cords 喉科医生

◇ **laryngology** *noun* study of diseases of the larynx, throat and vocal cords 喉科学

◇ **laryngopharynx** *noun* part of the pharynx below the hyoid bone 咽喉

◇ **laryngoscope** *noun* instrument for examining the inside of the larynx, using a light and mirrors 咽喉镜

◇ **laryngospasm** *noun* muscular spasm which suddenly closes the larynx 喉痉挛

◇ **laryngostenosis** *noun* narrowing of the lumen of the larynx 喉狭窄

◇ **laryngotomy** *noun* surgical operation to make an opening in the larynx through the membrane (especially in an emergency, when the throat is blocked) 喉切开术(在咽喉阻塞急救时用)

◇ **laryngotracheobronchitis** *noun* inflammation of the larynx, trachea and bronchi, as in croup 喉气管支气管炎

◇ **larynx** *or* **voice box** *noun* organ in the throat which produces sounds 喉 ◊ 见图 THROAT

> COMMENT: The larynx is a hollow passage made of cartilage, containing the vocal cords, situated behind the Adam's apple. It is closed by the epiglottis when swallowing or before coughing.
> 注释:喉是由软骨构成的中空的管道,内有位于喉结后的声带,在吞咽和咳嗽时由会厌封闭。

laser *noun* instrument which produces a highly concentrated beam of light, which can be used to cut or attach tissue, as in operations for detached retina 激光器,产生激光用于切割或附着组织,如剥离视网膜手术; **argon laser** = laser which uses argon as its medium 氩激光器; **laser probe** = metal probe which is inserted into the body and through which a laser beam can be passed to remove a blockage in an artery 激光探针,插入体内的金属探针,激光从中间穿过,可祛除动脉栓塞; **laser surgery** = surgery using lasers (such as removal of tumours, sealing blood vessels, etc.) 激光手术

Lassa fever *noun* highly infectious virus disease found in Central and West Africa 拉沙热,在中、西非发现的一种高传染性病毒性疾病

> COMMENT: The symptoms are high fever, pains, and ulcers in the mouth. It is often fatal.
> 注释:症状有高热、疼痛和口腔溃疡,常为致死性的。

Lassar's paste *noun* ointment made of zinc oxide, used to treat eczema 拉萨尔糊剂,氧化锌软膏,用于治疗湿疹

lassitude *noun* state where a person does not want to do anything, sometimes because he is depressed 倦怠

lata 拉塔病 *see* 见 FASCIA

latent *adjective* (disease) which is present in the body, but does not show any signs 潜伏的: ***The children were tested for latent viral infection.*** 儿童被检查是否有潜伏的病毒感染。

lateral *adjective* (i) further away from the midline of the body 外侧的 (ii) referring to one side of the body 一侧的; **lateral aspect** *or* **view** = view of the side of part of the body 侧面观; **lateral malleolus** = prominence on the outer surface of the ankle joint 外踝 *compare* 比较 MEDIAL

◇ **lateralis**外侧的 *see* 见 VASTUS

◇ **laterally** *adv* towards *or* on the side of the body 侧面的

◇ **lateroversion** *noun* turning (of an organ) to one side 侧倾

latissimus dorsi *noun* large flat triangular muscle covering the lumbar region and the lower part of the chest 背阔肌

laugh 1 *noun* sound made by the throat when a person is amused 笑声:

He said it with a laugh. 他笑着说。*She gave a hysterical laugh.* 她发出了歇斯底里的笑声。**2** *verb* to make a sound which shows amusement 笑: *He started to laugh hysterically.* 他开始歇斯底里地大笑。

◇ **laughing gas** *noun* nitrous oxide (N_2O), colourless gas with a sweet smell, used in combination with other gases as an anaesthetic in dentistry and surgery 笑气,一氧化二氮,有甜味儿的无色气体,与其他气体混合可用于牙科和手术麻醉

laundry *noun* (**a**) place where clothes, etc. are washed 洗衣店: *The bed clothes will be sent to the hospital laundry to be sterilized.* 被褥将送到医院洗衣房消毒。(**b**) clothes, etc. which need to be washed or which have been washed 将要洗或已经洗好的衣物: *The report criticized the piles of dirty laundry left lying in the wards.* 报告对病房内堆积的脏衣物提出了批评。

lavage *noun* washing out *or* irrigating an organ, such as the stomach 灌洗

lavatory *noun* toilet, a place or room where one can get rid of water or solid waste from the body 盥洗室,厕所: *The ladies' lavatory is to the right.* 女士卫生间在右面。*There are three lavatories for the ward of ten people.* 这10人的病房内有3个卫生间。

laxative *noun & adjective* (medicine) which causes a bowel movement 泻药(的)

> COMMENT: Laxatives are very commonly used without prescription to treat constipation, although they should only be used as a short term solution. Change of diet and regular exercise are better ways of treating most types of constipation.
> 注释:尽管泻药仅能暂时缓解症状,但因其可治疗便秘,作为非处方药应用地极为普遍。改变饮食和运动是治疗大多数便秘更有效的方法。

layer *noun* flat area *or* sheet of a substance under or over another area 层: *They put three layers of cotton wadding over his eye.* 他们在他的眼睛上覆盖了3层棉垫。

lazy *adjective* not wanting to do any work 懒惰的; **lazy eye** = eye which does not focus properly 弱视

lb 磅 *see* 见 POUND

LD = LETHAL DOSE 致死剂量

LDL = LOW DENSITY LIPOPROTEIN 低密度脂蛋白

L-dopa *or* **levodopa** *noun* amino acid used in the treatment of Parkinson's disease 左旋多巴,治疗帕金森病

l.e. *or* **LE** *abbreviation for* (缩写) LUPUS ERYTHEMATOSUS 红斑狼疮的简写; **LE cells** = white blood cells which show that a patient has lupus erythematosus 狼疮细胞,提示患有红斑狼疮的白细胞

lead *noun* very heavy soft metallic element, which is poisonous in compounds 铅; **lead line** = blue line seen on the gums in cases of lead poisoning 铅线,铅中毒时牙龈上可见的蓝线(NOTE: chemical symbol is **Pb**)

◇ **lead-free** *adjective* with no lead in it 无铅的; *lead-free paint* 无铅涂料; *lead-free petrol* 无铅汽油

◇ **lead poisoning** *or* **plumbism** *or* **saturnism** *noun* poisoning caused by taking in lead salts 铅中毒

> COMMENT: Lead salts are used externally to treat bruises or eczema, but if taken internally produce lead poisoning, which can also be caused by paint (children's toys must be painted in lead-free paint) or by lead fumes from car engines (which can be avoided by using lead-free petrol).
> 注释:铅盐外用可治疗青肿或湿疹,一旦内服可造成铅中毒。铅中毒也可因涂料(儿童的玩具必须用无铅涂料)或汽车尾气(用无铅汽油可避免)引起。

leak *verb* (*of liquids*) to flow out by accident *or* by mistake 渗漏: *Blood leaked into the subcutaneous layers.* 血液渗进了皮下层。

lecithins *noun* constituents of all animal and plant cells, involved with the transport and absorption of fats 卵磷脂，构成所有动植物细胞的成分，参与脂肪的转运和吸收

leech *noun* type of parasitic worm which lives in water and sucks the blood of animals by attaching itself to the skin 水蛭，生活在水中的寄生虫，通过吸附在动物皮肤上吸取血液；**medicinal leech** = leech which is raised specially for use in medicine 医用水蛭

> COMMENT: Leeches were formerly commonly used in medicine to remove blood from a patient. Today they are used in special cases, where it is necessary to make sure that blood does not build up in part of the body (as in a severed finger which has been sewn back on).
> 注释：水蛭以前普遍应用于祛除患者体内的血液。如今它们仅用于明确血液不是体内循环的一部分（如断指缝合）时的特殊病例。

left *adverb*, *adjective* & *noun* referring to the side of the body which usually has the weaker hand 左侧的，左侧：***He can't write with his left hand.*** 他不能用左手写字。***The heart is on the left side of the body.*** 心脏位于身体的左面。

◇ **left-hand** *adjective* on the left side 左手的，左面的：***Look in the left-hand drawer of the desk.*** 看看桌子左手面的抽屉。***The tablets are on the top left-hand shelf in the cupboard.*** 药片在药柜左手上面的一层。

◇ **left-handed** *adjective* using the left hand more often than the right for writing 左利的，左撇子的：***She's left-handed.*** 她是左撇子。***Left-handed people need special scissors.*** 左撇子需要特殊的剪刀。***About five percent of the population is left-handed.*** 大约5%的人是左撇子。

◇ **left-handedness** *noun* condition of a person who is left-handed 左利

leg *noun* part of the body with which a person or animal walks and stands 腿：***She made him stand on one leg and lift the other leg up.*** 她让他单腿直立，抬起另一条腿。***He is limping from a leg injury which he received playing football.*** 他因为打橄榄球一条腿受伤而瘸了。***His left leg is slightly shorter than the right.*** 他的左腿比右腿略短。***She complained of pains in her right leg.*** 她主诉右腿疼痛。***She fell off the wall and broke her leg.*** 她从墙上掉了下来，摔断了腿。

> COMMENT: The leg is formed of the thigh (with the thigh bone or femur), the knee (with the kneecap or patella), and the lower leg (with two bones - the tibia and fibula).
> 注释：腿由大腿（大腿骨或股骨）、膝（膝盖骨或髌骨）和小腿（胫骨和腓骨）组成。

legal *adjective* which is allowed by law 合法的；**legal abortion** = abortion carried out according to the law 合法流产

Legg-Calvé-Perthes disease *noun* degeneration of the upper end of the thigh bone in young boys, which prevents the bone growing properly and can result in a permanent limp 累－卡－佩三氏病，幼年变性形骨软骨炎，年轻男孩儿股骨上端变性，使骨发育不良，引起永久性跛足

legionnaires' disease *noun* bacterial disease similar to pneumonia 军团菌病

> COMMENT: The disease is thought to be transmitted in droplets of moisture in the air, and so the bacterium is found in central air-conditioning systems. It can be fatal to old or sick people, and so is especially dangerous if present in a hospital.
> 注释：本病由空气飞沫传播，细菌位于中央空调系统。老人或病人感染此病可以是致命的，尤以院内感染最为危险。

leiomyoma *noun* tumour of smooth muscle, especially the smooth muscle coating the uterus 平滑肌瘤

◇ **leiomyosarcoma** *noun* sarcoma in which large bundles of smooth muscle are found 平滑肌肉瘤

Leishmania *noun* tropical parasite which is passed to humans by the bites of sandflies 利什曼原虫

◇ **leishmaniasis** *noun* any of several diseases (such as Delhi boil *or* kala-azar) caused by the parasite *Leishmania*, one form giving disfiguring ulcers, another attacking the liver and bone marrow 利什曼病,由利什曼原虫引起的多种疾病,可以是毁容性溃疡,也可以侵犯肝和骨髓; **mucocutaneous leishmaniasis** = disorder affecting the skin and mucous membrane 皮肤粘膜型利什曼病

Lembert's suture *noun* suture used to close a wound in the intestine which includes all the coats of the intestine 郎贝尔缝术,闭合肠伤口的缝术,包括肠壁各层

Lempert operation *noun* fenestration, a surgical operation to relieve deafness by making a small opening in the inner ear 内耳开窗术,用以减轻耳聋

length *noun* measurement of how long something is 长度: ***The small intestine is about 5 metres in length.*** 小肠约5米长。

lens *noun* (**a**) part of the eye behind the iris and pupil, which focuses light coming from the cornea onto the retina (眼)晶体◇见图 EYE (**b**) piece of shaped glass *or* plastic which forms part of a pair of spectacles *or* microscope 镜片; **contact lens** = tiny glass *or* plastic lens which fits over the eyeball and is worn instead of spectacles 接触镜,隐形眼镜

◇ **lenticular** *adjective* referring to a lens *or* like a lens 晶体的,像晶体的

> COMMENT: The lens in the eye is elastic, and can change its shape under the influence of the ciliary muscle, to allow the eye to focus on objects at different distances.
> 注释:眼内晶体是有弹性的,在睫状肌调控下可改变形状,使眼睛对不同距离的物体聚焦。

lentigo *noun* freckle, a small brown spot on the skin often caused by exposure to sunlight 着色斑,皮肤上小的棕色斑点,常因日晒引起

leper *noun* person suffering from leprosy 麻风病患者: ***He works in a leper hospital.*** 他在麻风病医院工作。

lepidosis *noun* skin eruption, where pieces of skin fall off in flakes 鳞屑病,表现为皮疹,其皮屑呈片状剥脱

leproma *noun* lesion of the skin caused by leprosy 麻风结节

◇ **leprosy** *or* **Hansen's disease** *noun* infectious bacterial disease of skin and peripheral nerve tracts caused by *Mycobacterium leprae*, which destroys the tissues and can cripple the patient if left untreated 麻风病,皮肤和周围神经被麻风分枝杆菌感染,如不治疗,可破坏组织使患者病残

> COMMENT: Leprosy attacks the nerves in the skin, and finally the patient loses all feeling in a limb, and parts, such as fingers or toes, can drop off.
> 注释:麻风病侵及皮肤神经,使肢体或部分肢体如指、趾感觉丧失,最终脱落。

lepto- *prefix* meaning thin 薄的

◇ **leptocyte** *noun* thin red blood cell found in anaemia 薄红细胞

◇ **leptomeninges** *noun* two inner meninges (pia mater and arachnoid) 柔脑脊膜(软脑膜和蛛网膜)

◇ **leptomeningitis** *noun* inflammation of the leptomeninges 柔脑脊膜炎

◇ **leptospirosis** *or* **Weil's disease** *noun* infectious disease caused by the spirochaete *Leptospira* transmitted to humans from rats, giving jaundice and kidney damage 钩端螺旋体病,从鼠传给人的感染性疾病,表现为黄疸和肾脏损害

leresis *noun* uncoordinated speech, a sign of dementia 冗谈,饶舌

lesbian *noun* & *adjective* woman who experiences sexual attraction towards other women 女性同性恋者(的)

◇ **lesbianism** *noun* sexual attraction in one woman for another 女性同性恋 *compare* 比较 HOMOSEXUAL

lesion *noun* wound *or* sore *or* damage to the body 损害(NOTE: lesion is used to refer to any damage to the body, from the fracture of a bone to a cut on the skin)

lessen *verb* to make less strong 使减

轻,使减弱: ***The injection will lessen the pain.*** 这针可缓解疼痛。 ***Modern antibiotics lessen the chance of a patient getting gangrene.*** 现代的抗生素减少了患者发生坏疽的机率。

lesser *adjective* smaller 小的; **lesser trochanter** = projection on the femur which is the insertion of the psoas major muscle 小转子

lethal *adjective* which can kill 可致死的: ***she took a lethal dose of aspirin.*** 她服用了致死剂量的阿司匹林。 ***These fumes are lethal if inhaled.*** 这些气体一旦吸入将会致命。**lethal gene** = gene which can kill the person who inherits it 致死基因,一旦遗传将会使人死亡的基因

lethargic *adjective* showing lethargy 昏睡的; **lethargic encephalitis** *or* **encephalitis lethargica** = a common type of virus encephalitis occurring in epidemics in the 1920s 昏睡性脑炎,20 世纪 20 年代流行的一种病毒性脑炎

◇ **lethargy** *noun* mental torpor *or* tired feeling, when the patient has slow movements and is almost inactive 昏睡

leucine *noun* essential amino acid 亮氨酸

leuco- *or* **leuko-** *prefix* meaning white 白的

◇ **leucocyte** *or* **leukocyte** *noun* white blood cell which contains a nucleus but has no haemoglobin 白细胞

◇ **leucocytolysis** *noun* destruction of leucocytes 白细胞溶解

◇ **leucocytosis** *noun* increase in numbers of leucocytes in the blood above the normal upper limit (in order to fight an infection) 白细胞增多症

COMMENT: In normal conditions the blood contains far fewer leucocytes than erythrocytes (red blood cells), but their numbers increase rapidly when infection is present in the body. Leucocytes are either granular (with granules in the cytoplasm) or nongranular. The main types of leucocyte are : lymphocytes and monocytes which are nongranular, and neutrophils, eosinophils and basophils which are granular (granulocytes). Granular leucocytes are produced by the bone marrow, and their main function is to remove foreign particles from the blood and fight infection by forming antibodies.

注释:正常情况下,血内的白细胞远远少于红细胞,但感染时可增多。白细胞分为有颗粒的(胞浆内有颗粒)和无颗粒的。主要的白细胞有:淋巴细胞和单核细胞(无颗粒),中性粒细胞、嗜酸性粒细胞和嗜碱性粒细胞(颗粒细胞)。颗粒细胞由骨髓产生,其主要功能是清除血液内的异物和产生抗体抵抗感染。

◇ **leucoderma** *or* **vitiligo** *noun* condition where white patches appear on the skin 白斑病,皮肤出现白斑

◇ **leucolysin** *noun* protein which destroys white blood cells 白细胞溶素

◇ **leucoma** *noun* white scar of the cornea 角膜白斑

◇ **leuconychia** *noun* white marks on the fingernails 指甲上的白斑

◇ **leucopenia** *noun* reduction in the number of leucocytes in the blood, usually as a result of a disease 白细胞减少症

◇ **leucoplakia** *noun* condition where white patches form on mucous membranes (such as on the tongue or inside of the mouth) 粘膜白斑(如舌或口腔内粘膜)

◇ **leucopoiesis** *noun* production of leucocytes 白细胞生成

◇ **leucorrhoea** *or* **whites** *noun* excessive discharge of white mucus from the vagina 白带

◇ **leucotomy** *noun* **prefrontal leucotomy** = operation to divide some of the white matter in the prefrontal lobe, formerly used as a treatment for schizophrenia 额叶前部切断术,脑白质切断术,以前用于治疗精神分裂症

◇ **leukaemia** *noun* any of several malignant diseases where an abnormal number of leucocytes form in the blood 白血病,白细胞异常增多的血液恶性疾病

COMMENT: Apart from the increase in the number of leucocytes, the symptoms include swelling of the spleen and the lymph glands. There are several forms of leukaemia: the commonest is acute lymphoblastic leukaemia which occurs in children and can be treated by radiotherapy. 注释:除白细胞增多外,其他症状包括脾、淋巴结肿大。白血病有几种类型:最常见的是儿童急性淋巴细胞白血病,可用放疗治疗。

levator *noun* (**a**) surgical instrument for lifting pieces of fractured bone 上提骨折片的手术器械 (**b**) muscle which lifts a limb *or* a part of the body 提肌

level 1 *adjective* flat *or* horizontal *or* not rising and falling 平的,水平的,稳定的: ***Her temperature has remained level for the last hour.*** 过去的一小时中她的体温保持稳定。**2** *noun* amount 数量: ***He has a very high level of cholesterol in his blood.*** 他血中胆固醇水平很高。

levodopa *or* **L-dopa** *noun* drug used in the treatment of Parkinson's disease 左旋多巴

Leydig cells *or* **interstitial cells** *noun* testosterone-producing cells between the tubules in the testes 莱迪氏细胞,间质细胞,睾丸精管间的分泌睾酮的细胞

l. g. v. = LYMPHOGRANULOMA VENEREUM 性病性淋巴肉芽肿

LH = LUTEINIZING HORMONE 黄体生成素

liable to *adjective* likely to 倾向于: ***People in sedentary occupations are liable to have digestive disorders.*** 坐着工作的人易患消化系统疾病。

libido *noun* (**a**) sexual urge 性欲; **loss of libido** = loss of sexual urge 性欲丧失 (**b**) (*in psychology*) force which drives the unconscious mind, used especially referring to the sexual urge 欲望(精神病学),常指性欲

lice 虱 *see* 见 LOUSE

licence *or US* **license** *noun* official document which allows someone to do something (such as allowing a doctor to practise, a pharmacist to make and sell drugs or, in the USA, allowing a nurse to practise) 执照: ***He was practising as a doctor without a licence.*** 他无照行医。***She is sitting her registered nurse license examination.*** 她在参加注册护士执照考试。

◇ **license** *verb* to give someone a licence to do something 发执照: ***He is licensed to sell dangerous drugs.*** 他有销售危险药品的执照。

◇ **licentiate** *noun* person who has been given a licence to practise as a doctor 持照医生

◇ **licensure** *noun US* act of licensing a nurse to practise nursing 发给护士营业执照

lichen *noun* type of skin disease with thick skin and small lesions 苔藓,皮肤增厚和小皮损; **lichen planus** = skin disease where itchy purple spots appear on the arms and thighs 扁平苔藓,手臂和大腿上出现痒性紫癜

◇ **lichenification** *noun* thickening of the skin at the site of a lesion 苔藓化,病损处皮肤变厚

◇ **lichenoid** *adjective* like a lichen 苔藓样的

lick *verb* to make the tongue move over something to taste it *or* to wet it 舔

lid *noun* top which covers a container 盖子: ***Put the lid back on the jar.*** 把盖子盖回罐上。***A medicine bottle with a child-proof lid.*** 药瓶有防儿童打开的盖子。

lie 1 *noun* way in which a fetus is present in the womb 胎位; **longitudinal lie** = normal position of the fetus lying along the axis of the mother's body 纵位,正常胎位与母体长轴一致; **transverse lie** = position of the fetus across the body of the mother 横位 **2** *verb* to be in a flat position 平躺: ***The accident victim was lying on the pavement.*** 事故的受害者躺在人行道上。***Make sure the patient lies still and does not move.*** 保证患者躺着不动。(NOTE: **lies - lying - lay - has lain**)

◇ **lie down** *verb* to put yourself in a flat position 躺下: ***She lay down on the***

floor** or **on the bed**.* 她躺在地板(床)上。The doctor asked him to lie down on the couch**.* 医生让他躺在诊床上。***When I was lying down he asked me to lift my legs in the air**.* 我躺下后他让我把腿抬到空中。

Lieberkühn's glands *or* **crypts of Lieberkühn** *noun* tubular glands found in the mucous membrane of the small and large intestine, especially those between the bases of the villi in the small intestine 利贝昆氏腺,位于大小肠粘膜的管状腺体,尤其是小肠绒毛基底处

lientery *or* **lienteric diarrhoea** *noun* form of diarrhoea where the food passes through the intestine rapidly without being digested 消化不良性腹泻

life *noun* being alive *or* not being dead 生命: ***The surgeons saved the patient's life**.* 外科医师挽救了患者的生命。***His life is in danger because the drugs are not available**.* 因为没有药物,他的生命很危险。***The victim showed no sign of life**.* 受害者没有生命体征。**life expectancy** = number of years a person of a certain age is likely to live 预期寿命; **life insurance** = insurance against death 人寿保险; **life-threatening disease** = disease which may kill the patient 威胁生命的疾病

◇ **lifebelt** *noun* large ring which helps a person to float in water 救生圈

◇ **life-saving equipment** *noun* equipment (such as boats *or* stretchers *or* first-aid kit) kept ready in case of an emergency 救生设备

lift **1** *noun* (**a**) machine which takes people from one floor to another in a tall building 电梯 (**b**) way of carrying an injured person 救护法; **fireman's lift** = way of carrying an unconscious person on the shoulders of one carrier with the carrier's right arm passing between or around the patient's legs and holding the patient's right hand, allowing the carrier's left hand to remain free 消防员救护法,将昏迷者扛在肩上,右臂绕过或从患者的两腿之间穿过抓住其右手,救护者的左手空置; **shoulder lift** = way of carrying a heavy person, where the upper part of his body rests on the shoulders of two carriers 肩扛法,搬运重患者时,将其上部放于两位救护者的肩上 **2** *verb* to raise to a higher position 提升; to pick something up 捡起: ***This box is so heavy he can't lift it off the floor**.* 盒子太沉了,他提不起来。***She hurt her back lifting a box down from the shelf**.* 她把盒子从书架上搬下来时伤了背。

ligament *noun* thick band of fibrous tissue which connects the bones at a joint and forms the joint capsule 韧带 *see also* 参见 BROAD, EXTRINSIC, INTRINSIC, ROUND, SACRO UTERINE

ligate *verb* to tie with a ligature, as to tie a blood vessel to stop bleeding 结扎

◇ **ligation** *noun* surgical operation to tie up a blood vessel 结扎术

◇ **ligature** *noun* thread used to tie vessels or a lumen, such as a blood vessel to stop bleeding 结扎线

light **1** *adjective* (**a**) not heavy 轻的: ***She can carry this box easily — it's quite light**.* 她很容易就搬走了盒子——它相当轻。***He's not fit, so he can only do light work**.* 他身体不好,只能做一些轻松的工作。(**b**) bright so that one can see well 亮的: ***At six o'clock in the morning it was just getting light**.* 早晨6点,天刚亮。(**c**) (hair *or* skin) which is nearer white in colour rather than dark 浅色的: ***She has a very light complexion**.* 她的肤色白皙。***He has light coloured hair**.* 他的头发颜色很浅。(NOTE: **light - lighter - lightest**) **2** *noun* (**a**) thing which shines and helps one to see 光线: ***The light of the sun makes plants green**.* 阳光使植物变绿。***There's not enough light in here to take a photo**.* 在这里拍照光线不足。**light adaptation** = changes in the eye to adapt to an abnormally bright or dim light *or* to adapt to normal light after being in darkness 明适应,眼睛从暗环境下到亮处时发生的改变; **light reflex** = reflex of the pupil of the eye which contracts when exposed to bright light 光反射,光线刺激时瞳孔收缩; **light therapy** *or* **light treatment** = treatment of a disorder by exposing the patient to light (sunlight *or* infrared light, etc.) 光疗,用日光和红外线进行治疗; **light waves** = waves travelling in all directions from a source of light which stimulate the retina and are visible 光线 (**b**) object (usually a glass bulb) which gives out light 灯: ***Switch on the lights — it's getting dark.*** 把灯打开,天黑了。***The car was travelling with no lights.*** 汽车行驶时没有开灯。***The endoscope has a small light at the end.*** 内镜的末端有一小灯。

◇ **lighting** *noun* way of giving light 光线: ***The lighting in the operating theatre has to be very good.*** 手术室的照明很好。

◇ **lightly** *adverb* without using much pressure 轻轻的: ***The doctor pressed lightly round the swollen area with the tips of his fingers.*** 医生用手指轻压肿胀部位的边缘。

lightening *noun* late stage in pregnancy where the fetus goes down into the pelvic cavity 孕腹轻松,妊娠末期,胎儿进入盆腔时的轻松感

lightning pains *plural noun* sharp pains in the legs in a patient suffering from locomotor ataxia 闪电样痛,运动性共济失调患者腿部的剧痛

lignocaine *or US* **lidocaine** *noun* drug used as a local anaesthetic 利多卡因(局麻药)

limb *noun* one of the legs or arms 四肢之一; **lower limbs** = legs 下肢; **upper limbs** = arms 上肢; **limb lead** = electrode attached to an arm *or* leg when taking an electrocardiogram 肢导联,做心电图时连于上下肢的电极

◇ **limbless** *adjective* lacking one or more limbs 无肢的; ***a limbless ex-soldier*** 无肢的退伍军人

limbic system *noun* system of nerves in the brain, including the hippocampus, the amygdala and the hypothalamus, which are associated with emotions such as fear and anger 边缘系统,脑内的神经系统,包括海马、松果体和下丘脑,与恐惧、愤怒等情感有关

limbus *noun* edge, especially the edge of the cornea where it joins the sclera 缘,角膜缘 (NOTE: plural is **limbi**)

liminal *adjective* (stimulus) at the lowest level which can be sensed 下阈的

limit 1 *noun* furthest point *or* place beyond which you cannot go 界限: ***There is a speed limit of 30 miles per hour in towns.*** 镇上限速每小时30英里。***There is no age limit for joining the club.*** = People of all ages can join. 加入俱乐部没有年龄限制。***45 is the upper age limit for childbearing.*** = 45 is the oldest age at which a woman can have a child. 45岁是生育年龄的上限。**2** *verb* to set a limit to something 制定界限: ***You must limit your intake of coffee to two cups a day.*** 你必须将每天的咖啡摄入量限于两杯。

limp 1 *noun* way of walking awkwardly because of pain, stiffness *or* deformity in a leg or foot 跛足: ***He walks with a limp.*** 他走路一瘸一拐的。***The operation has left him with a limp.*** 手术使他留下了跛足的后遗症。**2** *verb* to walk awkwardly because of pain, stiffness *or* deformity in a leg or foot 跛行: ***He was still limping three weeks after the accident.*** 事故后3周他走路还一瘸一拐的。

linctus *noun* sweet cough medicine 舐膏剂

line 1 *noun* ridge *or* mark which connects two points 线 **2** *verb* to provide an inner coat to something 内衬; ***The intestine is lined with mucus.*** 肠壁覆有粘膜。***The inner ear is lined with fine hairs.*** 内耳覆有纤毛。

linea *noun* thin line 细线; **linea alba** = tendon running from the breastbone to the pubic area, to which abdominal muscles are attached 白线,从胸骨至耻骨区的肌腱,有腹肌附着; **linea nigra** = dark line on the skin from the navel to the pubis which appears during the later months of pregnancy 黑线,妊娠后期皮肤上从脐到耻骨的深色线

lingual *adjective* referring to the tongue 舌的; **lingual artery** = artery which supplies blood to the tongue 舌动脉; **lingual tonsil** = lymphoid tissue on the top surface of the back of the tongue 舌扁桃体 ◊ 见图 TONGUE; **lingual vein** = vein which takes blood from the tongue 舌静脉

liniment *noun* embrocation or oily liquid rubbed on the skin, which eases the pain *or* stiffness of a sprain *or* bruise by acting as a vasodilator *or* counterirritant 搽剂

lining *noun* substance *or* tissue on the inside of an organ 器官内面的组织,内衬; ***the thick lining of the aorta*** 主动脉内层

link *verb* to join things together 连接: ***The ankle bone links the bones of the lower leg to the calcaneus.*** 踝骨将下肢骨与跟骨相连。

◊ **linkage** *noun* (*of genes*) being close together on a chromosome, and therefore likely to be inherited together 联锁,基因在染色体上相邻很近,很可能一起遗传

linoleic acid *noun* one of the essential fatty acids which cannot be synthesized and has to be taken into the body from food (such as vegetable oil) 亚油酸,人体不能合成,必须从食物中摄取的必需脂肪酸之一

linolenic acid *noun* one of the essential fatty acids 亚麻酸

lint *noun* thick flat cotton wadding, used as a surgical dressing 绒布,用作手术敷料: ***She put some lint on the wound before bandaging it.*** 在包扎前她放了些绒布在伤口上。

liothyronine *noun* hormone produced by the thyroid gland which can be artificially synthesized for use as a rapid-acting treatment for hypothyroidism 三碘甲状腺氨酸,甲状腺分泌的激素,可人工合成用于快速治疗甲状腺功能减退

lip *noun* (i) one of two fleshy muscular parts round the edge of the mouth 口唇 (ii) flesh round the edge of an opening 唇: ***Her lips were cracked from the cold.*** 她的嘴唇因寒冷而皲裂。(NOTE: for terms referring to lips, see words beginning with **cheil-**, **lab-**, **labi**)

lipaemia *noun* excessive amount of fat (such as cholesterol) in the blood 高脂血症

lipase *noun* enzyme which breaks down fats in the intestine 脂酶

lipid *noun* fat *or* fatlike substance which exists in human tissue and forms an important part of the human diet 脂肪,脂质: **lipid metabolism** = chemical changes where lipids are broken down into fatty acids 脂代谢

> COMMENT: Lipids are not water soluble. They float in the blood and can attach themselves to the walls of arteries causing atherosclerosis.
> 注释:脂质不溶于水,他们漂浮在血液中,可沉积于动脉壁引起动脉硬化。

◊ **lipidosis** *noun* disorder of lipid metabolism, where subcutaneous fat is not present in some parts of the body 脂沉积症,脂代谢疾病,在身体的某些部位无皮下脂肪

◊ **lipochondrodystrophy** *noun* congenital disorder of the lipid metabolism, the bones and main organs, causing mental deficiency and physical deformity 脂肪软骨营养不良,脂代谢、骨和主要器官的先天性疾病,导致智力缺陷和身体畸形

◊ **lipodystrophy** *noun* disorder of lipid metabolism 脂肪营养不良,脂肪代谢障碍

◊ **lipogenesis** *noun* production *or* making deposits of fat 脂肪生成

◊ **lipoid** *noun & adjective* compound lipid *or* fatty substance (such as cholesterol) which is like a lipid 脂样的,脂类

◊ **lipoidosis** *noun* group of diseases with reticuloendothelial hyperplasia and abnormal deposits of lipoids in the cells 脂沉积症,网状内皮组织增生和脂质在细胞内异常沉积的一类疾病

◊ **lipolysis** *noun* process of breaking down fat by lipase 脂肪分解

◇ **lipolytic enzyme** = LIPASE 脂酶
◇ **lipoma** *noun* benign tumour formed of fatty tissue 脂肪瘤
◇ **lipomatosis** *noun* excessive deposit of fat in the tissues in tumour-like masses 脂肪过多症
lipoprotein *noun* protein which combines with lipids and carries them in the bloodstream and lymph system; lipoproteins are classified according to the percentage of protein which they carry 脂蛋白,结合脂质携带其在血液和淋巴系统流动的蛋白,脂蛋白根据携带蛋白的百分比分类; **high-density lipoproteins** (**HDLs**) = lipoproteins wich a lower percentage of cholesterol 高密度脂蛋白,胆固醇含量低; **low-density lipoproteins** (**LDLs**) = lipoproteins with a large percentage of cholesterol which deposit fats in muscles and arteries 低密度脂蛋白,携带有大量的胆固醇,可使脂肪沉积在肌肉和动脉
liposarcoma *noun* lipoma and sarcoma 脂肉瘤
◇ **lipotrophic** *adjective* (substance) which increases the amount of fat present in the tissues 脂肪增多的
Lippes loop *noun* type of intrauterine device 宫内节育器的一种
lipping *noun* condition where bone tissue grows over other bones 唇状突出
lipuria *noun* presence of fat *or* oily emulsion in the urine 脂肪尿
liquid *adjective* & *noun* matter (like water) which is not solid and is not a gas 液体(的): ***Sick patients need a lot of liquids***. 重病患者需要大量的液体。***He was put on a liquid diet***. 他吃流食。**liquid paraffin** = oil used as a laxative 液体石蜡
liquor *noun* (*in pharmacy*) solution, usually aqueous, of a pure substance 液体,溶液
lisp 1 *noun* speech defect where the patient has difficulty in pronouncing 's' sounds and replaces them with 'th' 咬舌音 **2** *verb* to talk with a lisp 咬舌发音
list 1 *noun* number of things written down one after the other 表,名单: ***There is a list of names in alphabetical order***. 有张以字母顺序排列的名单。***The names of duty nurses are on the list in the office***. 值班护士的名字列在办公室的名单上。***He's on the danger list***. = He is critically ill. 他列在重病名单上,他病得很厉害。***She's off the danger list***. = She is no longer critically ill 她被从重病名单上除名了,她的病情好转了。**2** *verb* to write something in the form of a list 列表,写名单: ***The drugs are listed at the back of the book***. 药物列表于书后。***The telephone numbers of the emergency services are listed in the Yellow Pages***. 急救服务的电话号码列于黄页上。
listen *verb* to pay attention to something heard 听诊: ***The doctor listened to the patient's chest***. 医生对患者的胸部进行听诊。
Listeria *noun* genus of bacteria found on domestic animals, which can cause uterine infection or meningitis 李斯特菌属
listless *adjective* weak and tired 虚弱的,疲乏的
◇ **listlessness** *noun* being generally weak and tired 虚弱,疲乏
lith- *prefix* meaning stone 石
◇ **lithaemia** *or* **uricacidaemia** *noun* abnormal amount of uric acid in the blood 尿酸盐血症
◇ **lithiasis** *noun* forming of stones in an organ 结石病
◇ **litholapaxy** *or* **lithotrity** *noun* evacuation of pieces of a stone in the bladder after crushing it with a lithotrite 碎石洗出术
◇ **lithonephrotomy** *noun* surgical removal of a stone in the kidney 肾石切除术
◇ **lithotomy** *noun* surgical removal of a stone from the bladder 膀胱结石取除术; **lithotomy position** = position of a patient for some medical examinations, where the patient lies on his back with his legs flexed and his thighs on his abdomen 截石位,患者仰卧腿屈曲,大腿贴于腹

部

◇ **lithotrite** *noun* surgical instrument which crushes a stone in the bladder 碎石器

◇ **lithotrity** = LITHOLAPAXY 碎石术

◇ **lithuresis** *noun* passage of small stones from the bladder during urination 石尿症

◇ **lithuria** *noun* presence of excessive amounts of uric acid *or* urates in the urine 尿酸盐尿

litmus *noun* substance which turns red in acid and blue in alkali 石蕊,酸性时变红,碱性时变蓝; **litmus paper** = small piece of paper impregnated with litmus, used to test for acidity *or* alkalinity 石蕊试纸,用于检测酸碱度

litre *US* **liter** *noun* unit of measurement of liquids (= 1. 76 pints) 升 (NOTE: with figures usually written **l** but it can be written in full to avoid confusion with the numeral **1**)

little *adjective* (**a**) small *or* not big 小的; **little finger** *or* **little toe** = smallest finger on the hand *or* smallest toe on the foot 小指(趾): ***He has a ring on his little finger.*** 他的小指戴有戒指。***Her little toe was crushed by the door.*** 她的小趾被门挤了。(**b**) not much 少的: ***She eats very little bread.*** 她吃了很少一点儿面包。

Little's area *noun* area of blood vessels in the nasal septum 李特尔氏区,鼻中隔上的血管区

◇ **Little's disease** = SPASTIC DIPLEGIA 李特尔氏病,痉挛性双侧瘫

live 1 *adjective* (**a**) living *or* not dead 活的: ***graft using live tissue*** 活体组织移植 (**b**) carrying electricity 带电的: ***He was killed when he touched a live wire.*** 他因碰上了带电的电线被电死了。**2** *verb* to be alive 活: ***He is very ill, and the doctor doesn't think he will live much longer.*** 他病得很厉害,医生认为他活不了多久了。

livedo *noun* discoloured spots on the skin 青斑

liver *noun* large gland in the upper part of the abdomen 肝: ***She has been suffering from liver trouble.*** 她患有肝病。***He has been having treatment for a liver infection.*** 他因为肝炎接受治疗。**liver extract** = food made from animal livers, used as an injection to treat anaemia 肝浸膏,动物肝脏提取物,用于治疗贫血。**liver fluke** = parasitic flatworm which can infest the liver 肝吸虫; **liver spot** = little brown spot on the skin 雀斑 ◇ 见图 DIGESTIVE SYSTEM (NOTE: for other terms referring to the liver, see words beginning with **hepat-**)

COMMENT: The liver is situated in the top part of the abdomen on the right side of the body next to the stomach. It is the largest gland in the body, weighing almost 2 kg. Blood carrying nutrients from the intestines enters the liver by the hepatic portal vein; the nutrients are removed and the blood returned to the heart through the hepatic vein. The liver is the major detoxicating organ in the body; it destroys harmful organisms in the blood, produces clotting agents, secretes bile, stores glycogen and metabolizes proteins, carbohydrates and fats. Diseases affecting the liver include hepatitis and cirrhosis; the symptom of liver disease is often jaundice.

注释:肝位于右上腹与胃相邻,它是体内最大的腺体,重约 2 千克。血液携带小肠吸收的营养从门静脉进入肝,营养被吸收后,血液由肝静脉流回心脏。肝是体内重要的解毒器官,它可破坏血中的毒性有机物,产生凝血因子,分泌胆汁,储存糖原,分解蛋白、碳水化合物和脂肪。肝脏疾病包括肝炎、肝硬化,肝病的常见症状是黄疸。

livid *adjective* (skin) with a blue colour because of being bruised *or* because of asphyxiation 青紫的

Loa loa *noun* tropical threadworm which digs under the skin, especially around and into the eye, causing loa loa and loiasis 罗阿丝虫,眼丝虫

◇ **loa loa** *noun* tropical disease of the

eye caused when the threadworm *Loa loa enters the eye or* the skin around the eye 罗阿丝虫病,眼丝虫病,眼丝虫进入眼或眼周围的皮肤引起的热带疾病

lobar *adjective* referring to a lobe 叶的; **lobar bronchi** *or* **secondary bronchi** = air passages supplying a lobe of a lung 肺叶支气管,二级支气管; **lobar pneumonia** = infection in one or more lobes of the lung 大叶性肺炎

◇ **lobe** *noun* (i) rounded section of an organ, such as the brain *or* lung *or* liver(脑、肺、肝)叶 (ii) soft fleshy part at the bottom of the ear 耳垂(iii) cusp on the crown of a tooth 牙尖; **frontal lobe** = front lobe of each cerebral hemisphere 额叶; **occipital lobe** = lobe at the back of each cerebral hemisphere 枕叶; **parietal lobe** = lobe at the side and to the top of each cerebral hemisphere 顶叶; **prefrontal lobe** = part of the brain in the front part of each hemisphere, in front of the frontal lobe, which is concerned with memory and learning 额前叶,与记忆和学习有关; **temporal lobe** = lobe above the ear in each cerebral hemisphere 颞叶 ◊ 见图 LUNGS

◇ **lobectomy** *noun* surgical removal of one of the lobes of an organ such as the lung 叶切除术

◇ **lobotomy** *noun* formerly, surgical operation to treat mental disease by cutting into a lobe of the brain to cut the nerve fibres 叶切断术,以前通过切断脑叶的神经纤维治疗精神病变 *see* 见 LEUCOTOMY

lobule *noun* small section of a lobe in the lung, formed of acini 小叶

local *adjective* referring to a separate place; confined to one part 局限的,局部的; **local anaesthesia** = loss of feeling in a single part of the body 局麻; **local anaesthetic** *or* **a local** = anaesthetic which removes the feeling in a certain part of the body only 局麻药: ***He had a local for the operation for an ingrowing toenail.*** 他在局麻下接受了内生甲手术治疗。***The surgeon removed the growth under local anaesthetic.*** 术者在局麻下切除了肿物。

◇ **localize** *verb* to locate something *or* to find where something is; to restrict the spread of something to a particular area 局限,集中

◇ **localized** *adjective* (infection) which occurs in one part of the body only 局限的(NOTE: the opposite is **generalized**)

locate *verb* (i) to find where something is 定位 (ii) to situate *or* to be situated in a place 位于

QUOTE: These patients may be candidates for embolization of their bleeding point, particularly as angiography will often be necessary to localize that point.
引文:这些患者可接受出血部位的栓塞治疗,特别是需血管造影明确出血部位的患者。
British Medical Journal 英国医学杂志

QUOTE: Few parts of the body are inaccessible to modern catheter techniques, which are all performed under local anaesthesia.
引文:现代导管技术在局麻下可达机体的任何部位。
British Medical Journal 英国医学杂志

QUOTE: Ultrasonography is helpful in determining sites of incompetence and in locating the course of veins in more obese patients.
引文:超声检查对明确过度肥胖患者功能不全的部位和静脉走行很有帮助。
British Journal of Hospital Medicine 英国医院医学杂志

QUOTE: The target cells for adult myeloid leukaemia are located in the bone marrow, and there is now evidence that childhood leukaemias also arise in the bone marrow.
引文:成人髓性白血病的靶细胞位于骨髓,现有证据表明儿童白血病也起源于骨髓。
British Medical Journal 英国医学杂志

lochia *noun* discharge from the vagina after childbirth or abortion 恶露，分娩或流产后的阴道排泄物

◇ **lochial** *adjective* referring to lochia 恶露的

lock *verb* (**a**) to close a door *or* box, etc. so that it has to be opened with a key 锁：***The drugs have to be kept in a locked cupboard.*** 药品应保存在上锁的柜子里。(**b**) to fix in a position 卡住，绞锁；**locked knee** = displaced piece of cartilage of the knee *or* condition where a piece of the cartilage in the knee slips (the symptom is a sharp pain, and the knee remains permanently bent) 膝闭锁，关节软骨错位或软骨位于关节内（症状为剧痛和膝关节持久性弯曲）；**locking of the knee** = condition where the knee joint suddenly becomes rigid 膝关节绞锁，膝关节突然强直

◇ **lockjaw** = TETANUS 破伤风

locomotion *noun* being able to move 运动

◇ **locomotor ataxia** = TABES DORSALIS 运动性共济失调

loculus *noun* small space (in an organ) 小腔

◇ **locum (tenens)** *noun* doctor who takes the place of another doctor for a time 代理医生

◇ **locus** *noun* area *or* point (of infection *or* disease) (感染、疾病) 部位；position on a chromosome where a gene is present 位点

lodge *verb* to stay *or* to stick 停留，粘附：***The piece of bone lodged in her throat.*** 一块骨头卡在了她的喉咙里。***The larvae of the tapeworm lodge in the walls of the intestine.*** 绦虫的蚴虫定居于肠壁。

logrolling *noun* method of moving a patient who is lying down into another position 滚动法，使平卧的患者改变体位的一种方法

loiasis *noun* tropical disease of the eye caused when the threadworm *Loa loa* enters the eye *or* the skin around the eye 罗阿丝虫病，眼丝虫病

loin *noun* lower back part of the body above the buttocks 腰部

long-acting *adjective* (drug *or* treatment) which has an effect that lasts a long time 长效的

longitudinal *adjective* lengthwise *or* in the direction of the long axis of the body 纵轴；**longitudinal arch** = part of the sole of the foot which curves upwards, running along the length of the foot from the heel to the ball of the foot 纵弓，从足跟到足掌的纵行突起

longsighted *adjective* able to see clearly things which are far away, but not things which are close 远视的

◇ **longsightedness** = HYPERMETROPIA 远视

◇ **long-stay** *adjective* staying a long time in hospital 长期住院的：***patients in long-stay units*** *or* ***long-stay patients*** 长期住院的患者

longus 长的 *see* 见 MUSCLE

look after *verb* to take care of *or* to attend to the needs of (a patient) 照顾：***The nurses looked after him very well*** *or* ***he was very well looked after in hospital.*** 护士对他照顾得很好。***She is off work looking after her children who have mumps.*** 她请假照顾患腮腺炎的孩子。***Some patients need a lot of looking after.*** = They need continual attention. 一些患者需要不断的照顾。

loop *noun* (**a**) curve *or* bend in a line, especially one of the particular curves in a fingerprint 袢；**loop of Henle** = curved tube which forms the main part of a nephron in the kidney 亨利袢，形成肾小体主要部分的弯曲的管道；**blind loop syndrome** *or* **stagnant loop syndrome** = condition which occurs in cases of diverticulosis or of Crohn's disease, with steatorrhoea, abdominal pain and megaloblastic anaemia 盲袢综合征，憩室炎或克隆氏病引起，伴有脂肪痢、腹痛和巨幼细胞性贫血 (**b**) curved piece of wire placed in the uterus to prevent contraception 宫内环，避孕工具

loose *adjective* not fixed *or* not attached *or* not tight 宽松的，不固定的：*One of my molars has come loose.* 我的一颗磨牙松动了。(NOTE：**loose - looser - loosest**)

◇ **loosely** *adverb* not tightly 宽松地：*The bandage was loosely tied round her wrist.* 绷带松宽地缠在她腕部。

◇ **loosen** *verb* to make loose 使松驰：*Loosen the tie round the victim's neck.* 放松遇害者颈部的领带。

lordosis *noun* excessive forward curvature of the lower part of the spine 脊柱前凸 *see also* 参见 KYPHOSIS

◇ **lordotic** *adjective* referring to lordosis 脊柱前凸的

lose *verb* not to have something any longer 丢失，丧失：*He lost the ability to walk.* 他丧失了行走的能力。*When you have a cold you can easily lose all sense of smell and taste.* 感冒时，你可以丧失所有的嗅觉和味觉。*She has lost weight since last summer.* = She has got thinner. 她从上个夏天起，体重就开始减轻。(NOTE：**loses - losing - lost - has lost**)

loss *noun* not having something any more 丢失，丧失；**loss of appetite** = not having as much appetite as before 丧失食欲；**loss of sensation** = not being able to feel the limbs any more 感觉丧失；**loss of weight** *or* **weight loss** = not weighing as much as before 体重减轻

lotion *noun* medicinal liquid used to rub on the skin *or* to use on the body 洗剂：*He bathed his eyes in a mild antiseptic lotion.* 他用温和的抗菌洗剂洗眼。*Use this lotion on your eczema.* 用这洗剂治疗你的湿疹。

louse *noun* small insect of the *Pediculus* genus, which sucks blood and lives on the skin as a parasite on animals and humans 虱 (NOTE：plural is **lice**)

> COMMENT：There are several forms of louse：the commonest are the body louse, the crab louse and the head louse and some diseases can be transmitted by lice.
> 注释：有几种类型的虱子：最常见的是体虱、阴虱和头虱，有些疾病是由虱子传播的。

low *adjective & adverb* near the bottom *or* towards the bottom 底部的；not high 不高：*He hit his head on the low ceiling.* 他头碰在了低矮的顶棚上。*The temperature is too low here for oranges to grow.* 这儿的温度对橘子生长来说太低了。**low blood pressure** *or* **hypotension** = condition where the pressure of the blood is abnormally low 低血压；**low-calorie diet** = diet with few calories (to help a person to lose weight) 低卡路里膳食(有助于减肥)；**low-fat diet** = diet with little animal fat which can help reduce the risk of heart disease and alleviate some skin conditions 低脂膳食，可减低发生心脏病的危险性，改善一些皮肤病；**low-risk patient** = patient not likely to catch a certain disease 低危人群，不易得某种疾病的人；**low-salt diet** = diet with little salt which has been shown to help reduce high blood pressure 低盐膳食，有助于降低高血压 *see also* 参见 NEURONE (NOTE：**low - lower - lowest.** Note also that the opposite of **low** is **high**)

◇ **lower 1** *adjective* further down 更低的；**lower jaw** = bottom jaw 下颌；**lower limbs** = legs 下肢 (NOTE：the opposite of **lower** is **upper**) **2** *verb* to make something go down 使下降；to reduce 减少：*They covered the patient with wet cloth to try to lower his body temperature.* 他们用湿敷料盖住患者以降低体温。

lozenge *noun* sweet medicinal tablet 糖剂，糖锭：*She was sucking a cough lozenge.* 她在喝咳嗽糖浆。

LPN *US* = LICENSED PRACTICAL NURSE 执照开业护士

LRCP = LICENTIATE OF THE ROYAL COLLEGE OF PHYSICIANS 皇家内科学会领照者

LSD *or* **lysergic acid diethylamide** *noun* powerful hallucinogenic drug 麦角二乙胺，强力的致幻药

lubb-dupp *noun* two sounds made by the heart, which represent each cardiac cycle when heard through a stethoscope 第一、二心音

lubricate *verb* to make smooth with oil *or* liquid 润滑

◇ **lubricant** *noun* fluid which lubricates 润滑剂

lucid *adjective* with a clearly working mind 清醒的: ***In spite of the pain, he was still lucid.*** 尽管疼痛,他仍然很清醒。

lucidum 透明的,清醒的 *see* 见 STRATUM

Ludwig's angina *noun* cellulitis of the mouth and some parts of the neck which causes the neck to swell and may obstruct the airway 路德维希氏咽峡炎,口腔和颈部的蜂窝织炎,导致颈部肿胀,可以阻塞呼吸道

lues *noun* former name for syphilis *or* the plague 瘟疫,梅毒

lumbago *noun* pain in the lower back 腰痛: ***She has been suffering from lumbago for years.*** 她腰痛已经好几年了。***He has had an attack of lumbago.*** 他腰痛发作了。

> COMMENT: Mainly due to rheumatism, but can be brought on by straining the back muscles, lesions of the intervertebral discs or bad posture.
> 注释:主要是因为风湿病,但也可因腰肌扭伤、椎间盘病变或不良的姿势引起。

lumbar *adjective* referring to the lower part of the back 腰的; **lumbar arteries** = five arteries altogether, which supply blood to the back muscles and skin 腰动脉,共有5条动脉,供应背部肌肉和皮肤的血液; **lumbar cistern** = subarachnoid space in the spinal cord, where the dura mater ends, filled with cerebrospinal fluid 腰池,脊索硬脑膜终止处的蛛网膜下腔,充满了脑脊液; **lumbar enlargement** = wider part of the spinal cord in the lower spine, where the nerves of the lower limbs are attached 腰膨大,脊索下部膨大处,下肢神经附着于此; **lumbar plexus** = point where several nerves which supply the thighs and abdomen join together, lying in the upper psoas muscle 腰丛,腰大肌上方支配大腿和腹部的神经交汇处; **lumbar puncture** 腰穿 *see* 见 PUNCTURE; **lumbar region** = two parts of the abdomen on either side of the umbilical region 腰区,脐区两侧的腹部; **lumbar vertebrae** = five vertebrae between the thoracic vertebrae and the sacrum 腰椎,位于胸椎和骶椎之间

lumbosacral *adjective* referring to the lumbar vertebrae and the sacrum 腰骶椎的; **lumbosacral joint** = joint at the bottom of the back between the lumbar vertebrae and the sacrum 腰骶关节

lumbricus *noun* earthworm 蚯蚓,蛔虫

lumen *noun* (**a**) SI unit of light emitted per second 流明,光的国际单位 (**b**) (i) inside width of a passage in the body *or* of an instrument(such as an endoscope) 腔 (ii) hole at the end of an instrument (such as an endoscope)孔

lump *noun* mass of hard tissue which rises on the surface *or* under the surface of the skin 肿块: ***He has a lump where he hit his head on the low door.*** 他头撞到矮门上后起了个包。***She noticed a lump in her right breast and went to see the doctor.*** 她在右乳摸到了个肿块,去看医生。

lunate (bone) *noun* one of the eight small carpal bones in the wrist 月状骨 ◇ 见图 HAND

lung *noun* one of two organs of respiration in the body into which air is sucked when a person breathes 肺: ***The doctor listened to his chest to see if his lungs were all right.*** 医生对他的胸部进行听诊,看肺是否有病。**lung cancer** = cancer in the lung 肺癌; **lung trouble** = disorder in the lung, such as bronchitis *or* pneumonia, etc. 肺病; **artificial lung** = machine through which the patient's deoxygenated blood is passed to absorb oxygen to take back to the bloodstream 人工肺,进行血液气体交换,吸收氧的仪器; **farmer's lung** = type of asthma caused by an allergy to rotting hay 农民肺,对腐烂的干草过敏引起的哮喘; **shock lung** = serious condition after a blow, where the patient's lungs fail to work 休克肺 (NOTE: for other terms referring to the lungs, see words beginning with **bronch-**, **pneumo-**, **pneumon-**, **pulmo-**, **pulmon-**)

COMMENT: The two lungs are situated in the chest cavity, protected by the ribcage. The heart lies between the lungs. The right lung has three lobes, the left lung only two. Air goes down into the lungs through the trachea and bronchi. It passes to the alveoli where its oxygen is deposited in the blood in exchange for waste carbon dioxide which is exhaled (gas exchange). Lung cancer can be caused by smoking tobacco, and is commonest in people who are heavy smokers.
注释:肺位于胸腔,有肋骨保护,心脏在两肺之间。右肺分为3叶,左肺有2叶。空气通过气管、支气管进入肺,在肺泡进行气体交换,氧气入血,二氧化碳被排出。吸烟可以引起肺癌,在抽烟很凶的人中最常见。

lunula *noun* curved white mark at the base of a fingernail 弧影,指甲基底部弧形的白色标志

lupus *noun* type of chronic skin disease 狼疮; **lupus erythematosus acutus** (**LE**) = one of several collagen diseases, a form of lupus, involving the heart and blood vessels 急性红斑狼疮,胶原病之一,侵及心血管; **lupus vulgaris** = form of tuberculosis of the skin, where red spots appear on the face and become infected 寻常狼疮,皮肤的结核病,表现为面部的红色斑点,可传染 *see also* 参见 DISSEMINATED, SYSTEMIC

lutein *noun* yellow pigment in the corpus luteum 黄体素; **luteinizing hormone** (**LH**) *or* **interstitial cell stimulating hormone** = hormone produced by the pituitary gland, which stimulates the formation of the corpus luteum in females and of testosterone in males 黄体生成激素,垂体分泌,刺激女性黄体形成和男性睾酮分泌的激素

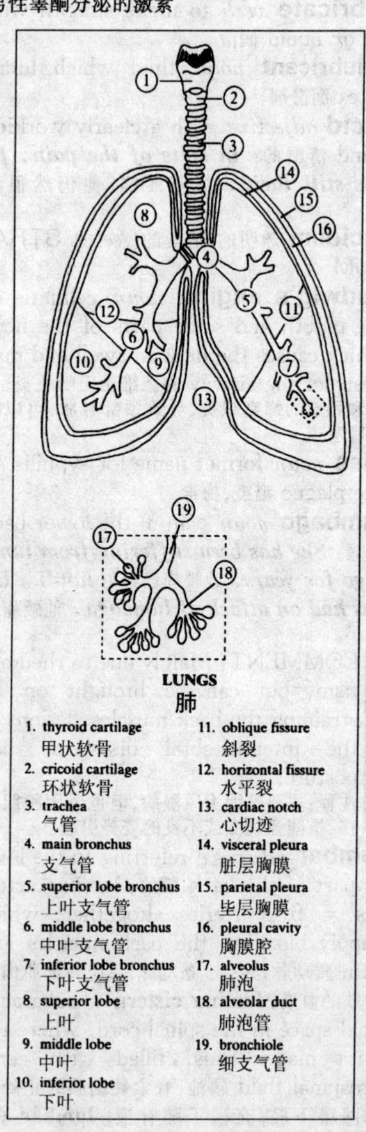

LUNGS
肺

1. thyroid cartilage 甲状软骨
2. cricoid cartilage 环状软骨
3. trachea 气管
4. main bronchus 支气管
5. superior lobe bronchus 上叶支气管
6. middle lobe bronchus 中叶支气管
7. inferior lobe bronchus 下叶支气管
8. superior lobe 上叶
9. middle lobe 中叶
10. inferior lobe 下叶
11. oblique fissure 斜裂
12. horizontal fissure 水平裂
13. cardiac notch 心切迹
14. visceral pleura 脏层胸膜
15. parietal pleura 壁层胸膜
16. pleural cavity 胸膜腔
17. alveolus 肺泡
18. alveolar duct 肺泡管
19. bronchiole 细支气管

◇ **luteum** *noun* **corpus luteum** 黄体 *see* 见 CORPUS, MACULA LUTEA

lux *noun* SI unit of brightness of light shining on a surface 勒克司,光亮的国际单位

luxation *noun* dislocation, a condition where a bone is displaced from its normal position 脱位

Lyme disease *noun* viral disease transmitted by bites from deer ticks (*Borrelia burgdorferi*). It causes rashes, nervous pains, paralysis and, in extreme cases, death 莱姆病,经鹿蜱叮咬传播的病毒性疾病,可引起皮疹、神经痛、瘫痪,严重时可致死

lymph (fluid) *noun* colourless liquid containing white blood cells, which circulates in the lymph system from all body tissues, carrying waste matter away from tissues to the veins 淋巴液,含有白细胞的无色液体,在全身组织的淋巴系统循环,将废物带回静脉; **lymph duct** = any channel carrying lymph 淋巴管; **lymph nodes** *or* **lymph glands** = collections of lymphoid tissue situated in various points of the lymphatic system (especially under the armpits and in the groin) through which lymph passes and in which lymphocytes are produced 淋巴结,淋巴系统的淋巴组织集中区,有淋巴通过并产生淋巴细胞,腋窝和腹股沟多见; **lymph vessels** = tubes which carry lymph round the body from the tissues to the veins 淋巴管

COMMENT: Lymph drains from the tissues through capillaries into lymph vessels. It is formed of water, protein and white blood cells (lymphocytes). Waste matter (such as infection) in the lymph is filtered out and destroyed as it passes through the lymph nodes, which then add further lymphocytes to the lymph before it continues in the system. It eventually drains into the brachiocephalic (innominate) veins, and joins the venous bloodstream. Lymph is not pumped round the body like blood but moves by muscle pressure on the lymph vessels and by the negative pressure of the large veins into which the vessels empty. Lymph is an essential part of the body's defence against infection.
注释:淋巴液经毛细血管从组织流入淋巴管,淋巴液由水、蛋白和白细胞(淋巴细胞)组成。淋巴液中的废物(如感染物)在经过淋巴结时被破坏、过滤掉,并有新的淋巴细胞加入。最终回流到头臂静脉,进入静脉血流。淋巴液不像血液是由泵推动在全身流动的,而是通过肌肉加在淋巴管壁上的压力和大静脉排空时产生的负压流动。淋巴液是机体抵抗感染的重要组成部分。

◇ **lymphadenectomy** *noun* surgical removal of a lymph node 淋巴结切除术

◇ **lymphadenitis** *noun* inflammation of the lymph nodes 淋巴结炎

◇ **lymphadenoma** *noun* hypertrophy of a lymph node 淋巴结增生,淋巴瘤

◇ **lymphadenopathy** *noun* any condition of the lymph nodes 淋巴结病

◇ **lymphangiectasis** *noun* swelling of the smaller lymph vessels as a result of obstructions in larger vessels 淋巴管扩张

◇ **lymphangiography** *noun* X-ray examination of the lymph vessels following introduction of radio-opaque material 淋巴管造影术

◇ **lymphangioma** *noun* tumour formed of lymph tissues 淋巴管瘤

◇ **lymphangioplasty** *noun* surgical operation to make artificial lymph channels 淋巴管成形术

◇ **lymphangiosarcoma** *noun* malignant tumour of the endothelial cells lining the lymph vessels 淋巴管肉瘤

◇ **lymphangitis** *noun* inflammation of the lymph vessels 淋巴管炎

◇ **lymphatic 1** *adjective* referring to lymph 淋巴的; **lymphatic capillaries** = capillaries which lead from tissue and join lymphatic vessels 淋巴毛细管; **lymphatic duct** = main channel for carrying lymph 淋巴管; **right lymphatic duct** = one of the main terminal channels for carrying lymph, draining the right side of the head and neck and entering the junction of the right subclavian and internal jugular veins. It is the smaller of the two main discharge points of the lymphatic system into the venous system, the larger being the thoracic duct 右淋巴管,终末淋巴管之一,收集头、颈右侧的淋巴液进入右锁骨下静脉和颈内静脉汇合处。它是较小的一条终末淋巴管,更大的一条是胸导管; **lymphatic nodes** *or* **lymphatic glands** = glands situated in various points of the lymphatic system, especially under the armpits and in the groin where they produce lymphocytes 淋巴结; **lymphatic nodule** = small lymph node found in clusters in tissues 淋巴小结; **lymphatic system** = series of vessels which transport lymph from the tissues through the lymph nodes and into the bloodstream 淋巴系统; **lymphatic vessel** = tube which carries lymph round the body from the tissue to the veins 淋巴管 **2** *noun* **the lymphatics** = lymph vessels 淋巴管

◇ **lymphoblast** *noun* abnormal cell which forms in acute lymphatic leukaemia, a cell formed by the change which takes place in a lymphocyte on contact with an antigen 幼稚淋巴细胞,原始淋巴细胞

◇ **lymphoblastic** *adjective* referring to lymphoblasts *or* forming lymphocytes 幼稚淋巴细胞的,淋巴母细胞的

◇ **lymphocyte** *noun* type of mature leucocyte *or* white blood cell formed by the lymph nodes, and concerned with the production of antibodies 淋巴细胞,淋巴结产生的一种成熟白细胞,可产生抗体; **T-lymphocyte** = lymphocyte formed in the thymus gland T 淋巴细胞,由胸腺产生

◇ **lymphocytosis** *noun* increased number of lymphocytes in the blood 淋巴细胞增多症

◇ **lymphoedema** *or US* **lymphedema** *noun* swelling caused by obstruction of the lymph vessels or abnormalities in the development of lymph vessels 淋巴水肿

◇ **lymphogranuloma inguinale** *or* **lymphogranuloma venereum** (**l.g.v.**) *noun* venereal disease which causes a swelling of the lymph glands in the groin, occurring in tropical countries 腹股沟淋巴肉芽肿,热带国家的一种性病,有腹股沟淋巴结肿大

◇ **lymphography** *noun* making images of the lymphatic system, after having introduced a radio-opaque substance 淋巴系统造影术

◇ **lymphoid tissue** *noun* tissue in the lymph nodes, the tonsils and the spleen where masses of lymphocytes are supported by a network of reticular fibres and cells 淋巴样组织,淋巴结、扁桃体和脾,大量的淋巴细胞被网状纤维和细胞构成的网架支撑

◇ **lymphoma** *noun* tumour arising from lymphoid tissue 淋巴瘤

◇ **lymphopenia** *or* **lymphocytopenia** *noun* reduction in the number of lymphocytes in the blood 淋巴细胞减少症

◇ **lymphopoiesis** *noun* production of lymphocytes *or* lymphoid tissue 淋巴细胞生成,淋巴组织生成

◇ **lymphorrhagia** *or* **lymphorrhoea** *noun* escape of lymph from ruptured *or* severed lymphatic vessels 淋巴溢

◇ **lymphosarcoma** *noun* malignant growth arising from lymphocytes and their cells of origin in the lymph nodes 淋巴肉瘤

◇ **lymphuria** *noun* presence of lymph in the urine 淋巴尿

lyophilize *verb* to preserve tissue *or* plasma *or* serum, etc. by freeze-drying in a vacuum 冻干

◇ **lyophilization** *noun* preserving tissue *or* plasma *or* serum, etc. by freeze-drying in a vacuum 冻干法

lysergic acid diethylamide (**LSD**) *noun* powerful hallucinogenic drug, used in the treatment of severe mental disorders 麦角二乙胺

lysin *noun* protein in the blood which destroys the cell against which it is directed *or* toxin which causes the lysis of cells 溶素 *see also* 参见 BACTERIOLYSIS, HAEMOLYSIN, LEUCOLYSIN

lysine *noun* essential amino acid 赖氨酸

lysis *noun* (**a**) destruction of a cell by a lysin, where the membrane of the cell is destroyed 溶解 (**b**) reduction in a fever *or* disease over a period of time 渐退,消散

COMMENT: In diseases such as typhoid fever, the patient's condition only improves gradually. The opposite where a patient gets rapidly better or worse, is called crisis. 注释:在副伤寒等疾病,患者的病情是逐渐改善的。相反的,如果患者的病情迅速好转或恶化则称为危象。

lysol *noun* strong disinfectant, made of cresol and soap 来苏儿,一种强力消毒剂,由甲酚和肥皂组成

lysosome *noun* particle in a cell which contains enzymes which break down substances (such as bacteria) which enter the cell 溶酶体,一种含有酶的细胞内小体,可降解进入细胞的物质(细菌)

lysozyme *noun* enzyme found in whites of eggs and in tears, and which destroys certain bacteria 溶菌酶,在蛋清和眼泪中发现的一种酶,可以破坏某些细菌

Mm

M *symbol for* mega- 表示大

m (**a**) = METRE 米 (**b**) *symbol for* milli-表示毫,千分之一

macerate *verb* to make something soft by letting it lie in a liquid for a time 浸渍,泡软

◊ **maceration** *noun* softening of a solid by letting it lie in a liquid so that the soluble matter dissolves 浸渍,泡软;**neonatal maceration** = softening *or* rotting of fetal tissue after the fetus has died in the womb and has remained in the amniotic fluid 死胎软化

Macmillan nurse *noun* nurse who specializes in cancer care, employed by the organization Macmillan Cancer Relief 麦克米伦护士(专门照顾癌症患者的护士)

macro- *prefix* meaning large 表示大 (NOTE: opposite is **micro-**)

macrobiotic *adjective* (food) which is healthy *or* which has been produced naturally without artificial additives *or* preservatives 健康食品(天然食品,没有人造添加剂或防腐剂)

> COMMENT: Macrobiotic diets are usually vegetarian and are prepared in a special way; they consist of beans, coarse flour, fruit and vegetables. They may not contain enough protein or trace elements, especially to satisfy the needs of children.
> 注释:健康饮食通常是由特殊方法调制的蔬菜类食品,由豆类、面粉、水果和蔬菜组成,所含蛋白质或微量元素往往不足,尤其不能满足儿童生长发育的需要。

◊ **macrocephaly** *noun* having an abnormally large head 巨头

◊ **macrocheilia** *noun* having large lips 巨唇

macrocyte *noun* abnormally large red blood cell found in patients suffering from pernicious anaemia 巨红细胞;

◊ **macrocytic** *adjective* referring to macrocytes 巨红细胞的;**macrocytic anaemia** = anaemia where the patient has abnormally large red blood cells 巨红细胞性贫血

◊ **macrocytosis** *or* **macrocythaemia** *noun* having macrocytes in the blood 巨红细胞血症

macrodactyly *noun* hypertrophy of the fingers *or* toes 巨指(趾)畸形;

◊ **macrogenitosoma** *noun* premature development of the body with the genitals being of an abnormally large size 巨大生殖器畸形

◊ **macroglobulin** *noun* immunoglobulin, a globulin protein of high molecular weight, which serves as an antibody 巨球蛋白

◊ **macroglossia** *noun* having an abnormally large tongue 巨舌畸形

◊ **macrognathia** *noun* condition in which the jaw is larger than normal 下颌肥大

◊ **macromastia** *noun* overdevelopment of breasts 巨乳症

◊ **macromelia** *noun* having abnormally large limbs 巨肢畸形

◊ **macrophage** *noun* any of several large cells, which destroy inflammatory tissue, found in connective tissue, wounds, lymph nodes and other parts 巨噬细胞

◊ **macropsia** *noun* seeing objects larger than they really are, caused by a defect in the retina 视物显大症

◊ **macroscopic** *adjective* which can be seen with the naked eye 裸眼可见的

macula *noun* (i) change in the colour of a small part of the body without changing the surface (as in freckles) 斑 (ii) area of hair cells inside the utricle and saccule of the ear 听斑;**macula lutea** = yellow spot on the retina, surrounding the fovea, the part of the eye which sees most clearly 黄斑 (NOTE: plural is **maculae**)

◊ **macular** *adjective* referring to a macula 斑的;**macular degeneration** =

eye disorder in elderly patients, where fluid leaks into the retina and destroys cones and rods, reducing central vision 黄斑变性; **macular oedema** = disorder of the eye where fluid gathers in the fovea 黄斑水肿

◇ **macule** *noun* small flat coloured spot on the skin 斑,斑点 (NOTE: a spot which is raised above the surface of the skin is a **papule**)

◇ **maculopapular** *adjective* (rash) made up of macules and papules 斑丘疹的

mad *adjective* (person) who is suffering from a mental disorder 发疯的,发狂的 (NOTE: not a medical term)

maduromycosis *or* **Madura foot** *or* **maduromycetoma** *noun* tropical fungus infection in the feet, which can destroy tissue and infect bones 马杜拉足分支菌病(足部的热带真菌感染,可破坏组织感染骨)

Magendie's foramen *noun* opening in the fourth ventricle of the brain which allows cerebrospinal fluid to flow 马让迪氏孔,第四脑室孔

magna 小脑延髓的 *see* 见 CISTERNA

magnesium *noun* chemical element found in green vegetables, which is essential especially for the correct functioning of muscles 镁; **magnesium sulphate** = Epsom salts, magnesium salt used as a laxative 硫酸镁(用于导泻); **magnesium trisilicate** = magnesium compound used to treat peptic ulcers 三矽酸镁(用于治疗消化性溃疡) (NOTE: chemical symbol is **Mg**)

◇ **Magnesia**苦土,氧化镁 *see* 见 MILK

magnetic *adjective* having the attraction of a magnet 有磁性的; **magnetic field** = area round a body which is under the influence of its attraction 磁场; **magnetic resonance imaging (MRI)** = scanning technique for examining soft body tissue and cells 磁共振成像 *see also* 参见 NUCLEAR MAGNETIC RESONANCE

> QUOTE: Magnetic Resonance Imaging scans produce more sensitive images than X-rays, so they are more useful in determining pathophysiology. Although MRI scans are similar to CT scans, they work differently.
> 引文:磁共振成像扫描能产生比X线扫描更精密的图像,因此在确定病理生理改变上更有帮助。虽然磁共振成像与CT扫描相似,但它们的工作原理是不同的。
> **Nursing 87 护理 87**

magnum 大,头状骨 *see* 见 FORAMEN

maidenhead *noun* hymen, the membrane which partially covers the vaginal passage in a virgin 处女膜

maim *verb* to incapacitate someone with a major injury 致残: ***The car crash maimed him for life.*** 车祸使他成为终生残疾。

maintain *verb* to keep up 维持,保持: ***The heart beats regularly to maintain the supply of oxygen to the tissues.*** 心脏有节律地跳动维系着组织的供氧。

major *adjective* greater *or* important *or* serious 大的,重要的,严重的: ***He had to undergo major surgery on his heart.*** 他不得不做心脏大手术。***The operation was a major one.*** 这是个大手术。**labia majora** = two large fleshy folds at the edge of the vulva 大阴唇 ◊ 见图 UROGENITAL SYSTEM (female) (NOTE: the opposite is **minor**)

mal *noun* illness *or* disease 疾病; **grand mal** = commonest form of epilepsy, where the patient loses consciousness and falls to the ground with convulsions; urinary incontinence is common 癫痫大发作; **petit mal** = less severe form of epilepsy, where loss of consciousness happens suddenly but lasts a few seconds only and the patient does not fall or urinate 癫痫小发作

mal- *prefix meaning bad or* abnormal 坏的,异常的

malabsorption *noun* defective absorption by the intestines of fluids and nutrients in food 吸收不良; **malabsorption syndrome** = group of symptoms and signs resulting from steatorrhoea and malabsorption of vitamins, protein, carbohydrates and water, including malnutrition, anaemia, oedema, dermatitis 吸收不良综合征

malacia *noun & suffix* pathological softening of an organ *or* tissue 软化,软化症

maladjusted *adjective* (child) who has difficulty fitting into society or family 适应不良的

malaise *noun* feeling of discomfort 不适

malaligned *adjective* (bone) which is not correctly aligned (骨)排列不齐

malar *adjective* referring to the cheek 颧的,颊的; **malar bone** = zygoma *or* zygomatic bone, the cheekbone which forms the prominent part of the cheek and the lower part of the eye socket 颧骨

malaria *noun* paludism, tropical disease caused by a parasite *Plasmodium* which enters the body after a bite from the female anopheles mosquito 疟疾

COMMENT: Malaria is a recurrent disease which produces regular periods of shivering, vomiting, sweating and headaches as the parasites develop in the body; the patient also develops anaemia.
注释:疟疾是一种反复发作的疾病,疟原虫在体内生长发育造成周期性的寒战、呕吐、出汗和头痛,病人还可以发生贫血。

◇ **malarial** *adjective* referring to malaria 疟疾的; **malarial parasite** = parasite transmitted into the human bloodstream by the bite of the female anopheles mosquito 疟原虫

◇ **malarious** *adjective* (region) where malaria is endemic 疟疾流行的

male *noun & adjective* referring to a man *or* of the same sex as a man 男子,男性的,雄性的; **male sex hormone** = testosterone, the hormone produced by the testes, which causes physical changes to take place in males as they become sexually mature 雄性激素; **male sex organs** = the testes, epididymis, vasa deferentia, seminal vesicles, ejaculatory ducts and penis 男性性器官

malformation *noun* abnormal development of a structure 畸形; **congenital malformation** = malformation (such as cleft palate) which is present at birth 先天畸形

◇ **malformed** *adjective* (part of the body) which has been badly formed 畸形的

malfunction 1 *noun* abnormal working of an organ 功能不良: ***His loss of consciousness was due to a malfunction of the kidneys** or **to a kidney malfunction.*** 他失去知觉是由于肾功能不良。2 *verb* to work badly 不能正常执行功能: ***During the operation his heart began to malfunction.*** 手术中他的心脏功能开始恶化。

malignant *adjective* threatening life *or* tending to cause death *or* virulent (tumour) 恶性的; **malignant hypertension** = dangerously high blood pressure 恶性高血压; **malignant melanoma** = dark tumour, which develops on the skin from a mole, caused by exposure to strong sunlight 恶性黑素瘤; **malignant tumour** = cancer, a tumour which is cancerous and can reappear or spread into other tissue, even if removed surgically 恶性肿瘤 (NOTE: the opposite is **benign** *or* **non-malignant**)

◇ **malignancy** *noun* state of being malignant 恶性: ***The tests confirmed the malignancy of the growth.*** 实验证实生长物是恶性的。

QUOTE: Without a functioning immune system to ward off germs, the patient now becomes vulnerable to becoming infected by bacteria, protozoa, fungi and other viruses and malignancies which may cause life-threatening illness.
引文:免疫系统失去了对微生物的屏蔽功能,目前患者易受细菌、原虫、真菌和其他病毒侵袭,并且易患威胁生命的其他恶性疾病。

Journal of the American Medical Association 美国医学会杂志

malingerer *noun* person who pretends to be ill 诈病者

◇ **malingering** *adjective* pretending to be ill 诈病的

malleolus *noun* one of two bony prominences at each side of the ankle 脚踝; **lateral malleolus** = part of the end of the fibula which protrudes on the outside of the ankle 外踝; **medial malleolus** = part of the end of the tibia which protrudes on the inside of the ankle 内踝 (NOTE: plural is **malleoli**)

◇ **malleolar** *adjective* referring to a malleolus 脚踝的

mallet finger *noun* finger which cannot be straightened because the tendon attaching the top joint has been torn 槌状指

malleus *noun* largest of the three ossicles in the middle ear, shaped like a hammer 锤骨 ◊ 见图 EAR

Mallory-Weiss tears *plural noun* tearing of the mucous membrane at the junction of the oesophagus and the stomach 马－魏氏撕裂(食管和胃交界处的粘膜撕裂)

Mallory's stain *noun* trichrome stain, used in histology to distinguish collagen, cytoplasm and nuclei 马洛里氏染色(一种三色组织学染色,用来区别胶原、胞浆和细胞核)

malnourished *adjective* (person) who does not have enough to eat 营养不良的

malnutrition *noun* (i) bad nutrition, as a result of starvation *or* wrong diet *or* bad absorption of food 营养不良 (ii) not having enough to eat 进食不足,饥饿状态

malocclusion *noun* condition where the teeth in the upper and lower jaws do not meet properly when the patient's mouth is closed 错位咬合,错殆 *see also* 参见 OCCLUSION

malodorous *adjective* with a strong unpleasant smell 有难闻气味的,有恶臭的

Malpighian body *or* **Malpighian corpuscle** *or* **renal corpuscle** 马耳皮基氏小体 *see* 见 CORPUSCLE

◇ **Malpighian glomerulus** *noun* expanded end of a renal tubule, surrounding a glomerular tuft 马耳皮基氏小球(肾小管膨大的远端,环绕肾小球血管袢)

◇ **Malpighian layer** *noun* deepest layer of the epidermis 马耳皮基氏层(上皮中最深的一层)

malposition *noun* wrong position (as of the fetus in the womb *or* of fractured bones) (胎异位或骨折)不正,错位

malpractice *noun* (i) acting in an unprofessional *or* illegal way 非专业行为,违法行为 (ii) wrong treatment of a patient (by a doctor *or* surgeon *or* dentist, etc.) for which the doctor may be tried in court 医疗差错,治疗失当: ***The surgeon was found guilty of malpractice.*** 这个外科医师犯治疗失当罪。

malpresentation *noun* abnormal presentation of the fetus in the womb 先露异常

Malta fever = BRUCELLOSIS 马耳他热(布氏杆菌病)

maltase *noun* enzyme in the small intestine which converts maltose into glucose 麦芽糖酶

◇ **maltose** *noun* sugar formed by digesting starch or glycogen 麦芽糖

malunion *noun* incorrect union of pieces of a broken bone (骨折)错位愈合

mamma *noun* the breast, one of two glands on the chest of a woman which secrete milk 乳房

◇ **mammal** *noun* type of animal (such as the human being) which gives birth to live young, secretes milk to feed them, keeps a constant body temperature and is covered with hair 哺乳动物

◇ **mammary** *adjective* referring to the breast 乳房的; **mammary gland** = gland in females which produces milk 乳腺

◇ **mamilla** *or* **mammilla** *noun* nipple, protruding part in the centre of the breast, containing the milk ducts through which the milk flows 乳头

◇ **mamillary** *or* **mammillary** *adjective* referring to the nipple 乳头的; **mamillary bodies** = two little projections on the base of the hypothalamus 乳头体(下丘脑基底部的两个小突起)

◇ **mammogram** *noun* picture of a breast made using soft-tissue radiography 乳腺 X 线片

◇ **mammography** *noun* examination of the breast, using a special X-ray technique 乳腺 X 线检查

◇ **mammoplasty** *noun* plastic surgery to reduce the size of the breasts 乳房成形术

◇ **mammothermography** *noun* thermography of a breast 乳腺拍(像)图检查

> QUOTE: Mammography is the most effective technique available for the detection of occult (non-palpable) breast cancer. It has been estimated that mammography can detect a carcinoma two years before it becomes palpable.
> 引文:乳腺 X 线检查是目前发现潜在(触摸不到的)乳腺癌最有效的技术。据估计,乳腺 X 线检查能在癌症病灶可摸到前两年就发现它。
> **Southern Medical Journal** 南部医学杂志

manage *verb* (**a**) to control; to be in charge of 处理,管理: ***She manages the ward very efficiently.*** 她把病房管理得井井有条。***We want to appoint someone to manage the group of hospitals.*** 我们想指派一个人来管理这些医院。***Bleeding can usually be managed, but sometimes an operation may be necessary.*** 出血一般是能止住的,但有时需要做手术。(**b**) to be able to do something; to succeed in doing something 能做,能做好: ***Did you manage to phone the doctor?*** 你能设法给医生打个电话吗? ***Can she manage at home all by herself?*** 她一个人在家行吗? ***How are we going to manage without the nursing staff?*** 没有护理人员我们怎么工作呢? ***I managed to get him back into bed.*** 我设法让他回到病床上去。

◇ **management** *noun* (i) organization *or* running (of a hospital *or* clinic *or* health authority, etc.) 管理 (ii) organization of a series of different treatments for a patient 组织、策划治疗方案

◇ **manager** *noun* person in charge of a department in the health service *or* person in charge of a group of hospitals 经理; **nurse manager** = nurse who has administrative duties in a hospital *or* the health service 护理部主任

mandible *noun* lower bone in the jaw 下颌骨 ◇ 见图 SKULL

> COMMENT: The jaw is formed of two bones, the mandible which is attached to the skull with a hinge joint and can move up and down, and the maxillae which are fixed parts of the skull.
> 注释:颌骨由两块骨头组成,下颌骨由铰链关节相连附着在颅骨上,并能上下活动,上颌骨则是颅骨上固着的一个部分。

◇ **mandibular** *adjective* referring to the lower jaw 下颌骨的; **mandibular fossae** = sockets in the skull into which the ends of the lower jaw fit 下颌凹; **mandibular nerve** = sensory nerve which supplies the teeth in the lower jaw, the temple, the floor of the mouth and the back part of the tongue 下颌神经

mane *Latin word meaning* 'during the daytime': used on prescriptions[拉丁语] 白天(处方用语) (NOTE: the opposite is **nocte**)

> QUOTE: He was diagnosed as having diabetes mellitus at age 14, and was successfully controlled on insulin 15 units mane and 10 units nocte.
> 引文:14 岁时他被诊断患糖尿病,采用胰岛素治疗,白天 15 个单位,夜间 10 个单位成功地控制了病情。
> **British Journal of Hospital Medicine** 英国医院医学杂志

manganese *noun* metallic trace element 锰 (NOTE: chemical symbol is **Mn**)

mania *noun* state of manic-depressive psychosis where the patient is in a state of excitement, very sure of his own abilities and has increased energy 躁狂

◇ **-mania** *suffix* 后缀 obsession with something 对某事强迫; **dipsomania** = addiction to alcohol 嗜酒狂;**kleptomania** = obsessive stealing of objects 偷窃狂

◇ **maniac** *noun* person suffering from an obsession 躁狂患者

◇ **manic** *adjective* referring to mania 躁狂的; **manic depression** = MANIC-DEPRESSIVE ILLNESS 躁狂抑郁性精神病

◇ **manic-depressive** *adjective* (person) suffering from manic depression 躁狂抑郁患者; **manic-depressive illness** *or* **manic-depressive psychosis** = bipolar disorder, a psychological condition where a patient moves between mania and depression and experiences delusion 躁狂抑郁性精神病

manifestation *noun* sign *or* indication *or* symptom (of a disease) 表现

> QUOTE: The reason for this susceptibility is a profound abnormality of the immune system in children with sickle cell disease. The major manifestations of pneumococcal infection in SCD are septicaemia, meningitis and pneumonia.
> 引文:镰状细胞贫血患儿容易感染的原因在于免疫系统存在严重异常。肺炎球菌感染这些患儿主要表现为败血症、脑膜炎和肺炎。
>
> **Lancet** 柳叶刀

manipulate *verb* to rub *or* to move parts of the body with the hands to treat a joint *or* a slipped disc *or* a hernia手法操作,推拿

◇ **manipulation** *noun* moving *or* rubbing parts of the body with the hands to treat a disorder of a joint *or* a hernia 手法操作,推拿

manner *noun* way of doing something *or* way of behaving 方式、态度: ***He was behaving in a strange manner.*** 他的行为很古怪。**doctor with a good bedside manner** = doctor who comforts and reassures patients when he examines them in hospital 临床态度优秀的医生

mannitol *noun* diuretic substance, used to treat oedema 甘露醇(有利尿作用,用于治疗水肿)

manometer *noun* instrument for comparing pressures 测压计,压力计

Mantoux test *noun* test for tuberculosis, where the patient is given an intracutaneous injection of tuberculin 芒图氏试验,结核菌素试验 *compare* 比较 PATCH TEST

manual *adjective* done by hand 手工的

manubrium (sterni) *noun* top part of the breastbone 胸骨柄

MAO = MONOAMINE OXIDASE 单胺氧化酶; **MAO inhibitor** = drug used to treat depression by inhibiting the action of MAO, but which also prevents the breakdown of tyramine in the brain and can cause high blood pressure 单胺氧化酶抑制剂

map out *verb* to show clearly in a diagram 图解,图示: ***To map out the extent of a tumour.*** 描绘出肿瘤的范围。

marasmus *or* **failure to thrive** *noun* wasting disease which affects small children who have difficulty in absorbing nutrients *or* who are suffering from malnutrition 消瘦病(亦称婴儿萎缩症)

marble bone disease = OSTEOPETROSIS 骨质石化症

Marburg virus disease *or* **green monkey disease** *noun* virus disease of green monkeys which is transmitted to humans 绿猴病,马尔堡病毒病

> COMMENT: Because monkeys are used in laboratory experiments, the disease mainly affects laboratory workers. Symptoms include headaches and bleeding from mucous membras; the disease is often fatal.
> 注释:由于实验室用猴子做试验,这种疾病主要感染实验室工作人员,症状有头痛和粘膜出血,这种疾病往往是致命的。

march fracture *noun* fracture of one

of the metatarsal bones in the foot, caused by excessive exercise to which the body is not accustomed 跖骨劳累性骨折

Marfan's syndrome *noun* hereditary condition where the patient has extremely long fingers and toes, with abnormalities of the heart, aorta and eyes 马方综合征,马凡氏综合征(一种遗传疾病,病人手指和脚趾奇长,并有心脏、主动脉及眼睛的异常。)

margarine *noun* vegetable fat which looks like butter and is used instead of butter 人造黄油

marijuana *or* **cannabis** *noun* (i) addictive drug made from the leaves *or* flowers of the Indian hemp plant 大麻(药品)(ii) tropical plant from whose leaves *or* flowers an addictive drug is produced 大麻(植物)

mark 1 *noun* spot *or* small area of a different colour 斑点: ***There's a red mark where you hit your head.*** 你头部受伤的地方有一个红点。***The rash has left marks on the chest and back.*** 皮疹在胸背留下了斑点。**2** *verb* to make a mark 作标记: ***The tin is marked 'dangerous'.*** = It has the word 'dangerous' written on it. 这个罐子上标着"危险"。

◊ **marked** *adjective* obvious *or* noticeable 明显的,能引起注意的: ***There has been a marked improvement in his condition.*** 他的状况有了明显改观。

◊ **marker** *noun* (i) label *or* thing which marks a place 标记,标志,标记物 (ii) substance which is part of a chromosome and gives it a genetic mark which can be used as a point of reference 染色体上的基因标记 (iii) substance introduced into the body to make internal structures clearer to X-rays 显影剂

market 交易 *see* 见 INTERNAL

marrow *or* **bone marrow** *noun* soft tissue in cancellous bone 骨髓; **bone marrow transplant** = transplant of marrow from a donor to a recipient 骨髓移植 ◊ 见图 BONE STRUCTURE (NOTE: for other terms referring to bone marrow, see words beginning with **myel-**, **myelo-**)

> COMMENT: Two types of bone marrow are to be found: red bone marrow or myeloid tissue, which forms red blood cells and is found in cancellous bone in the vertebrae, the sternum and other flat bones; as a person gets older, fatty yellow bone marrow develops in the central cavity of long bones.
> 注释:有两种骨髓:红骨髓或髓样组织,它是生成红细胞的地方,可以存在于椎骨、胸骨和其他扁平骨的海绵状骨质中;随年龄增长,长骨中央的空腔中长出富含脂肪的黄骨髓。

masculinization *noun* development of male characteristics (such as body hair and a deep voice) in a woman, caused by hormone deficiency *or* by treatment with male hormones 男性化

mask *noun* (i) metal and rubber frame that fits over the patient's nose and mouth and is used to administer an anaesthetic 麻醉面罩 (ii) piece of gauze which fits over the mouth and nose to prevent droplet infection 口罩 (iii) cover which fits over the face of a person who has been disfigured in an accident 面具(用于因事故毁容者)

masochism *noun* abnormal sexual condition where a person takes pleasure in being hurt *or* badly treated 受虐狂

◊ **masochist** *noun* person suffering from masochism 受虐狂患者

◊ **masochistic** *adjective* referring to masochism 受虐狂的 *compare* 比较 SADISM, SADIST, SADISTIC

mass *noun* (**a**) (i) body of matter 团块 (ii) mixture for making pills 用于制造药丸的混合剂 (iii) main solid part of bone 骨质 (**b**) large quantity, such as a large number of people 大量: ***The patient's back was covered with a mass of red spots.*** 病人的背部有大量红点。**mass radiography** = taking X-ray photographs of large numbers of people to check for tuberculosis 群体X线筛查(结核); **mass**

screening = testing large numbers of people for the presence of a disease 群体筛查

massage 1 *noun* treatment of muscular conditions which involves rubbing *or* stroking *or* pressing a patient's body with the hands 按摩; **external cardiac massage** = method of making a patient's heart start beating again by rhythmic pressing on the breastbone 心外按摩; **internal cardiac massage** = method of making a patient's heart start beating again by pressing on the heart itself 开胸心脏按摩 (NOTE: no plural, but **a massage** is used to refer to a single treatment : **he had a hot bath and a massage**) **2** *verb* to rub *or* stroke *or* press a patient's body with the hands 按摩

masseter (muscle) *noun* muscle which clenches the lower jaw making it move up 咬肌

massive *adjective* very large 很多,大量: ***He was given a massive injection of penicillin.*** 给他注射了大量青霉素。***She had a massive heart attack.*** 她经历了一次严重的心脏病发作。

mast- *prefix referring to a breast* 乳房

◇ **mastalgia** *noun* pain in the mammary gland 乳房疼痛

◇ **mastatrophy** *noun* atrophy of the mammary gland 乳腺萎缩

mast cell *noun* large cell in connective tissue, which carries histamine and reacts to allergens 肥大细胞(结缔组织中一种含有组胺的大细胞,可对过敏原起反应)

mastectomy *noun* surgical removal of a breast 乳房切除术; **radical mastectomy** = removal of the breast, and also the associated lymph nodes and muscles 根治性乳房切除术

masticate *verb* to chew food 咀嚼

◇ **mastication** *noun* chewing food 咀嚼

mastitis *noun* inflammation of the breast 乳腺

mastoid *adjective* (i) shaped like a nipple 乳头形的 (ii) belonging to the mastoid part of the temporal bone 颞骨乳突的; **mastoid antrum** 鼓窦 *see* 见 ANTRUM; **mastoid (air) cells** = air cells in the mastoid process 乳突细胞; **mastoid process** *or* **mastoid** = part of the temporal bone which protrudes at the side of the head behind the ear 乳突(颞骨的一部分) ⇨ 见图 SKULL

◇ **mastoidectomy** *noun* surgical operation to remove part of the mastoid process, as a treatment for mastoiditis 乳突切除术

◇ **mastoiditis** *noun* inflammation of the mastoid process and air cells 乳突炎

> COMMENT: Symptoms are fever, and pain in the ears. The mastoid process can be infected by infection from the middle ear through the mastoid antrum. Mastoiditis can cause deafness and can affect the meninges if not treated.
> 注释:症状有发热和耳痛,是中耳的感染经鼓窦传至乳突所致,如不经治疗可导致耳聋并影响脑膜。

◇ **mastoidotomy** *noun* surgical operation to make a cut into the mastoid process to treat infection 乳突切开术(用于治疗感染)

masturbate *verb* to excite one's own genitals so as to produce an orgasm 手淫

◇ **masturbation** *noun* stimulation of one's own genitals to produce an orgasm 手淫

match *verb* (**a**) to examine two things to see if they are similar *or* to see if they fit together 匹配,比较: ***They are trying to match the donor to the recipient.*** 他们努力找相匹配的捐献者给接受者。(**b**) to fit together in a certain way 相配: ***The two samples don't match.*** 这两个样本不相配。

> QUOTE: Bone marrow from donors has to be carefully matched with the recipient or graft-versus-host disease will ensue.
> 引文:来自捐献者的骨髓必须与接受者仔细匹配,否则会引发移植物抗宿主疾病。
> **Hospital Update** 现代化医院

mater 脑(脊)膜 *see* 见 ARACHNOID, DURA MATER, PIA MATER

materia medica *Latin words meaning* 'medical substance': study of drugs *or* dosages as used in treatment[拉丁语]药物,药物学

material *noun* (**a**) matter which can be used to make something 材料 (**b**) cloth 敷料: ***The wound should be covered with gauze*** *or* ***other light material.*** 伤口应当用纱布或其它轻软敷料覆盖。(**c**) all that is necessary in surgery 手术材料

maternal *adjective* referring to a mother 母亲的,母系的; **maternal death** = death of a mother during pregnancy, childbirth or up to twelve months after childbirth 产妇死亡(特指孕、产期或生后12个月内母亲的死亡); **maternal deprivation** 丧母 *see* 见 DEPRIVATION; **maternal instincts** = instinctive feelings in a woman to look after and protect her child 母爱

◇ **maternity** *noun* childbirth *or* becoming a mother 分娩,产妇; **maternity case** = woman who is about to give birth 临产妇; **maternity clinic** = clinic where expectant mothers are taught how to look after babies, do exercises and have medical checkups 产科门诊; **maternity hospital** *or* **maternity ward** *or* **maternity unit** = hospital *or* ward *or* unit which deals only with women giving birth 产科医院、产科病房或产房

matrix *or* **ground substance** *noun* amorphous mass of cells forming the basis of connective tissue 基质

matron *noun* woman in charge of the nurses in a hospital 总护士长,护理部主任: ***She has been made matron of the maternity hospital.*** 她已经成为产科医院的总护士长。***Such cases should be reported to the matron.*** 这类病例应当向总护士长报告。(NOTE matron can be used with names **Matron Jones**; the official title is '**Nursing officer**)

matter *noun* (**a**) substance 物质; **grey matter** = nerve tissue which is of a dark grey colour and forms part of the central nervous system 灰质; **white matter** = nerve tissue in the central nervous system which contains more myelin than grey matter 白质 (**b**) (**infected**) **matter** = pus 脓

mattress *noun* thick soft part of a bed which you lie on 床垫,褥子; **mattress suture** = suture made with a loop on each side of the incision 褥状缝合

maturation *noun* becoming mature *or* fully developed 成熟

◇ **mature** *adjective* fully developed 成熟的; **mature follicle** = Graafian follicle just before ovulation 成熟卵泡

◇ **maturing** *adjective* becoming mature 成熟的; **maturing egg** *or* **ovum** = ovum contained by a Graafian follicle 成熟卵子

◇ **maturity** *noun* (**a**) being fully developed 成熟 (**b**) (*in psychology*) being a responsible adult 成人(指心理上的成熟,即成为能负起责任的成人)

maxilla (**bone**) *noun* upper jaw bone 上颌骨 ◇ 见图 SKULL (NOTE: plural is **maxillae.** It is more correct to refer to the upper jaw as the **maxillae** as it is in fact formed of two bones which are fused together)

◇ **maxillary** *adjective* referring to the maxilla 上颌骨的; **maxillary air sinus** *or* **maxillary antrum** *or* **antrum of Highmore** = one of two sinuses behind the cheekbones in the upper jaw 上颌窦

MB = BACHELOR OF MEDICINE 医学学士

McBurney's point *noun* point which indicates the normal position of the appendix on the right side of the abdomen, between the hip bone and the navel, which is extremely painful if pressed when the patient has appendicitis 麦氏点

MCP = METACARPOPHALANGEAL 掌指骨的

MD = DOCTOR OF MEDICINE 医学博士

ME = MYALGIC ENCEPHALOMYELITIS 肌痛性脑脊髓炎

meal *noun* eating food at a particular time 餐: ***We have three meals a day — breakfast, lunch and dinner.*** 我们一日三餐—早、中、晚。***You should only have a light meal in the evening.*** 你晚间应当只吃清淡的食物。**barium meal** = liquid solution containing barium sulphate which a patient drinks so that an X-ray can be taken of his stomach 钡餐

measles *or* **morbilli** *or* **rubeola** *noun* infectious disease of children, where the body is covered with a red rash 麻疹: ***She's in bed with measles.*** 她因麻疹而卧床。***Have you had measles?*** 你得过麻疹吗? ***He's got measles.*** 他得了麻疹。***They caught measles from their friend at school.*** 他从学校的朋友那儿传染了麻疹。*see also* 参见 GERMAN MEASLES, KOPLIK'S SPOTS

> COMMENT: Measles can be a serious disease as it weakens the body's resistance to other diseases, especially bronchitis and ear infections; it can be prevented by immunization. If caught by an adult it can be very serious.
> 注释:麻疹会削弱身体对其他疾病的抵抗力,特别是对支气管炎和耳部感染,因而是一种严重的疾病,可以通过免疫接种来预防它。如果是成年人得了麻疹,病情常非常严重。

measure 1 *noun* (**a**) unit of size *or* quantity *or* degree 量度: ***A metre is a measure of length.*** 米是长度单位。(**b**) **tape measure** = long tape with centimetres, inches, etc. marked on it 卷尺 **2** *verb* to find out the size of something; to be a certain size 测量: ***The room measures 3 metres by 2 metres.*** 这个房间3米长,2米宽。***A thermometer measures temperature.*** 温度计是用来量温度的。

◇ **measurement** *noun* size, length, etc. of something which has been measured 尺寸,大小

meat *noun* animal flesh which is eaten (可食用的)肉 (NOTE: no plural **some meat, a piece** *or* **a slice of meat; he refuses to eat meat**)

meatus *noun* opening leading to an internal passage in the body, such as the urethra *or* the nasal cavity 道,口; **external auditory meatus** = tube in the skull leading from the outer ear to the eardrum 外耳道; **internal auditory meatus** = channel which takes the auditory nerve through the temporal bone 内耳道 ◊ 见图 EAR, SKULL

mechanism *noun* physical *or* chemical changes by which a function is carried out *or* system in the body which functions in a particular way 机制,机构: ***The inner ear is the body's mechanism for the sense of balance.*** 内耳是身体感知平衡的器官。

Meckel's diverticulum 麦克尔憩室 *see* 见 DIVERTICULUM

meconium *noun* first dark green faeces produced by a newborn baby 胎粪

media *or* **tunica media** *noun* middle layer of the wall of an artery *or* vein (血管壁)中膜

◇ **medial** *adjective* nearer to the central midline of the body or to the centre of an organ 中间的,内侧的,接近中线的; **medial arcuate ligament** = fibrous arch to which the diaphragm is attached 内侧弓状韧带; **medial malleolus** = bone at the end of the tibia which protrudes at the inside of the ankle 内踝; **medial rectus** = muscle arising from the medial part of the common tendinous ring and inserted into the sclera anterior of the eyeball 内直肌 *compare* 比较 LATERAL

◇ **medialis** 中间的,内的 *see* 见 VASTUS

◇ **medially** *adverb* towards *or* on the sagittal plane of the body 内侧地,朝向矢状面地

◇ **median** *adjective* towards the central midline of the body *or* placed in the middle 正中的,中线的; **median nerve** = one of the main nerves of the forearm and hand 正中神经; **median plane** =

midline at right angles to the coronal plane and dividing the body into right and left parts 中线平面

mediastinal *adjective* referring to the mediastinum 纵隔的: ***the mediastinal surface of pleura** or **of the lungs*** 胸膜或肺的纵隔面

◊ **mediastinitis** *noun* inflammation of the mediastinum 纵隔炎

◊ **mediastinum** *noun* section of the chest between the lungs, where the heart, oesophagus, and phrenic and vagus nerves are situated 纵隔

medical 1 *adjective* (i) referring to the study of diseases 医学的 (ii) referring to treatment of disease which does not involve surgery 内科的 (iii) (treatment) given by a doctor (as opposed to a surgeon) in a hospital *or* in his surgery 医疗的: ***a medical student*** 医学生; ***Medical help was provided by the Red Cross.*** 医疗救助是由红十字会提供的。 **medical assistance** = help provided by a nurse *or* by an ambulance man *or* by a member of the Red Cross, etc. 医疗援助; **medical certificate** = official document signed by a doctor, giving a patient permission to be away from work *or* not to do certain types of work 医疗证明; **medical committee** = committee of doctors in a hospital who advise the management on medical matters 医疗委员会; **medical doctor** (**MD**) = doctor who practises medicine, but not usually a surgeon 医师(一般不用来指外科医生); **medical examination** = examination of a patient by a doctor 体格检查; **medical history** = details of a patient's medical records over a period of time 病史; **chief medical officer** = government official responsible for all aspects of public health 卫生局局长; **Medical Officer of Health** (**MOH**) = formerly, local government official in charge of the health service in a certain district 卫生官员; **medical practitioner** = person qualified in medicine (a doctor *or* surgeon) 开业医生; **Medical Research Council** (**MRC**) = government body which organizes and pays for medical research 医学研究委员会; **medical secretary** = qualified secretary who specializes in medical documentation, either in a hospital or in a doctor's surgery 医学秘书; **medical social worker** = person who helps patients with their family problems *or* problems related to their work, which may have an effect on their response to treatment 医学社会工作者; **medical ward** = ward for patients who do not have to undergo surgical operations 内科病房 **2** *noun* official examination of a person by a doctor 体检: ***He wanted to join the army, but failed his medical.*** 他想参军,但没有通过体检。 ***You will have to have a medical if you take out an insurance policy.*** 如果你要投保,你得进行一次体检。

Medic-Alert bracelet *noun* bracelet worn by a person to show that he suffers from a certain condition (such as diabetes or an allergy) 医用警示手镯(标明患有某种疾病或对某些物质过敏)

Medicare *noun* system of public health insurance in the USA 美公共健康保险系统

medication *noun* (i) method of treatment by giving drugs to a patient 给药 (ii) medicine *or* drug taken by a patient 病人所服的药: ***He was given medication by the ambulancemen.*** 急救人员给他用了药。 ***What sort of medication has she been taking?*** 她吃了哪种药? ***80% of elderly patients admitted to geriatric units are on medication.*** 老年病房的老年病人 80% 都在服药。 *see also* 参见 PREMEDICATION

◊ **medicated** *adjective* (talcum powder *or* cough sweet, etc.) which contains a medicinal drug 含药的; **medicated shampoo** = shampoo containing a chemical which is supposed to prevent dandruff 药用香波

medicine *noun* (**a**) drug *or* preparation taken to treat a disease *or* condition

药物：*Take some cough medicine if your cough is bad.* 如果你咳嗽的厉害就服用咳嗽药。*You should take the medicine three times a day.* 这药你一天要吃三次。**medicine bottle** = special bottle which contains medicine 药瓶；**medicine cabinet** *or* **medicine chest** = cupboard where medicines, bandages, thermometers, etc. can be left locked up, but ready for use in an emergency 药柜，药箱 (**b**) (i) study of diseases and how to cure or prevent them 医学 (ii) study and treatment of diseases which does not involve surgery 内科学：*He is studying medicine because he wants to be a doctor.* 他正在学医，因为他想当医生。**clinical medicine** = study and treatment of patients in a hospital ward *or* in the doctor's surgery (as opposed to the operating theatre *or* laboratory) 临床医学 (NOTE: no plural in this meaning)

◇ **medicinal** *adjective* referring to medicine 医疗的；(substance) with healing properties 有药用价值的(物质)：*He has a drink of whisky before he goes to bed for medicinal purposes.* 为治病，他睡前喝杯威士忌。**medicinal drug** = drug used to treat a disease as opposed to hallucinatory *or* addictive drugs 医疗用药

◇ **medicinally** *adverb* used as a medicine 医学地，医疗上：*The herb can be used medicinally.* 这种草药能用于临床。

medico *noun* (*informal* 非正式) doctor 医生：*My medico said I was perfectly fit.* 我的医生说我很健康。

medico- *prefix* referring to medicine *or* to doctors 与医学、医生有关的

◇ **medicochirurgical** *adjective* referring to both medicine and surgery 内外科的

medium 1 *adjective* average *or* in the middle *or* at the halfway point 中间 2 *noun* substance through which something acts 介质；**contrast medium** = radio-opaque dye introduced into an organ *or* part of the body so that soft tissue will show clearly on an X-ray photograph 造影剂；**culture medium** = jelly (such as agar) in which a bacterial culture is grown in a laboratory 培养基

medroxyprogesterone *noun* synthetic female sex hormone used as a contraceptive 甲羟孕酮，一种合成女性激素，用于避孕

medulla *noun* (i) soft inner part of an organ (as opposed to the outer cortex) 髓质 (ii) bone marrow 骨髓 (iii) any structure similar to bone marrow 髓样结构；**medulla oblongata** = continuation of the spinal cord going through the foramen magnum into the brain 延髓；**renal medulla** = inner part of a kidney containing no glomeruli 肾髓质 ◊ 见图 KIDNEY；**adrenal medulla** *or* **suprarenal medulla** = inner part of the adrenal gland which secretes adrenaline and noradrenaline 肾上腺髓质

◇ **medullary** *adjective* (i) similar to marrow 髓样的 (ii) referring to a medulla 髓质的；**medullary cavity** = hollow centre of a long bone, containing bone marrow 骨髓腔 ◊ 见图 BONE STRUCTURE；**medullary cord** = epithelial fibre found near the hilum of the fetal ovary 髓索

◇ **medullated nerve** *noun* nerve surrounded by a myelin sheath 有髓神经

◇ **medulloblastoma** *noun* tumour which develops in the medulla oblongata and the fourth ventricle of the brain in children 成神经管细胞瘤

mega- *or* **megalo-** *prefix* (**a**) meaning large 大 (NOTE: the opposite is **micro-**) (**b**) meaning one million (10^6) 一百万，兆；**megajoule** = unit of measurement of energy (= one million joules) 一百万焦耳，兆焦 (NOTE: symbol is **M**)

◇ **megacolon** *noun* condition where the lower colon is very much larger than normal, because part of the colon above is constricted, making bowel movements impossible 巨结肠症

◇ **megakaryocyte** *noun* bone marrow cell which produces blood platelets 巨核

细胞

◇ **megaloblast** *noun* abnormally large blood cell found in the bone marrow of patients suffering from certain types of anaemia caused by vitamin B_{12} deficiency 巨幼红细胞

◇ **megaloblastic** *adjective* referring to megaloblasts 巨幼红细胞的; **megaloblastic anaemia** = anaemia caused by vitamin B_{12} deficiency 巨幼红细胞性贫血

◇ **megalocephaly** *noun* having an abnormally large head 巨颅症

◇ **megalocyte** *noun* abnormally large red blood cell, found in pernicious anaemia 巨红细胞

meibomian cyst *noun* chalazion, swelling of a sebaceous gland in the eyelid 睑板腺囊

◇ **meibomian gland** *or* **tarsal gland** *noun* sebaceous gland on the edge of the eyelid which secretes a liquid to lubricate the eyelid 睑板腺

meiosis *or US* **miosis** *noun* process of cell division which results in two pairs of haploid cells (cells with only one set of chromosomes) 减数分裂 *compare* 比较 MITOSIS

Meissner's plexus *noun* network of nerve fibres in the wall of the alimentary canal 麦氏丛

◇ **Meissner's corpuscle** *noun* receptor cell in the skin which is thought to be sensitive to touch 麦氏小体 ◊ 见图 SKIN & SENSORY RECEPTORS

melaena *or* **melena** *noun* black faeces where the colour is caused by bleeding in the intestine 黑便

melancholia *noun* (i) severe depressive illness occurring usually between the ages of 45 and 65 更年期忧郁症 (ii) clinical syndrome with tendency to delusion, fixed personality, and agitated movements 忧郁症,激越性抑郁; **involutional melancholia** = depression which occurs in people (mainly women) after middle age, probably caused by a change of endocrine secretions 衰老性忧郁症

melanin *noun* dark pigment which gives colour to skin and hair, also found in the choroid of the eye and in certain tumours 黑色素

◇ **melanism** *or* **melanosis** *noun* (i) abnormally depositing of dark pigment 黑变 (ii) staining of all body tissue with melanin in a form of carcinoma 黑变病

◇ **melanocyte** *noun* any cell which carries pigment 黑色素细胞

◇ **melanocyte-stimulating hormone** (**MSH**) *noun* hormone produced by the pituitary gland which causes darkening in the colour of the skin 促黑素

◇ **melanoderma** *noun* (i) abnormally large amount of melanin in the skin 黑皮病 (ii) discoloration of patches of the skin 皮肤片状脱色

◇ **melanoma** *noun* tumour formed of dark pigmented cells 黑色素瘤; **malignant melanoma** = dark tumour which develops on the skin from a mole, caused by exposure to strong sunlight 恶性黑色素瘤

◇ **melanophore** *noun* cell which contains melanin 黑色素细胞

◇ **melanoplakia** *noun* areas of pigment in the mucous membrane inside the mouth(口)粘膜黑斑

◇ **melanosis**黑变病 *see* 见 MELANISM

◇ **melanuria** *noun* (i) presence of dark colouring in the urine 深色尿 (ii) condition where the urine turns black after being allowed to stand (as in cases of malignant melanoma) 恶性黑素瘤时黑色尿

melasma *noun* presence of little brown, yellow or black spots on the skin 黑斑病

melatonin *noun* hormone produced by the pineal gland during the hours of darkness, which makes animals sleep during the winter months(动物)褪黑激素

> COMMENT: Bright light hitting the eye has the effect of stopping the production of melatonin.

注释:亮光照射眼睛可阻止褪黑激素产生。

melena = MELAENA 黑便

mellitus 糖尿 *see* 见 DIABETES

membrane *noun* thin layer of tissue which lines *or* covers an organ 膜,被膜; **membrane bone** = bone which develops from tissue and not from cartilage 膜成骨; **basement membrane** = membrane at the base of an epithelium 基底膜; **mucous membrane** = membrane which lines internal passages in the body (such as nose *or* mouth) and secretes mucus 粘膜; **serous membrane** = membrane which lines an internal cavity which does not come into contact with air (such as the peritoneum *or* pericardium) 浆膜; **synovial membrane** = smooth membrane which forms the inner lining of the capsule covering a joint, and secretes the fluid which lubricates the joint 滑膜; **tectorial membrane** = spiral membrane in the inner ear above the organ of Corti, which contains the hair cells which transmit impulses to the auditory nerve 耳蜗覆膜; **tympanic membrane** = eardrum 鼓膜 ◊ 见图 EAR

◊ **membranous** *adjective* referring to membrane 膜的; **membranous labyrinth** = canals round the cochlea 膜迷路

memory *noun* ability to remember 记忆力: ***He has a very good memory for dates.*** 他对日期有非常好的记忆力。***I have no memory for names.*** 我记不住名字。***He said the whole list from memory.*** 他凭记忆说出整个名单。**loss of memory** = not being able to remember anything 失去记忆力,失忆; ***She was found wandering in the street suffering from loss of memory.*** 有人发现她失去了记忆,在街上转悠。***He lost his memory after the accident.*** 事故后他失去了记忆力。

menarche *noun* start of menstrual periods 初潮

mend *verb* to repair; to make something perfect which has a fault in it 修理,修补: ***The surgeons are trying to mend the defective heart valves.*** 外科医师在尽力修补有缺损的瓣膜。

Mendel's laws *noun* laws of heredity 孟德尔定律

Mendelson's syndrome *noun* sometimes fatal condition where acid fluid from the stomach is brought up into the windpipe and passes into the lungs, occurring mainly in obstetric patients 门德尔森氏综合征(胃内容物误吸入气道,可致命,主要发生于产科病人)

Ménière's disease *or* **syndrome** *noun* disease of the middle ear, where the patient becomes dizzy, hears ringing in the ears and may vomit and becomes progressively deaf 美尼尔氏病(综合征)

COMMENT: The causes are not certain, but may include infections or allergies, which increase the fluid contents of the labyrinth in the middle ear.
注释:病因不明,可能与感染或过敏有关,感染与过敏增加内耳迷路内的液体含量。

mening- *or* **meningo-** *prefix* referring to the meninges 脑膜

◊ **meninges** *plural noun* membranes which surround the brain and spinal cord 脑脊膜 (NOTE: the singular is **meninx**)

COMMENT: The meninges are divided into three layers: the tough outer layer (dura mater) which protects the brain and spinal cord, the middle layer (arachnoid mater) and the delicate inner layer (pia mater) which contains the blood vessels. The cerebrospinal fluid flows in the space (subarachnoid space) between the arachnoid mater and pia mater.
注释:脑脊膜分为三层:坚硬的外层(硬脑膜)保护着脑和脊髓,中层(蛛网膜)和娇嫩的内层(软脑膜),软脑膜上有血管。脑脊液在蛛网膜和软脑膜之间的腔隙(蛛网膜下腔)中流动。

◊ **meningeal** *adjective* referring to the meninges 脑(脊)膜的; **meningeal haemorrhage** = haemorrhage from a meningeal artery 脑（脊）膜出血; **meningeal sarcoma** = malignant tumour in the meninges 脑(脊)膜肉瘤

◇ **meningioma** *noun* benign tumour in the meninges 脑(脊)膜瘤

◇ **meningism** *noun* condition where there are signs of meningeal irritation suggesting meningitis, but where there is no pathological change in the cerebrospinal fluid 假性脑(脊)膜炎

◇ **meningitis** *noun* inflammation of the meninges, where the patient has violent headaches, fever, and stiff neck muscles, and can become delirious 脑膜炎; **aseptic meningitis** = relatively mild viral form of meningitis 非细菌性脑膜炎 *see also* 参见 HIB, MENINGOCOCCAL

> COMMENT: Meningitis is a serious viral or bacterial disease which can cause brain damage and even death. The bacterial form can be treated with antibiotics. The most common forms of bacterial meningitis are Hib and meningococcal.
> 注释:脑膜炎是由病毒或细菌引起的严重疾病,可以导致脑损伤甚至死亡。细菌性脑膜炎可用抗生素治疗,最常见的细菌性脑膜炎是由乙型流感嗜血杆菌和脑膜炎球菌引起。

◇ **meningocele** *noun* condition where the meninges protrude through the vertebral column or skull 脑脑脊膜膨出

◇ **meningococcal** *adjective* referring to meningococcus 脑膜炎球菌的; **meningococcal disease** = disease caused by a meningococcus 脑膜炎球菌病; **meningococcal meningitis** = cerebrospinal fever *or* cerebrospinal meningitis *or* spotted fever, the commonest epidemic form of meningitis, caused by a bacterium *Neisseria meningitidis*, where the meninges become inflamed causing headaches and fever 脑膜炎球菌性脑膜炎

◇ **meningococcus** *noun* bacterium *Neisseria meningitidis* which causes meningococcal meningitis 脑膜炎球菌,奈瑟菌属 (NOTE: plural is **meningococci**)

◇ **meningoencephalitis** *noun* inflammation of the meninges and the brain 脑膜脑炎

◇ **meningoencephalocele** *noun* condition where part of the meninges and the brain push through a gap in the skull 脑脑膜膨出

◇ **meningomyelocele** *noun* hernia of part of the meninges and the spinal cord 脊髓脊膜疝

◇ **meningovascular** *adjective* referring to the meningeal blood vessels 脑(脊)膜血管的

meniscectomy *noun* surgical removal of a cartilage from the knee 半月板切除

◇ **meniscus** *noun* semilunar cartilage, one of two pads of cartilage (lateral meniscus and medial meniscus) between the femur and tibia in a knee joint 半月板 (NOTE: the plural is **menisci**)

meno- *prefix referring to menstruation* 与月经有关的

◇ **menopause** *noun* period (usually between 45 and 55 years of age) when a woman stops menstruating and can no longer bear children 停经,闭经; **male menopause** = non-medical term given to a period in a man's life in middle age (男性)中年 (NOTE: also called **climacteric** *or* **change of life**)

◇ **menopausal** *adjective* referring to the menopause 闭经的

◇ **menorrhagia** *noun* very heavy bleeding during menstruation 月经过多

◇ **menses** *plural noun* = MENSTRUATION 行经

◇ **menstrual** *adjective* referring to menstruation 月经期的; **menstrual cramp** = cramp in the muscles round the uterus during menstruation 痛经; **menstrual cycle** = period (usually 28 days) during which a woman ovulates, then the walls of the uterus swell and bleeding takes place if the ovum has not been fertilized 月经周期; **menstrual flow** = discharge of blood from the womb during menstruation 经血

◇ **menstruate** *verb* to bleed from the

uterus during menstruation 行经
◇ **menstruation** *noun* bleeding from the uterus which occurs in a woman each month when the lining of the womb is shed because no fertilized egg is present 月经
◇ **menstruum** *noun* liquid used in the extract of active principles from an unrefined drug 溶媒,溶剂

mental *adjective* (**a**) referring to the mind 精神的,心理的,心灵的; **mental age** = age of a person's mental development, measured by intelligence tests 心理年龄: ***She has a mental age of three.*** 她的心理年龄是3岁。**mental block** = temporary inability to remember something, caused by the effect of nervous stress on the mental processes 心理阻隔; **mental deficiency** *or* **defect** *or* **handicap** *or* **retardation** *or* **subnormality** = condition where a person's mind has not developed as fully as the body, so that he is not so mentally advanced as others of the same age 心理缺陷、智力残障、精神发育迟滞; **mental development** = development of the mind 心理发育: ***Although physically handicapped her mental development is higher than normal for her age.*** 虽然她身体上有残疾,她的心理发育是超过她的实际年龄的。**mental hospital** = special hospital for the treatment of mentally ill patients 精神病院; **mental illness** = any disorder which affects the mind 精神疾患,心理疾病; **mental patient** = patient suffering from a mental illness 精神病患者 (**b**) referring to the chin 颏的,下巴的; **mental nerve** = nerve which supplies the chin 颏神经
◇ **mentalis muscle** *noun* muscle attached to the front of the lower jaw and the skin of the chin 颏肌
◇ **mentally** *adverb* in the mind *or* referring to the mind 精神上的,心理上的: ***Mentally, she is very advanced for her age.*** 在心理上,她是大大超前于自己的年龄。**mentally defective** *or* **mentally retarded** = (person) with a mental ability which is less than normal for his age 心理上有缺陷,精神发育迟滞: ***By the age of four he was showing signs of being mentally retarded.*** 4岁时,他表现出精神发育迟滞的征象。

menthol *noun* strongly scented compound, produced from peppermint oil, used in cough medicines and in the treatment of neuralgia 薄荷醇
◇ **mentholated** *adjective* impregnated with menthol 浸薄荷醇的

mentum *noun* chin 颏,下巴

meralgia (paraesthetica) *noun* pain in the top of the thigh (caused by a pinched nerve) 股痛

mercury *noun* poisonous liquid metal, used in thermometers 水银,汞; **mercury poisoning** = poisoning by drinking mercury *or* mercury compounds *or* by inhaling mercury vapour 汞中毒 (NOTE: the chemical symbol is Hg)
◇ **mercurialism** *noun* mercury poisoning 汞中毒病
◇ **mercurochrome** *noun* red antiseptic solution 红汞(俗称:红药水)
◇ **mercurous chloride** (Hg_2Cl_2) *noun* calomel, a poisonous substance used to treat pinworms in the intestine 氯化亚汞,甘汞

mercy killing *noun* euthanasia, the killing of a sick person to put an end to suffering 安乐死

Merkel's cells *or* **discs** *noun* epithelial cells in the deeper part of the dermis which form touch receptors 默克氏触盘,默克氏细胞

merocrine *or* **eccrine** *adjective* (gland, especially a sweat gland) which does not disintegrate and remains intact during secretion 部分分泌的,局泌的

mes- *or* **meso-** *prefix* meaning middle 中
◇ **mesaortitis** *noun* inflammation of the media of the aorta 主动脉中层炎
◇ **mesarteritis** *noun* inflammation of the media of an artery 动脉中层炎
◇ **mesencephalon** *or* **midbrain**

noun small section of the brain stem, above the pons, between the hindbrain and the cerebrum 中脑

mesentery *noun* double layer peritoneum which attaches the small intestine and other abdominal organs to the abdominal wall 肠系膜

◇ **mesenteric** *adjective* referring to the mesentery 肠系膜的; **superior** *or* **inferior mesenteric arteries** = arteries which supply the small intestine *or* the transverse colon and rectum 肠系膜上/下动脉; **mesenteric vein** = vein in the portal system running from the intestine to the portal vein 肠系膜静脉

◇ **mesenterica** 肠系膜的 *see* 见 TABES

mesoappendix *noun* fold of peritoneum which links the appendix and the ileum 阑尾系膜

◇ **mesocolon** *noun* fold of peritoneum which supports the colon (in an adult it supports the transverse and sigmoid sections only) 结肠系膜

◇ **mesoderm** *or* **embryonic mesoderm** *noun* middle layer of an embryo, which develops into muscles, bones, blood, kidneys, cartilages, urinary ducts, and the cardiovascular and lymphatic systems 中胚层

◇ **mesodermal** *adjective* referring to the mesoderm 中胚层的

◇ **mesometrium** *noun* muscle layer of the uterus 子宫肌层

◇ **mesomorph** *noun* type of person of average height but strong build 中胚层体型的人,中型身材

◇ **mesomorphic** *adjective* like a mesomorph 中胚层体型的,中型身材的 *see also* 参见 ECTOMORPH, ENDOMORPH

◇ **mesonephros** *noun* Wolffian body, kidney tissue which exists in a human embryo 中肾

◇ **mesosalpinx** *noun* upper part of the broad ligament around the Fallopian tubes 输卵管系膜

◇ **mesotendon** *noun* synovial membrane connecting the lining of the fibrous sheath to that of a tendon 肌腱系膜

◇ **mesothelioma** *noun* tumour of the serous membrane, which can be benign or malignant 间皮瘤; **pleural mesothelioma** = tumour of the pleura, due to inhaling asbestos dust 胸膜间皮瘤

◇ **mesothelium** *noun* layer of cells lining a serous membrane 间皮 *see also* 参见 EPITHELIUM, ENDOTHELIUM

◇ **mesovarium** *nou n* fold of peritoneum around the ovaries 卵巢系膜

messenger *noun* person who brings a message 信使; **messenger RNA** = type of ribonucleic acid which transmits the genetic code from the DNA to the ribosomes which form the proteins coded on the DNA 信使核糖核酸,信使 RNA

meta- *prefix* which changes 改变

◇ **metabolism** *noun* chemical processes which are continually taking place in the human body and which are essential to life 新陈代谢; **basal metabolism** = minimum amount of energy needed to keep the body functioning and the temperature normal when at rest 基础代谢

◇ **metabolic** *adjective* referring to metabolism 新陈代谢的; **basal metabolic rate (BMR)** = amount of energy used by a body in exchanging oxygen and carbon dioxide when at rest, i.e. energy needed to keep the body functioning and the temperature normal (formerly used as a way of testing the thyroid gland) 基础代谢率 *see also* 参见 ACIDOSIS, ALKALOSIS

◇ **metabolite** *noun* substance produced by metabolism *or* substance taken into the body in food and then metabolized 代谢产物

◇ **metabolize** *verb* to change the nature of something by metabolism 代谢: ***The liver metabolizes proteins and carbohydrates.*** 肝脏代谢蛋白质和碳水化合物。

COMMENT: Metabolism covers all changes which take place in the body:

the building of tissue (anabolism); the breaking down of tissue (catabolism); the conversion of nutrients into tissue; the elimination of waste matter; the action of hormones, etc. 注释:新陈代谢涵盖了人体发生的所有变化:组织的构建(合成代谢),组织的降解(分解代谢),将营养物质转化为组织,清除废物,激素的作用等等。

metacarpus *noun* the five bones in the hand between the fingers and the wrist 掌骨 ◊ 见图 HAND

◊ **metacarpal** *noun & adjective* **metacarpal bone** *or* **metacarpal** = one of the five bones in the metacarpus 掌骨(指任一掌骨)

◊ **metacarpophalangeal joint** (**MCP** *or* **MP joint**) *noun* joint between a metacarpal bone and a finger 掌指关节

QUOTE: Replacement of the MCP joint is usually undertaken to relieve pain, deformity and immobility due to rheumatoid arthritis.
引文:通常用置换掌指关节的办法缓解类风湿关节炎带来的疼痛、畸形和僵硬。
Nursing Times 护理时代

metal *noun* material (either an element *or* a compound) which can carry heat and electricity (some metals are essential for life) 金属

◊ **metallic** *adjective* like a metal *or* referring to a metal 金属的; **metallic element** = chemical element which is a metal 金属元素

metamorphopsia *noun* condition where the patient sees objects in distorted form, usually due to inflammation of the choroid 视物变形(通常由脉络膜炎引起)

metaphase *noun* one of the stages in mitosis *or* meiosis 中期(有丝分类或减数分裂的一个阶段)

metaphysis *noun* end of the central section of a long bone, where the bone grows and where it joins the epiphysis 骨骺

metaplasia *noun* change of one tissue to another 化生

metastasis *noun* spreading of a malignant disease from one part of the body to another through the bloodstream *or* the lymph system(恶性肿瘤)转移 (NOTE: plural is **metastases**)

◊ **metastasize** *noun* to spread by metastasis(恶性肿瘤)扩散

◊ **metastatic** *adjective* referring to metastasis(恶性肿瘤)转移的: ***Metastatic growths developed in the liver.*** 肝内发生了转移瘤。

QUOTE: He suddenly developed problems with his balance and a solitary brain metastasis was diagnosed.
引文:他突然发生了平衡问题,经诊断发现了脑内孤立转移灶。
British Journal of Nursing 英国护理杂志

metatarsus *noun* the five long bones in the foot between the toes and the tarsus 跖骨 (NOTE: plural is **metatarsi**)

◊ **metatarsal** *noun & adjective* one of the five bones in the metatarsus 跖骨(五块中的任何一块),跖骨的; **metatarsal arch** = arched part of the sole of the foot, running across the sole of the foot from side to side 跖弓,足弓

◊ **metatarsalgia** *noun* pain in the heads of the metatarsal bones 脚掌痛,跖(骨)痛

◊ **metatarsophalangeal joint** *noun* joint between a metatarsal bone and a toe 跖趾关节

meteorism *noun* tympanites, condition where gas is present in the stomach or intestines, causing dilatation and pain 腹胀,胃肠胀气

methaemoglobin *noun* dark brown substance formed from haemoglobin which develops during illness *or* following treatment with certain drugs 高铁血红蛋白

COMMENT: Methaemoglobin can not transport oxygen round the body, and so causes cyanosis.
注释:高铁血红蛋白不能将氧运送到身体各部分,因此导致紫绀。

◊ **methaemoglobinaemia** *noun* presence of methaemoglobin in the blood 高

铁血红蛋白血症

methionine *noun* essential amino acid 甲硫氨酸,蛋氨酸

method *noun* way of doing something 方法

methyl alcohol *noun* wood alcohol (a poisonous alcohol used as fuel) 甲醇

◇ **methylated spirits** *noun* almost pure alcohol, with wood alcohol and colouring added 甲基化酒精

◇ **methylene blue** *noun* blue dye, formerly used as a mild urinary antiseptic, now used to treat drug-induced methaemoglobinaemia 亚甲蓝,美蓝

metr- *or* **metro-** *prefix* referring to the uterus 子宫

◇ **metralgia** *noun* pain in the uterus 子宫疼痛

metre *or US* **meter** *noun* SI unit of length 米(长度单位): ***The room is four metres by three.*** 这个房间 4 米长 3 米宽。(NOTE: metre is usually written **m** with **figures: the colon is 1.3 m long**)

metritis *noun* inflammation of the myometrium 子宫炎

◇ **metrocolpocele** *noun* condition where the uterus protrudes into the vagina 子宫坠入阴道

◇ **metropathia haemorrhagica** *noun* essential uterine haemorrhage, abnormal condition of the uterus, where the lining swells and there is heavy menstrual bleeding 自发性子宫出血

◇ **metroptosis** *noun* prolapsed womb *or* prolapse of the uterus, condition where the womb has moved downwards out of its normal position 子宫脱垂

◇ **metrorrhagia** *noun* abnormal bleeding from the vagina between the menstrual periods 子宫渗血,血崩

◇ **metrostaxis** *noun* continual light bleeding from the uterus 子宫出血,淋漓不尽

Mg *chemical symbol for* magnesium 镁的化学元素符号

mg = MILLIGRAM 毫克

MI = MITRAL INCOMPETENCE 二尖瓣关闭不全

micelle *noun* tiny particle formed by the digestion of fat in the small intestine 脂滴

Michel's clips 密歇尔氏夹 *see* 见 CLIP

micro- *prefix* (**a**) meaning very small 微,极小的 (NOTE: the opposite is **macro-** *or* **mega-** *or* **megalo-**) (**b**) meaning one millionth (10^6) 百万分之一; **microgram** = unit of measurement of weight (= one millionth of a gram) 微克; **micromole** = unit of measurement of the amount of substance (= one millionth of a mole) 微摩尔 (NOTE: symbol is **μ**)

◇ **microaneurysm** *noun* tiny swelling in the wall of a capillary in the retina 微动脉瘤

◇ **microangiopathy** *noun* any disease of the capillaries 微血管病

microbe *noun* microorganism, such as a bacterium, which may cause disease and which can only be seen with a microscope 微生物

◇ **microbial** *adjective* referring to microbes 微生物的; **microbial disease** = disease caused by a microbe 微生物所致疾病; **microbial ecology** = study of the way in which microbes develop in nature 微生物生态学

◇ **microbiological** *adjective* referring to microbiology 微生物学的

◇ **microbiologist** *noun* scientist who specializes in the study of microorganisms 微生物学家

◇ **microbiology** *noun* scientific study of microorganisms 微生物学

Microcephaly *noun* condition where a person has an abnormally small head 小头畸形

◇ **Microcephalic** *adjective* suffering from microcephaly 小头畸形的

> COMMENT: Microcephaly in a baby can be caused by the mother having had German measles during pregnancy.
> 注释:婴儿小头畸形可能是母亲怀孕时感染了风疹所致。

◇ **microcheilia** *noun* having abnormally small lips 小唇畸形

◇ **Micrococcus** *noun* genus of bacterium, some species of which cause arthritis, endocarditis and meningitis 微球菌

◇ **microcyte** *noun* abnormally small red blood cell 小红细胞

◇ **microcytic** *adjective* referring to microcytes 小红细胞的

◇ **microcytosis** *or* **microcythaemia** *noun* presence of excess microcytes in the blood 小红细胞血症

◇ **microdactylia** *noun* having abnormally small *or* short fingers or toes 短指(趾)畸形

◇ **microdontism** *noun* having abnormally small teeth 小齿畸形

◇ **microglia** *noun* tiny cells in the central nervous system which destroy other cells 小胶质细胞

◇ **microglossia** *noun* having an abnormally small tongue 小舌畸形

◇ **micrognathia** *noun* condition where one jaw is abnormally smaller than the other 小颌畸形

◇ **micromastia** *noun* having abnormally small breasts 乳房过小

◇ **micromelia** *noun* having abnormally small arms *or* legs 小肢畸形

◇ **micrometer** *noun* (**a**) instrument for taking very small measurements, such as measuring the width *or* thickness of very thin pieces of tissue 测微计，千分尺 (**b**) *US* = MICROMETRE 微米

micrometre *or* **micron** *noun* unit of measurement of thickness (= one millionth of a metre) 微米 (NOTE: with figures usually written μm)

microorganism *noun* very small organism which may cause disease and which can only be seen under a microscope 微生物

> COMMENT: Viruses, bacteria, protozoa and fungi are all forms of microorganism.
> 注释：病毒、细菌、原虫和真菌是不同形式的微生物。

micropsia *noun* seeing objects smaller than they really are, caused by a defect in the retina 视物显小症(由视网膜病损引起)

microscope *noun* scientific instrument with lenses, which makes very small objects appear larger 显微镜：***The tissue was examined under the microscope.*** 用显微镜对组织进行检查。***Under the microscope it was possible to see the cancer cells.*** 显微镜下可能看到癌细胞。

electron microscope (**EM**) = microscope which uses a beam of electrons instead of light 电子显微镜

> COMMENT: In an ordinary or light microscope the image is magnified by lenses. In an electron microscope the lenses are electromagnets and a beam of electrons is used instead of light, thereby achieving much greater magnifications
> 注释：光镜的图像是由透镜放大；电子显微镜的透镜是由电磁体场构成的，一束电子代替了光线，由此可获得很大的放大倍数。

◇ **microscopic** *noun* so small that it can only be seen through a microscope 显微水平

◇ **microscopy** *noun* science of the use of microscopes 显微学

microsecond *noun* unit of measurement of time (= one millionth of a second) 百万分之一秒，微秒 (NOTE: with figures usually written **us**)

Microsporum *noun* type of fungus which causes ringworm of the hair, skin and sometimes nails 小孢子菌属

◇ **microsurgery** *noun* surgery on very small parts of the body, using tiny instruments and a microscope 显微外科

> COMMENT: Microsurgery is used in operations on eyes and ears, and also to connect severed nerves and blood vessels.
> 注释：显微外科用于眼及耳的手术，也用于连接离断的神经和血管。

◇ **microvillus** *noun* very small process found on the surface of many cells, especially the epithelial cells in the intestine 微绒毛(NOTE: plural is **microrilli**)

micturate *verb* to urinate, to pass urine from the body 排尿

◇ **micturition** *noun* urination, passing of urine from the body 排尿

mid- *prefix* meaning middle 中间

◇ **midbrain** *or* **mesencephalon** *noun* small section of the brain stem, above the pons, between the cerebrum and the hindbrain 中脑

◇ **midcarpal** *adjective* between the two rows of carpal bones 腕骨间的

middle *noun* (**a**) centre *or* central point of something 中间 (**b**) waist 腰部: ***The water came up to my middle.*** 水漫过了我的腰部。

◇ **middle-aged** *adjective* not very young and not very old 中年的: ***A disease which affects middle-aged women.*** 一种侵及中年妇女的疾病。

◇ **middle ear** *noun* section of the ear between the eardrum and the inner ear 中耳;**middle ear infection** *or* **otitis media** = infection of the middle ear, usually accompanied by headaches and fever 中耳炎(中耳的感染,通常伴有头疼和发热)

COMMENT: The middle ear contains the three ossicles which receive vibrations from the eardrum and transmit them to the cochlea. The middle ear is connected to the throat by the Eustachian tube.
注释:中耳有三块听小骨,它们接受鼓膜传来的震动并将其传到耳蜗,中耳借咽鼓管与喉咙相连。

◇ **middle finger** *noun* the longest of the five fingers 中指

midgut *noun* middle part of the gut in an embryo, which develops into the small intestine 中肠

mid-life crisis = MENOPAUSE 闭经

midline *noun* imaginary line drawn down the middle of the body from the head through the navel to the point between the feet 中线

QUOTE: Patients admitted with acute abdominal pains were referred for study. Abdominal puncture was carried out in the midline immediately above or below the umbilicus.
引文:因急性腹痛收入院的病人选为研究对象,在紧靠脐上或下的中线位置进行了腹腔穿刺。
Lancet 柳叶刀

midriff *noun* the diaphragm 横膈

midstream specimen *or* **midstream urine** *noun* urine sample taken in the middle of a flow of urine 中段尿

midtarsal *adjective* between the tarsal bones 跖骨间的

midwife *noun* professional person who helps a woman give birth to a child (often at home) 助产士; **community midwife** = midwife who works in a community as part of a primary health care team 社区助产士 (NOTE: plural is **midwives**)

◇ **midwifery** *noun* (i) profession of a midwife 助产学 (ii) study of practical aspects of obstetrics 产科学; **midwifery course** = training course to teach nurses the techniques of being a midwife 助产士课程

COMMENT: To become a Registered Midwife (RM), a Registered General Nurse has to take a further 18 month course, or alternatively can follow a full 3 year course.
注释:要成为一名注册助产士,一个注册的全科护士必须再上 18 个月的课,或继续完成 3 年的专门课程的学习。

migraine *noun* sharp severe recurrent headache, often associated with vomiting and visual disturbances 偏头痛: ***He had an attack of migraine and could not come to work.*** 他的偏头痛发作了,不能来工作。***Her migraine attacks seem to be worse in the summer.*** 她的偏头痛发作似乎夏天更重些。

◇ **migrainous** *adjective* (person) who is subject to migraine attacks 偏头痛的

COMMENT: The cause of migraine is

not known. Attacks are often preceded by an 'aura', where the patient sees flashing lights or the eyesight becomes blurred. The pain is normally intense and affects one side of the head only.
注释：偏头痛的病因不明，发作前常有"前兆"，病人看到闪光或视物模糊，疼痛一般是剧烈的，并且只影响头的一侧。

mild *adjective* not severe *or* not cold *or* gentle 轻度的，轻微的，温和的：***we had a very mild winter.*** 这个冬天非常和暖。***She's had a mild attack of measles.*** 她患了轻型麻疹。***He was off work with a mild throat infection.*** 他因为咽喉轻微感染没来工作。（NOTE：**mild - milder - mildest**）

◊ **mildly** *adverb* slightly *or* not strongly 轻微地，和缓地：***a mildly infectious disease*** 一种和缓的感染性疾病；***a mildly antiseptic solution*** 一种作用温和的消毒液

miliaria *or* **prickly heat** *or* **heat rash** *noun* itchy red spots which develop on the chest, under the armpits and between the thighs in hot countries, caused by blocked sweat glands 痱子，汗疹

◊ **miliary** *adjective* small in size, like a seed 粟粒状的；**miliary tuberculosis** = tuberculosis which occurs as little nodes in various parts of the body including the meninges of the brain and spinal cord 粟粒性结核

◊ **milium** *noun* (i) white pinhead-sized tumour on the face in adults 粟粒疹 (ii) retention cyst in infants 婴儿潴留囊肿 (iii) cyst on the skin 皮肤囊肿（NOTE：plural is **milia**）

milk *noun* (**a**) white liquid produced by female mammals to feed their young 乳汁：***Can I have a glass of milk, please?*** 我能来杯奶吗？***Have you enough milk?*** 你的奶够吗？***The patient can only drink warm milk.*** 这个病人只能喝热牛奶。(**b**) milk produced by a woman 母乳：***The milk will start to flow a few days after childbirth.*** 产后几天便会开始泌乳。（NOTE：no plural **some milk**, **a bottle of milk** *or* **a glass of milk**）

◊ **milk leg** *or* **white leg** *or* **phlegmasia alba dolens** *noun* acute oedema of the leg, a condition which affects women after childbirth, where a leg becomes pale and inflamed as a result of lymphatic obstruction 股白肿

◊ **Milk of Magnesia** *noun* trade name for a mixture of magnesium hydroxide and water taken as an antacid and a laxative 镁乳（商品名，氢氧化镁与水的混合物，用作抗酸剂和导泻剂）

◊ **milk sugar** = LACTOSE 乳糖

◊ **milk teeth** *or* **deciduous teeth** *noun* a child's first twenty teeth, which are gradually replaced by permanent teeth 乳牙

◊ **milky** *adjective* (liquid) which is white like milk 乳白色的（NOTE：for other terms referring to milk, see words beginning with **galact-**, **lact**）

milli- *prefix* meaning one thousandth (10^3)千分之一，毫（NOTE：symbol is **m**）

◊ **milligram** *noun* unit of measurement of weight (= one thousandth of a gram) 毫克（NOTE：with figures usually written **mg**）

◊ **millilitre** *or US* **milliliter** *noun* unit of measurement of liquid (= one thousandth of a litre) 毫升（NOTE：with figures usually written **ml**）

◊ **millimetre** *or US* **millimeter** *noun* unit of measurement of length (= one thousandth of a metre) 毫米（NOTE：with figures usually written **mm**）

◊ **millimole** *noun* unit of measurement of the amount of substance (= one thousandth of a mole) 毫摩尔（NOTE：with figures usually written **mmol**）

◊ **millisievert** *noun* unit of measurement of radiation 毫希(沃特)（测量放射线量的单位）；**millisievert/year** (**mSv/year**) = number of millisieverts per year 每年接受放射线的毫希数（NOTE：with figures usually written **mSv**）

QUOTE: Radiation limits for workers should be cut from 50 to 5 millisieverts, and those for members of the public from 5 to 0.25.
引文:工作场合的放射线量应从50毫希降到5毫希,公共场合则应从5毫希降到0.25毫希。

Guardian 卫报

Milroy's disease *noun* hereditary condition where the lymph vessels are blocked and the legs swell 遗传性下肢淋巴水肿米尔罗伊病

Minamata disease *noun* form of mercury poisoning from eating polluted fish, found first in Japan 水俣病(食用被污染的鱼而汞中毒导致的疾病,首先在日本水俣县被发现)

mind *noun* part of the brain which controls memory *or* consciousness *or* reasoning 心灵,心智: ***He's got something on his mind.*** = He's worrying about something. 他心里有事,他在为某事担心。 ***Let's try to take her mind off her exams.*** = Try to stop her worrying about them. 尽力使她不想考试的事,尽量使她不为考试而烦恼。 **state of mind** = general feeling 心理状态,普遍感觉: ***He's in a very miserable state of mind*** 他的心理状态很糟。(NOTE: for terms referring to mind, see **mental**, and words beginning with **psych-**)

miner *noun* person who works in a coal mine 煤矿工人; **miner's elbow** = inflammation of the elbow caused by pressure 矿工肘

mineral *noun* inorganic substance 矿物质; **mineral water** = water taken out of the ground and sold in bottles 矿泉水

COMMENT: The most important minerals required by the body are: calcium (found in cheese, milk and green vegetables) which helps the growth of bones and encourages blood clotting; iron (found in bread and liver) which helps produce red blood cells; phosphorus (found in bread and fish) which helps in the growth of bones and the metabolism of fats; iodine (found in fish) is essential to the functioning of the thyroid gland.
注释:人体需要的矿物质中最重要的有:钙(奶酪、牛奶和绿叶蔬菜中富含),它能促进骨骼生长和凝血;铁(面包和动物肝脏中富含),能促进红细胞生成;磷(面包和鱼类中富含),能促进骨骼生长和脂肪代谢;碘(海鱼中富含),对甲状腺正常发挥功能至关重要。

minim *noun* liquid measure used in pharmacy (one sixtieth of a drachm) 量滴(药剂学上液体测量单位,一打兰的六十分之一)

minimum 1 *adjective* smallest possible 最小的 **2** *noun* smallest possible amount 最小量(NOTE: plural is **minimums** *or* **minima**)

◇ **minimal** *adjective* very small 很小,很少

minor *adjective* not important 轻的,不重要的; **minor illness** = illness which is not serious 小病; **minor surgery** = surgery which can be undertaken even when there are no hospital facilities 小手术; **labia minora** = two small fleshy folds at the edge of the vulva 小阴唇(NOTE: the opposite is **major**)

QUOTE: Practice nurses play a major role in the care of patients with chronic disease and they undertake many preventive procedures. They also deal with a substantial amount of minor trauma.
引文:开业护士在慢性病人的护理上起着重要作用,她们还承担着许多预防工作,而且还负责处理大量轻微创伤。

Nursing Times 护理时代

minute 1 *adjective* very small 很小,很少: ***A minute piece of dust got in my eye.*** 一粒小灰尘进了我的眼睛。 **2** *noun* unit of time equal to 60 seconds 分钟

miosis *or* **myosis** *noun* **(a)** contraction of the pupil of the eye (as in bright light) 瞳孔缩小 **(b)** *US* = MEIOSIS

◇ **miotic** *noun* drug which makes the pupil of the eye become smaller 缩瞳药

mis- *prefix* meaning wrong 错误的

miscarriage *noun* spontaneous abortion, situation where an unborn baby leaves the womb before the end of the pregnancy, especially during the first seven months of pregnancy 自然流产,小产: *She had two miscarriages before having her first child*.她生第一个孩子前曾两次小产。

◇ **miscarry** *verb* to have a miscarriage 自然流产,小产: *The accident made her miscarry*.事故使她流产了。*She miscarried after catching the infection*.感染后她小产了。

misconduct *noun* wrong action by a professional person, such as a doctor 处置不当; **professional misconduct** = actions which are considered to be wrong by the body which regulates a profession (such as an action by a doctor which is considered wrong by the Professional Conduct Committee of the General Medical Council) 处置不当,医疗差错

misdiagnose *verb* to make an incorrect diagnosis 误诊

mismatch *verb* to match tissues wrongly 失配

> QUOTE: Finding donors of correct histocompatible type is difficult but necessary because results using mismatched bone marrow are disappointing.
> 引文:找到组织相容性相配的捐献者并不容易,但又是必须的,因为用了不匹配的骨髓,结果会令人失望。
> **Hospital Update** 现代化医院

mist. *or* **mistura** 合剂 *see* 见 RE. MIST.

misuse 1 *noun* wrong use 滥用: *He was arrested for misuse of drugs*.他因滥用药物被逮捕。2 *verb* to use (a drug) wrongly 滥用

mite *noun* very small parasite, which causes dermatitis 螨; **harvest mite** *or* **chigger** = tiny parasite which enters the skin near a hair follicle and travels under the skin, causing intense irritation 恙螨

mitochondrion *noun* tiny rod-shaped part of a cell's cytoplasm responsible for cell respiration 线粒体(细胞的呼吸器官) (NOTE: plural is **mitochondria**)

◇ **mitochondrial** *adjective* referring to mitochondria 线粒体的

mitosis *noun* process of cell division, where the mother cell divides into two identical daughter cells 有丝分裂 *compare* 比较 MEIOSIS

mitral *adjective* referring to the mitral valve 二尖瓣的; **mitral incompetence** (**MI**) = situation where the mitral valve does not close completely so that blood goes back into the atrium 二尖瓣关闭不全; **mitral stenosis** = condition where the opening in the mitral valve is made smaller because the cusps have stuck together 二尖瓣狭窄; **mitral valve** *or* **bicuspid valve** = valve in the heart which allows blood to flow from the left atrium to the left ventricle but not in the opposite direction 二尖瓣; **mitral valvotomy** = surgical operation to detach the cusps of the mitral valve in mitral stenosis 二尖瓣切开,二尖瓣分离术

mittelschmerz *noun* pain felt by women in the lower abdomen at ovulation 月经间期痛

mix *verb* to put things together 混合: *The pharmacist mixed the chemicals in a bottle*.药剂师在一个瓶子里混合药物。

◇ **mixture** *noun* chemical substances mixed together 混合物: *The doctor gave me an unpleasant mixture to drink*.医生给了我一种很难喝的混合物。*Take one spoonful of the mixture every three hours*.每三个小时服一勺混合物。**cough mixture** = medicine taken to stop you coughing 咳嗽合剂

ml = MILLILITRE 毫升

mm = MILLIMETRE 毫米

mmol = MILLIMOLE 毫摩尔

MMR = MEASLES, MUMPS AND RUBELLA 麻疹、流行性腮腺炎和风疹

Mn *chemical symbol for* manganese 锰

的化学元素符号

Mo *chemical symbol for* molybdenum 钼的化学元素符号

MO = MEDICAL OFFICER 医政官员

mobile *adjective* able to move about 能动的,可动的: ***It is important for elderly patients to remain mobile.*** 保持运动对老年病人来说是重要的。

◇ **mobility** *noun* (*of patients*) being able to move about 运动能力; **mobility allowance** = government benefit to help disabled people pay for transport(残疾人)交通补助

◇ **mobilization** *noun* making something mobile 使运动; **stapedial mobilization** = operation to relieve deafness by detaching the stapes from the fenestra ovalis 镫骨松动术

moderate *adjective* not high or low 中度的

◇ **moderately** *adverb* not at one or other extreme 中度地,一般地: ***The patient had a moderately comfortable night.*** 病人这晚过得还算舒服。

modiolus *noun* central stalk in the cochlea 蜗轴

MOH = MEDICAL OFFICER OF HEALTH 卫生官员

moist *adjective* slightly wet *or* damp 潮湿的,湿润的: ***The compress should be kept moist.*** 压缩器应当保持湿润。**moist gangrene** = condition where dead tissue decays and swells with fluid because of infection 湿性坏疽

◇ **moisten** *verb* to make something damp 加湿,弄湿,沾湿

◇ **moisture** *noun* water *or* other liquid 潮湿,湿气,潮气: ***Moisture can collect in the scar tissue.*** 瘢痕组织能聚集湿气。***There is moisture in the air on a humid day.*** 阴湿的天气空气是潮润的。**moisture content** = amount of water *or* other liquid which a substance contains 潮湿量

mol = MOLE (b)摩尔

molar 1 *adjective* (**a**) referring to the large back teeth 臼齿的 (**b**) referring to the mole, the SI unit of amount of a substance 摩尔的 **2** *noun* one of the large back teeth, used for grinding food 臼齿; **third molar** *or* **wisdom tooth** = one of the four molars at the back of the jaw, which only appears at about the age of 20 and sometimes does not appear at all 第三臼齿,智齿 ◊ 见图 TEETH

> COMMENT: In milk teeth there are eight molars and in permanent teeth there are twelve.
> 注释:乳牙有 8 个臼齿,恒牙有 12 个臼齿。

◇ **molarity** *noun* strength of a solution shown as the number of moles of a substance per litre of solution 摩尔浓度

molasses *noun* dark sweet substance made of sugar before it has been refined 糖浆

mole *noun* (**a**) dark raised spot on the skin 黑痣: ***She has a large mole on her chin.*** 她下巴上有颗黑痣。(**b**) SI unit of measurement of the amount of substance 摩尔(物质量的单位) (NOTE: with figures usually written **mol**)

molecule *noun* smallest independent mass of a substance 分子

◇ **molecular** *adjective* referring to a molecule 分子的; **molecular biology** = study of the molecules of living matter 分子生物学; **molecular weight** = weight of one molecule of a substance 分子量

molluscum *noun* soft round skin tumour 软疣; **molluscum contagiosum** = contagious viral skin infection which gives a small soft sore 传染性软疣; **molluscum fibrosum** = skin tumours of neurofibromatosis 纤维性软疣(皮肤的神经纤维瘤病); **molluscum sebaceum** = benign skin tumour which disappears after a short time 脂性软疣

molybdenum *noun* metallic trace element 钼 (NOTE: the chemical symbol is **Mo**)

monaural *adjective* referring to the use of one ear only 单耳的

Mönckeberg's arteriosclerosis *noun* condition of old people, where the media of the arteries in the legs harden, causing limping 门克伯氏动脉硬化,动脉中层硬化

mongolism *noun* former name for Down's syndrome 先天愚型(Down 综合征的旧称)

◇ **mongol** *noun* former word for a person suffering from Down's syndrome 先天愚型患者(Down 综合征患者的旧称)

Monilia = CANDIDA 念珠菌属

◇ **moniliasis** = CANDIDIASIS 念珠菌病

monitor 1 *noun* screen (like a TV screen) on a computer 显示器,监测仪; **cardiac monitor** = instrument which checks the functioning of the heart in an intensive care unit 心电监测 **2** *verb* to check *or* to examine how a patient is progressing 监测

◇ **monitoring** *noun* regular examination and recording of a patient's temperature *or* weight *or* blood pressure, etc. 监测

mono- *prefix* meaning single *or* one 单一的

◇ **monoamine oxidase** (**MAO**) *noun* enzyme which breaks down the catecholamines to their inactive forms 单胺氧化酶; **monoamine oxidase inhibitor** *or* **MAO inhibitor** = drug which inhibits monoamine oxidase (used to treat depression, it can also cause high blood pressure) 单胺氧化酶抑制剂

◇ **monoblast** *noun* cell which produces a monocyte 成单核细胞

◇ **monochromat** *noun* colour-blind person 色盲患者

◇ **monocular** *adjective* referring to one eye 单眼的,独眼的; **monocular vision** = seeing with one eye only, so that the sense of distance is impaired 单眼视觉 *compare* 比较 BINOCULAR

◇ **monocyte** *noun* type of nongranular leucocyte, a white blood cell with a nucleus shaped like a kidney, which destroys bacterial cells 单核细胞

◇ **monocytosis** *or* **mononucleosis** *noun* glandular fever, condition in which there is an abnormally high number of monocytes in the blood 单核细胞增多症

> COMMENT: Symptoms include sore throat, swelling of the lymph nodes and fever; it is probably caused by the Epstein-Barr virus.
> 注释:症状包括嗓子疼,淋巴结肿大和发热;可能由 EB 病毒感染引起。

◇ **monodactylism** *noun* congenital condition in which only one finger or toe is present on the hand or foot 单指(趾)

◇ **monomania** *noun* deranged state where a person concentrates attention on one idea 偏执狂

◇ **mononeuritis** *noun* neuritis which affects one nerve 单神经炎

◇ **mononuclear** *adjective* (cell, such as a monocyte) which has one nucleus 单核的

◇ **mononucleosis**单核细胞增多症 *see* 见 MONOCYTOSIS

◇ **monoplegia** *noun* paralysis of one part of the body only (i. e. one muscle, one limb) 单瘫,部分麻痹

◇ **monorchism** *noun* condition in which only one testis is visible 单睾症

◇ **monosodium glutamate** *noun* a salt, often used to make food taste better 谷氨酸钠(味精的主要成分) *see also* 参见 CHINESE RESTAURANT SYNDROME

◇ **monosomy** *noun* condition where a person has a chromosome missing from one or more pairs 单体性

◇ **monosynaptic** *adjective* (nervous pathway) with only one synapse 单突触的

◇ **monovalent** *adjective* having a valency of one 一价的

◇ **monozygotic twins** = IDENTICAL TWINS 同卵双胞胎

◇ **monoxide**一氧化 *see* 见 CARBON

mons pubis *or* **mons veneris** *noun* cushion of fat covering the pubis 阴阜

monster *noun* deformed fetus which cannot live 畸胎

Montezuma's revenge *noun* (*informal* 非正式) diarrhoea which affects people travelling in foreign countries, eating unwashed fruit *or* drinking water which has not been boiled 墨西哥腹泻(外出食用不洁食物所致腹泻)

Montgomery's glands *noun* sebaceous glands around the nipple which become more marked in pregnancy 蒙哥马利氏腺(乳晕上的浆液腺,妊娠时更明显)

mood *noun* a person's mental state (of excitement, depression, euphoria, etc.) 情绪,心境

Mooren's ulcer *noun* chronic ulcer of the cornea, found in elderly patients 莫伦氏溃疡(老年人的慢性角膜溃疡)

morbid *adjective* (i) showing symptoms of being diseased 有症状的 (ii) referring to disease 病态的 (iii) unhealthy (mental faculty)(心理上)不健康的: ***The X-ray showed a morbid condition of the kidneys.*** ***X*** 线检查发现肾脏有病变。**morbid anatomy** *or* **pathology** = visual study of a diseased body and the changes which the disease has caused to the body 病理解剖学

◇ **morbidity** *noun* being diseased *or* sick 病态; **morbidity rate** = number of cases of a disease per hundred thousand of population 患病率

> QUOTE: Apart from death, coronary heart disease causes considerable morbidity in the form of heart attack, angina and a number of related diseases.
> 引文:除死亡外,冠心病还可引发大量病理状态,有心脏病发作、心绞痛及很多相关疾病。
> **Health Education Journal** 健康教育杂志

> QUOTE: Adults are considered morbidly obese when they are 45 kg or 100% above their ideal weight.
> 引文:成年人体重比理想体重多 45 公斤或超出 100% 则被视为病理性肥胖。
> **Southern Medical Journal** 南部医学杂志

morbilli *or* **rubeola** = MEASLES 麻疹

◇ **morbilliform** *adjective* (rash) similar to measles 麻疹样的

moribund *noun* & *adjective* dying (person) 濒临死亡,濒死的

morning *noun* first part of the day before 12 o'clock noon 上午; **morning sickness** = illness (including nausea and vomiting) experienced by women in the early stages of pregnancy when they get up in the morning 晨吐;(*informal* 非正式) **morning-after feeling** = HANGOVER 宿醉后第二天早晨的不适感; **morning-after pill** = contraceptive pill which is effective if taken after sexual intercourse 房事后避孕药

Moro reflex *noun* reflex of a newborn baby when it hears a loud noise (the baby is laid on a table and raises its arms if the table is struck) 莫罗氏反射(新生儿对声音刺激的一种反射)

morphea *or* **morphoea** *noun* form of scleroderma, a disease where the skin is replaced by thick connective tissue 硬皮病

morphine *noun* alkaloid made from opium, used to relieve pain 吗啡: ***The doctor gave him a morphine injection.*** 医生给他注射了吗啡。

morphology *noun* study of the structure and shape of living organisms 形态学

mortality (rate) *noun* number of deaths per year, shown per hundred thousand of population 死亡率

mortis 尸体的 *see* 见 RIGOR

mortuary *noun* room in a hospital where dead bodies are kept until removed by an undertaker for burial 太平间

morula *noun* early stage in the development of an embryo, where the cleavage of the ovum creates a mass of cells 桑葚胚

mosquito *noun* insect which sucks human blood, some species of which can pass viruses or parasites into the bloodstream 蚊子

COMMENT: In northern countries a

mosquito bite merely produces an itchy spot; in tropical countries dengue, filariasis, malaria and yellow fever are transmitted in this way. Mosquitoes breed in water and they spread rapidly in lakes or canals created by dams and other irrigation schemes. Because irrigation is more widely practised in tropical countries, mosquitoes are increasing and diseases such as malaria are spreading
注释:在北方,蚊子咬一下只引起个痒疹;在热带地区,登革热、丝虫病、疟疾和黄热病都是由蚊叮传播的。蚊子生长在水中,它们在水坝和其他灌溉设施形成的湖、渠中快速孳生,由于热带地区灌溉设施应用得更广泛,蚊子数量增多,如疟疾这样的疾病也便播散开来。

mother *noun* female parent 母亲; **mother cell** = original cell which splits into daughter cells by mitosis 母细胞; **mother-fixation** = condition where a patient's development has been stopped at a stage where the adult remains like a child, dependent on the mother 恋母情结

motile *adjective* (cell *or* microbe) which can move spontaneously 能自行移动的: ***Sperm cells are extremely motile.*** 精子细胞特别好动。

◇ **motility** *noun* (*of cells or microbes*) being able to move about 运动性能

motion *noun* (**a**) faeces, the matter which is evacuated in a bowel movement 粪便,大肠排空物: ***He passed blood with his motions.*** 他便血了。(**b**) movement 运动; **motion sickness** *or* **travel sickness** = illness and nausea felt when travelling 晕动病,旅行病

◇ **motionless** *noun* not moving 静止不动: ***Catatonic patients can sit motionless for hours.*** 紧张症病人可以一连好几个小时坐着不动。

COMMENT: The movement of liquid inside the labyrinth of the middle ear causes motion sickness, which is particularly noticeable in vehicles which are closed, such as planes, coaches, hovercraft.
注释:内耳迷路内液体的流动引起晕动病,这在封闭的运输工具中特别明显,如飞机、客车、气垫船中。

motor *adjective* referring to movement *or* which produces movement 运动的; **motor area** *or* **motor cortex** *or* **pyramidal area** = part of the cortex in the brain which controls voluntary muscle movement by sending impulses to the motor nerves 运动区,运动皮质,锥体区(大脑皮质司运动的区域); **motor end plate** = end of a motor nerve where it joins muscle fibre 运动终板; **motor nerve** = nerve which carries impulses from the brain to muscles and causes voluntary movement 运动神经; **motor neurone** = neurone which forms part of a motor nerve pathway leading from the brain to a muscle 运动神经元; **motor neurone disease** = disease of the nerve cells which control the movement of the muscles 运动神经元病; **motor pathway** = series of motor neurones leading from the motor cortex to a muscle 运动(神经)通路

COMMENT: Motor neurone disease has three forms: progressive muscular atrophy (PMA), which affects movements of the hands, lateral sclerosis, which is a form of spasticity, and bulbar palsy, which affects the mouth and throat
注释:运动神经原病有三种形式:进行性肌萎缩,影响手的运动;侧索硬化,一种痉挛性疾病;还有球麻痹,影响口咽部。

mottled *adjective* (skin) with patches of different colours(皮肤)颜色斑驳的

mountain fever = BRUCELLOSIS 布氏杆菌病

◇ **mountain sickness** *noun* altitude sickness, condition where a person suffers from oxygen deficiency from being at a high altitude (as on a mountain) where the level of oxygen in the air is low 高山反应,高原反应

mouth *noun* opening at the head of the alimentary canal, through which food and drink are taken in, and through which a person speaks and can breathe 口,嘴: ***She was sleeping with her mouth open*.** 她张着嘴睡觉。**roof of the mouth** = the palate, the top part of the inside of the mouth, which is divided into a hard front part and soft back part 腭; **mouth-to-mouth breathing** *or* **mouth-to-mouth ventilation** = method of making a patient start to breathe again, by blowing air through his mouth into his lungs 口对口呼吸

◇ **mouthful** *noun* amount which you can hold in your mouth 一口: ***He had a mouthful of soup*.** 他含着一口汤。

◇ **mouthwash** *noun* antiseptic solution used to treat infection in the mouth 漱口液 (NOTE: for terms referring to the mouth, see **oral** and words beginning with **stomat**)

movement *noun* (**a**) act of moving 运动; **active movement** = movement made by a patient using his own will 主动活动,主动运动 (**b**) **bowel movement** = defecation, evacuation of solid waste matter from the bowel through the anus 排便: ***The patient had a bowel movement this morning*.** 患者今晨排便了。

moxybustion *noun* treatment used in the Far East, where dried herbs are placed on the skin and set on fire 艾灸

MP = METACARPOPHALANGEAL (JOINT) 掌指(关节)

MPS = MEMBER OF THE PHARMACEUTICAL SOCIETY 药学会会员

MRC = MEDICAL RESEARCH COUNCIL 医学研究委员会

MRCGP = MEMBER OF THE ROYAL COLLEGE OF GENERAL PRACTITIONERS 皇家全科医师学会会员

MRCP = MEMBER OF THE ROYAL COLLEGE OF PHYSICIANS 皇家内科医师学会会员

MRCS = MEMBER OF THE ROYAL COLLEGE OF SURGEONS 皇家外科医师学会会员

MRI = MAGNETIC RESONANCE IMAGING 磁共振成像

> QUOTE: During a MRI scan, the patient lies within a strong magnetic field as selected sections of his body are stimulated with radio frequency waves . Resulting energy changes are measured and used by the MRI computer to generate images.
> 引文:磁共振成像扫描时,病人躺在一个强磁场中,用一定放射频率的波激发选定检查的身体部位。测量由此导致的能量变化,并以磁共振成像计算机产生图像。
> **Nursing 87** 护理 87

MS = MULTIPLE SCLEROSIS, MITRAL STENOSIS 多发性硬化

MSH = MELANOCYTE-STIMULATING HORMONE 促黑素

mSv = MILLISIEVERT 毫希(沃特)

mucin *noun* compound of sugars and protein which is the main substance in mucus 粘蛋白

muco- *prefix* referring to mucus 粘液的

◇ **mucocele** *noun* cavity containing an accumulation of mucus 粘液囊肿

◇ **mucocutaneous** *adjective* referring to mucous membrane and the skin 皮肤粘膜的

◇ **mucoid** *adjective* similar to mucus 粘液样的

◇ **mucolytic** *noun* substance which dissolves mucus 粘液溶媒

◇ **mucomembranous colitis** = MUCOUS COLITIS 粘膜结肠炎,粘液性结肠炎

◇ **mucoprotein** *noun* form of protein found in blood plasma 粘蛋白

◇ **mucopurulent** *adjective* consisting of a mixture of mucus and pus 粘液脓性的

◇ **mucopus** *noun* mixture of mucus and pus 粘液性脓

mucormycosis *noun* disease of the ear and throat caused by the fungus *Mucor* 毛霉菌病

mucosa *noun* mucous membrane 粘膜

◇ **mucosal** *adjective* referring to a mucous membrane 粘膜的

◇ **mucous** *adjective* referring to mucus *or* covered in mucus 粘液的; **mucous cell** = cell which contains mucinogen which secretes mucin 粘液细胞; **mucous colitis** *or* **irritable bowel syndrome** *or* **irritable colon** *or* **spastic colon** = inflammation of the mucous membrane in the intestine, where the patient suffers pain caused by spasms in the muscles of the walls of the colon 粘液性结肠炎,过敏性结肠综合征,过敏性结肠,痉挛性结肠; **mucous membrane** *or* **mucosa** = wet membrane which lines internal passages in the body (such as the nose, mouth, stomach and throat) and secretes mucus 粘膜; **mucous plug** = plug of mucus which blocks the cervical canal during pregnancy 粘液栓

◇ **mucoviscidosis** *noun* cystic fibrosis, hereditary disease in which there is malfunction of the exocrine glands, such as the pancreas, in particular those which secrete mucus(胰腺)纤维性囊肿病

◇ **mucus** *noun* slippery liquid secreted by mucous membranes inside the body, which protects those membranes 粘液 (NOTE: for other terms referring to mucus, see words beginning with **blenno-**)

muddled *adjective* (person) whose thought processes are confused 头脑糊涂的(指人)

Müllerian duct = PARAMESONEPHRIC DUCT 苗勒管,副中肾管

multi- *prefix* meaning many 多

◇ **multicentric** *adjective* in several centres 多中心的; **multicentric trial** *or* **testing** = trials carried out in several centres at the same time 多中心试验

◇ **multifocal lens** *noun* lens in spectacles whose focus changes from top to bottom so that the person wearing the spectacles can see objects clearly at different distances 变焦透镜 *compare* 比较 BIFOCAL

◇ **multiforme** 多形性 *see* 见 ERYTHEMA

◇ **multigravida** *noun* pregnant woman who has been pregnant two or more times before 经产孕妇

◇ **multinucleated** *adjective* (cell) with several nuclei, such as a megakaryocyte 多核的

◇ **multipara** *noun* woman who has given birth to two or more live children (mainly used for a woman in labour for the second time) 经产妇; **gravides multiparae** = women who have had a least four live births 多产妇 (NOTE: plural is **multiparae**)

multiple *adjective* which occurs several times *or* in several places 多数的,多次的; **multiple birth** = giving birth to more than one child at the same time 多胎产的(一次分娩多个婴儿); **multiple fracture** = condition where a bone is broken in several places 多发骨折; **multiple myeloma** = malignant tumour in bone marrow, most often affecting flat bones 多发性骨髓瘤; **multiple pregnancy** = pregnancy where the mother is going to produce more than one baby (i. e. twins, triplets, etc.) 多胎怀孕; **multiple sclerosis (MS)** *or* **disseminated sclerosis** = disease of the central nervous system which gets progressively worse, where patches of fibres lose their myelin, causing numbness in the limbs, progressive weakness and paralysis 多发性硬化

◇ **multipolar** *adjective* (neurone) with several processes 多极的 *see also* 参见 BIPOLAR, UNIPOLAR

◇ **multiresistant** *adjective* (disease) which is resistant against several types of antibiotic 耐多种抗生素的

mumps *or* **infectious parotitis** *plural noun* infectious disease of children, with fever and swellings in the salivary glands, caused by a paramyxovirus 腮腺炎: ***He caught mumps from the children next door.*** 他从隔壁孩子那里传染了腮腺炎。***She's in bed with mumps.*** 她因腮腺炎而卧床。***He can't go***

to school — he's got mumps. 他不能上学了,他得了腮腺炎。

> COMMENT: Mumps is a relatively mild disease in children; in adult males it can have serious complications and cause inflammation of the testicles (mumps orchitis).
> 注释:在儿童,腮腺炎是一种较轻的疾病;在成年男性则可引起严重的并发症,引起睾丸发炎(腮腺炎后睾丸炎)。

Münchhausen's syndrome *noun* condition where the patient pretends to be ill in order to be admitted to hospital 闵希豪生综合征(一种表现人为制造体征以求住院的精神障碍,与诈病的区别是,这种障碍患者只以住院为目的,而不是求得赔偿或逃避责任)

murder **1** *noun* (**a**) killing someone illegally and intentionally 谋杀: ***He was charged with murder*** *or* ***he was found guilty of murder.*** 起诉他谋杀或发现他犯有谋杀罪。***The murder rate has fallen over the last year.*** 去年,谋杀率下降了。(**b**) an act of killing someone illegally and intentionally 谋杀: ***Three murders have been committed during the last week.*** 上周发生了三起谋杀。***The police are looking for the knife used in the murder.*** 警察在寻找谋杀时用过的刀。**2** *verb* to kill someone illegally and intentionally 谋杀

murmur *noun* sound (usually the sound of the heart), heard through a stethoscope 杂音; **friction murmur** = sound of two serous membranes rubbing together, heard with a stethoscope in patients suffering from pericarditis, pleurisy 摩擦音

Murphy's sign *noun* sign of an inflamed gall bladder, where the patient will experience pain if the abdomen is pressed while he inhales 墨菲氏征

muscae volitantes *noun* spots *or* shapes which can be seen before the eyes 飞蝇幻视,飞蝇症(我国多用飞蚊症)

muscle *noun* organ in the body, which contracts to make part of the body move 肌肉: ***If you do a lot of exercises you develop strong muscles.*** 如果你做大量运动,你的肌肉就会很健壮。***The muscles in his legs were still weak after he had spent two months in bed.*** 他躺了两个月后腿部肌肉很虚弱。***He had muscle cramp after going into the cold water.*** 他浸入冷水后,肌肉痉挛了。**muscle fatigue** = tiredness in the muscles after strenuous exercise 肌肉疲劳; **muscle fibre** = component fibre of muscles (there are two types of fibre which form striated and smooth muscles) 肌纤维; **muscle relaxant** = drug which reduces contractions in the muscles 肌松剂; **muscle spasm** = sudden sharp contraction of a muscle 肌肉痉挛; **muscle spindles** = sensory receptors which lie along striated muscle fibres 肌梭; **muscle tissue** = tissue which forms the muscles and which is able to expand and contract 肌肉组织; **muscle wasting** = condition where the muscles lose weight and become thin 肌肉萎缩; **cardiac muscle** = muscle in the heart which makes the heart beat 心肌; **skeletal muscle** = muscle attached to a bone, which makes a limb move 骨骼肌; **smooth muscle** *or* **unstriated muscle** = type of muscle found in involuntary muscles 平滑肌,非横纹肌; **striated muscle** *or* **striped muscle** = type of muscle found in skeletal muscles whose movements are controlled by the central nervous system 横纹肌; **visceral muscle** = muscle in the walls of the intestines which makes the intestine contract 内脏肌肉 (NOTE: for other terms referring to muscles, see words beginning with **my-, myo-**)

> COMMENT: There are two types of muscle: voluntary (striated) muscles, which are attached to bones and move parts of the body when made to do so by the brain, and involuntary (smooth) muscles which move essential organs such as the intestines and bladder automatically. The heart muscle also works automatically.
> 注释:肌肉有两种:随意肌(横纹肌),它附

着在骨骼上，根据大脑发出的命令移动身体的某些部分；不随意肌（平滑肌），它自动地使重要脏器运动，如肠道、膀胱，心肌也是自动工作的。

◇ **muscular** *adjective* referring to muscle 肌肉的；**muscular branch** = branch of a nerve to a muscle carrying efferent impulses to produce contraction 肌肉支（支配肌肉运动的神经分支）；**muscular defence** = rigidity of muscles associated with inflammation such as peritonitis 肌肉保护，肌卫；**muscular disorders** = disorders (such as cramp *or* strain) which affect the muscles 肌动紊乱；**muscular dystrophy** = type of muscle disease where some muscles become weak and are replaced with fatty tissue 肌营养不良 *see also* 参见 DUCHENNE；**muscular relaxant** = drug which relaxes the muscles 肌松剂；**muscular rheumatism** = pains in the back *or* neck, usually caused by fibrositis or inflammation of the muscles 肌风湿病；**muscular system** = the muscles in the body, usually applied only to striated muscles 肌肉系统；**muscular tissue** = tissue which forms the muscles and which is able to expand and contract 肌肉组织

◇ **muscularis** *noun* muscular layer of an internal organ 肌层

◇ **musculocutaneous** *noun* referring to muscle and skin 肌皮的；**musculocutaneous nerve** (**in the upper limb**) = nerve in the brachial plexus which supplies the muscles in the arm 肌皮神经

◇ **musculoskeletal** *adjective* referring to muscles and bone 肌（与）骨骼的

◇ **musculotendinous** *adjective* referring to both muscular and tendinous tissue 肌腱的

mutant *noun & adjective* (i) (gene) in which mutation has occurred 突变的（基因）(ii) (organism) carrying a mutant gene 含突变基因的（生物）

◇ **mutate** *verb* to undergo a genetic change 突变：***Bacteria can mutate suddenly, and become increasingly able to infect.*** 细菌可以发生突变，感染力提高。

◇ **mutation** *noun* change in the DNA which changes the physiological effect of the DNA on the cell 突变

mutism *noun* dumbness *or* being unable to speak 自闭症

MW = MOLECULAR WEIGHT 分子量

my- *or* **myo-** *prefix* referring to muscle 肌肉

◇ **myalgia** *noun* muscle pain 肌痛

◇ **myalgic encephalomyelitis** (**ME**) = postviral fatigue syndrome, a long-term condition affecting the nervous system, where the patient feels tired and depressed and has pain and weakness in the muscles 肌痛性脑脊髓炎

◇ **myasthenia** (**gravis**) *noun* general weakness and dysfunction of the muscles, caused by defective conduction at the motor end plates（重症）肌无力

myc- *prefix* referring to fungus 真菌

◇ **mycelium** *noun* mass of threads which forms the main part of a fungus 菌丝体

◇ **mycetoma** = MADUROMYCOSIS 足分支菌病

◇ **Mycobacterium** *noun* one of a group of bacteria, including those which cause leprosy and tuberculosis 分枝杆菌

◇ **mycology** *noun* study of fungi 真菌学

◇ **Mycoplasma** *noun* type of microorganism similar to a bacterium, associated with diseases such as pneumonia and urethritis 支原体

◇ **mycosis** *noun* any disease (such as athlete's foot) caused by a fungus 真菌病；**mycosis fungoides** = form of skin cancer, with irritating nodules 蕈样真菌病

mydriasis *noun* enlargement of the pupil of the eye 散瞳

◇ **mydriatic** *noun* drug which makes the pupil of the eye become larger 散瞳剂

myectomy *noun* surgical removal of part *or* all of a muscle 肌切除

myel- *or* **myelo-** *prefix* referring (i)

to bone marrow 骨髓的 (ii) to the spinal cord 脊髓,脊索

◇ **myelin** *noun* protective white substance which is formed into a covering (myelin sheath) round nerve fibres by Schwann cells 髓鞘 ◇ 见图 NEURONE

◇ **myelinated** *adjective* (nerve fibre) covered by a myelin sheath 有(髓)鞘的

◇ **myelination** *noun* process by which a myelin sheath forms round nerve fibres 髓鞘生成

◇ **myelitis** *noun* (i) inflammation of the spinal cord 脊髓炎 (ii) inflammation of bone marrow 骨髓炎

◇ **myeloblast** *noun* precursor of a granulocyte 成髓细胞,原始粒细胞

◇ **myelocele** *noun* form of spina bifida where part of the spinal cord passes through a gap in the vertebrae 脊柱裂

◇ **myelocyte** *noun* cell in bone marrow which develops into a granulocyte 髓细胞,中幼粒细胞

◇ **myelofibrosis** *noun* fibrosis of bone marrow, associated with anaemia 骨髓纤维变性

◇ **myelogram** *noun* record of the spinal cord taken by myelography 脊髓X线造影片

◇ **myelography** *noun* X-ray examination of the spinal cord and subarachnoid space after a radio-opaque substance has been injected 脊髓X线造影术

◇ **myeloid** *adjective* referring to bone marrow *or* to the spinal cord *or* produced by bone marrow 骨髓的,脊髓的; **myeloid leukaemia** = acute form of leukaemia in adults 髓性白血病; **myeloid tissue** = red bone marrow 髓样组织

◇ **myeloma** *noun* malignant tumour in bone marrow *or* at the ends of long bones or in the jaw 骨髓瘤

◇ **myelomalacia** *noun* softening of tissue in the spinal cord 脊髓软化

◇ **myelomatosis** *noun* disease where malignant tumours infiltrate the bone marrow 骨髓瘤病,多发性骨髓瘤

◇ **myelopathy** *noun* any disorder of the spinal cord *or* bone marrow 骨髓疾病,脊髓疾病

myenteron *noun* layer of muscles in the small intestine, which produces peristalsis 肠肌层

myiasis *noun* infestation by larvae of flies 蝇蛆病

mylohyoid *noun* & *adjective* referring to the molar teeth in the lower jaw and the hyoid bone 下臼齿与舌骨的; **mylohyoid line** = line running along the outside of the lower jawbone, dividing the upper part of the bone which forms part of the mouth from the lower part which is part of the neck 下颌线

myo- *prefix* meaning muscle 肌肉

◇ **myoblast** *noun* embryonic cell which develops into muscle 成肌细胞

◇ **myoblastic** *adjective* referring to myoblast 成肌细胞的

◇ **myocardial** *adjective* referring to the myocardium 心肌的; **myocardial infarction** = death of part of the heart muscle after coronary thrombosis 心肌梗死

◇ **myocarditis** *noun* inflammation of the heart muscle 心肌炎

◇ **myocardium** *noun* middle layer of the wall of the heart, formed of heart muscle 心肌 ◇ 见图 HEART

◇ **myocele** *noun* condition where a muscle pushes through a gap in the surrounding membrane 肌膨出

◇ **myoclonic** *adjective* referring to myoclonus 肌阵挛; **myoclonic epilepsy** = form of epilepsy where the limbs jerk frequently 肌阵挛性癫痫

◇ **myoclonus** *noun* muscle spasm which makes a limb give an involuntary jerk 肌阵挛

◇ **myodynia** *noun* pain in muscles 肌痛

◇ **myofibril** *noun* long thread of striated muscle fibre 肌纤维

◇ **myofibrosis** *noun* condition where muscle tissue is replaced by fibrous tissue 肌纤维变性

◇ **myogenic** *adjective* (movement)

which comes from an involuntary muscle 肌源性的

◇ **myoglobin** *noun* muscle haemoglobin, which takes oxygen from blood and passes it to the muscle 肌红蛋白

◇ **myoglobinuria** *noun* presence of myoglobin in the urine 肌红蛋白尿

◇ **myogram** *noun* record showing how a muscle is functioning 肌动图

◇ **myograph** *noun* instrument which records the degree and strength of a muscle contraction 肌动描记仪

◇ **myography** *noun* recording the degree and strength of a muscle contraction with a myograph 肌动描记

◇ **myokymia** *noun* twitching of a certain muscle 肌颤

◇ **myology** *noun* study of muscles and their associated structures and diseases 肌学

◇ **myoma** *noun* benign tumour in a smooth muscle 肌瘤

◇ **myomectomy** *noun* (i) surgical removal of a benign growth from a muscle, especially removal of a fibroid from the uterus 肌瘤切除 (ii) myectomy 肌切除

◇ **myometritis** *noun* inflammation of the myometrium 子宫肌炎

◇ **myometrium** *noun* muscular tissue in the uterus 子宫肌层

◇ **myoneural junction** = NEUROMUSCULAR JUNCTION 肌肉神经接头

◇ **myopathy** *noun* disease of a muscle, especially where the muscle wastes away 肌病; **focal myopathy** = destruction of muscle tissue caused by the substance injected 局部肌肉坏死(由注射物质引起); **needle myopathy** = destruction of muscle tissue caused by using a large needle in intramuscular injections 注射所致肌肉坏死

myopia *noun* shortsightedness *or* nearsightedness, condition where a patient can see clearly objects which are close, but not ones which are further away 近视

◇ **myopic** *adjective* shortsighted *or* nearsighted, able to see close objects clearly, but not objects which are further away 近视的 (NOTE: the opposite is **longsightedness** *or* **hypermetropia**)

myoplasm *or* **sarcoplasm** *noun* cytoplasm of muscle cells 肌浆

◇ **myoplasty** *noun* plastic surgery to repair a muscle 肌修复术

◇ **myosarcoma** *noun* (i) malignant tumour containing unstriated muscle 肉瘤 (ii) combined myoma and sarcoma 肌肉瘤

◇ **myosin** *noun* protein in the A bands of muscle fibre which makes muscles elastic肌浆球蛋白,肌球蛋白

myosis, myotic 缩瞳剂,缩瞳的 *see* 见 MIOSIS, MIOTIC

myositis *noun* inflammation and degeneration of a muscle 肌炎

◇ **myotactic** *adjective* referring to the sense of touch in a muscle 肌触觉的; **myotactic reflex** = reflex action in a muscle which contracts after being stretched 牵张反射

myotomy *noun* surgical operation to cut a muscle 肌切除

◇ **myotonia** *noun* difficulty in relaxing a muscle after exercise 肌张力过高,肌强直

◇ **myotonic** *adjective* referring to tone in a muscle 肌张力的,肌强直的; **myotonic dystrophy** *or* **dystrophia myotonica** = hereditary disease with muscle stiffness leading to atrophy of the muscles of the face and neck 强直性肌萎缩

◇ **myotonus** *noun* muscle tone 肌张力,肌强直

myringa *noun* the eardrum, membrane at the end of the external auditory meatus leading from the outer ear, which vibrates with sound and passes the vibrations on to the ossicles in the middle ear 鼓膜

◇ **myringitis** *noun* inflammation of the eardrum 鼓膜炎

◇ **myringoplasty** *noun* plastic surgery

to correct a defect in the eardrum 鼓膜修复术

◇ **myringotome** *noun* sharp knife used in myringotomy 鼓膜刀

◇ **myringotomy** *noun* surgical operation to make an opening in the eardrum 鼓膜切开术

myxoedema *noun* condition caused when the thyroid gland does not produce enough thyroid hormone 粘液水肿

> COMMENT: The patient (usually a middle-aged woman) becomes fat, moves slowly and develops coarse skin; the condition can be treated with thyroxine.

> 注释：病人（通常是中年妇女）变得肥胖，行动迟缓，皮肤粗糙，这种病可以用甲状腺素治疗。

◇ **myxoedematous** *adjective* referring to myxoedema 粘液水肿的

myxoma *noun* benign tumour of mucous tissue, usually found in subcutaneous tissue of the limbs and neck 粘液瘤

myxosarcoma *noun* malignant tumour of mucous tissue 粘液肉瘤

myxovirus *noun* any virus which has an affinity for the mucoprotein receptors in red blood cells (one of which causes influenza) 粘液病毒

Nn

N (**a**) *chemical symbol for nitrogen* 氮的化学元素符号 (**b**) = NEWTON 牛顿

n *symbol for nano-* 毫微的符号

Na *chemical symbol for sodium* 钠的化学符号

nabothian cyst *or* **nabothian follicle** *or* **nabothian gland** *noun* cyst which forms in the cervix of the uterus when the ducts in the cervical glands are blocked 纳博特囊肿,子宫颈腺囊肿

naevus *noun* birthmark, a mark on the skin which a baby has at birth and which cannot be removed 痣,胎记 *see also* 参见 HAEMANGIOMA, PORT WINE STAIN, STRAWBERRY (NOTE: plural is **naevi**)

Naga sore *noun* tropical ulcer, large area of infection which forms round a wound in tropical countries 热带溃疡,(非洲)锥虫病

nagging pain *noun* dull, continuous throbbing pain 跳痛,抽痛

nail *or* **unguis** *noun* hard growth, formed of keratin, which forms on the top surface at the end of each finger and toe 甲,爪; **nail biting** = obsessive chewing of the fingernails, usually a sign of stress 咬指甲; **nail scissors** = special curved scissors for cutting nails 指甲剪 *see also* 参见 FINGERNAIL, TOENAIL (NOTE: for terms referring to nail, see words beginning with **onych-**)

nano- *prefix* meaning one thousand millionth (10^{-9}) 纤,毫微 (NOTE: symbol is n)

◇ **nanometre** *noun* unit of measurement of length (= one thousand millionth of a metre) 纳米 (NOTE: with figures usually written **nm**)

◇ **nanomole** *noun* unit of measurement of the amount of substance (= one thousand millionth of a mole) 纳摩尔 (NOTE: with figures usually written **nmol**)

◇ **nanosecond** *noun* unit of measurement of time (= one thousand millionth of a second) 纳秒 (NOTE: with figures usually written **ns**)

nape *or* **nucha** *noun* back of the neck 项,(俗)后脖颈子

napkin *noun* soft cloth, used for wiping or absorbing 纸巾; **sanitary napkin** *or* **sanitary towel** = wad of absorbent cotton material attached by a woman over the vulva to absorb the menstrual flow 卫生巾; **napkin rash** = NAPPY RASH 尿布疹

◇ **nappy** *noun* cloth used to wrap round a baby's bottom and groin to keep clothing clean and dry 尿布; **disposable nappy** = paper nappy which is thrown away when dirty, and not washed and used again 一次性尿布; **nappy rash** = sore red skin on a baby's buttocks and groin, caused by reaction to long contact with ammonia in a wet nappy 尿布疹 (NOTE: the US English is **diaper**)

narco- *prefix* meaning sleep *or* stupor 睡眠,昏迷,麻醉

◇ **narcoanalysis** *noun* use of narcotics to induce a comatose state in a patient about to undergo psychoanalysis which may be emotionally disturbing 麻醉分析

◇ **narcolepsy** *noun* condition where the patient has an uncontrollable tendency to fall asleep at any time 发作性睡病

◇ **narcoleptic** *noun & adjective* (substance) which causes narcolepsy; (patient) suffering from narcolepsy 发作性睡病患者,引起发作性睡病的物质

narcosis *noun* state of stupor induced by a drug 麻醉; **basal narcosis** = making a patient completely unconscious by administering a narcotic before a general anaesthetic 基础麻醉

◇ **narcotic** *noun & adjective* (pain-relieving drug) which makes a patient sleep *or* become unconscious 麻醉药,麻

醉品,麻醉剂: ***The doctor put her to sleep with a powerful narcotic*.** 医生用麻醉药使她进入睡眠。***the narcotic side-effects of an antihistamine*** 抗组胺药的困倦副作用

COMMENT: Although narcotics are used medicinally as pain-killers, they are highly addictive. The main narcotics are barbiturates, cocaine, and opium and drugs derived from opium, such as morphine, codeine and heroin. Addictive narcotics are widely used for the relief of pain in terminally ill patients.
注释:虽然麻醉剂在医学上用于镇痛,但也具有很高的成瘾性。主要的麻醉品有巴比妥类、可卡因、鸦片和鸦片衍生物,如吗啡、可待因和海洛因。成瘾性麻醉品广泛应用于解除临终病人痛苦上。

nares *plural noun* nostrils, two passages in the nose through which air is breathed in or out 鼻孔; **anterior nares** *or* **external nares** = the two nostrils 前鼻孔,外鼻孔; **internal nares** *or* **posterior nares** *or* **choanae** = two openings shaped like funnels leading from the nasal cavity to the pharynx 后鼻孔,内鼻孔(NOTE: singular is **naris**)

narrow 1 *adjective* not wide 狭窄的: ***The blood vessel is a narrow channel which takes blood to the tissues*.** 血管是向组织输送血液的狭长管道。***The surgeon inserted a narrow tube into the vein*.** 外科医师将一根狭长的管子插入了静脉。(NOTE: **narrow - narrower - narrowest.** Note also the opposite is **broad**) **2** *verb* to become narrow 变狭窄: ***The bronchial tubes are narrowed causing asthma*.** 支气管狭窄引起哮喘。

nasal *adjective* referring to the nose 鼻子的; **nasal apertures** *or* **choanae** = two openings shaped like funnels leading from the nasal cavity to the pharynx 后鼻孔; **nasal bones** = two small bones which form the bridge at the top of the nose 鼻骨◇见图 SKULL; **nasal cavity** = cavity behind the nose between the cribriform plates above and the hard palate below, divided in two by the nasal septum and leading to the nasopharynx 鼻腔◇见图 THROAT; **nasal cartilage** = two cartilages in the nose (the upper is attached to the nasal bone and the front of the maxilla, the lower is thinner and curls round each nostril to the septum) 鼻软骨; **nasal conchae** *or* **turbinate bones** = three ridges of bone (superior, middle and inferior conchae) which project into the nasal cavity from the side walls 鼻甲; **nasal congestion** = condition where the nose is blocked by inflamed and congested mucous membrane and mucus 鼻充血; **nasal drops** = drops of liquid inserted into the nose 滴鼻剂; **nasal septum** = division between the two parts of the nasal cavity, formed of the vomer and the nasal cartilage 鼻中隔; **nasal spray** = spray of liquid into the nose 鼻腔用气雾剂(鼻喷剂)

naso- *prefix* referring to the nose 鼻

◇ **nasogastric** *adjective* referring to the nose and stomach 鼻胃的; **nasogastric tube** = tube passed through the nose into the stomach 鼻胃管

◇ **nasogastrically** *adverb* (to feed a patient) via a tube passed through the nose into the stomach 鼻饲地

QUOTE: All patients requiring nutrition are fed enterally, whether nasogastrically or directly into the small intestine.
引文:所有病人均需胃肠道营养,可鼻饲,也可直接送入小肠。
British Journal of Nursing 英国护理杂志

nasolacrimal *adjective* referring to the nose and the tear glands 鼻泪腺的; **nasolacrimal duct** = duct which drains tears from the lacrimal sac into the nose 鼻泪管

◇ **nasopharyngeal** *adjective* referring to the nasopharynx 鼻咽的

◇ **nasopharyngitis** *noun* inflammation of the mucous membrane of the nasal part of the pharynx 鼻咽炎

◇ **nasopharynx** *noun* top part of the

pharynx which connects with the nose 鼻咽部

nasty *adjective* unpleasant 令人作呕的，令人难受的：***This medicine has a nasty taste***. 这种药有令人作呕的味道。***Drink some orange juice to take away the nasty taste***. 喝点儿橘汁去掉那种令人作呕的味道。***This new drug has some nasty side-effects***. 这种新药有些令人难受的副作用。(NOTE：**nasty - nastier - nastiest**)

nates *plural noun* buttocks 臀部

National Health Service (**NHS**) *noun* government service in the UK which provides medical services free of charge, or at reduced cost, to the whole population 国家保健事业；**a NHS doctor** = a doctor who works in the National Health Service 国家保健事业的医生；**NHS glasses** = cheap spectacles provided by the National Health Service 国家保健事业提供的眼镜；**on the NHS** = free *or* paid for by the NHS 国家保健事业付款：***He had his operation on the NHS***. 国家保健事业负担他的手术费用。***She went to see a specialist on the NHS***. 她找专家看病的费用由国家保健事业付款。(NOTE：the opposite of '**on the NHS**' is '**privately**')

> QUOTE：Figures reveal that 5% more employees in the professional and technical category were working in the NHS compared with three years before.
> 引文：数字显示受雇于国家保健事业的专业技术人员比3年前上升了5%。
> **Nursing Times** 护理时代

nature *noun* (**a**) (i) essential quality of something 本质，本性 (ii) kind *or* sort 种类 (iii) plants and animals 动植物；**nature study** = learning about plant and animal life at school 自然研究 (**b**) **human nature** = general behavioural characteristics of human beings 天性

◇ **natural** *adjective* (**a**) normal *or* not surprising 自然的：***His behaviour was quite natural***. 他的行为很自然。***It's natural for old people to go deaf***. 老年人失聪是自然规律。**natural childbirth** = childbirth where the mother is not given pain-killing drugs but is encouraged to give birth to the baby with as little medical assistance as possible 自然顺产；**natural immunity** = immunity from disease a newborn baby has from birth, which is inherited, acquired in the womb or from the mother's milk 天然免疫 (**b**) not made by men; (thing) which comes from nature 自然的，天然的，非人工的；**natural gas** = gas which is found in the earth and not made in a factory 天然气；**natural history** = study of nature 自然史

◇ **naturopathy** *noun* treatment of diseases and disorders which does not use medical or surgical means, but natural forces such as light, heat, massage, eating natural foods and using herbal remedies 自然疗法(不借助于现代医学的疗法，而借助自然的力量如利用晒太阳、热敷、按摩、食疗、草药等的一种疗法)

nausea *noun* feeling sick *or* feeling that you want to vomit 恶心：***She suffered from nausea in the morning***. 她患有晨吐。***He felt slight nausea in getting onto the boat***. 上了船，他感到轻微的恶心。

◇ **nauseated** *or US* **nauseous** *adjective* feeling sick *or* feeling about to vomit 恶心的：***The casualty may feel nauseated***. 伤员也许会感到恶心。

> COMMENT：Nausea can be caused by eating habits, such as eating too much rich food or drinking too much alcohol; it can also be caused by sensations such as unpleasant smells or motion sickness. Other causes include stomach disorders, such as gastritis, ulcers and liver infections. Nausea is commonly experienced by women in the early stages of pregnancy, and is called 'morning sickness'.
> 注释：某些饮食习惯可以导致恶心，如吃过于油腻的食物或饮酒过多；另外，令人不快的味道或晕车也可以引起恶心；其他原因包括：胃病如胃炎、溃疡或肝脏的感染；女性怀孕通常早期也可以感到恶心，称为晨

吐。

navel *or* **umbilicus** *noun* scar with a depression in the middle of the abdomen where the umbilical cord was detached after birth 脐 (NOTE: for terms referring to the navel, see words beginning with **omphal-**)

navicular bone *noun* one of the tarsal bones in the foot 舟状骨 ◊ 见图 FOOT

nearsightedness = MYOPIA 近视

◊ **nearsighted** = MYOPIC 近视的

nebula *noun* (i) slightly cloudy spot on the cornea 角膜云翳 (ii) spray of medicinal solution, applied to the nose or throat using a nebulizer 喷雾剂

◊ **nebulizer** = ATOMIZER 喷雾器

Necator *noun* genus of hookworm which infests the small intestine 板口线虫属

◊ **necatoriasis** *noun* infestation of the small intestine by the parasite Necator 板口线虫病

neck *noun* (**a**) part of the body which joins the head to the body 颈,脖子(俗): ***He is suffering from pains in the neck.*** 他脖子疼。***The front of the neck is swollen with goitre.*** 颈前因甲状腺肿而变粗了。***The jugular veins run down the side of the neck.*** 颈静脉自颈部的侧面下行。**stiff neck** = condition where moving the neck is painful, usually caused by a strained muscle *or* by sitting in a cold draught 颈强直; **neck collar** = special strong collar to support the head of a patient with neck injuries or a condition such as cervical spondylosis 护颈 (**b**) narrow part (of a bone *or* organ) 颈; **neck of tooth** = point where a tooth narrows slightly, between the crown and the root 牙颈; **neck of the uterus** = **CERVIX** 子宫颈部,宫颈 (NOTE: for terms referring to the neck, see **cervical**)

> COMMENT: The neck is formed of the seven cervical vertebrae, and is held vertical by strong muscles. Many organs pass through the neck, including the oesophagus, the larynx and the arteries and veins which connect the brain to the bloodstream. The front of the neck is usually referred to as the throat.
> 注释:颈部由七块颈椎构成,并有强健的肌肉使它保持正直。许多器官取道颈部,包括食管、喉,以及连接大脑、输送血流的动脉和静脉,颈前部通常称作咽喉。

necro- *prefix* meaning death 坏死

◊ **necrobiosis** *noun* (i) death of cells surrounded by living tissue 坏死组织 (ii) gradual localized death of a part or tissue 渐进性坏死

◊ **necrology** *noun* scientific study of mortality statistics 死亡统计学

◊ **necrophilia** *or* **necrophilism** *noun* (i) abnormal pleasure in corpses 恋尸癖 (ii) sexual attraction to dead bodies 恋尸

◊ **necropsy** = POST MORTEM 尸检

◊ **necrosed** *adjective* dead (tissue *or* bone)坏死的

◊ **necrosis** *noun* death of a part of the body, such as a bone *or* tissue *or* an organ 坏死: ***Gangrene is a form of necrosis.*** 坏疽是一种坏死。

◊ **necrospermia** *noun* condition where dead sperm exist in the semen 死精症

◊ **necrotic** *adjective* referring to necrosis; dead (tissue)坏死的

◊ **necrotomy** *noun* dissection of a dead body 尸体解剖; **osteoplastic necrotomy** = surgical removal of a piece of necrosed bone tissue 骨成形性死骨切除

needle *noun* (i) thin metal instrument with a hole at one end for attaching a thread, and a sharp point at the other end, used for sewing up surgical incisions 缝合针 (ii) thin hollow metal instrument with a point at one end, attached to a hypodermic syringe and used for giving injections 注射针头: ***It is important that needles used for injections should be sterilized.*** 注射用针头的消毒是重要的。***AIDS can be transmitted by using non-sterile needles.*** 用没有消毒过的针头可以传染艾滋病。**stop nee-**

dle = needle with a ring round it, so that it can only be pushed a certain distance into the body 有档针;**surgical needle** = needle for sewing up surgical incisions 外科针;**needle myopathy** = destruction of muscle tissue caused by using a large needle for intramuscular injections 穿刺导致的肌病

◇ **needlestick** *noun* accidental pricking of one's own skin by a needle (as by a nurse picking up a used syringe)针刺伤

◇ **needling** *noun* puncture of a cataract with a needle 针术(用针拨白内障),针刺

negative *adjective & noun* showing 'no'负的,阴性的,否定的,负,阴性: ***The answer is in the negative.*** = The answer is 'no' 回答是否定的。***The test was negative.*** = The test showed that the patient did not have the disease. 检查结果是阴性的。**negative feedback** = situation where the result of a process represses the process which caused it 负反馈

◇ **negativism** *noun* attitude of a patient who opposes what someone says 违拗症

> COMMENT: There are two types of negativism: active, where the patient does the opposite of what a doctor tells him, and passive, where the patient does not do what he has been asked to do.
> 注释:违拗症有两种形式:主动型,病人做的与医生说的刚好相反;被动型,病人不按要求的去做。

negra 黑的 *see* 见 LINEA

Negri bodies *plural noun* particles found in the cerebral cells of patients suffering from rabies 内格里小体(狂犬病患者脑神经细胞内的原虫样小体)

Neil Robertson stretcher 罗宾逊氏担架 *see* 见 STRETCHER

Neisseria *noun* genus of bacteria, including gonococcus which causes gonorrhoea, and meningococcus which causes meningitis 奈瑟菌属(引起淋病的淋球菌和引起脑膜炎的脑膜炎双球菌都是这一属的细菌)

nematode *noun* type of parasitic roundworm, such as hookworms, pinworms and threadworms 线虫

neo- *prefix* meaning new 新

◇ **neocerebellum** *noun* middle part of the cerebellum 新小脑

◇ **neomycin** *noun* type of antibiotic used for treatment of skin disease 新霉素

◇ **neonatal** *noun* referring to the first few weeks after birth 新生儿的;**neonatal death rate** = number of newborn babies who die, shown per thousand babies born 新生儿死亡率

◇ **neonate** *noun* newborn baby, less than four weeks old 新生儿

◇ **neonatorum** 新生儿的 *see* 见 ASPHYXIA

◇ **neoplasm** *noun* any new and morbid formation of tissue 新生物

> QUOTE: One of the most common routes of neonatal poisoning is percutaneous absorption following topical administration.
> 引文:局部用药后经皮吸收是新生儿中毒最常见的途径之一。
> **Southern Medical Journal** 南部医学杂志

> QUOTE: Testicular cancer comprises only 1% of all malignant neoplasms in the male, but it is one of the most frequently occurring types of tumours in late adolescence.
> 引文:睾丸癌只占男性恶性肿瘤的1%,但它却是青春期末最常发生的肿瘤之一。
> **Journal of American College Health** 美国卫生学会杂志

nephr- *prefix* referring to the kidney 肾

◇ **nephralgia** *noun* pain in the kidney 肾痛

◇ **nephrectomy** *noun* surgical removal of the whole kidney 肾切除

◇ **nephritis** *noun* inflammation of the kidney 肾炎

> COMMENT: Acute nephritis can be caused by a streptococcal infection. Symptoms can include headaches,

swollen ankles, and fever.
注释：链球菌感染可以引起急性肾炎，症状包括头疼、脚踝肿胀和发烧。

◇ **nephroblastoma** *noun* Wilms' tumour, malignant tumour in the kidneys in young children, usually under the age of 10, leading to swelling of the abdomen, which is treated by removal of the affected kidney 肾母细胞瘤

◇ **nephrocalcinosis** *noun* condition where calcium deposits are found in the kidney 肾钙质沉着

◇ **nephrocapsulectomy** *noun* surgical removal of the capsule round a kidney 肾被膜剥离术

◇ **nephrolithiasis** *noun* condition where stones form in the kidney 肾石病

◇ **nephrolithotomy** *noun* surgical removal of a stone in the kidney 肾石切除术

◇ **nephrologist** *noun* doctor who specializes in the study of the kidney and its diseases 肾病学家

◇ **nephrology** *noun* study of the kidney and its diseases 肾病学

◇ **nephroma** *noun* tumour in the kidney *or* tumour derived from renal substances 肾瘤

◇ **nephron** *noun* tiny structure in the kidney, through which fluid is filtered 肾单位

COMMENT: A nephron is formed of a series of tubules, the loop of Henle, Bowman's capsule and a glomerulus. Blood enters the nephron from the renal artery, and waste materials are filtered out by the Bowman's capsule. Some substances return to the bloodstream by reabsorption in the tubules. Urine is collected in the ducts leading from the tubules to the ureters.
注释：肾单位由肾小管、亨利袢、肾小球囊及肾小球等一系列结构组成。血液自肾动脉进入肾单位，废物由肾小球囊滤出，一些物质经肾小管的重吸收返回血流。从肾小管到输尿管的管道系统收集尿液。

◇ **nephropexy** *noun* surgical operation to attach a mobile kidney 肾固定术

◇ **nephroptosis** *or* **floating kidney** *noun* condition where the kidney is mobile 肾下垂

◇ **nephrosclerosis** *noun* kidney disease due to vascular change 肾硬化

◇ **nephrosis** *noun* degeneration of the tissue of a kidney 肾病

◇ **nephrostomy** *noun* surgical operation to make a permanent opening into the pelvis of the kidney from the surface 肾造瘘

◇ **nephrotic syndrome** *noun* increasing oedema, albuminuria and raised blood pressure 肾病综合征

◇ **nephrotomy** *noun* surgical operation to cut into a kidney 肾切开术

◇ **nephroureterectomy** *or* **ureteronephrectomy** *noun* surgical removal of all or part of a kidney and the ureter attached to it 肾输尿管切除术

nerve *noun* (**a**) bundle of fibres in a body which take impulses from one part of the body to another (each fibre being the axon of a nerve cell) 神经; **cranial nerves** = twelve pairs of nerves which are connected directly to the brain, and govern mainly the structures of the head and neck 颅神经 *see also* 参见 *the list at* CRANIAL; **spinal nerves** = thirty-one pairs of nerves which lead from the spinal cord, and govern mainly the trunk and limbs 脊神经; **motor nerve** *or* **efferent nerve** = nerve which carries impulses from the brain and spinal cord to muscles and causes movements 运动神经，传出神经; **peripheral nerves** = parts of motor and sensory nerves which branch from the brain and spinal cord 周围神经; **sensory nerve** *or* **afferent nerve** = nerve which registers a sensation, such as heat *or* taste *or* smell, etc., and carries impulses to the brain and spinal cord 感觉神经，传入神经; **vasomotor nerve** = nerve whose impulses make the arterioles become narrower 血

管运动神经 (**b**) (*names of nerves*) 神经; **abducent nerve** = sixth cranial nerve which controls the muscle which makes the eyeball turn 外展神经; **accessory nerve** = eleventh cranial nerve which supplies the muscles in the neck and shoulders 副神经; **acoustic nerve** *or* **auditory nerve** *or* **vestibulocochlear nerve** = eighth cranial nerve which governs hearing and balance 听神经,前庭耳蜗神经; **circumflex nerve** = sensory and motor nerve in the upper arm 腋神经; **cochlear nerve** = division of the auditory nerve 耳蜗神经; **facial nerve** = seventh cranial nerve which governs the muscles of the face, the taste buds on the front of the tongue and the salivary and lacrimal glands 面神经; **femoral nerve** = nerve which governs the muscle at the front of the thigh 股神经; **glossopharyngeal nerve** = ninth cranial nerve which controls the pharynx, the salivary glands and part of the tongue 舌咽神经; **hypoglossal nerve** = twelfth cranial nerve which governs the muscles of the tongue 舌下神经; **oculomotor nerve** = third cranial nerve which controls the eyeballs and eyelids 动眼神经; **olfactory nerve** = first cranial nerve which controls the sense of smell 嗅神经; **optic nerve** = second cranial nerve which takes sensation of sight from the eye to the brain 视神经; **phrenic nerve** = nerve which controls the muscles in the diaphragm 膈神经; **pneumogastric nerve** *or* **vagus nerve** = tenth cranial nerve which controls swallowing and nerve fibres in the heart and chest 肺胃神经,迷走神经; **radial nerve** = main motor nerve of the arm 桡神经; **sacral nerves** = nerves which branch from the spinal cord in the sacrum and govern the legs, the arms and the genital area 骶神经; **trigeminal nerve** = fifth cranial nerve which controls the sensory nerves in the forehead and face and the muscles in the jaw 三叉神经; **trochlear nerve** = fourth cranial nerve which controls the muscles of the eyeball 滑车神经; **ulnar nerve** = nerve running from the neck to the elbow, which controls the muscles in the forearm and fingers 尺神经; **vestibulocochlear nerve** = eighth cranial nerve which governs hearing and balance 前庭耳蜗神经 (**c**) **nerve block** = stopping the function of a nerve by injecting an anaesthetic 神经阻滞; **nerve cell** *or* **neurone** = cell in the nervous system, consisting of a cell body, axon(s) and dendrites, which transmits nerve impulses 神经细胞,神经原; **nerve centre** = point at which nerves come together 神经中枢; **nerve ending** = terminal at the end of a nerve fibre, where a nerve cell connects with another nerve or with a muscle 神经末梢; **nerve fibre** = axon, a thread-like structure which is part of a nerve cell and carries nerve impulses 神经纤维; **nerve gas** = gas which attacks the nervous system 神经毒气; **nerve impulse** = electrochemical impulse which is transmitted by nerve cells 神经冲动; **nerve root** = first part of a nerve as it leaves or joins the spinal column (the dorsal nerve root is the entry for a sensory nerve, and the ventral nerve root is the exit for a motor nerve) 神经根; **nerve tissue** = tissue which forms nerves, and which is able to transmit the nerve impulses 神经组织

> COMMENT: Nerves are the fibres along which impulses are carried. Motor nerves or efferent nerves take messages between the central nervous system and muscles, making the muscles move. Sensory nerves or afferent nerves transmit impulses (such as sight or pain) from the sense organs to the brain.
> 注释:神经是传导冲动的纤维。运动神经,或称传出神经将信号从中枢传到肌肉,使肌肉运动。感觉神经,或称传入神经将感官的冲动(如视觉信号或痛觉信号)传到大脑。

◇ **nervosa** 神经性的 *see* 见 ANOREXIA

◇ **nervous** *adjective* (**a**) referring to nerves 神经的; **nervous breakdown** = non-medical term for a sudden mental illness, where a patient becomes so depressed and worried that he is incapable of doing anything 神经崩溃; **nervous system** = nervous tissues of the body, including the peripheral nerves, spinal cord, ganglia and nerve centres 神经系统; **autonomic nervous system** = nervous system which regulates the automatic functioning of the structures of the body, such as the heart and lungs 自主神经系统; **central nervous system** (**CNS**) = brain and spinal cord which link together all the nerves 中枢神经系统; **peripheral nervous system** (**PNS**) = nervous tissue outside the central nervous system 周围神经系统 *see also* 参见 PARASYMPATHETIC, SYMPATHETIC (**b**) very easily worried 神经质的, 紧张不安的, 担心焦急的: ***She's nervous about her exams.*** 她担心自己的考试结果。***Don't be nervous - the operation is a very simple one.*** 别担心, 这只是个很小的手术。

◇ **nervousness** *noun* state of being nervous 神经质, 紧张不安, 担心

◇ **nervy** *adjective* (*informal* 非正式) worried and nervous 担心的, 焦急的 (NOTE: for other terms referring to nerves, see words beginning with **neur**)

nettle rash *noun* urticaria, affection of the skin, with white or red weals which sting or itch, caused by an allergic reaction (often to plants) 荨麻疹

network *noun* interconnecting system of lines and spaces, like a net 网络: ***a network of fine blood vessels*** 小血管网

neur- *or* **neuro-** *prefix* referring to a nerve *or* the nervous system 神经

◇ **neural** *adjective* referring to a nerve *or* the nervous system 神经的; **neural arch** = curved part of a vertebra, which forms the space through which the spinal cord passes 神经弓; **neural crest** = ridge of cells in an embryo which forms nerve cells of the sensory and autonomic ganglia 神经嵴; **neural groove** = groove on the back of an embryo, formed as the neural plate closes to form the neural tube 神经沟; **neural plate** = thickening of an embryonic disc which folds over to form the neural tube 神经板; **neural tube** = tube lined with ectodermal cells running the length of an embryo, which develops into the brain and spinal cord 神经管; **neural tube defect** = congenital defect (such as spina bifida) which occurs when the edges of the neural tube do not close up properly 神经管缺损

◇ **neuralgia** *noun* spasm of pain which runs along a nerve 神经痛; **trigeminal neuralgia** = pain in the trigeminal nerve, which sends intense pains shooting across the face 三叉神经痛

◇ **neurapraxia** *noun* lesion of a nerve which leads to paralysis for a very short time, giving a tingling feeling and loss of function 神经失用症, 功能性麻痹

◇ **neurasthenia** *noun* type of neurosis where the patient is mentally and physically irritable and extremely fatigued 神经衰弱

◇ **neurasthenic** *noun & adjective* (person) suffering from neurasthenia 神经衰弱的

◇ **neurectasis** *noun* surgical operation to stretch a peripheral nerve 神经牵伸术

◇ **neurectomy** *noun* surgical removal of all or part of a nerve 神经切除术

◇ **neurilemma** *or* **neurolemma** *noun* outer sheath formed of Schwann cells, which covers the myelin sheath covering a nerve fibre 神经鞘

◇ **neurilemmoma** *or* **neurinoma** *noun* benign tumour of a nerve, formed from the neurilemma 神经鞘瘤

◇ **neuritis** *noun* inflammation of a nerve, giving a constant pain 神经炎

◇ **neuroanatomy** *noun* scientific study

of the structure of the nervous system 神经解剖

◇ **neuroblast** *noun* cell in the embryonic spinal cord which forms a nerve cell 成神经细胞

◇ **neuroblastoma** *noun* malignant tumour formed from the neural crest, found mainly in young children 成神经细胞瘤

◇ **neurocranium** *noun* part of the skull which encloses and protects the brain 脑颅

◇ **neurodermatitis** *noun* inflammation of the skin caused by psychological factors 神经性皮炎

◇ **neurodermatosis** *noun* nervous condition involving the skin 神经性皮肤病

◇ **neuroendocrine system** *noun* system where some organs are controlled by both the nervous system and by hormones 神经内分泌系统

◇ **neuroepithelium** *noun* epithelial cells forming part of the lining of the mucosa of the nose or the labyrinth of the middle ear 神经上皮

◇ **neuroepithelial** *adjective* referring to the neuroepithelium 神经上皮的

◇ **neuroepithelioma** *noun* malignant tumour in the retina 神经上皮瘤

◇ **neurofibril** *noun* fine thread in the cytoplasm of a neurone 神经纤维

◇ **neurofibroma** *noun* benign tumour of a nerve, formed from the neurilemma 神经纤维瘤; **acoustic neurofibroma** = tumour in the sheath of the auditory nerve 听神经纤维瘤

◇ **neurofibromatosis** (**NF**) *noun* hereditary condition where the patient has neurofibromata on the nerve trunks, limb plexuses or spinal roots, and pale brown spots appear on the skin 神经纤维瘤病 (NOTE: also called **molluscum fibrosum** *or* **von Recklinghausen's disease**)

◇ **neurogenesis** *noun* development and growth of nerves and nervous tissue 神经发生

◇ **neurogenic** *adjective* (i) coming from the nervous system 神经原性的 (ii) referring to neurogenesis 神经发生的; **neurogenic bladder** = any disturbance of the bladder function caused by lesions in the nerve supply to the bladder 神经原性膀胱

◇ **neuroglandular junction** *noun* point where a nerve joins the gland which it controls 神经腺体联接

◇ **neuroglia** *noun* supporting cells of the spinal cord and brain 神经胶质

◇ **neurohormone** *noun* hormone produced in some nerve cells and secreted from the nerve endings 神经激素

◇ **neurohypophysis** *noun* lobe at the back of the pituitary gland, which secretes oxytocin and vasopressin 神经垂体

◇ **neurolemma** *noun* = NEURILEMMA 神经鞘

◇ **neuroleptic** *noun* tranquillizer, drug which calms a patient and stops him worrying 神经松弛剂

◇ **neurological** *adjective* referring to neurology 神经病学的

◇ **neurologist** *noun* doctor who specializes in the study of the nervous system and the treatment of its diseases 神经病学家

◇ **neurology** *noun* scientific study of the nervous system and its diseases 神经病学

◇ **neuroma** *noun* benign tumour formed of nerve cells and nerve fibres 神经瘤; **acoustic neuroma** = tumour in the sheath of the auditory nerve 听神经瘤

◇ **neuromuscular** *adjective* referring to nerves and muscles 神经肌肉的; **neuromuscular junction** *or* **myoneural junction** = point where a motor nerve joins muscle fibre 神经肌肉联接

◇ **neuromyelitis optica** *noun* Devic's disease, condition similar to multiple sclerosis, where the patient has acute myelitis and the optic nerve is also affected 视神经脊髓炎

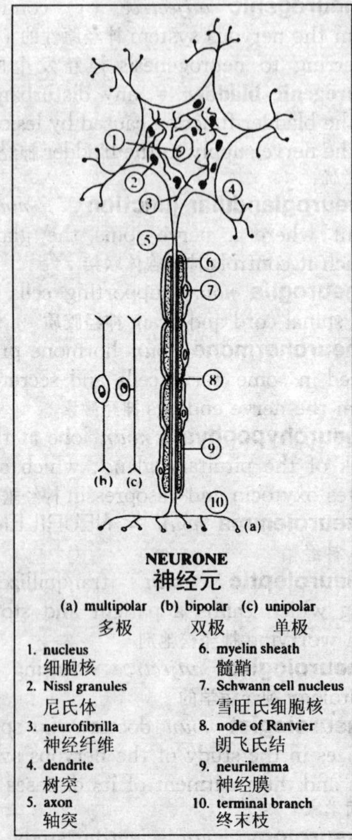

◇ **neurone** *or* **neuron** *or* **nerve cell** *noun* cell in the nervous system which transmits nerve impulses 神经元; **bipolar neurone** = neurone with two processes (found in the retina) 双极神经元; **motor neurone** = neurone which is part of a nerve pathway transmitting impulses from the brain to a muscle or gland 运动神经元; **upper motor neurone** = neurone which takes impulses from the cerebral cortex 上运动神经元; **lower motor neurone** = linked neurones which carry motor impulses from the spinal cord to the muscles 下运动神经元; **multipolar neurone** = neurone with several processes 多极神经元; **sensory neurone** = sensory neurone which receives its stimulus directly from the receptor, and passes the impulse to the sensory cortex 感觉神经元; **unipolar neurone** = neurone with a single process 单极神经元

neuropathology *noun* study of diseases of the nervous system 神经病理学

◇ **neuropathy** *noun* disease involving destruction of the tissues of the nervous system 神经病

◇ **neurophysiologist** *noun* scientist who studies the physiology of the nervous system 神经生理学家

◇ **neurophysiology** *noun* study of the physiology of nerves 神经生理学

◇ **neuroplasty** *noun* surgery to repair damaged nerves 神经修复术

◇ **neuropsychiatric** *adjective* referring to neuropsychiatry 神经精神病学的

◇ **neuropsychiatrist** *noun* doctor who specializes in the study and treatment of mental and nervous disorders 神经精神病学家

◇ **neuropsychiatry** *noun* study of mental and nervous disorders 神经精神病学

◇ **neurorrhaphy** *noun* surgical operation to join by suture a nerve which has been cut 神经缝合术

◇ **neuroscientist** *noun* scientist who studies the nervous system 神经科学家

◇ **neurosecretion** *noun* (i) substance secreted by a nerve cell 神经分泌物 (ii) secretion of active substance by nerve cells 神经分泌

neurosis *noun* illness of the personality, in which a patient becomes obsessed with something and experiences strong emotions towards it, such as fear of empty spaces, jealousy of a sibling, etc. 神经症; **anxiety neurosis** = neurotic condition where the patient is anxious and has morbid fears 焦虑性神经症 (NOTE: plural is **neuroses**)

◇ **neurotic** *noun & adjective* (i) (person) who suffers from neurosis 神经症的(患者) (ii) (any person) who is worried or obsessed with something 精神紧张的

(者)

◇ **neurotically** *adverb* in a neurotic way 神经质地: ***She is neurotically obsessed with keeping herself clean.*** 她神经质地执着于保持个人卫生。

neurosurgeon *noun* surgeon who operates on the nervous system, including the brain 神经外科医师

◇ **neurosurgery** *noun* surgery on the nervous system, including the brain and spinal cord 神经外科

◇ **neurosyphilis** *noun* syphilis which attacks the nervous system 神经梅毒

◇ **neurotmesis** *noun* cutting a nerve completely 神经断离

◇ **neurotomy** *noun* surgical operation to cut a nerve 神经切断术

◇ **neurotoxic** *adjective* (substance) which can harm or be poisonous to nerve cells 神经毒性的

◇ **neurotransmitter** *noun* chemical substance which transmits nerve impulses from one neurone to another 神经递质

◇ **neurotripsy** *noun* surgical bruising *or* crushing of a nerve 神经压轧术

◇ **neurotropic** *adjective* (bacterium) which is attracted to and attacks nerves 亲神经的

neuter *adjective* neither male nor female 中性的(非雌非雄)

◇ **neutral** *adjective* neither acid nor alkali 中性的(非酸非碱): ***A pH factor of 7 is neutral.*** *pH* 值等于7时为中性的。

neutralize *verb* to counteract the effect of something (*in bacteriology*) to make a toxin harmless by combining it with the correct amount of antitoxin 中和: ***Alkali poisoning can be neutralized by applying acid solution.*** 碱的毒性可以用酸溶液来中和。

neutropenia *noun* condition where there are fewer neutrophils than normal in the blood 中性粒细胞减少症

◇ **neutrophil** *adjective* polymorph, type of white blood cell with an irregular nucleus, which can attack and destroy bacteria 中性粒细胞

nevus *US* = NAEVUS 痣

newborn *adjective* & *noun* (baby) which has been born recently 新生儿,新生儿的

newton *noun* SI unit of measurement of force 牛顿 (NOTE: usually written **N** with figures **the muscle exerted a force of 5N**)

> COMMENT: 1 newton is the force required to move 1 kilogram at the speed of 1 metre per second.
> 注释:1 牛顿指把1千克的物体加速到1米/秒需要的力。

nexus *noun* link *or* point where two organs *or* tissues join 结合,联合

NF = NEUROFIBROMATOSIS 神经纤维瘤病

NHS = NATIONAL HEALTH SERVICE 国家卫生保健事业

niacin *or* **nicotinic acid** ($C_6H_5NO_2$) *noun* vitamin of the vitamin B complex found in milk, meat, liver, kidney, yeast, beans, peas and bread (lack of niacin can cause mental disorders and pellagra) 烟酸

nick 1 *noun* little cut 小伤口: ***He had a nick in his ear lobe which bled.*** 他耳廓上有一个流着血的小伤口。**2** *verb* to make a little cut 切一个小口,划破一个小口: ***He nicked his chin while shaving.*** 他剃须时划了个小口子。

nicotine ($C_{10}H_{14}N_2$) *noun* main alkaloid substance found in tobacco 尼古丁,烟碱; **nicotine addiction** = addiction to nicotine, derived from smoking tobacco 尼古丁成瘾; **nicotine patch** = patch containing nicotine which is released slowly into the bloodstream, as a method of curing nicotine addiction 尼古丁贴片; **nicotine poisoning** *or* **nicotinism** = poisoning of the autonomic nervous system with large quantities of nicotine 尼古丁中毒

◇ **nicotinic acid** *noun* = NIACIN 烟酸

nictation *or* **nictitation** *noun* act of winking 眨眼,瞬目

nidation *noun* (**a**) building of the endometrial layers of the uterus between menstrual periods 子宫内膜复生（**b**）implantation, the point in the development of an embryo, when the fertilized ovum reaches the uterus and implants in the wall of the uterus 着床

nidus *noun* centre of infection *or* site where bacteria can settle and breed 病灶

Nielsen 尼耳森氏 *see* 见 HOLGER

night *noun* period between sunset and sunrise *or* part of the day when it is dark 晚上，夜里：***I don't like going out alone late at night.*** 我不喜欢深夜独自外出。***There are two nurses on duty each night.*** 每晚有两名护士值班。**night blindness** = NYCTALOPIA 夜盲症；**night duty** = being on duty at night 夜班；**night nurse** = nurse who is on duty at night 夜班护士；**night sweat** = heavy sweating when asleep at night 夜间盗汗；**night terror** = disturbed sleep, which a child does not remember 梦惊

◇ **nightmare** *noun* dream which frightens 梦魇，噩梦：***The little girl had a nightmare and woke up screaming.*** 小女孩做了个噩梦，尖叫着醒了。

◇ **nightshade** 茄属植物 *see* 见 BELLADONNA

nigra 黑质 *see* 见 LINEA

ninety-nine（**99**）*number* number which a doctor asks someone to say, so that he can inspect the back of the throat 医生让病人说出英文 99，以检查其咽部，相当于中国医生让病人"啊"：***The doctor told him to open his mouth wide and say ninety-nine.*** 医生让他张大嘴，说"啊"。

nipple *or* **mammilla** *noun* protruding darker part in the centre of the breast, containing the milk ducts through which the milk passes 乳头

Nissl granules *or* **Nissl bodies** *noun* coarse granules surrounding the nucleus in the cytoplasm of nerve cells 尼斯尔体，尼氏体 ◊ 见图 NEURONE

nit *noun* egg or larva of a louse 虱卵

nitrogen *noun* chemical element, a gas which is the main component of air and is an essential part of protein 氮（NOTE：chemical symbol is **N**）

◇ **nitrous oxide** *or* **laughing gas**（N_2O）*noun* colourless gas with a sweet smell, used in combination with other gases as an anaesthetic in dentistry and surgery 一氧化二氮，笑气

> COMMENT：Nitrogen is taken into the body by digesting protein-rich foods; excess nitrogen is excreted in urine. When the intake of nitrogen and the excretion rate are equal, the body is in nitrogen balance or protein balance.
> 注释：人体通过消化富含蛋白质的食物摄入氮；多余的氮从尿液排出体外。如果氮的摄入和排出量是相等的，身体处于氮平衡或称蛋白质平衡。

nm = NANOMETRE 纳米

nmol = NANOMOLE 纳摩尔

NMR = NUCLEAR MAGNETIC RESONANCE 核磁共振

Nocardia *noun* genus of bacteria found in soil, some species of which cause nocardiosis and Madura foot 诺卡菌属，放线菌属

◇ **nocardiosis** *or* **nocardiasis** *noun* lung infection which may metastasize to other tissue, caused by *Nocardia* 放线菌病

nociceptive *adjective*（nerves）which carry pain to the brain 感受伤害的

◇ **nociceptor** *noun* sensory nerve which carries pain to the brain 伤害感受器

nocte *Latin word meaning* 'at night'（written on prescriptions）在夜里（处方用语）（NOTE：opposite is **mane**）

◇ **nocturia** *noun* passing abnormally large quantity of urine during the night 夜尿

◇ **nocturnal** *adjective* at night 夜间的；**nocturnal enuresis** *or* **bedwetting** = passing urine when asleep in bed at night（especially used of children）遗尿，尿床

nod 1 *noun* moving the head forward（as to show agreement）点头：***When the***

nurse asked him if he wanted a drink, he gave a nod. 护士问他是否要喝水时,他点了一下头。**2** *verb* to move the head forward (as to show agreement) 点头: ***When she asked if anyone wanted an ice cream, all the children nodded.*** 当她问有没有人要冰淇淋时,所有的孩子都点了头。

◇ **nod off** *verb* (*informal* 非正式) to begin to go to sleep 打瞌睡: ***He nodded off in his chair.*** 他坐在椅子上打瞌睡。

nodal *adjective* referring to nodes 结的; **nodal tachycardia** = sudden attack of rapid heartbeats 窦性心动过速

node *noun* (i) small mass of tissue 结节 (ii) group of nerve cells 神经结; **atrioventricular node** *or* **AV node** = mass of conducting tissue in the right atrium, which continues as the bundle of His and passes impulses from the atria to the ventricles 房室结; **axillary nodes** = part of the lymphatic system in the arm 腋窝淋巴结; **cervical nodes** = lymph nodes in the neck 颈淋巴结; **Heberden's node** = (手指骨关节炎时隆起的结节) small bony lump which develops on the terminal phalanges of fingers in osteoarthritis 希伯登结节; **lymph nodes** = glands of lymphoid tissue situated at various points of the lymphatic system (especially under the armpits and in the groin), through which lymph passes and in which lymphocytes are produced 淋巴结; **Osler's nodes** = tender swellings at the ends of fingers and toes in patients suffering from subacute bacterial endocarditis 奥斯勒结节(亚急性细菌性心内膜炎时指端的结节); **node of Ranvier** = one of a series of points along the length of a nerve, where the myelin sheath round the nerve fibre ends and connective tissue touches the axon 朗飞氏结

◇ **nodosa** 结节性 *see* 见 PERIARTERITIS

◇ **nodosum** 结节性 *see* 见 ERYTHEMA

◇ **nodule** *noun* small node or group of cells; anterior part of the inferior vermis 小结节 *see also* 参见 BOHN

◇ **nodular** *adjective* formed of nodules 小结节状的

noma *noun* cancrum oris, severe ulcers in the mouth, leading to gangrene 走马疳,坏疽性口炎

nomen proprium 药名 *see* 见 N.P.

non- *prefix* meaning not 不,否,非; **non-absorbable suture** = suture made of a substance which cannot be absorbed into the body, and which eventually has to be removed 不可吸收的缝线; **non-allergenic** = (cosmetic, etc.) which will not aggravate an allergy 非致敏的; **non-contagious** = not contagious 无沾染的,无污染的; **non-emergency surgery** *or* **non-urgent surgery** = operation, such as a joint replacement, for a condition which is not life-threatening and which, therefore, does not need to be performed immediately 非急诊手术; **non-nucleated** = (cell) with no nucleus 无细胞核的; **non-smoker** = person who does not smoke 不吸烟的人; **non-venereal disease** = disease which is not a venereal disease 非性病

non compos mentis *Latin phrase meaning* 'not of sound mind': (person) who is mentally incapable of managing his own affairs[拉丁语] 精神不健全

nongranular leucocytes *noun* leucocytes (such as lymphocytes *or* monocytes) which have no granules 非粒白细胞

non-invasive *adjective* (inspection *or* treatment) which does not involve entering the body by making an incision 非介入性的,无创性 *see also* 参见 INVASIVE

non-malignant *adjective* not malignant 良性的; **a non-malignant growth** 良性增生

non-medical *adjective* (word) which is not used in specialized medical speech 非医学专业的: ***'Nervous breakdown' is a non-medical term for a type of sudden mental illness.*** "神经崩溃"是对突发精神

病的一种外行说法。

non-secretor *noun* person who does not secrete indicators of blood grouping into body fluids 不分泌血型抗原的人

non-specific *adjective* (condition) which is not caused by any single identifiable cause 非特异的; **non-specific urethritis (NSU)** = formerly, sexually transmitted inflammation of the urethra not caused by gonorrhea 非特异性尿道炎(非淋病性尿道炎)

non-sterile *adjective* (dressing) which is not sterile *or* (instrument) which has not been sterilized 未消毒的

non-union *noun* condition where the two parts of a fractured bone do not join together and do not heal(骨折)未愈合

noradrenaline *or US* **norepinephrine** *noun* hormone secreted by the medulla of the adrenal glands which acts as a vasoconstrictor and is used to maintain blood pressure in shock or haemorrhage or hypotension 去甲肾上腺素

norma *noun* in anatomy, the skull as seen from a certain angle[拉丁语](颅骨)外观

normal *adjective* usual *or* ordinary *or* according to a standard 正常的: ***After taking the tablets, his blood pressure went back to normal.*** 服药后，他的血压恢复正常了。***Her temperature is two degrees above normal.*** 她的体温高于正常水平2度。***He had an above normal pulse rate.*** 他的脉搏比正常快。***It is normal for a person with myopia to suffer from headaches.*** 近视的人常头痛。

◊ **normally** *adverb* in a normal *or* ordinary way 正常地: ***The patients are normally worried before the operation.*** 病人对手术有些担心是正常的。***He was breathing normally.*** 他呼吸正常。

normoblast *noun* early form of a red blood cell, normally found only in bone marrow but found in the blood in certain types of leukaemia and anaemia 幼红细胞

normocyte *noun* normal red blood cell 正常红细胞

◊ **normocytic** *adjective* referring to a normocyte 正常红细胞的

◊ **normocytosis** *noun* having the normal number of red blood cells in the peripheral blood 血液中红细胞正常

normotension *noun* normal blood pressure 血压正常

◊ **normotensive** *adjective* (blood pressure) at normal level 血压正常的

nose *noun* organ through which a person breathes and smells 鼻子: ***She must have a cold - her nose is running.*** = Liquid mucus is dripping from her nose 她正在流鼻涕一定是感冒了。***He blew his nose.*** = He blew air through his nose into a handkerchief to get rid of mucus in his nose. 擤鼻涕。**to speak through your nose** = to speak as if your nose is blocked, so that you say 'b' instead of 'm' and 'd' instead of 'n' 鼻音

◊ **nosebleed** *noun* epistaxis, bleeding from the nose, usually caused by a blow *or* by sneezing *or* by blowing the nose hard *or* by high blood pressure 流鼻血: ***She had a headache, followed by a violent nosebleed.*** 她一阵头疼，紧接着猛流鼻血。(NOTE: for other terms referring to the nose, see words beginning with naso-, **rhin-**, **rhino**)

> COMMENT: The nose is formed of cartilage and small bones making the bridge at the top. It leads into two passages (the nostrils) which in turn lead to the nasal cavity, divided in two by the septum. The nasal passages connect with the sinuses, with the ears through the Eustachian tubes, and with the pharynx. The receptors which detect smell are in the top of the nasal passage.
> 注释：鼻子由软骨和小骨头构成鼻梁，它有2个通道(鼻孔)，通入鼻腔，鼻腔间被鼻中隔分开。鼻道与鼻窦和咽相连，并通过咽鼓管与耳道相通，感受味道的受体位于鼻腔的顶部。

noso- *prefix* referring to diseases 病

◇ **nosocomial** *adjective* referring to hospitals 医院的; **nosocomial infection** = infection which is passed on to someone in a hospital 医院内感染

◇ **nosology** *noun* classification of diseases 疾病分类学

nostril *or* **naris** *nou* one of the two passages in the nose through which air is breathed in or out 鼻孔: ***His right nostril is blocked.*** 他的右鼻孔堵了。

notch *noun* depression on a surface, usually on a bone, but sometimes on an organ 切迹; **cardiac notch** = (i) point in the left lung, where the right inside wall is bent 肺的心脏切迹 (ii) notch at the point where the oesophagus joins the greater curvature of the stomach 胃的心脏切迹; **occipital notch** = point on the lower edge of the cerebral hemisphere, where the surface has a notch 枕骨切迹

notice 1 *noun* (**a**) piece of writing giving information, usually put in a place where everyone can see it 通知: ***He pinned up a notice about the meeting.*** 他贴了一张开会通知。***Notices warning the public about the angers of rabies are posted at every port and airport.*** 每个港口和机场都张贴了警告狂犬病的通告。(**b**) warning 警告,提醒,预先通知: ***They had to leave with ten minutes' notice.*** 事先提醒他们在 *10* 分钟内离开。***It had to be done at short notice.*** = with very little warning time 做这事的时间很紧。(**c**) attention 注意,在意: ***Take no notice of what he says.*** = pay no attention to it *or* don't worry about it. 别在意他说什么。***She took no notice of what the doctor suggested.*** 她没在意医生的忠告。**2** *verb* to see *or* to take note of 注意,发现: ***Nobody noticed that the patient was sweating.*** 没人注意到病人在出汗。***Did you notice the development of any new symptoms?*** 你发现产生新症状了吗?

◇ **noticeable** *adjective* which can be noticed 能觉察到的: ***The disease has no easily noticeable symptoms.*** 这种病没有易于识别的症状。

◇ **noticeboard** *noun* flat piece of wood, etc., on a wall, on which notices can be pinned 布告栏

notify *verb* to inform someone officially 正式通知,正式通报: ***The local doctor notified the Health Service of the case of cholera.*** 当地医生向卫生部门报告了一例霍乱病例。(NOTE: you notify someone **of something**)

◇ **notifiable disease** *noun* serious infectious disease which in Great Britain has to be reported by a doctor to the Department of Health so that steps can be taken to stop it spreading 应上报的疾病

> COMMENT: The following are notifiable diseases: cholera, diphtheria, dysentery, encephalitis, food poisoning, jaundice, malaria, measles, meningitis, ophthalmia neonatorum, paratyphoid, plague, poliomyelitis, relapsing fever, scarlet fever, smallpox, tuberculosis, typhoid, typhus, whooping cough, yellow fever.
> 注释:应上报的疾病有:霍乱、白喉、痢疾、脑炎、食物中毒、黄疸、疟疾、麻疹、脑膜炎、新生儿眼炎、副伤寒、鼠疫、脊髓灰质炎、回归热、猩红热、天花、结核病、伤寒、斑疹伤寒、百日咳、黄热病。

nourish *verb* to give food *or* nutrients to (someone) 滋养,营养; **nourishing food** = food (such as liver *or* brown bread) which supplies nourishment 有营养的食品

◇ **nourishment** *noun* (i) act of supplying nutrients 营养供给 (ii) nutrients (such as proteins, fats or vitamins) 营养品

noxious *adjective* harmful (drug *or* gas) 有毒的

n. p. *abbreviation for* (缩写) *the Latin phrase* 'nomen proprium': the name of the drug (written on the label of the container) [拉丁语] 药名

NPO *abbreviation for* (缩写) *the Latin phrase* 'nil per oram': nothing by the mouth (used to refer to patients being kept without food) [拉丁语] 禁食: ***The patient should be kept NPO for five hours before the operation.*** 手术前5小时病人应当禁食。

NSU = NON-SPECIFIC URETHRITIS 非特异性尿道炎

nucha *or* **nape** *noun* back of the neck 项,颈部后面,后脖颈子

◇ **nuchal** *adjective* referring to the nape 项的,颈后部的

nuclear *adjective* referring to nuclei 核的; **nuclear magnetic resonance (NMR)** = scanning technique, using magnetic fields and radio waves, which reveals abnormalities in soft tissue *or* body fluids, etc. 核磁共振 *see also* 参见 MAGNETIC RESONANCE IMAGING; **nuclear medicine** = use of radioactive substances for detecting and treating disorders 核医学; **nuclear radiation** 核辐射 *see* 见 RADIATION

◇ **nuclease** *noun* enzyme which breaks down the nucleic acids 核酸酶

◇ **nucleic acids** *noun* organic acids combined with proteins (DNA or RNA) which exist in the nucleus and protoplasm of all cells 核酸

◇ **nucleolus** *noun* structure inside a cell nucleus containing RNA 核仁

◇ **nucleoprotein** *noun* compound of protein and nucleic acid, such as chromosomes or ribosomes 核蛋白

◇ **nucleus** *noun* (**a**) central body in a cell, containing DNA and RNA, and controlling the function and characteristics of the cell 细胞核 (**b**) group of nerve cells in the brain or spinal cord 核团; **basal nuclei** = masses of grey matter at the bottom of each cerebral hemisphere 基底核; **nucleus pulposus** = soft central part of an intervertebral disc which disappears in old age 髓核 ◊ 见图 NEURONE (NOTE: the plural is **nuclei**)

nullipara *noun & adjective* (woman) who has never had a child 未产妇女,没生过孩子的

numb *adjective* (limb) which has no feeling 麻木的: ***Her fingers were numb with cold.*** 她的手指冻麻木了。 ***The tips of his ears went numb*** *or* **became numb.** 他的耳垂麻木了。

◇ **numbness** *noun* loss of feeling 麻木

nurse 1 *noun* person (usually a woman) who looks after sick people in a hospital *or* helps a doctor in his surgery 护士: ***She works as a nurse in the local hospital.*** 她在当地医院当护士。 ***She's training to be a nurse.*** 她在接受当护士的培训。 **charge nurse** = nurse who is in charge of a group of patients, a ward or a department in a hospital 主管护士; **district nurse** *or* **home nurse** = nurse who visits and treats patients in their homes 地区护士,家庭护士; **escort nurse** = nurse who goes with a patient to the operating theatre and back to the ward 护送护士; **practice nurse** *or* **nurse practitioner** = nurse employed by a clinic *or* doctor's practice who can give advice to patients 开业护士; **staff nurse** = nurse who is on the permanent staff of a hospital 医院护士; **theatre nurse** = nurse who is specially trained to assist a surgeon during an operation 手术室护士; **ward nurse** = nurse who works in a hospital ward 病房护士; **nurse manager** = nurse who has administrative duties in the health service *or* in a hospital 护理部主任 (NOTE: although the term nurse applies to both men and women, in popular speech it is used more frequently to refer to women, and **male nurse** is used for men. Nurse can be used as a title before a name: **Nurse Jones**) **2** *verb* to look after sick people 护理,照顾: ***When he was ill his mother nursed him until he was better.*** 他得病时由母亲照顾,直到他好起来。

> COMMENT: In the UK qualified nurses are either ENs (Enrolled Nurses) or RNs (Registered Nurses). Registered nurses follow a three year course and have to pass the ENB examinations before becoming RGN, RMN or RNMH.

RSCNs have a further 6 months or 4 term course before they qualify. Enrolled nurses follow 2 year courses.
注释:英国合格的护士有两种:登记护士和注册护士。注册护士要学习三年的课程并通过 ENB 考试才能成为注册全科护士、注册心理护士或注册精神残疾专科护士。若要成为合格的注册儿科护士则要再上 6 个月或 4 个学期的课。登记护士需要上 2 年的课。

◇ **nursery school** *noun* school for little children 幼儿园; **day nursery** = place where small children can be looked after during the daytime, and go home in the evenings 日托幼儿园

◇ **nursing 1** *noun* work *or* profession of being a nurse 护理工作: ***She enjoys nursing.*** 她喜爱护理工作。***He is taking a nursing course.*** 他正在学习护理课程。***He has chosen nursing as his career.*** 他已经选定护理为自己的职业。**nursing home** = house where convalescents or old people can live under medical supervision by a qualified nurse 疗养院; **nursing practice** = treatment given by nurses 护理操作; **nursing process** = standard method of treatment carried out by nurses and its documentation 护理经过 **2** *adjective* providing care as a nurse 照顾,看护; **nursing mother** = mother who breast-feeds her baby 哺乳母亲; **nursing officer** = nurse who has administrative duties in the National Health Service 护理官员

QUOTE: Few would now dispute the need for clear, concise nursing plans to guide nursing practice, provide educational tools and give an accurate legal record.
引文:现在不再有人争论清晰、简洁的护理计划在指导护理操作、提供教育工具和使病历记录准确合法上的必要性了。
Nursing Times 护理时代

QUOTE: All relevant sections of the nurses' care plan and nursing process records had been left blank.
引文:护士的护理计划和护理过程记录都是空白。
Nursing Times 护理时代

nutans 点头的 *see* 见 SPASMUS

nutation *noun* involuntary nodding of the head 点头(尤指不随意点头)

nutrient *noun* substance (such as protein *or* fat *or* vitamin) in food which is necessary to provide energy or to help the body grow 营养素

◇ **nutrition** *noun* (i) study of the supply of nutrients to the body from digesting food 营养学 (ii) nourishment *or* food 营养品

◇ **nutritional** *adjective* referring to nutrition 营养学的,营养品的; **nutritional anaemia** = anaemia caused by an imbalance in the diet 营养性贫血; **nutritional disorder** = disorder (such as obesity) related to food and nutrients 营养紊乱

◇ **nutritionist** *noun* dietitian *or* person who specializes in the study of nutrition and advises on diets 营养师

nyctalopia *noun* night blindness, being unable to see in bad light 夜盲症

◇ **nyctophobia** *noun* fear of the dark 恐黑

nymphae *noun* the labia minora, two small fleshy folds at the edge of the vulva 小阴唇

◇ **nymphomania** *noun* obsessive sexual urge in a woman 女性色情狂,慕男狂 (NOTE: in a man, called **satyriasis**)

◇ **nymphomaniac** *noun* woman who has an abnormally obsessive sexual urge 色情女

nystagmus *noun* rapid movement of the eyes up and down or from side to side 眼震

COMMENT: Nystagmus can be congenital, but is also a symptom of multiple sclerosis and Ménière's disease.
注释:眼震可以是先天性的,也可以是多发性硬化或梅尼尔氏病的症状。

Oo

O *chemical symbol for* 'oxygen' 氧的化学元素符号

oat cell carcinoma *noun* type of cancer of the bronchi, with distinctive small cells 燕麦细胞癌

obese 1 *adjective* (person who is) too fat *or* too heavy 肥胖的 **2** *plural noun* **the obese** = overweight people 胖子

◇ **obesity** *noun* being overweight 肥胖

> COMMENT: Obesity is caused by excess fat accumulating under the skin and around organs in the body. It is sometimes due to glandular disorders, but it is usually caused by eating or drinking too much. A tendency to obesity can be hereditary.
> 注释:肥胖是由于脂肪过度堆积于皮下或器官周围所致,腺体分泌异常可导致肥胖,但通常是由于进食过量或饮料喝得过多引起的,而且肥胖有遗传倾向。

obey *verb* to do what someone *or* a rule says you should do 服从: ***You ought to obey the doctor's instructions and go to bed.*** 你应当遵照医嘱去睡觉。***Patients must obey the hospital rules.*** 病人必须遵守医院的规定。

obligate *adjective* (organism) which exists and develops in only one way (as viruses which are parasites only inside cells) 专性的,必需的

oblique *noun* & *adjective* (muscle) which lies at an angle 斜的; **oblique fissure** = groove between the lobes of the lungs(肺)斜裂; **oblique fracture** = fracture where the bone is not broken directly across its axis 斜行骨折; **oblique muscle** = (i) muscle which controls the eyeball 眼斜肌(如控制眼动的上斜肌,下斜肌) (ii) muscle which controls the abdominal wall 腹斜肌(如腹内斜肌,腹外斜肌); **external oblique** = outer abdominal muscle 腹外斜肌; **internal oblique** = muscle covering the abdomen beneath the external oblique 腹内斜肌

> QUOTE: There are four recti muscles and two oblique muscles in each eye, which coordinate the movement of the eyes and enable them to work as a pair.
> 引文:每只眼睛有四条直肌和两条斜肌,它们协调眼球的运动,使双眼能配合发挥功能。
>
> **Nursing Times** 护理时代

obliterans 闭塞性 *see* 见 ENDARTERITIS

obliterate *verb* to remove a cavity completely 消灭,去除(腔隙)

◇ **obliteration** *noun* complete removal *or* eradication (of a cavity, etc.)消除,消失,去除(腔隙)

oblongata 延髓 *see* 见 MEDULLA

observe *verb* to notice *or* to see something and understand it 观察: ***The nurses observed signs of improvement in the patient's condition.*** 护士观察到病人状况改善。***The girl's mother observed symptoms of anorexia and reported them to her doctor.*** 母亲注意到女孩的厌食症状并把这一情况报告了医生。

◇ **observation** *noun* examining something over a period of time 观察: ***He was admitted to hospital for observation.*** 收他住院观察。

obsession *noun* mental disorder where the patient has a fixed idea *or* emotion which he cannot get rid of, even if he knows it is wrong or unpleasant 强迫(症): ***She has an obsession about cats.*** 她对猫有强迫症状。

◇ **obsessional** *adjective* referring to an obsession 强迫的: ***He is suffering from an obsessional disorder.*** 他患了强迫症。

◇ **obsessed** *adjective* suffering from an obsession(被)强迫的: ***He is obsessed with the idea that his wife is trying to kill him.*** 他强迫认为妻子要杀死他。

◇ **obsessive** *adjective* showing an obsession 有强迫症状的,强迫性的: ***He has an obsessive desire to steal little objects.***

他强迫性渴望偷盗小东西。**obsessive action** = repeated actions (such as washing) which indicate a mental disorder 强迫行为

obstetrics *noun* branch of medicine and surgery dealing with pregnancy, childbirth and the period immediately after childbirth 产科,产科学

◊ **obstetric(al)** *adjective* referring to obstetrics 产科的,产科学的; **obstetrical forceps** = type of large forceps used to hold a baby's head during childbirth 产钳; **obstetric patient** = woman who is being treated by an obstetrician 产妇

◊ **obstetrician** *noun* doctor who specializes in obstetrics 产科医师

obstruct *verb* to block 阻塞: ***The artery was obstructed by a blood clot.*** 血栓阻塞了动脉。

◊ **obstruction** *noun* (i) something which blocks (a passage *or* a blood vessel) 阻塞物 (ii) blocking of a passage *or* blood vessel 阻塞; **intestinal obstruction** *or* **obstruction of the bowels** = blockage of the intestine 肠梗阻; **urinary obstruction** = blockage of the urethra, which prevents urine being passed 尿路梗阻

◊ **obstructive** *adjective* caused by an obstruction 梗阻的,阻塞的; **obstructive jaundice** = jaundice caused by an obstruction in the bile ducts 阻塞性黄疸; **obstructive lung disease** = bronchitis and emphysema 阻塞性肺病

obtain *verb* to get 得到,获得: ***Some amino acids are obtained from food.*** 某些氨基酸可以从食物中获得。***Where did he obtain the drugs?*** 他从哪搞到的药物?

obtrusive *adjective* (scar) which is very noticeable 突出的

obturator *noun* (i) one of two muscles in the pelvis which govern the movement of the hip and thigh 闭孔肌 (ii) device which closes an opening, such as a dental prosthesis which covers a cleft palate 充填器 (iii) metal bulb which fits into a bronchoscope *or* sigmoidoscope 内窥镜的金属快门; **obturator foramen** = opening in the hip bone near the acetabulum 闭孔

obtusion *noun* condition where perception and feelings become dulled 感觉迟钝

occiput *noun* lower part of the back of the head or skull(头颅)枕部

◊ **occipital** *adjective* referring to the back of the head 枕部的,枕骨的; **occipital bone** *or* **occipital** = one of the bones in the skull, the bone at the back of the head 枕骨; **occipital condyle** = round part of the occipital bone which joins it to the atlas 枕骨髁; **occipital lobe** = lobe at the back of each cerebral hemisphere 枕叶; **occipital notch** = point on the lower edge of the cerebral hemisphere where the surface has a notch 枕骨切迹

◊ **occipito-anterior** *adjective* (position of a baby at birth) where the baby faces the mother's back 枕前位

◊ **occipito-posterior** *adjective* (position of a baby at birth) where the baby faces the front 枕后位

occluded *adjective* closed *or* blocked 闭锁的

◊ **occlusion** *noun* (**a**) blockage *or* thing which blocks a passage *or* which closes an opening 闭锁,闭塞; **coronary occlusion** = blood clot in the coronary arteries leading to heart failure 冠脉闭塞 (**b**) the way in which the teeth in the upper and lower jaws fit together when the jaws are closed 咬合 (NOTE: a bad fit between the teeth is **a malocclusion**)

◊ **occlusive** *adjective* referring to occlusion *or* to blocking 闭锁的,闭塞的; **occlusive stroke** = stroke caused by a blood clot 闭塞性脑卒中; **occlusive therapy** = treatment of a squint where the good eye is covered up in order to encourage the squinting eye to become straight(斜视)遮盖疗法

occult *adjective* (i) not easy to see with the naked eye 不易用肉眼看见的 (ii) (symptom *or* sign) which is hidden (症状,体征)潜隐的; **occult blood** = very small quantities of blood in the faeces, which can only be detected by tests 潜血 (NOTE: the opposite is **overt**)

◇ **occulta**隐性 *see* 见 SPINA BIFIDA

occupancy rate *noun* number of beds occupied in a hospital, shown as a percentage of all the beds 床位占有率

occupation *noun* job *or* work 职业,工作: ***What is his occupation?*** 他是做什么工作的? ***People in sedentary occupations are liable to digestive disorders.*** 经常坐着工作的人易产生消化不良。

◇ **occupational** *adjective* referring to work 职业的,工作的; **occupational asthma** *or* **occupational dermatitis** = asthma *or* dermatitis caused by materials with which one comes into contact at work 职业性哮喘,职业性皮炎; **occupational disease** = disease which is caused by the type of work *or* the conditions in which someone works (such as disease caused by dust *or* chemicals in a factory) 职业病; **occupational health (OH) nurse** = nurse who deals with health problems of people at work 职业保健护士; **occupational therapist** = qualified therapist who treats people with mental or physical handicaps by using activities such as light work, hobbies, etc. 职业治疗师; **occupational therapy** = light work or hobbies used as a means of treatment, especially for handicapped or mentally ill patients and during the recovery period after an illness or operation 工娱治疗

occur *verb* to happen *or* to take place; to be found 发生,出现: ***Thrombosis occurred in the artery.*** 动脉血栓形成。***A form of glaucoma which occurs in infants.*** 一种发生于婴儿期的青光眼。***One of the most frequently occurring types of tumour.*** 最常见的肿瘤类型之一。

◇ **occurrence** *noun* taking place *or* happening 发生: ***Neuralgia is a common occurrence after shingles.*** 带状疱疹后常发生神经痛。

ochronosis *noun* condition where cartilage, ligaments and other fibrous tissue become dark as a result of a metabolic disorder, and also the urine turns black on exposure to air 褐黄病

ocular *adjective* referring to the eye 眼睛的: ***Opticians are trained to detect all kinds of ocular imbalance.*** 验光师被训练得能发现各种眼球运动的不协调。

◇ **oculi** 眼 *see* 见 ALBUGINEA, ORBICULARIS

◇ **oculist** *noun* qualified physician or surgeon who specializes in the treatment of eye disorders 眼科医师

◇ **oculogyric** *adjective* which causes eye movements 动眼的

◇ **oculomotor** *adjective* referring to movements of the eyeball 动眼的; **oculomotor nerve** = third cranial nerve which controls the eyeball and upper eyelid 动眼神经

◇ **oculonasal** *adjective* referring to the eye and the nose 眼鼻的

o.d. (**a**) *abbreviation for* (缩写) *the Latin phrase* 'omni die': every day (written on a prescription) 每天(用于处方书写) (**b**) *abbreviation for* (缩写) overdose 过量

ODA = OPERATING DEPARTMENT ASSISTANT 手术室助手

odont- *prefix* meaning teeth 牙齿

◇ **odontalgia** *noun* toothache 牙疼

◇ **odontitis** *noun* inflammation of the pulpy interior of a tooth 牙龈炎

◇ **odontoid process** *noun* projecting part of a vertebra, shaped like a tooth 齿状突

◇ **odontology** *noun* study of teeth and associated structures, and their disorders 牙科学

◇ **odontoma** *or* **odontome** *noun* (i) structure like a tooth which has an abnormal arrangement of its component tissues 牙齿样组织 (ii) solid or cystic tumour derived from cells concerned with the development of a tooth 牙瘤

odour *or US* **odor** *noun* smell 味道; **body odour** = unpleasant smell caused by perspiration 体味,体臭

◇ **odourless** *adjective* (liquid, etc.) with no smell 无味的

odynophagia *noun* condition where pain occurs when food is swallowed 吞咽痛

oe- (NOTE: words beginning with **oe-** are written **e-** in American English)

oedema *or US* **edema** *noun* dropsy, swelling of part of the body caused by accumulation of fluid in the intercellular tissue spaces 水肿: ***Her main problem is oedema of the feet.*** 她的主要问题是足部水肿。**macular oedema** = disorder of the eye where fluid gathers in the fovea 黄斑水肿; **pulmonary oedema** = collection of fluid in the lungs as in left-sided heart failure 肺水肿; **subcutaneous oedema** = fluid collecting under the skin, usually at the ankles 皮下水肿

◇ **oedematous** *adjective* referring to oedema 水肿的

Oedipus complex *noun* (*in psychology*) condition where a boy feels sexually attracted to his mother and sees his father as an obstacle (心理学)恋母情结

oesophageal *adjective* referring to the oesophagus 食管的; **oesophageal hiatus** = opening in the diaphragm through which the oesophagus passes 食管裂孔; **oesophageal spasm** = spasm in the oesophagus 食道痉挛; **oesophageal ulcer** = ulcer in the oesophagus 食管溃疡; **oesophageal varices** = varicose veins in the oesophagus 食管静脉曲张

◇ **oesophagectomy** *noun* surgical removal of part of the oesophagus 食管切除

◇ **oesophagitis** *noun* inflammation of the oesophagus (caused by acid juices from the stomach *or* by infection) 食管炎

◇ **oesophagocele** *noun* condition where the mucous membrane lining the oesophagus protrudes through the wall 食管粘膜膨出

◇ **oesophagoscope** *noun* thin tube with a light at the end, which is passed down the oesophagus to examine it 食管镜

◇ **oesophagoscopy** *noun* examination of the oesophagus with an oesophagoscope 食管内窥镜检查

◇ **oesophagostomy** *noun* surgical operation to make an opening in the oesophagus to allow the patient to be fed, usually after an operation on the pharynx 食管造口术

◇ **oesophagotomy** *noun* surgical operation to make an opening in the oesophagus to remove something which is blocking it 食管切开术

◇ **oesophagus** *US* **esophagus** *noun* tube down which food passes from the pharynx to the stomach 食管 ◊ 见图 STOMACH, THROAT

oestradiol *noun* type of oestrogen secreted by an ovarian follicle, which stimulates the development of secondary sexual characteristics in females at puberty (a synthetic form is given as treatment for oestrogen deficiency) 雌二醇

◇ **oestriol** *noun* placental hormone with oestrogenic properties, found in the urine of pregnant women 雌三醇

◇ **oestrogen** *noun* any substance with the physiological activity of oestradiol 雌激素

◇ **oestrogenic hormone** *noun* oestrogen used to treat conditions which develop during menopause 雌性激素

◇ **oestrone** *noun* type of oestrogen 雌酮

> COMMENT: Synthetic oestrogens form most oral contraceptives, and are also used in the treatment of menstrual and menopausal disorders.
> 注释:大多数口服避孕药是合成雌激素,它也可用来治疗月经紊乱和闭经。

official *adjective* (i) accepted by an authority 官方的,正式的 (ii) (drug) which is permitted by an authority 官方批准的(药物)

◇ **officially** *adverb* (accepted *or* permitted) by an authority 官方认可地,正式地: ***The drug has been officially listed as a dangerous drug.*** 这种药已被正式列为危险药品。

OH = OCCUPATIONAL HEALTH 职业保健; **an OH nurse** 一名职业保健护士

oil *noun* liquid which cannot be mixed with water (there are three types: fixed vegetable *or* animal oils; volatile oils; mineral oils) 油; **cod liver oil** = oil from the liver of the cod fish, which is rich in calories and in vitamins A and D 鱼肝油; **essential oils** = oils from scented plants used in cosmetics and as antiseptics 精炼油,香料油; **fixed oil** = oil which is liquid at 20 °C不挥发油

◇ **oily** *adjective* containing oil 油腻腻的,油糊糊的

ointment *noun* smooth oily medicinal preparation which can be spread on the skin to soothe *or* to protect 药膏,软膏

olecranon (process) *noun* curved process at the end of the ulna(尺骨)鹰嘴 (NOTE: called also **funny bone**)

oleic *adjective* referring to oil 油的; **oleic acid** = one of the fatty acids, present in most oils 油酸

◇ **oleaginous** *adjective* oily 油脂性的,油状的

◇ **oleum** *noun* (*term used in pharmacy*) oil[拉丁语]油(药剂学用语)

olfaction *noun* (i) sense of smell 嗅觉 (ii) way in which a person's sensory organs detect smells 嗅

◇ **olfactory** *adjective* referring to the sense of smell 嗅觉的; **olfactory bulb** = end of the olfactory tract, where the processes of the sensory cells in the nose are linked to the fibres of the olfactory nerve 嗅球; **olfactory nerve** = first cranial nerve which controls the sense of smell 嗅神经; **olfactory tract** = nerve tract which takes the olfactory nerve from the nose to the brain 嗅束

olig- *or* **oligo-** *prefix* meaning few *or* little 寡,少

◇ **oligaemia** *noun* condition where the patient has too little blood in his circulatory system 血量减少

◇ **oligodactylism** *noun* congenital condition where a baby is born without some fingers or toes 指(趾)缺少症

◇ **oligodipsia** *noun* condition where a patient does not want to drink 渴感缺乏

◇ **oligodontia** *noun* state in which most of the teeth are lacking 缺齿

◇ **oligohydramnios** *noun* condition where the amnion surrounding the fetus contains too little amniotic fluid 羊水过少

◇ **oligomenorrhoea** *noun* condition where the patient menstruates infrequently 月经稀少

◇ **oligospermia** *noun* condition where there are too few spermatozoa in the semen 精子缺乏症,少精症

◇ **oliguria** *noun* condition where the patient does not produce enough urine 少尿

olive *noun* (**a**) fruit of a tree, which gives an edible oil 橄榄 (**b**) swelling containing grey matter, on the side of the pyramid of the medulla oblongata(延髓)橄榄部

o. m. *abbreviation for* (缩写) *the Latin phrase* 'omni mane': every morning (written on a prescription)每天早晨(处方用语)

-oma *suffix* meaning tumour 瘤 (NOTE: plural is **-omata**)

Ombudsman 保健事业督察员 *see* 见 HEALTH SERVICE COMMISSIONER

oment- *prefix* referring to the omentum 网膜

◇ **omental** *adjective* referring to the omentum网膜的

◇ **omentectomy** *noun* surgical removal of part of the omentum 网膜切除术

◇ **omentopexy** *noun* surgical operation to attach the omentum to the abdominal wall 网膜固定术

◇ **omentum** *or* **epiploon** *noun* double fold of peritoneum hanging down over the intestines 网膜(NOTE: the plural is **omenta**, Note that for the terms referring to the omentum see words beginning with **epiplo**)

> COMMENT: The omentum is in two sections: the greater omentum which covers the intestines, and the lesser omentum which hangs between the liver and the stomach and the liver and the duodenum
> 注释:网膜分两部分:大网膜,覆盖小肠;小网膜,张于肝脏和胃以及肝脏和十二指肠之间。

omphal- *prefix* referring to the navel 脐

◇ **omphalitis** *noun* inflammation of the navel 脐炎

◇ **omphalocele** *noun* hernia where part of the intestine protrudes through the abdominal wall near the navel 脐疝

◇ **omphalus** *or* **navel** *or* **umbilicus** *noun* scar with a depression in the middle of the abdomen where the umbilical cord was detached after birth 脐

o. n. *abbreviation for* (缩写) *the Latin phrase* 'omni nocte': every night (written on a prescription) 每晚(处方用语)

onanism *noun* masturbation 手淫

Onchocerca *noun* genus of tropical parasitic threadworm 盘尾属

◇ **onchocerciasis** *noun* infestation with *Onchocerca* where the larvae can move into the eye, causing river blindness 盘尾丝虫病

onco- *prefix* referring to tumours 肿瘤

◇ **oncogene** *noun* part of the genetic system which causes malignant tumours to develop 瘤基因

◇ **oncogenesis** *noun* origin and development of a tumour 肿瘤形成,肿瘤发生

◇ **oncogenic** *adjective* (substance *or* virus) which causes tumours to develop 致肿瘤的

◇ **oncology** *noun* scientific study of new growths 肿瘤学

◇ **oncolysis** *noun* destruction of a tumour *or* of tumour cells 瘤细胞溶解

◇ **oncotic** *adjective* referring to a tumour 肿瘤的

> QUOTE: All cancers may be reduced to fundamental mechanisms based on cancer risk genes or oncogenes within ourselves. An oncogene is a gene that encodes a protein that contributes to the malignant phenotype of the cell.
> 引文:所有癌症都可以溯源到我们体内的癌高危基因或称瘤基因这一基本机制上。癌基因是编码调控细胞表型恶性转化蛋白的基因。
> **British Medical Journal** 英国医学杂志

onset *noun* beginning 发作,发病: ***The onset of the illness is marked by sudden high temperature.*** 这种病的发作以突起高热为标志。

> QUOTE: A follow-up study of 84 patients with early onset pre-eclampsia (before 37 weeks' gestation) showed a high prevalence of renal disease.
> 引文:对 84 名早发型(孕 37 周以前)先兆子痫患者的随访研究发现她们的肾病患病率较高。
> **British Medical Journal** 英国医学杂志

ontogeny *noun* origin and development of an individual organism 个体发生

onych- *prefix* referring to nails 指(趾)甲

◇ **onychauxis** *noun* overgrowth of the nails of the fingers or toes 甲肥厚

◇ **onychia** *noun* abnormality of the nails, caused by inflammation of the matrix 甲沟炎

◇ **onychogryphosis** *noun* condition where the nails are bent or curved over the ends of the fingers or toes 甲弯曲

◇ **onycholysis** *noun* condition where a nail becomes separated from its bed, without falling out 甲剥离

◇ **onychomadesis** *noun* condition where the nails fall out 甲缺失

◇ **onychomycosis** *noun* infection of the nail with a fungus 甲癣

◇ **onychosis** *noun* any disease of the nails 甲病

o'nyong-nyong fever *or* **joint-breaker fever** *noun* infectious virus disease prevalent in East Africa, spread by mosquitoes 关节断裂热,东非的一种由蚊子传播的病毒感染性疾病

> COMMENT: The symptoms are high fever, inflammation of the lymph nodes and excruciating pains in the joints.
> 注释:症状为高热、淋巴结炎和关节剧痛。

oo- *prefix* referring to an ovum *or* to an embryo 卵;孕卵

◇ **oocyesis** *noun* pregnancy which develops in the ovary 卵巢妊娠

◇ **oocyte** *noun* cell which forms from an oogonium and becomes an ovum by meiosis 卵母细胞

◇ **oogenesis** *noun* formation and development of ova 卵子发生

◇ **oogenetic** *adjective* referring to oogenesis 卵子发生的,卵子形成的

◇ **oogonium** *noun* cell produced at the beginning of the development of an ovum 卵原细胞 (NOTE: the plural is **oogonia**)

> COMMENT: In oogenesis, an oogonium produces an oocyte which develops through several stages to produce a mature ovum. Polar bodies are also formed which do not develop into ova.
> 注释:在卵子发生过程中,一个卵原细胞产生一个卵母细胞,卵母细胞再经过几个阶段发育成一个成熟的卵子。也可形成不发育成卵子的极体。

oopho- *or* **oophoro-** *prefix* referring to the ovaries 卵巢

◇ **oophoralgia** *noun* pain in the ovaries 卵巢痛

◇ **oophorectomy** *or* **ovariectomy** *noun* surgical removal of an ovary 卵巢切除术

◇ **oophoritis** *or* **ovaritis** *noun* inflammation in an ovary, which can be caused by mumps 卵巢炎

◇ **oophoroma** *noun* rare ovarian tumour, occurring in middle age 恶性卵巢瘤

◇ **oophoron** *or* **ovary** *noun* one of two organs in a woman which produce ova *or* egg cells and secrete the female hormone oestrogen 卵巢

◇ **oophoropexy** *noun* surgical operation to attach an ovary 卵巢固定术

◇ **oophorosalpingectomy** *noun* surgical removal of an ovary and the Fallopian tube attached to it 卵巢输卵管切除术

ooze *verb* (*of pus or blood*) to flow slowly(脓或血)渗出

OP = OUTPATIENT 门诊患者

opacity *noun* (i) not allowing light to pass through 浑浊,不透明 (ii) area in the eye which is not clear 浑浊斑

◇ **opaque** *adjective* not transparent 不透明的;**radio-opaque dye** = liquid which appears on an X-ray, and which is introduced into soft organs (such as the kidney) so that they show up clearly on an X-ray photograph 不透X线的染料(用作造影剂)

open *adjective* not closed 开放的;**open fracture** *or* **compound fracture** = fracture where the skin surface is damaged *or* where the broken bone penetrates the surface of the skin 开放性骨折,有创骨折;**open-heart surgery** = surgery to repair part of the heart *or* one of the coronary arteries, performed while the heart has been bypassed and the blood is circulated by a pump 需心脏转流的手术,需心脏切开的手术;**open visiting** = arrangement in a hospital where visitors can enter the wards at any time 开放探视

◇ **opening** *noun* place where something opens 开口

operation *noun* (i) way in which a drug acts 药物起作用的方式 (ii) surgical intervention *or* act of cutting open a patient's body to treat a disease *or* disorder 手术:***She's had an operation on her foot.*** 她做了一次足部手术。***The operation***

to remove the cataract was successful*.**去除白内障的手术成功了。A team of surgeons performed the operation*.**手术由手术小组完成。***Heart operations are always difficult*.**心脏手术总是有难度的。(NOTE: a surgeon **performs** an operation **on** a patient)

◇ **operable** *adjective* (condition) which can be treated by an operation 可以施行手术的: ***The cancer is still operable*.**这个癌瘤还可以手术切除。

◇ **operate** *verb* (**a**) **to operate on a patient** = to treat a patient's condition by cutting open his body and removing a part which is diseased *or* repairing a part which is not functioning correctly 给某位病人做手术: ***The patient was operated on yesterday*.**这个病人昨天接受了手术。***The surgeons decided to operate as the only way of saving the baby's life*.**外科医师认为,手术是挽救这个婴儿生命的惟一方法。**operating department assistant** (**ODA**) = nurse working in the operating department 手术室助手; **operating microscope** = special microscope with two eyepieces and a light, used in very delicate surgery 手术显微镜; **operating theatre** *US* **operating room** (**OR**) = special room in a hospital where surgeons carry out operations 手术室; **operating table** = special table on which the patient is placed to undergo a surgical operation 手术台 (**b**) **operating gene** = the gene in an operon which regulates the functions of the others 操纵子基因

◇ **operative** *or* **peroperative** *adjective* taking place during a surgical operation 手术过程中的,手术的 *see also* 参见 POSTOPERATIVE, PREOPERATIVE

◇ **operator** *noun* surgeon who operates 术者; **operator gene** = OPERATING GENE 操纵子基因

operculum *noun* (i) part of the cerebral hemisphere which overlaps the insula 大脑被盖 (ii) plug of mucus which can block the cervical canal during pregnancy 宫颈粘液栓

operon *noun* group of genes which controls the production of enzymes 操纵子

ophth- *prefix* referring to the eye 眼

◇ **ophthalmectomy** *noun* surgical removal of an eye 眼球摘除术

◇ **ophthalmia** *noun* inflammation of the eye 眼炎; **ophthalmia neonatorum** = conjunctivitis of a newborn baby, beginning 21 days after birth, caused by infection in the birth canal 新生儿眼炎; **Egyptian ophthalmia** *or* **trachoma** = virus disease of the eyes, common in tropical countries 埃及眼炎,沙眼

◇ **ophthalmic** *adjective* referring to the eye 眼睛的; **ophthalmic practitioner** *or* **optician** = qualified person who specializes in testing eyes and prescribing lenses 验光师; **ophthalmic surgeon** = surgeon who specializes in surgery to treat eye disorders 眼科医师; **ophthalmic nerve** = branch of the trigeminal nerve, supplying the eyeball, the upper eyelid, the brow and one side of the scalp 三叉神经眼支

◇ **ophthalmitis** *noun* inflammation of the eye 眼炎

◇ **ophthalmological** *adjective* referring to ophthalmology 眼科学的

◇ **ophthalmologist** *noun* doctor who specializes in the study of the eye and its diseases 眼科学家

◇ **ophthalmology** *noun* study of the eye and its diseases 眼科学

◇ **ophthalmoplegia** *noun* paralysis of the muscles of the eye 眼肌麻痹

◇ **ophthalmoscope** *noun* instrument containing a bright light and small lenses, used by a doctor to examine the inside of an eye 检眼镜

◇ **ophthalmoscopy** *noun* examination of the inside of an eye using an ophthalmoscope 用检眼镜检查

◇ **ophthalmotomy** *noun* surgical operation to make a cut in the eyeball 眼球切开术

◇ **ophthalmotonometer** *noun*

tonometer, instrument which measures pressure inside the eye 眼压仪

-opia *suffix* referring to a defect in the eye 眼,视力; **myopia** = being short-sighted 近视

opiate *noun* sedative which is prepared from opium, such as morphine or codeine 阿片制剂

◇ **opium** *noun* substance made from poppies, used in the preparation of codeine and heroin 阿片

opinion *noun* what someone thinks about something 观点,看法: ***What's the surgeon's opinion of the case***? 外科医师对这个病例有什么看法? ***The doctor asked the consultant for his opinion as to the best method of treatment***. 医生向会诊医师询问对最佳治疗方法。***She has a very high or very low opinion of her doctor***. = She thinks he is very good *or* very bad. 她很重视或轻视她的医生。**to ask for a second opinion** = to ask another doctor *or* consultant to examine a patient and give his opinion on diagnosis *or* treatment 征询会诊意见

opponens *noun* muscles of the fingers which tend to draw these fingers opposite to other fingers 对掌肌,对跖肌 *see* 见 OPPOSITION

opportunist(ic) *adjective* (parasite *or* microbe) which senses that an organism is weak and then attacks it 机会致病菌的,机会主义者的

opposition *noun* movement of the hand muscles where the tip of the thumb is made to touch the tip of another finger so as to hold something 对指

opsonic index *noun* number which gives the strength of an individual's serum reaction to bacteria 调理指数

◇ **opsonin** *noun* substance, usually an antibody, in blood which sticks to the surface of bacteria and helps to destroy them 调理素

optic *adjective* referring to the eye *or* to sight 视力的,视觉的;眼的,光学的;**optic chiasma** = structure where some of the optic nerves from each eye partially cross each other in the hypothalamus 视交叉;**optic disc** *or* **optic papilla** = point on the retina where the optic nerve starts 视盘,视乳头;**optic nerve** = second cranial nerve which transmits the sensation of sight from the eye to the brain 视神经 ◇ 见图 EYE; **optic neuritis** = inflammation of the optic nerve, which makes objects appear blurred 视神经炎; **optic radiations** = nerve tracts which take the optic impulses from the optic tracts to the visual cortex 视放射;**optic tracts** = nerve tracts which take the optic nerves from the optic chiasma to the optic radiations 视束

◇ **optical** *adjective* referring to optics 眼的,视力的,光学的;**optical illusion** = something which is seen wrongly so that it appears to be something else 视错觉

◇ **optician** *noun* **dispensing optician** = person who fits and sells glasses but does not test eyes 配镜师; **ophthalmic optician** = qualified person who specializes in making glasses and in testing eyes and prescribing lenses 验光配镜师 (NOTE: in US English an **optician** is a technician who makes lenses and fits glasses, but cannot test patient's eyesight)

COMMENT: In the UK qualified ophthalmic opticians must be registered by the General Optical Council before they can practise.
注释:在英国,合格的验光配镜师必须先在眼科总会登记注册后才能开业。

◇ **optics** *noun* study of light rays and sight 光学; **fibre optics** 光纤 *see* 见 FIBRE

◇ **optometer** = REFRACTOMETER 视力计

◇ **optometrist** *noun mainly US* person who specializes in testing eyes and prescribing lenses 验光师(主要用于美国)

◇ **optometry** *noun* testing of eyes and prescribing of lenses to correct defects in sight 验光

OR *US* = OPERATING ROOM 手术室;***an OR nurse*** 一名手术室护士

oral *adjective* referring to the mouth 口;**oral cavity** = the mouth 口腔;**oral contraceptive** = contraceptive pill which is swallowed 口服避孕药;**oral hygiene** = keeping the mouth clean by gargling and mouthwashes 口腔卫生;**oral medication** = medicine which is taken by swallowing 口服药;**oral thermometer** = thermometer which is put into the mouth to take a patient's temperature 口含体温计

◇ **orally** *adverb* (medicine taken) by the mouth 经口地:***The lotion cannot be taken orally.*** 洗液不能口服。*compare* 比较 PARENTERAL

orbicularis *adjective* circular muscle in the face 轮匝肌;**orbicularis oculi** = muscle which opens and closes the eye 眼轮匝肌;**orbicularis oris** = muscle which closes the lips tight 口轮匝肌

orbit *noun* eye socket, the hollow bony depression in the front of the skull in which each eye and lacrimal gland are situated 眼眶 ◊ 见图 SKULL

◇ **orbital** *adjective* referring to the orbit 眼眶的

orchi- *prefix* referring to the testes 睾丸

◇ **orchidalgia** *noun* neuralgic-type pain in a testis 睾丸痛

◇ **orchidectomy** *noun* surgical removal of a testis 睾丸切除术

◇ **orchidopexy** *or* **orchiopexy** *noun* surgical operation to place an undescended testis in the scrotum 睾丸固定术

◇ **orchidotomy** *noun* surgical operation to make a cut into a testis 睾丸切开术

◇ **orchis** *noun* testis 睾丸

◇ **orchitis** *noun* inflammation of the testes, characterized by hypertrophy, pain and a sensation of weight 睾丸炎

orderly *noun* person who does general work 工人;**hospital orderly** = person who does heavy work in a hospital, such as wheeling patients into the operating theatre, moving equipment about, etc. 护理员

organ *noun* part of the body which is distinct from other parts and has a particular function (such as the liver *or* an eye *or* the ovaries, etc.)器官;**organ of Corti** *or* **spiral organ** = membrane in the cochlea which takes sounds and converts them into impulses sent to the brain along the auditory nerve 科蒂器,耳蜗螺旋器;**organ transplant** = transplanting of an organ from one person to another 器官移植

◇ **organic** *adjective* (**a**) referring to organs in the body 器质性的,某一器官的;**organic disorder** = disorder caused by changes in body tissue *or* in an organ 器质性障碍 (**b**) (i) (substance) which comes from an animal *or* plant 有机的 (ii) (food) which has been cultivated naturally, without any chemical fertilizers *or* pesticides 自然(食品),绿色(食品)

◇ **organically** *adverb* (food) grown using natural fertilizers and not chemicals(食物)自然生成地

◇ **organism** *noun* any single living plant, animal, bacterium or fungus 微生物

◇ **organotherapy** *noun* treatment of a disease by using an extract from the organ of an animal (such as using liver extract to treat anaemia)器官疗法,内脏制剂疗法

orgasm *noun* climax of the sexual act, when a person experiences a moment of great excitement 性高潮

oriental sore *noun* Leishmaniasis, skin disease of tropical countries caused by the parasite *Leishmania* 皮肤利什曼病,东方疖

orifice *noun* opening 开口;**cardiac orifice** = opening where the oesophagus joins the stomach 贲门;**ileocaecal orifice** = opening where the small intestine joins the large intestine 回盲部,小肠和大

肠的接口；**pyloric orifice** = opening where the stomach joins the duodenum 幽门，胃与十二指肠的接口

origin *noun* place where a muscle is attached *or* where the branch of a nerve or blood vessel begins 肌肉附着处，血管神经分支处

◇ **original** *adjective* as in the first place 原本的，原来的：***The surgeon was able to move the organ back to its original position.*** 外科医师能将器官移回原来的位置。

◇ **originate** *verb* to start (in a place) 开始；to begin *or* to make something begin 创始：***The treatment originated in China.*** 这种治疗源于中国。***Drugs which originated in the tropics.*** 源于热带的药物。

oris 口的 *see* 见 CANCRUM ORIS, ORBICULARIS ORIS

ornithine *noun* amino acid produced by the liver 鸟氨酸(2,5－二氨基戊酸)

ornithosis *noun* disease of birds which can be passed to humans as a form of pneumonia 鸟疫 *see also* 参见 PSITTACOSIS

oropharynx *noun* part of the pharynx below the soft palate at the back of the mouth 口咽

ortho- *prefix* meaning correct *or* straight 正，直，矫正

◇ **orthodiagraph** *noun* X-ray photograph of an organ taken using only a thin stream of X-rays which allows accurate measurements of the organ to be made X线正影描记器

◇ **orthodontic** *adjective* which corrects badly formed *or* placed teeth; referring to orthodontics 口腔正畸的：***He had to undergo a course of orthodontic treatment.*** 他不得不进行口腔正畸治疗。

◇ **orthodontics** *or US* **orthodontia** *noun* branch of dentistry which deals with correcting badly placed teeth 口腔正畸学，口腔正畸科

◇ **orthodontist** *noun* dental surgeon who specializes in correcting badly placed teeth 口腔正畸医师

◇ **orthopaedic** *adjective* which corrects badly formed bones *or* joints; referring to *or* used in orthopaedics 矫形的，正畸的；**orthopaedic collar** = special strong collar to support the head of a patient with neck injuries or a condition such as cervical spondylosis 矫形护领；**orthopaedic hospital** = hospital which specializes in operations to correct badly formed joints *or* bones 矫形医院，正畸医院；**orthopaedic surgeon** = surgeon who specializes in orthopaedics 矫形外科医师

◇ **orthopaedics** *noun* branch of surgery dealing with abnormalities, diseases and injuries of the locomotor system 矫形外科学，正畸外科学

◇ **orthopaedist** *noun* surgeon who specializes in orthopaedics 矫形外科医师

◇ **orthopnoea** *noun* condition where the patient has great difficulty in breathing while lying down 端坐呼吸 *see also* 参见 DYSPNOEA

◇ **orthopnoeic** *adjective* referring to orthopnoea 端坐呼吸的

◇ **orthopsychiatry** *noun* science and treatment of behavioural and personality disorders 行为精神病学

◇ **orthoptics** *noun* methods used to treat squints 斜视矫正

◇ **orthoptist** *noun* eye specialist working in an eye hospital, who treats squints and other disorders of eye movement 视轴矫正专家

◇ **orthosis** *noun* device which is fitted to the outside of the body to support a weakness *or* correct a deformity (such as a surgical collar, leg braces, etc.) 矫形器 (NOTE: plural is **orthoses**)

◇ **orthostatic** *adjective* referring to the position of the body when standing up straight 直立的；**orthostatic hypotension** = common condition where the blood pressure drops when someone stands up suddenly, causing dizziness 直立性低血压

◇ **orthotist** *noun* qualified person who

fits orthoses 矫形器修配师

Ortolani's sign *noun* test for congenital dislocation of the hip, where the hip makes a clicking noise if the joint is rotated 奥氏征(检查先天性髋脱臼)

os *Latin noun* (**a**) bone[拉丁语]骨 (NOTE: plural is **ossa**) (**b**) mouth 口 (NOTE: plural is **ora**)

osculum *noun* small opening *or* pore 小开口,小孔

-osis *suffix* referring to disease 病

Osler's nodes *noun* tender swellings at the ends of fingers and toes in patients suffering from subacute bacterial endocarditis 厄司勒结节(亚急性细菌性心内膜炎时指、趾末端的痛性肿胀)

osmosis *noun* movement of solvent from one part of the body through a semipermeable membrane to another part where there is a higher concentration of molecules 渗透

◇ **osmoreceptor** *noun* cell in the hypothalamus which checks the level of osmotic pressure in the blood and regulates the amount of water in the blood 渗透压感受器

◇ **osmotic pressure** *noun* pressure required to stop the flow of the solvent through a membrane 渗透压

osseous *adjective* bony *or* referring to bones 骨头的; **osseous labyrinth** = hard part of the temporal bone surrounding the inner ear 骨迷路

◇ **ossicle** *noun* small bone 小骨; **auditory ossicles** = three little bones (the malleus, the incus and the stapes) in the middle ear 听小骨

> COMMENT: The auditory ossicles pick up the vibrations from the eardrum and transmit them through the oval window to the cochlea in the inner ear. The three bones are articulated together; the stapes is attached to the membrane of the oval window, and the malleus to the eardrum, and the incus lies between the other two.
>
> 注释:听小骨接纳鼓膜传来的震动,并通过卵圆窗把它传递到内耳的耳蜗。三块听小骨连在一起:镫骨附着于卵圆窗的膜上,锤骨与鼓膜相接,锤骨与镫骨之间是砧骨。

◇ **ossification** *noun* osteogenesis, formation of bone 骨化

◇ **ossium**骨的 *see* 见 FRAGILITAS

ost- *or* **osteo-** *prefix* referring to bone 骨

◇ **osteitis** *noun* inflammation of a bone due to injury *or* infection 骨炎; **osteitis deformans** *or* **Paget's disease** = disease which gradually softens bones in the spine, legs and skull, so that they become curved 畸形性骨炎,佩吉特病; **osteitis fibrosis cystica** = generalized weakness of bones, associated with formation of cysts, where bone tissue is replaced by fibrous tissue, caused by excessive activity of the thyroid gland (the localized form is osteitis fibrosis localista)囊性纤维性骨炎

◇ **osteoarthritis** *or* **osteoarthrosis** *noun* chronic degenerative arthritic disease of middle-aged and elderly people, where the joints are inflamed and become stiff and painful 骨关节炎(病)

◇ **osteoarthropathy** *noun* disease of the bone and cartilage at a joint, particularly the ankles, knees or wrists, associated with carcinoma of the bronchi 骨关节炎

◇ **osteoarthrosis** *noun* = OSTEOARTHRITIS 骨关节炎

◇ **osteoarthrotomy** *noun* surgical removal of the articular end of a bone 骨关节端切除术

◇ **osteoblast** *noun* cell in an embryo which forms bone 成骨细胞

◇ **osteochondritis** *noun* degeneration of epiphyses 骨软骨炎; **osteochondritis dissecans** = painful condition where pieces of articular cartilage become detached from the joint surface 分离性骨软骨炎

◇ **osteochondroma** *noun* tumour containing both bony and cartilagious cells 骨软骨瘤

◇ **osteoclasia** *or* **osteoclasis** *noun*

(i) destruction of bone tissue by osteoclasts 骨破坏 (ii) surgical operation to fracture or refracture bone to correct a deformity 折骨术

◇ **osteoclast** *noun* (i) cell which destroys bone 破骨细胞 (ii) surgical instrument for breaking bones 折骨器

◇ **osteoclastoma** *noun* usually benign tumour occurring at the ends of long bones 破骨细胞瘤

◇ **osteocyte** *noun* bone cell 骨细胞

◇ **osteodystrophia** *or* **osteodystrophy** *noun* bone disease, especially one caused by disorder of the metabolism 骨营养不良

◇ **osteogenesis** *noun* formation of bone 骨发生,骨形成; **osteogenesis imperfecta** *or* **fragilitas ossium** = congenital condition where bones are brittle and break easily due to abnormal bone formation 成骨不全

◇ **osteogenic** *adjective* made of bone tissue *or* starting from bone tissue 骨发生的,成骨的

◇ **osteology** *noun* study of bones and their structure 骨科学

◇ **osteolysis** *noun* (i) destruction of bone tissue by osteoclasts 骨质溶解 (ii) removal of bone calcium 脱钙

◇ **osteolytic** *adjective* referring to osteolysis 骨质溶解的

◇ **osteoma** *noun* benign tumour in a bone 骨瘤

◇ **osteomalacia** *noun* condition in adults, where the bones become soft because of lack of calcium and vitamin D 骨软化

◇ **osteomyelitis** *noun* inflammation of the interior of bone, especially the marrow spaces 骨髓炎

◇ **osteon** *noun* = HAVERSIAN SYSTEM 骨单位,哈弗系统

◇ **osteopath** *noun* person who practises osteopathy 接骨师

◇ **osteopathy** *noun* (i) way of treating diseases and disorders by massage and manipulation of bones and joints 接骨术 (ii) any disease of bone 骨病

◇ **osteopetrosis** *noun* marble bone disease, disease where bones become condensed 骨硬化病,骨石化病

◇ **osteophony** 骨传导 *see* 见 CONDUCTION

◇ **osteophyte** *noun* bony growth 骨赘

◇ **osteoplasty** *noun* plastic surgery on bones 骨成型术

◇ **osteoporosis** *noun* condition where the bones become thin, porous and brittle, because of lack of calcium and lack of physical exercise 骨质疏松症

◇ **osteosarcoma** *noun* malignant tumour of bone cells 骨肉瘤

◇ **osteosclerosis** *noun* condition where the bony spaces become hardened as a result of chronic inflammation 骨硬化

◇ **osteotome** *noun* type of chisel used by surgeons to cut bone 骨凿

◇ **osteotomy** *noun* surgical operation to cut a bone, especially to relieve pain in a joint 骨(关节)切开术

ostium *noun* opening into a passage 开口,门口

-ostomy *suffix* referring to an operation to make an opening 造口术,造瘘术

◇ **ostomy** *noun* (*informal* 非正式) colostomy *or* ileostomy 结肠或回肠切除

ot- *or* **oto-** *prefix* referring to the ear 耳

◇ **otalgia** *noun* earache *or* pain in the ear 耳痛

OT = OCCUPATIONAL THERAPIST 职业治疗师

OTC *abbreviation* (缩写) 'over the counter': (drug) which can be bought freely at the chemist's shop, and does not need a prescription 非处方药

otic *adjective* referring to the ear 耳的

◇ **otitis** *noun* inflammation of the ear 耳炎; **otitis externa** *or* **external otitis** = any inflammation of the external auditory meatus to the eardrum 外耳炎; **otitis interna** *or* **labyrinthitis** = inflammation of the inner ear 内耳炎,迷

路炎; **otitis media** *or* **tympanitis** = inflammation of the middle ear 中耳炎; **secretory otitis media** *or* **glue ear** = condition where fluid forms behind the eardrum and causes deafness 分泌性中耳炎,耳流脓 *see also* 参见 PANOTITIS

◇ **otolaryngologist** *noun* doctor who specializes in treatment of diseases of the ear and throat 耳鼻喉科医师

◇ **otolaryngology** *noun* study of diseases of the ear and throat 耳鼻喉学

◇ **otolith** *noun* (i) stone which forms in the inner ear 耳石 (ii) tiny piece of calcium carbonate attached to the hair cells in the saccule and utricle of the inner ear 耳砂; **otolith organs** = two pairs of sensory organs (the saccule and the utricle) in the inner ear which pass information to the brain about the position of the head 含耳砂的器官,内耳平衡觉感知器,球囊和卵圆囊

◇ **otologist** *noun* doctor who specializes in the study of the ear 耳科医师

◇ **otology** *noun* scientific study of the ear and its diseases 耳科学

◇ **otomycosis** *noun* infection of the external auditory meatus by a fungus 耳真菌病

◇ **otoplasty** *noun* plastic surgery of the external ear to repair damage *or* deformity 耳整形术

◇ **otorhinolaryngologist** *noun* ENT specialist, doctor who specializes in the study of the ear, nose and throat 耳鼻喉科医师

◇ **otorhinolaryngology** (**ENT**) *noun* study of the ear, nose and throat 耳鼻喉科学

◇ **otorrhagia** *noun* bleeding from the external ear 耳出血

◇ **otorrhoea** *noun* discharge of pus from the ear 耳流脓

◇ **otosclerosis** *noun* condition where the ossicles in the middle ear become thicker, the stapes becomes fixed to the oval window, and the patient becomes deaf 耳硬化

◇ **otoscope** = AURISCOPE 耳镜

outbreak *noun* series of cases of a disease which start suddenly 爆发: ***There is an outbreak of typhoid fever or a typhoid outbreak in the town.*** 镇子上伤寒爆发。

outer *adjective* (part) which is outside 外面的,靠外的; **outer ear** *or* **pinna** = part of the ear on the outside of the head, with a channel leading into the eardrum 外耳(鼓膜以外); **outer pleura** = membrane attached to the diaphragm and covering the chest cavity 壁层胸膜 (NOTE: opposite is **inner**)

outlet *noun* opening *or* channel through which something can go out 出口; **thoracic outlet** = large opening at the base of the thorax 胸廓出口

out of hours *adverb* not during the normal opening hours of a doctor's surgery 不在工作时间的: ***There is a special telephone number if you need to call the doctor out of hours.*** 如果在非工作时间需要找医生,请拨打特殊电话号码。

outpatient *noun* patient living at home, who comes to the hospital for treatment 门诊病人: ***She goes for treatment as an outpatient.*** 她去接受门诊治疗。 **outpatient department** *or* **outpatients' department** *or* **clinic** = department of a hospital which deals with outpatients 门诊部: ***He cut his hand badly in the accident and the police took him to the outpatients' department to have it dressed.*** 他的手在事故中严重受伤,警察把他带到门诊部包扎伤口。 ***25 patients were selected from the outpatient department for testing.*** 从门诊病人中选了25名进行检测。 *see also* 参见 INPATIENT

outreach *noun* services provided for patients *or* the public outside a hospital *or* clinic *or* local government department 医疗部门的外延机构

ova 卵 *see* 见 OVUM

oval window *or* **fenestra ovalis** *noun* oval opening between the middle ear and the inner ear 卵圆窗 ◊ 见图 EAR; **foramen ovale** = opening between the two parts of the heart in a fetus 卵圆孔

ov- *or* **ovar-** *prefix* referring to the ovaries 卵巢的

◇ **ovaralgia** *or* **ovarialgia** *noun* pain in the ovaries 卵巢痛

◇ **ovarian** *adjective* referring to the ovaries 卵巢的；**ovarian cyst** = cyst which develops in the ovaries 卵巢囊肿；**ovarian follicle** *or* **Graafian follicle** = cell which contains an ovum 卵泡

◇ **ovariectomy** *or* **oophorectomy** *noun* surgical removal of an ovary 卵巢切除术

◇ **ovariocele** *noun* hernia of an ovary 卵巢疝

◇ **ovariotomy** *noun* surgical removal of an ovary *or* a tumour in an ovary 卵巢切开术

◇ **ovaritis** *or* **oophoritis** *noun* inflammation of an ovary or both ovaries 卵巢炎

◇ **ovary** *noun* one of two organs in a woman, which produce ova *or* egg cells and secrete the female hormone oestrogen 卵巢 ◊ 见图 UROGENITAL SYSTEM（female）（NOTE：for other terms referring to ovaries, see words beginning with **oophor-**）

over- *prefix* too much 过分

◇ **overbite** *noun* normal formation of the teeth, where the top incisors come down over and in front of the bottom incisors when the jaws are closed 覆𬌗

◇ **overcome** *verb*（**a**）to fight something and win 战胜：***She overcame her disabilities and now leads a normal life.*** 她战胜了自身残疾，现在过上了正常的生活。（**b**）to make someone lose consciousness 使意识丧失，晕了过去：***Two people were overcome by smoke in the fire.*** 着火产生的烟把两个人呛晕了。（NOTE：**overcomes - overcoming - overcame - has overcome**）

◇ **overcompensate** *verb* to try to cover the effects of a handicap by making too strenuous efforts 过分代偿

◇ **overdo（things）** *verb*（*informal* 非正式）to work too hard *or* to do too much exercise 过劳：***He has been overdoing things and has to rest.*** 他做的太多，不得不休息。***She overdid it, working until 9 o'clock every evening.*** 她每晚工作到 9 点钟，太过劳了。（NOTE：**overdoes - overdoing - overdid - has overdone**）

◇ **overdose** *noun* dose（of a drug）which is larger than normal 过量：***She went into a coma after an overdose of heroin or after a heroin overdose.*** 她因海洛因过量而昏迷了。

◇ **overeating** *noun* eating too much food 吃的太多

◇ **overexertion** *noun* doing too much physical work *or* taking too much exercise 过劳

◇ **overgrow** *verb* to grow over a tissue 过度生长

◇ **overgrowth** *noun* growth of tissue over another tissue 生长过度

◇ **overjet** *noun* space which separates the top incisors from the bottom incisors when the jaws are closed 咬合间隙

◇ **overlap** *verb*（*of bandages, etc.*）to lie partly on top of another 覆压，重叠

◇ **overprescribe** *verb* to issue too many prescriptions 处方过量：***Some doctors seriously overprescribe tranquillizers.*** 有些医生开出的安定剂太多。

◇ **overproduction** *noun* producing too much 产生过多：***The condition is caused by overproduction of thyroxine by the thyroid gland.*** 这种状况是甲状腺产生的甲状腺素过多引起的。

◇ **oversew** *verb* to sew a patch of tissue over a perforation 补片缝合（NOTE：**oversews - oversewing - oversewed - has oversewn**）

◇ **overweight** *adjective* too fat and heavy 超重：***He is several kilos overweight for his age and height.*** 相对于他的年龄和身高，他超重了几千克。

◇ **overwork 1** *noun* doing too much work 过劳：***He collapsed from overwork.*** 他因过劳而拖垮了。**2** *verb* to work too much *or* to make something work too much 过劳，使用过度：***He has been overworking his heart.*** 他使自己心脏负担过重

了。

◇ **overwrought** *adjective* very tense and nervous 过分紧张: ***He is rather overwrought because of troubles at work.*** 他因为工作中的麻烦弄得精神过分紧张。

overt *adjective* easily seen with the naked eye 明显的 (NOTE: the opposite is **occult**)

oviduct = FALLOPIAN TUBE 输卵管

ovulate *verb* to release a mature ovum into a Fallopian tube 排卵

◇ **ovulation** *noun* release of an ovum from the mature ovarian follicle into the Fallopian tube 排卵

◇ **ovum** *noun* female egg cell which, when fertilised by a spermatazoon, begins to develop into an embryo 卵子 (NOTE: the plural is **ova**. Note that for other terms referring to ova, see words beginning with **oo-**)

oxidase *noun* enzyme which encourages oxidation by removing hydrogen 氧化酶 *see also* 参见 MONOAMINE

◇ **oxidation** *noun* action of making oxides by combining with oxygen or removing hydrogen 氧化

> COMMENT: Carbon compounds form oxides when metabolised with oxygen in the body, producing carbon dioxide.
> 注释:含碳化合物在体内有氧代谢时产生二氧化碳。

◇ **oxide** *noun* compound formed with oxygen 氧化物; **zinc oxide** (**ZnO**) = compound of zinc and oxygen, which forms a soft white soothing powder used in creams and lotions 氧化锌(霜剂或药膏中的添加物)

oxycephalic *adjective* referring to oxycephaly 尖头的

◇ **oxycephaly** *noun* turricephaly, condition where the skull is deformed into a point, with exophthalmos and defective sight 尖头畸形

oxygen *noun* chemical element, a common colourless gas which is present in the air and essential to human life 氧; **oxygen cylinder** = heavy metal tube which contains oxygen and is connected to a patient's oxygen mask 氧气瓶; **oxygen mask** = mask connected to a supply of oxygen, which can be put over the face to help a patient with breathing difficulties 氧气面罩; **oxygen tent** = type of cover put over a patient so that he can breathe in oxygen 氧气帐篷; **oxygen therapy** = any treatment involving the administering of oxygen, as in an oxygen tent, in emergency treatment for heart failure, etc. 氧疗 (NOTE: chemical symbol is **O**)

> COMMENT: Oxygen is absorbed into the bloodstream through the lungs and is carried to the tissues along the arteries; it is essential to normal metabolism and given to patients with breathing difficulties.
> 注释:氧气经肺吸收入血,沿动脉运至器官组织;它是正常代谢必需的,有呼吸困难的病人更是需要补充氧气。

◇ **oxygenate** *verb* to treat (blood) with oxygen 充氧,氧合; **oxygenated** *or* **arterial blood** = blood which has received oxygen in the lungs and is being carried to the tissues along the arteries (it is brighter red than venous deoxygenated blood) 氧合血,动脉血

◇ **oxygenation** *noun* becoming filled with oxygen 氧合: ***Blood is carried along the pulmonary artery to the lungs for oxygenation.*** 血液经肺动脉到肺部进行氧合。

◇ **oxygenator** *noun* machine which puts oxygen into the blood, used as an artificial lung in surgery 氧合器

◇ **oxyhaemoglobin** *noun* compound of haemoglobin and oxygen, which is the way oxygen is carried in arterial blood from the lungs to the tissues 氧合血红蛋白 *see also* 参见 HAEMOGLOBIN

oxyntic cell *noun* parietal cell, cell in the gastric gland which secretes hydrochloric acid(胃)壁细胞

oxytocin *noun* hormone secreted by

the pituitary gland, which controls the contractions of the uterus and encourages the flow of milk 催产素

COMMENT: An extract of oxytocin is used as an injection to start contractions of the uterus.
注释:注射催产素的提取物可发动子宫收缩。

oxyuriasis = ENTEROBIASIS 蛲虫病

◇ **Oxyuris** = ENTEROBIUS 尖尾线虫属

ozaena *noun* (i) disease of the nose, where the nasal passage is blocked and mucus forms, giving off an unpleasant smell 臭鼻症 (ii) any unpleasant discharge from the nose 脏鼻涕

Pp

P *chemical symbol for* phosphorus 磷的化学元素符号

Pa = PASCAL 帕

pacemaker *noun* (**a**) sinoatrial node *or* SA node, node in the heart which regulates the heartbeat 起搏点; **ectopic pacemaker** = abnormal focus of the heart muscle which takes the place of the SA node 异位起搏点 (**b**) (**cardiac**) **pacemaker** = electronic device implanted on a patient's heart or which a patient wears attached to his chest, which stimulates and regulates the heartbeat (心脏)起搏器: ***The patient was fitted with a pacemaker.*** 这个病人身上装了一个起搏器。**endocardial pacemaker** = pacemaker attached to the lining of the heart 心内膜起搏器; **epicardial pacemaker** = pacemaker attached to the surface of the ventricle 心外膜起搏器

> COMMENT: An electrode is usually attached to the epicardium and linked to the device which can be implanted in various positions in the chest.
> 注释:电极通常附着在心外膜上,并与可植入胸壁任何部位的装置相连。

pachy- *prefix* meaning thickening 增厚

◇ **pachydactyly** *noun* condition where the fingers and toes become thicker than normal 指(趾)肥大

◇ **pachydermia** *or* **pachyderma** *noun* condition where the skin becomes thicker than normal 皮肤增厚

◇ **pachymeningitis** *noun* inflammation of the dura mater 硬脑(脊)膜炎

◇ **pachymeninx** *noun* the dura mater, thicker outer layer covering the brain and spinal cord 硬脑(脊)膜

◇ **pachysomia** *noun* condition where soft tissues of the body become abnormally thick 躯体肥厚

pacifier *noun US* rubber teat given to a baby to suck, to prevent it crying 橡皮奶头(用于使婴儿安静) (NOTE: GB English is **dummy**)

Pacinian corpuscle 帕西尼氏小体,环层小体 *see* 见 CORPUSCLE

pacing *noun* surgical operation to implant *or* attach a cardiac pacemaker 安置起搏器

pack 1 *noun* (**a**) (i) tampon of gauze *or* cotton wool, used to fill an orifice such as the nose *or* vagina 填塞物 (ii) wet material folded tightly, used to press on the body 叠紧的湿敷料,用于压迫 (iii) treatment where a blanket or sheet is used to wrap round the patient's body 包扎法; **cold pack** *or* **hot pack** = cold *or* hot wet cloth put on a patient's body to reduce *or* increase his body temperature 冷/热敷法; **ice pack** = cold compress made of lumps of ice wrapped in a cloth, and pressed on a swelling *or* bruise to reduce the pain 冰敷法 (**b**) box *or* bag of goods for sale 包,盒: ***a pack of sticking plaster*** 一盒橡皮膏; ***She bought a sterile dressing pack.*** 她买了一个消毒敷料包。***The cough tablets are sold in packs of fifty.*** 这种咳嗽药片每50片一盒。**2** *verb* (**a**) to fill an orifice with a tampon (of cotton wool) 填塞: ***The ear was packed with cotton wool to absorb the discharge.*** 耳朵里塞上了药棉以吸排出液。(**b**) to put things in cases *or* boxes 包装,打包: ***The transplant organ arrived at the hospital packed in ice.*** 用冰包装的移植器官送到了医院。**packed cell volume** (**haematocrit**) = volume of red blood cells in a patient's blood shown against the total volume of blood 细胞压积

◇ **packing** *noun* absorbent material put into a wound or part of the body to abosrb fluids 填塞物

◇ **pack up** *verb* (*informal* 非正式) to stop working 卷铺盖走人,交卸了,停工: ***His heart simply packed up under the strain.*** 在这样的压力下他的心脏干脆歇工了。

pad *noun* (i) soft absorbent material,

placed on part of the body to protect it 垫儿 (ii) thickening of part of the skin 皮肤增厚处: ***She wrapped a pad of soft cotton wool round the sore.*** 她用一块软棉垫包扎伤口。

paed- *or* **paedo-** *prefix* referring to children 儿童,孩子 (NOTE: words beginning with the prefix paed- *or* paedo- are written **ped-** *or* **pedo-** in US English)

◇ **paediatric** *adjective* referring to the treatment of the diseases of children 儿科的: ***A new paediatric hospital has been opened.*** 新开了一家儿童医院。 ***Parents can visit children in the paediatric wards at any time.*** 任何时间,父母都可以到儿科病房看自己的孩子。

◇ **paediatrician** *noun* doctor who specializes in the treatment of diseases of children 儿科医师

◇ **paediatrics** *noun* study of children, their development and diseases 儿科学 *compare* 比较 GERIATRICS

> QUOTE: Paediatric day surgery minimizes the length of hospital stay and therefore is less traumatic for both child and parents.
> 引文:儿科日间手术缩短了住院时间,因此对患儿及其父母的打击都减小了。
> **British Journal of Nursing** 英国护理杂志

Paget's disease *noun* (**a**) osteitis deformans, a disease which gradually softens and thickens the bones in the spine, skull and legs, so that they become curved 佩吉特病,变形性骨炎 (**b**) form of breast cancer which starts as an itchy rash round the nipple 乳晕癌

pain *noun* feeling which a person has when hurt 疼痛: ***She had pains in her legs after playing tennis.*** 打完网球她双腿疼了起来。 ***The doctor gave him an injection to relieve the pain.*** 医生给他打针止痛。 ***She is suffering from back pain.*** 她背痛。 **to be in great pain** = to have very sharp pains which are difficult to bear 剧痛; **abdominal pain** = pain in the abdomen, caused by indigestion or serious disorder 腹痛; **chest pains** = pains in the chest which may be caused by heart disease 胸痛; **labour pains** = pains felt at regular intervals by a woman as the muscles of the uterus contract during childbirth 分娩阵痛; **nagging pain** = dull, continuous throbbing pain 跳痛,抽痛; **throbbing pain** = pain which continues in repeated short attacks 刺痛; **referred pain** = SYNALGIA 牵涉痛; **pain pathway** = series of linking nerve fibres and neurones which carry impulses of pain from the site to the sensory cortex 痛觉通路; **pain receptor** = nerve ending which is sensitive to pain 痛觉感受器; **pain relief** = easing pain by using analgesics 止痛,释痛; **pain threshold** = point at which a person finds it impossible to bear pain without crying 痛阈 (NOTE: pain can be used in the plural to show that it recurs **she has pains in her left leg**)

◇ **painful** *adjective* which hurts 疼痛的: ***She has a painful skin disease.*** 她的皮肤病很疼。 ***His foot is so painful he can hardly walk.*** 他的脚疼得使他几乎不能走路。 ***Your eye looks very red — is it very painful?*** 你的眼睛看上去红红的,很疼吗?

◇ **painkiller** *or* **painkilling drug** *or* **pain-relieving drug** *or* **analgesic** *noun* drug which stops a patient feeling pain 止痛药,镇痛药

◇ **painless** *adjective* which does not hurt *or* which gives no pain 无痛的: ***a painless method of removing warts*** 祛除疣的无痛方法

> COMMENT: Pain is carried by the sensory nerves to the central nervous system; from the site it travels up the spinal column to the medulla and through a series of neurones to the sensory cortex. Pain is the method by which a person knows that part of the body is damaged or infected, though the pain is not always felt in the affected part (see synalgia).
> 注释:痛觉由感觉神经传入中枢神经系统;从痛点经脊髓到延髓,通过一系列神经元

到达感觉皮质。痛觉是人赖以了解自己身体某部位受损伤或被感染的方式,尽管而受损的部位不一定疼病(见牵涉痛)。

paint 1 *noun* coloured antiseptic *or* analgesic *or* astringent liquid which is put on the surface of the body 涂剂(用于皮肤消毒、镇痛、收敛等) 2 *verb* to cover (a wound) with an antiseptic *or* analgesic *or* astringent liquid or lotion 涂抹(外用药): ***She painted the rash with calamine.*** 她用炉甘石洗剂涂在皮疹上。

◇ **painter's colic** *noun* form of lead poisoning caused by working with paint 铅绞痛(铅中毒的表现)

palate *noun* roof of the mouth and floor of the nasal cavity (formed of the hard and soft palates) 腭,上颚,上牙膛(俗); **hard palate** = front part of the palate between the upper teeth, made of the horizontal parts of the palatine bone and processes of the maxillae 硬腭; **soft palate** = back part of the palate leading to the uvula 软腭 ◇ 见图 THROAT

◇ **cleft palate** *noun* congenital defect, where there is a fissure in the hard palate allowing the mouth and nasal cavities to be linked 腭裂

COMMENT: A cleft palate is usually associated with a harelip. Both are due to incomplete fusion of the maxillary processes. Both can be successfully corrected by surgery.
注释:腭裂通常伴有兔唇,二者都是由于上颌突融合不全所致,可通过手术成功矫正。

◇ **palatine** *adjective* referring to the palate 腭的; **palatine arches** = folds of tissue between the soft palate and the pharynx 软腭弓; **palate bones** *or* **palatine bones** = two bones which form part of the hard palate, the orbits of the eyes and the cavity behind the nose 腭骨; **palatine tonsil** *or* **tonsil** = lymphoid tissue at the back of the throat, between the soft palate, the tongue and the pharynx 腭扁桃体

◇ **palato-** *prefix* referring to the palate 腭

◇ **palatoglossal arch** *noun* fold between the soft palate and the tongue, anterior to the tonsil 舌腭弓

◇ **palatopharyngeal arch** *noun* fold between the soft palate and the pharynx, posterior to the tonsil 咽腭弓

◇ **palatoplasty** *noun* plastic surgery of the roof of the mouth, such as to repair a cleft palate 腭成形术

◇ **palatoplegia** *noun* paralysis of the soft palate 腭麻痹

◇ **palatorrhaphy** *noun* surgical operation to suture and close a cleft palate 腭修补术,腭裂缝合术 (NOTE: also called **staphylorrhaphy** *or* **uraniscorrhaphy**)

pale *adjective* light coloured *or* white 苍白: ***After her illness she looked pale and tired.*** 病后她显得苍白憔悴。***With his pale complexion and dark rings round his eyes, he did not look at all well.*** 他面色苍白,眼圈发黑,看上去不大好。 **to turn pale** = to become white in the face, because the flow of blood is reduced 脸色变白: ***Some people turn pale at the sight of blood.*** 有些人一见血脸就发白。

◇ **paleness** *or* **pallor** *noun* being pale 面色苍白

pali- *or* **palin-** *prefix* which repeats 反复出现

◇ **palindromic** *adjective* (disease) which recurs 复发,再发

◇ **palilalia** *noun* speech defect where the patient repeats words 口吃,结巴(俗)

palliative *noun* & *adjective* treatment *or* drug which relieves the symptoms, but does nothing to cure the disease which causes the symptoms (a pain killer can reduce the pain in a tooth, but will not cure the caries which causes the pain) 姑息治疗(仅缓解症状而不治疗疾病本身的一种治疗方法)

QUOTE: Coronary artery bypass grafting is a palliative procedure aimed at the relief of persistent angina pectoris.
引文:冠状动脉搭桥术是一种姑息疗法,旨在缓解持续性心绞痛。
British Journal of Hospital Medicine
英国医院医学杂志

pallor *noun* paleness *or* being pale 面色苍白

palm *noun* soft inside part of the hand 掌

◊ **palmar** *adjective* referring to the palm 掌的；**palmar arch** = one of two arches in the palm formed by two arteries which link together 掌弓；**palmar interosseus** = deep muscle between the bones in the hand 骨间肌；**palmar region** = area of skin around the palm 手掌 (NOTE: in the hand **palmar** is the opposite of **dorsal**)

palpable *adjective* which can be felt when touched; which can be examined with the hand 可触及的

◊ **palpate** *verb* to examine part of the body by feeling it with the hand 触诊

◊ **palpation** *noun* examination of part of the body by feeling it with the hand 触诊；**breast palpation** = feeling a breast to see if a lump is present which might indicate breast cancer 乳房触诊；**digital palpation** = pressing part of the body with the fingers 指诊

> QUOTE: Mammography is the most effective technique available for the detection of occult (non-palpable) breast cancer. It has been estimated that mammography can detect a carcinoma two years before it becomes palpable.
> 引文：乳腺 X 线摄影是目前可发现潜在(触摸不到的)乳腺癌最有效的技术。据估计，乳腺 X 线摄影能在癌症病灶可摸到前两年就发现它。
> **Southern Medical Journal** 南部医学杂志

palpebra *noun* eyelid 眼睑 (NOTE: plural is **palpebrae**)

◊ **palpebral** *adjective* referring to the eyelids 眼睑的

palpitation *noun* awareness that the heart is beating abnormally, caused by stress *or* by a disease 心悸

◊ **palpitate** *verb* to beat rapidly *or* to throb *or* to flutter 心悸

palsy *noun* paralysis 麻痹，瘫痪；**cerebral palsy** = disorder of the brain, mainly due to brain damage occurring before birth, or due to lack of oxygen during birth 脑瘫；**Erb's palsy** = condition where an arm is paralysed because of birth injuries to the brachial plexus 欧勃氏瘫痪(臂丛产伤后所致上肢瘫痪) *see also* 参见 BELL'S PALSY

> COMMENT: Cerebral palsy is the disorder affecting spastics. The patient may have bad coordination of muscular movements, impaired speech, hearing and sight, and sometimes mental retardation.
> 注释：脑瘫是一种导致痉挛的疾病。病人肌肉运动共济差，存在听、说及看的功能障碍，有时还造成精神发育迟滞。

◊ **palsied** *adjective* suffering from palsy 瘫痪的：***cerebral palsied children*** 脑瘫患儿

paludism = MALARIA 疟疾

pan- *or* **pant-** *or* **panto-** *prefix* meaning generalized *or* affecting everything 泛，全

◊ **panacea** *noun* medicine which is supposed to cure everything 万应灵药，包治百病

◊ **panarthritis** *noun* inflammation of all the tissues of a joint *or* of all the joints in the body 全(身)关节炎

◊ **pancarditis** *noun* inflammation of all the tissues in the heart, i. e. the heart muscle, the endocardium and the pericardium 全心炎(涉及心肌、心内膜、心包)

pancreas *noun* gland which lies across the back of the body between the kidneys 胰腺

◊ **pancreatectomy** *noun* surgical removal of all *or* part of the pancreas 胰腺切除术；**partial pancreatectomy** = removal of part of the pancreas 胰腺部分切除；**subtotal pancreatectomy** = removal of most of the pancreas 胰腺次全切除；**total pancreatectomy** *or* **Whipple's operation** = removal of the whole pancreas together with part of the duodenum 胰腺全切

◇ **pancreatic** *adjective* referring to the pancreas 胰腺的; **benign pancreatic disease** = chronic pancreatitis 良性胰腺疾病; **pancreatic duct** = duct leading through the pancreas to the duodenum 胰腺导管; **pancreatic fibrosis** = CYSTIC FIBROSIS 胰腺纤维化; **pancreatic juice** *or* **pancreatic secretion** = digestive juice formed of enzymes produced by the pancreas which digests fats and carbohydrates 胰液

◇ **pancreatin** *noun* substance made from enzymes secreted by the pancreas and used to treat a patient whose pancreas does not produce pancreatic enzymes 胰酶

◇ **pancreatitis** *noun* inflammation of the pancreas 胰腺炎; **acute pancreatitis** = inflammation after pancreatic enzymes have escaped into the pancreas, causing symptoms of acute abdominal pain 急性胰腺炎; **chronic pancreatitis** = chronic inflammation, after repeated attacks of acute pancreatitis, where the gland becomes calcified 慢性胰腺炎; **relapsing pancreatitis** = form of pancreatitis where the symptoms recur, but in a less painful form 复发性胰腺炎

◇ **pancreatomy** *or* **pancreatotomy** *noun* surgical operation to open the pancreatic duct 胰切开术

COMMENT: The pancreas has two functions: the first is to secrete the pancreatic juice which goes into the duodenum and digests proteins and carbohydrates; the second function is to produce the hormone insulin which regulates the use of sugar by the body. This hormone is secreted into the bloodstream by the islets of Langerhans which are in the pancreas.
注释:胰腺有两种功能:首先是向十二指肠分泌胰液,消化蛋白质和碳水化合物;其次是产生胰岛素调节身体对糖的利用。胰岛素由胰岛的郎氏细胞分泌入血。

pancytopenia *noun* condition where the numbers of red and white blood cells and blood platelets are all reduced together 全血细胞缺乏

◇ **pandemic** *noun* & *adjective* (epidemic disease) which affects many parts of the world 大流行的,大流行病 *compare with* 比较 ENDEMIC, EPIDEMIC

pang *noun* sudden sharp pain (especially in the intestine) 突发剧痛(特别是肠道的突发疼痛,肚子痛): ***After not eating for a day, he suffered pangs of hunger.*** 一天没吃东西,他饿得肚子一阵剧痛。

panhysterectomy *noun* surgical removal of all the womb and the cervix 子宫全切

panic 1 *noun* sudden great fear which cannot be stopped and which sometimes results in irrational behaviour 惊恐: ***He was in a panic as he sat in the consultant's waiting room.*** 他惊恐地坐在咨询室等候。**panic attack** = sudden attack of panic 惊恐发作 **2** *verb* to be suddenly afraid 惊吓: ***He panicked when the surgeon told him he might have to have an operation.*** 当外科医师通知他可能得做个手术时,他惊恐不已。

panniculitis *noun* inflammation of the panniculus adiposus, producing tender swellings on the thighs and breasts 脂膜炎

◇ **panniculus** *noun* layer of membranous tissue 膜; **panniculus adiposus** = fatty layer of tissue underneath the skin 脂膜

pannus *noun* growth on the cornea containing tiny blood vessels 角膜血管翳

panophthalmia *or* **panophthalmitis** *noun* inflammation of the whole of the eye 全眼球炎

◇ **panosteitis** *or* **panostitis** *noun* inflammation of all of a bone 全骨炎

◇ **panotitis** *noun* inflammation affecting all of the ear, but especially the middle ear 全耳炎

◇ **panproctocolectomy** *noun* surgical removal of the whole of the rectum and the colon 全直肠结肠切除术

pant *verb* to take short breaths because of overexertion *or* to gasp for breath 气喘吁吁：***He was panting when he reached the top of the stairs.*** 到楼顶时他气喘吁吁。

pantothenic acid *noun* vitamin of the vitamin B complex, found in liver, yeast and eggs 泛酸

pantotropic *or* **pantropic** *adjective* (virus) which attacks many different parts of the body 泛向的(病毒可侵犯机体各部的)

Papanicolaou test *or* **Pap test** *or* **Pap smear** *noun* method of staining smears from various body secretions to test for malignancy, such as testing a cervical smear sample to see if cancer is present 帕氏涂片检查

papilla *noun* small swelling which protrudes above the normal surface level 乳头：***The upper surface of the tongue is covered with papillae.*** 舌上面有乳头覆盖。**hair papilla** = part of the skin containing capillaries which feed blood to the hair 毛乳头；**optic papilla** *or* **optic disc** = point on the retina where the optic nerve starts 视乳头 ◊ 见图 TONGUE *see also* 参见，CIRCUMVALLATE, FILIFORM, FUNGIFORM, VALLATE (NOTE: plural is **papillae**)

◊ **papillary** *adjective* referring to papillae 乳头的

◊ **papillitis** *noun* inflammation of the optic disc at the back of the eye 视乳头炎

◊ **papilloedema** *noun* oedema of the optic disc at the back of the eye 视乳头水肿

◊ **papilloma** *noun* benign tumour on the skin *or* mucous membrane 乳头(状)瘤

◊ **papillomatosis** *noun* (i) being affected with papillomata 乳头瘤病 (ii) formation of papillomata 乳头形成

papovavirus *noun* family of viruses which start tumours, some of which are malignant, and some of which, like warts, are benign 乳头瘤病毒

Pap test *or* **Pap smear** 帕氏试验 *see* 见 PAPANICOLAOU TEST

papule *noun* small coloured spot raised above the surface of the skin as part of a rash 丘疹 (NOTE: a flat spot is a **macule**)

◊ **papular** *adjective* referring to a papule 丘疹的

◊ **papulopustular** *adjective* (rash) with both papules and pustules 丘疹脓疱性的

◊ **papulosquamous** *adjective* (rash) with papules and a scaly skin 丘疹鳞屑性的

para- *prefix* meaning (i) similar to *or* near 类似 (ii) changed *or* beyond 错乱

◊ **paracentesis** *noun* draining of fluid from a cavity inside the body, using a hollow needle, either for diagnostic purposes or because the fluid is harmful 穿刺术

◊ **paracetamol** *noun* pain-killing drug 扑热息痛、醋氨酚

◊ **paracolpitis** = PERICOLPITIS 阴道周围炎

◊ **paracusis** *or* **paracousia** *noun* disorder of hearing 听觉倒错

◊ **paradoxical breathing** *or* **respiration** *noun* condition of a patient with broken ribs, where the chest appears to move in when the patient breathes in, and appears to move out when he breathes out 反常呼吸

◊ **paradoxus** 相反的，反常的 *see* 见 PULSUS

◊ **paraesthesia** *noun* numbness and tingling feeling, like pins and needles 感觉异常 (NOTE: plural is **paraesthesiae**)

> QUOTE: The sensory symptoms are paraesthesiae which may spread up the arm over the course of about 20 minutes.
> 引文：感觉异常的症状约 20 分钟播散到整个胳膊。
> **British Journal of Hospital Medicine**
> 英国医院医学杂志

paraffin *noun* oil produced from petroleum, forming the base of some ointments, and also used for heating and light 石蜡；**liquid paraffin** = oil used as a laxative 液体石蜡(用来导泻); **paraffin gauze** = gauze covered with solid paraffin,used as a dressing 石蜡纱布

parageusia *noun* (i) disorder of the sense of taste 味觉异常 (ii) unpleasant taste in the mouth 口内异味

◇ **paragonimiasis** *noun* endemic haemoptysis, tropical disease where the patient's lungs are infested with a fluke and he coughs up blood 肺吸虫病

paraguard stretcher 加缚单架 *see* 见 STRETCHER

para-influenza virus *noun* virus which causes upper respiratory tract infection (in its structure it is identical to paramyxoviruses and the measles virus) 副流感病毒

paralysis *noun* condition where the muscles of part of the body become weak and cannot be moved because the motor nerves have been damaged 麻痹, 瘫痪: ***The condition causes paralysis of the lower limbs.*** 这种病导致下肢瘫痪。***He suffered temporary paralysis of the right arm.*** 他得了一过性右臂瘫痪。**bulbar paralysis** = form of motor neurone disease which affects the muscles of the mouth, jaw and throat 球麻痹; **facial paralysis** = BELL'S PALSY 面神经麻痹; **infantile paralysis** = POLIOMYELITIS 婴儿瘫; **paralysis agitans** = PARKINSON'S DISEASE 震颤麻痹; **general paralysis of the insane** (**GPI**) = very serious condition marking the final stages of syphilis 麻痹性痴呆; **spastic paralysis** *or* **cerebral palsy** = disorder of the brain affecting spastics, caused by brain damage before birth or lack of oxygen at birth 痉挛性麻痹,脑瘫 *see also* 参见 DIPLEGIA, HEMIPLEGIA, MONOPLEGIA, PARAPLEGIA, QUADRIPLEGIA

> COMMENT: Paralysis can have many causes: the commonest are injuries to or diseases of the brain or the spinal column
> 注释:很多原因都可以引起瘫痪:最常见的是脑或脊柱的损伤或疾病。

◇ **paralyse** *or US* **paralyze** *verb* to weaken (muscles) so that they cannot function 瘫痪: ***His arm was paralysed after the stroke.*** 中风后他的胳膊瘫痪了。***She is paralysed from the waist down.*** 她腰以下瘫痪了。

◇ **paralytic** *adjective* referring to paralysis; (person) who is paralysed 瘫痪的; **paralytic ileus** = obstruction in the ileum caused by paralysis of the muscles of the intestine 麻痹性肠梗阻

◇ **paralytica**麻痹的 *see* 见 DEMENTIA PARALYTICA

paramedian *adjective* near the midline of the body 正中旁的; **paramedian plane** = plane near the midline of the body, parallel to the sagittal plane and at right angles to the coronal plane 旁正中面(与矢状面平行,冠状面垂直)

paramedic *noun* person in a profession linked to that of nurse, doctor or surgeon 医务辅助人员

◇ **paramedical** *adjective* referring to services linked to those given by nurses, doctors and surgeons 医务辅助人员的 (NOTE: paramedic is used to refer to all types of services and staff, from therapists and hygienists, to ambulancemen and radiographers, but does not include doctors, nurses or midwives)

paramesonephric duct *noun* Müllerian duct, one of the two ducts in an embryo which develop into the uterus and Fallopian tubes 副中肾管(苗勒管,后发育成子宫及输卵管的结构)

parameter *noun* measurement of something (such as blood pressure) which may be an important factor in treating the condition which the patient is suffering from 参数

parametritis *noun* inflammation of the parametrium 子宫旁炎

◇ **parametrium** *noun* connective tissue around the womb 子宫旁组织

◇ **paramnesia** *noun* disorder of the memory where the patient remembers events which have not happened 记忆倒错

◇ **paramyxovirus** *noun* one of a group of viruses, which cause mumps, measles and other infectious diseases 副粘液病毒

◇ **paranasal** *adjective* by the side of the nose 鼻旁的; **paranasal air sinus** = one of the four sinuses in the skull near the nose 鼻旁窦

COMMENT: The four pairs of paranasal sinuses are the frontal, maxillary, ethmoidal, and sphenoidal.
注释:4 对鼻旁窦是额窦、上颌窦、筛窦和蝶窦。

paranoia *noun* mental disorder where the patient has fixed delusions, usually that he is being persecuted *or* attacked 偏执狂,妄想狂

◇ **paranoiac** *noun* person suffering from paranoia 偏执狂患者

◇ **paranoid** *adjective* suffering from a fixed delusion 类偏执狂的; **paranoid schizophrenia** = form of schizophrenia where the patient believes he is being persecuted 偏执狂型精神分裂症

paraparesis *noun* incomplete paralysis of the legs 下肢轻瘫

◇ **paraphasia** *noun* speech defect where the patient uses a wrong sound in the place of the correct word or phrase 言语错乱

◇ **paraphimosis** *noun* condition where the foreskin is tight and has to be removed by circumcision 嵌顿性包茎

◇ **paraphrenia** *noun* paranoid psychosis, where the patient has delusions and the personality disintegrates 妄想痴呆

paraplegia *noun* paralysis which affects the lower part of the body and the legs, usually caused by an injury to the spinal cord 截瘫; **spastic paraplegia** = paraplegia caused by disturbed nutrition of the cortex in elderly people 痉挛性截瘫

◇ **paraplegic** *noun & adjective* (person) suffering from paraplegia 截瘫患者;截瘫的

parapsoriasis *noun* group of skin diseases with scales, similar to psoriasis 类牛皮癣

parasagittal *adjective* near the midline of the body 旁矢状面的; **parasagittal plane** = plane near the midline of the body, parallel to the sagittal plane and at right angles to the coronal plane 旁矢状面

parasite *noun* plant *or* animal which lives on or inside another organism and draws nourishment from that organism 寄生虫,寄生植物

◇ **parasitic** *adjective* referring to parasites 寄生虫的; **parasitic cyst** = cyst produced by a parasite, usually in the liver 寄生虫囊

◇ **parasiticide** *noun & adjective* (substance) which kills parasites 杀寄生虫药

◇ **parasitology** *noun* scientific study of parasites 寄生虫学

COMMENT: The commonest parasites affecting humans are lice on the skin, and various types of worms in the intestines. Many diseases (such as malaria and amoebic dysentery) are caused by infestation with parasites.
注释:影响人类的最常见的寄生虫是皮肤上的虱子,以及各种肠道寄生虫。许多疾病(如疟疾和阿米巴痢疾)都是由寄生虫感染引起的。

parasuicide *noun* act where the patient tries to kill himself, but without really intending to do so, rather as a way of drawing attention to his psychological condition 自杀企图,假自杀

parasympathetic nervous system *noun* one of two systems in the autonomic nervous system 副交感神经系统

COMMENT: The parasympathetic nervous system originates in some of the cranial and sacral nerves. It acts in opposition to the sympathetic nervous system, slowing down the action of the heart, reducing blood pre

ssure, and increasing the rate of digestion.
注释:副交感神经系统源自某些颅神经和骶神经。它的作用与交感神经系统相反,减缓心脏工作、降低血压、加快消化系统的运转。

parathormone *noun* parathyroid hormone, the hormone secreted by the parathryoid glands which regulates the level of calcium in blood plasma 甲状旁腺素

◊ **parathyroid(gland)** *noun & adjective* one of four glands in the neck, near the thyroid gland, which secrete parathyroid hormones 甲状旁腺,甲状旁腺的; **parathyroid hormone** = hormone secreted by the parathyroid gland which regulates the level of calcium in blood plasma 甲状旁腺素

◊ **parathyroidectomy** *noun* surgical removal of a parathyroid gland 甲状旁腺切除术

paratyphoid (fever) *noun* infectious disease which has similar symptoms to typhoid and is caused by bacteria transmitted by humans or animals 副伤寒

COMMENT: There are three forms of paratyphoid fever, known by the letters A, B, and C. They are caused by three types of bacterium *Salmonella paratyphi* A, B, and C. TAB injections give immunity against paratyphoid A and B, but not against C.
注释:副伤寒有三种形式,标作A、B、C,是由沙门副伤寒菌A, B, C三型细菌引起的。伤寒副伤寒三联菌苗注射可以对副伤寒A和B产生免疫,但不能对副伤寒C产生免疫。

paravertebral *adjective* near the vertebrae *or* beside the spinal column 椎旁的; **paravertebral injection** = injection of local anaesthetic into the back near the vertebrae 椎旁注射

parenchyma *noun* tissues which contain the working cells of an organ as opposed to the stoma or supporting tissue 实质

parent *noun* mother or father 父母; **single parent family** = family which consists of a child or children and only one parent (because of death, divorce or separation) 单亲家庭; **parent cell** *or* **mother cell** = original cell which splits into daughter cells by mitosis 母细胞

◊ **parenthood** *noun* state of being a parent 作为父母; **planned parenthood** = situation where two people plan to have a certain number of children and take contraceptives to limit the number of children in the family 计划生育的父母

QUOTE: In most paediatric wards today open visiting is the norm, with parent care much in evidence. Parents who are resident in the hospital also need time spent with them.
引文:今天,大多数儿科病房已形成开放探视的常规,很显然是因为父母挂念孩子。父母是医院的住院医也要花时间和孩子在一起。

Nursing Times 护理时代

parenteral *adjective* (drug) which is not given orally and so not by way of the digestive tract, but given in the form of injections *or* suppositories 肠道外给药的; **parenteral nutrition** *or* **feeding** = feeding of a patient by means other than by way of the digestive tract, especially giving injections of glucose to a critically ill patient 肠道外营养 *compare* 比较 ENTERAL

paresis *noun* partial paralysis 轻瘫

paresthesia = PARAESTHESIA 感觉异常

paries *noun* (i) superficial parts of a structure of organ 器官表面 (ii) wall of a cavity 壁 (NOTE: plural is **parietes**)

◊ **parietal** *adjective* referring to the wall of a cavity *or* any organ 器官壁层的; **parietal bones** *or* **parietals** = two bones which form the sides of the skull 顶骨; **parietal cell** = OXYNTIC CELL 壁细胞; **parietal lobe** = middle lobe of the cerebral hemisphere, which is associated with language and other mental processes, and also contains the postcentral gyrus 顶叶; **parietal pericardium** = outer layer of the serous pericardium not in direct contact with the heart muscle, which lies inside and is attached to the fibrous pericardium 心包壁层; **parietal peritoneum** = part of the peritoneum which lines the abdominal cavity and covers the abdominal viscera 腹膜壁层; **parietal pleura** = membrane attached to the diaphragm, and covering the chest cavity and lungs 胸膜壁层

Paris 巴黎 *see* 见 PLASTER

parkinsonism *or* **Parkinson's disease** *noun* slow progressive disorder affecting elderly people 帕金森氏病

◇ **parkinsonian** *adjective* referring to Parkinson's disease 帕金森病的; **parkinsonian tremor** 帕金森震颤

> COMMENT: Parkinson's disease affects the parts of brain which control movement. The symptoms include trembling of the limbs, a shuffling walk and difficulty in speaking. Some cases can be improved by treatment with levodopa.
> 注释:帕金森病影响脑控制运动的部分,症状包括肢体震颤、步态不稳及言语困难,一些病例用左旋多巴治疗有效。

paronychia *noun* inflammation near the nail which forms pus, caused by an infection in the fleshy part of the tip of a finger 甲沟炎 *see also* 参见 WHITLOW

parosmia *noun* disorder of the sense of smell 嗅觉倒错

parotid *adjective & noun* near the ear 耳旁,耳旁的; **parotid glands** *or* **parotids** = glands which produce saliva, situated in the neck behind the joint of the jaw and ear 腮腺 ◊ 见图 THROAT

◇ **parotitis** *noun* inflammation of the parotid glands 腮腺炎

> COMMENT: Mumps is the commonest form of parotitis, where the parotid gland becomes swollen and the sides of the face become fat.
> 注释:流行性腮腺炎是腮腺炎的最常见形式,发病时腮腺肿胀,一侧脸颊好像变胖了。

parous *adjective* (woman) who has given birth to one or more children 经产的

paroxysm *noun* (i) sudden movement of the muscles 发作,阵发 (ii) sudden appearance of symptoms of the disease 突发,症状突然出现 (iii) sudden attack of coughing *or* sneezing 阵咳、打喷嚏: ***He suffered paroxysms of coughing during the night.*** 他夜间阵发性咳嗽。

◇ **paroxysmal** *adjective* referring to a paroxysm; similar to a paroxysm 阵发的; **paroxysmal dyspnoea** = attack of breathlessness at night, caused by heart failure 阵发性呼吸困难; **paroxysmal tachycardia** = sudden attack of rapid heartbeats 阵发性心动过速

Parrot disease = PSITTACOSIS 鹦鹉热

pars *Latin word meaning* part 部分

part *noun* piece *or* one of the sections which make up a whole organ *or* body 部分; **spare part surgery** = surgery where parts of the body (such as bones or joints) are replaced by artificial pieces 置换术

◇ **partial** *adjective* not complete *or* affecting only part of something 部分的: ***He only made a partial recovery.*** 他只是部分恢复。**partial amnesia** = being unable to remember certain facts, such as the names of people 部分遗忘; **partial deafness** = being able to hear some sounds but not all 部分性耳聋; **partial gastrectomy** *or* **partial mastectomy** = operations to remove part of the stomach *or* part of a breast 胃或乳房部分切除; **partial vision** = being able to see only a part of the total field of vision *or* not being able to see anything very clearly 视野缺损、弱视

◇ **partially** *adverb* not completely 部分地: ***He is partially paralysed in his right side.*** 他的右侧部分瘫痪。**the partially sighted** = people who have only partial vision 弱视患者

◇ **partly** *adverb* not completely 部分地：***She is partly paralysed.*** 她部分瘫痪。

particle *noun* very small piece of matter 颗粒

◇ **particulate** *adjective* (i) referring to particles 粒子的 (ii) made up of separate particles 由粒子组成的

parturition *noun* childbirth 分娩

◇ **parturient** *adjective & noun* (i) referring to childbirth 产妇的 (ii) (woman) who is in labour 临产的

pascal *noun* SI unit of measurement of pressure 帕，压力的国际单位（NOTE: with figures usually written **Pa**）

> COMMENT：1 pascal is the pressure exerted on an area of 1 square metre by a force of 1 newton.
> 注释：1 帕是 1 平方米上施以 1 牛顿的压力。

Paschen bodies *plural noun* particles which occur in the skin lesions of smallpox patients 帕兴氏小体(天花病人皮损上的小颗粒)

pass *verb* to allow (faeces or urine) to come out of the body 排(泄)，排(遗)：***He passed blood in his bowel movement.*** 他便血。***She had pains when she passed water.*** 她尿痛。***He passed a small stone in his urine.*** 他尿中排出了一个小结石。

◇ **pass away** *or* **pass on** *verb* to die 死亡

◇ **pass on** *verb* to give to someone 传给(某人)：***Haemophilia is passed on by a woman to her sons.*** 血友病是由母亲传给儿子的。***The disease was quickly passed on by carriers to the rest of the population.*** 这种病很快由携带者传给了人群中的其他人。

◇ **pass out** *verb* to faint 晕厥：***When we told her her father was ill, she passed out.*** 我们告诉她她父亲病了，她当时就晕了过去。

passage *noun* (i) long narrow channel inside the body 管道，腔道 (ii) moving from one place to another 移动 (iii) evacuation of the bowels 结肠排空 (iv) introduction of an instrument into a cavity 在腔内插入器械；**air passage** = tube which takes air to the lungs 呼吸道；**anal passage** *or* **back passage** = the anus 肛门；**front passage** = (i) the urethra 尿道 (ii) the vagina 阴道

passive *adjective* not active 被动的，不活跃的；**passive immunity** = immunity which is acquired by a baby in the womb *or* by a patient through an injection with an antitoxin 被动免疫；**passive movement** = movement of a joint by a doctor *or* therapist, not by the patient himself 被动运动

past *adjective* (time) which has passed 过去的；**past history** = records of earlier illnesses 既往史：***He has no past history of renal disease*** 他既往无肾病史。

paste *noun* medicinal ointment which is quite solid and is spread or rubbed onto the skin 药膏

Pasteurella *noun* genus of parasitic bacteria, one of which causes the plague 巴斯德菌属

◇ **pasteurization** *noun* heating of food *or* food products to destroy bacteria 巴斯德消毒法

◇ **pasteurize** *verb* to kill bacteria in food by heating it 巴斯德消毒(加热消毒)：***The government is telling people to drink only pasteurized milk.*** 政府告诫市民只能喝消毒的牛奶。

> COMMENT：Pasteurization is carried out by heating food for a short time at a lower temperature than that used for sterilization: the two methods used are heating to 72℃ for fifteen seconds (the high temperature short time method) or to 65℃ for half an hour, and then cooling rapidly. This has the effect of killing tuberculosis bacteria.
> 注释：巴斯德消毒法是将食物在较低的温度短时间加热，加热温度比消毒灭菌低：常用的两种方法是在 72℃ 加热 15 分钟(高热短时法)或在 65℃ 加热半小时，然后迅速冷却，这样有杀灭结核菌的效果。

pastille *noun* (i) sweet jelly with medication in it, which can be sucked to relieve a sore throat 锭剂 (ii) small paper disc covered with barium platinocyanide, which changes colour when exposed to radiation 射线测试纸碟

pat *verb* to hit lightly 轻拍: ***She patted the baby on the back to make it burp.*** 她拍着婴儿的背部让他打嗝。

patch *noun* piece of plaster with a substance on it, which is stuck to the skin of a patient to allow the substance to be gradually absorbed into the system through the skin (as in HRT)贴剂; **nicotine patch** = patch containing nicotine which is released slowly into the bloodstream, as a method of curing nicotine addiction 尼古丁贴片; **patch test** = test for allergies *or* tuberculosis, where a piece of plaster containing an allergic substance *or* tuberculin is stuck to the skin to see if there is a reaction 斑贴试验(检测过敏原或结核) *compare* 比较 MANTOUX TEST

> COMMENT: Patches are available on prescription for various treatments, especially for administering hormone replacement therapy. They are also used for treating nicotine addiction and can be bought without a prescription.
> 注释:医生处方后可以得到用于多种治疗特别是激素替代治疗的贴片。贴片也可以用来治疗尼古丁成瘾并不用医生处方就能买到。

patella *or* **kneecap** *noun* small bone in front of the knee joint 髌骨,膝盖

◇ **patellar** *noun* referring to the kneecap 髌骨的,膝盖的; **patellar reflex** *or* **knee jerk** = jerk made as a reflex action by the knee, when the legs are crossed and the patellar tendon is tapped sharply 膝反射; **patellar tendon** = tendon just below the kneecap 髌韧带

◇ **patellectomy** *noun* surgical operation to remove the kneecap 髌骨摘除

patent *adjective* (**a**) open; exposed 开放的,未关闭的: ***The presence of a pulse shows that the main blood vessels from the heart to the site of the pulse are patent.*** 脉搏存在表明从心脏到有脉处的主要血管没有阻塞。**patent ductus arteriosus** = congenital condition where the ductus arteriosus does not close, allowing blood into the circulation without having passed through the lungs 动脉导管未闭 (**b**) **patent medicine** = medicinal preparation with special ingredients which is made and sold under a trade name 专利药品

◇ **patency** *noun* being open 开放,通畅: ***They carried out an examination to determine the patency of the Fallopian tubes.*** 他们做了一个检查来确定输卵管的通畅与否。***A salpingostomy was performed to restore the patency of the Fallopian tube.*** 施行输卵管再通术以恢复输卵管的通畅。

path- *or* **patho-** *prefix* referring to disease 病

◇ **pathogen** *noun* germ *or* microorganism which causes a disease 病原体

◇ **pathogenesis** *noun* origin *or* production *or* development of a morbid *or* diseased condition 疾病发生学,发病机制

◇ **pathogenetic** *adjective* referring to pathogenesis 发病的,致病的

◇ **pathogenic** *adjective* which can cause *or* produce a disease 致病的

◇ **pathogenicity** *noun* ability of a pathogen to cause a disease 致病力

◇ **pathognomonic** *adjective* (symptom) which is typical and characteristic, and which indicates that a patient has a particular disease 疾病特异性的

◇ **pathological** *adjective* referring to a disease *or* which is caused by a disease; which indicates a disease 病理学的,病理的; **pathological fracture** = fracture of a diseased bone 病理性骨折

◇ **pathologist** *noun* (**a**) doctor who specializes in the study of diseases and the changes in the body caused by disease; he examines tissue specimens from patients and reports on the presence or absence of disease in them 病理学家 (**b**) doctor who examines dead bodies to find out the cause of death 病

理解剖学家

◇ **pathology** *noun* study of diseases and the changes in structure and function which diseases cause in the body 病理学; **clinical pathology** = study of disease as applied to treatment of patients 临床病理学; **pathology report** = report on tests carried out to find the cause of a disease 病理报告

◇ **pathophysiology** *noun* study of abnormal or diseased organs 病理生理学

pathway *noun* series of linked neurones along which nerve impulses travel 通路; **final common pathway** = linked neurones which take all impulses from the central nervous system to a muscle 最终共同通路; **motor pathway** = series of motor neurones leading from the brain to the muscles 运动神经通路

-pathy *suffix* (i) diseased 病 (ii) treatment of a disease 治病

patient 1 *adjective* being able to wait a long time without getting annoyed 有耐心的: ***You will have to be patient if you are waiting for treatment — the doctor is late with his appointments.*** 等待治疗时你不得不耐下心来——医生比预约的晚到。**2** *noun* person who is in hospital *or* who is being treated by a doctor 病人: ***The patients are all asleep in their beds.*** 病人都在床上睡着了。***The doctor is taking the patient's temperature.*** 医生正在试病人的体温。**private patient** = patient who is paying for treatment, and who is not being treated under the National Health Service 就诊于私立医疗系统的病人,自费病人

◇ **patiently** *adverb* without getting annoyed 耐心地: ***They waited patiently for two hours before the consultant could see them.*** 他们在会诊医生看病之前耐心地等了两个小时。

patulous *adjective* stretched open *or* patent 开放的,扩展的

Paul-Bunnell reaction *or* **Paul-Bunnell test** *noun* blood test to see if a patient has glandular fever, where the patient's blood is tested against a solution containing glandular fever bacilli 保罗-邦内氏反应(检测传染性单核细胞增多症的试验)

Paul's tube *noun* glass tube used to remove the contents of the bowel after an opening has been made between the intestine and the abdominal wall 保罗氏管(用于小肠造瘘术后清除结肠内容物)

pavement epithelium *noun* squamous epithelium, a simple type of epithelium with flattened cells like scales, forming the lining of the serous membrane of the pericardium, the peritoneum and the pleura 鳞状上皮,扁平上皮

pay bed *noun* bed (usually in a separate room) in a National Health Service hospital for which a patient pays separately 自费病床

Pb *chemical symbol for* lead 铅的化学元素符号

PBI test = PROTEIN-BOUND IODINE TEST 蛋白结合碘试验

p.c. *abbreviation for* (缩写) *the Latin phrase* 'post cibium': after food (written on prescriptions) 餐后用(处方用语)

PCC = PROFESSIONAL CONDUCT COMMITTEE 专业指导委员会

pearl 珠 *see* 见 BOHN

Pearson bed *noun* type of bed with a Balkan frame, used for patients with fractures 皮尔逊床,用于骨折病人的带支架的床

peau d'orange *French phrase meaning* 'orange peel': thickened skin with many little depressions caused by lymphoedema which forms over a breast tumour or in elephantiasis [法语] 橘皮样变(淋巴水肿引起,见于乳腺肿瘤或象皮病)

pecten *noun* (i) middle section of the wall of the anal passage 肛门梳 (ii) hard ridge on the pubis 耻骨梳

◇ **pectineal** *adjective* (i) referring to the pecten of the pubis 耻骨梳的 (ii) (structure) with ridges like a comb 梳

pectoral 1 *noun* (**a**) therapeutic substance which has a good effect on respiratory disease 祛痰剂,舒胸理肺药 (**b**) = PECTORAL MUSCLE 胸肌 **2** *adjective* referring to the chest 胸部的; **pectoral girdle** *or* **shoulder girdle** = shoulder bones (the scapulae and clavicles) to which the upper arm bones are attached 肩胛带,上肢带; **pectoral muscle** *or* **chest muscle** = one of two muscles which lie across the chest and control movements of the shoulder and arm 胸肌

◇ **pectoralis** *noun* chest muscle 胸肌; **pectoralis major** = large chest muscle which pulls the arm forward or rotates it 胸大肌; **pectoralis minor** = small chest muscle which allows the shoulder to be depressed 胸小肌

◇ **pectoris** 心胸的 *see* 见 ANGINA

◇ **pectus** *noun* anterior part of the chest 前胸; **pectus excavatum** = FUNNEL CHEST 漏斗胸

ped- *or* **pedo-** 儿童 *US see* 见 PAED-

◇ **pediatrics**, **pediatrician** *US* 儿科学,儿科医师 *see* 见 PAEDIATRICS, PAEDIATRICIAN

pedicle *noun* (i) long thin piece of skin which attaches a skin graft to the place where it was growing originally 皮瓣 (ii) piece of tissue which connects a tumour to healthy tissue 连接肿瘤和健康组织的蒂 (iii) bridge which connects the lamina of a vertebra to the body 椎弓根

Pediculus *noun* louse, little insect which lives on humans and sucks blood 虱属; **Pediculus capitis** = head louse 头虱; **Pediculus corporis** = body louse 体虱; **Pediculus pubis** = pubic louse 阴虱 (NOTE: plural is **Pediculi**)

◇ **pediculosis** *noun* skin disease caused by being infested with lice 虱病

pediodontia *noun* study of children's teeth 儿童牙科学

◇ **pediodontist** *noun* dentist who specializes in the treatment of children's teeth 儿科牙医

peduncle *noun* stem *or* stalk 干,茎; **cerebellar peduncle** = band of nerve tissue connecting parts of the cerebellum 小脑脚; **cerebral peduncle** = mass of nerve fibres connecting the cerebral hemispheres to the midbrain 大脑脚 ◊ 见图 BRAIN

◇ **pedunculate** *adjective* having a stem *or* stalk 有干、茎的 (NOTE: the opposite is **sessile**)

PEEP = POSITIVE END-EXPIRATORY PRESSURE 呼气末正压呼吸

peel *verb* to take the skin off a fruit or vegetable 剥皮; (*of skin*) to come off in pieces 皮肤蜕皮: ***After getting sunburnt his skin began to peel.*** 太阳灼伤后,他开始脱皮。

Pel-Ebstein fever *noun* fever (associated with Hodgkin's disease) which recurs regularly 佩－埃二氏热(霍杰金氏病氏引起的周期热)

pellagra *noun* disease caused by deficiency of nicotinic acid, riboflavine and pyridoxine from the vitamin B complex, where patches of skin become inflamed, and the patient has anorexia, nausea and diarrhoea 糙皮病(缺乏 B 族维生素所致,症状有皮损、厌食、恶心及腹泻等)

> COMMENT: In some cases the patient's mental faculties can be affected, with depression, headaches and numbness of the extremities. Treatment is by improving the patient's diet.
> 注释:有些病人的精神会受到影响,可伴有抑郁、头痛及肢端麻木,治疗的方法是改善病人的饮食。

pellet *noun* (i) pill of steroid hormone, usually either oestrogen or testosterone 激素糖丸(通常含雌激素或睾酮) (ii) solid sediment at base of container after centrifuging 离心后的固体沉淀

pellicle *noun* thin layer of skin tissue 表皮

Pellegrini-Stieda disease *noun* disease where an injury to a knee causes the ligament to become calcified 佩－施二氏病(膝关节受伤后导致的韧带钙化)

pellucida 透明的 *see* 见 ZONA

pelvic *adjective* referring to the pelvis 骨盆的; **pelvic brim** = line on the ilium which separates the false pelvis from the true pelvis 骨盆缘; **pelvic cavity** = space below the abdominal cavity above the pelvis 盆腔; **pelvic floor** = lower part of the space beneath the pelvic girdle formed of muscle 骨盆底; **pelvic fracture** = fracture of the pelvis 骨盆骨折; **pelvic girdle** *or* **hip girdle** = ring formed by the two hip bones to which the thigh bones are attached 骨盆带

◊ **pelvimeter** *noun* instrument to measure the diameter and capacity of the pelvis 骨盆测量器

◊ **pelvimetry** *noun* measuring the pelvis, especially to see if the internal ring is wide enough for a baby to pass through in childbirth 骨盆测量

◊ **pelvis** *noun* (**a**) (i) group of bones and cartilage which form a ring and connect the thigh bones to the spine 骨盆 (ii) the internal space inside the pelvic girdle 盆腔 (**b**) **renal pelvis** *or* **pelvis of the kidney** = main central tube leading into the kidney from where the ureter joins it 肾盂 ◊ 见图 KIDNEY (NOTE: the plural is **pelves** *or* **pelvises.** Note also that for terms referring to the renal pelvis, see words beginning with **pyel-** *or* **pyelo-**)

COMMENT: The pelvis is a bowl-shaped ring, formed of the two hip bones, with the sacrum and the coccyx at the back. The hip bones are each in three sections: the ilium, the ischium and the pubis and are linked in front by the pubic symphysis. The pelvic girdle is shaped in a different way in men and women, the internal space being wider in women. The top part of the pelvis, which does not form a complete ring, is called the 'false pelvis'; the lower part is the 'true pelvis'.
注释：骨盆是一个碗形的圈，由两块髋骨及后面的骶骨和尾骨构成。两髋骨又各由三部分组成：髂骨、坐骨和耻骨，两边的髋骨在前面借耻骨联合相接。骨盆带的形状男女有别，女性的内骨盆较宽。骨盆的上部并未形成一个闭合的环，因此称作"假骨盆"；下部则是"真骨盆"。

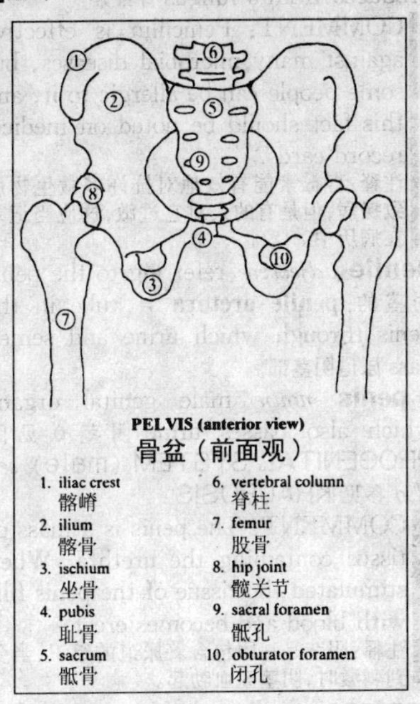

PELVIS (anterior view)
骨盆（前面观）

1. iliac crest 髂嵴
2. ilium 髂骨
3. ischium 坐骨
4. pubis 耻骨
5. sacrum 骶骨
6. vertebral column 脊柱
7. femur 股骨
8. hip joint 髋关节
9. sacral foramen 骶孔
10. obturator foramen 闭孔

pemphigoid *adjective* & *noun* (skin disease) which is similar to pemphigus 天疱疮样的，类天疱疮

◊ **pemphigus** *noun* rare disease where large blisters form inside the skin 天疱疮

penetrate *verb* to go through something *or* to go into something 穿透，穿入: ***The end of the broken bone has penetrated the liver.*** 骨折的断端刺破了肝脏。***The ulcer burst, penetrating the wall of the duodenum.*** 溃疡发作，穿透了十二指肠壁。

◊ **penetration** *noun* act of penetrating 穿透，穿入: ***the penetration of the vagina by the penis*** 阴茎插入阴道; ***penetration of an ovum by a spermatozoon*** 卵子被精子穿透

-penia *suffix* meaning lack *or* not enough of something 缺乏; **cytopenia** = lack of cellular elements in the blood 血细胞减少

Penicillium *noun* fungus from which penicillin is derived 青霉菌

◇ **penicillin** *noun* common antibiotic produced from a fungus 青霉素

> COMMENT: Penicillin is effective against many microbial diseases, but some people can be allergic to it, and this fact should be noted on medical record cards.
> 注释:青霉素能有效地对抗许多微生物所致疾病,但是有的人对它过敏,这应当记录在病历中。

penile *adjective* referring to the penis 阴茎的; **penile urethra** = tube in the penis through which urine and semen pass 尿道阴茎部

◇ **penis** *noun* male genital organ, which also passes urine 阴茎 ◊ 见图 UROGENITAL SYSTEM (male) *see also* 参见 KRAUROSIS

> COMMENT: The penis is a mass of tissue containing the urethra. When stimulated the tissue of the penis fills with blood and becomes erect.
> 注释:阴茎是一团包含着尿道的组织,当受到刺激时,阴茎充血勃起。

pentose *noun* sugar containing five carbon atoms 戊糖

◇ **pentosuria** *noun* abnormal condition where pentose is present in the urine 戊糖尿

pep *verb* (*informal* 非正式) to give (someone) a feeling of well-being 安慰: ***These pills will pep you up.*** 这些药丸会使你好起来的。

◇ **pep pill** = AMPHETAMINE 苯丙胺

pepsin *noun* enzyme in the stomach which breaks down the proteins in food into peptones 胃蛋白酶

◇ **pepsinogen** *noun* secretion from the gastric gland which is the inactive form of pepsin 胃蛋白酶原

◇ **peptic** *adjective* referring to digestion *or* to the digestive system 消化的; **peptic ulcer** = benign ulcer in the duodenum *or* in the stomach 消化性溃疡

◇ **peptidase** *noun* enzyme which breaks down proteins in the intestine into amino acids 肽酶

◇ **peptide** *noun* compound formed of two or more amino acids 肽

◇ **peptone** *noun* substance produced by the action of pepsins on proteins in food 蛋白胨

◇ **peptonuria** *noun* abnormal condition where peptones are present in the urine 蛋白胨尿

per *preposition* out of *or* for each 出于,超,每…; **ten per thousand** = ten out of every thousand 每千个之中有十个: ***The number of cases of cervical cancer per thousand patients tested.*** 每千名宫颈癌病人中接受试验的例数。

◇ **per cent** *adverb* & *noun* in *or* for every hundred 百分之: ***Fifty per cent (50%) of the tests were positive.*** 百分之五十的试验呈阳性。***Seventy-five per cent (75%) of hospital cases remain in hospital for less than four days.*** 75%的住院病人留院时间少于4天。***There has been a five per cent increase in applications.*** = The number of applications has gone up by five in every hundred. 申请的数量上升了5%。(NOTE: usually written % with figures: **we need to increase output by 5%**)

◇ **percentage** *noun* proportion rate in every hundred *or* for every hundred 百分率: ***What is the percentage of long-stay patients in the hospital?*** 长期住院病人的百分数是多少?

perception *noun* impression formed in the brain as a result of information about the outside world which is passed back by the senses 知觉

◇ **perceptive deafness** *noun* deafness caused by a disorder of the auditory nerves *or* the brain centres which receive nerve impulses 感受性耳聋

percussion *noun* test (usually on the heart and lungs) in which the doctor taps part of the patient's body and listens to the sound produced 叩诊

percutaneous *adjective* through the skin 经皮的

per diem *Latin phrase meaning* 'per day' (written on prescriptions)每天(处方用语)

perennial *adjective* which continues all the time, for a period of years 常年累月的,常年的:***She suffers from perennial bronchial asthma.*** 她常年患有支气管哮喘。

perforation *noun* hole through the whole thickness of a tissue *or* membrane (such as a hole in the intestine or in the eardrum)穿孔

◇ **perforate** *verb* to make a hole through something 穿孔:***The ulcer perforated the duodenum.*** 溃疡穿透了十二指肠。**perforated eardrum** = eardrum with a hole in it 穿孔的鼓膜;**perforated ulcer** = ulcer which has made a hole in the wall of the intestine 穿孔的溃疡

perform *verb* (**a**) to do (an operation) 施行:***A team of three surgeons performed the heart transplant operation.*** 三名外科医师组成的手术小组施行了那次心脏移植。(**b**) to work 运转,发挥功能:***The new heart has performed very well.*** 新(移植)的心脏工作良好。***The kidneys are not performing as well as they should.*** 双肾功能不佳。

◇ **performance** *noun* way in which something works 表现:***The doctors are not satisfied with the performance of the transplanted heart.*** 医生们对移植心脏的表现不满意。

perfusion *noun* passing of a liquid through vessels *or* an organ *or* tissue, especially the flow of blood into lung tissue 灌注;**hypothermic perfusion** = method of preserving donor organs by introducing a preserving solution and storing the organ at a low temperature 低温灌注

peri- *prefix* meaning near *or* around *or* enclosing 周匝

◇ **periadenitis** *noun* inflammation of tissue round a gland 腺体周围炎

◇ **perianal** *adjective* around the anus 肛周的;**perianal haematoma** = small painful swelling outside the anus caused by forcing a bowel movement 肛周血肿

◇ **periarteritis** *noun* inflammation of the outer coat of an artery and the tissue round it 动脉周围炎;**periarteritis nodosa** *or* **polyarteritis nodosa** = collagen disease, where the walls of the arteries become inflamed, causing asthma, high blood pressure and kidney failure 结节性动脉周围炎,结节性多动脉炎

◇ **periarthritis** *noun* inflammation of the tissue round a joint 关节周围炎;**chronic periarthritis** *or* **scapulohumeral arthritis** = inflammation of tissues round the shoulder joint 肩周炎

pericard- *prefix* referring to the pericardium 心包的

◇ **pericardectomy** *or* **pericardiectomy** *noun* surgical removal of the pericardium 心包切除

◇ **pericardial** *adjective* referring to the pericardium 心包的;**pericardial effusion** = fluid which forms in the pericardial sac during pericarditis 心包渗出;**pericardial friction** = rubbing together of the two parts of the pericardium in pericarditis 心包摩擦;**pericardial sac** *or* **serous pericardium** = the inner part of the pericardium forming a sac which contains fluid to prevent the two parts of the pericardium rubbing together 心包腔

◇ **pericardiocentesis** *noun* puncture of the pericardium to remove fluid 心包穿刺

◇ **pericardiorrhaphy** *noun* surgical operation to repair a wound in the pericardium 心包缝合术

◇ **pericardiostomy** *noun* surgical operation to open the pericardium through the thoracic wall to drain off fluid 心包造口术

◇ **pericarditis** *noun* inflammation of the pericardium 心包炎;**acute pericarditis** = sudden attack of fever and pains in the chest, caused by the two parts of the pericardium rubbing together 急性心包炎;**chronic pericarditis** *or* **constrictive pericarditis** = condition where the pericardium becomes thickened and prevents the heart from functioning normally 慢性心包炎,缩窄性心包炎

◇ **pericardium** *noun* membrane which surrounds and supports the heart 心包; **fibrous pericardium** = outer part of the pericardium which surrounds the heart and is attached to the main blood vessels 心包纤维层(壁层); **parietal pericardium** = outer layer of serous pericardium attached to the fibrous pericardium 壁层心包; **serous pericardium** *or* **pericardial sac** = the inner part of the pericardium, forming a double sac which contains fluid to prevent the two parts of the pericardium from rubbing together 浆液性心包,心包腔; **visceral pericardium** = inner layer of serous pericardium, attached to the wall of the heart 脏层心包

◇ **pericardotomy** *or* **pericardiotomy** *noun* surgical operation to open the pericardium 心包切开术

perichondritis *noun* inflammation of cartilage, especially in the outer ear 软骨膜炎

◇ **perichondrium** *noun* fibrous connective tissue which covers cartilage 软骨膜

◇ **pericolpitis** *or* **paracolpitis** *noun* inflammation of the connective tissue round the vagina 阴道周围炎

◇ **pericranium** *noun* connective tissue which covers the surface of the skull 颅骨膜

◇ **pericystitis** *noun* inflammation of the structures round the bladder, usually caused by infection in the uterus 膀胱周围炎

◇ **perifolliculitis** *noun* inflammation of the skin round hair follicles 毛囊周围炎

◇ **perihepatitis** *noun* inflammation of the membrane round the liver 肝脏周围炎

◇ **perilymph** *noun* fluid found in the labyrinth of the inner ear 外淋巴

perimeter *noun* (**a**) instrument to measure the field of vision 视野计 (**b**) length of the outside line around an enclosed area 周边

◇ **perimetry** *noun* measurement of the field of vision 视野检查

perimetritis *noun* inflammation of the perimetrium 子宫浆膜炎

◇ **perimetrium** *noun* membrane round the uterus 子宫外膜,子宫浆膜

◇ **perimysium** *noun* sheath which surrounds a bundle of muscle fibres 肌束膜

◇ **perinatal** *adjective* referring to the period just before and after childbirth 围产期的; **perinatal mortality rate** = number of babies born dead *or* who die during the period immediately after childbirth, shown per thousand babies born 围产期死亡率; **perinatal period** = period of time before and after childbirth (from the 28th week after conception to the first week after delivery) 围产期

perineal *adjective* referring to the perineum 会阴的; **perineal body** = mass of muscle and fibres between the anus and the vagina or prostate 会阴体; **perineal muscles** = muscles which lie in the perineum 会阴肌

◇ **perineoplasty** *noun* surgical operation to repair the perineum by grafting tissue 会阴成形术

◇ **perineorrhaphy** *noun* surgical operation to stitch up a perineum which has torn during childbirth 会阴缝合术

◇ **perinephric** *adjective* around the kidney 肾周围的

◇ **perinephritis** *noun* inflammation of tissue round the kidney, which spreads from an infected kidney 肾脏周围炎

◇ **perineum** *noun* skin and tissue between the opening of the urethra and the anus 会阴

◇ **perineurium** *noun* connective tissue which surrounds bundles of nerve fibres 神经束膜

period *noun* (**a**) length of time 时期: ***The patient regained consciousness after a short period of time.*** 病人很快就恢复了意识。***She is allowed out of bed for two periods each day.*** 允许她一天有两次下床活动时间。**safe period** = time during the menstrual cycle when conception is not likely to occur (used as a method of contraception)安全期(避孕方法之一) *see also* 参见 RHYTHM METHOD (**b**) menstruation *or* the menses *or* bleeding from the uterus which occurs in a woman each month when the lining of the womb is shed because no fertilized egg is present 月经期,月经,月经量: ***She always has heavy periods.*** 她经量总是很多。***Some women experience abdominal pain during their periods.*** 有些妇女有经期腹痛。***She has bleeding between periods.*** 她月经间期出血。

◇ **periodic** *adjective* which occurs from time to time 周期性的: ***He has periodic attacks of migraine.*** 他周期性偏头痛发作。***She has to go to the clinic for periodic checkups.*** 她不得不到诊所去做定期检查。**periodic fever** = disease of the kidneys, common in Mediterranean countries 周期热; **periodic paralysis** = recurrent attacks of weakness where the level of potassium in the blood is low 周期性麻痹

◇ **periodicity** *noun* timing of recurrent attacks of a disease 周期性

periodontal *or* **periodontic** *adjective* referring to the area around the teeth 牙周的; **periodontal disease** = PERIODONTITIS 牙周病; **periodontal membrane** *or* **periodontal ligament** = membrane which attaches a tooth to the bone of the jaw 牙周膜或韧带 ◇ 见图 TOOTH

◇ **periodontics** *or* **periodontia** *noun* study of diseases of the periodontal membrane 牙周病学

◇ **periodontist** *noun* dentist who specializes in the treatment of gum diseases 牙周病专家

◇ **periodontitis** *noun* infection of the periodontal membrane leading to pyorrhoea, and resulting in the teeth falling out if untreated 牙周炎

◇ **periodontium** *noun* periodontal membrane, but also used to refer to the gums and bone around a tooth 牙周组织;

perionychia *or* **perionyxis** *noun* painful swelling round a fingernail 甲周炎

perioperative *adjective* before and after a surgical operation 围手术期的

> QUOTE: During the perioperative period little attention is given to thermoregulation.
> 引文:围手术期间很少注意体温调节。
> **British Journal of Nursing** 英国护理杂志

periosteal *adjective* referring to the periosteum 骨膜的; attached to the periosteum 附着于骨膜的

◇ **periosteotome** *noun* surgical instrument used to cut the periosteum 骨膜刀

◇ **periosteum** *noun* dense layer of connective tissue around a bone 骨膜 ◇ 见图 BONE STRUCTURE

◇ **periostitis** *noun* inflammation of the periosteum 骨膜炎

peripheral *adjective* at the edge 外周的,周边的; **peripheral nerves** = pairs of motor and sensory nerves which branch out from the brain and spinal cord 外周神经; **peripheral nervous system (PNS)** = all the nerves in different parts of the body which are linked and governed by the central nervous system 外周神经系统; **peripheral vasodilator** = chemical substance which acts to widen the blood vessels in the arms and legs and so improves bad circulation 外周血管扩张剂; **peripheral vascular disease** = disease affecting the blood vessels which supply the arms and legs 周围血管病

periphlebitis *noun* (i) inflammation of the outer coat of a vein 静脉外膜炎 (ii) inflammation of the connective tissue round a vein 静脉周围炎

◇ **perisalpingitis** *noun* inflammation of the peritoneum and other parts round a Fallopian tube 输卵管腹膜炎

◇ **perisplenitis** *noun* inflammation of the peritoneum and other parts round the spleen 脾周炎

peristalsis *noun* movement (like waves) produced by alternate contraction and relaxation of muscles along an organ such as the intestine *or* oesophagus, which pushes the contents of the organ along it automatically 蠕动 *compare* 比较 ANTIPERISTALSIS

◇ **peristaltic** *adjective* occurring in waves, as in peristalsis 蠕动的

peritendinitis *noun* painful inflammation of the sheath round a tendon 腱鞘炎

◇ **peritomy** *noun* (i) surgical operation on the eye, where the conjunctiva is cut in a circle round the cornea 球结膜环状切开术 (ii) circumcision 包皮环切术

peritoneal *adjective* referring to the peritoneum; belonging to the peritoneum 腹膜的; **peritoneal cavity** = space between the layers of the peritoneum, containing the major organs of the abdomen 腹腔; **peritoneal dialysis** = removing waste matter from a patient's blood by introducing fluid into the peritoneum which then acts as a filter (as opposed to haemodialysis)腹膜透析

◇ **peritoneoscope** = LAPAROSCOPE 腹腔镜

◇ **peritoneoscopy** = LAPAROSCOPY 腹腔镜检查

◇ **peritoneum** *noun* membrane which lines the abdominal cavity and covers the organs in it 腹膜; **parietal peritoneum** = part of the peritoneum which lines the inner abdominal wall 壁层腹膜; **visceral peritoneum** = part of the peritoneum which covers the organs in the abdominal cavity 脏层腹膜

◇ **peritonitis** *noun* inflammation of the peritoneum as a result of bacterial infection 腹膜炎; **primary peritonitis** = peritonitis caused by direct infection from the blood *or* the lymph 原发性腹膜炎; **secondary peritonitis** = peritonitis caused by infection from an adjoining tissue, such as the rupturing of the appendix 继发性腹膜炎

> COMMENT: Peritonitis is a serious condition and can have many causes. One of its effects is to stop the peristalsis of the intestine so making it impossible for the patient to eat and digest.
> 注释:腹膜炎是一种严重的疾病,可以由许多原因引起。腹膜炎的结果之一是使肠道蠕动停止,致使病人不能进食和消化。

peritonsillar *adjective* around the tonsils 扁桃体周围的; **peritonsillar abscess** = QUINSY 扁桃体周围脓肿

peritrichous *adjective* (bacteria) where the surface of the cell is covered with flagella(细菌)有周毛的

◇ **periumbilical** *adjective* around the navel 脐周的

◇ **periureteritis** *noun* inflammation of the tissue round a ureter, usually caused by inflammation of the ureter itself 输尿管周围炎

◇ **periurethral** *adjective* around the urethra 尿道周围的

perlèche *noun* (i) cracks in dry skin at the corners of the mouth, often caused by riboflavine deficiency 传染性口角炎 (ii) candidiasis 念珠菌病

permanent *adjective* which exists always 永恒的,永久性的: ***The accident left him with a permanent disability.*** 事故给他造成了永久性残疾。 **permanent teeth** = teeth in an adult, which replace the child's milk teeth during late childhood 恒牙

> COMMENT: The permanent teeth consist of eight incisors, four canines, eight premolars and twelve molars, the last four molars (one on each side of the upper and lower jaw) being called the wisdom teeth.
> 注释:恒牙由 8 个切牙、4 个犬齿、8 个前臼齿和 12 个臼齿组成,最后 4 个臼齿(上下左右各一)称作智齿。

◇ **permanently** *adverb* always *or* for ever 永久地: ***He was permanently disabled in the accident.*** 他因事故导致了永久性残疾。

permeability *noun* (*of a membrane*) ability to allow certain substances in a fluid to pass through 通透性

◇ **permeable membrane** *noun* membrane which allows certain substances in a fluid to pass through it 通透膜

pernicious *adjective* harmful *or* dangerous (disease) *or* abnormally severe (disease) which is likely to end in death 恶性的; **pernicious anaemia** *or* **Addison's anaemia** = disease where an inability to absorb vitamin B_{12} prevents the production of red blood cells and damages the spinal cord 恶性贫血

pernio *noun* **erythema pernio** *or* **chilblain** = condition where the skin of the fingers, toes, nose or ears reacts to cold by becoming red, swollen and itchy 冻疮

◇ **perniosis** *noun* any condition caused by cold which affects blood vessels in the skin 冻伤

pero- *prefix* meaning deformed *or* defective 残缺

◇ **peromelia** *noun* congenital deformity of the limbs 四肢不全

peroneal *adjective* referring to the outside of the leg 腓骨的, 腓侧的; **peroneal muscle** *or* **peroneus** = one of three muscles (brevis, longus, tertius) on the outside of the lower leg which make the leg turn outwards 腓骨肌群

peroperative *adjective* taking place during a surgical operation 手术期间的

peroral *adjective* through the mouth 经口的

persecute *verb* to make someone suffer all the time 被迫害妄想: ***In paranoia, the patient feels he is being persecuted.*** 病人患偏执狂觉得被迫害。

◇ **persecution** *noun* being made to suffer 被迫害妄想: ***He suffers from persecution mania.*** 他患有被迫害妄想症。

perseveration *noun* repeating actions *or* words without any stimulus 重复言语, 重复动作

persist *verb* to continue for some time 持续: ***The weakness in the right arm persisted for two weeks.*** 右臂无力持续了两周。

◇ **persistent** *adjective* which continues for some time 持续的: ***She suffered from a persistent cough.*** 她患有持续咳嗽。 ***Treatment aimed at the relief of persistent angina.*** 治疗目标是解除持续性心绞痛。

person *noun* man *or* woman 人

◇ **personal** *adjective* (i) referring to a person 个人的 (ii) belonging to a person 属于个人的: ***Only certain senior members of staff can consult the personal records of the patients.*** 只有某些高级工作人员可以查阅病人的个人档案记录。

◇ **personality** *noun* way in which one person is mentally different from another 人格; **personality disorder** = disorder which affects the way a person behaves, especially in relation to other people 人格障碍

> QUOTE: Alzheimer's disease is a progressive disorder which sees a gradual decline in intellectual functioning and deterioration of personality and physical coordination and activity.
> 引文:阿尔茨海默病是一种渐进性疾病,可以见到智力逐渐下降,人格、躯体协调性和活动能力的破坏。
>
> **Nursing Times** 护理时代

personnel *noun* members of staff 人员: ***All hospital personnel must be immunized against hepatitis.*** 所有医院工作人员必须经过肝炎免疫。 ***Only senior personnel can inspect the patients' medical records.*** 只有高级工作人员能查看病人的病历。(NOTE: **personnel** is singular)

perspiration *noun* (i) action of sweating *or* of producing moisture through the sweat glands 出汗 (ii) sweat *or* moisture produced by the sweat glands 汗: ***Perspiration broke out on his forehead.*** 他前额出汗了。 **Sensible perspiration** = drops of sweat which can be seen on the skin, secreted by the sweat glands 可感知的出汗, 显性出汗

◇ **perspire** *verb* to sweat *or* to produce moisture through the sweat glands 出汗: ***After the game of tennis he was perspiring.*** 网球运动之后他出汗了。

> COMMENT: Perspiration is formed in the sweat glands under the epidermis and cools the body as the moisture evaporates from the skin. Sweat contains salt, and in hot countries it may be necessary to take salt tablets to replace the salt lost through perspiration.
> 注释:汗是表皮下的汗腺分泌的,汗液蒸发可以冷却身体。汗液中含有盐,在气候炎热的国家有时必须服用盐片来补充出汗丢失的盐分。

Perthes' disease *or* **Perthes' hip** *noun* disease (found in young boys) where the upper end of the femur degenerates and does not develop normally, sometimes resulting in a permanent limp 佩特兹病(骨骺的骨软骨病)

pertussis = WHOOPING COUGH 百日咳

perversion *noun* any abnormal behaviour 倒错,乖舛: ***He is suffering from a form of sexual perversion.*** 他得了一种性倒错病。

pes *noun* foot 足; **pes cavus** = CLAW FOOT 弓形足; **pes planus** = FLAT FOOT 扁平足

pessary *noun* (**a**) vaginal suppository *or* drug in soluble material which is pushed into the vagina and absorbed into the blood there 阴道栓剂 (**b**) contraceptive device worn inside the vagina to prevent spermatozoa entering 子宫托 (**c**) device like a ring, which is put into the vagina as treatment for prolapse of the womb 阴道环

pest *noun* animal which carries disease *or* attacks plants and animals and harms or kills them 害虫: ***a spray to remove insect pests*** 驱除传染疾病昆虫的喷剂

◇ **pesticide** *noun* substance which kills pests 杀虫剂

petechia *noun* small red spot, where blood has entered the skin 瘀血点 (NOTE: the plural is **petechiae**)

petit mal *noun* (less severe form of epilepsy, where loss of consciousness attacks last only a few seconds and the patient appears simply to be thinking deeply) 癫痫小发作

Petri dish *noun* small glass *or* plastic dish with a lid, in which a culture is grown 佩特里培养皿

petrosal *adjective* referring to the petrous part of the temporal bone(颞骨)岩部的

◇ **petrositis** *noun* inflammation of the petrous part of the temporal bone 颞骨岩部炎

◇ **petrous** *adjective* (i) like stone 岩石样的 (ii) petrosal(颞骨)岩部的: **petrous bone** = part of the temporal bone which forms the base of the skull and the inner and middle ears 颞骨岩部

-pexy *suffix* referring to fixation of an organ by surgery 固定术

Peyer's patches *noun* patches of lymphoid tissue on the mucous membrane of the small intestine 派依尔氏淋巴结

Peyronie's disease *noun* condition where hard fibre develops in the penis which becomes painful when erect (associated with Dupuytren's contracture) 佩罗尼氏病(纤维性海绵体炎)

pH *noun* concentration of hydrogen ions in a solution, which determines its acidity 酸碱度; **pH factor** = factor which indicates acidity or alkalinity pH 值; **pH test** = test to see how acid or alkaline a solution is pH 测定

> COMMENT: The pH factor is shown as a number; pH 7 is neutral; pH 8 and above show that the solution is alkaline and pH 6 and below show that the solution is acid.
> 注释:pH 值以数字来表示:pH 7 是中性的,pH 8 以上是碱性的,pH 6 以下是酸性的。

phaco- *or* **phako-** *prefix* referring to the lens of the eye 晶状体

phaeochromocytoma *noun* tumour

of the adrenal glands which affects the secretion of hormones such as adrenaline, which in turn results in hypertension and hyperglycaemia 嗜铬细胞瘤

phag- *or* **phago-** *prefix* referring to eating 吞咽

◊ **-phage** *suffix* which eats 吞咽

◊ **-phagia** *suffix* referring to eating 吞咽

◊ **phagocyte** *noun* cell, especially a white blood cell, which can surround and destroy other cells, such as bacteria cells 吞噬细胞

◊ **phagocytic** *adjective* (i) referring to phagocytes 吞噬细胞的 (ii) which destroys cells 破坏细胞的: ***Monocytes become phagocytic during infection.*** 感染时单核细胞变成吞噬细胞。

◊ **phagocytosis** *noun* destruction of bacteria cells and foreign bodies by phagocytes 吞噬作用

phako- *or* **phaco-** *prefix* referring to the lens of the eye 晶状体

◊ **phakic** *adjective* (eye) which has its natural lens(眼)带有本身晶状体的

phalangeal *adjective* referring to the phalanges 指(趾)骨的

◊ **phalanges** *plural of* PHALANX 指(趾)骨的复数形式

◊ **phalangitis** *noun* inflammation of the fingers or toes caused by infection of tissue 指(趾)骨炎

◊ **phalanx** *noun* bone in a finger or toe 指(趾)骨 ◊ 见图 HAND, FOOT

> COMMENT: The fingers and toes have three phalanges each, except the thumb and big toe, which have only two.
> 注释:指和趾各有三节指(趾)骨,拇指和踇趾除外,它只有两节。

phalloplasty *noun* surgical operation to repair a damaged *or* deformed penis 阴茎成形术

◊ **phallus** *noun* penis *or* male genital organ 阴茎

phantom *noun* (**a**) model of the whole body *or* part of the body, used to practise or demonstrate surgical operations 模型 (**b**) ghost, something which is not there but seems to be there 幻象; **phantom limb** = condition where a patient seems to feel sensations in a limb which has been amputated 幻肢; **phantom pregnancy** = PSEUDOCYESIS 假孕; **phantom tumour** = condition where a swelling occurs which imitates a swelling caused by a tumour 假瘤

pharmaceutical 1 *adjective* referring to pharmacy *or* drugs 药剂学的; **the Pharmaceutical Society** = professional association for pharmacists in Great Britain 药学会 **2** *noun* **pharmaceuticals** = drugs 药品

◊ **pharmacist** *noun* trained person who is qualified to prepare medicines according to the instructions on a doctor's prescription 药剂师; **community pharmacist** *or* **retail pharmacist** = person who makes medicines and sells them in a chemist's shop 社区药剂师,零售药剂师

> COMMENT: Qualified pharmacists must be registered by the Pharmaceutical Society of Great Britain before they can practise.
> 注释:合格的药剂师在开业前必须在大不列颠药学会登记。

◊ **pharmaco-** *prefix* referring to drugs 药

◊ **pharmacodynamic** *adjective* (property of a drug) which affects the part where it is applied 药效学的

◊ **pharmacokinetic** *adjective* (property of a drug) which has an effect over a period of time 药代动力学的

◊ **pharmacological** *adjective* referring to pharmacology 药理学的

◊ **pharmacologist** *noun* doctor who specializes in the study of drugs 药理学家

◊ **pharmacology** *noun* study of drugs *or* medicines, and their actions, properties and characteristics 药理学

◊ **pharmacopoeia** *noun* official list of drugs, their methods of preparation, dosages and the ways in which they should be used 药典

COMMENT: The British Pharmocopoeia is the official list of drugs used in the United Kingdom. The drugs listed in it have the letters BP after their name. In the USA the official list is the United States Pharmacopeia or USP.
注释:英国药典是联合王国内的法定药物清单,上面开列的药物在药名后有 BP 字样。在美国,法定清单是美国药典或USP。

◇ **pharmacy** *noun* (**a**) study of making and dispensing of drugs 药学: ***The six pharmacy students are taking their diploma examinations this year.*** 今年药学系有 6 个学生要进行执照考试。***He has a qualification in pharmacy.*** 他有药学合格证书。(**b**) shop *or* department in a hospital where drugs are prepared 药房,药店

◇ **Pharmacy Act** *or* **Poisons Act** *noun* one of several Acts of the British Parliament (Pharmacy and Poisons Act 1933, Misuse of Drugs Act 1971, Poisons Act 1972) which regulate the making *or* prescribing *or* selling of drugs 药物法,毒物法

pharyng- *or* **pharyngo-** *prefix* referring to the pharynx 咽

◇ **pharyngeal** *adjective* referring to the pharynx 咽部的: **pharyngeal pouch** *or* **visceral pouch** = one of the pouches in the side of the throat of an embryo 咽囊; **pharyngeal tonsil** = adenoidal tonsil, lymphoid tissue at the back of the throat where the passages from the nose join the pharynx 咽扁桃体

◇ **pharyngectomy** *noun* surgical removal of part of the pharynx, especially in cases of cancer of the pharynx 咽(部分)切除

◇ **pharyngismus** *or* **pharyngism** *noun* spasm which contracts the muscles of the pharynx 咽痉挛

◇ **pharyngitis** *noun* inflammation of the pharynx 咽炎

◇ **pharyngocele** *noun* (i) cyst which opens off the pharynx 咽突出 (ii) hernia of part of the pharynx 咽疝

◇ **pharyngolaryngeal** *adjective* referring to the pharynx and the larynx 咽喉的

◇ **pharyngoscope** *noun* instrument with a light attached, used by a doctor to examine the pharynx 咽镜

◇ **pharyngotympanic tube** *noun* Eustachian tube, one of two tubes which connect the back of the throat to the middle ear 咽鼓管

◇ **pharynx** *noun* muscular passage leading from the back of the mouth to the oesophagus 咽

COMMENT: The nasal cavity (or nasopharynx) leads to the back of the mouth (or oropharynx) and then into the pharynx proper, which in turn becomes the oesophagus when it reaches the sixth cervical vertebra. The pharynx is the channel both for air and food; the trachea (or windpipe) leads off it before it joins the oesophagus. The upper part of the pharynx (the nasopharynx) connects with the middle ear through the Eustachian tubes. When air pressure in the middle ear is not equal to that outside (as when going up or down in a plane), the tube becomes blocked and pressure can be reduced by swallowing.
注释:鼻腔(鼻咽)通向口的后部(口咽),进而到咽,咽部到达第六颈椎水平再演进为食管。咽既是空气的通道,也是食物的通道,气管(气道)在咽和食管汇合前先从咽部分出。咽的上部(鼻咽)借咽鼓管与中耳相通。当中耳的气压不等于外界气压时(如飞机起飞或降落时),咽鼓管闭合,压力可以通过吞咽降下来。

phase *noun* stage *or* period of development 期,相: ***If the cancer is diagnosed in its early phase, the chances of complete cure are much greater.*** 如果癌症在早期就诊断出来,完全治愈的机会就大得多。

phenobarbitone *noun* barbiturate drug, used as a sedative 苯巴比妥

phenol *or* **carbolic acid** *noun* strong disinfectant used for external use

酚,石炭酸

phenotype *noun* the particular characteristics of an organism 表型 *compare* 比较 GENOTYPE

QUOTE: All cancers may be reduced to fundamental mechanisms based on cancer risk genes or oncogenes within ourselves. An oncogene is a gene that encodes a protein that contributes to the malignant phenotype of the cell.
引文:所有癌症都可以归结为以体内癌基因为基础的根本机制。癌基因是编码致细胞恶性表型的蛋白质的基因。
British Medical Journal 英国医学杂志

phenylalanine *noun* essential amino acid 苯丙氨酸

phenylketonuria *noun* hereditary defect which affects the way in which the body breaks down phenylalanine, which in turn concentrates toxic metabolites in the nervous system causing brain damage 苯丙酮酸尿症

COMMENT: To have phenylketonuria, a child has to inherit the gene from both parents. The condition can be treated by giving the child a special diet but early diagnosis is essential to avoid brain damage.
注释:孩子患苯丙酮酸尿症的前提是自父母双方获得致病基因。可以通过给患儿提供特殊饮食来治疗此病,但要避免发生脑损害必须早期诊断。

phial *noun* small medicine bottle 小药瓶,管形瓶

-philia *suffix* meaning attraction *or* liking for something 嗜好,亲

philtrum *noun* (i) groove in the centre of the top lip 人中 (ii) drug believed to stimulate sexual desire 春药

phimosis *noun* condition where the foreskin is tight and has to be removed by circumcision 包茎

phleb- *or* **phlebo-** *prefix* referring to a vein 静脉

◇ **phlebectomy** *noun* surgical removal of a vein *or* part of a vein 静脉剥脱术

◇ **phlebitis** *noun* inflammation of a vein 静脉炎

◇ **phlebogram** *noun* venogram, an X-ray picture of a vein or system of veins 静脉造影片

◇ **phlebography** *noun* venography, X-ray examination of a vein using a radio-opaque dye so that the vein will show up on the film 静脉造影术

◇ **phlebolith** *noun* stone which forms in a vein as a result of an old thrombus becoming calcified 静脉石

◇ **phlebothrombosis** *noun* blood clot in a deep vein in the legs or pelvis, which can easily detach and form an embolus in a lung 静脉血栓

◇ **phlebotomy** *noun* operation where a vein or an artery is cut so that blood can be removed (as when taking blood from a donor)静脉切开术,放血术

phlegm *or* **sputum** *noun* mucus found in an inflamed nose, throat or lung and coughed up by the patient 粘液,痰: ***She was coughing up phlegm into her handkerchief.*** 她向手绢里咳痰。

◇ **phlegmasia alba dolens** *noun* milk leg *or* white leg, acute oedema of the leg, a condition which affects women after childbirth, where a leg becomes pale and inflamed as a result of lymphatic obstruction 股白肿(常见于产褥期)

phlyctenule *noun* (i) tiny blister on the cornea *or* conjunctiva 角膜或结膜的小水疱 (ii) any small blister 小水疱

phobia *noun* abnormal fear 恐怖症,恐惧症: ***He has a phobia about or of dogs.*** 他有恐犬症。***Fear of snakes is one of the commonest phobias.*** 怕蛇是常见的恐怖症之一。

◇ **-phobia** *suffix* meaning neurotic fear of something 怕,…恐怖; **agoraphobia** = fear of open spaces 聚会恐怖症,广场恐怖症,旷野恐怖症; **claustrophobia** = fear of enclosed spaces 幽闭恐怖症

◇ **phobic** *adjective* referring to a phobia 恐怖症的; **phobic anxiety** = state of worry caused by a phobia 恐怖症性焦虑

◇ **-phobic** *suffix* person who has a phobia of something…恐怖症患者; **agoraphobic** = person who is afraid of open spaces 聚会恐怖症患者

phocomelia *or* **phocomely** *noun* (i) congenital condition where the upper part of the limbs do not develop, leaving the hands or feet directly attached to the body 短肢畸形,海豹肢畸形 (ii) congenital condition in which the legs develop normally, but the arms are absent or underdeveloped 上肢短肢畸形

phon- *or* **phono-** *prefix* referring to sound *or* voice 声音

◇ **phonocardiogram** *noun* chart of the sounds made by the heart 心音图

◇ **phonocardiography** *noun* recording the sounds made by the heart 心音描记法

phosphataemia *noun* presence of excess phosphates (such as calcium *or* sodium) in the blood 高磷酸盐血症

◇ **phosphatase** *noun* group of enzymes which are important in the cycle of muscle contraction and in the calcification of bones 磷酸酶

◇ **phosphate** *noun* salt of phosphoric acid, used in tonics 磷酸盐

◇ **phosphaturia** *noun* condition where excess phosphates are present in the urine 磷酸盐尿症

> COMMENT: The urine becomes cloudy, which can indicate stones in the bladder or kidney.
> 注释:尿变混浊,提示膀胱或肾中有结石。

◇ **phospholipid** *noun* compound with fatty acids, which is one of the main components of membranous tissue 磷脂

◇ **phosphonecrosis** *noun* necrotic condition affecting the kidneys, liver and bones, usually seen in people who work with phosphorus 磷中毒性坏死

◇ **phosphorescent** *adjective* which shines without producing heat 磷光的

◇ **phosphoric acid** *noun* acid which forms phosphates 磷酸

◇ **phosphorus** *noun* toxic chemical element which is present in minute quantities in bones and nerve tissue; it causes burns if it touches the skin, and can poison if swallowed 磷 (NOTE: chemical symbol is **P**)

◇ **phossy jaw** *noun* type of phosphonecrosis resulting in disintegration of the bones of the lower jaw, caused by inhaling phosphorus fumes (the disease was once common among workers in match factories) 磷中毒性下颌坏死

phot- *or* **photo-** *prefix* referring to light 光,亮

◇ **photalgia** *noun* (i) pain in the eye caused by bright light 光敏致痛 (ii) severe photophobia 严重的光恐怖症

◇ **photocoagulation** *noun* process where tissue coagulates from the heat caused by light 光凝

> COMMENT: Photocoagulation is used to treat a detached retina.
> 注释:光凝术用于治疗视网膜脱离。

◇ **photodermatosis** *noun* lesion of the skin after exposure to bright light 日光性皮炎,光照性皮炎

◇ **photogenic** *adjective* (i) which is produced by the action of light 光所导致的 (ii) which produces light 发光的

◇ **photograph 1** *noun* picture taken with a camera, which uses the chemical action of light on sensitive film 照片; **X-ray photograph** = picture produced by exposing sensitive film to X-rays X 线片,X 光片: ***He was examining the X-ray photographs of the patient's chest.*** 他给病人拍了胸片。**2** *verb* to take a picture with a camera 照相,拍照

◇ **photography** *noun* taking pictures with a camera 照相术: ***The development of X-ray photography has meant that internal disorders can be more easily diagnosed.*** X 线照相术的进展意味着诊断体内疾病容易了。

◇ **photophobia** *noun* (i) condition where the eyes become sensitive to light and conjunctivitis may be caused (it can be associated with measles and some other infectious diseases) 畏光 (ii)

morbid fear of light 光恐怖症

◇ **photophthalmia** *noun* inflammation of the eye caused by bright light, as in snow blindness 强光眼炎

◇ **photopic vision** *noun* vision which is adapted to bright light (as in daylight) by using the cones in the retina instead of the rods, as in scotopic vision 明适应,光适应 *see also* 参见 LIGHT ADAPTATION

◇ **photoreceptor neurone** *noun* rod or cone in the retina, which is sensitive to light or colour 感光神经元

◇ **photoretinitis** *or* **sun blindness** *noun* damaged retina caused by looking at the sun 光照/日射性视网膜炎

◇ **photosensitive** *adjective* (skin *or* lens) which is sensitive to light *or* which is stimulated by light 光敏的

◇ **photosensitivity** *noun* being sensitive to light 光敏性

◇ **phototherapy** *noun* treatment of jaundice and vitamin D deficiency, which involves exposing a patient to rays of ultraviolet light 光疗

◇ **photuria** *noun* phosphorescent urine 磷光尿

phren- *or* **phreno-** *prefix* referring to (i) the brain 脑 (ii) the phrenic nerve 膈神经

◇ **phrenemphraxis** *noun* surgical operation to crush the phrenic nerve in order to paralyse the diaphragm 膈神经压轧术

◇ **-phrenia** *suffix* meaning disorder of the mind 精神障碍

phrenic *adjective* (i) referring to the diaphragm 膈的 (ii) referring to the mind *or* intellect 精神的,心灵的,心智的; **phrenic nerve** = pair of nerves which controls the muscles in the diaphragm 膈神经; **phrenic avulsion** 膈神经抽出术 *see* 见 AVULSION

◇ **phrenicectomy** *noun* surgical removal of all *or* part of the phrenic nerve 膈神经切除术

◇ **phreniclasia** *noun* operation to clamp the phrenic nerve 膈神经压轧术

◇ **phrenicotomy** *noun* operation to divide the phrenic nerve 膈神经分离术

Phthirius pubis *noun* pubic louse *or* crab louse *or* louse which infests the pubic region 阴虱

◇ **phthiriasis** *noun* infestation with the crab louse 阴虱病

phthisis *noun* old term for tuberculosis 痨病(结核的旧称)

phycomycosis *noun* acute infection of the lungs, central nervous system and other organs by a fungus 急性脏器真菌感染,藻菌病

physi- *or* **physio-** *prefix* referring to (i) physiology 生理 (ii) physical 体力

◇ **physic** *noun* old term for medicine 医学的旧称

physical 1 *adjective* referring to the body, as opposed to the mind 身体的,躯体的(与心灵的相对); **physical dependence** = state where a person is addicted to a drug such as heroin and suffers physical effects if he stops taking the drug 躯体依赖; **physical education** = teaching of sports and exercises in school 体育; **physical examination** = examination of a patient's body to see if he is healthy 体检; **physical medicine** = branch of medicine which deals with physical disabilities *or* with treatment of disorders after they have been diagnosed 躯体医学; **physical sign** = symptom which can be seen on the patient's body *or* which can be produced by percussion and palpation 体征; **physical therapy** = treatment of disorders by heat *or* by massage *or* by exercise and other physical means 理疗 **2** *noun* physical examination 体检: ***He has to pass a physical before being accepted by the police force.*** 被警察部队接收前他必须通过体检。

◇ **physically** *adverb* referring to the body 身体方面,躯体上: ***Physically he is very weak, but his mind is still alert.*** 他身体非常虚弱,但仍旧精神矍铄。

physician *noun* registered doctor who is not a surgeon 医生,内科医师 (NOTE: in GB English, **physician** refers to a specialist doctor, though not usually a surgeon, while in US English it is used for any qualified doctor)

physiological *adjective* referring to physiology *or* to the normal functions of the body 生理的; **physiological saline** *or* **solution** = any solution used to keep cells *or* tissue alive 生理盐水

◇ **physio** *noun* (*informal* 非正式) (i) session of physiotherapy treatment 理疗 (ii) physiotherapist 理疗师

◇ **physiologist** *noun* scientist who specializes in the study of the functions of living organisms 生理学家

◇ **human physiology** *noun* study of the human body and its normal functions 人体生理学

physiotherapy *noun* treatment of a disorder or condition by exercise *or* massage *or* heat treatment *or* infrared lamps, etc., to restore strength, to restore function after a disease or injury, to correct a deformity 理疗; **physiotherapy clinic** = clinic where patients can have physiotherapy 理疗门诊

◇ **physiotherapist** *noun* trained specialist who gives physiotherapy 理疗师

phyt- *or* **phyto-** *prefix* referring to plants *or* coming from plants 植物

pia mater *noun* delicate inner layer of the meninges, the membrane which covers the brain and spinal cord 软脑(脊)膜

pian = YAWS 雅司病

pica *noun* desire to eat things (such as wood *or* paper) which are not food, often found in pregnant women and small children 异食癖

pick *verb* to take away small pieces of something with the fingers *or* with a tool 拣拾: ***She picked the pieces of glass out of the wound with tweezers.*** 她用镊子夹出伤口中的玻璃片。**to pick one's nose** = to take pieces of mucus out of the nostrils 挖鼻子; **to pick one's teeth with a pin** = to take away pieces of food which are stuck between the teeth 剔牙

◇ **pick up** *verb* (*informal* 非正式) (**a**) to catch a disease 得(病): ***He must have picked up the disease when he was travelling in Africa.*** 他肯定是在非洲旅行时得上这种病的。(**b**) to get stronger *or* better 好起来,痊愈: ***He was ill for months, but he's picking up now.*** 他病了几个月,现在痊愈了。

Pick's disease *noun* (**a**) rare condition, where a disorder of the lipoid metabolism causes retarded mental development, anaemia, loss of weight and swelling of the spleen and liver 皮克病(一种类脂代谢障碍引起的罕见疾病,造成精神发育迟滞、贫血、消瘦及肝脾肿大) (**b**) constrictive pericarditis 缩窄性心包炎

pico- *prefix* meaning one million millionth (10^{-12})微微,毫纤 (NOTE: symbol is **P**)

◇ **picomole** *noun* unit of measurement of the amount of substance (= one million millionth of a mole)皮摩尔 (NOTE: with figures usually written **pmol**)

picornavirus *noun* virus containing RNA, such as enteroviruses and rhinoviruses 微小 RNA 病毒

PID = PROLAPSED INTERVERTEBRAL DISC 椎间盘脱出

pigeon chest *noun* deformity of the chest, where the breastbone sticks out 鸡胸

◇ **pigeon toes** *noun* condition where the feet turn towards the inside when a person is standing upright 鸽趾,内收足

pigment *noun* (i) substance which gives colour to part of the body such as blood *or* the skin *or* hair 色素 (ii) (*in pharmacy*) a paint (药物上)染料; **bile pigment** = yellow colouring matter in bile 胆色素; **blood pigment** = HAEMOGLOBIN 血色素; **respiratory pigment** = blood pigment which can carry oxygen collected in the lungs and release it in tissues 呼吸色素(从肺带走氧的血红蛋白)

◇ **pigmentation** *noun* colouring of the body, especially that produced by deposits of pigment 色素沉着

◇ **pigmented** *adjective* coloured *or* showing an abnormal colour 色素沉着的,有色素的; **pigmented epithelium** *or* **pigmented layer** = coloured tissue at the back of the retina 色素上皮,色素层

COMMENT: The body contains several substances which control colour: melanin gives dark colour to the skin and hair; bilirubin gives yellow colour to bile and urine; haemoglobin in the blood gives the skin a pink colour; carotene can give a reddish-yellow colour to the skin if the patient eats too many tomatoes or carrots. Some pigment cells can carry oxygen and are called 'respiratory pigments'.
注释:体内有几种物质可以控制颜色:黑色素使皮肤和头发呈黑色;胆色素使胆汁和尿呈黄色;血红蛋白使皮肤显粉色;如果病人食用过多的西红柿或胡萝卜,胡萝卜素使皮肤呈橘黄色。有些色素可以携带氧,称为"呼吸色素"。

piles = HAEMORRHOIDS 痔疮

pill *noun* small hard round ball of drug which is to be swallowed whole 药丸: ***He has to take the pills twice a day.*** 他每天必须吃两次药丸。 ***The doctor put her on a course of vitamin pills.*** 医生让她服用维生素药丸。 **the pill** = oral contraceptive 口服避孕药: ***She's on the pill.*** = She is taking a regular course of contraceptive pills. 她定期服用口服避孕药。 **morning-after pill** *or* **next-day pill** = contraceptive pill taken after intercourse 房事后女性服用的避孕药

◇ **pill-rolling** *noun* nervous action of the fingers, in which the patient seems to be rolling a very small object, associated with Parkinson's disease 搓丸样动作(见于帕金森病)

pillow *noun* soft cushion on a bed which the head lies on when the patient is lying down 枕头: ***The nurse gave her an extra pillow to keep her head raised.*** 护士给她加了个枕头使她的头部抬高。

pilo- *prefix* referring to hair 头发

◇ **pilomotor nerve** *noun* nerve which supplies the arrector pili muscles attached to hair follicles 竖毛神经

◇ **pilonidal cyst** *noun* cyst containing hair, usually found at the bottom of the spine near the buttocks(骶部)毛囊

◇ **pilonidal sinus** *noun* small depression with hairs at the base of the spine (骶部)毛窦

◇ **pilosebaceous** *adjective* referring to the hair follicles and the glands attached to them 毛囊与皮脂腺的

◇ **pilosis** *or* **pilosism** *noun* condition where someone has an abnormal amount of hair or where hair is present in an abnormal place 多毛症

◇ **pilus** *noun* (i) one hair(一根)毛发 (ii) hair-like process on the surface of a bacterium 菌体纤毛 *see also* 参见 ARRECTOR PILI

pimple *noun* papule *or* pustule (small swelling on the skin, containing pus)小脓疱: ***He had pimples on his neck.*** 他颈部有小脓疱。 ***Is that red pimple painful?*** 那个红色的小脓疱疼吗? **goose pimples** = reaction of the skin to being cold *or* frightened, where the skin is raised into many little bumps by the action of the arrector pili muscles 鸡皮疙瘩

◇ **pimply** *adjective* covered with pimples 多脓疱的

pin 1 *noun* (**a**) small sharp piece of metal for attaching things together 别针: ***The nurse fastened the bandage with a pin.*** 护士用别针固定绷带。 **safety pin** = special type of bent pin with a guard which protects the point, used for attaching nappies or bandages 安全别针(用于固定尿布或绷带) (**b**) metal nail used to attach broken bones(骨科)针,钉: ***He has had a pin inserted in his hip.*** 他的髋关节中有颗骨钉。 **2** *verb* to attach with a pin 用别针别住: ***She pinned the bandages carefully to stop them slipping.*** 她小心地用别针别好绷带以防滑动。 ***The bone had fractured in several places and needed***

***pinning*.** 这根骨头多处骨折,需要钢针固定。

pinch 1 *noun* (i) squeezing the thumb and first finger together 捏 (ii) quantity of something which can be held between the thumb and first finger 一小撮: ***She put a pinch of salt into the water*.** 她捏起一小撮盐放到水里。**2** *verb* (**a**) to squeeze something tightly between the thumb and first finger 捏,掐 (**b**) to squeeze 挤压: ***She developed a sore on her ankle where her shoe pinched*.** 她的脚踝被鞋子挤出了疱。

pineal (body) *or* **pineal gland** *noun* small cone-shaped gland situated below the corpus callosum in the brain, which produces melatonin and is believed to be associated with the circadian rhythm 松果体,松果腺 ◊ 见图 BRAIN

pinguecula *or* **pinguicula** *noun* condition affecting old people, where the conjunctiva in the eyes has small yellow growths near the edge of the cornea, usually on the nasal side 结膜黄斑(见于老人)

pink *adjective* of a colour like very pale red 粉红色; **pink disease** *or* **erythroedema** *or* **acrodynia** = children's disease where the child's hands, feet and face swell and become pink, with a fever and loss of appetite, caused by an allergy to mercury 红皮病,红皮性水肿(儿童对水银过敏所致,表现为手、脚和面部肿胀发红,伴有发热、纳差); **pink eye** *or* **epidemic conjunctivitis** = inflammation of the conjunctiva, where the eyelids become swollen and sticky and discharge pus, common in schools and other institutions, caused by the Koch-Weeks bacillus 红眼病,流行性结膜炎

pinna *or* **outer ear** *noun* part of the ear which is outside the head, connected by a passage to the eardrum 耳廓 ◊ 见图 EAR

pinocytosis *noun* process by which a cell surrounds and takes in fluid 胞饮作用,饮液作用

pins and needles *noun* non-medical term for paraesthesia, an unpleasant tingling feeling, caused when a nerve is irritated, as when a limb has become numb after the circulation has been blocked for a short time 针扎感,发麻

pint *noun* unit of measurement of liquids (= about 0.56 of a litre) 品脱(容量单位 = 0.56 升): ***He was given six pints of blood in blood transfusions during the operation*.** 手术中给他输了 6 品脱血。

pinta *noun* skin disease of the tropical regions of America, caused by a spirochaete *Treponema* 品他病(一种密螺旋体造成的皮肤病,见于非洲热带地区)

> COMMENT: The skin on the hands and feet swells and loses its colour.
> 注释:手脚的皮肤肿胀脱色。

pinworm *noun US* threadworm *or* thin nematode worm *Enterobius vermicularis* which infests the large intestine 线虫或蛲虫

PIP = PROXIMAL INTERPHALANGEAL JOINT 近端指(趾)间关节

pipette *noun* thin glass tube used in the laboratory for taking or measuring samples of liquid 吸量管,移液管

piriform fossae *plural noun* two hollows at the sides of the upper end of the larynx 梨状凹

pisiform (bone) *noun* one of the eight small carpal bones in the wrist 豌豆骨 ◊ 见图 HAND

pit *noun* hollow place on a surface 小凹; **the pit of the stomach** *or* **epigastrium** = part of the upper abdomen between the ribcage above the navel 胃窝,上腹部 *see also* 参见 ARMPIT

pitcher's elbow *US* = TENNIS ELBOW 网球肘

pithiatism *noun* way of influencing the patient's mind by persuading him of something, as when the doctor treats a condition by telling the patient that he is in fact well 说服疗法,暗示疗法

pitted *adjective* covered with small hollows 有小凹的,坑洼不平的: ***His skin was pitted by acne*.** 他的皮肤由于粉刺而坑

洼不平。

◇ **pitting** *noun* formation of hollows in the skin 皮肤变得坑洼不平

pituitary body *or* **pituitary gland** *or* **hypophysis cerebri** *noun* main endocrine gland in the body 垂体 ◇ 见图 BRAIN; **pituitary fossa** *or* **sella turcica** = hollow in the upper surface of the sphenoid bone in which the pituitary gland sits 垂体窝,蝶鞍

◇ **pituitrin** *noun* hormone secreted by the pituitary gland 垂体素

> COMMENT: The pituitary gland is about the size of a pea and hangs down from the base of the brain, inside the sphenoid bone, on a stalk which attaches it to the hypothalamus. The front lobe of the gland (the adenohypophysis) secretes several hormones (TSH, ACTH) which stimulate the adrenal and thyroid glands, or which stimulate the production of sex hormones, melanin and milk. The posterior lobe of the pituitary gland (the neurohypophysis) secretes the antidiuretic hormone (ADH) and oxytocin. The pituitary gland is the most important gland in the body because the hormones it secretes control the functioning of the other glands.
> 注释:垂体有豌豆大小,自脑底部垂下,它位于蝶骨之内,有柄与下丘脑相连。垂体前叶(腺垂体)分泌几种激素包括刺激甲状腺和肾上腺的甲状刺激素,促肾上腺皮质激素,及刺激性激素、黑色素和乳汁产生的激素。垂体后叶(神经垂体)分泌抗利尿激素和催产素。垂体是人体最重要的腺体,因为它所分泌的激素控制着其他腺体的功能。

pityriasis *noun* any skin disease where the skin develops thin scales 糠疹; **pityriasis alba** = disease of children with flat white patches on the cheeks 白糠疹; **pityriasis capitis** = dandruff, a condition where pieces of dead skin form on the scalp and fall out when the hair is combed 头皮糠疹; **pityriasis rosea** = mild irritating rash affecting young people, which appears especially in the early part of the year and has no known cause 玫瑰糠疹,蔷薇糠疹; **pityriasis rubra** = serious, sometimes fatal, skin disease, a type of exfoliative dermatitis, where the skin turns dark red and is covered with white scales 红糠疹,剥脱性皮炎

pivot 1 *noun* stem used to attach an artificial crown to the root of a tooth 桩,柱 2 *verb* to rest and turn on a point 作为枢轴: ***The atlas bone pivots on the second vertebra*** . 寰椎以第二颈椎为枢轴。**pivot joint** *or* **trochoid joint** = joint where a bone can rotate freely 枢轴关节

placebo *noun* tablet which appears to be a drug, but has no medicinal substance in it 安慰剂; **placebo effect** = apparently beneficial effect of telling a patient that he is having a treatment, even if this is not true, caused by the patient's hope that the treatment will be effective 安慰剂效应

> COMMENT: Placebos may be given to patients who have imaginary illnesses; placebos can also help in treating real disorders by stimulating the patient's psychological will to be cured. Placebos are also used on control groups in tests of new drugs (a placebo-controlled study).
> 注释:对疑病患者可以给予安慰剂;安慰剂还可通过激发病人要求治愈的心理愿望而对疾病起辅助治疗作用;在试验新药时还可用于对照组(安慰剂对照研究)。

placenta *noun* tissue which grows inside the uterus during pregnancy and links the baby to the mother 胎盘; **placenta praevia** = condition where the fertilized egg becomes implanted in the lower part of the uterus, which means that the placenta lies across the cervix and may become detached during childbirth and cause brain damage to the baby 前置胎盘; **battledore placenta** = placenta where the umbilical cord is attached to the edge and not the centre 球拍状胎盘(脐带在胎盘一侧而不是中

间)

◇ **placental** *adjective* referring to the placenta 胎盘的; **placental insufficiency** = condition where the placenta does not provide the fetus with the necessary oxygen and nutrients 胎盘功能不足

◇ **placentography** *noun* X-ray examination of the placenta of a pregnant woman after a radio-opaque dye has been injected 胎盘造影

> COMMENT: The vascular system of the fetus is not directly connected to that of the mother. The placenta allows an exchange of oxygen and nutrients to be passed from the mother to the fetus to which she is linked by the umbilical cord. It stops functioning when the baby breathes for the first time and is then passed out of the womb as the afterbirth.
> 注释:胎儿的血管系统并不直接与母亲的相通。胎盘使母亲和胎儿之间能够进行氧和营养的交换。当婴儿第一次呼吸时胎盘停止工作,而后以胎衣形式娩出子宫。

Placido's disc *or* **keratoscope** *noun* instrument for examining the cornea to see if it has an abnormal curvature 普莱西多氏盘,角膜镜

plagiocephaly *noun* condition where a person has a distorted head 斜头畸形

plague *noun* infectious disease which occurs in epidemics where many people are killed 鼠疫,瘟疫; **bubonic plague** = fatal disease caused by *Pasteurella pestis* in the lymph system transmitted to humans by fleas from rats 腺鼠疫(由鼠疫巴斯德菌由跳蚤从老鼠传到人,侵及淋巴系统); **pneumonic plague** = form of bubonic plague where mainly the lungs are affected 肺鼠疫; **septicaemic plague** = form of bubonic plague where the symptoms are generalized 鼠疫败血症; ***The hospitals cannot cope with all the plague victims.*** 医院不能接受治疗所有的鼠疫患者。***Thousands of people are dying of plague.*** 成千上万的人死于鼠疫。

> COMMENT: Bubonic plague was the Black Death of the Middle Ages; its symptoms are fever, delirium, prostration, rigor and swellings on the lymph nodes.
> 注释:腺鼠疫就是中世纪的黑死病;它的症状有发热、谵妄、衰竭、强直和淋巴结肿大。

plan 1 *noun* arrangement of how something should be done 计划; **care plan** = plan drawn up by the nursing staff for the treatment of an individual patient 护理计划 **2** *verb* to arrange how something is going to be done 计划,安排: ***They are planning to have a family.*** = They expect to have children and so are not taking contraceptives. 他们打算要孩子,无需避孕。

◇ **planned parenthood** *noun* situation where two people plan to have a certain number of children, and take contraceptives to control the number of children in the family 计划生育的父母

◇ **planning** *noun* arranging how something should be done 计划,打算; **family planning** = using contraceptives to control the number of children in a family 计划生育; **family planning clinic** = clinic which gives advice on contraception 计划生育门诊

> QUOTE: One issue has arisen — the amount of time and effort which nurses need to put into the writing of detailed care plans. Few would now dispute the need for clear, concise nursing plans to guide nursing practice, provide educational tools and give an accurate legal record.
> 引文:有一个问题——护士需要花多少时间和精力来写详细的护理计划。无需质疑一个清晰、简洁的护理计划可指导护理实践、提供教育工具和给出准确的法律上有效的记录。
>
> **Nursing Times** 护理时代

plane *noun* flat surface, especially that of the body seen from a certain angle 平面 *see* 见 CORONAL, MEDIAN, SAGITTAL

planta *noun* the sole of the foot 足底,

趾

◇ **plantar** *adjective* referring to the sole of the foot 足底的; **plantar arch** = curved part of the sole of the foot running along the length of the foot 足弓; **deep plantar arch** = curved artery crossing the sole of the foot 足深弓; **plantar flexion** = bending of the toes downwards 足趾弯曲; **plantar reflex** *or* **plantar response** = normal downward movement of the toes when the sole of the foot is stroked in Babinski test 趾反射; **plantar region** = the sole of the foot 足底区; **plantar surface** = the skin of the sole of the foot 脚底板; **plantar wart** = wart on the sole of the foot 趾疣

planus 扁平的 *see* 见 LICHEN, PES

plaque *noun* flat area 板,斑; **bacterial plaque** = hard smooth bacterial deposit on teeth 牙菌斑; **atherosclerotic plaque** = deposit on the walls of arteries 动脉硬化斑

-plasia *suffix* which develops *or* grows 增生

plasm- *or* **plasmo-** *prefix* referring to blood plasma 血浆

◇ **plasma** *noun* (i) yellow watery liquid which makes up the main part of blood 血浆 (ii) lymph with no corpuscles 淋巴液 (iii) cytoplasm 胞浆: ***The accident victim was given plasma.*** 给事故受难者输血浆。 **plasma cell** = lymphocyte which produces a certain type of antibody 浆细胞; **plasma protein** = protein in plasma (such as albumin, gamma globulin and fibrinogen) 血浆蛋白

◇ **plasmacytoma** *noun* malignant tumour of plasma cells, normally found in lymph nodes *or* bone marrow 浆细胞瘤

◇ **plasmapheresis** *noun* operation to take blood from a patient, then to separate the red blood cells from the plasma, and to return the red blood cells suspended in a saline solution to the patient through a transfusion 去血浆红细胞回输法

◇ **plasmin** *noun* fibrinolysin, enzyme which digests fibrin 纤维蛋白溶酶

◇ **plasminogen** *noun* substance in blood plasma which becomes activated and forms plasmin 纤溶酶原

> COMMENT: If blood does not clot it separates into blood corpuscles and plasma, which is formed of water and proteins, including the clotting agent fibrinogen. If blood clots, the corpuscles separate from serum, which is a watery liquid similar to plasma, but not containing fibrinogen. Dried plasma can be kept for a long time, and is used, after water has been added, for transfusions.
> 注释:如果血液不凝固,会分成血细胞和血浆,后者由水和蛋白质组成,包括凝血成分纤维蛋白原。如果血液凝固了,血细胞从血清中分离出来,血清是与血浆类似的水样液体,但是不含纤维蛋白原。干血浆可以保存很长时间,加水溶解后可用于输血。

Plasmodium *noun* type of parasite which infests red blood cells and causes malaria 疟原虫

plasmolysis *noun* contraction of a cell protoplasm by dehydration, where the surrounding cell wall becomes smaller 胞浆皱缩

plaster *noun* (**a**) white powder which is mixed with water and used to make a solid support to cover a broken limb 石膏: ***After his accident he had his leg in plaster for two months.*** 出车祸后,他的腿打了两个月石膏。 **plaster of Paris** = fine white plaster used to make plaster casts 巴黎石膏,煅石膏,干燥硫酸钙; **frog plaster** = plaster cast made to keep the legs in the correct position after an operation to correct a dislocated hip 蛙形石膏; **plaster cast** = hard support made of bandage soaked in liquid plaster of Paris, which is allowed to harden after being wrapped round a broken limb and which prevents the limb moving while the bone heals 石膏模具 (**b**) **sticking plaster** = adhesive plaster *or* sticky tape used to cover a small wound *or* to attach a pad of dressing to the skin 创可贴: ***Put a***

plaster on your cut. 在你的伤口上贴上创可贴。

plastic 1 *noun* artificial material made from petroleum, and used to make many objects, including replacement organs 塑料 **2** *adjective* which can be made in different shapes 可塑的; **plastic lymph** *or* **inflammatory lymph** = yellow liquid produced by an inflamed wound and which helps the healing process 可塑性淋巴, 炎症性淋巴; **plastic surgery** = surgery which repairs defective *or* deformed parts of the body 整形手术; **plastic surgeon** = surgeon who specializes in plastic surgery 整形外科医师

> COMMENT: Plastic surgery is especially important in treating accident victims or people who have suffered burns. It is also used to correct congenital deformities such as a cleft palate. When the object is simply to improve the patient's appearance, it is usually referred to as 'cosmetic surgery'.
> 注释:整形外科在事故受害者或烧伤患者的治疗中非常重要。它还可以用来矫正先天畸形,如腭裂。如果目标只是改进病人的外貌,则通常叫做美容外科。

-plasty *suffix* referring to plastic surgery 整形外科

plate *noun* **(a)** flat round piece of china for putting food on 盘子: ***The nurses brought round sandwiches on a plate for lunch.*** 护士们在盘子上盛了圆形三明治作午餐。***Pass your dirty plates to the person at the end of the table.*** 把脏盘子递给桌子顶头的那个人。**(b)** (i) flat sheet of metal *or* bone, etc. 板, 骨板 (ii) flat piece of metal attached to a fractured bone to hold the broken parts together 用于骨折内固定的钢板: ***The surgeon inserted a plate in her skull.*** 外科医师在她的头骨里钉入了一块钢板。**cribriform plate** = top part of the ethmoid bone which forms the roof of the nasal cavity and part of the top of the eye sockets 筛板; **dental plate** = prosthesis made to the shape of the mouth, which holds artificial teeth 牙板

platelet *noun* thrombocyte, a small blood cell which releases thromboplastin and which multiplies rapidly after an injury, encouraging the coagulation of blood 血小板; **platelet count** = test to count the number of platelets in a certain quantity of blood 血小板计数

platy- *prefix* meaning flat 平的

◇ **platysma** *noun* flat muscle running from the collarbone to the lower jaw (颈)阔肌

-plegia *suffix* meaning paralysis 麻痹, 瘫痪

pleio- *or* **pleo-** *prefix* meaning too many 过多

◇ **pleocytosis** *noun* condition where there are an abnormal number of leucocytes in the cerebrospinal fluid 脑脊液中白细胞增多

pleoptics *noun* treatment to help the partially sighted 弱视治疗

plessor *noun* little hammer with a rubber tip, used by doctors to tap tendons to test for reflexes or for percussion of the chest 叩诊槌

plethora *noun* old term meaning too much blood in the body 多血(症)

◇ **plethoric** *adjective* (appearance) due to dilatation of superficial blood vessels 多血的(表浅血管扩张所致)

plethysmography *noun* method of recording the changes in the volume of organs, mainly used to measure blood flow in the limbs 体积描记器

pleur- *or* **pleuro-** *prefix* referring to the pleura 胸膜

◇ **pleura** *noun* one of two membranes lining the chest cavity and covering each lung 胸膜; **parietal pleura** *or* **outer pleura** = membrane attached to the diaphragm and covering the chest cavity 壁层胸膜, 外层胸膜; **visceral pleura** *or* **inner pleura** = membrane attached to the surface of the lung 脏层胸膜, 内层胸膜 ⇨ 见图 LUNGS (NOTE: plural is pleurae)

◇ **pleuracentesis** 胸腔穿刺术 *see* 见 PLEUROCENTESIS

◇ **pleural** *adjective* referring to the pleura 胸膜的; **pleural cavity** = space between the inner and outer pleura 胸膜腔; **pleural effusion** = excess fluid formed in the pleural sac 胸膜渗出; **pleural fluid** = fluid which forms between the layers of the pleura in pleurisy 胸膜液; **pleural membrane** = PLEURA 胸膜

◇ **pleurectomy** *noun* surgical removal of part of the pleura which has been thickened or made stiff by chronic empyema 胸膜切除术

pleurisy *noun* inflammation of the pleura, usually caused by pneumonia 胸膜炎; **diaphragmatic pleurisy** = inflammation of the outer pleura only 膈胸膜炎

> COMMENT: The symptoms of pleurisy are coughing, fever, and sharp pains when breathing, caused by the two layers of pleura rubbing together.
> 注释:胸膜炎的症状包括咳嗽、发热和呼吸时锐痛,这是由两层胸膜摩擦所致。

pleuritis = PLEURISY 胸膜炎

◇ **pleurocele** *noun* (i) condition where part of the lung *or* pleura is herniated 胸膜突出,胸膜疝 (ii) fluid in the pleural cavity 胸膜液

◇ **pleurocentesis** *or* **pleuracentesis** *noun* operation where a hollow needle is put into the pleura to drain liquid 胸腔穿刺术

◇ **pleurodesis** *noun* treatment for a collapsed lung, where the inner and outer pleura are stuck together 胸膜固定术

◇ **pleurodynia** *noun* pain in the muscles between the ribs, due to rheumatic inflammation 胸肌痛; **epidemic pleurodynia** *or* **Bornholm disease** = virus disease affecting the intestinal muscles, with symptoms like influenza, fever, headaches and pains in the chest 流行性胸膜痛,流行性胸肌痛

◇ **pleuropneumonia** *noun* acute lobar pneumonia (the classic type of pneumonia) 胸膜肺炎

plexor 叩诊槌 *see* 见 PLESSOR

plexus *noun* network of nerves *or* blood vessels *or* lymphatics 丛; **Auerbach's plexus** = group of nerve fibres in the intestine 奥氏神经丛(位于小肠壁内); **brachial plexus** = group of nerves at the armpit and base of the neck which lead to the nerves in the arms and hands; injury to the brachial plexus at birth leads to Erb's palsy 臂丛; **cervical plexus** = group of nerves in front of the vertebrae in the neck, which lead to nerves supplying the skin and muscles of the neck, and also the phrenic nerve which controls the diaphragm 颈丛; **choroid plexus (of the lateral ventricle)** = part of the pia mater, a network of small blood vessels in the ventricles of the brain which produce cerebrospinal fluid 脉络丛; **lumbar plexus** = point near the spine above the pelvis where several nerves supplying the thigh and abdomen are joined together 腰丛; **sacral plexus** = group of nerves inside the pelvis near the sacrum which lead to nerves in the buttocks, back of the thigh and lower leg and foot 骶丛; **solar plexus** *or* **coeliac plexus** = network of nerves in the abdomen, behind the stomach 腹腔丛

pliable *adjective* which can bend easily 易弯曲的

plica *noun* fold 皱襞,褶

◇ **plicate** *adjective* folded 有皱襞的

◇ **plication** *noun* (i) surgical operation to reduce the size of a muscle *or* a hollow organ by making folds in its walls and attaching them 折叠术 (ii) the action of folding 折叠 (iii) a fold 皱褶

plombage *noun* (i) packing bone cavities with antiseptic material 骨腔充填术 (ii) packing of the lung *or* pleural cavities with inert material 肺或胸腔充填术

plumbism *noun* lead poisoning 铅中毒

Plummer-Vinson syndrome *noun* type of iron-deficiency anaemia, where the tongue and mouth become inflamed and the patient cannot swallow 普－文二氏综合征(缺铁性贫血所致,口舌肿胀,病人不能吞咽)

plunger *noun* part of a hypodermic syringe which slides up and down inside the tube, either sucking liquid into the syringe or forcing the contents out 针栓

PM = POST MORTEM 尸检: ***What are the results of the PM?*** 尸检的结果如何?

PMA = PROGRESSIVE MUSCULAR ATROPHY 进行性肌萎缩

pmol = PICOMOLE 皮摩尔

PMT = PREMENSTRUAL TENSION 经前紧张: ***She is being treated for PMT.*** 她因经前紧张在接受治疗。***The hospital has a special clinic for PMT sufferers.*** 医院设有针对经前紧张的专科门诊。

-pnea *or* **-pnoea** *suffix* referring to breathing 呼吸

pneum- *or* **pneumo-** *prefix* referring to air *or* to the lungs *or* to breathing 空气,呼吸,肺

◊ **pneumatocele** *noun* (i) sac *or* tumour filled with gas 气瘤,气囊 (ii) herniation of the lung 肺膨出

◊ **pneumaturia** *noun* passing air or gas in the urine 含气尿

◊ **pneumocephalus** *noun* presence of air *or* gas in the brain 颅腔积气

◊ **pneumococcal** *adjective* referring to pneumococci 肺炎球菌的

◊ **pneumococcus** *noun* genus of bacteria which causes respiratory tract infections, including pneumonia 肺炎球菌 (NOTE: plural is **pneumococci**)

◊ **pneumoconiosis** *noun* lung disease where fibrous tissue forms in the lungs because the patient has inhaled particles of stone *or* dust over a long period of time 尘肺

◊ **pneumoencephalography** *noun* X-ray examination of the ventricles and spaces of the brain taken after air has been injected into the cerebrospinal fluid by lumbar puncture 气脑造影术

> COMMENT: The air takes the place of the cerebrospinal fluid and makes it easier to photograph the ventricles clearly. This technique has been superseded by CAT and MRI.
> 注释:气体占据了脑脊液的位置,使脑室更易清晰地显影。这一技术已经被 CT 和磁共振成像取代。

◊ **pneumogastric** *adjective* referring to the lungs and the stomach 肺胃的; **pneumogastric nerve** *or* **vagus nerve** = tenth cranial nerve, which controls swallowing and nerve fibres in the heart and chest 肺胃神经,迷走神经

◊ **pneumograph** *noun* instrument which records chest movements during breathing 呼吸描记器

◊ **pneumohaemothorax** *or* **haemopneumothorax** *noun* blood *or* air in the pleural cavity 血气胸

◊ **pneumomycosis** *noun* infection of the lungs caused by a fungus 肺真菌感染

pneumon- *or* **pneumono-** *prefix* referring to the lungs 肺

◊ **pneumonectomy** *noun* surgical removal of all *or* part of a lung 肺(叶)切除术

pneumonia *noun* inflammation of a lung, where the tiny alveoli of the lung become filled with fluid 肺炎: ***He developed pneumonia and had to be hospitalized.*** 他得了肺炎,不得不住院。***She died of pneumonia.*** 她死于肺炎。**bacterial pneumonia** = form of pneumonia caused by pneumococcus 细菌性肺炎 *see also* 参见 BRONCHOPNEUMONIA; **double pneumonia** *or* **bilateral pneumonia** = pneumonia affecting both lungs 双侧肺炎; **hypostatic pneumonia** = pneumonia caused by fluid which accumulates in the posterior bases of the lungs of a bedridden patient 坠积性肺炎 **lobar pneumonia** = pneumonia which affects one or more lobes of the lung 大叶性肺炎; **viral** *or* **virus pneumonia** = type of inflammation of the lungs caused by a virus 病

毒性肺炎 *see also* 参见 ASPIRATION

> COMMENT: The symptoms of pneumonia are shivering, pains in the chest, high temperature and sputum brought up by coughing.
> 注释:肺炎的症状是寒战、胸痛、高热和咳痰。

pneumonic plague *noun* form of bubonic plague which mainly affects the lungs 肺鼠疫

◇ **pneumonitis** *noun* inflammation of the lungs 肺炎

◇ **pneumoperitoneum** *noun* air in the peritoneal cavity 气腹症

◇ **pneumoradiography** *noun* X-ray examination of part of the body after air *or* a gas has been inserted to make the organs show more clearly 充气造影术

◇ **pneumothorax** *noun* collapsed lung, condition where air *or* gas is in the thorax 气胸; **artificial pneumothorax** = former method of treating tuberculosis, where air was introduced between the layers of the pleura to make the lung collapse 人工气胸; **spontaneous pneumothorax** = pneumothorax caused by a rupture of an abnormal condition on the surface of the pleura 自发性气胸; **tension pneumothorax** = pneumothorax where rupture of the pleura forms an opening like a valve, through which air is forced during coughing but cannot escape 张力性气胸; **traumatic pneumothorax** = pneumothorax which results from damage to the lung surface *or* wall of the chest, which allows air to leak into the space between the pleurae 创伤性气胸

-pnoea *suffix* referring to breathing 呼吸

PNS = PERIPHERAL NERVOUS SYSTEM 周围神经系统

pock *noun* (i) localized lesion on the skin, due to smallpox *or* chickenpox 疱 (ii) infective focus on the membrane of a fertile egg, caused by a virus 痘

◇ **pockmark** *noun* scar left by a pustule, as in smallpox 痘痕

◇ **pockmarked** *adjective* (face) with scars from smallpox 有痘痕的

pocket *noun* (i) small bag attached to the inside to a coat, etc. in which money, handkerchief, keys, etc., can be kept 口袋 (ii) cavity in the body 体腔; **pocket of infection** = place where an infection remains 感染灶

pod- *prefix* referring to the foot 足

podagra = GOUT 痛风

podalic version *noun* turning of the fetus in the womb by the feet 胎足倒转术

podiatrist *noun US* person who specializes in the care of the foot and its diseases 足病治疗师

◇ **podiatry** *noun US* study of minor diseases and disorders of the feet 足病学

-poiesis *suffix* which forms 产生,造

poikilo- *prefix* meaning irregular *or* varied 不规则的,变异的

◇ **poikilocyte** *noun* abnormally large red blood cell with an irregular shape 异形红细胞

◇ **poikilocytosis** *noun* condition where poilkilocytes exist in the blood 异形红细胞症

poikilothermic *adjective* (animal) with cold blood *or* cold-blooded (animal) 变温的,冷血的(动物),冷血的 *compare* 比较 HOMOIOTHERMIC

> COMMENT: The body temperature of cold-blooded animals changes with the outside temperature.
> 注释:冷血动物的体温随外界温度而变化。

point *noun* (**a**) sharp end 尖儿: ***Surgical needles have to have very sharp points.*** 外科针必须有很锋利的尖。(**b**) dot used to show the division between whole numbers and parts of numbers 小数点 (NOTE: **3.256**: say 'three point two five six'; **his temperature was 38.7**: say 'thirty-eight point seven) (**c**) mark in a series of numbers 点: ***What's the freezing point of water?*** 水的冰点是多少?

◇ **pointed** *adjective* with a sharp point 有尖儿的; **a pointed rod** 带尖儿的杆

poison 1 *noun* substance which can

kill *or* harm body tissues if eaten or drunk 毒物: ***He died after someone put poison in his coffee.*** 有人在他的咖啡里投毒后，他死了。 ***Poisons must be kept locked up.*** 毒物必须锁好保存。 **poison ivy** *or* **poison oak** = American plants whose leaves can cause a painful rash if touched 有毒常春藤，毒橡树; **Poisons Act** 毒物法 *see* 见 PHARMACY ACT **2** *verb* to give someone a poison *or* a substance which can harm or kill 投毒，毒害，损害: ***The workers were poisoned by toxic fumes.*** 工人们毒气中毒了。 ***The wound was poisoned by bacterial infection.*** 细菌感染使伤口恶化了。

◇ **poisoning** *noun* condition where a person is made ill *or* is killed by a poisonous substance 中毒; **blood poisoning** = condition where bacteria are present in blood and cause illness 败血症，菌血症; **Salmonella poisoning** = poisoning by Salmonellae which develop in the intestines 沙门氏菌中毒; **staphylococcal poisoning** = poisoning by staphylococci in food 葡萄球菌中毒

◇ **poisonous** *or* **toxic** *adjective* (substance) which is full of poison *or* which can kill or harm 有毒的: ***Some mushrooms are good to eat and some are poisonous.*** 有些蘑菇可食用，有些蘑菇有毒。 **poisonous gas** = gas which can kill *or* which can make someone ill 毒气

> COMMENT: The commonest poisons, of which even a small amount can kill, are arsenic, cyanide and strychnine. Many common foods and drugs can be poisonous if taken in large doses. Common household materials such as bleach, glue and insecticides can also be poisonous. Some types of poisoning, such as Salmonella, can be passed to other people through lack of hygienic conditions.
> 注释：最常见的毒物是砷、氰化物和马钱子碱，很少量就能致死。许多普通的食物和药物如果大量食用也可以中毒。通常的家居材料，如漂白剂、胶水和杀虫剂也是有毒的。有些中毒，如沙门菌中毒，因卫生条件欠佳而传给他人。

polar *adjective* with a pole 有极的; **polar body** = small cell which is produced from an oocyte but does not develop into an ovum 极体

◇ **pole** *noun* (i) end of an axis 极 (ii) end of a rounded organ, such as the end of a lobe in the cerebral hemisphere 圆形器官的边缘

poli- *or* **polio-** *prefix* referring to grey matter in the nervous system 灰质

◇ **polio** (*informal* 非正式) 脊髓灰质炎 *see* 见 POLIOMYELITIS

◇ **polioencephalitis** *noun* type of viral encephalitis, an inflammation of the grey matter in the brain caused by the same virus as poliomyelitis 脑灰质炎

◇ **polioencephalomyelitis** *noun* polioencephalitis which also affects the spinal cord 脑脊髓灰质炎

◇ **poliomyelitis** *or* **polio** *or* **infantile paralysis** *noun* infection of the anterior horn cells of the spinal cord caused by a virus which attacks the motor neurones and can lead to paralysis 脊髓灰质炎，小儿麻痹; **abortive poliomyelitis** = mild form of poliomyelitis which only affects the throat and intestines 顿挫型脊髓灰质炎; **bulbar poliomyelitis** = type of polio affecting the brain stem, which makes it difficult for a patient to swallow or breathe 延髓型脊髓灰质炎; **nonparalytic poliomyelitis** = form of poliomyelitis similar to the abortive form but which also affects the muscles to a certain degree 非瘫痪性脊髓灰质炎; **paralytic poliomyelitis** = poliomyelitis which affects the patient's muscles 瘫痪性脊髓灰质炎

◇ **poliovirus** *noun* virus which causes poliomyelitis 脊髓灰质炎病毒

> COMMENT: Symptoms of poliomyelitis are paralysis of the limbs, fever and stiffness in the neck. The bulbar form may start with difficulty in swallowing. Poliomyelitis can be

prevented by immunization and two vaccines are used: the Sabin vaccine is formed of live polio virus and is taken orally on a piece of sugar; Salk vaccine is given as an injection of dead virus.
注释:脊髓灰质炎的症状有肢体瘫痪、发热和颈项僵硬。延髓型可以以吞咽困难开始。脊髓灰质炎可以通过免疫来预防,有两种疫苗可用:萨宾疫苗是活病毒制成的口服糖丸;索尔克疫苗是注射用死病毒。

Politzer bag *noun* rubber bag which is used to blow air into the middle ear to unblock a Eustachian tube 波利泽尔咽鼓管吹气袋

pollen *noun* tiny cells from flowers which float in the air in spring and summer, and which cause hay fever 花粉; **pollen count** = figure which shows the amount of pollen in a sample of air 花粉计数

pollex *noun* thumb 拇指 (NOTE: the plural is **pollices**)

pollinosis = HAY FEVER 花粉病,枯草热

pollute *verb* to make the air *or* a river *or* the sea dirty, especially with industrial waste 污染

◇ **pollutant** *noun* substance which pollutes 污染物

◇ **pollution** *noun* making dirty 污染; **atmospheric pollution** = pollution of the air 大气污染

poly- *prefix* meaning many *or* much *or* touching many organs 多

◇ **polyarteritis nodosa** *or* **periarteritis nodosa** *noun* collagen disease where the walls of the arteries in various parts of the body become inflamed, leading to asthma, high blood pressure and kidney failure 结节性多动脉炎

◇ **polyarthritis** *noun* inflammation of several joints, such as rheumatoid arthritis 多关节炎

◇ **polycystitis** *noun* congenital disease where several cysts form in the kidney at the same time 多囊肾

◇ **polycythaemia** *noun* blood disease where the number of red blood cells increases often due to difficulties which the patient has in breathing 红细胞增多症; **polycythaemia vera** *or* **erythraemia** = blood disease where the number of red blood cells increases, together with an increase in the number of white blood cells, making the blood thicker and slowing its flow 真性红细胞增多症

◇ **polydactylism** *or* **hyperdactylism** *noun* condition where a person has more than five fingers or toes 多指(趾)

◇ **polydipsia** *noun* condition (often caused by diabetes insipidus) where the patient is abnormally thirsty 烦渴

◇ **polygraph** *noun* instrument which records the pulse in several parts of the body at the same time 多种波动描记器

◇ **polymorph** *or* **neutrophil** *noun* type of leucocyte or white blood cell with an irregular nucleus 多形核粒细胞

◇ **polymyalgia rheumatica** *noun* disease of elderly people where the patient has pain and stiffness in the shoulder and hip muscles making them weak and sensitive 风湿性多肌痛

◇ **polyneuritis** *noun* inflammation of many nerves 多神经炎

◇ **polyneuropathy** *noun* any disease which affects several nerves 多神经病

◇ **polyopia** *or* **polyopsia** *or* **polyopy** *noun* condition where the patient sees several images of one object at the same time 视物显多症(三个以上) *compare* 比较 DIPLOPIA

polyp *or* **polypus** *noun* tumour, growing on a stalk in mucous membrane, which can be cauterized, often found in the nose, mouth or throat 息肉 (NOTE: plural of **polypus** is **polypi**)

◇ **polyposis** *noun* condition where a patient has a number of polyps 息肉病 *see also* 参见 FAMILIAL ADENOMATOUS POLYPOSIS

polypeptide *noun* type of protein formed of linked amino acids 多肽

◇ **polyphagia** *noun* (i) condition where a patient eats too much 多食 (ii) morbid desire for every kind of food 贪食症

◇ **polypharmacy** *noun* prescribing several drugs to be taken at the same time 联合用药

◇ **polyploid** *adjective* (cell) where there are more than three sets of the haploid number of chromosomes 多倍体 *compare with* 比较 DIPLOID, HAPLOID

◇ **polyposis** *noun* condition where many polyps form in the mucous membrane of the colon 息肉病

◇ **polypus** = POLYP 息肉

◇ **polyradiculitis** *noun* disease of the nervous system which affects the roots of the nerves 多神经根炎

◇ **polysaccharide** *noun* type of carbohydrate 多糖

◇ **polyserositis** *noun* inflammation of the membranes lining the abdomen, chest and joints and exudation of serous fluid 多浆膜炎

◇ **polyspermia** *or* **polyspermism** *or* **polyspermy** *noun* (i) excessive seminal secretion 精液过多 (ii) fertilization of one ovum by several spermatozoa 多精子受精

◇ **polyunsaturated fat** *noun* fatty acid capable of absorbing more hydrogen (typical of vegetable and fish oils) 多不饱和脂肪

◇ **polyuria** *noun* condition where a patient passes a large quantity of urine, usually as a result of diabetes insipidus 多尿

◇ **polyvalent** *adjective* having more than one valency 多价的

pompholyx *noun* (i) type of eczema with many irritating little blisters on the hands and feet 汗疱 (ii) morbid skin condition with bulbous swellings 汗疱疹

pons *noun* (**a**) bridge of tissue joining parts of an organ 组织间的桥联 (**b**) **pons (Varolii)** = part of the hindbrain, formed of fibres which continue the medulla oblongata 脑桥 ◊ 见图 BRAIN (NOTE: plural is **pontes**)

◇ **pontine** *noun* referring to a pons 脑桥的; **pontine cistern** = subarachnoid space in front of the pons, containing the basilar artery 脑桥池

poor *adjective* not very good 糟糕,差: ***He's in poor health.*** 他身体状况很糟。***She suffers from poor circulation.*** 她血循环很差。

◇ **poorly** *adjective* (*informal* 非正式) not very well 糟糕地: ***Her mother has been quite poorly recently.*** 最近她的母亲情况很糟。***He felt poorly and stayed in bed.*** 他感觉不舒服,卧床未起。

POP = PROGESTERONE ONLY PILL 孕酮片

popeyes *plural noun US* protruding eyes 突眼

popliteal *adjective* referring to the back of the knee 腘窝的; **popliteal artery** = artery which branches from the femoral artery behind the knee and leads into the tibial arteries 腘动脉; **popliteal fossa** *or* **popliteal space** = space behind the knee between the hamstring and the calf muscle 腘窝

◇ **popliteus** *or* **popliteal muscle** *noun* muscle at the back of the knee 腘肌

population *noun* (**a**) number of people living in a country *or* town 人口: ***Population statistics show that the birth rate is slowing down.*** 人口统计显示出生率在下降。***The government has decided to screen the whole population of the area.*** 政府已经决定筛查该地区的所有人口。(**b**) number of patients in hospital 病人数: ***The hospital population in the area has fallen below ten thousand.*** 这一地区的住院病人数已经下降到不足一万。

pore *noun* (i) tiny hole in the skin through which the sweat passes 毛孔 (ii) small communicating passage between cavities 孔,门 ◊ 见图 SKIN & SENSORY RECEPTORS

porencephaly *or* **porencephalia**

or **porencephalus** *noun* abnormal cysts in the cerebral cortex, as a result of defective development 脑孔洞畸形

porous *adjective* (i) containing pores 有孔的 (ii) (tissue) which allows fluid to pass through 渗水的: ***Porous bone surrounds the Eustachian tubes.*** 咽鼓管周围包绕着松质骨。

porphyria *noun* hereditary disease affecting the metabolism of porphyrin pigments 血卟啉病

◇ **porphyrin** *noun* family of biological pigments (the commonest is protoporphyrin IX) 卟啉

◇ **porphyrinuria** *noun* presence of excess porphyrins in the urine, a sign of porphyria or of metal poisoning 卟啉尿

COMMENT: Porphyria causes abdominal pains and attacks of mental confusion. The skin becomes sensitive to light and the urine becomes coloured and turns dark brown when exposed to the light.
注释:血卟啉病引起腹痛和精神错乱。病人皮肤对光过敏,尿颜色改变,见光后变成深棕色。

porta *noun* opening which allows blood vessels to pass into an organ 门; **porta hepatis** = opening in the liver through which the hepatic artery, hepatic duct and portal vein pass 肝门

portable *adjective* which can be carried 便携的: ***He keeps a portable first aid kit in his car.*** 他在汽车中放了一个便携式的急救包。***The ambulance team carried a portable blood testing unit.*** 救护队带了一套便携式血液检测装置。

portal *adjective* referring to a porta, especially the portal system *or* the portal vein 门的,特别指门静脉系统的; **portal hypertension** = high pressure in the portal vein, caused by cirrhosis of the liver or a clot in the vein, causing internal bleeding 门脉高压 *see also* 参见 BANTI'S SYNDROME; **portal pyaemia** = infection of the portal vein in the liver, giving abscesses 化脓性门静脉炎; **portal system** = group of veins which have capillaries at both ends and do not go to the heart, such as the portal vein 门脉系统; **portal vein** = vein which takes blood from the stomach, pancreas, gall bladder, intestines and spleen to the liver 门静脉

porter *noun* person who does general work in a hospital, such as wheeling a patient's trolley into the operating theatre, moving heavy equipment, etc. 护理员

portocaval *adjective* linking the portal vein to the inferior vena cava 门腔静脉的; **portocaval anastomosis** = surgical operation to join the portal vein to the inferior vena cava 门腔静脉吻合术; **portocaval shunt** = artificial passage made between the portal vein and the inferior vena cava to relieve portal hypertension 门腔静脉分流术

◇ **porto-systemic encephalopathy** *noun* mental disorder and coma caused by liver disorder due to portal hypertension 门脉系统脑病 (NOTE: for terms referring to the portal vein, see words beginning with **pyl-** or **pyle-**)

port wine stain *noun* naevus *or* purple birthmark 胎痣(紫色)

position 1 *noun* (**a**) place (where something is) 位置: ***The exact position of the tumour is located by an X-ray.*** X线确定了肿瘤的确切位置。(**b**) the way a patient stands *or* sits *or* lies 体位; **genupectoral position** = kneeling with the chest on the floor 膝胸卧位; **lithotomy position** = lying on the back with the hips and knees bent 截石位; **recovery position** *or* **semiprone position** = lying face downwards, with one knee and one arm bent forwards and the face turned to one side 半俯卧位 *see also* 参见 TRENDELENBURG'S **2** *verb* to place in a certain position 占位: ***The fetus is correctly positioned in the uterus.*** 胎儿在子宫内位置正确。

positive *adjective* which indicates the

answer 'yes' or which shows the presence of something 阳性的: ***Her cervical smear was positive.*** 她的宫颈涂片结果是阳性的。***She gave a positive test for cervical cancer.*** 她的宫颈癌试验呈阳性。**positive end-expiratory pressure (PEEP)** = forcing the patient to breathe through a mask in cases where fluid has collected in the lungs 呼气末正压通气; **positive feedback** = situation where the result of a process stimulates the process which caused it 正反馈; **positive pressure ventilation (PPV)** = forcing air into the lungs to encourage the lungs to expand 正压通气; **positive pressure respirator** = machine which forces air into a patient's lungs through a tube inserted in the mouth 正压呼吸

◇ **positively** *adverb* in a positive way 积极地, 正确地: ***She reacted positively to the test.*** 她积极地对待试验。

posology *noun* study of doses of medicine 药物剂量学

posseting *noun* (*in babies*) bringing up small quantities of curdled milk into the mouth after feeding (婴儿)溢奶

Possum *noun* device using electronic switches which helps a severely paralysed patient to work a machine such as a telephone or typewriter 助动器 (NOTE: the name is derived from the first letters of **Patient-Operated Selector Mechanism**)

post- *prefix* meaning after *or* later 之后

◇ **postcentral gyrus** *noun* sensory area of the cerebral cortex, which receives impulses from receptor cells and senses pain, heat, touch, etc. 中央后回

◇ **post-cibal** *adjective* after having eaten food 餐后的

◇ **postconcussional** *adjective* (symptoms) which follow after a patient has had concussion 脑震荡后的

◇ **post-epileptic** *adjective* after an epileptic fit 癫痫发作后的

posterior *adjective* at the back 后面的: ***The cerebellum is posterior to the medulla oblongata.*** 小脑位于延髓后面。**posterior approach** = (operation) carried out from the back 后入路(手术从背部开口); **posterior aspect** = view of the back of the body *or* of part of the body 后面观; **posterior chamber (of the eye)** = part of the aqueous chamber which is behind the iris 后房; **posterior synechia** = condition of the eye where the iris sticks to the anterior surface of the lens 虹膜后粘连

◇ **posteriorly** *adverb* behind 从后面地: ***An artery leads to a posteriorly placed organ.*** 有一根动脉伸入到后位的器官。***Rectal biopsy specimens are best taken posteriorly.*** 直肠活检最好从后壁取标本。(NOTE: the opposite is **anterior**)

postganglionic *adjective* placed after a ganglion (神经)节后的; **postganglionic fibre** = axon of a nerve cell which starts in a ganglion and extends beyond the ganglion 节后纤维; **postganglionic neurone** = neurone which starts in a ganglion and ends in a gland *or* unstriated muscle 节后神经元

◇ **posthepatic** *adjective* after the liver 肝后的; **posthepatic bilirubin** = bilirubin which enters the plasma after being treated by the liver 肝后性胆红素; **posthepatic jaundice** *or* **obstructive jaundice** = jaundice caused by an obstruction in the bile ducts 肝后性黄疸, 梗阻性黄疸

◇ **post herpetic neuralgia** *noun* pains felt after an attack of shingles 带状疱疹后神经痛

◇ **posthitis** *noun* inflammation of the foreskin 包皮炎

◇ **posthumous** *adjective* after death 遗腹的; **posthumous birth** = (i) birth of a baby after the death of the father 产下遗腹子 (ii) birth of a baby by Caesarean section after the mother has died 孕妇死后做剖宫产

◇ **post-irradiation** *adjective* (pain *or* disorder) caused by X-rays 放射后的

◇ **postmature baby** *noun* baby born

more than nine months after conception 过期产婴儿

◇ **postmaturity** *noun* pregnancy which lasts longer than nine months 过期孕娃

◇ **postmenopausal** *adjective* after the menopause 绝经后的: ***She experienced some postmenopausal bleeding.*** 她有些绝经后出血。

◇ **post mortem**(**PM**) *noun* examination of a dead body by a pathologist to find out the cause of death 尸检: ***The post mortem (examination) showed that he had been poisoned.*** 尸检显示他曾中毒。

◇ **postnasal** *noun* behind the nose 鼻后的; **postnasal drip** = condition where mucus from the nose runs down into the throat and is swallowed 鼻涕倒流

◇ **postnatal** *adjective* after the birth of a child 出生后的; **postnatal depression** = depression which sometimes affects a woman after childbirth 产后抑郁

◇ **postnecrotic cirrhosis** *noun* cirrhosis of the liver caused by viral hepatitis 坏死性肝硬化

◇ **post-op** (*informal* 非正式) = POSTOPERATIVE, POSTOPERATIVELY 术后的

◇ **postoperative** *adjective* after a surgical operation 术后的: ***The patient has suffered postoperative nausea and vomiting.*** 病人术后恶心呕吐。***Occlusion may appear as postoperative angina pectoris.*** (冠脉)阻塞可以表现为术后心绞痛。**the second postoperative day** = the second day after an operation 术后第二天; **postoperative pain** = pain felt by a patient after an operation 术后疼痛

◇ **postoperatively** *adverb* after a surgical operation 术后地: **At twelve months post-op** *or* **postoperatively** = twelve months after the operation 术后12个月

> QUOTE: The nurse will help ensure that the parent is physically fit to cope with the postoperative child.
> 引文:护士会帮助确保父母在体力上能胜任孩子的术后照顾。
> **British Journal of Nursing** 英国护理杂志

◇ **postpartum** *adjective* postnatal *or* after the birth of a child 产后的; **postpartum haemorrhage** (**PPH**) = heavy bleeding after childbirth 产后大出血

◇ **postprandial** *adjective* after eating a meal 餐后的

◇ **post-primary tuberculosis** *noun* reappearance of tuberculosis in a patient who has been infected with it before 复发性结核病

◇ **postsynaptic** *adjective* after a synapse 突触后的; **postsynaptic axon** = nerve leaving one side of a synapse 突触后轴突

◇ **post-traumatic** *adjective* after a trauma (such as an accident, rape, fire, etc.) 创伤后的; **post-traumatic amnesia** = amnesia which follows a trauma 创伤后遗忘

posture *noun* way of standing *or* sitting 姿势,体位: ***Bad posture can cause pain in the back.*** 不良姿势可以引起背痛。***She has to do exercises to correct her bad posture*** *or* ***she has to do posture exercises.*** 她不得不通过练习来纠正自己的坏姿势或她不得不做姿势练习。

◇ **postural** *adjective* referring to posture 姿势的,体位的: ***a study of postural disorders*** 一项对体位障碍的研究; **postural drainage** = removing matter from infected lungs by making the patient lie down with his head lower than his feet, so that he can cough more easily 体位引流; **postural hypotension** = low blood pressure when standing up suddenly, causing dizziness 体位性低血压

postviral *adjective* after a virus 病毒(感染)后的; **postviral fatigue syndrome** = myalgic encephalomyelitis, a long-term condition affecting the nervous system, where the patient feels tired and depressed and has pain and weakness in the muscles 病毒后肌痛性脑脊髓炎

potassium *noun* metallic element 钾 (NOTE: chemical symbol is **K**)

◇ **potassium permanganate** （**$KMnO_4$**）*noun* purple-coloured poisonous salt, used as a disinfectant 高锰酸钾(用于消毒)

Pott's disease *or* **Pott's caries** *noun* tuberculosis of the spine, causing paralysis 波特氏病,波特氏骨疡(脊柱结核,造成瘫痪)

◇ **Pott's fracture** *noun* fracture of the lower end of the fibula together with displacement of the ankle and foot outwards 波特氏骨折(腓骨下端骨折合并踝和足外翻)

pouch *noun* small sac *or* pocket attached to an organ 囊,窝,凹陷; **branchial pouch** = pouch on the side of the neck of an embryo 鳃囊

poultice *noun* fomentation, compress made of hot water and flour paste *or* other substances which is pressed on to an infected part to draw out pus *or* to relieve pain *or* to encourage the circulation 泥敷剂,糊状药剂

pound *noun* measure of weight (about 450 grams) 磅（约 450 克）: ***The baby weighed only four pounds at birth.*** 这个婴儿出生时只有 4 磅重。(NOTE: with numbers **pound** is usually written **lb**; **the baby weighs 6lb**)

Poupart's ligament *noun* inguinal ligament, ligament in the groin, running from the spine to the pubis 普帕尔韧带(腹股沟韧带)

powder *noun* medicine like fine dry dust made from particles of drugs 药粉: ***He took a powder to help his indigestion or he took an indigestion powder.*** 他服用一种药粉来帮助改善消化不良或他服用了一种治疗消化不良的药粉。

◇ **powdered** *adjective* crushed so that it forms a fine dry dust 制成粉末状的: ***The medicine is available in tablets or in powdered form.*** 这种药有片剂和粉剂两种剂型。

pox *noun* (i) old name for syphilis 梅毒的旧称 (ii) disease with eruption of vesicles *or* pustules 痘

◇ **poxvirus** *noun* any of a group of viruses, such as those which cause cowpox and smallpox 痘病毒

> QUOTE: Molluscum contagiosum is a harmless skin infection caused by a poxvirus that affects mainly children and young adults.
> 引文:传染性软疣是一种无害的皮肤感染,由痘病毒引起,主要感染儿童和青壮年。
> **British Medical Journal** 英国医学杂志

PPD = PURIFIED PROTEIN DERIVATIVE 纯化蛋白衍化物

PPH = POSTPARTUM HAEMORRHAGE 产后大出血

PPV = POSITIVE PRESSURE VENTILATION 正压通气

p. r. *abbreviation for* (缩写) *the Latin phrase* 'per rectum': examination by the rectum 经直肠的,肛诊

practice *noun* (**a**) patients of a doctor *or* dentist; work of a doctor *or* dentist 从业,执业,开业,行医: ***He has been in practice for six years.*** 他已经行医 6 年了。***After qualifying he joined his father's practice.*** 取得行医资格后,他跟着父亲开业。**general practice** = doctor's practice where patients from an area are treated for all types of disease 全科医疗: ***He left the hospital and went into general practice.*** 他离开了医院,到全科领域行医。***She is in general practice in the North of London or she has a general practice in North London.*** 她在伦敦北区做全科医师。**group practice** = medical practice where several doctors *or* dentists share the same office building and support services 集体开业,集体行医; **practice leaflet** = leaflet produced by the doctors in a practice, giving details of the telephone numbers, hours when the surgery is open, etc. 导医手册; **practice nurse** = nurse employed by a clinic *or* doctor's practice who can give help and advice to patients 开业护士 (**b**) actual working 实践,实习: ***It's a good idea, but will it work in practice?*** 这是一个好主意,但在实践中能行得通吗?

QUOTE: Practice nurses play a major role in the care of patients with chronic disease and they undertake many preventive procedures.
引文:开业护士在照顾慢性病人上起着主要作用,而且他们承担了许多预防工作。
Nursing Times 护理时代

QUOTE: Patients presenting with symptoms of urinary tract infection were recruited in a general practice survey.
引文:全科医生调查的对象是有尿路感染症状的患者。
Journal of the Royal College of General Practitioners 皇家全科医师学会杂志

◇ **practise** *verb* to work as a doctor 行医: ***He practises in North London.*** 他在伦敦北部行医。***She practises homeopathy.*** 她在从事顺势医疗。***A doctor must be registered before he can practise.*** 医生在行医前必须登记。

◇ **practitioner** *noun* doctor, a qualified person who practises 开业医; **general practitioner (GP)** = doctor who treats many patients in an area for all types of illness and does not specialize 全科医师; **nurse practitioner** = (i) nurse employed by a clinic *or* doctor's practice who can give advice to patients 开业护士(被开业医雇佣的护士) (ii) *US* trained nurse who has not been licensed (美式)无执照的实习护士; **ophthalmic practitioner** = qualified person who specializes in testing eyes and prescribing lenses开业验光师 *see also* 参见 FAMILY

praecox 早发的 *see* 见 DEMENTIA, EJACULATIO

praevia 前置的,在前的 *see* 见 PLACENTA

pre- *prefix* meaning before *or* in front of 前; **preadmission information** = information given to a patient before he is admitted to hospital 入院须知; **pre-anaesthetic round** = examination of patients by the surgeon before they are anaesthetized 麻醉前查房

◇ **precancer** *noun* growth *or* cell which is not malignant but which may become cancerous 癌前病变

◇ **precancerous** *adjective* (growth) which is not malignant now, but which can become cancerous later 癌前病变的

precaution *noun* action taken before something happens 预防: ***She took the tablets as a precaution against seasickness.*** 她服了几片药预防晕船。**to take safety precautions** = to do things which will make yourself safe 采取安全预防手段

precede *verb* to happen before *or* earlier 领先,前兆: ***The attack was preceded by a sudden rise in body temperature.*** 发作的前兆是体温突然升高。

precentral gyrus *noun* motor area of the cerebral cortex 中央前回

precipitate 1 *noun* substance which is precipitated during a chemical reaction 沉淀物 2 *verb* (a) to make a substance separate from a chemical compound and fall to the bottom of a liquid during a chemical reaction 使沉淀: ***Casein is precipitated when milk comes into contact with an acid.*** 酪蛋白在牛奶遇酸时沉淀下来。(b) to make something start suddenly 诱发,引发

◇ **precipitation** *noun* action of forming a precipitate 沉淀作用

◇ **precipitin** *noun* antibody which reacts to an antigen and forms a precipitate, used in many diagnostic tests 沉淀素

QUOTE: It has been established that myocardial infarction and sudden coronary death are precipitated in the majority of patients by thrombus formation in the coronary arteries.
引文:已经确认,冠脉内血栓形成是大多数病人发生心肌梗死和冠脉猝死的诱因。
British Journal of Hospital Medicine 英国医院医学杂志

precise *adjective* very exact *or* correct 精确的: ***The instrument can give precise measurements of changes in heartbeat.*** 这台仪器能精确地测定心跳的变化。

preclinical *adjective* (**a**) before diagnosis 诊断前的: ***the preclinical stage of an infection*** 感染的临床前期 (**b**) first part of a medical course, before the students are allowed to examine real patients 临床前的(医学生正式接触病人前的阶段): ***a preclinical student*** 临床前阶段的学生

precocity *noun* being precocious 早熟

◇ **precocious** *adjective* more physically *or* mentally developed than is normal for a certain age 早熟的

precordial *adjective* referring to the precordium 心前区的

◇ **precordium** *noun* part of the thorax over the heart 心前区

precursor *noun* substance *or* cell from which another substance *or* cell is developed 前体

predict *verb* to say what will happen in the future 预言,预计: ***Doctors are predicting a rise in cases of whooping cough.*** 医生们预计百日咳病例要增多。

◇ **prediction** *noun* saying what you expect will happen in the future 预言: ***The Health Ministry's prediction of a rise in cases of hepatitis B.*** 卫生部预言乙型肝炎病例要增多。

◇ **predictive** *adjective* which predicts 估计的,预计的; **the predictive value of a test** = the accuracy of the test in predicting a medical condition 一项试验的预期值

predigestion *noun* artificial starting of the digestive process before food is eaten 预消化

◇ **predigested food** *noun* food which has undergone predigestion 预消化食物

predisposed to *adjective* with a tendency to 有某种倾向的: ***All the members of the family are predisposed to vascular diseases.*** 这个家族的所有成员都有得血管疾病的倾向。

◇ **predisposition** *noun* tendency 倾向性: ***She has a predisposition to obesity.*** 她有发胖的倾向。

predominant *adjective* which is more powerful than others 主导的,占优势的

pre-eclampsia *noun* condition of pregnant women towards the end of the pregnancy, which may lead to eclampsia 先兆子痫; **early onset pre-eclampsia** = pre-eclampsia which appears before 37 weeks' gestation 早发型先兆子痫(发生在孕37周以前)

> COMMENT: Symptoms are high blood pressure, oedema and protein in the urine.
> 注释:症状有高血压、水肿和蛋白尿。

preemie *noun US* (*informal* 非正式) premature infant 早产儿

prefrontal *adjective* in the front part of the frontal lobe 额叶前的; **prefrontal leucotomy** = operation to divide some of the white matter in the prefrontal lobe, formerly used as a treatment for schizophrenia 额叶前白质切除(旧时用于治疗精神分裂症); **prefrontal lobe** = part of the brain in the front part of each hemisphere, in front of the frontal lobe, which is concerned with memory and learning 额叶前叶(与记忆和学习有关)

◇ **preganglionic** *adjective* near to and in front of a ganglion 神经节前的; **preganglionic fibre** = nerve fibre which ends in a ganglion where it is linked in a synapse to a postganglionic fibre 节前纤维; **preganglionic neurone** = neurone which ends in a ganglion 节前神经元

pregnancy *noun* (i) time between conception and childbirth when a woman is carrying the unborn child in her womb 孕期,妊娠期 (ii) condition of being pregnant 怀孕,妊娠; **extrauterine** *or* **ectopic pregnancy** = pregnancy where the embryo develops outside the uterus, usually in one of the Fallopian tubes 宫外孕,异位妊娠; **multiple pregnancy** = pregnancy where the mother is going to give birth to more than one child 多胎妊娠; **phantom pregnancy** *or* **pseudocyesis** = psychological condition where a woman has all the symptoms of pregnancy without being pregnant 假孕;**tubal pregnancy** = the most common form of ectopic pregnancy, where the fetus develops in a Fallopian tube instead of the uterus 输卵管妊娠;**unwanted pregnancy** = condition where a woman becomes pregnant without wanting to have a child 意外受孕;**pregnancy-associated hypertension** = high blood pressure which is associated with pregnancy 妊娠高血压;**pregnancy test** = test to see if a woman is pregnant or not 妊娠试验

◇ **pregnant** *adjective* (woman) with an unborn child in her uterus 怀孕的,妊娠的:***She is six months pregnant.*** 她怀孕6个月了。

prehepatic *adjective* before the liver 肝前的;**prehepatic bilirubin** = bilirubin in plasma before it passes through the liver 肝前性胆红素;**prehepatic jaundice** = jaundice which occurs because of haemolysis before the blood reaches the liver 肝前性黄疸

premature *adjective* early *or* before the normal time 过早的:***The baby was born five weeks premature.*** 这个婴儿早产了5周。**premature baby** = baby born earlier than 37 weeks from conception, or weighing less than 2.5 kilos, but capable of independent life 早产儿;**premature beat** *or* **ectopic beat** = abnormal extra beat of the heart which can be caused by caffeine or other stimulants 期前收缩,异搏;**premature birth** = birth of a baby earlier than 37 weeks from conception 早产;**premature ejaculation** = situation where a man ejaculates too early during sexual intercourse 早泄;**premature labour** = starting to give birth earlier than 37 weeks from conception 早产:***After the accident she went into premature labour.*** 事故后,她早产了。

◇ **prematurely** *adverb* early *or* before the normal time 过早地:***The baby was born two weeks prematurely.*** 这个婴儿早产了2周。***A large number of people die prematurely from ischaemic heart disease.*** 有很多人因缺血性心脏病而过早去世。

◇ **prematurity** *noun* situation where something occurs early, before the normal time 过早

> COMMENT: Babies can survive even if born several weeks premature. Even babies weighing less than one kilo at birth can survive in an incubator, and develop normally. 注释:婴儿早产几周也能存活下来。甚至出生体重不足1千克的婴儿也能在孵育箱内存活并正常发育。

premed *noun* (*informal* 非正式) stage of being given premedication 术前用药阶段:***The patient is in premed.*** 病人处于术前用药阶段。

◇ **premedication** *or* **premedicant drug** *noun* drug (such as a sedative) given to a patient before an operation begins in order to block the parasympathetic nervous system and prevent vomiting during the operation 术前用药

premenstrual *adjective* before menstruation 月经前的;**premenstrual tension (PMT)** = nervous stress experienced by a woman for one or two weeks before a menstrual period starts 经前紧张

◇ **premolar** *noun* tooth with two points, situated between the canines and the first proper molar 双尖牙,前磨牙 ⇨见图 TEETH

◇ **prenatal** *adjective* during the period between conception and childbirth 产前的;**prenatal diagnosis** *or* **antenatal diagnosis** = medical examination of a pregnant woman to see if the fetus is developing normally 产前诊断(用于诊断胎儿是否正常发育)

◇ **pre-op** (*informal* 非正式) = PRE-OPERATIVE 术前的

preoperative *adjective* before a surgical operation 术前的;**preoperative medication** = drug (such as a sedative) given to a patient before an operation begins 术前用药

◇ **preoperatively** *adverb* before a surgical operation 术前地

prep (*informal* 非正式) **1** *noun* preparing *or* getting a patient ready for an operation 术前准备: ***The prep is finished, so the patient can be taken to the operating theatre.*** 术前准备做完了,病人可以带到手术室去了。**2** *verb* to prepare *or* get a patient ready for an operation 术前准备: ***Has the patient been prepped?*** 给这个病人做术前准备了吗?

prepare *verb* to get something ready; to make something 准备: ***He prepared a soothing linctus.*** 他准备了一贴安神舐膏。***Six rooms in the hospital were prepared for the accident victims.*** 医院准备出6间病房给事故受害者。***The nurses were preparing the patient for the operation.*** 护士们正在给病人做术前准备。

◇ **preparation** *noun* (**a**) act of preparing a patient before an operation 术前准备 (**b**) medicine *or* liquid containing a drug 制剂: ***He was given a preparation containing an antihistamine.*** 给他开了一种抗组胺制剂。

prepatellar bursitis *noun* housemaid's knee, condition where the fluid sac at the knee becomes inflamed, caused by kneeling on hard surfaces 髌骨前滑囊炎

◇ **prepubertal** *adjective* referring to the period before puberty 发育前的,青春期前的

◇ **prepuberty** *noun* period before puberty 发育前,青春期前

prepuce *noun* foreskin, skin covering the top of the penis, which can be removed by circumcision 包皮

presby- *or* **presbyo-** *prefix* referring to old age 老年

◇ **presbyacusis** *noun* condition where an old person's hearing fails gradually, due to degeneration of the internal ear 老年性耳聋

◇ **presbyopia** *noun* condition where an old person's sight fails gradually, due to hardening of the lens 老视,老花眼

prescribe *verb* to give instructions for a patient to get a certain dosage of a drug *or* a certain form of therapeutic treatment 开处方: ***The doctor prescribed a course of antibiotics.*** 医生开了一个疗程的抗生素。

◇ **prescription** *noun* order written by a doctor to a pharmacist asking for a drug to be prepared and given or sold to a patient 处方

presence *noun* being there 存在: ***Tests showed the presence of sugar in the urine.*** 试验表明尿中含糖。

presenile *adjective* (i) prematurely old 早老 (ii) (condition) which affects people of early or middle age, but has characteristics of old age 老年前期; **presenile dementia** = form of mental degeneration affecting adults before old age (as in Alzheimer's disease) 早老性痴呆

◇ **presenility** *noun* ageing of the body *or* brain before the normal time, with the patient showing symptoms which are normally associated with old people 早老

present 1 *verb* (**a**) to show *or* to be present 有,存在: ***The patient presented with severe chest pains.*** 病人剧烈胸痛。***The doctors' first task is to relieve the presenting symptoms.*** 医生的第一个任务就是解除现有症状。***The condition may also present in a baby.*** 这种状况也可以出现在婴儿身上。(**b**) (*in obstetrics*) to appear (in the vaginal channel) 先露; **the presenting part** = the part of the fetus which appears first 先露部分 **2** *adjective* which is there 现存的,现有的: ***All the symptoms of the disease are present.*** 这种疾病的所有症状都存在。

◇ **presentation** *noun* way in which a baby will be born, i. e. the part of the baby's body which will appear first in the vaginal channel 先露; **breech presentation** = position of the baby in the womb, where the buttocks will appear first 臀先露; **cephalic presentation** = normal presentation, where the baby's head will appear first 头先露; **face**

presentation = position of the baby in the womb, where the face will appear first 面先露; **shoulder presentation** = position of the baby in the womb, where the shoulder will appear first 肩先露; **transverse presentation** = position of the baby in the womb, where the baby's side will appear first, normally requiring urgent manipulation or Caesarean section to prevent complications 横位先露

> QUOTE: 26 patients were selected from the outpatient department on grounds of disabling breathlessness present for at least five years.
> 引文:从门诊选出 26 名呼吸困难影响生活至少 5 年的患者。
> **Lancet** 柳叶刀

> QUOTE: Chlamydia in the male commonly presents a urethritis characterized by dysuria.
> 引文:男性衣原体感染常表现为尿道炎,其特征是排尿困难。
> **Journal of American College Health** 美国健康协会杂志

> QUOTE: Sickle cell chest syndrome is a common complication of sickle cell disease, presenting with chest pain, fever and leucocytosis.
> 引文:镰状细胞性胸部综合征是镰状细胞(贫血)病的常见并发症,表现为胸痛、发热和白细胞增多。
> **British Medical Journal** 英国医学杂志

> QUOTE: A 24 year-old woman presents with an influenza-like illness of five days' duration.
> 引文:24 岁女性,患流感样疾病 5 天。
> **British Journal of Hospital Medicine** 英国医院医学杂志

> QUOTE: The presenting symptoms of Crohn's disease may be extremely variable.
> 引文:克隆氏病的症状极其多变。
> **New Zealand Medical Journal** 新西兰医学杂志

preserve *verb* to keep *or* to stop (tissue sample) from rotting 保存,保有,保藏,防腐

◊ **preservation** *noun* keeping of tissue sample *or* donor organ in good condition 保存,保藏,防腐

press *verb* to push *or* to squeeze 压迫: ***The tumour is pressing against a nerve.*** 肿瘤压迫神经了。

◊ **pressor** *adjective* (nerve) which increases the action of part of the body 增加活力的; (substance) which raises blood pressure 增加血压的

◊ **pressure** *noun* (i) action of squeezing *or* of forcing 压 (ii) force of something on its surroundings 压力 (iii) mental *or* physical stress caused by external events 精神压力; **blood pressure** 血压 *see* 见 BLOOD; **diastolic pressure** = low point of blood pressure during the diastole 舒张压; **osmotic pressure** = pressure by which certain molecules in a fluid go through a membrane into another part of the body 渗透压; **pulse pressure** = difference between the diastolic and systolic pressure 脉压; **systolic pressure** = high point of blood pressure during the systole 收缩压; **pressure area** = area of the body where a bone is near the surface of the skin, so that if the skin is pressed the circulation will be cut off 压迫(止血)区; **pressure point** = place where an artery crosses over a bone, so that the blood can be cut off by pressing with the finger 压迫(止血)点; **pressure sore** = ulcer which forms on the skin at a pressure area *or* where something presses on it 压迫性溃疡

presynaptic *adjective* before a synapse 突触前的; **presynaptic axon** = nerve leading to one side of a synapse 突触前轴突

presystole *noun* period before systole in the cycle of heartbeats 收缩期前

preterm *adjective* (birth of a child) taking place before the normal time 早产

prevalent *adjective* common (in

comparison to something) 流行的: ***The disease is prevalent in some African countries.*** 此病流行于非洲某些国家。***A condition which is more prevalent in the cold winter months.*** 一种多发于寒冬季节的疾病。

◇ **prevalence** *noun* percentage *or* number of cases of a disease in a certain place at a certain time 患病率: ***the prevalence of malaria in some tropical countries*** 某些热带国家的疟疾患病率; ***the prevalence of cases of malnutrition in large towns*** 大城镇的营养不良患病率; ***a high prevalence of renal disease*** 肾病患病率高

prevent *verb* to stop something happening 预防,防止: ***The treatment is given to prevent the patient's condition from getting worse.*** 采取治疗措施以防病人病情恶化。***Doctors are trying to prevent the spread of the outbreak of legionnaires' disease.*** 医生们正全力以赴防止军团菌病的暴发流行。(NOTE: you prevent something **from** happening or simply **prevent something happening**)

◇ **prevention** *noun* stopping something happening 预防; **accident prevention** = taking steps to prevent accidents happening 事故预防

◇ **preventive** *adjective* which prevents 预防的,防患于未然的; **preventive medicine** = medical action to prevent a disease from occurring 预防医学; **preventive measure** = step taken to prevent a disease from occurring 预防措施

> COMMENT: Preventive measures include immunization, vaccination, sterilization, quarantine and improving standards of housing and sanitation. Health education also has an important role to play in the prevention of disease.
> 注释:预防措施包括免疫、疫苗接种、消毒灭菌、检疫以及改善住房和卫生条件。健康教育在疾病预防上也起重要作用。

prevertebral *adjective* in front of the spinal column *or* a vertebra 椎体前的

priapism *noun* erection of the penis without sexual stimulus, caused by a blood clot in the tissue of the penis *or* injury to the spinal cord *or* stone in the urinary bladder 阴茎异常勃起

prick *verb* to make a small hole with a sharp point 刺破: ***The nurse pricked the patient's finger to take a blood sample.*** 护士刺破病人的手指取血样。***She pricked her finger on the needle and the spot became infected.*** 她的手指被针划破了,破口的地方还感染了。

prickle cell *noun* cell with many processes connecting it to other cells, found in the inner layer of the epidermis 棘细胞(上皮内层的一种细胞,有很多突起与其它细胞相连)

prickly heat = MILIARIA 痱子

primary *adjective* (**a**) (condition) which is first, and leads to another (the secondary condition) 原发的; **primary complex** = first lymph node to be infected by tuberculosis 原发综合征(指肺结核); **primary haemorrhage** = bleeding which occurs immediately after an injury has been suffered 原发出血; **primary tubercle** = first infected spot where tuberculosis starts in a lung 原发结核灶; **primary tuberculosis** = infection of a patient with tuberculosis for the first time 原发性结核 *see also* 参见 AMENORRHOEA (**b**) which is most important 首要的,初级的; **primary health care** *or* **primary medical care** = treatment provided by a general practitioner 初级卫生保健,初级医疗保健 *compare with* 比较 SECONDARY

> QUOTE: Among primary health care services, 1.5% of all GP consultations are due to coronary heart disease.
> 引文:初级卫生保健服务中,由于冠心病到全科医师那里就医者占所有病人的1.5%。
> **Health Services Journal** 保健事业杂志

> QUOTE: Primary care is largely concerned with clinical management of individual patients, while community medicine tends to view the whole population as its patient.

引文：初级保健多观注对个案病例的临床处理；而社区医疗则倾向于把整个人群作为服务对象。

Journal of the Royal College of General Practitioners 皇家全科医师学会杂志

primigravida *or* **primigravid patient** *noun* woman who is pregnant for the first time 初次妊娠的妇女

◇ **primipara** *noun* woman who has given birth to one child 初产妇 (NOTE: also called **unipara**)

primordial *adjective* in the very first stage of development 原始的，初级的；**primordial follicle** = first stage of development of an ovarian follicle 原始卵泡

principle *noun* rule *or* theory 原则；**active principle** = main ingredient of a drug which makes it have the required effect on a patient 有效成分

private *adjective* (i) belonging to one person, not to the public 私人的 (ii) which is paid for by a person 私立的，个人负担的：***He runs a private clinic for alcoholics***. 他开了一家私立戒酒诊所。***She is in private practice as an orthopaedic consultant***. 她在一家私立医疗机构当矫形外科医师。**private patient** = patient who is paying for his treatment, not having it done through the National Health Service 自费病人；**private practice** = services of a doctor *or* surgeon *or* dentist which are paid for by the patients themselves (or by a medical insurance), but not by the National Health Service 私人开业

◇ **privately** *adverb* (paid by the patient, not by the National Health Service) 自费地：***She decided to have the operation done privately***. 她决定自费做手术。(NOTE: the opposite is '**on the National Health**')

p. r. n. *abbreviation for* (缩写) *the Latin phrase* 'pro re nata': as and when required (written on a prescription) 必要时(处方用语)

pro- *prefix* meaning before *or* in front of 在…之前

probang *noun* surgical instrument, like a long rod with a brush at one end, formerly used to test and find strictures in the oesophagus and to push foreign bodies into the stomach 食管探子

probe 1 *noun* (i) instrument used to explore inside a cavity *or* wound 探针 (ii) device inserted into a medium to obtain information 探头；**laser probe** = metal probe which is inserted into the body and through which a laser beam can be passed to remove a blockage in an artery 激光探头；**ultrasonic** *or* **ultrasound probe** = instrument which locates organs *or* tissues inside the body, using ultrasound 超声探头 **2** *verb* to investigate the inside of something 刺探，探查：***The surgeon probed the wound with a scalpel***. 外科医师用解剖刀探查伤口。

problem *noun* (**a**) something which is difficult to find an answer to 医学问题，难题：***Scientists are trying to find a solution to the problem of drug-related disease***. 科学家正在努力寻找解决药物相关疾病的答案。**problem child** = child who is difficult to control 问题儿童 (**b**) medical disorder, usually an addiction 医学问题 (通常指药物成瘾)：***He has an alcohol problem or a drugs problem***. = He is addicted to alcohol *or* drugs. 他酒精成瘾，他药物成瘾。**problem drinking** = alcoholism which has a bad effect on a person's behaviour or work 酗酒

procedure *noun* (i) type of treatment 疗法 (ii) treatment given at one time 治疗：***The hospital has developed some new procedures for treating Parkinson's disease***. 这家医院创建了一些治疗帕金森病的新疗法。***We are hoping to increase the number of procedures carried out per day***. 我们希望增加每天的治疗次数。**surgical procedure** = one surgical operation 外科操作

QUOTE: Disposable items now available for medical and nursing procedures range from cheap syringes to expensive cardiac pacemakers.

引文:医疗和护理操作中可便捷使用的器具有多种,从便宜的注射器到昂贵的心脏起搏器。

Nursing Times 护理时代

QUOTE: The electromyograms and CT scans were done as outpatient procedures.
引文:肌电图和CT扫描列为门诊项目。

Southern Medical Journal 南部医学杂志

process 1 *noun* **(a)** projecting part of the body 突起; **articulating process** = piece of bone which sticks out of the neural arch in a vertebra and articulates with the next vertebra 关节突; **ciliary processes** = series of ridges behind the iris to which the lens of the eye is attached 睫状突 ◊ 见图 EYE; **mastoid process** = part of the temporal bone which protrudes at the side of the head behind the ear 乳突 ◊ 见图 SKULL; **transverse process** = part of a vertebra which protrudes at the side 横突; **xiphoid process** = bottom part of the breastbone which is originally cartilage but becomes bone by middle age 剑突 **(b)** technical *or* scientific action 方法: ***A new process for testing serum samples has been developed in the research laboratory.*** 试验室研究开发了一种检测血清样本的新方法。**(c)** **nursing process** = standard method of treatment carried out by nurses, and the documents which go with it 护理程序 **2** *verb* to examine *or* to test samples 加工,处理: ***The blood samples are being processed by the laboratory.*** 血样由试验室处理。

QUOTE: The nursing process serves to divide overall patient care into that part performed by nurses and that performed by the other professions.
引文:护理程序把全部的病人护理分成由护士具体执行的部分和由其他专业人员执行的部分。

Nursing Times 护理时代

QUOTE: All relevant sections of the nurses' care plan and nursing process records had been left blank.
引文:所有护士护理计划和护理程序记录都是空白。

Nursing Times 护理时代

procidentia *noun* movement of an organ downwards 脱垂; **uterine procidentia** = condition where the womb has passed through the vagina 子宫脱垂

proct- *or* **procto-** *prefix* referring to the anus *or* rectum 肛门,直肠

◊ **proctalgia** *noun* pain in the lower rectum *or* anus, caused by neuralgia 直肠痛,肛痛; **proctalgia fugax** = condition where the patient suffers sudden pains in the rectum during the night, usually relieved by eating or drinking 痉挛性肛痛

◊ **proctatresia** *noun* imperforate anus, condition where the anus does not have an opening 肛门闭锁

◊ **proctectasia** *noun* condition where the rectum *or* anus is dilated because of continued constipation 肛裂

◊ **proctectomy** *noun* surgical removal of the rectum 直肠切除

◊ **proctitis** *noun* inflammation of the rectum 直肠炎

◊ **proctocele** *noun* **vaginal proctocele** = condition associated with prolapse of the womb, where the rectum protrudes into the vagina 阴道内直肠膨出

◊ **proctoclysis** *noun* introduction of a lot of fluid into the rectum slowly 直肠滴注法

◊ **proctocolectomy** *noun* surgical removal of the rectum and the colon 大肠切除术(含结肠和直肠)

◊ **proctocolitis** *noun* inflammation of the rectum and part of the colon 直肠结肠炎

◊ **proctodynia** *noun* sensation of pain in the anus 肛门痛

◊ **proctology** *noun* scientific study of the rectum and anus and their associated diseases 直肠病学

◊ **proctorrhaphy** *noun* surgical operation to stitch up a tear in the rectum *or* anus 直肠缝合术

◇ **proctoscope** *noun* surgical instrument consisting of a long tube with a light in the end, used to examine the rectum 直肠镜

◇ **proctoscopy** *noun* examination of the rectum using a proctoscope 直肠镜检查

◇ **proctosigmoiditis** *noun* inflammation of the rectum and the sigmoid colon 直肠乙状结肠炎

◇ **proctotomy** *noun* (i) surgical operation to divide a structure of the rectum *or* anus 直肠切开术 (ii) opening of an imperforate anus 直肠造口术

prodromal *adjective* (time) between when the first symptoms of a disease appear, and the appearance of the major effect, such as a fever *or* rash 前驱症状的; **prodromal rash** = early rash *or* rash which appears as a symptom of a disease before the major rash 先锋疹

◇ **prodrome** *or* **prodroma** *noun* early symptom of an attack of a disease 前驱症状

> QUOTE: In classic migraine a prodrome is followed by an aura, then a headache, and finally a recovery phase. The prodrome may not be recognised.
> 引文:典型偏头痛的发作过程:前驱症状之后是先兆期,然后是头痛期,最后是缓解期。前驱症状有时未能辨识。
> **British Journal of Hospital Medicine**
> 英国医院医学杂志

produce *verb* to make 产生: ***The drug produces a sensation of dizziness.*** 这种药会产生头晕眼花的感觉。***Doctors are worried by the side-effects produced by the new painkiller.*** 医生们为新镇痛药的副作用而担忧。

◇ **product** *noun* (i) thing which is produced 产品 (ii) result *or* effect of a process 结果; **pharmaceutical products** = medicines *or* pills *or* lozenges *or* creams which are sold in chemists' shops 药品

proenzyme *or* **zymogen** *noun* first mature form of an enzyme, before it develops into an active enzyme 前酶,酶原

profession *noun* (i) type of job for which special training is needed 专业 (ii) all people working in a specialized type of employment for which they have been trained 专业人员: ***the medical profession*** = all doctors 医务人员; ***He's a doctor by profession.*** = His job is being a doctor. 他是个医生。

◇ **professional** *adjective* referring to a profession 专业的; **professional body** = organization which acts for all the members of a profession 专业团体; **Professional Conduct Committee (PCC)** = committee of the General Medical Council which decides on cases of professional misconduct 职业行为委员会; **professional misconduct** = action which is thought to be wrong by the body which regulates a profession (such as an action by a doctor which is considered wrong by the General Medical Council) 专业失误

profound *adjective* serious 严重的: ***a profound abnormality of the immune system*** 免疫系统严重异常

profunda *adjective* (blood vessels) which lie deep in tissues 深部(血管)

profuse *adjective* very large quantity 大量的: ***Fever accompanied by profuse sweating.*** 发热伴大汗淋漓。***Pains with profuse internal bleeding.*** 疼痛伴有大量内出血。

progeria *noun* premature senility 早老,早衰 (NOTE: also called **Hutchinson-Gilford syndrome**)

progesterone *noun* hormone produced in the second part of the menstrual cycle by the corpus luteum and which stimulates the formation of the placenta if an ovum is fertilized (it is also produced by the placenta itself) 孕酮,黄体酮

◇ **progestogen** *noun* any substance which has the same effect as progesterone 孕激素

COMMENT: Because natural progesterones prevent ovulation during pregnancy, synthetically produced progestogens are used to make contraceptive pills.
注释:由于天然孕酮在孕期有阻止排卵的作用,合成孕激素被用来制造避孕药。

prognathism *noun* condition where one jaw (especially the lower) or both jaws protrude 突颌

◇ **prognathic jaw** *noun* jaw which protrudes further than the other 兜齿,下颌前突

prognosis *noun* opinion of how a disease *or* disorder will develop 预后: ***This cancer has a prognosis of about two years.*** = The patient will die within two years unless this cancer is eradicated. 这种癌症预计生存期是2年。*compare* 比较 DIAGNOSIS

◇ **prognostic** *adjective* referring to prognosis 预后的; **prognostic test** = test to decide how a disease will develop *or* how long a patient will survive an operation 预后试验

programme *noun* series of medical treatments given in a set way at set times 疗程: ***The doctor prescribed a programme of injections.*** 医生开了一个疗程的针剂。***She took a programme of steroid treatment.*** 她用了一个疗程的类固醇。

progress 1 *noun* development *or* way in which a person is becoming well 进展: ***The doctors seem pleased that she has made such good progress since her operation.*** 医生们为她术后能恢复的这么好而高兴。**2** *verb* to develop *or* to continue to do well 进展: ***The patient is progressing well.*** 病人病情控制很好。***The doctor asked how the patient was progressing.*** 医生询问病人病情进展如何。

◇ **progression** *noun* development 进展,进步; **progression of a disease** = way in which a disease develops 疾病的进展

◇ **progressive** *adjective* which develops all the time 进行性的: ***Alzheimer's disease is a progressive disorder which sees a gradual decline in intellectual functioning.*** 阿尔茨海默病是一种进行性障碍,智力功能逐渐下降。**progressive deafness** = condition where the patient becomes more and more deaf 进行性耳聋; **progressive muscular atrophy** = any form of muscular dystrophy, with progressive weakening of the muscles, particularly in the pelvic and shoulder girdles 进行性肌萎缩

◇ **progressively** *adverb* more and more 进行性地,越来越: ***He became progressively more disabled.*** 他的残障越来越重。

proinsulin *noun* substance produced by the pancreas, then converted to insulin 前胰岛素

project *verb* to protrude *or* to stick out 突出,伸出

◇ **projection** *noun* (**a**) piece of a part which protrudes 突出部分; **projection tract** = fibres connecting the cerebral cortex with the lower parts of the brain and spinal cord 投射束 (**b**) (*in psychology*) mental action, where the patient blames another person for his own faults 推诿(心理防御机制之一,即归咎于他人)

prolactin *or* **lactogenic hormone** *noun* hormone secreted by the pituitary gland which stimulates the production of milk 催乳素

prolapse *noun* condition where an organ has moved downwards out of its normal position 脱垂: **rectal prolapse** *or* **prolapse of the rectum** = condition where mucous membrane of the rectum moves downwards and passes through the anus 直肠脱垂; **prolapsed intervertebral disc (PID)** *or* **slipped disc** = condition where an intervertebral disc becomes displaced where the soft centre of a disc passes through the hard cartilage of the exterior and presses onto a nerve 椎间盘脱出; **prolapsed womb** *or* **prolapse of the uterus** = UTERINE PROLAPSE 子宫脱垂

proliferate *verb* to produce many similar cells or parts, and so grow 增生，增殖

◇ **proliferation** *noun* process of proliferating 增生，增殖

◇ **proliferative** *adjective* which multiplies 增生的，增殖的；**proliferative phase** = period when a disease is spreading fast 增殖期

proline *noun* amino acid found in proteins, especially in collagen 脯氨酸

prolong *verb* to make longer 延长：***The treatment prolonged her life by three years.*** 治疗使她的生命延长了3年。

◇ **prolonged** *adjective* very long 延长了的：***She had to undergo a prolonged course of radiation treatment.*** 她不得不延长放疗时间。

prominent *adjective* which stands out *or* which is very visible 显著的，明显的，显而易见的：***She had a prominent scar on her neck which she wanted to have removed.*** 她脖子上有一道明显的伤疤，她想去掉它。

◇ **prominence** *noun* projection, part of the body which stands out 显著；**the laryngeal prominence** = the Adam's apple 喉结

promontory *noun* projection, section of an organ (especially the middle ear and sacrum) which stands out above the rest 岬

promote *verb* to help something take place 促进：***The drug is used to promote blood clotting.*** 这种药物用来促进凝血。

pronate *verb* (i) to lie face downwards 俯卧 (ii) to turn the hand so that palm faces downwards 旋前

◇ **pronation** *noun* turning the hand round so that the palm faces downwards 旋前

◇ **pronator** *noun* muscle which makes the hand turn face downwards 旋前肌

◇ **prone** *adjective* (i) lying face downwards 俯卧 (ii) (arm) with the palm facing downwards(前臂)旋前位 (NOTE: the opposite is **supination**, **supine**)

pronounced *adjective* very obvious *or* marked 非常显著的，非常明显的：***She has a pronounced limp.*** 她的腿瘸得非常明显。

prop up *verb* to support a patient (as with pillows) 支撑(如用枕头垫起病人)

propagate *verb* to multiply 繁殖，培养

◇ **propagation** *noun* increasing *or* causing something to spread 传播，繁殖

properdin *noun* protein in blood plasma which can destroy Gram-negative bacteria and neutralize viruses when acting together with magnesium 备解素，裂解素

prophase *noun* first stage of mitosis when the chromosomes are visible as long thin double threads 前期

prophylactic *noun & adjective* (substance) which helps to prevent the development of a disease 预防，预防的

◇ **prophylaxis** *noun* (i) prevention of disease 疾病预防 (ii) preventive treatment 预防性治疗

> QUOTE: Most pacemakers are inserted prophylactically for either atrioventricular block or sick sinus syndrome.
> 引文：大多数起搏器是针对房室传导阻滞或病窦综合征而预防性植入的。
> **British Journal of Hospital Medicine** 英国医院医学杂志

proportion *noun* Quantity of something, especially as compared to the whole 比例：***A high proportion of cancers can be treated by surgery.*** 大部分癌症可用外科手术治疗。***The proportion of outpatients to inpatients is increasing.*** 门诊病人与住院病人的比例在上升。

> QUOTE: The target cells for adult myeloid leukaemia are located in the bone marrow, and there is now evidence that a substantial proportion of childhood leukaemias also arise in the bone marrow.
> 引文：成年人髓样白血病的靶细胞定位于骨髓，现有证据表明相当比例的儿童白血病也来自骨髓。
> **British Medical Journal** 英国医学杂志

proprietary *adjective* which belongs to a commercial company 专利的; **proprietary drug** = drug which is sold under a trade name 专利药; **proprietary name** = trade name for a drug 专利名 *compare* 比较 GENERIC

proprioceptor *noun* end of a sensory nerve which reacts to stimuli from muscles and tendons as they move 本体感受器

◇ **proprioception** *noun* reaction of nerves to body movements and relation of information about movements to the brain 本体感觉

◇ **proprioceptive** *adjective* referring to sensory impulses from the joints, muscles and tendons, which relate information about body movements to the brain 本体感觉的

proptosis *noun* forward displacement of the eyeball(眼球)前突

prosop- *or* **prosopo-** *prefix* referring to the face 脸,面部

prostaglandins *noun* fatty acids present in many parts of the body, which are associated with the sensation of pain and have an effect on the nervous system, blood pressure and in particular the uterus at menstruation 前列腺素(分布于机体许多部位的脂肪酸,与痛觉、神经系统、血压调节及月经期子宫状况都有关系)

prostate (gland) *noun* gland in men which produces a secretion in which sperm cells float 前列腺: ***He has prostate trouble.*** = He is suffering from prostatitis *or* he has an enlarged prostate gland. 他患有前列腺疾病。◇见图 UROGENITAL SYSTEM (MALE)

◇ **prostatectomy** *noun* surgical removal of all *or* part of the prostate gland 前列腺切除术; **retropubic prostatectomy** = prostatectomy where the operation is performed through the membrane surrounding the prostate gland 耻骨后前列腺切除术; **transurethral prostatectomy** *or* **transurethral resection** = prostatectomy where the operation is performed through the urethra 经尿道前列腺切除术; **transvesical prostatectomy** = prostatectomy where the operation is performed through the bladder 经膀胱前列腺切除术 *see also* 参见 HARRIS'S OPERATION

◇ **prostatic** *adjective* referring to the prostate gland; belonging to the prostate gland 前列腺的; **prostatic hypertrophy** = enlargement of the prostate gland 前列腺肥大; **prostatic massage** = removing fluid from the prostate gland through the rectum 前列腺按摩; **prostatic urethra** = section of the urethra which passes through the prostate 尿道前列腺部; **prostatic utricle** = sac branching from the prostatic urethra 前列腺囊

◇ **prostatitis** *noun* inflammation of the prostate gland 前列腺炎

◇ **prostatocystitis** *noun* inflammation of the prostatic part of the urethra and the bladder 前列腺膀胱炎

◇ **prostatorrhoea** *noun* discharge of fluid from the prostate gland 前列腺溢液

> COMMENT: The prostate gland lies under the bladder and surrounds the urethra (the tube leading from the bladder to the penis). It secretes a fluid containing enzymes. As a man grows older, the prostate gland tends to enlarge and constrict the point at which the urethra leaves the bladder, making it difficult to pass urine.
> 注释:前列腺位于膀胱下面,包绕着尿道(从膀胱到阴茎的管道),它分泌的液体含有酶。当男性年老时,前列腺增大,缩窄尿道出膀胱的位置,造成排尿困难。

prosthesis *noun* device which is attached to the body to take the place of a part which is missing (such as an artificial leg *or* glass eye, etc.) 假体; **dental prosthesis** = one or more false teeth 义齿 (NOTE: plural is **prostheses**)

◇ **prosthetic** *adjective* (artificial limb) which replaces a part of the body which has been amputated *or* removed 假体的: ***He was fitted with a prosthetic hand.*** 他

装了一只假手。

◇ **prosthetics** *noun* study and making of prostheses 假体学

◇ **prosthetist** *noun* qualified person who fits prostheses 假体技师

> QUOTE: The average life span of a joint prosthesis is 10 - 15 years.
> 引文:人工关节的平均寿命为10~15年。
> **British Journal of Nursing** 英国护理杂志

prostration *noun* extreme tiredness of body *or* mind 衰竭

protamine *noun* simple protein found in fish, used with insulin to slow down the insulin absorption rate 精蛋白,鱼精蛋白

protanopia = DALTONISM 红色盲

protease *or* **proteolytic enzyme** *noun* digestive enzyme which breaks down protein in food by splitting the peptide link 蛋白酶,蛋白水解酶

protect *verb* to keep something safe from harm 保护: ***The population must be protected against the spread of the virus.*** 必须保护人群不受病毒传播的侵袭。

◇ **protection** *noun* thing which protects 保护: ***Children are vaccinated as a protection against disease.*** 给儿童种疫苗是为了保护他们不受疾病侵害。

◇ **protective** *adjective* which protects 保护性的; **protective cap** = condom, a rubber sheath put over the penis before intercourse as a contraceptive or as a protection against venereal disease 阴茎套,避孕套

protein *noun* nitrogen compound which is present in and is an essential part of all living cells in the body, formed by the condensation of amino acids 蛋白质; **protein balance** = situation when the nitrogen intake in protein is equal to the excretion rate (in the urine) 蛋白质平衡; **protein deficiency** = lack of enough proteins in the diet 蛋白质缺乏

◇ **protein-bound iodine** *noun* compound of thyroxine and iodine 蛋白结合碘; **protein-bound iodine test (PBI test)** = test to measure if the thyroid gland is producing adequate quantities of thyroxine 蛋白结合碘试验

◇ **proteinuria** *noun* proteins in the urine 蛋白尿

◇ **proteolysis** *noun* breaking down of proteins in food by proteolytic enzymes 蛋白水解

◇ **proteolytic** *adjective* referring to proteolysis 蛋白水解的; **proteolytic enzyme** = PROTEASE 蛋白水解酶

> COMMENT: Proteins are necessary for growth and repair of the body's tissue; they are mainly formed of carbon, nitrogen and oxygen in various combinations as amino acids. Certain foods (such as beans, meat, eggs, fish and milk) are rich in protein.
> 注释:蛋白质是生长和修复身体组织所必需的;它们主要由碳、氮和氧以不同形式结合的各种氨基酸构成。某些食物(如豆类、肉、蛋、鱼和乳类)富含蛋白质。

Proteus *noun* genus of bacteria commonly found in the intestines 变形杆菌属

prothrombin *noun* Factor II, a protein in blood which helps blood to coagulate and which needs vitamin K to be effective 凝血酶原; **prothrombin time** = time taken (in Quick's test) for clotting to take place 凝血酶原时间

proto- *prefix* meaning first *or* at the beginning 原,初

◇ **protopathic** *adjective* (i) referring to nerves which are able to sense only strong sensations 神经迟钝的 (ii) referring to a first symptom *or* lesion 原发的 (iii) referring to the first sign of partially restored function in an injured nerve 受损神经功能恢复的苗头 *see also* 参见 EPICRITIC

protoplasm *noun* substance like a jelly which makes up the largest part of each cell 原浆,厚生质

◇ **protoplasmic** *adjective* referring to protoplasm 原生质的

protoporphyrin IX *noun* commonest form of porphyrin, found in haemoglobin and chlorophyll 原卟啉 IX

Protozoa *plural noun* tiny simple organisms with a single cell 原生动物门 (NOTE: the singular is **protozoon**)

◊ **protozoan** *adjective* referring to the Protozoa 原生动物的

COMMENT: Parasitic Protozoa can cause several diseases, such as amoebiasis, malaria and other tropical diseases.
注释:寄生性原生动物可以引起几种疾病,如阿米巴病、疟疾和其它热带病。

protrude *verb* to stick out 伸出: ***She wears a brace to correct her protruding teeth.*** 她带着矫正牙齿突出的支架。 ***Protruding eyes are associated with some forms of goitre.*** 突眼与某些形式的甲状腺肿有关。

protuberance *noun* rounded part of the body which projects above the rest 隆突

proud flesh *noun* new vessels and young fibrous tissue which form when a wound *or* incision *or* lesion is healing 肉芽

provide *verb* to supply *or* to give 提供: ***A balanced diet should provide the necessary protein required by the body.*** 平衡膳食应提供机体必需的蛋白质。 ***A dentist's surgery should provide adequate room for patients to wait in.*** 牙科诊室应给候诊的患者提供足够的房间。 ***The hospital provides an ambulance service to the whole area.*** 医院面向整个地区提供救护服务。

◊ **provision** *noun* act of providing 提供,供给: ***The provision of aftercare facilities for patients recently discharged from hospital.*** 对新近出院病人提供出院后护理设施。

◊ **provisional** *adjective* temporary *or* which may be changed 临时的: ***The hospital has given me a provisional date for the operation.*** 医院给我确定了临时手术日期。 ***The paramedical team attached sticks to the broken leg to act as provisional splints.*** 辅助医疗队将棍子绑缚在断腿上作为临时夹板。

◊ **provisionally** *adverb* in a temporary way *or* not certainly 临时地,暂时地: ***She has provisionally accepted the offer of a bed in the hospital.*** 她暂时同意接受医院提供的病房。

provoke *verb* to stimulate *or* make something happen 引发: ***The medication provoked a sudden rise in body temperature.*** 药物引发了体温的突然升高。 ***The fit was provoked by the shock of the accident.*** 抽搐发作是事故所致休克诱发的。

proximal *adjective* near the midline *or* the central part of the body 接近的,临近的,近中线的; **proximal convoluted tubule** = part of the kidney filtering system, between the loop of Henle and the glomerulus 近曲小管; **proximal interphalangeal joint** (**PIP**) = joint nearest the point of attachment of a finger *or* toe 近端指(趾)间关节

◊ **proximally** *adverb* placed further towards the centre *or* point of attachment 接近地,近中线地 (NOTE: the opposite is **distal**, **distally**)

prurigo *noun* itchy eruption of papules 痒疹; **Besnier's prurigo** = irritating form of prurigo on the backs of the knees and the insides of the elbows 贝尼埃痒疹(肘内侧和腘部的痒疹)

◊ **pruritus** *noun* irritation of the skin which makes a patient want to scratch 瘙痒; **pruritus ani** = itching round the anal orifice 肛门瘙痒; **pruritus vulvae** = itching round the vulva 外阴瘙痒

prussic acid = CYANIDE 氢氰酸

pseud- *or* **pseudo-** *prefix* meaning false *or* similar to something, but not the same 假,伪

◊ **pseudoangina** *noun* pain in the chest, caused by worry but not indicating heart disease 假性心绞痛

◊ **pseudoarthrosis** *noun* false joint, as when the two broken ends of a fractured bone do not bind together but heal separately 假关节(不是关节的地方异常地形成类似关节的弯曲,如骨折的断端分别愈合)

◇ **pseudocoxalgia** *noun* Legg-Calv-Perthes disease, degeneration of the upper end of the femur (in young boys) which prevents the femur from growing properly and can result in a permanent limp 假性髋关节痛(男孩股骨上端变形性骨软骨炎)

◇ **pseudocrisis** *noun* sudden fall in the temperature of the patient with fever, but which does not mark the end of the fever 假性退热

◇ **pseudocroup** *noun* (i) laryngismus stridulus 喘鸣性喉痉挛 (ii) form of asthma, where contractions take place in the larynx 喉痉挛性哮喘

◇ **pseudocyesis** *noun* phantom pregnancy, condition where a woman has the physical symptoms of pregnancy, but is not pregnant 假妊娠

◇ **pseudocyst** *noun* (i) false cyst 假囊 (ii) space which fills with fluid in an organ, but without the walls which would form a cyst, as a result of softening *or* necrosis of the tissue 假性囊肿(由组织软化或坏死形成)

◇ **pseudodementia** *noun* condition of extreme apathy found in hysterical people (where their behaviour corresponds to what they imagine to be insanity, though they show no signs of true dementia)假性痴呆

◇ **pseudohypertrophic muscular dystrophy** *noun* Duchenne muscular dystrophy, a hereditary disease affecting the muscles, which swell and become weak, beginning in early childhood 假性肥大性肌萎缩

◇ **pseudohypertrophy** *noun* overgrowth of fatty *or* fibrous tissue in a part *or* organ, which results in the part *or* organ being enlarged 假性增生

◇ **pseudomyxoma** *noun* tumour rich in mucus 假性粘液瘤

◇ **pseudoplegia** *or* **pseudoparalysis** *noun* (i) loss of muscular power in the limbs, but without true paralysis 假性瘫痪 (ii) paralysis caused by hysteria 癔病性瘫痪

◇ **pseudopolyposis** *noun* condition where polyps are found in many places in the intestine, usually resulting from an earlier infection 假性息肉病

psilosis *noun* sprue, disease of the small intestine, which prevents the patient from absorbing food properly 口炎性腹泻

> COMMENT: The condition is often found in the tropics, and results in diarrhoea and loss of weight.
> 注释:本病常见于热带,造成腹泻和体重下降。

psittacosis *noun* parrot disease, disease of parrots which can be transmitted to humans 鹦鹉热

> COMMENT: The disease is similar to typhoid fever, but atypical pneumonia is present; symptoms include fever, diarrhoea and distension of the abdomen.
> 注释:本病与伤寒相似,但存在非典型肺炎;症状包括发热、腹泻和腹胀。

psoas major *noun* muscle in the groin which flexes the hip 腰大肌;**psoas minor** = small muscle, similar to the psoas major, but which is not always present 腰小肌

psoriasis *noun* common inflammatory skin disease where red patches of skin are covered with white scales 牛皮癣,银屑病

◇ **psoriatic** *adjective* referring to psoriasis 牛皮癣的,银屑病的;**psoriatic arthritis** = form of psoriasis which is associated with arthritis 牛皮癣性关节炎

psych- *or* **psycho-** *prefix* referring to the mind 心灵,精神

◇ **psychasthenia** *noun* (i) any psychoneurosis, except hysteria 精神衰弱(指除癔病外的所有神经症) (ii) psychoneurosis characterized by fears and phobias 以害怕和恐怖为特征的神经症

◇ **psyche** *noun* the mind 心灵,精神

◇ **psychedelic** *adjective* (drug, such as LSD) which expands a person's consciousness 致幻的

◇ **psychiatric** *adjective* referring to psychiatry 精神病学的,精神科的: ***He is undergoing psychiatric treatment.*** 他在接受精神科治疗。**psychiatric hospital** = hospital which specializes in the treatment of patients with mental disorders 精神病医院

◇ **psychiatrist** *noun* doctor who specializes in the diagnosis and treatment of mental disorders and behaviour 精神病学家,精神科医师

◇ **psychiatry** *noun* branch of medicine concerned with diagnosis and treatment of mental disorders and behaviour 精神病学

◇ **psychoanalysis** *noun* treatment of mental disorder, where a specialist talks to the patient and analyses with him his condition and the past events which have caused it 精神分析

◇ **psychoanalyst** *noun* doctor who is trained in psychoanalysis 精神分析学家

◇ **psychogenic** *or* **psychogenetic** *or* **psychogenous** *adjective* (illness) which starts in the mind, rather than in a physical state 精神性的,心理性的

◇ **psychogeriatrics** *adjective* study of the mental disorders of old people 老年精神病学的

◇ **psychological** *adjective* referring to psychology; caused by a mental state 心理学的; **psychological dependence** = state where a person is addicted to a drug (such as cannabis) but does not suffer physical effects if he stops taking it 心理依赖(对毒品)

◇ **psychologically** *adverb* in a way which is caused by a mental state 心理上地,从心理角度地: ***She is psychologically incapable of making decisions.*** 她在心理上不能作决定。***He is psychologically addicted to tobacco.*** 他在心理上依赖烟草。

◇ **psychologist** *noun* person who specializes in the study of the mind and mental processes 心理学家; **clinical psychologist** = psychologist who studies and treats sick patients in hospital 临床心理学家; **educational psychologist** = psychologist who studies the problems of education 教育心理学家

◇ **psychology** *noun* study of the mind and mental processes 心理学

◇ **psychometrics** *noun* way of measuring intelligence and personality where the result is shown as a number on a scale 心理测量学

◇ **psychomotor** *adjective* referring to muscle movements caused by mental activity 精神运动性的; **psychomotor disturbance** = muscles movements (such as twitching) caused by mental disorder 精神运动性紊乱; **psychomotor epilepsy** = epilepsy in which fits are characterized by blurring of consciousness and accompanied by coordinated but wrong movements 精神运动性癫痫; **psychomotor retardation** = slowing of thought and action 精神运动性迟滞

◇ **psychoneurosis** *or* **neurosis** *noun* any of a group of mental disorders in which a patient has a faulty response to the stresses of life 精神神经症,神经症(对生活应激不恰当反应的一组精神障碍)

◇ **psychopath** *noun* person whose behaviour is abnormal and may be violent and antisocial 精神变态者,变态人格者

◇ **psychopathic** *adjective* referring to psychopathy 精神变态的变态人格的

◇ **psychopathological** *adjective* referring to psychopathology 精神病理学的

◇ **psychopathology** *noun* branch of medicine concerned with the pathology of mental disorders and diseases 精神病理学

◇ **psychopathy** *noun* any disease of the mind 精神变态,变态人格

◇ **psychopharmacology** *noun* study of the actions and applications of drugs which have a powerful effect on the mind and behaviour 精神药理学

◇ **psychophysiological** *adjective* referring to psychophysiology 精神生理学的

◇ **psychophysiology** *noun* physiology of the mind and its functions 精神生

理学

◇ **psychosis** *noun* general term for any serious mental disorder where the patient shows lack of insight 精神病(病人本人缺乏自知力的一种严重精神障碍)

◇ **psychosocial** *adjective* concerning the interaction of psychological and social factors 心理社会的

> QUOTE: Recent efforts to redefine nursing have moved away from the traditional medically dominated approach towards psychosocial care and forming relationships with patients.
> 引文:新近对护理的重新定义已经将护理从传统的医学为主的导向转为心理社会护理以及和病人建立关系方面。
> **British Journal of Nursing** 英国护理杂志

◇ **psychosomatic** *adjective* referring to the relationship between body and mind 身心的

> COMMENT: Many physical disorders, such as duodenal ulcers or high blood pressure, can be caused by mental conditions like worry or stress, and are then termed psychosomatic in order to distinguish them from the same conditions having physical or hereditary causes.
> 注释:许多躯体障碍,如十二指肠溃疡或高血压,可由烦恼或应激等心理状态引起,被叫做身心障碍,以区别于由躯体或遗传引起的同样的状况。

◇ **psychosurgery** *noun* brain surgery, used as a treatment for psychological disorders 精神外科学

◇ **psychosurgical** *adjective* referring to psychosurgery 精神外科学的

◇ **psychotherapeutic** *adjective* referring to psychotherapy 心理治疗的

◇ **psychotherapist** *noun* person trained to give psychotherapy 心理治疗师

◇ **psychotherapy** *noun* treatment of mental disorders by psychological methods, as when a psychotherapist talks to the patient and encourages him to talk about his problems 心理治疗 *see also* 参见 THERAPY

◇ **psychotic** *adjective* (i) referring to psychosis 精神病的 (ii) characterized by mental disorder 有精神病特征的

◇ **psychotropic** *adjective* (drug) which affects a patient's mood (such as a stimulant or a sedative)(药物)影响精神状态的

pt = PINT 品脱

pterion *noun* point on the side of the skull where the frontal, temporal parietal and sphenoid bones meet 翼点

pterygium *noun* degenerative condition where a triangular growth of conjunctiva covers part of the cornea, with its apex towards the pupil 翼状胬肉

pterygo- *suffix* referring to the pterygoid process 翼状突的

◇ **pterygoid process** *noun* one of two projecting parts on the sphenoid bone 翼状突; **pterygoid plate** = small flat bony projection on the pterygoid process 翼状板; **pterygoid plexus** = group of veins and sinuses which join together behind the cheek 翼状丛

◇ **pterygomandibular** *adjective* referring to the pterygoid process and the mandible 翼突下颌的

◇ **pterygopalatine fossa** *noun* space between the pterygoid process and the upper jaw 翼突腭窝

ptomaine *noun* group of nitrogenous substances produced in rotting food, which gives the food a special smell 尸碱,尸毒 (NOTE: **ptomaine poisoning** was the term formerly used to refer to any form of food poisoning)

ptosis *noun* (i) prolapse of an organ 下垂 (ii) drooping of the upper eyelid which makes the eye stay half closed 上睑下垂

◇ **-ptosis** *suffix* meaning prolapse *or* fallen position of an organ 下垂,脱垂

ptyal- *or* **ptyalo-** *prefix* referring to the saliva 唾液,涎

◇ **ptyalin** *noun* enzyme in saliva which cleanses the mouth and converts starch into sugar 唾液淀粉酶

◇ **ptyalism** *noun* production of an excessive amount of saliva 流涎,涎液分泌过多

◇ **ptyalith** *or* **sialolith** *noun* stone in the salivary gland 涎石

◇ **ptyalography** *or* **sialography** *noun* X-ray examination of the ducts of the salivary gland 涎管造影术

pubertal *or* **puberal** *adjective* referring to puberty 发育的,青春期的

◇ **puberty** *noun* physical and psychological changes which take place when childhood ends and adolescence and sexual maturity begin and the sex glands become active 发育,青春期

COMMENT: Puberty starts at about the age of 10 in girls, and slightly later in boys.
注释:女孩青春期大约在10岁开始,男孩则晚些。

pubes *noun* part of the body just above the groin, where the pubic bones are found 阴阜

◇ **pubis** *noun* bone forming the front part of the pelvis 耻骨 (NOTE: the plural is **pubes**)

◇ **pubic** *adjective* referring to the area near the genitals 耻骨的; **pubic bone** = pubis, the bone in front of the pelvis 耻骨; **pubic hair** = tough hair growing in the genital region 阴毛; **pubic louse** *or* **Phthirius** = louse which infests the pubic regions 阴虱; **pubic symphysis** = piece of cartilage which joins the two sections of the pubic bone 耻骨联合

COMMENT: In a pregnant woman, the pubic symphysis stretches to allow the pelvic girdle to expand so that there is room for the baby to pass through.
注释:孕妇的耻骨联合伸展开,使骨盆带扩张以留出空间让婴儿通过。

pudendal *adjective* referring to the pudendum 阴部的; **pudendal block** = operation to anaesthetize the pudendum during childbirth 阴部阻滞麻醉

◇ **pudendum** *noun* external genital organ of a woman 阴部(女性) (NOTE: the plural is **pudenda**)

puerpera *noun* woman who has recently given birth *or* is giving birth, and whose womb is still distended 产妇,产褥期妇女

◇ **puerperal** *or* **puerperous** *adjective* (i) referring to the puerperium 产妇的 (ii) referring to childbirth 分娩的,产褥期的 (iii) which occurs after childbirth 产后的; **puerperal fever** = form of septicaemia, which was formerly common in mothers immediately after childbirth and caused many deaths 产褥热

◇ **puerperalism** *noun* illness of a baby or its mother resulting from *or* associated with childbirth 产褥病

◇ **puerperium** *noun* period of about six weeks which follows immediately after the birth of a child, during which the mother's sexual organs recover from childbirth 产褥期

puke *verb* (*informal* 非正式) to vomit *or* to be sick 恶心,呕吐

Pulex *noun* genus of human fleas 虱子,虱属

pull *verb* to strain *or* to make a muscle move in a wrong direction 牵张,拉伤: ***He pulled a muscle in his back.*** 他后背肌肉拉伤了。

◇ **pull through** *verb* (*informal* 非正式) to recover from a serious illness 挺过来,熬过来: ***The doctor says she is strong and should pull through.*** 医生说她很强壮会挺过来的。

◇ **pull together** *verb* **to pull yourself together** = to become calmer 使心绪宁静: ***Although he was very angry he soon pulled himself together.*** 虽然他很生气,但他很快就使自己平静下来了。

pulley *noun* device with rings through which wires *or* cords pass, used in traction to make wires tense 滑车

pulmo- *or* **pulmon-** *or* **pulmono-** *prefix* referring to the lungs 肺

◇ **pulmonale** 肺的 *see* 见 COR PULMONALE

◇ **pulmonary** *adjective* referring to the lungs 肺的; **pulmonary arteries** =

arteries which take deoxygenated blood from the heart to the lungs for oxygenation 肺动脉 ◇ 见图 HEART; **pulmonary circulation** = circulation of blood from the heart through the pulmonary arteries to the lungs for oxygenation and back to the heart through the pulmonary veins 肺循环; **pulmonary embolism** = blockage of a pulmonary artery by a blood clot 肺动脉栓塞; **pulmonary hypertension** = high blood pressure in the blood vessels supplying blood to the lungs 肺动脉高压; **pulmonary insufficiency** *or* **incompetence** = dilatation of the main pulmonary artery and stretching of the valve ring, due to pulmonary hypertension 肺灌注不足; **pulmonary oedema** = collection of fluid in the lungs, as occurs in left-sided heart failure 肺水肿; **pulmonary stenosis** = condition where the opening of the right ventricle becomes narrow 肺动脉瓣狭窄; **pulmonary valve** = valve at the opening of the pulmonary artery 肺动脉瓣; **pulmonary vein** = vein which takes oxygenated blood from the lungs to the atrium of the heart 肺静脉

◇ **pulmonectomy** *or* **pneumonectomy** *noun* surgical removal of a lung *or* part of a lung 肺(叶)切除术

pulp *noun* soft tissue, especially when surrounded by hard tissue such as the inside of a tooth 髓; **pulp cavity** = centre of a tooth containing soft tissue 牙髓腔 ◇ 见图 TOOTH

◇ **pulpy** *adjective* made of pulp 髓的: ***the pulpy tissue inside a tooth*** 牙内的髓样组织

pulsation *noun* action of beating regularly, such as the visible pulse which can be seen under the skin in some parts of the body 脉搏搏动

◇ **pulse** *noun* (**a**) (i) any regular recurring variation in quantity 搏动 (ii) pressure wave which can be felt in an artery each time the heart beats to pump blood 脉搏; **to take** *or* **to feel someone's pulse** = to place fingers on an artery to feel the pulse and count the number of beats per minute 把脉: ***Has the patient's pulse been taken***? 给病人测脉搏了吗? ***Her pulse is very irregular***. 她的脉搏很不规律。**carotid pulse** = pulse in the carotid artery at the side of the neck 颈动脉搏动; **femoral pulse** = pulse taken in the groin 股动脉搏动; **radial pulse** = main pulse in the wrist, taken near the outer edge of the forearm, just above the wrist 桡动脉搏动; **ulnar pulse** = secondary pulse in the wrist, taken near the inner edge of the forearm 尺动脉搏动; **pulse point** = place on the body where the pulse can be taken 脉搏点; **pulse pressure** = difference between the diastolic and systolic pressure 脉压差 *see also* 参见 CORRIGAN (**b**) (*food*)(食品) **pulses** = beans and peas 豆子,豆类食物: ***Pulses provide a large amount of protein***. 豆类提供大量蛋白质。

◇ **pulseless** *adjective* (patient) who has no pulse because the heart is beating very weakly 无脉的

◇ **pulsus** *noun* the pulse 脉搏; **pulsus alternans** = pulse with a beat which is alternately strong and weak 交替脉; **pulsus bigeminus** = double pulse, with an extra ectopic beat 二联脉; **pulsus paradoxus** = condition where there is a sharp fall in the pulse when a patient breathes in 奇脉(吸气时脉搏明显变弱)

> COMMENT: The normal, adult pulse is about 72 beats per minute, but it is higher in children. The pulse is normally taken by placing the fingers on the patient's wrist, at the point where the radial artery passes through the depression just below the thumb.
> 注释:正常成年人脉搏大约是每分钟 72 跳,儿童的则快些。把脉一般是将手指放在病人的腕部桡动脉通过的地方,即拇指根部下方凹下去的地方。

pulvis *noun* powder 散剂,粉剂

pump 1 *noun* machine which forces

liquids *or* air into or out of something 泵;**stomach pump** = instrument for sucking out the contents of a patient's stomach, especially if he has just swallowed a poison 洗胃泵 **2** *verb* to force liquid *or* air along a tube 泵出: ***The heart pumps blood round the body.*** 心脏泵出血液周流全身。***The nurses tried to pump the poison out of the stomach.*** 护士们力图用泵将毒物从胃里洗出。

punch drunk syndrome *noun* condition of a patient (usually a boxer) who has been hit on the head many times, and develops impaired mental faculties, trembling limbs and speech disorders 拳击手综合征

punctum *noun* point 点,尖; **puncta lacrimalia** = small openings at the corners of the eyes through which tears drain into the nose 泪点 (NOTE: plural is **puncta**)

puncture 1 *noun* (i) neat hole made by a sharp instrument 穿刺点 (ii) making a hole in an organ *or* swelling to take a sample of the contents *or* to remove fluid 穿刺术: **lumbar puncture** *or* **spinal puncture** = surgical operation to remove a sample of cerebrospinal fluid by inserting a hollow needle into the lower part of the spinal canal 腰穿,脊髓穿刺 (NOTE: US English is also **spinal tap**);**sternal puncture** = surgical operation to remove a sample of bone marrow from the breastbone for testing 胸骨穿刺术(为取骨髓标本); **puncture wound** = wound made by a sharp instrument which makes a hole in the tissue 穿刺伤 **2** *verb* to make a hole in tissue with a sharp instrument 穿刺

pupil *noun* central opening in the iris of the eye, through which light enters the eye 瞳孔 ◊ 见图 EYE

◊ **pupillary** *adjective* referring to the pupil 瞳孔的;**pupillary reaction** *or* **light reflex** = reflex where the pupil changes size according to the amount of light going into the eye 瞳孔反射,对光反射

pure *adjective* very clean *or* not mixed with other substances 纯净的;**pure alcohol** *or* **alcohol BP** = alcohol with 5% water 纯酒精

purgation *noun* using a drug to make a bowel movement 催泻

◊ **purgative** *noun & adjective* laxative; (medicine) which causes evacuation of the bowels 催泻的,催泻剂

◊ **purge** *verb* to induce evacuation of a patient's bowels 催泻

purify *verb* to make pure 纯化; **purified protein derivative** (**PPD**) = pure form of tuberculin, used in tuberculin tests 纯化蛋白衍生物(用于检测结核)

Purkinje cells *noun* neurones in the cerebellar cortex 普肯耶细胞(小脑皮层的一种细胞)

◊ **Purkinje fibres** *noun* bundle of fibres which form the atrioventricular bundle and pass from the AV node to the septum 普肯耶纤维(心脏传导束中的一段)

◊ **Purkinje shift** *noun* change in colour sensitivity which takes place in the eye in low light when the eye starts using the rods in the retina because the light is too weak to stimulate the cones 普肯耶移动(人眼在昏暗条件下启动视杆细胞致色觉敏感性改变,原因是光线太暗时视锥细胞无法被激动)

purpura *noun* purple colouring on the skin, similar to a bruise, caused by blood disease and not by trauma 紫癜; **Henoch's purpura** = blood disorder of children, where the skin becomes purple and bleeding takes place in the intestine 神经性紫癜;**Schönlein's purpura** = blood disorder of children, where the skin becomes purple and the joints are swollen and painful 过敏性紫癜

pursestring 缩窄 *see* 见 SHIRODKAR

purulent *adjective* suppurating, containing *or* producing pus 脓性的

pus *noun* yellow liquid composed of blood serum, pieces of dead tissue, white blood cells and the remains of bacteria, formed by the body in reaction to infection 脓 (NOTE: for terms referring to pus, see words beginning with **py- or pyo-**)

pustule *noun* small pimple filled with pus 脓疱

◇ **pustular** *adjective* (i) covered with *or* composed of pustules 有脓疱的,长脓疱的 (ii) referring to pustules 脓疱的

put up *verb* to arrange (a drip for a patient)安置(输液器)

putrefaction *noun* decompositon of organic substances by bacteria, making an unpleasant smell 腐败

◇ **putrefy** *verb* to rot *or* to decompose 腐败

p.v. *abbreviation for* (缩写) *the Latin phrase* 'per vaginam': by way of the vagina 经阴道的

PVS = PERMANENT VEGETATIVE STATE 永久性植物人状态

PWA *noun* person with AIDS 艾滋病患者

py- *or* **pyo-** *prefix* referring to pus 脓

◇ **pyaemia** *noun* invasion of blood with bacteria, which then multiply and form many little abscesses in various parts of the body 脓血症

◇ **pyarthrosis** *noun* acute suppurative arthritis, a condition where a joint becomes infected with pyogenic organisms and fills with pus 关节积脓

pyel- *or* **pyelo-** *prefix* referring to the pelvis of the kidney *or* renal pelvis 肾盂

◇ **pyelitis** *noun* inflammation of the central part of the kidney 肾盂炎

◇ **pyelocystitis** *noun* inflammation of the pelvis of the kidney and the urinary bladder 肾盂膀胱炎

◇ **pyelogram** *noun* X-ray photograph of a kidney and the urinary tract 肾盂造影片; **intravenous pyelogram** = X-ray photograph of a kidney using intravenous pyelography 静脉肾盂造影片

◇ **pyelography** *noun* X-ray examination of a kidney after introduction of a contrast medium 肾盂造影; **intravenous pyelography** = X-ray examination of a kidney after opaque liquid has been injected intravenously into the body and taken by the blood into the kidneys 静脉肾盂造影; **retrograde pyelography** = X-ray examination of the kidney where a catheter is passed into the kidney and the opaque liquid is injected directly into it 逆行性肾盂造影

◇ **pyelolithotomy** *noun* surgical removal of a stone from the pelvis of the kidney 肾盂结石摘除术

◇ **pyelonephritis** *noun* inflammation of the kidney and the pelvis of the kidney 肾盂肾炎

◇ **pyeloplasty** *noun* any surgical operation on the pelvis of the kidney 肾盂成形术

◇ **pyelotomy** *noun* surgical operation to make an opening in the pelvis of the kidney 肾盂造口术

pyemia = PYAEMIA 脓血症

pyknolepsy *noun* former name for a type of frequent attack of petit mal epilepsy, affecting children 癫痫小发作(旧称)

pyl- *or* **pyle-** *prefix* referring to the portal vein 门静脉

◇ **pylephlebitis** *noun* thrombosis of the portal vein 门静脉栓塞

◇ **pylethrombosis** *noun* condition where blood clots are present in the portal vein or any of its branches 门静脉血栓

pylor- *or* **pyloro-** *prefix* referring to the pylorus 幽门

◇ **pylorectomy** *noun* surgical removal of the pylorus and the antrum of the stomach 幽门切除术(含胃窦部)

◇ **pyloric** *adjective* referring to the pylorus 幽门的; **pyloric antrum** = space at the bottom of the stomach before the pyloric sphincter 幽门胃窦; **pyloric orifice** = opening where the stomach joins the duodenum 幽门口; **pyloric sphincter**

= muscle which surrounds the pylorus, makes it contract and separates it from the duodenum 幽门括约肌; **pyloric stenosis** = blockage of the pylorus, which prevents food from passing from the stomach into the duodenum 幽门狭窄

◇ **pyloroplasty** *noun* surgical operation make the pylorus larger, sometimes combined with treatment for peptic ulcers 幽门成形术

◇ **pylorospasm** *noun* muscle spasm which closes the pylorus so that food cannot pass through into the duodenum 幽门痉挛

◇ **pylorotomy** *noun* Ramstedt's operation, surgical operation to cut into the muscle surrounding the pylorus to relieve pyloric stenosis 幽门切开术

◇ **pylorus** *noun* opening at the bottom of the stomach leading into the duodenum 幽门(胃与十二指肠的接口)

pyo- *prefix* referring to pus 脓

◇ **pyocele** *noun* enlargement of a tube *or* cavity due to accumulation of pus 脓肿

◇ **pyocolpos** *noun* accumulation of pus in the vagina 阴道积脓

◇ **pyoderma** *noun* eruption of pus in the skin 脓皮病

◇ **pyogenic** *adjective* which produces *or* forms pus 生脓的

◇ **pyometra** *noun* accumulation of pus in the uterus 子宫积脓

◇ **pyomyositis** *noun* inflammation of a muscle caused by staphylococci *or* streptococci 脓性肌炎(常由葡萄球菌或链球菌引起)

◇ **pyonephrosis** *noun* distension of the kidney with pus 肾盂积脓

◇ **pyopericarditis** *noun* bacterial pericarditis, an inflammation of the pericardium due to infection with staphylococci *or* streptococci *or* pneumococci 脓性心包炎

◇ **pyorrhoea** *noun* discharge of pus 流脓; **pyorrhoea alveolaris** = suppuration from the supporting tissues round the teeth 牙槽溢脓

◇ **pyosalpinx** *noun* inflammation and formation of pus in a Fallopian tube 输卵管积脓

◇ **pyosis** *noun* formation of pus *or* suppuration 化脓

◇ **pyothorax** = EMPYEMA 脓胸

pyr- *or* **pyro-** *prefix* referring to burning *or* fever 火,热

pyramid *noun* cone-shaped part of the body, especially a cone-shaped projection on the surface of the medulla oblongata *or* in the medulla of the kidney 锥体(如肾锥体,延髓锥体束) ◊ 见图 KIDNEY

◇ **pyramidal** *adjective* referring to a pyramid 锥体的; **pyramidal cell** = cone-shaped cell in the cerebral cortex 锥体细胞; **pyramidal tracts** = tracts in the brain and spinal cord which carry the motor neurone fibres from the cerebral cortex 锥体束(运动神经纤维下传的传导束之一)

pyrexia *noun* fever, a rise in body temperature, or a sickness when the temperature of the body is higher than normal 发热

pyridoxine = VITAMIN B_6 吡哆醇,维生素 B_6

pyrogen *noun* substance which causes a fever 致热原

◇ **pyrogenic** *adjective* which causes a fever 致热原的

pyrosis = HEARTBURN 胃灼热

pyruvic acid *noun* substance formed from muscle glycogen when it is broken down to release energy 丙酮酸(由肌糖原分解产热生成)

pyuria *noun* pus in the urine 脓尿

Qq

q.d.s. *or* **q.i.d.** *abbreviation for* (缩写) *the Latin phrase* 'quater in die sumendus': four times a day (written on prescriptions)每天 4 次(处方用语)

Q fever *noun* infectious rickettsial disease of sheep and cows caused by *Coxiella burnetti* transmitted to humans 寇热(一种由牛、羊传染给人的立克次体病)

COMMENT: Q fever mainly affects farm workers and workers in the meat industry. The symptoms are fever, cough and headaches.
注释:Q 热主要感染农场工人和肉联厂工人,症状有发热、咳嗽及头痛。

q.s. *abbreviation for* (缩写) *the Latin phrase* 'quantum sufficiat': as much as necessary (written on prescriptions) 按所需剂量(处方用语)

quad = QUADRUPLET 四胞胎之一

quadrant *noun* quarter of a circle; sector of the body 四分之一象限: ***tenderness in the right lower quadrant*** 右下象限压痛

◇ **quadrantanopia** *noun* blindness in a quarter of the field of vision 象限盲

quadrate lobe *noun* lobe on the lower side of the liver 方叶(肝脏的一叶,在下方)

◇ **quadratus** *noun* any muscle with four sides 方形肌肉; **quadratus femoris** = muscle at the top of the femur, that rotates the thigh 股方肌

quadri- *prefix* referring to four 四

◇ **quadriceps femoris** *noun* large muscle in the front of the thigh, which extends to the leg 股四头肌

COMMENT: The quadriceps femoris is divided into four parts: the rectus femoris, vastus lateralis, vastus medialis, and the vastus intermedius. It is the sensory receptors in the quadriceps which react to give a knee jerk when the patellar tendon is tapped.
注释:股四头肌分为四个部分:股直肌、股外侧肌、股内侧肌和股中间肌。叩击髌韧带时引起膝跳反射正是由于股四头肌内的感受器对击打的反应。

◇ **quadriplegia** *noun* paralysis of all four limbs: both arms and both legs 四肢瘫

◇ **quadriplegic** *noun & adjective* (person) paralysed in all four arms and legs 四肢瘫痪的

quadruple *adjective* four times *or* in four parts 四倍,四联的; **quadruple vaccine** = vaccine which immunizes against four diseases: diphtheria, whooping cough, poliomyelitis, and tetanus 四联疫苗(对白喉、百日咳、脊髓灰质炎和破伤风免疫的疫苗)

quadruplet *or* **quad** *noun* one of four babies born to a mother at the same time 四胞胎之一: ***She had quadruptlets or quads.*** 她生了四胞胎。*see also* 参见 QUINTUPLET, SEXTUPLET, TRIPLE-T, TWIN

quadrupod *noun* walking stick which ends in four little legs 四爪手杖

qualify *verb* to pass a course of study and be accepted as being able to practise 取得资格: ***He qualified as a doctor two years ago.*** 他两年前取得了医生资格。

◇ **qualification** *noun* being qualified 合格: ***She has a qualification in pharmacy.*** 她取得了药剂师资格。***Are his qualifications recognized in Great Britain?*** 他的资格被大不列颠承认吗?

quarantine 1 *noun* period (originally forty days) when an animal *or* person *or* ship just arrived in a country has to be kept separate in case a serious disease may be carried, to allow the disease time to develop 检疫期: ***The animals were put in quarantine on arrival at the port.*** 动物到港时隔离检疫。***A ship in quarantine shows a yellow flag called the quarantine flag.*** 检疫中的船只插有黄旗称作检疫旗。**2** *verb* to put a person *or* animal in quarantine 检疫

COMMENT: Animals coming into

Great Britain are quarantined for six months because of the danger of rabies. People who are suspected of having an infectious disease can be kept in quarantine for a period which varies according to the incubation period of the disease. The main diseases concerned are cholera, yellow fever and typhus.
注释:来到大不列颠的动物因为有狂犬病的危险要检疫6个月。被怀疑有传染病的人也可以被稽留检疫一段时间,长短随疾病的潜伏期而定。主要的疾病有霍乱、黄热病和斑疹伤寒。

quartan fever *noun* infectious disease *or* form of malaria caused by *Plasmodium malariae* where the fever returns every four days 三日疟 *see also* 参见 TERTIAN

Queckenstedt's test *noun* test done during a lumbar puncture where pressure is applied to the jugular veins, to see if the cerebrospinal fluid is flowing correctly 奎肯斯提试验(用于估计脑脊液压力)

quickening *noun* first sign of life in an unborn baby, usually after about four months of pregnancy, when the mother can feel it moving in her uterus 胎动初感

Quick test *noun* test to identify the clotting factors in a blood sample 魁克试验(检查血样中的凝血因子)

quiescent *adjective* inactive; (disease) with symptoms reduced either by treatment *or* in the normal course of the disease 静息的,静止的

quin = QUINTUPLET 五胞胎之一

quinidine *noun* drug similar to quinine, used to treat tachycardia 奎尼丁(用于治疗心动过速)

quinine *noun* alkaloid drug made from the bark of a South American tree (the cinchona) 奎宁(提取自南美一种树皮); **quinine poisoning** = illness caused by taking too much quinine 奎宁中毒

◇ **Quininism** *or* **quinism** *noun* quinine poisoning 奎宁中毒

COMMENT: Quinine was formerly used to treat the fever symptoms of malaria, but is not often used now because of its side-effects. Symptoms of quinine poisoning are dizziness and noises in the head. Small amounts of quinine have a tonic effect and are used in tonic water.
注释:以前用奎宁治疗疟疾的发热症状,但是因为它的副作用现已不常用了。奎宁中毒的症状有头晕和耳鸣。小剂量奎宁有强身作用,用于健胃水。

quinsy *noun* peritonsillar abscess, acute throat inflammation with an abscess round a tonsil 扁桃体周围脓肿

quintuplet *or* **quin** *noun* one of five babies born to a mother at the same time 五胞胎之一 *see also* 参见 QUADRUPLET, SEXTUPLET, TRIPLET, TWIN

quotidian *adjective* recurring daily 每日的; **quotidian fever** = violent form of malaria where the fever returns at daily or even shorter intervals 日发疟

quotient *noun* result when one number is divided by another 商数; **intelligence quotient** (**IQ**) = ratio of the result of an intelligence test shown as a relationship of the mental age to the actual age of the person tested (the average being 100) 智商; **respiratory quotient** = ratio of the amount of carbon dioxide passed from the blood into the lungs to the amount of oxygen absorbed into the blood from the air 呼吸商

Rr

R = ROENTGEN 伦琴

R/ *abbreviation for* (缩写) *the Latin word* 'recipe': prescription 处方

Ra *chemical symbol for* radium 镭的化学元素符号

rabbit fever = TULARAEMIA 兔热病

rabid *adjective* referring to rabies *or* suffering from rabies 狂犬病的,得狂犬病的: ***He was bitten by a rabid dog.*** 他被疯狗咬了。**rabid encephalitis** = fatal encephalitis resulting from the bite of a rabid animal 狂犬病脑炎

◊ **abies** *or* **hydrophobia** *noun* frequently fatal viral disease transmitted to humans by infected animals 狂犬病,恐水症

> COMMENT: Rabies affects the mental balance, and the symptoms include difficulty in breathing or swallowing and an intense fear of water (hydrophobia) to the point of causing convulsions at the sight of water.
> 注释:狂犬病影响精神状态的平衡,症状包括呼吸或吞咽困难、对水的强烈恐惧(恐水症),甚至到见水即诱发惊厥的程度。

rachi- *or* **rachio-** *prefix* referring to the spine"脊柱"

◊ **rachianaesthesia** = SPINAL ANAESTHESIA 脊髓麻醉法

◊ **rachiotomy** *noun* laminectomy, surgical operation to cut through a vertebra in the spine to reach the spinal cord 脊柱切开术

◊ **rachis** = BACKBONE 脊柱

◊ **rachischisis** = SPINA BIFIDA 脊柱裂

◊ **rachitic** *adjective* (child) with rickets 佝偻病的

◊ **rachitis** = RICKETS 佝偻病

rad *noun* unit of measurement of absorbed radiation dose 拉德(放射性度量单位) *see also* 参见 BECQUEREL, GRAY (NOTE: **gray** is now used to mean one hundred rads)

radial *adjective* (i) referring to something which branches 辐射的,放射状的 (ii) referring to the radius, one of the bones in the forearm 桡骨的; **radial artery** = artery which branches from the brachial artery, running near the radius, from the elbow to the palm of the hand 桡动脉; **radial nerve** = main motor nerve in the arm, running down the back of the upper arm and the outer side of the forearm 桡神经; **radial pulse** = main pulse in the wrist, taken near the outer edge of the forearm, just above the wrist 桡动脉搏动; **radial recurrent** = artery in the arm which forms a loop beside the brachial artery 桡动脉袢(肱动脉以外的臂上的动脉回路); **radial reflex** = jerk made by the forearm when the insertion in the radius of one of the muscles (the brachioradialis) is hit 桡骨反射(叩击桡骨的肌腱受后引发的前臂反射)

radiate *verb* (**a**) to spread out in all directions from a central point 放射: ***The pain radiates from the site of the infection.*** 疼痛从感染的地方放射开来。(**b**) to send out rays 辐射: ***Heat radiates from the body.*** 热从身体辐射出来。

◊ **radiation** *noun* waves of energy which are given off by certain substances, especially radioactive substances 放射,辐射; **radiation burn** = burning of the skin caused by exposure to large amounts of radiation 放射性灼伤; **radiation enteritis** = enteritis caused by X-rays 放射性肠炎; **radiation sickness** = illness caused by exposure to radiation from radioactive substances 放射病; **radiation treatment** = RADIOTHERAPY 放射治疗 *see also* 参见 OPTIC RADIATION, SENSORY RADIATION

> COMMENT: Prolonged exposure to many types of radiation can be harmful. Nuclear radiation is the most obvious, but exposure to X-rays

(either as a patient being treated, or as a radiographer) can cause radiation sickness. First symptoms of the sickness are diarrhoea and vomiting, but radiation can also be followed by skins burns and loss of hair. Massive exposure to radiation can kill quickly, and any person exposed to radiation is more likely to develop certain types of cancer than other members of the population.
注释：长时间暴露于多种放射线是有害的。核辐射是最明显的例子，但暴露于X线(作为病人接受放射治疗或作为放射科医生)也可以导致放射病。这种病的最早的症状是腹泻和呕吐，放射后也可以出现皮肤灼伤和脱发。暴露于大剂量放射线可以迅速致死，而且任何暴露于放射线的人都比人群中的其他人更易得某些类型的癌症。

radical *adjective* (i) very serious *or* which deals with the root of a problem 根本的 (ii) (operation) which removes the whole of a part or of an organ, together with its lymph system and other tissue 根治性(手术); **radical mastectomy** = surgical removal of a breast and the lymph nodes and muscles associated with it 根治性乳腺切除术; **radical mastoidectomy** = operation to remove all of the mastoid process 根治性乳突切除术; **radical treatment** = treatment which aims at complete eradication of a disease 根治性治疗

radicle *noun* (i) a small root *or* vein 细小静脉 (ii) tiny fibre which forms the root of a nerve 细小神经根

◇ **radicular** *adjective* referring to a radicle 根的

◇ **radiculitis** *noun* inflammation of a radicle of a cranial *or* spinal nerve 脊(颅)神经根炎 *see also* 参见 POLYRADICULITIS

radio- *prefix* referring to (i) radiation 放射 (ii) radioactive substances 放射性物质 (iii) the radius in the arm 桡骨

radioactive *adjective* (substance) whose nucleus disintegrates and gives off energy in the form of radiation which can pass through other substances 有放射活性的; **radioactive isotope** 放射性同位素 *see* 见 RADIOISOTOPE

◇ **radioactivity** *noun* energy in the form of radiation emitted by a radioactive substance 放射活性

COMMENT: The commonest naturally radioactive substances are radium and uranium. Other substances can be made radioactive for medical purposes by making their nuclei unstable, so forming radioactive isotopes. Radioactive iodine is used to treat conditions such as thyrotoxicosis. Radioactive isotopes of various chemicals are used to check the functioning of or disease in internal organs.
注释：最常见的天然放射性物质是镭和铀。医疗上通过另一些放射性物质的核稳定性使之具有放射活性，做成有放射活性的同位素，如放射性碘用来治疗甲状腺毒症。许多放射性同位素被用来检查内脏的功能或疾病。

◇ **radiobiologist** *noun* doctor who specializes in radiobiology 放射生物学家

◇ **radiobiology** *noun* scientific study of radiation and its effects on living things 放射生物学

radiocarpal joint *noun* wrist joint, the joint where the radius articulates with the scaphoid (one of the carpal bones) 桡腕关节

radiodermatitis *noun* inflammation of the skin caused by exposure to radiation 放射性皮炎

◇ **radiograph** *noun* X-ray photograph 放射线摄片

◇ **radiographer** *noun* (i) person specially trained to operate a machine to take X-ray photographs *or* radiographs (diagnostic radiographer) 放射科摄片技师 (ii) person specially trained to use X-rays *or* radioactive isotopes in treatment of patients (therapeutic radiographer) 放射治疗师

◇ **radiography** *noun* examining the

internal parts of a patient by taking X-ray photographs 放射检查

◇ **radioimmunoassay** *noun* process of finding out if antibodies are present by injecting radioactive tracers into the bloodstream 放免法

◇ **radioisotope** *noun* isotope of a chemical element which is radioactive 放射性同位素

COMMENT: Radioisotopes are used in medicine to provide radiation for radiation treatment. Radioactive isotopes of various chemicals are used to check how organs function or if they are diseased: for example, radioisotopes of iodine are used to investigate thyroid activity.
注释:放射性同位素用于医疗提供放射治疗所需的射线。多种元素的放射性同位素被用来检查器官的功能状况或器官是否有病,例如,碘的放射性同位素被用来检查甲状腺活性。

◇ **radiologist** *noun* doctor who specializes in radiology 放射学家

◇ **radiology** *noun* use of radiation to diagnose disorders (as in the use of X-rays or radioactive tracers) *or* to treat diseases such as cancer 放射学

◇ **radionuclide** *noun* element which gives out radiation 放射性核素; **radionuclide scan** = scan (especially of the brain) where radionuclides are put in compounds which are concentrated in certain parts of the body 放射性核素扫描

◇ **radio-opaque** *adjective* (substance) which absorbs all or most of a radiation 不透射线的

COMMENT: Radio-opaque substances appear dark on X-rays and are used to make it easier to have clear radiographs of certain organs.
注释:不透射线的物质在 X 线片上是暗影,利用它更容易地得到某些器官清晰的图像。

◇ **radiopharmaceutical** *noun* radioisotope used in medical diagnosis *or* treatment 放射性药物

◇ **radio pill** *noun* tablet with a tiny radio transmitter 同位素颗粒

COMMENT: The patient swallows the pill and as it passes through the body it gives off information about the digestive system.
注释:病人吞下同位素颗粒,当它通过体内时就能提供消化道有关的信息。

◇ **radioscopy** *noun* examining an X-ray photograph on a fluorescent screen 放射透视检查

◇ **radiosensitive** *adjective* (cancer cell) which is sensitive to radiation and can be treated by radiotherapy 对放射线敏感的(指某种肿瘤细胞)

◇ **radiosensitivity** *noun* sensitivity of a cell to radiation 对放射线的敏感性

◇ **radiotherapy** *noun* treating a disease by exposing the affected part to radioactive rays such as X-rays *or* gamma rays 放射治疗

COMMENT: Many forms of cancer can be treated by directing radiation at the diseased part of the body.
注释:多种癌症可以用直接照射疾病部位来治疗。

radium *noun* radioactive metallic element 镭 (NOTE: chemical symbol is **Ra**)

radius *noun* the shorter and outer of the two bones in the forearm between the elbow and the wrist (the other bone is the ulna) 桡骨 ◊ 见图 HAND, SKELETON (NOTE: plural is **radii**)

radix *or* **root** *noun* (i) point from which a part of the body grows 根 (ii) part of a tooth which is connected to a socket in the jaw 牙根

radon *noun* radioactive gas, formed from the radioactive decay of radium, and used in capsules (known as radon seeds) to treat cancers inside the body 氡 (NOTE: chemical symbol is **Rn**)

COMMENT: Radon occurs naturally in soil, in construction materials and even in ground water. It can seep into houses and causes radiation sickness.
注释:自然状态的土壤中就有氡存在,建筑材料乃至地下水中也有氡,它可以渗到房屋里并引起放射病。

raise *verb* (**a**) to lift 抬起: ***Lie with your legs raised above the level of your head.*** 平躺,将腿抬举过头。(**b**) to increase 增加: ***Anaemia causes a raised level of white blood cells in the body.*** 贫血引起体内白细胞水平上升。

rale = CREPITATION 罗音

Ramstedt's operation = PYLOROTOMY 幽门切除术

ramus *noun* (**a**) branch of a nerve *or* artery *or* vein(神经,动脉或静脉的)支 (**b**) the ascending part on each side of the mandible 下颌骨的升支 (NOTE: plural is **rami**)

randomized *adjective* which has been selected *or* carried out at random 随机的: ***a double-blind randomized trial*** 一项随机双盲试验

range *noun* (i) series of different but similar things 系列 (ii) difference between lowest and highest values in a series of data 区间: ***The drug offers protection against a wide range of diseases.*** 这种药保护作用的范围很宽,对多种疾病有效。***Doctors have a range of drugs which can be used to treat arthritis.*** 医生有一系列药物可以治疗关节炎。

ranula *noun* small cyst under the tongue, on the floor of the mouth, which forms when a salivary duct is blocked 舌下囊肿

Ranvier 郎飞氏 *see* 见 NODE

raphe *noun* long thin fold which looks like a seam, along a midline such as on the dorsal face of the tongue 缝

rapid *adjective* fast 快; **rapid eye movement (REM) sleep** = phase of normal sleep with fast movements of the eyeballs which occur at intervals 快动眼睡眠

> COMMENT: During REM sleep, a person dreams, breathes lightly and has a raised blood pressure and an increased rate of heartbeat. The eyes may be half-open, and the sleeper may make facial movements.
> 注释:人在快动眼睡眠期做梦、呼吸轻、血压和心率增加。眼睛可以是半睁的,睡眠者可以有面部运动。

◇ **rapid-acting** *adjective* (drug *or* treatment) which has an effect very quickly 起效快的,速效的

rare *adjective* not common *or* (disease) of which there are very few cases 罕见的: ***He is suffering from a rare blood disorder.*** 他得了一种罕见的血液病。***AO is not a rare blood group.*** AO不是一种罕见血型。

rarefy *verb* (*of bones*) to become less dense 使(骨质)疏松

◇ **rarefaction** *noun* condition where bone tissue becomes more porous and less dense because of lack of calcium 骨质疏松

rash *noun* mass of small spots which stays on the skin for a period of time, and then disappears 皮疹; **to break out in a rash** = to have a rash which starts suddenly 急疹: ***She had a high temperature and then broke out in a rash.*** 她高热,出急疹。**nappy** *US* **diaper rash** = sore red skin on a baby's buttocks and groin, caused by long contact with ammonia in a wet nappy 尿布疹

> COMMENT: Many common diseases such as chickenpox and measles have a special rash as their main symptom. Rashes can be very irritating, but the itching can be relieved by applying calamine lotion.
> 注释:许多常见病,如水痘、麻疹,以特殊的皮疹为其主要症状。皮疹可以有非常强的刺激性,但瘙痒可用炉甘石洗剂缓解。

raspatory *noun* surgical instrument like a file, which is used to scrape the surface of a bone 骨锉

rat-bite fever *or* **disease** *noun* fever caused by either of two bacteria *Spirillum minor* or *Streptobacillus moniliformis* and transmitted to humans by rats 鼠咬热

rate *noun* (**a**) amount *or* proportion of something compared to something else 比率; **birth rate** = number of children born per 1000 of population 出生率(每千

人口中婴儿出生数)；**fertility rate** = number of births per year calculated per 1000 females aged between 15 and 44 生育率(每千名15～44岁的妇女分娩数)；(**b**) number of times something happens 频度,频率：***The heart was beating at a rate of only 59 per minute.*** 心脏跳动的频率仅为每分钟59次。**heart rate** = number of times the heart beats per minute 心率；**pulse rate** = number of times the pulse beats per minute 脉率

> COMMENT：Pulse rate is the heart rate felt at various parts of the body.
> 注释：脉率是在身体不同位置感受到的心率。

ratio *noun* number which shows a proportion *or* which is the result of one number divided by another 比率：***An IQ is the ratio of the person's mental age to his chronological age.*** 智商是一个人的智力年龄与其实际年龄的比率。

Rauwolfia *noun* tranquillizing drug extracted from a plant 萝芙木；***Rauwolfia serpentina*** sometimes used to treat high blood pressure 印度萝芙木(用于治疗高血压) *see also* 参见 RESERPINE

raw *adjective* (**a**) not cooked 生的,未煮过的 (**b**) (i) sensitive (skin)(皮肤)敏感的 (ii) (skin) scraped *or* partly removed 擦破皮的,露肉的：***The scab came off leaving the raw wound exposed to the air.*** 痂掉了,露出新鲜的伤口暴露在空气中。

ray *noun* line of light *or* radiation *or* heat 射线；**infrared rays** = long invisible rays, below the visible red end of the spectrum, used to warm body tissue 红外线；**ultraviolet rays** (**UV rays**) = short invisible rays beyond the violet end of the spectrum, which form the element in sunlight which tans the skin 紫外线 *see also* 参见 X-RAY

Raynaud's disease *noun* condition where the fingers and toes become cold, white and numb at temperatures that would not affect a normal person, commonly called 'dead man's fingers' 雷诺氏病(手指或脚趾遇凉时异常发白、麻木、刺痛,通常又叫作"指")

RBC = RED BLOOD CELL 红细胞

RCGP = ROYAL COLLEGE OF GENERAL PRACTITIONERS 皇家全科医师学会

◇ **RCN** = ROYAL COLLEGE OF NURSING 皇家护理学会

◇ **RCOG** = ROYAL COLLEGE OF OBSTETRICIANS AND GYNAECOLOGISTS 皇家妇产科医师学会

◇ **RCP** = ROYAL COLLEGE OF PHYSICIANS 皇家内科医师学会

reabsorb *verb* to absorb again 再吸收,重吸收：***Glucose is reabsorbed by the tubules in the kidney.*** 肾小管重吸收葡萄糖。

◇ **reabsorption** *noun* process of being reabsorbed 再吸收,重吸收：***Some substances which are filtered into the tubules of the kidney, then pass into the bloodstream by tubular reabsorption.*** 某些被过滤到肾小管的物质通过小管的重吸收作用回到血流中。

reach 1 *noun* distance which one can stretch a hand; distance which one can travel easily 伸手可及的距离,能轻易达到的距离：***Medicines should be kept out of the reach of children.*** 药物应当保存在孩子拿不到的地方。***The hospital is in easy reach of the railway station.*** 从火车站到医院很方便。2 *verb* to arrive at a point 到达：***Infection has reached the lungs.*** 感染已达肺部。

react *verb* (**a**) **to react to something** = to act because of something else *or* to act in response to something 反应：***The tissues reacted to the cortisone injection.*** 组织对可的松注射起了反应。***The patient reacted badly to the penicillin.*** 病人对青霉素的反应不好。***She reacted positively to the Widal test.*** 她肥达试验反应阳性(用于检测伤寒)。(**b**) (*of a chemical substance*) **to react with something** = to change because of the presence of another substance 起化学反应

◇ **reaction** *noun* (**a**) (i) action which takes place because of something which has happened earlier 反应 (ii) effect produced by a stimulus 对刺激产生反应: ***A rash appeared as a reaction to the penicillin injection.*** 出皮疹是对注射青霉素的一种反应。***The patient suffers from an allergic reaction to oranges.*** 这位患者对橘子起了过敏反应。**immune reaction** = reaction of a body to an antigen 免疫反应 (**b**) particular response of a patient to a test 特异性反应; **Wassermann reaction** = reaction to a blood test for syphilis 瓦氏反应(检测梅毒)

◇ **reactive** *or* **reactionary** *adjective* which takes place because of a reaction 反应性的; **reactionary haemorrhage** = bleeding which follows an operation 反应性出血; **reactive hyperaemia** = congestion of blood vessels after an occlusion has been removed 反应性充血

◇ **reactivate** *verb* to make active again 再活化,激活: ***His general physical weakness has reactivated the dormant virus.*** 他全身状况虚弱激活了休眠的病毒。

reading *noun* note taken of figures, especially of degrees on a scale 读数: ***The sphygmomanometer gave a diastolic reading of 70.*** 血压计舒张压的读数是70。

reagent *noun* chemical substance which reacts with another substance (especially when used to detect the presence of the second substance) 试剂

◇ **reagin** *noun* antibody which reacts against an allergen 反应素(对过敏原产生反应的抗体)

reappear *verb* to appear again 再现

◇ **reappearance** *noun* appearing again 再现: ***The reappearance of the symptoms happens after a period of several months.*** 几个月后症状再次出现。

reason *noun* (**a**) thing which explains why something happens 原因: ***What was the reason for the sudden drop in the patient's pulse rate?*** 病人脉率突然下降的原因是什么? (**b**) being mentally stable 理智: ***Her reason was beginning to fail.*** 她已经开始失去理智。

reassure *verb* to make someone sure *or* to give someone hope 安慰: ***The doctor reassured her that the drug had no unpleasant side-effects.*** 医生安慰她说药物没有令人不快的副作用。***He reassured the old lady that she should be able to walk again in a few weeks.*** 他安慰老妇人说她几周以后她就又能走路了。

◇ **reassurance** *noun* act of reassuring 安慰

rebore *noun* (*informal* 非正式) endarterectomy, the surgical removal of the lining of a blocked artery 动脉内膜切除术(用以使血管再通)

rebuild *verb* to reconstruct a defective *or* damaged part of the body 再构筑,重建: ***After the accident, she had several operations to rebuild her pelvis.*** 事故之后,她经历了几次手术以重建她的骨盆。

recalcitrant *adjective* (condition) which does not respond to treatment 对治疗无反应的,难治的,顽固的

recall 1 *noun* act of remembering something from the past 回忆; **total recall** = being able to remember something in complete detail 完全回忆 **2** *verb* to remember something which happened in the past 回忆

receive *verb* to get something (especially a transplanted organ) 接受: ***She received six pints of blood in a transfusion.*** 她输了6品脱血。***He received a new kidney from his brother.*** 他从自己兄弟那儿接受了一个新肾。

receptaculum *noun* part of a tube which is expanded to form a sac 球囊

receptor *noun* nerve ending which senses a change (such as cold *or* heat) in the surrounding environment *or* in the body and reacts to it by sending an impulse to the central nervous system 受体(感受某种刺激的神经信号并向中枢传递的一种神经末梢) *see also* 参见 ADRENERGIC, CHEMORECEPTOR, EXTEROCEPTOR, INTEROCEPTOR, THERMORECEPTOR, VISCERRECEPTOR

recess *noun* hollow part in an organ 隐窝

◇ **recessive** *adjective* & *noun* (trait)

which is weaker than and hidden by a dominant gene 隐性(基因),隐性的

COMMENT: Since each physical characteristic is governed by two genes, if one is dominant and the other recessive, the resulting trait will be that of the dominant gene. Traits governed by recessive genes will appear if both genes are recessive.
注释:由于每个躯体特征由两个基因控制,如果一个基因是显性的而另一个是隐性的,那么最终的特性是那个显性基因决定的。由隐性基因决定的特征只有两个基因都是隐性基因时才表现出来。

recipient *noun* person who receives something, such as a transplant *or* a blood transfusion from a donor 受体

QUOTE: Bone marrow from donors has to be carefully matched with the recipient or graft-versus-host disease will ensue.
引文:捐献者的骨髓必须与受者的仔细匹配,否则会引发移植物抗宿主反应。
Hospital Update 现代化医院

Recklinghausen 雷克林豪森 *see* 见 VON RECKLINGHAUSEN

recognize *verb* (**a**) to sense something (as to see a person *or* to taste a food) and remember it from an earlier sensing 认识: ***She did not recognize her mother.*** 她没有认出自己的妈妈。(**b**) to approve of something officially (正式)认可: ***The diploma is recognized by the Department of Health.*** 这个执照是卫生部认可的。

recommend *verb* to suggest that it would be a good thing if someone did something 推荐: ***The doctor recommended that she should stay in bed.*** 医生建议她卧床。***I would recommend following a diet to try to lose some weight.*** 我建议(你)遵循节食原则试着减轻体重。

reconstruct *verb* to rebuild a defective *or* damaged part of the body 重建,修复

◇ **reconstruction** *noun* rebuilding a defective *or* damaged part of the body 重建,修复

◇ **reconstructive surgery** *noun* plastic surgery, surgery which rebuilds a defective *or* damaged part of the body 重建手术,修复手术

reconvert *verb* to convert back into an earlier form 恢复,复原再转化: ***The liver reconverts some of its stored glycogen into glucose.*** 肝脏把它存储的一些糖原再转化为葡萄糖。

record 1 *verb* to note information 记录: ***The chart records the variations in the patient's blood pressure.*** 此图记录了病人的血压变化。***You must take the patient's temperature every hour and record it in this book.*** 你必须每小时给病人测一次体温并记录在这个本子上。**2** *noun* piece of information about something 记录; **medical records** = information about a patient's medical history 医疗记录,病历

COMMENT: Patients are not usually allowed to see their medical records because the information in them is confidential to the doctor.
注释:一般不允许病人看自己的病历,因为里面有只供医生看的保密信息。

recover *verb* (**a**) to get better after an illness *or* operation *or* accident 恢复: ***She recovered from her concussion in a few days.*** 几天后她从脑震荡中恢复了过来。***It will take him weeks to recover from the accident.*** 他得用几周才能从事故中恢复过来。(NOTE: you recover **from** an illness) (**b**) to get back something which has been lost 回复: ***Will he ever recover the use of his legs?*** 他还能回复到(自如)运动双腿的状态吗? ***She recovered her eyesight after all the doctors thought she would be permanently blind.*** 在所有医生都认为她会永久失明时候,她的视力却恢复了。

◇ **recovery** *noun* getting better after an illness *or* accident *or* operation 康复: ***He is well on the way to recovery.*** = He is getting better. 他处于康复之中。***She made only a partial recovery.*** = She is better, but will never be completely well. 她只是部分康复了。***She has made a***

complete** or **splendid recovery. = She is completely well. 她完全恢复了。**recovery room** = room in a hospital where a patient who has had an operation is placed until the effects of the anaesthetic have worn off and he can be moved into an ordinary ward 术后恢复室

◊ **recovery position** *noun* lying face downwards, with one knee and one arm bent forwards and the face turned to one side 康复位

> COMMENT: Called the recovery position because it is recommended for accident victims or for people who are suddenly ill, while waiting for an ambulance to arrive. The position prevents the patient from swallowing and choking on blood or vomit.
> 注释:之所以叫做康复位是因为它是推荐给事故受害人或急症患者在等待救护车到来时采取的体位。这种体位防止病人误吞出血或呕吐物以防哽噎。

recrudescence *noun* reappearance of symptoms (of a disease which seemed to have got better) 复发

◊ **recrudescent** *adjective* (symptom) which has reappeared 复发的

recruit *verb* to get people to join the staff *or* a group 招募: ***We are trying to recruit more nursing staff***. 我们正在尽力招募更多的护理人员。

> QUOTE: Patients presenting with symptoms of urinary tract infection were recruited in a general practice surgery.
> 引文:以泌尿道感染症状来就诊的患者被分诊到普外科。
> **Journal of the Royal College of General Practitioners** 皇家全科医师学会杂志

rect- *or* **recto-** *prefix* referring to the rectum 直肠

◊ **rectal** *adjective* referring to the rectum 直肠的; **rectal fissure** = crack in the wall of the anal canal 直肠裂; **rectal prolapse** = condition where part of the rectum moves downwards and passes through the anus 直肠脱垂; **rectal temperature** = temperature in the rectum, taken with a rectal thermometer 直肠温度; **rectal thermometer** = thermometer which is inserted into the patient's rectum to take the temperature 直肠温度计; **rectal triangle** *or* **anal triangle** = posterior part of the perineum 直肠三角,肛门三角

◊ **rectally** *adverb* through the rectum 通过直肠地: ***The temperature was taken rectally***. 这个温度是通过直肠测得的。

◊ **rectocele** *or* **proctocele** *noun* condition associated with prolapse of the womb, where the rectum protrudes into the vagina 直肠膨出

◊ **rectopexy** *noun* surgical operation to attach a rectum which has prolapsed 直肠固定术

◊ **rectoscope** *noun* instrument for looking into the rectum 直肠镜

◊ **rectosigmoidectomy** *noun* surgical removal of the sigmoid colon and the rectum 直肠乙状结肠切除术

◊ **rectovaginal examination** *noun* examination of the rectum and vagina 直肠阴道检查

◊ **rectovesical** *adjective* referring to the rectum and the bladder 直肠膀胱的

rectum *noun* end part of the large intestine leading from the sigmoid colon to the anus 直肠 ◊ 见图 DIGESTIVE SYSTEM, UROGENITAL TRACT (NOTE: for terms referring to the rectum, see words beginning with **procto-**)

rectus *noun* straight muscle 直肌; **rectus abdominis** = long straight muscle which runs down the front of the abdomen 腹直肌; **rectus femoris** = flexor muscle in the front of the thigh, one of the four parts of the quadriceps femoris 股直肌 *see also* 参见 MEDIAL (NOTE: plural is **recti**)

> QUOTE: There are four recti muscles and two oblique muscles in each eye, which coordinate the movement of the eyes and enable them to work as a pair.

> 引文：每只眼睛有 4 条直肌和 2 条斜肌，它们协调眼球的运动，使双眼能够成对地发挥作用。
>
> **Nursing Times** 护理时代

recumbent *adjective* lying down 躺着的

recuperate *verb* to recover *or* to get better after an illness *or* accident 复原，康复：***He is recuperating after an attack of flu***. 感冒之后他正在恢复中。***She is going to stay with her mother while she recuperates***. 在母亲恢复期间她想去陪着她。

◇ **recuperation** *noun* getting better after an illness 恢复，复原：***His recuperation will take several months***. 他需要几个月时间恢复。

recur *verb* to return 复发，再发：***The headaches recurred frequently, but usually after the patient had eaten chocolate***. 头疼经常复发，但通常是在病人吃了巧克力之后。

◇ **recurrence** *noun* act of returning 复发，再发：***He had a recurrence of a fever which he had caught in the tropics***. 他在热带传上了一种反复发热的病。

◇ **recurrent** *adjective* (**a**) which occurs again 复发的；**recurrent abortion** = condition where a woman has abortions with one pregnancy after another 反复发生流产(习惯性流产)；**recurrent fever** = fever (like malaria) which returns at regular intervals 回归热 (**b**) (vein *or* artery *or* nerve) which forms a loop 血管或神经袢；**radial recurrent** = artery in the arm which forms a loop beside the brachial artery 桡动脉袢

red *adjective* & *noun* (of) a colour like the colour of blood 红色，红色的：***Blood in an artery is bright red, but venous blood is darker***. 动脉血是鲜红的，静脉血则是暗红。**red blood cell** (**RBC**) *or* **erythrocyte** = blood cell which contains haemoglobin and carries oxygen 红细胞；**red eye** = PINK EYE 红眼病

◇ **Red Crescent** *noun* organization similar to the Red Cross, working in Muslim countries 红新月会(穆斯林国家中与红十字会相似的组织)

◇ **Red Cross** *noun* **International Committee of the Red Cross** (**ICRC**) = international organization which provides mainly emergency medical help, but also relief to victims of earthquakes, floods, etc., or to prisoners of war 红十字会国际委员会：***Red Cross officials or officials of the Red Cross arrived in the disaster area this morning***. 今晨红十字会官员抵达受灾现场。

◇ **redness** *noun* being red *or* red colour 红色，变成红色，发红：***The redness showed where the skin had reacted to the injection***. 皮肤发红的地方指示对注射有反应。

reduce *verb* (**a**) to make something smaller *or* lower 减少，缩减，降低：***They used ice packs to try to reduce the patient's temperature***. 他们试图用冰袋给病人降温。(**b**) to put (a dislocated *or* a fractured bone, a displaced organ *or* part *or* a hernia) back into its proper position so that it can heal 复原

◇ **reducible** *adjective* (hernia) where the organ can be pushed back into place without an operation 可复原的

◇ **reduction** *noun* (**a**) making less *or* becoming less 减少，降低：***They noted a reduction in body temperature***. 他们注意到体温下降了。(**b**) putting (a hernia *or* dislocated joint *or* a broken bone) back into the correct position 复原，使回复原位

> QUOTE: Blood pressure control reduces the incidence of first stroke and aspirin appears to reduce the risk of stroke after transient ischaemic attacks by some 15%.
>
> 引文：控制血压可减少初次卒中的发生率，阿司匹林将一过性缺血发作后的脑卒中发生的危险性减少了大约 15%。
>
> **British Journal of Hospital Medicine** 英国医院医学杂志

re-emerge *verb* to come out again 再浮现

◇ **re-emergence** *noun* coming out again 再浮现

refer *verb* (**a**) to mention *or* to talk about something 涉及,提及: ***The doctor referred to the patient's history of sinus problems.*** 医生提到了病人的鼻窦炎病史。(**b**) to suggest that someone should consult something 参见,参引,参考: ***For method of use, please refer to the manufacturer's instructions.*** 使用方法请参见制造商提供的使用说明。***The user is referred to the page giving the results of the tests.*** 使用者应参考列出试验结果的那一页。(**c**) to pass on information about a patient to someone else 转诊: ***She was referred to a gynaecologist.*** 她被转诊给妇科医师。***The GP referred the patient to a consultant.*** = He passed details about the patient's case to the consultant so that the consultant could examine him. 全科医师将病人转诊到会诊医生那里。(**d**) to send to another place 送; **referred pain** = SYNALGIA 牵涉痛

◇ **referral** *noun* sending a patient to a specialist 转诊: ***She asked for a referral to a gynaecologist.*** 她请求转诊到妇科医师。

QUOTE: 27 adult patients admitted to hospital with acute abdominal pains were referred for study because their attending clinicians were uncertain whether to advise an urgent laparotomy.
引文:以急性腹痛收入院的患者有27人被转诊到观察室,因为他们的主治医对是否建议急诊开腹手术没有把握。
Lancet 柳叶刀杂志

QUOTE: Many patients from outside districts were referred to London hospitals by their GPs.
引文:许多外省病人是经他们的全科医师转诊到伦敦的医院来的。
Nursing Times 护理时代

QUOTE: He subsequently developed colicky abdominal pain and tenderness which caused his referral.
引文:他后来出现了痉挛性腹痛并有压痛,因此被转诊。
British Journal of Hospital Medicine 英国医院医学杂志

reflex *noun* automatic reaction to something (such as a knee jerk) 反射; **accommodation reflex** = reaction of the pupil when the eye focuses on an object which is close 调节反射; **light reflex** = reaction of the pupil of the eye which changes size according to the amount of light going into the eye 光反射; **reflex action** = automatic reaction to a stimulus (such as a sneeze) 反射性动作; **reflex arc** = basic system of a reflex action, where a receptor is linked to a motor neurone which in turn is linked to an effector muscle 反射弧 *see also* 参见 PATELLAR, PLANTAR, RADIAL

◇ **reflexologist** *noun* person specializing in reflexology 足底反射治疗师

◇ **reflexology** *noun* treatment to relieve tension by massaging the soles of the feet and thereby stimulating the nerves and increasing the blood supply 足底反射治疗学

reflux *noun* flowing backwards (of a liquid) in the opposite direction to normal flow 返流: ***The valves in the veins prevent blood reflux.*** 静脉瓣的作用就是防止血液返流。**reflux oesophagitis** = inflammation of the oesophagus caused by regurgitation of acid juices from the stomach 返流性食管炎 *see also* 参见 VESICOURETERIC

refract *verb* to make light rays change direction as they go from one medium (such as air) to another (such as water) at an angle 折射: ***The refracting media in the eye are the cornea, the aqueous humour, the vitreous humour and the lens.*** 眼的折射介质包括角膜、房水、玻璃体液和晶状体。

◇ **refraction** *noun* (i) change of direction of light rays as they enter a medium (such as the eye) 折射 (ii) measuring the angle at which the light rays bend, as a test to see if someone needs to wear glasses 屈光

◇ **refractometer** *noun* optometer, instrument which measures the refraction of the eye 屈光仪

refractory *adjective* which it is difficult *or* impossible to treat *or* (condition) which does not respond to treatment 难治的; **refractory period** = short space of time after the ventricles of the heart have contracted, when they cannot contract again 不应期

refrigerate *verb* to make something cold 冷冻: ***The serum should be kept refrigerated*.** 血清应冷冻保存。

◇ **refrigeration** *noun* (i) making something cold 冷冻 (ii) making part of the body very cold, to give the effect of an anaesthetic 冷冻局麻

◇ **refrigerator** *noun* machine which keeps things cold 冰箱

regain *verb* to get back something which was lost 重获: ***He has regained the use of his left arm*.** 他又能使用自己的左臂了。***She went into a coma and never regained consciousness*.** 她昏迷了,再也没有恢复意识。

regenerate *verb* to grow again 再生

◇ **regeneration** *noun* growing again of tissue which has been destroyed 再生

regimen *noun* fixed course of treatment (such as a course of drugs or a special diet) 疗程

region *noun* area *or* part which is around something 区,部位: ***She experienced itching in the anal region*.** 她肛门部位瘙痒。***The rash started in the region of the upper thigh*.** 皮疹是从大腿上部开始的。***The plantar region is very sensitive*.** 足底区是非常敏感的。

◇ **regional** *adjective* in *or* referring to a particular region 地区的,某一部位的,节段性的; **Regional Health Authority (RHA)** = administrative unit in the National Health Service which is responsible for the planning of health services in a large part of the country 地区卫生当局; **regional ileitis** *or* **regional enteritis** *or* **Crohn's disease** 节段性肠炎 *see* 见 ILEITIS

register 1 *noun* official list 花名册; **The Medical Register** = list of doctors approved by the General Medical Council 医生花名册: ***The committee ordered his name to be struck off the register*.** 委员会决定将他从花名册中除名。2 *verb* to write a name on an official list, especially to put one's name on the official list of patients treated by a GP *or* dentist *or* on the list of patients suffering from a certain disease 注册,上花名册: ***She registered with her local GP*.** 她在地方全科医师那里注册了。***He is a registered heroin addict*.** 他是登记在册的海洛因成瘾者。***They went to register the birth with the Registrar of Births, Marriages and Deaths*.** 他们到出生、婚姻及死亡登记官那里给新生儿登记。***Before registering with the GP, she asked if she could visit him*.** 在全科医师那里登记前,她询问可否拜访他一下。***All practising doctors are registered with the General Medical Council*.** 所有开业医生都是在医学总会注册的。**registered midwife** = qualified midwife who is registered to practise 注册助产士; **Registered Nurse (RN)** *or* **Registered General Nurse (RGN)** 注册护士或注册全科护士; **Registered Theatre Nurse (RTN)** = nurses who have been registered by the UKCC 注册手术室护士 *see also* 参见 *note at* NURSE

◇ **registrar** *noun* (**a**) qualified doctor *or* surgeon in a hospital who supervises house officers 管注册的医生 (**b**) person who registers something officially 登记员; **Registrar of Births, Marriages and Deaths** = official who keeps the records of people who have been born, married or who have died in a certain area 负责登记出生、婚姻和死亡的官员

◇ **registration** *noun* act of registering 注册、登记: ***A doctor cannot practise without registration by the General Medical Council*.** 没有到医学总会注册的医生不能开业。

regress *verb* to return to an earlier stage *or* condition 退化,回归

◇ **regression** *noun* (i) stage where symptoms of a disease are disappearing and the patient is getting better 消退 (ii) (*in psychiatry*) returning to a mental state which existed when the patient was younger(精神病学上)退行

regular *adjective* which takes place again and again after the same period of time; which happens at the same time each day 规律的,定期的: ***He was advised to make regular visits to the dentist.*** 建议他定期去看牙医师。***She had her regular six-monthly checkup.*** 她每6个月做一次体检。

◇ **regularly** *adverb* happening repeatedly after the same period of time 有规律地: ***The tablets must be taken regularly every evening.*** 必须每天晚上规律服药。***You should go to the dentist regularly.*** 你应当定期去看牙医师。

regulate *verb* to make something work (in a regular way) 调节,调整: ***The heartbeat is regulated by the sinoatrial node.*** 心跳是由窦房结调节的。

◇ **regulation** *noun* act of regulating 调节,调整: ***the regulation of the body's temperature*** 体温调节

regurgitate *verb* to bring into the mouth food which has been partly digested in the stomach 食糜返流

◇ **regurgitation** *noun* flowing back in the opposite direction to the normal flow, especially bringing up partly digested food from the stomach into the mouth 返流; **aortic regurgitation** = flow of blood backwards, caused by a defective heart valve 主动脉返流

rehabilitate *verb* to make someone fit to work *or* to lead a normal life 康复

◇ **rehabilitation** *noun* making a patient fit to work *or* to lead a normal life again 康复

rehydration *noun* giving water *or* liquid to a patient suffering from dehydration 补液

reinfect *verb* to infect again 再感染,二次感染

Reiter's syndrome *or* **Reiter's disease** *noun* illness which may be venereal, with arthritis, urethritis and conjunctivitis at the same time, affecting mainly men 莱特尔氏综合征(同时患关节炎、尿道炎及结膜炎,性病的一种,主要侵及男性)

reject *verb* not to accept 排斥: ***The new heart was rejected by the body.*** 身体排斥新移植的心脏。***They gave the patient drugs to prevent the transplant being rejected.*** 他们给病人用药以防发生移植物被排斥问题。

◇ **rejection** *noun* act of rejecting tissue 排斥: ***The patient was given drugs to reduce the possibility of tissue rejection.*** 给病人用药以减少组织排斥的可能。

relapse 1 *noun* (*of patient or disease*) becoming worse *or* reappearing (after seeming to be getting better) (病情)复发,加重 **2** *verb* to become worse *or* to return 复发,加重: ***He relapsed into a coma.*** 他病情加重昏迷了。**relapsing fever** = disease caused by a bacterium, where attacks of fever recur at regular intervals 回归热; **relapsing pancreatitis** = form of pancreatitis where the symptoms recur, but in a milder form 复发性胰腺炎

relate *verb* to connect to 与…有关: ***The disease is related to the weakness of the heart muscles.*** 这种病与心肌衰弱有关。

◇ **-related** *suffix* connected to 相关; **drug-related diseases** 药物相关性疾病

◇ **relationship** *noun* way in which someone *or* something is connected to another 关系: ***The incidence of the disease has a close relationship to the environment.*** 此病发病率与环境密切相关。***He became withdrawn and broke off all relationships with his family.*** 他变得孤僻退缩,与所有家人断绝了关系。

relax *verb* to become less tense *or* less strained 放松: ***He was given a drug to relax the muscles.*** 他用药使肌肉放松。***After a hard day in the clinic the nurses like to relax by playing tennis.*** 在临床

辛苦工作一天之后，护士们喜欢打网球来放松。*The muscle should be fully relaxed.* 肌肉应当完全放松。

◇ **relaxant** *adjective* (substance) which relieves strain 松弛剂的; **muscle relaxant** = drug which reduces contractions in muscles 肌松剂

◇ **relaxation** *noun* (i) reducing strain in a muscle 肌肉放松 (ii) reducing stress in a person 精神放松; **relaxation therapy** = treatment of a patient where he is encouraged to relax his muscles to reduce stress 放松疗法

◇ **relaxative** *noun US* drug which reduces stress 松驰药

◇ **relaxin** *noun* hormone which may be secreted by the placenta to make the cervix relax and open fully in the final stages of pregnancy before childbirth 松弛素

release 1 *noun* allowing something to go out 释放: ***the slow release of the drug into the bloodstream*** 药物缓慢释放入血 **2** *verb* to let something out *or* to let something go free 释放: ***Hormones are released into the body by glands.*** 激素是由腺体释放到体内的。**release hormones** = hormones secreted by the hypothalamus which make the pituitary gland release certain hormones 释放激素(控制其它激素释放的激素，一般由下丘脑分泌，作用于垂体)

relieve *verb* to make better *or* to make easier 减轻，减缓: ***Nasal congestion can be relieved by antihistamines.*** 抗组胺药可以减轻鼻充血。***The patient was given an injection of morphine to relieve the pain.*** 给病人注射了一针吗啡以缓解疼痛。***The condition is relieved by applying cold compresses.*** 用冷敷法可以使这种病减轻。

◇ **relief** *noun* making better *or* easier 减轻: ***The drug provides rapid relief for patients with bronchial spasms.*** 药物可以使病人的支气管痉挛迅速缓解。

QUOTE: Complete relief of angina is experienced by 85% of patients subjected to coronary artery bypass surgery.
引文：冠脉旁路搭桥术后85%的病人心绞痛完全缓解。
British Journal of Hospital Medicine 英国医院医学杂志

QUOTE: Replacement of the metacarpophalangeal joint is mainly undertaken to relieve pain, deformity and immobility due to rheumatoid arthritis.
引文：掌指关节置换主要用以缓解类风湿关节炎引起的疼痛、变形和僵硬不能活动。
Nursing Times 护理时代

REM = RAPID EYE MOVEMENT 快速动眼

remedy *noun* cure *or* drug which will cure 药物，治疗: ***Honey and glycerine is an old remedy for sore throats.*** 蜂蜜和甘油是治疗嗓子疼的传统药物。

◇ **remedial** *adjective* which cures 治疗的

remember *verb* to bring back into the mind something which has been seen *or* heard before 记起，回想起: ***He remembers nothing*** *or* ***he can't remember anything about the accident.*** 他什么也回忆不起来了，事故的有关情况他一点儿也想不起来了。

remission *noun* period when an illness *or* fever is less severe 缓解期

◇ **remittent fever** *noun* fever which goes down for a period each day, like typhoid fever 弛张热

re. mist. *abbreviation for* (缩写) *the Latin phrase* 'repetatur mistura': repeat the same mixture (written on a prescription) 重复上次剂量(处方用语)

remove *verb* to take away 移开，挪开，去掉: ***He will have an operation to remove an ingrowing toenail.*** 将给他做手术以去掉内生甲。

◇ **removal** *noun* action of removing 去掉，移开: ***An appendicectomy is the surgical removal of an appendix.*** 阑尾切除术是用外科方法把阑尾去掉。

ren- *or* **reni-** *or* **reno-** *prefix* referring to the kidneys 肾

◇ **renal** *adjective* referring to the kidneys 肾脏的;**renal arteries** = pair of arteries running from the abdominal aorta to the kidneys 肾动脉;**renal calculus** = stone in the kidney 肾结石;**renal capsule** = fibrous tissue surrounding a kidney 肾被膜;**renal colic** = sudden pain caused by kidney stone or stones in the ureter 肾绞痛;**renal corpuscle** = part of a nephron in the cortex of a kidney 肾小体;**renal cortex** = outer covering of the kidney, immediately beneath the capsule 肾皮质;**renal hypertension** = high blood pressure linked to kidney disease 肾性高血压;**renal pelvis** = upper and wider part of the ureter leading from the kidney where urine is collected before passing down the ureter into the bladder 肾盂;**renal rickets** = form of rickets caused by kidneys which do not function properly 肾性佝偻病;**renal sinus** = cavity in which the renal pelvis and other tubes leading into the kidney fit 肾窦;**renal transplant** = kidney transplant 肾移植;**renal tubule** *or* **uriniferous tubule** = tiny tube which is part of a nephron 肾小管

◇ **renin** *noun* enzyme secreted by the kidney to prevent loss of sodium, and which also affects blood pressure 肾素

renew *verb* **to renew a prescription** = to get a new prescription for the same drug as before 新开一张处方

rennin *noun* enzyme which makes milk coagulate in the stomach, so as to slow down the passage of the milk through the digestive system 凝乳酶

renography *noun* examination of a kidney after injection of a radioactive substance, using a gamma camera 肾造影术

reovirus *noun* virus which affects both the intestine and the respiratory system, but does not cause serious illness 呼肠孤病毒 *compare* 比较 ECHOVIRUS

rep *abbreviation of* (缩写) *the Latin word* 'repetatur': repeat (written on a prescription)重复(处方用语)

repair *verb* to mend *or* to make something good again 修补: ***Surgeons operated to repair a hernia or defective heart valve.*** 外科医师在修补疝气或修补心脏瓣膜缺损。

repeat *verb* to say *or* do something again 重复: ***The course of treatment was repeated after two months.*** 两个月后再重复这一疗程。**repeat prescription** = prescription which is exactly the same as the previous one, and is often given without examination of the patient by the doctor and may sometimes be requested by telephone 重开处方

repel *verb* to make something go away 驱除: ***If you spread this cream on your skin it will repel insects.*** 如果你把这种药膏涂在皮肤上,它能起驱虫作用。

repetitive strain injury *or* **repetitive stress injury** (**RSI**) *noun* pain in the arm felt by someone who performs the same movement many times over a certain period, as when operating a computer terminal or playing a musical instrument 反复应力性损伤

replace *verb* (i) to put back 复原 (ii) to exchange one part for another 取代,置换: ***an operation to replace a prolapsed uterus*** 脱子宫垂复位术; ***The surgeons replaced the diseased hip with a metal one.*** 外科医师以金属关节取代了生病的髋关节。

◇ **replacement** *noun* operation to replace part of the body with an artificial part 置换术;**replacement transfusion** *or* **exchange transfusion** = treatment for leukaemia *or* erythroblastosis where almost all the abnormal blood is removed from the body and replaced by normal blood 置换性输血;**hip replacement** = surgical operation to replace a defective *or* arthritic hip with an artificial one 髋关节置换;**total hip replacement** = replacing both the head of the femur and the acetabulum with an artificial joint 全髋关节置换

replicate *verb* (*of a cell*) to make a copy of itself 复制

◇ **replication** *noun* process in the division of a cell, where the DNA makes copies of itself 复制

report 1 *noun* official note stating what action has been taken *or* what treatment given *or* what results have come from a test, etc. 报告: ***The patient's report card has to be filled in by the nurse.*** 病人的报告卡须由护士填写。***The inspector's report on the hospital kitchens is good.*** 检查人员有关医院厨房的报告写的不错。**2** *verb* to make an official report about something 报告: ***The patient reported her doctor to the FPC for misconduct.*** 病人向家庭医生协会上报她的医生的医疗失误。***Occupational diseases or serious accidents at work must be reported to the local officials.*** 职业病和严重工伤事故必须向地方当局报告。**reportable diseases** = diseases (such as asbestosis *or* hepatitis *or* anthrax) which may be caused by working conditions or may infect other workers and must be reported to the District Health Authority 需上报的疾病

repositor *noun* surgical instrument used to push a prolapsed organ back into its normal position 复位器

repress *verb* to hide in the back of the mind feelings *or* thoughts which may be unpleasant *or* painful 抑制,压抑

◇ **repression** *noun* (*in psychiatry*) hiding feelings *or* thoughts which might be unpleasant 抑制,压抑

reproduce *verb* (**a**) to produce children (*of bacteria*, *etc.*) to produce new cells 生殖 (**b**) to do a test again in exactly the same way 重做

◇ **reproduction** *noun* process of making children *or* derived cells, etc 生殖; **organs of reproduction** = REPRODUCTIVE ORGANS 生殖器官

◇ **reproductive** *adjective* referring to reproduction 生殖的; **reproductive organs** = parts of the bodies of men and women which are involved in the conception and development of a fetus 生殖器官; **reproductive system** = arrangement of organs and ducts in the bodies of men and women which produces spermatozoa and ova 生殖系统; **reproductive tract** = series of tubes and ducts which carry spermatozoa and ova from one part of the body to another 生殖道

COMMENT: In the human male, the testes produce the spermatozoa which pass through the vasa efferentia and the vasa deferentia where they receive liquid from the seminal vesicles, then out of the body through the urethra and penis on ejaculation. In the female, an ovum, produced by one of the two ovaries, passes through the Fallopian tube where it is fertilized by a spermatozoon from the male. The fertilized ovum moves down into the uterus where it develops into an embryo.

注释:男性睾丸产生精子,精子通过输精管和射精管并在此接受从精囊来的液体,然后通过尿道及阴茎在射精时排出体外。女性的卵子由卵巢产生,通过输卵管并在此遇到来自男性的精子而受精。受精卵下行到子宫并在子宫发育成胚胎。

require *verb* to need 需求,需要: ***His condition may require surgery.*** 他的病需要手术治疗。***Is it a condition which requires immediate treatment?*** 这是需要立即处理的情况吗? **required effect** = effect which a drug is expected to have 预期效应: ***If the drug does not produce the required effect, the dose should be increased.*** 如果药物不能发挥预期效果,就应当加量。

◇ **requirement** *noun* something which is necessary 需要: ***One of the requirements of the position is a qualification in pharmacy.*** 对此项职务的要求之一是有药剂师资格。

RES = RETICULOENDOTHELIAL SYSTEM 网状内皮系统

research 1 *noun* scientific study

which investigates something new 研究: ***He is the director of a medical research unit*.** 他是一个医学研究单位的负责人。***She is doing research into finding a cure for leprosy*.** 她正在致力于寻找治愈麻风病的研究。***Research workers or research teams are trying to find a vaccine against AIDS*.** 研究工作者(研究小组)正努力寻找对抗艾滋病的疫苗。**the Medical Research Council** (**MRC**) = governmental body which organizes and pays for medical research 医学研究委员会 **2** *verb* to carry out scientific study 研究: ***He is researching the origins of cancer*.** 他在研究癌症的起因。

resect *verb* to remove part of the body by surgery 切除

◇ **resection** *noun* surgical removal of part of an organ 切除术; **submucous resection** = removal of bent cartilage from the nasal septum 粘膜下切除; **transurethral resection** (**TUR**) *or* **resection of the prostate** = surgical removal of the prostate gland through the urethra 经尿道前列腺切除

◇ **resectoscope** *noun* surgical instrument used to carry out a transurethral resection 经尿道前列腺切除器

reserpine *noun* tranquillizing drug derived from Rauwolfia, used in the treatment of high blood pressure and nervous tension 利血平

reset *verb* to break a badly set bone and set it again correctly 再安置,重新接骨: ***His arm had to be reset*.** 他的胳膊不得不重新接骨。

resident *noun & adjective* (**a**) (person) who lives in a place 居民,居民的: ***All the residents of the old people's home were tested for food poisoning*.** 养老院的所有居民都做了食物中毒检查。**resident doctor** *or* **nurse** = doctor *or* nurse who lives in a certain building (such as an old people's home) 家庭医生或护士 (**b**) *US* qualified doctor who is employed by a hospital and sometimes lives in the hospital 住院医 *compare* 比较 INTERN

◇ **residential** *adjective* living in a hospital *or* at home 居住的; **residential care** = care of patients either in a hospital or at home (but not as outpatients) 病床护理(含家庭病床)

residual *adjective* remaining *or* which is left behind 剩余的; **residual urine** = urine left in the bladder after a person has passed as much water as possible 剩余尿; **residual air** *or* **residual volume** = air left in the lungs after a person has breathed out as much air as possible 残气,残气量

resin *noun* sticky juice which comes from some types of tree 树脂

resist *verb* to be strong enough to fight against a disease *or* to avoid being killed *or* attacked by a disease 抵抗: ***A healthy body can resist some infections*.** 健康的身体可以抵抗某些感染。

◇ **resistance** *noun* (i) ability of a person not to get a disease 抵抗力 (ii) ability of a germ not to be affected by antibiotics 耐药性(指细菌): ***The bacteria have developed a resistance to certain antibiotics*.** 细菌对某些抗生素产生了耐药性。***After living in the tropics his resistance to colds was low*.** 在热带地区居住后他对寒冷的抵抗力减弱了。**penicillin resistance** = ability of bacteria to resist penicillin(细菌)对青霉素耐药 (**b**) opposition to force 阻力; **peripheral resistance** = ability of the peripheral blood vessels to slow down the flow of blood inside them 外周阻力

◇ **resistant** *adjective* able not to be affected by something 有抵抗力的: ***The bacteria are resistant to some antibiotics*.** 这种细菌对某些抗生素耐药。**resistant strain** = strain of bacterium which is not affected by antibiotics 耐药株

resolution *noun* (i) amount of detail which can be seen in a microscope *or* on a computer monitor(显微镜或计算机显示器的)分辨率 (ii) point in the development of a disease where the inflammation begins to disappear 消散,消退

◇ **resolve** *verb* (*of inflammation*) to begin to disappear(炎症) 消退,消散

QUOTE: Valve fluttering disappears as the pneumothorax resolves. Always confirm resolution with a physical examination and X-ray.
引文:在气胸消退之后瓣膜的翕动也消失了。通常用体检和 X 射线检查的方法来确定气胸是否消退。
American Journal of Nursing
美国护理杂志

resonance *noun* sound made by a hollow part of the body when hit 反响,叩响 *see also* 参见 MAGNETIC

resorption *noun* absorbing again of a substance already produced back into the body 重吸收

respiration *noun* action of breathing 呼吸; **artificial respiration** = way of reviving someone who has stopped breathing (as by mouth-to-mouth resuscitation) 人工呼吸; **assisted respiration** = breathing with the help of a machine 辅助呼吸; **controlled respiration** = control of a patient's breathing by an anaesthetist during an operation, if normal breathing has stopped 控制呼吸; **external respiration** = part of respiration concerned with oxygen in the air being exchanged in the lungs for carbon dioxide from the blood 外呼吸(肺内氧气与二氧化碳的交换); **internal respiration** = part of respiration concerned with the passage of oxygen from the blood to the tissues, and the passage of carbon dioxide from the tissues to the blood 内呼吸(组织对氧的摄取并放出二氧化碳); **respiration rate** = number of times a person breathes per minute 呼吸频率

◇ **respirator** *noun* (**a**) machine which gives artificial respiration 呼吸机; **cuirass respirator** = type of iron lung, where the patient's limbs are not enclosed 胸甲式呼吸机; **Drinker respirator** *or* **iron lung** = machine which encloses all a patient's body, except the head, and in which air pressure is increased and decreased in turn, so forcing the patient to breathe 铁肺; **positive pressure respirator** = machine which forces air into a patient's lungs through a tube inserted in the mouth *or* in the trachea (after a tracheostomy), and then let out by releasing pressure 正压呼吸机; ***The patient was put on a respirator.*** = The patient was attached to a machine which forced him to breathe. 给病人安上了呼吸机。(**b**) mask worn to prevent someone breathing harmful gas *or* fumes 防毒面具

◇ **respiratory** *adjective* referring to breathing 呼吸的; **respiratory bronchiole** = end part of a bronchiole in the lung, which joins the alveoli 呼吸细支气管; **respiratory centre** = nerve centre in the brain which regulates the breathing 呼吸中枢; **respiratory distress syndrome** *or* **hyaline membrane disease** = condition of newborn babies, where the lungs do not expand properly, due to lack of surfactant (the condition is common among premature babies) 呼吸窘迫综合征,肺透明膜病; **respiratory failure** = failure of the lungs to oxygenate the blood correctly 呼吸衰竭; **respiratory illness** = illness which affects the patient's breathing 呼吸疾病; **upper respiratory infection** = infection in the upper part of the respiratory system 上呼吸道感染; **respiratory pigment** = blood pigment which can carry oxygen collected in the lungs and release it in tissues 呼吸色素; **respiratory quotient** (**RQ**) = ratio of the amount of carbon dioxide taken into the alveoli of the lungs from the blood to the amount the oxygen which the alveoli take from the air 呼吸商; **respiratory syncytial virus** (**RSV**) = virus which causes infections of the nose and throat in adults but serious bronchiolitis in children 呼吸道合胞病毒; **respiratory system** *or* **respiratory tract** = series of organs and passages which take air into the lungs, and exchange oxygen for carbon dioxide 呼吸系统,呼吸道

COMMENT: Respiration includes two stages: breathing in (inhalation) and breathing out (exhalation). Air is taken into the respiratory system through the nose or mouth, and goes down into the lungs through the pharynx, larynx, and windpipe. In the lungs, the bronchi take the air to the alveoli (air sacs) where oxygen in the air is passed to the bloodstream in exchange for waste carbon dioxide which is then breathed out.
注释:呼吸包括两个相:吸气相和呼气相。空气通过口鼻进入呼吸系统,然后经咽、喉和气管下行到肺,支气管再将空气送到肺泡,在那里空气中的氧进入血液与作为废物的二氧化碳交换,然后二氧化碳被呼出体外。

respond *verb* to react to something *or* to begin to get better because of a treatment 反应: ***The cancer is not responding to drugs.*** 癌症对药物没有反应。 ***She is responding to treatment.*** 她对治疗有反应了(在好转中)。

◊ **response** *noun* reaction by an organ *or* tissue *or* a person to an external stimulus 反应; **immune response** = (i) reaction of a body to an antigen 身体对抗原的免疫反应 (ii) reaction of a body which rejects a transplant 身体对移植物的排斥性免疫反应

◊ **responsible** *adjective* which is the cause of something 负责的,可归因于的: ***The allergen is responsible for the patient's reaction.*** 过敏原是病人起反应的原因。 ***This is one of several factors which can be responsible for high blood pressure.*** 这是造成高血压的几个因素之一。

◊ **responsiveness** *noun* being able to respond to other people *or* to sensations 反应性

QUOTE: Many severely confused patients, particularly those in advanced stages of Alzheimer's disease, do not respond to verbal communication.
引文:许多严重意识混浊的病人,特别是阿尔茨海默病进展期的病人,对言语交流没有反应。
Nursing Times 护理时代

QUOTE: Anaemia may be due to insufficient erythrocyte production, in which case the reticulocyte count will be low, or to haemolysis or haemorrhage, in which cases there should be a reticulocyte response.
引文:贫血可能由红细胞生成不足引起,这种情况下网织红细胞计数是低的,而由溶血或出血引起贫血时网织红细胞反应性上升。
Southern Medical Journal 南部医学杂志

rest 1 *noun* lying down *or* being calm 休息: ***What you need is a good night's rest.*** 你需要好好休息一晚上。 ***I had a few minutes' rest and then I started work again.*** 我休息了几分钟,然后又开始工作。 ***The doctor prescribed a month's total rest.*** 医生开了全休一个月的假。 **2** *verb* to lie down *or* to be calm 休息: ***Don't disturb your mother - she's resting.*** 别打扰你妈,她在休息呢。

◊ **restless** *adjective* not still *or* not calm 不安的: ***The children are restless in the heat.*** 孩子们热得烦躁不安。 ***She had a few hours' restless sleep.*** 她有几个小时睡不安稳。

restore *verb* to give back 恢复: ***She needs vitamins to restore her strength.*** 她需要维生素来恢复她的体力。 ***The physiotherapy should restore the strength of the muscles.*** 理疗应当能够恢复肌肉的力量。 ***A salpingostomy was performed to restore the patency of the Fallopian tube.*** 做了输卵管造口术以恢复其开放。

restrict *verb* (i) to make less *or* smaller 缩减 (ii) to set limits to something 限制: ***The blood supply is restricted by the tight bandage.*** 勒紧的绷带限制了血液供应。 ***The doctor suggested she should restrict her intake of alcohol.*** 医生建议她必须减少酒的摄入。

◊ **restrictive** *adjective* which restricts *or* which makes smaller 限制性的

result 1 *noun* figures at the end of a calculation *or* at the end of a test 结果: ***What was the result of the test?*** 试验的结果是什么? ***The doctor told the patient the result of the pregnancy test.*** 医生告诉

病人妊娠试验的结果。*The result of the operation will not be known for some weeks*. 几周内不会知道手术的结果。2 *verb* to happen because of something 结果，导致：*The cancer resulted from exposure to radiation at work*. 癌症是由工作时暴露于射线造成的。*His illness resulted in his being away from work for several weeks*. 他的病使他几周都不能工作。

resuscitate *verb* to make someone who appears to be dead start breathing again, and to restart the circulation of blood 复苏

◇ **resuscitation** *noun* reviving someone who seems to be dead, by making him breathe again and restarting the heart 复苏术；**cardiopulmonary resuscitation (CPR)** = method of reviving someone where stimulation is applied to both heart and lungs 心肺复苏

> COMMENT: The commonest methods of resuscitation are artificial respiration and cardiac massage.
> 注释：最常用的复苏方法是人工呼吸和心脏按摩。

retain *verb* to keep *or* to hold 保留：*He was incontinent and unable to retain urine in his bladder*. 他小便失禁，不能把尿留在膀胱内。*see also* 参见 RETENTION

retard *verb* to make something slower *or* to slow down the action of a drug 推迟，阻滞：*The drug will retard the onset of the fever*. 药物能阻滞发热的出现。*The injections retard the effect of the anaesthetic*. 注射推迟了麻药的作用。

◇ **retardation** *noun* making slower 阻滞；**mental retardation** = condition where a person's mind has not developed as fully as normal, so that he is not as advanced mentally as others of the same age 精神发育迟滞；**psychomotor retardation** = slowing of movement and speech, caused by depression 精神运动迟滞

◇ **retarded** *adjective* (person) who has not developed mentally as far as others of the same age 精神发育迟滞的：*a school for retarded children* 精神发育迟滞儿童的学校；*By the age of four, he has showing signs of being mentally retarded*. 四岁时他出现了精神发育迟滞的征象。

retch *verb* to try to vomit without bringing any food up from the stomach 干呕

◇ **retching** *noun* attempting to vomit without being able to do so 干呕

rete *noun* structure, formed like a net, made up of tissue fibres *or* nerve fibres *or* blood vessels 网；**rete testis** = network of channels in the testis which take the sperm to the epididymis 睾丸网 *see also* 参见 RETICULAR (NOTE: the plural is **retia**)

retention *noun* holding back (such as holding back urine in the bladder) 保持，保留，潴留；**retention cyst** = cyst which is formed when a duct from a gland is blocked 潴留囊；**retention of urine** = condition where passing urine is difficult *or* impossible because the urethra is blocked *or* because the prostate gland is enlarged 尿潴留

reticular *adjective* made like a net *or* (fibres) which criss-cross or branch 网状的；**reticular fibres** *or* **reticular tissue** = fibres in connective tissue which support organs *or* blood vessels, etc. 网状纤维，网状组织

◇ **reticulin** *noun* fibrous protein which is one of the most important components of reticular fibres 网霉素

◇ **reticulocyte** *noun* red blood cell which has not yet fully developed 网织红细胞

◇ **reticulocytosis** *noun* condition where the number of reticulocytes in the blood increases abnormally 网织红细胞血症

◇ **reticuloendothelial system (RES)** *noun* series of phagocytic cells in the body (found especially in bone marrow, lymph nodes, liver and spleen) which attack and destroy bacteria and form antibodies 网状内皮系统; **reticuloendothelial cell** = phagocytic cell in the RES 网状内皮细胞

◇ **reticuloendotheliosis** *noun* condition where cells in the RES grow large and form swellings in bone marrow *or* destroy bones 网状内皮系统增殖

◇ **reticulosis** *noun* any of several conditions where cells in the reticuloendothelial system grow large and form usually malignant tumours 网状细胞增多

◇ **reticulum** *noun* series of small fibres *or* tubes forming a network 网状组织; **endoplasmic reticulum** (**ER**) = network in the cytoplasm of a cell 内质网; **sarcoplasmic reticulum** = network in the cytoplasm of striated muscle fibres 肌浆网

retina *noun* inside layer of the eye which is sensitive to light 视网膜; **detached retina** = RETINAL DETACHMENT 视网膜脱离 ◇ 见图 EYE

retinaculum *noun* band of tissue which holds a structure in place, as found in the wrist and ankle over the flexor tendons 系带

retinal *adjective* referring to the retina 视网膜的; **retinal artery** = sole artery of the retina (it accompanies the optic nerve) 视网膜动脉; **retinal detachment** = condition where the retina is partly detached from the choroid 视网膜脱离

◇ **retinitis** *noun* inflammation of the retina 视网膜炎; **retinitis pigmentosa** = hereditary condition where inflammation of the retina can result in blindness 色素性视网膜炎

◇ **retinoblastoma** *noun* rare tumour in the retina, affecting infants 视网膜母细胞瘤

◇ **retinol** *noun* vitamin A, vitamin (found in liver, vegetables, eggs and cod liver oil) which is essential for good vision 维生素 A, 视黄醇

◇ **retinopathy** *noun* any disease of the retina 视网膜病; **diabetic retinopathy** = defect in vision linked to diabetes 糖尿病性视网膜病变

◇ **retinoscope** *noun* instrument with various lenses, used to measure the refraction of the eye 视网膜镜

> COMMENT: Light enters the eye through the pupil and strikes the retina. Light-sensitive cells in the retina (cones and rods) convert the light to nervous impulses; the optic nerve sends these impulses to the brain which interprets them as images. The point where the optic nerve joins the retina has no light-sensitive cells, and is known as the blind spot.
> 注释:光通过瞳孔进入眼睛并到达视网膜。视网膜上的光敏感细胞(视杆细胞和视锥细胞)将光刺激转换成神经脉冲;视神经将这些脉冲传到大脑,由大脑释义为图像。视神经与视网膜相接的地方没有光敏感细胞,即所谓的盲点。

retire *verb* to stop work at a certain age 退休: ***Most men retire at 65, but women only go on working until they are 60.*** 多数男性 65 岁退休,但妇女只工作到 60 岁。*Although she has retired, she still does voluntary work at the clinic.* 虽然她已经退休了,她仍在诊所做志愿工作。

◇ **retirement** *noun* act of retiring; being retired 退休: ***The retirement age for men is 65.*** 男性的退休年龄是 65 岁。

retraction *noun* moving backwards *or* becoming shorter 缩: ***There is retraction of the overlying skin.*** 覆盖的皮肤收缩了。**retraction ring** *or* **Bandl's ring** = groove round the womb, separating the upper and lower parts of the uterus, which, in obstructed labour, prevents the baby from moving forward normally into the cervical canal 收缩环

◇ **retractor** *noun* surgical instrument which pulls and holds back the edge of the incision in an operation 牵开器,拉钩儿

retro- *prefix* meaning at the back *or* behind 后,向后

◇ **retrobulbar neuritis** *noun* optic neuritis, inflammation of the optic nerve which makes objects appear blurred 球后神经炎

◇ **retroflexion** *noun* being bent backwards 后屈; **uterine retroflexion** *or* **retroflexion of the uterus** = condition where the uterus bends backwards away from its normal position 子宫后屈

◇ **retrograde** *adjective* going backwards 退行性的,逆行的; **retrograde pyelography** = X-ray examination of the kidney where a catheter is passed into the kidney through the ureter, and the opaque liquid is injected directly into it 逆行性肾盂造影

◇ **retrogression** *noun* returning to an earlier state 退行

◇ **retrolental fibroplasia** *noun* condition where fibrous tissue develops behind the lens of the eye, resulting in blindness 晶状体后纤维增生

> COMMENT: The condition is likely in premature babies if they are treated with large amounts of oxygen immediately after birth.
> 注释:这种状况易出现于生后立即接受大量氧气治疗的早产儿。

◇ **retro-ocular** *adjective* at the back of the eye 眼球后的

◇ **retroperitoneal** *adjective* at the back of the peritoneum 腹膜后的

◇ **retropharyngeal** *adjective* at the back of the pharynx 咽后的

◇ **retropubic** *adjective* at the back of the pubis 耻骨后的; **retropubic prostatectomy** = removal of the prostate gland which is carried out through a suprapubic incision and by cutting the membrane which surrounds the gland 耻骨后前列腺切除术

◇ **retrospection** *noun* recalling what happened in the past 回忆,追忆

◇ **retroversion** *noun* sloping backwards 后倾; **uterine retroversion** *or* **retroversion of the uterus** = condition where the uterus slopes backwards away from its normal position 子宫后倾

◇ **retroverted uterus** *noun* condition where the uterus slopes backwards away from its normal position 后倾子宫

◇ **retrovirus** *noun* virus whose genetic material contains RNA from which DNA is synthesized 逆转录病毒

> COMMENT: The AIDS virus and many carcinogenic viruses are retroviruses.
> 注释:艾滋病病毒和许多致癌病毒是逆转录病毒。

reveal *verb* to show 揭示,发现: ***Digital palpation revealed a growth in the breast.*** 手指扪诊发现乳腺有增生物。

revision *noun* subsequent examination of a surgical operation 术后检查: ***a revision of a radical mastoidectomy*** 乳突根治性切除术术后检查

revive *verb* to bring back to life *or* to consciousness 使复生,救活: ***They tried to revive him with artificial respiration.*** 他们想用人工呼吸救活他。***She collapsed on the floor and had to be revived by the nurse.*** 她瘫倒在地板上,不得不由护士来抢救。

Reye's syndrome *noun* encephalopathy affecting young children who have had a viral infection 雷亥综合征(一种病毒感染小孩的脑病)

RGN = REGISTERED GENERAL NURSE 注册全科护士

Rh *abbreviation for* (缩写) rhesus 恒河猴

RHA = REGIONAL HEALTH AUTHORITY 地区卫生当局

rhabdovirus *noun* any of a group of viruses containing RNA, one of which causes rabies 棒状病毒(RNA 病毒)

rhachio- *suffix* referring to the spine 脊柱

rhagades *noun* fissures, long thin scars in the skin round the nose, mouth or anus, seen in syphilis 皲裂

rhesus factor *or* **Rh factor** *noun* antigen in red blood cells, which is an element in blood grouping Rh 因子(一种红细胞抗原,用于血型分类); **rhesus baby** = baby with erythroblastosis fetalis Rh 婴儿(成红细胞增多症的婴儿); **Rh-negative**

= (person) who does not have the rhesus factor in his blood Rh 阴性；**Rh-positive** = (person) who has the rhesus factor in his blood Rh 阳性；**rhesus factor disease** *or* **Rh disease** = disease which occurs when the blood of a fetus is incompatible with that of the mother Rh 因子病(母婴血型不合造成的疾病)

> COMMENT：The rhesus factor is important in blood grouping, because although most people are Rh-positive, a Rh-negative patient should not receive a Rh-positive blood transfusion as this will cause the formation of permanent antibodies. If a Rh-negative mother has a child by a Rh-positive father, the baby will inherit Rh-positive blood, which may then pass into the mother's circulation at childbirth and cause antibodies to form. This can be prevented by an injection of anti D immunoglobulin immediately after the birth of the first Rh-positive child and any subsequent Rh-positive children. If a Rh-negative mother has formed antibodies to Rh-positive blood in the past, these antibodies will affect the blood of the fetus and may cause erythroblastosis fetalis.
> 注释：Rh 因子在血型分类上很重要，因为虽然大多数人是 Rh 阳性的，Rh 阴性的病人却不能接受 Rh 阳性的输血，因为这样会产生永久性抗体。如果 Rh 阴性的母亲和一个 Rh 阳性的父亲怀了孩子，婴儿会遗传 Rh 阳性的血液，在分娩时胎儿的血会进入母亲的循环导致抗体形成。要防止这一现象发生需在生出第一个 Rh 阳性孩子及以后每生下 Rh 阳性孩子后都立即注射抗 D 免疫球蛋白。如果 Rh 阴性的母亲血液中已经形成了抗 Rh 阳性的抗体，这些抗体会影响胎儿的血液，可以引起胎儿成红细胞增多症。

rheumatic *adjective* referring to rheumatism 风湿的；**rheumatic fever** *or* **acute rheumatism** = collagen disease of young people and children, caused by haemolytic streptococci, where the joints and also the valves and lining of the heart become inflamed 风湿热，急性风湿病

> COMMENT：Rheumatic fever often follows another streptococcal infection such as a strep throat or tonsillitis. Symptoms are high fever, pains in the joints, which become red, formation of nodules on the ends of bones, and difficulty in breathing. Although recovery can be complete, rheumatic fever can recur and damage the heart permanently.
> 注释：风湿热经常继发于另一起链球菌感染，如喉部链球菌感染或扁桃腺炎。症状包括高热、关节疼痛、发红，骨端形成小结节，还有呼吸困难。虽然可以完全恢复，但风湿热可以再发并对心脏造成永久性损害。

rheumatism *noun* general term for pains and stiffness in the joints and muscles 风湿病：***She has rheumatism in her hips.*** 她的髋关节有风湿病。***He has a history of rheumatism.*** 他有风湿病史。***She complained of rheumatism in her knees.*** 她主诉双膝有风湿病。**muscular rheumatism** = pains in muscles *or* joints, usually caused by fibrositis *or* inflammation of the muscles *or* osteoarthritis 肌肉风湿病 *see also* 参见 RHEUMATOID ARTHRITIS, RHEUMATIC FEVER, OSTEOARTHRITIS

◊ **rheumatoid** *adjective* similar to rheumatism 类风湿的；**rheumatoid arthritis** = general painful disabling collagen disease affecting any joint, but especially the hands, feet and hips, making them swollen and inflamed 类风湿关节炎；**rheumatoid erosion** = erosion of bone and cartilage in the joints caused by rheumatoid arthritis 类风湿破坏

◊ **rheumatologist** *noun* doctor who specializes in rheumatology 风湿病学家

◊ **rheumatology** *noun* branch of medicine dealing with rheumatic disease of muscles and joints 风湿病学

QUOTE: Rheumatoid arthritis is a chronic inflammatory disease which can affect many systems of the body, but mainly the joints. 70% of sufferers develop the condition in the metacarpophalangeal joints.
引文:类风湿关节炎是可以侵及身体多个系统的慢性炎症性疾病,但受累的主要器官是关节,70%的患者掌指关节受累。

Nursing Times 护理时代

Rh factor Rh 因子 *see* 见 RHESUS FACTOR

rhin- *or* **rhino-** *prefix* referring to the nose 鼻子

◇ **rhinitis** *noun* inflammation of the mucous membrane in the nose, which makes the nose run, caused by a virus infection (cold) *or* an allergic reaction to dust *or* flowers, etc. 鼻炎; **acute rhinitis** = common cold *or* a virus infection which causes inflammation of the mucous membrane in the nose and throat 急性鼻炎; **allergic rhinitis** = HAY FEVER 过敏性鼻炎,枯草热; **chronic catarrhal rhinitis** = chronic form of inflammation of the nose where excess mucus is secreted by the mucous membrane 慢性卡他性鼻炎

◇ **rhinology** *noun* branch of medicine dealing with diseases of the nose and the nasal passage 鼻科学

◇ **rhinomycosis** *noun* infection of the nasal passages by a fungus 鼻霉菌病

◇ **rhinophyma** *noun* condition caused by rosacea, where the nose becomes permanently red and swollen 肥大性酒渣鼻

◇ **rhinoplasty** *noun* plastic surgery to correct the appearance of the nose 鼻成形术

◇ **rhinorrhoea** *noun* watery discharge from the nose 流涕,鼻溢液

◇ **rhinoscope** *noun* instrument for examining the inside of the nose 鼻镜

◇ **rhinoscopy** *noun* examination of the inside of the nose 鼻镜检查

◇ **rhinosporidiosis** *noun* infection of the nose, eyes, larynx and genital organs by a fungus *Rhinosporidium seeberi* 鼻孢子虫病

◇ **rhinovirus** *noun* group of viruses containing RNA, which cause infection of the nose, including the virus which causes the common cold 鼻病毒

rhiz- *or* **rhizo-** *prefix* referring to a root 根

◇ **rhizotomy** *noun* surgical operation to cut *or* divide the roots of a nerve to relieve severe pain 脊神经根切断术

rhodopsin *noun* visual purple, light-sensitive purple pigment in the rods of the retina, which makes it possible to see in dim light 视紫红质

rhombencephalon *noun* the hindbrain, the part of the brain which contains the cerebellum, the medulla oblongata and the pons 菱脑(后脑,包括小脑、延髓和脑桥)

◇ **rhomboid** *noun* one of two muscles in the top part of the back which move the shoulder blades 菱形肌

rhonchus *noun* abnormal sound in the chest, heard through a stethoscope, caused by a partial blockage in the bronchi 干罗音 (NOTE: the plural is **rhonchi**)

rhythm *noun* regular movement *or* beat 节律 *see also* 参见 CIRCADIAN; **rhythm method** = method of birth control where sexual intercourse should take place only during the safe periods *or* when conception is least likely to occur, that is at the beginning and at the end of the menstrual cycle 节律避孕法(同安全期避孕)

COMMENT: This method is not as safe as other methods of contraception because the time when ovulation takes place cannot be accurately calculated if a woman does not have regular periods.
注释:这种方法不如其他避孕方法可靠,因为如果女性月经不规律排,卵发生的时间难以准确推算。

◇ **rhythmic** *adjective* regular *or* with

a repeated rhythm 有固定节律的

rib *noun* one of twenty-four curved bones which protect the chest 肋骨; **cervical rib** = extra rib sometimes found attached to the cervical vertebrae and which may cause thoracic inlet syndrome 颈肋(多出的附着于颈椎的肋骨,可以造成胸廓出口综合征); **false ribs** = bottom five ribs on each side which are not directly attached to the breastbone 假肋(下 5 对肋骨,因不与胸骨直接相连,故称之为假肋); **floating ribs** = two lowest false ribs on each side, which are not attached to the breastbone 浮肋(最低的两对肋骨,不与胸骨相连); **true ribs** = top seven pairs of ribs 真肋(上 7 对肋骨)

◇ **rib cage** *noun* the ribs and the space enclosed by them 胸廓 (NOTE: for other terms referring to the ribs, see words beginning with **cost-**)

> COMMENT: The rib cage is formed of twelve pairs of curved bones. The top seven pairs (the true ribs) are joined to the breastbone in front by costal cartilage; the other five pairs of ribs (the false ribs) are not attached to the breastbone, though the 8th, 9th and 10th pairs are each attached to the rib above. The bottom two pairs, which are not attached to the breastbone at all, are called the floating ribs.
> 注释:胸廓由 12 对弯曲的骨头形成。上 7 对(真肋)在前面经肋软骨与胸骨相连;另 5 对(假肋)不与胸骨接触,而是 8、9、10 对肋骨与它们上面的肋骨相连。最底下的 2 对肋骨则根本不与胸骨相接,所以叫做浮肋。

riboflavine = VITAMIN B_2 核黄素

ribonuclease *noun* enzyme which breaks down RNA 核糖核酸酶

ribonucleic acid (**RNA**) *noun* one of the nucleic acids in the nucleus of all living cells, which takes coded information form DNA and translates it into specific enzymes and proteins 核糖核酸 *see also* 参见 DNA

ribose *noun* type of sugar found in RNA 核糖

ribosomal *adjective* referring to ribosomes 核糖体的

◇ **ribosome** *noun* tiny particle in a cell, containing RNA and protein, where protein is synthesized 核糖体

rice *noun* common food plant, grown in hot countries, of which the whitish grains are eaten 大米

◇ **ricewater stools** *noun* typical watery stools, passed by patients suffering from cholera 米泔水样便,淘米水样便

rich *adjective* (**a**) **rich in** = having a lot of something 富含: ***Green vegetables are rich in minerals.*** 绿色蔬菜富含矿物质。***The doctor has prescribed a diet which is rich in protein** or **a protein-rich diet.*** 医生开具了高蛋白饮食。(**b**) (food) which has high calorific value 食物,高热量的

> QUOTE: The sublingual region has a rich blood supply derived from the carotid artery.
> 引文:舌下区有来自颈动脉的丰富血供。
> **Nursing Times** 护理时代

ricin *noun* highly toxic albumin found in the seeds of the castor oil plant 蓖麻(子)蛋白

rickets *or* **rachitis** *noun* disease of children, where the bones are soft and do not develop properly because of lack of vitamin D 佝偻病; **renal rickets** = form of rickets caused by poor kidney function 肾性佝偻病

> COMMENT: Initial treatment for rickets in children is a vitamin-rich diet, together with exposure to sunshine which causes vitamin D to form in the skin.
> 注释:开始治疗佝偻病患儿时用富含维生素的饮食,并同时多晒太阳,这样能促进皮肤生成维生素 D。

Rickettsia *noun* genus of microorganisms which causes several diseases including Q fever and typhus 立克次体(一类致病微生物)

◇ **rickettsial** *adjective* referring to

Rickettsia 立克次体的; **rickettsial pox** = disease found in North America, caused by *Rickettsia akari* passed to humans by bites from mites which live on mice 立克次体痘(北美的一种疾病,由小蛛立克次体引起,是经螨从鼠传染到人的)

rid *verb* **to get rid of something** = to make something go away 去掉; **to be rid of something** = not to have something unpleasant any more 无…之忧: ***He can't get rid of his cold — he's had it for weeks.*** 他去不掉自己的感冒,他已经感冒好几个星期了。***I'm very glad to be rid of my flu.*** 我非常高兴我的流感好了。

ridge *noun* long raised part on the surface of a bone *or* organ 嵴

right 1 *adjective & adverb & noun* not left *or* referring to the side of the body which usually has the stronger hand (which most people use to write with) 右: ***My right arm is stronger than my left.*** 我的右臂比左臂有劲儿。***He writes with his right hand.*** 他用右手写字。**2** *noun* what the law says a person is bound to have 权利: ***The patient has no right to inspect his medical records.*** 病人没有权利查看病历。***You always have the right to ask for a second opinion.*** 你始终有权利询问另一种意见。

◇ **right-hand** *adjective* on the right side 右手的: ***The stethoscope is in the right-hand drawer of the desk.*** 听诊器在右手边的抽屉里。

◇ **right-handed** *adjective* using the right hand more often than the left 右利手: ***He's right-handed.*** 他是右利手。***Most people are right-handed.*** 多数人是右利手。

rigid *adjective* stiff *or* not moving 僵硬的

◇ **rigidity** *noun* being rigid *or* bent *or* not able to be moved 僵硬,强直 *see also* 参见 SPASTICITY

◇ **rigor** *noun* attack of shivering, often with fever 寒战; **rigor mortis** = condition where the muscles of a dead body become stiff a few hours after death and then become relaxed again 尸僵

COMMENT: Rigor mortis starts about eight hours after death, and begins to disappear several hours later; environment and temperature play a large part in the timing.
注释:尸僵开始于死后8小时,几小时后消失;出现和消失的时间上受环境和温度的影响。

rima *noun* narrow crack *or* cleft 裂; **rima glottidis** = space between the vocal cords 声门裂

ring *noun* circle of tissue, tissue *or* muscle shaped like a circle 环; **ring finger** *or* **third finger** = the finger between the little finger and the middle finger 环指,无名指

◇ **ringing in the ear** 耳鸣 *see* 见 TINNITUS

◇ **ringworm** *noun* any of various infections of the skin by a fungus, in which the infection spreads out in a circle from a central point (ringworm is very contagious and difficult to get rid of) 癣 *see also* 参见 TINEA

Rinne's test *noun* hearing test 林内氏试验(听力试验)

COMMENT: A tuning fork is hit and its handle placed near the ear (to test for air conduction) and then on the mastoid process (to test for bone conduction). It is then possible to determine the type of lesion which exists by finding if the sound is heard for a longer period by air *or* by bone conduction.
注释:击打音叉并将音叉的柄放置在耳朵边上,(检查气传导),然后把音叉放到乳突上(检查骨传导)。根据声音气传导和骨传导的时间可以确定损伤的类型。

rinse out *verb* to wash the inside of something to make it clean 清洗容器内部,漱: ***She rinsed out the measuring jar.*** 她清洗了测量罐。***Rinse your mouth out with mouthwash.*** 用漱口液漱口。

ripple bed *noun* type of bed with an air-filled mattress divided into sections, in which the pressure is continuously being changed so that the patient's body can be massaged and bedsores can be avoided 气垫床

rise *verb* to go up 升高: ***His temperature rose sharply.*** 他的体温急剧升高。(NOTE: **rises - rising - rose - has risen**)

risk 1 *noun* (**a**) possible harm *or* possibility of something happening 危险: ***There is a risk of a cholera epidemic.*** 有霍乱流行的危险。***There is no risk of the disease spreading to other members of the family.*** 这个病不会传染到其他家庭成员。***Businessmen are particularly at risk of having a heart attack.*** 商人特别好发心脏病。**children at risk** = children who are more likely to be harmed *or* to catch a disease 高危儿童 *see also* 参见 HIGH-RISK, LOW-RISK **2** *verb* to do something which may possibly harm *or* have bad results 冒险: ***If the patient is not moved to an isolation ward, all the patients and staff in the hospital risk catching the disease.*** 如果这个病人不搬到隔离病房,医院里的所有病人和工作人员都要冒得病的危险。

QUOTE: Adenomatous polyps are a risk factor for carcinoma of the stomach.
引文:腺瘤型息肉是发生胃癌的一个危险因素。
Nursing Times 护理时代

QUOTE: Three quarters of patients aged 35 - 64 on GPs' lists have at least one major risk factor: high cholesterol, high blood pressure or addiction to tobacco.
引文:全科医师的病人名册上 35~64 岁的病人中有 3/4 至少存在一个主要的危险因素:高胆固醇、高血压或吸烟成瘾。
Health Services Journal 卫生保健杂志

risus sardonicus *noun* twisted smile which is a symptom of tetanus 痉挛笑(破伤风症状之一)

river blindness *noun* blindness caused by larvae getting into the eye in cases of onchocerciasis 河盲症(盘尾丝虫病引起)

RM = REGISTERED MIDWIFE 注册助产士

RMN = REGISTERED MENTAL NURSE 注册精神科护士

Rn *chemical symbol for* radon 氡的化学元素符号

RN = REGISTERED NURSE 注册护士

RNA = RIBONUCLEIC ACID 核糖核酸; **messenger RNA** = type of RNA which transmits information from DNA to form enzymes and proteins 信使 RNA; **RNMH** = REGISTERED NURSE FOR THE MENTALLY HANDICAPPED 精神残疾专业注册护士

Rocky Mountain spotted fever *noun* type of typhus caused by *Rickettsia rickettsii*, transmitted to humans by ticks 落基山斑疹热(蜱传斑疹伤寒)

rod *noun* (**a**) long thin round stick 杆: ***Some bacteria are shaped like rods or are rod-shaped.*** 有些细菌是杆状的。(**b**) one of two types of light-sensitive cell in the retina of the eye 视杆细胞 *see also* 参见 CONE

COMMENT: Rods are sensitive to poor light. They contain rhodopsin or visual purple, which produces the nervous impulse which the rod transmits to the optic nerve.
注释:视杆细胞对弱光敏感。细胞中含有视紫红质,由它产生神经冲动,视杆细胞再把冲动传给视神经。

Rodent ulcer *noun* basal cell carcinoma, a malignant tumour on the face 侵蚀性溃疡(面部皮肤基底细胞癌)

COMMENT: Rodent ulcers are different from some other types of cancer in that they do not spread to other parts of the body and do not metastasize, but remain on the face, usually near the mouth or eyes. Rodent ulcer is rare before middle age.
注释:侵蚀性溃疡与其它类型的癌症不同,它不传播到身体的其他部分而且也不转移,一直在脸上,通常是在口周或眼睛周围。侵蚀性溃疡很少在中年以前发生。

roentgen *noun* unit which measures the amount of exposure to X-rays *or* gamma rays 伦琴(X线单位)(NOTE: with figures usually written **R**); **roentgen rays** = X-rays *or* gamma rays which can pass through tissue and leave an image on a photographic film 伦琴射线 X线

◇ **roentgenogram** *noun* X-ray photograph X线照片

◇ **roentgenology** *noun* study of X-rays and their use in medicine X线学

rolled bandage *or* **roller bandage** *noun* bandage in the form of a long strip of cloth which is rolled up from one or both ends 绷带卷

Romberg's sign *noun* symptom of a sensory disorder in the position sense 罗姆伯格征(闭目难立征)

> COMMENT: If a patient cannot stand upright when his eyes are closed, this shows that nerves in the lower limbs which transmit position sense to the brain are damaged.
> 注释:如果病人闭目时难以站立,说明下肢向脑传导位置觉的神经有损坏。

rongeur *noun* strong surgical instrument like a pair of pliers, used for cutting bone 咬骨钳

roof *noun* top part of the mouth *or* other cavity(口腔或其它腔的)顶

root *or* **radix** *noun* (i) origin *or* point from which a part of the body grows 根 (ii) part of a tooth which is connected to a socket in the jaw 牙根; **root canal** = canal in the root of a tooth through which the nerves and blood vessels pass 根管 ◊ 见图 TOOTH

Rorschach test *noun* the ink blot test, used in psychological diagnosis, where the patient is shown a series of blots of ink on paper, and is asked to say what each blot reminds him of. The answers give information about the patient's psychological state 洛夏克测验(一种心理投射测验)

rosacea *noun* common skin disease affecting the face, and especially the nose, which becomes red because of enlarged blood vessels; the cause is not known 酒渣鼻,红斑狼疮

rosea 玫瑰的 *see* 见 PITYRIASIS

roseola *noun* any disease with a light red rash 玫瑰疹,蔷薇疹; **roseola infantum** *or* **exanthem subitum** = sudden infection of small children, with fever, swelling of the lymph glands and a rash 幼儿急疹

rostral *adjective* like the beak of a bird 喙样的

◇ **rostrum** *noun* projecting part of a bone *or* structure shaped like a beak 喙样突起(NOTE: plural is **rostra**)

rot *verb* to decay *or* to become putrefied 腐烂: ***The flesh was rotting round the wound as gangrene set in.*** 随着坏疽的进展,伤口周围的肉烂了。***The fingers can rot away in leprosy.*** 麻风病可以使手指烂掉。

rota *noun* **duty rota** = list of duties which have to be done and the names of the people who will do them 值班名册,任务名册

rotate *verb* to move in a circle 旋转

◇ **rotation** *noun* moving in a circle 旋转; **lateral and medial rotation** = turning part of the body to the side *or* towards the midline 外旋和内旋

◇ **rotator** *noun* muscle which makes a limb rotate 旋肌

rotavirus *noun* any of a group of viruses associated with gastroenteritis in children 轮状病毒

> QUOTE: Rotavirus is now widely accepted as an important cause of childhood diarrhoea in many different parts of the world.
> 引文:目前普遍认为轮状病毒是引起世界各地儿童腹泻的重要病因。
> **East African Medical Journal**
> 东非医学杂志

Roth spot *noun* pale spot which sometimes occurs on the retina of a person suffering from leukaemia or some other diseases 罗特斑(白血病或其它疾病时出现在视网膜上的白斑)

Rothera's test *noun* test to see if acetone is present in urine, a sign of ketosis which is a complication of diabetes mellitus 罗瑟雷试验(检验尿酮体的试验)

rotunda 蜗的 *see* 见 FENESTRA

rough *adjective* not smooth 粗糙的: ***She put cream on her hands which were rough from heavy work.*** 她在重体力劳动弄粗了的手上涂护肤霜。

◊ **roughage** *noun* dietary fibre, fibrous matter in food, which cannot be digested 粗糙食物(富含难以消化纤维的食物)

> COMMENT: Roughage is found in cereals, nuts, fruit and some green vegetables. It is believed to be necessary to help digestion and avoid developing constipation, obesity and appendicitis.
> 注释:谷物、坚果、水果和绿色蔬菜都是富含难消化纤维的食物。它们在辅助消化和防止发生便秘、肥胖及阑尾炎上是不可替代的。

rouleau *noun* roll of red blood cells which have stuck together like a column of coins 红细胞缗钱串 (NOTE: the plural is **rouleaux**)

round 1 *adjective* shaped like a circle 圆的; **round ligament** = band of ligament which stretches from the uterus to the labia 圆韧带(连接子宫与阴唇的韧带); **round window** *or* **fenestra rotunda** = round opening between the middle ear and the inner ear 圆窗(中耳和内耳之间的开口) 2 *noun* regular visit 查房; **to do the rounds of the wards** = to visit various wards in a hospital and talk to the nurses and check on patients' progress or condition 查房; **a health visitor's rounds** = regular series of visits made by a health visitor 保健访视员的巡视

◊ **roundworm** *noun* any of several common types of parasitic worms with round bodies, such as hookworms (as opposed to flatworms) 圆形体的寄生虫,线虫(如蛔虫、钩虫)

Rovsing's sign *noun* pain in the right iliac fossa when the left iliac fossa is pressed 罗符辛氏征(按压左髂窝而右髂窝疼痛)

> COMMENT: A sign of acute appendicitis.
> 注释:急性阑尾炎的体征之一。

Royal College of Nursing *noun* professional association which represents nurses 皇家护理学会

RQ = RESPIRATORY QUOTIENT 呼吸商

RR = RECOVERY ROOM 恢复室

-rrhage *or* **-rrhagia** *suffix* referring to abnormal flow *or* discharge of blood 流

-rrhaphy *suffix* referring to surgical sewing *or* suturing 缝合

-rrhexis *suffix* referring to splitting *or* rupture 裂

-rrhoea *suffix* referring to an abnormal flow *or* discharge of fluid from an organ 流

RSCN = REGISTERED SICK CHILDREN'S NURSE 注册的儿科护士

RSI = REPETITIVE STRAIN INJURY 反复应力性损伤

RSV = RESPIRATORY SYNCYTIAL VIRUS 呼吸道合胞病毒

RTN = REGISTERED THEATRE NURSE 注册手术室护士

rub 1 *noun* lotion used to rub on the skin 擦剂: ***The ointment is used as a rub.*** 这种膏是用来涂擦的。2 *verb* to move something (especially the hands) backwards and forwards over a surface. 擦: ***She rubbed her leg after she knocked it against the table.*** 她的腿碰到桌子上了,她用手揉了揉。***He rubbed his hands to make the circulation return.*** 他搓手以使循环恢复。

◊ **rub into** *verb* to make an ointment go into the skin by rubbing 涂擦使深入皮肤: ***Rub the liniment gently into the skin.*** 轻轻涂擦使擦剂渗入皮肤。

◊ **rubbing alcohol** *noun US* ethyl alcohol, used as a disinfectant *or* for rubbing on the skin 酒精擦剂(用作消毒)(NOTE: GB English is **surgical spirit**)

rubber *noun* material which can be stretched and compressed, made from the thick white liquid (latex) from a tropical tree 橡胶; **rubber sheet** = waterproof sheet put on hospital beds *or* on the bed of a child who suffers from bedwetting, to protect the mattress 橡胶床单(防止尿破坏床垫)

rubefacient *adjective* & *noun* (substance) which makes the skin warm, and pink or red 发红的,发红药(使皮肤红、暖的药)

rubella = GERMAN MEASLES 风疹

rubeola = MEASLES 麻疹

Rubin's test *noun* test to see if the Fallopian tubes are free from obstruction 鲁宾试验(检查输卵管是否通畅)

rubor *noun* redness (of the skin *or* tissue) 红,发红

rubra 红的 *see* 见 PITYRIASIS

rudimentary *adjective* which exists in a small form *or* which has not developed fully 痕迹器官的,残留器官的,发育不全的: ***The child was born with rudimentary arms.*** 这个孩子生来双臂发育不全。

Ruffini corpuscles *or* **Ruffini nerve endings** 鲁菲尼氏小体 *see* 见 CORPUSCLE

ruga *noun* fold *or* ridge (especially in mucous membrane such as the lining of the stomach) 皱褶 (NOTE: plural is **rugae**)

rule out *verb* to state a patient does not have a certain disease 除外: ***We can rule out shingles.*** 我们可以排除带状疱疹的诊断。

rumbling *noun* borborygmus, noise in the abdomen, caused by gas in the intestine 肠鸣音

run *verb* (*of the nose*) to drip with liquid secreted from the mucous membrane in the nasal passage(鼻子)流涕: ***His nose is running.*** 他在流鼻涕。***If your nose is running, blow it on a handkerchief.*** 如果你流鼻涕,用手绢擦擦。***One of the symptoms of a cold is a running nose.*** 感冒的症状之一是流鼻涕。

◇ **runny nose** *noun* nose which is dripping with liquid from the mucous membrane 流涕的鼻子

R-unit = ROENTGEN UNIT 伦琴单位

rupture 1 *noun* (**a**) breaking *or* tearing (of an organ such as the appendix) 破裂 (**b**) hernia, condition where the muscles *or* wall round an organ become weak and the organ bulges through the wall 疝 **2** *verb* to break *or* tear 破裂,撕裂; **ruptured spleen** = spleen which has been torn by piercing *or* by a blow 脾脏破裂

Russell traction *noun* type of traction with weights and slings used to straighten a femur which has been fractured 拉塞尔牵引(牵引骨折的股骨)

Ryle's tube *noun* thin tube which is passed into a patient's stomach through either the nose *or* mouth, used to pump out the contents of the stomach *or* to introduce a barium meal in the stomach 赖氏管,胃管

Ss

S *chemical symbol for* sulphur 硫的化学元素符号

SA node *or* **S-A node** = SINOATRIAL NODE 窦房结

Sabin vaccine *noun* vaccine against poliomyelitis 萨宾疫苗(脊髓灰质炎疫苗) *compare* 比较 SALR

COMMENT: The Sabin vaccine is given orally and consists of weak live polio virus.
注释:脊髓灰质炎疫苗是口服的,由弱的活脊髓灰质炎病毒组成。

sac *noun* part of the body shaped like a bag 囊; **amniotic sac** = thin sac which covers an unborn baby in the womb, containing the amniotic fluid 羊膜囊(包被胎儿,内含羊水); **hernial sac** = membranous sac of peritoneum where an organ has pushed through a cavity in the body 疝囊; **pericardial sac** = the serous pericardium 心包脏层

sacchar- *or* **saccharo-** *prefix* referring to sugar 糖

◇ **saccharide** *noun* form of carbohydrate 糖类

◇ **saccharin** *noun* sweet substance, used in place of sugar because although it is nearly 500 times sweeter than sugar it contains no carbohydrates 糖精

saccule *or* **sacculus** *noun* smaller of two sacs in the vestibule of the inner ear which is part of the mechanism which relates information about the position of the head in space 小囊

sacral *adjective* referring to the sacrum 骶骨的; **sacral foramina** = openings *or* holes in the sacrum through which pass the sacral nerves 骶孔 ◊ 见图 PELVIS; **sacral nerves** = nerves which branch from the spinal cord in the sacrum 骶神经; **sacral plexus** = plexus, a group of nerves inside the pelvis near the sacrum, which supply nerves in the buttocks, back of the thigh and lower leg, foot and the urogenital area 骶丛; **sacral vertebrae** = five vertebrae in the lower part of the spine which are fused together to form the sacrum 骶椎

◇ **sacralization** *noun* abnormal condition where the lowest lumbar vertebra fuses with the sacrum 腰椎骶化

◇ **sacro-** *prefix* referring to the sacrum 骶骨

◇ **sacrococcygeal** *adjective* referring to the sacrum and the coccyx 骶尾的

◇ **sacroiliac** *adjective* referring to the sacrum and the ilium 骶髂的; **sacroiliac joint** = joint where the sacrum joins the ilium 骶髂关节

◇ **sacroiliitis** *noun* inflammation of the sacroiliac joint 骶髂关节炎

◇ **sacrotuberous ligament** *noun* large ligament between the iliac spine, the sacrum, the coccyx and the ischial tuberosity 骶结节韧带

◇ **sacro-uterine ligament** *noun* ligament which goes from the neck of the uterus to the sacrum, passing on each side of the rectum 骶骨子宫韧带

◇ **sacrum** *noun* flat triangular bone, between the lumbar vertebrae and the coccyx with which it articulates, formed of five sacral vertebrae fused together; it also articulates with the hip bones 骶骨 ◊ 见图 PELVIS, VERTEBRAL COLUMN

SAD = SEASONAL AFFECTIVE DEPRESSION 季节性情感抑郁

saddle joint *noun* synovial joint where one element is concave and the other convex, like the joint between the thumb and the wrist 鞍状关节

saddle-nose *noun* deep bridge of the nose, normally a sign of injury but sometimes a sign of tertiary syphilis 鞍鼻

sadism *noun* abnormal sexual condition, where a person finds sexual pleasure in hurting others 性虐待狂

◇ **sadist** *noun* person whose sexual urge is linked to sadism 性虐待狂者

◇ **sadistic** *adjective* referring to sadism 性虐待的 *compare* 比较 MASOCHISM

safe *adjective* not likely to hurt or cause damage 安全的: ***Medicines should be kept in a place which is safe from children.*** 药物应当放在孩子够不到的安全地方。***This antibiotic is safe to be used on very small babies.*** 这种抗生素用于很小的婴儿也是安全的。***It is a safe painkiller, with no harmful side-effects.*** 这是一种安全的镇痛药,没有有害的副作用。***It is not safe to take the drug and also drink alcohol.*** 用这种药的时候喝酒是不安全的。**safe dose** = amount of a drug which can be taken without causing harm to the patient 安全剂量;**safe period** = time during the menstrual cycle, when conception is not likely to occur, and sexual intercourse can take place (used as a method of contraception)安全期(月经周期中不易受孕的一段时间,可用以避孕);**safe sex** = measures to reduce the possibility of catching a sexually transmitted disease, such as using a contraceptive sheath and having only one sexual partner(针对性病而言)安全的性生活(NOTE: **safe - safer - safest**)

◇ **safely** *adverb* without danger *or* without being hurt 安全地: ***You can safely take six tablets a day without any risk of side-effects.*** 你可以一天服6片药,而没有任何副作用。

◇ **safety** *noun* being safe *or* without danger 安全性; **to take safety precautions** = to do certain things which make your actions or condition safe 采取保障安全的预防措施; **safety belt** = belt which is worn in a car or a plane to help to stop a passenger being hurt if there is an accident 安全带; **safety pin** = special type of bent pin with a guard which covers the point, used for attaching nappies *or* bandages 安全别针

> QUOTE: A good collateral blood supply makes occlusion of a single branch of the coeliac axis safe.
> 引文:良好的侧支血供使腹动脉即使单支阻塞也是安全的。
> **British Medical Journal** 英国医学杂志

sagittal *adjective* which goes from the front of the body to the back, dividing it into right and left 矢状的; **sagittal plane** *or* **median plane** = division of the body along the midline, at right angles to the coronal plane, dividing the body into right and left parts 矢状面; **sagittal section** = any section *or* cut through the body, going from the front to the back along the length of the body 矢状切面; **sagittal suture** = joint along the top of the head where the two parietal bones are fused 矢状缝(颅骨上两侧顶骨融合形成的缝隙)

salicylic acid *noun* white antiseptic substance, which destroys bacteria and fungi and which is used in ointments to treat corns, warts and other skin disorders 水杨酸

◇ **salicylate** *or* **acetylsalicylic acid** *noun* pain-killing substance, derived from salicylic acid, used in the treatment of rheumatism, headaches and minor pains 水杨酸盐(解热镇痛药)

saline 1 *adjective* referring to salt 盐的: ***The patient was given a saline transfusion.*** 给病人输注了盐水。***She is on a saline drip.*** 她正在点滴盐水。**saline drip** = drip containing a saline solution 生理盐水点滴; **saline solution** = salt solution, made of distilled water and sodium chloride, which is introduced into the body intravenously through a drip 生理盐水溶液 **2** *noun* saline solution 盐水溶液

saliva *noun* fluid in the mouth, secreted by the salivary glands, which starts the process of digesting food 唾液

◇ **salivary** *adjective* referring to saliva 唾液的; **salivary calculus** = stone which forms in a salivary gland 唾液腺结石; **salivary gland** = gland which secretes saliva 唾液腺

◇ **salivate** *verb* to produce saliva 分泌

唾液

◇ **salivation** *noun* production of saliva 唾液分泌 (NOTE: for terms referring to saliva, see words beginning with **ptyal-, sial-**)

COMMENT: Saliva is a mixture of a large quantity of water and a small amount of mucus, secreted by the salivary glands. Saliva acts to keep the mouth and throat moist, allowing food to be swallowed easily. It also contains the enzyme ptyalin, which begins the digestive process of converting starch into sugar while food is still in the mouth. Because of this association with food, the salivary glands produce saliva automatically when food is seen, smelt or even simply talked about. The salivary glands are situated under the tongue (the sublingual glands), beneath the lower jaw (the submandibular glands) and in the neck at the back of the lower jaw joint (the parotid glands).
注释:唾液是唾液腺分泌的由大量水和少量粘液组成的混合物。唾液的作用是使口腔和咽喉湿润,使食物能被轻松咽下。它还含有唾液淀粉酶,在食物尚在口腔之中时便开始消化,即将淀粉转化成糖。因为这一过程与食物有关,所以当见到、闻到甚至谈到食物时唾液腺便自动分泌唾液。唾液腺分布在舌下(舌下腺),下颌骨下面(颌下腺)及下颌关节后面的颈部(腮腺)。

Salk vaccine *noun* vaccine against poliomyelitis 索尔克疫苗(脊髓灰质炎疫苗) *compare* 比较 SABIN

COMMENT: The Salk vaccine consists of dead polio virus and is given by injection.
注释:索尔克疫苗由死的脊髓灰质炎病毒组成而且是注射用的。

Salmonella *noun* genus of bacteria which are in the intestines, which are pathogenic, are usually acquired by eating contaminated food, and cause typhoid or paratyphoid fever, gastroenteritis or food poisoning 沙门氏菌属(引起伤寒、副伤寒及肠炎、食物中毒的一族致病菌): ***Five people were taken to hospital with Salmonella poisoning***. 有5个人因为沙门氏菌中毒而被送往医院。(NOTE: plural is **Salmonellae**)

◇ **salmonellosis** *noun* food poisoning caused by *Salmonella* in the digestive system 沙门氏菌食物中毒

salping- *or* **salpingo-** *prefix* referring to a tube 管 (i) the Fallopian tubes 输卵管 (ii) the auditory meatus 咽鼓管

◇ **salpingectomy** *noun* surgical operation to remove *or* cut a Fallopian tube (used as a method of contraception) 输卵管切除术

◇ **salpingitis** *noun* inflammation, usually of a Fallopian tube 输卵管炎

◇ **salpingography** *noun* X-ray examination of the Fallopian tubes 输卵管造影

◇ **salpingo-oophoritis** *or* **salpingo-oothecitis** *noun* inflammation of a Fallopian tube and the ovary connected to it 输卵管卵巢炎

◇ **salpingo-oophorocele** *or* **salpingo-oothecocele** *noun* hernia where a Fallopian tube and its ovary pass through a weak point in surrounding tissue 输卵管卵巢疝

◇ **salpingostomy** *noun* surgical operation to open up a blocked Fallopian tube 输卵管造口术,输卵管再通术

◇ **salpinx** = FALLOPIAN TUBE 输卵管

salt 1 *noun* (**a**) **common salt** = sodium chloride, a white powder used to make food, especially meat, fish and vegetables, taste better 食盐; **salt depletion** = loss of salt from the body, by sweating or vomiting, which causes cramp and other problems 盐缺失: ***A patient with heart failure is put on a salt restricted diet***. 心力衰竭的病人应给予限盐饮食。***He should reduce his intake of salt***. 他应当减少盐的摄入。(**b**) chemical compound formed from an acid and a metal 盐,由酸和金属组成的化合物; **bile salts** = alkaline salts in the bile 胆盐; **Epsom salts** = magnesium sulphate ($MgSO_4 \cdot 7H_2O$), white powder which when diluted in water is used as a laxative 硫酸镁(用于导泻) **2** *adjective* tasting of salt 咸的: ***Sea water is salt***. 海水是咸的。***Sweat tastes salt***. 汗是咸的。

COMMENT: Salt forms a necessary part of diet, as it replaces salt lost in sweating and helps to control the water balance in the body. It also improves the working of the muscles and nerves. Most diets contain more salt than each person actually needs, and although it has not been proved to be harmful, it is generally wise to cut down on salt consumption. Salt is one of the four tastes, the others being sweet, sour and bitter.
注释:盐是饮食中必不可少的一个组成部分,因为它补充出汗所丢失的盐分辅助身体对体液平衡的控制。盐还能提高肌肉和神经功能的发挥。多数饮食中含盐量超过身体的实际需要,尽管尚未证实这样对身体有害,但减少盐的摄入仍不失为一种明智的举动。盐的咸味是 4 种基本味道之一,其他几种是甜、酸和苦。

salve *noun* ointment 软膏, 油膏; **lip salve** = ointment, usually sold as a soft stick, used to rub on lips to prevent them cracking 唇膏

sample *noun* small quantity of something used for testing 样本: ***Blood samples were taken from all the staff in the hospital***. 从所有医院工作人员身上取血样。***The doctor asked her to provide a urine sample***. 医生让她提供尿样。

sanatorium *noun* institution (like a hospital) which treats certain types of disorder, such as tuberculosis, or offers special treatment such as hot baths, massage, etc. 疗养院 (NOTE: plural is **sanatoria**, **sanatoriums**)

sandflea *noun* the jigger, tropical insect which enters the skin between the toes and digs under the skin, causing intense irritation 沙蚤

sandfly fever *noun* virus infection like influenza, which is transmitted by the bite of the sandfly *Phlebotomus papatasii* and is common in the Middle East 白蛉热(由巴浦白蛉叮咬传播的病毒感染,常见于中东)

sanguineous *adjective* referring to blood *or* containing blood 多血的,血液的

sanies *noun* discharge from a sore *or* wound which has an unpleasant smell (伤口)脓液

sanitary *adjective* (i) clean 干净的 (ii) referring to hygiene *or* to health 卫生的,健康的; **sanitary napkin** *or* **sanitary towel** = wad of absorbent cotton placed over the vulva to absorb the menstrual flow 卫生巾

◇ **sanitation** *noun* being hygienic (especially referring to public hygiene) 环境卫生: ***Poor sanitation in crowded conditions can result in the spread of disease***. 拥挤的环境、糟糕的卫生状况可以导致疾病的传播。

saphenous nerve *noun* branch of the femoral nerve which connects with the sensory nerves in the skin of the lower leg 隐神经,股神经的分支与下肢皮肤的感觉神经相连; **saphenous opening** = hole in the fascia of the thigh through which the saphenous vein passes 隐静脉口(大腿筋膜上隐静脉通过的开口); **saphenous vein** *or* **saphena** = one of two veins which take blood from the foot up the leg 隐静脉

COMMENT: The long (internal) saphenous vein, the longest vein in the body, runs from the foot up the inside of the leg and joins the femoral vein. The short (posterior) saphenous vein runs up the back of the lower leg and joins the popliteal vein.
注释:大隐(内侧)静脉是体内最长的静脉,从足部上方腿的内侧开始直到与股静脉汇合。小隐(后侧)静脉沿下肢的后面向上走行,与腘静脉汇合。

sapraemia *noun* blood poisoning by saprophytes 腐血症

◇ **saprophyte** *noun* microorganism which lives on dead *or* decaying tissue 腐生生物

◇ **saprophytic** *adjective* (organism) which lives on dead *or* decaying tissue

腐生生物的

sarc- *or* **sarco-** *prefix* referring to (i) flesh 肉 (ii) muscle 肌

◇ **sarcoid** *noun* & *adjective* (tumour) which is like a sarcoma 结节病,结节病的

◇ **sarcoidosis** *noun* disease causing enlargement of the lymph nodes, where small nodules *or* granulomas form in certain tissues, especially in the lungs *or* liver and other parts of the body 结节病(导致淋巴结肿大的一种疾病,在特定组织,尤其是肺、肝及其他部位有小的结节或肉芽肿形成)(NOTE: also called **nymphomania Boeck's disease** *or* **Boeck's sarcoid**)

> COMMENT: The Kveim test confirms the presence of sarcoidosis.
> 注释:Kveim 试验能确认有结节病。

◇ **sarcolemma** *noun* membrane surrounding a muscle fibre 肉膜

◇ **sarcoma** *noun* cancer of connective tissue, such as bone, muscle or cartilage 肉瘤

◇ **sarcomatosis** *noun* condition where a sarcoma has spread through the bloodstream to many parts of the body 肉瘤病(肉瘤沿血流播散到身体的许多部位)

◇ **sarcomatous** *adjective* referring to a sarcoma 肉瘤的

◇ **sarcomere** *noun* filament in myofibril 肌节

◇ **sarcoplasm** *or* **myoplasm** *noun* semi-liquid cytoplasm in muscle membrane 肌浆

◇ **sarcoplasmic** *adjective* referring to sarcoplasm 肌浆的; **sarcoplasmic reticulum** = network in the cytoplasm of striated muscle fibres 肌浆网

◇ **sarcoptes** *noun* type of mite which causes scabies 疥螨

sardonicus 痉笑的 *see* 见 RISUS

sartorius *noun* very long muscle (the longest muscle) which runs from the anterior iliac spine, across the thigh down to the tibia 缝匠肌

saturated fat *noun* fat which has the largest amount of hydrogen possible 饱和脂肪(含有大量氢的脂肪)

> COMMENT: Animal fats such as butter and fat meat are saturated fatty acids. It is known that increasing the amount of unsaturated and polyunsaturated fats (mainly vegetable fats and oils, and fish oil), and reducing saturated fats in the food intake helps reduce the level of cholesterol in the blood, and so lessens the risk of atherosclerosis.
> 注释:动物脂肪,如黄油和肥肉,是饱和脂肪酸。众所周知,食中增加不饱和脂肪酸和多不饱和脂肪酸(主要存在于植物脂肪和植物油及鱼油中)的摄入,减少饱和脂肪酸的摄入有助于降低血液中胆固醇的水平,由此减少了动脉粥样硬化的危险。

saturnism *noun* lead poisoning 铅中毒

satyriasis *noun* abnormal sexual urge in a man 男性色情狂 (NOTE: in a woman, called **nymphomania**)

save *verb* to rescue someone *or* to stop someone from being hurt or killed *or* to stop something from being damaged 挽救,保有: ***The doctors saved the little boy from dying of cancer.*** 医生们从癌症的死亡线上挽救了这个小男孩。***The surgeons were unable to save the sight of their patient.*** 外科医师不能保住病人的视力。***The surgeons saved her life.*** = They stopped the patient from dying. 外科医师挽救了她的生命。

saw 1 *noun* tool with a long metal blade with teeth along its edge, used for cutting 锯 **2** *verb* to cut with a saw 用锯子锯 (NOTE: **saws - sawing - sawed - has sawn**)

Sayre's jacket *noun* plaster cast which supports the spine when vertebrae have been deformed by tuberculosis or spinal disease 塞尔背心(石膏背心)

s.c. = SUBCUTANEOUS 皮下

scab *noun* crust of dry blood which forms over a wound and protects it 痂,结痂

scabicide *noun* & *adjective* (solution) which kills mites 杀疥螨药(的)

◇ **scabies** *noun* very irritating infection of the skin caused by a mite which lives under the skin 疥螨病,疥疮

scala *noun* spiral canal in the cochlea 耳蜗螺旋管

COMMENT: The cochlea is formed of three spiral canals: the scala vestibuli which is filled with perilymph and connects with the oval window; the scala media which is filled with endolymph and transmits vibrations from the scala vestibuli through the basilar membrane to the scala tympani, which in turn transmits the sound vibrations to the round window.
注释:耳蜗由三个螺旋管组成:前庭螺旋管(前庭阶),充满前淋巴液,与卵圆窗相连;中阶,充满内淋巴液,通过基膜将来自前庭阶的震动通过基底膜传到鼓阶;鼓阶再将声音震动传到圆窗。

scald 1 *noun* injury to the skin caused by touching a very hot liquid *or* steam 烫伤 **2** *verb* to injure the skin with a very hot liquid *or* steam 烫(伤)

◇ **scalding** *adjective* (i) very hot (liquid)(液体)非常热的 (ii) (urine) which gives a burning sensation when passed 排尿烧灼感的

scale 1 *noun* (**a**) flake of dead tissue (as dead skin in dandruff) 鳞屑 (**b**) **scales** = machine for weighing 磅秤: ***The nurses weighed the baby on the scales.*** 护士给婴儿过磅。**2** *verb* to scrape teeth to remove plaque 刮治(清洁牙垢的一种治疗方法)

◇ **scale off** *verb* to fall off in scales 脱屑

scalenus *or* **scalene** *noun* one of a group of muscles in the neck which bend the neck forwards and sideways, and also help expand the lungs in deep breathing 斜角肌; **scalenus syndrome** = pain in an arm, caused by the scalenus anterior muscle pressing the subclavian artery and the brachial plexus against the vertebrae 斜角肌综合征(由前斜角肌压迫锁骨下动脉和臂神经丛所致的臂痛)

scaler *noun* surgical instrument for scaling teeth 刮器(牙科刮治用具)

scalp *noun* thick skin and muscle (with the hair) which covers the skull 头皮; **scalp wound** = wound in the scalp 头皮伤

scalpel *noun* small sharp pointed knife used in surgery 解剖刀,手术刀

scaly *adjective* covered in scales 鳞屑覆盖的: ***The pustules harden and become scaly.*** 脓疱变硬并为鳞屑所覆盖。

scan 1 *noun* (i) examination of part of the body using computer-interpreted X-rays to create a picture of the part on a screen 扫描 (ii) picture of part of the body created on a screen using computer-interpreted X-rays 扫描图; **CAT scan** = scan where a narrow X-ray beam, guided by a computer, photographs a thin section of the body *or* an organ from different angles; the results are fed into the computer which analyses them and produces a picture of a slice of the body *or* organ CT 扫描 **2** *verb* to examine part of the body, using computer-interpreted X-rays, and create a picture of the part on a screen 扫描

◇ **scanner** *noun* (**a**) machine which scans a part of the body 扫描器; **brain scanner** *or* **body scanner** = machines which scan only the brain *or* all the body 脑扫描器,躯干扫描器 (**b**) (i) person who examines a test slide 读片人(指切片) (ii) person who operates a scanning machine 扫描器操作者

◇ **scanning speech** *noun* defect in speaking, where each sound is spoken separately and given equal stress 断续言语

scaphocephaly *noun* condition where the skull is abnormally long and narrow 舟状头畸形

◇ **scaphocephalic** *adjective* having a long narrow skull 舟状头畸形的

scaphoid (bone) *noun* one of the carpal bones in the wrist 舟状骨(腕骨之一)

◇ **scaphoiditis** *noun* degeneration of the navicular bone in children 舟骨炎

scapula *noun* shoulder blade *or* one of two large flat bones covering the top part of the back 肩胛骨(NOTE: plural is **scapulae**)

◇ **scapular** *adjective* referring to the shoulder blade 肩胛骨的

◇ **scapulohumeral** *adjective* referring to the scapula and humerus 肩胛骨肱骨的; **scapulohumeral arthritis** = PERIARTHRITIS 肩胛骨肱骨关节炎,肩周炎

scar 1 *noun* cicatrix, the mark left on the skin after a wound *or* surgical incision has healed 疤痕: ***He still has the scar of his appendicectomy.*** 他还有阑尾切除术留下的疤痕。**scar tissue** = fibrous tissue which forms a scar 瘢痕组织 **2** *verb* to leave a scar on the skin 留疤,形成瘢痕: ***The burns have scarred him for life.*** 烧伤给他留下了终身疤痕。***Plastic surgeons have tried to repair the scarred arm.*** 整形外科医师已在试图修补那疤痕累累的胳臂。***Patients were given special clothes to reduce hypertrophic scarring.*** 给病人特殊的衣服以减少疤痕增生。

scarification *noun* scratching, making minute cuts on the surface of the skin (as for smallpox vaccination) 划痕,划破

scarlatina *or* **scarlet fever** *noun* infectious disease with a fever, sore throat and red rash, caused by a haemolytic streptococcus 猩红热(溶血性链球菌引起的感染性疾病,表现为发热、咽痛和猩红色皮疹)

> COMMENT: Scarlet fever can sometimes have serious complications if the kidneys are infected.
> 注释:如果感染侵及肾脏,猩红热可引起严重的并发症。

Scarpa's triangle *noun* femoral triangle, slight hollow in the groin; it contains the femoral vessels and nerve 斯卡帕三角,股三角(位于腹股沟,股血管和股神经通过的地方)

scat- *or* **scato-** *prefix* referring to the faeces 粪便

◇ **scatole** *noun* substance in faeces, formed in the intestine, which causes a strong smell 粪臭素

SCD = SICKLE-CELL DISEASE 镰状细胞病

> QUOTE: Even children with the milder forms of SCD have an increased frequency of pneumococcal infection.
> 引文:即使是轻型的镰状细胞病也会使患儿患肺炎球菌感染的几率上升。
> **Lancet** 柳叶刀

scent *noun* (i) pleasant smell 好闻的气味 (ii) cosmetic substance which has a pleasant smell 化妆品的香气 (iii) smell given off by a substance which stimulates the sense of smell 散发的刺激性气味: ***The scent of flowers makes me sneeze.*** 花香使我打喷嚏。

◇ **scented** *adjective* with a strong pleasant smell 香的: ***He is allergic to scented soap.*** 他对香皂过敏。

schema 图,图示 *see* 见 BODY SCHEMA

Scheuermann's disease *noun* inflammation of the bones and cartilage in the spine, usually affecting adolescents 绍依尔曼氏病,脊柱骨软骨病(脊柱的骨和软骨发炎,通常侵及青少年)

Schick test *noun* test to see if a person is immune to diphtheria 锡克试验(检验是否对白喉有免疫力)

> COMMENT: In this test, a small amount of diphtheria toxin is injected, and if the point of injection becomes inflamed it shows the patient is not immune to the disease (= positive reaction).
> 注释:此试验是注射小量的白喉毒素,如果注射的部位发炎说明病人对疾病没有免疫力(阳性反应)。

Schilling test *noun* test to see if a patient can absorb vitamin B_{12} through the intestines, to determine cases of pernicious anaemia 希林试验(检验病人能否通过肠道吸收维生素 B_{12},用于诊断恶性贫血)

-schisis *suffix* referring to a fissure *or* split 裂

◇ **schisto-** *or* **schizo-** *prefix* referring to something which is split 分开,分

裂

Schistosoma *or* **schistosome** = BILHARZIA 血吸虫

◇ **schistosomiasis** = BILHARZIASIS 血吸虫病

schiz- *or* **schizo-** *prefix* referring to something which is split 分裂,分开

◇ **schizoid 1** *adjective* referring to schizophrenia 分裂样的; **schizoid personality** *or* **split personality** = disorder where the patient is cold towards other people, thinks mainly about himself and behaves in an odd way 分裂人格(极端孤僻,冷淡,举止怪异的人) **2** *noun* person suffering from a less severe form of schizophrenia 分裂样精神障碍

◇ **schizophrenia** *noun* mental disorder where the patient withdraws from contact with other people, has delusions and seems to lose contact with the real world 精神分裂症; **catatonic schizophrenia** 紧张型精神分裂症 *see* 见 CATATONIC

◇ **schizophrenic** *noun* & *adjective* (person) suffering from schizophrenia 精神分裂症的,精神分裂症患者

Schlatter's disease *noun* inflammation in the bones and cartilage at the top of the tibia 施莱特病,胫骨粗隆的骨软骨病

Schlemm's canal *noun*) circular canal in the sclera of the eye, which drains the aqueous humour 施雷姆氏管,巩膜静脉窦

Schönlein's purpura 过敏性紫癜 *see* 见 PURPURA

school *noun* (**a**) place where children are taught 学校; **school health service** = special service, part of the Local Health Authority, which looks after the health of children in school 学校卫生服务 (**b**) specialized section of a university 学院; **medical school** = section of a university which teaches medicine 医学院: ***He is at medical school***. 他在医学院上学。***She is taking a course at the School of Dentistry***. 她正在口腔学院上课。

Schwann cells *noun* cells which form the myelin sheath round a nerve fibre 雪旺氏细胞(神经鞘细胞) ◇ 见图 NEURONE

◇ **schwannoma** *or* **neurofibroma** *noun* benign tumour of a peripheral nerve 神经纤维瘤

Schwartze's operation *noun* the original surgical operation to drain fluid and remove infected tissue from the mastoid process 施瓦茨手术,乳突引流术

sciatic *adjective* referring to (i) the hip 坐骨的 (ii) the sciatic nerve 坐骨神经的; **sciatic nerve** = one of two main nerves which run from the sacral plexus into the thighs, dividing into a series of nerves in the lower legs and feet; it is the largest nerve in the body 坐骨神经

◇ **sciatica** *noun* pain along the sciatic nerve, usually at the back of the thighs and legs 坐骨神经痛

> COMMENT: Sciatica can be caused by a slipped disc which presses on a spinal nerve, or can simply be caused by straining a muscle in the back.
> 注释:坐骨神经痛可以由滑脱的椎间盘压迫脊神经引起,也可以仅由拉伤背部肌肉导致。

science *noun* study based on looking at and noting facts, especially facts arranged into a system 科学

◇ **scientific** *adjective* referring to science 科学的: ***he carried out scientific experiments***. 他进行科学试验。

◇ **scientist** *noun* person who specializes in scientific studies 科学家

scintigram *noun* recording radiation from radioactive isotopes injected into the body 闪烁图

◇ **scintillascope** *noun* instrument which produces a scintigram 闪烁镜

◇ **scintillator** *noun* substance which produces a flash of light when struck by radiation 闪烁体

◇ **scintiscan** *noun* scintigram which shows the variations in radiation from one part of the body to another 闪烁扫描

scirrhus *noun* hard malignant tumour (especially in the breast)硬癌

◇ **scirrhous** *adjective* hard (tumour) 硬癌的

scissors *plural noun* instrument for cutting, made of two blades and two handles 剪刀; **scissor legs** = deformed legs, where one leg is permanently crossed over in front of the other 剪刀样腿 (NOTE: say **'a pair of scissors'** when referring to one instrument)

scler- *or* **sclero-** *prefix* (i) meaning hard *or* thick; referring to 硬,厚 (ii) sclera 巩膜 (iii) sclerosis 硬化

◇ **sclera** *or* **sclerotic (coat)** *noun* hard white outer covering of the eyeball 巩膜 ◇ 见图 EYE

> COMMENT: The front part of the sclera is the transparent cornea, through which the light enters the eye. The conjunctiva, or inner skin of the eyelids, connects with the sclera and covers the front of the eyeball.
> 注解:巩膜的前部是透明的角膜,光通过它进入眼睛。结膜或睑结膜与巩膜相连,覆盖在眼球前面。

◇ **scleral** *adjective* referring to the sclera 巩膜的; **scleral lens** = large contact lens which covers most of the front of the eye 巩膜镜(大的接触镜)

◇ **scleritis** *noun* inflammation of the sclera 巩膜炎

◇ **scleroderma** *noun* collagen disease which thickens connective tissue and produces a hard thick skin 硬皮病

◇ **scleroma** *noun* patch of hard skin *or* hard mucous membrane 硬结

◇ **scleromalacia (perforans)** *noun* condition of the sclera in which holes appear 穿通性巩膜软化

◇ **sclerosing** *adjective* which becomes hard *or* which makes tissue hard 硬化; **sclerosant agent** *or* **sclerosing agent** *or* **sclerosing solution** = irritating liquid injected into tissue to harden it 硬化剂

◇ **sclerosis** *noun* hardening of tissue 组织硬化; **multiple sclerosis** *or* **disseminated sclerosis** = nervous disease which gets progressively worse, where patches of the fibres of the central nervous system lose their myelin, causing numbness in the limbs and progressive weakness and paralysis 多发性硬化,弥漫性硬化(神经系统进行性脱髓鞘疾病,造成肢体麻木,进行性肌无力和瘫痪) *see also* 参见 ARTERIOSCLEROSIS, ATHEROSCLEROSIS, GEHRIG'S DISEASE

◇ **sclerotherapy** *noun* treatment of a varicose vein by injecting a sclerosing agent into the vein, and so encouraging the blood in the vein to clot 硬化疗法(静脉内注射硬化剂以治疗静脉曲张)

◇ **sclerotic 1** *adjective* referring to sclerosis; suffering from sclerosis 硬化的; 患有硬化的 **2** *noun* hard white covering of the eyeball 巩膜

◇ **sclerotome** *noun* sharp knife used in sclerotomy 巩膜刀

◇ **sclerotomy** *noun* surgical operation to cut into the sclera 巩膜切开术

scolex *noun* head of a tapeworm, with hooks which attach it to the wall of the intestine(绦虫)头节

scoliosis *noun* condition where the spine curves sideways 脊柱侧凸

◇ **scoliotic** *adjective* (spine) which curves sideways 脊柱侧凸的

scoop stretcher *noun* type of stretcher formed of two jointed sections which can slide under a patient and lock together 分体担架

-scope *suffix* referring to an instrument for examining by sight 镜

scorbutus *or* **scurvy** *noun* disease caused by lack of vitamin C *or* ascorbic acid which is found in fruit and vegetables 坏血病(维生素 C 缺乏引起)

◇ **scorbutic** *adjective* referring to scurvy 坏血病的 *see* 见 *note at* SCURVY

scoto- *prefix* meaning dark 黑,暗

◇ **scotoma** *noun* small area in the field of vision where the patient cannot see 盲点,暗点

◇ **scotometer** *noun* instrument used

to measure areas of defective vision 暗点计

◇ **scotopia** *noun* the power of the eye to adapt to poor lighting conditions and darkness 暗适应

◇ **scotopic** *adjective* referring to scotopia 暗适应的;**scotopic vision** = vision in the dark and in dim light (the rods of the retina are used instead of the cones which are used for photopic vision) 暗适应视觉 *see* 见 DARK ADAPTATION

scrape *verb* to remove the surface of something by moving a sharp knife across it 刮去

scratch 1 *noun* slight wound on the skin made when a sharp point is pulled across it 抓伤,抓破: ***She had scratches on her legs and arms.*** 她的胳膊上和腿上有抓伤。 ***Wash the dirt out of that scratch in case it gets infected.*** 把抓破处的脏东西洗掉以免发生感染。 **2** *verb* to harm the skin by moving a sharp point across it 抓,挠: ***The cat scratched the girl's face.*** 猫抓破了女孩的脸。 ***Be careful not to scratch yourself on the wire.*** 小心别让自己被电线刮伤。

scream 1 *noun* loud sharp cry 尖叫: ***You could hear the screams of the people in the burning building.*** 你可以听到着火楼房里人们的尖叫声。 **2** *verb* to make a loud sharp cry 尖叫: ***She screamed when a man suddenly opened the door.*** 当一个男人突然将门打开时她尖叫起来。

screen 1 *noun* (**a**) light wall, sometimes with a curtain, which can be moved about and put round a bed to shield the patient 屏风 (**b**) screening 筛查 **2** *verb* to examine large numbers of people to test them for a disease 筛查: ***The population of the village was screened for meningitis.*** 在一个村的人群中筛查脑膜炎。

◇ **screening** *noun* testing large numbers of people to see if any has a certain type of disease 筛查

> QUOTE: In the UK the main screen is carried out by health visitors at 6 – 10 months. With adequately staffed and trained community services, this method of screening can be extremely effective.
> 引文:在英国,主要的筛查工作由保健访视员每6~10个月施行一次。在恰当的人员配备和训练有素的社区服务机构配合下,这种筛查是极有效的。
> **Lancet** 柳叶刀

> QUOTE: GPs are increasingly requesting blood screening for patients concerned about HIV.
> 引文:全科医师对可能感染人类免疫缺陷病毒的病人越来越倾向做血样筛查。
> **Journal of the Royal College of General Practitioners** 皇家全科医师学会杂志

scrofula *noun* form of tuberculosis in the lymph nodes in the neck, formerly caused by unpasteurized milk, but now rare 淋巴结结核,瘰疬

◇ **scrofulous** *adjective* suffering from scrofula 淋巴结结核的,瘰疬的

◇ **scrofuloderma** *noun* form of tuberculosis of the skin, forming ulcers, and secondary to tuberculous infection of an underlying lymph gland *or* structure 皮肤结核,皮肤瘰疬

scrotal *adjective* referring to the scrotum 阴囊的

◇ **scrotum** *noun* bag of skin hanging from behind the penis, containing the testes, epididymides and part of the spermatic cord 阴囊 ◊ 见图 UROGENITAL SYSTEM (male)

scrub nurse *noun* nurse who cleans the operation site on a patient's body before an operation 备皮护士

◇ **scrub up** *verb* (*of surgeon or* theatre nurse) to wash the hands and arms carefully before an operation 刷手

scrub typhus *or* **tsutsugamushi disease** *noun* severe form of typhus caused by Rickettsia bacteria, passed to humans by mites, found in South East Asia 恙虫病(立克次体感染所致斑疹伤寒的

严重型,由螨传播给人,见于东南亚)

scurf *or* **dandruff** *or* **pityriasis capitis** *noun* pieces of dead skin which form on the scalp and fall out when the hair is combed 头皮屑

scurvy *or* **scorbutus** *noun* disease caused by lack of vitamin C *or* ascorbic acid which is found in fruit and vegetables 坏血病

COMMENT: Scurvy causes general weakness and anaemia, with bleeding from the gums, joints, and under the skin. In severe cases, the teeth drop out. Treatment consists of vitamin C tablets and a change of diet to include more fruit and vegetables.
注释:坏血病引起全身虚弱和贫血,还伴有牙龈、关节和皮下出血。在严重病例,可有牙齿脱落。治疗包括用维生素 C 片和改变饮食,多吃水果和蔬菜。

scybalum *noun* very hard faeces 硬粪块

Se *chemical symbol for* selenium 硒的化学元素符号

sea *noun* area of salt water which covers a large part of the earth 海: ***When the sea is rough he is often sick.*** 当海浪汹涌的时候他常感到恶心。

◇ **seasick** *adjective* feeling sick because of the movement of a ship 晕船: ***As soon as the ferry started to move she felt seasick.*** 一开船她就感到晕船。

◇ **seasickness** *or* **travel sickness** *or* **motion sickness** *noun* illness, with nausea, vomiting and sometimes headache, caused by the movement of a ship 晕船,晕车,晕动病: ***Take some seasickness tablets if you are going on a long journey.*** 如果你准备长途旅行就备些治疗晕船的药。

seasonal affective depression *or* **seasonal affective disorder (SAD)** = *noun* condition in which the patient becomes depressed and anxious during the winter when there are fewer hours of daylight: the precise cause is not known, but it is thought that the shortage of daylight may provoke a reaction between various hormones and neurotransmitters in the brain 季节性情感抑郁(在冬季日照减少时患者感觉抑郁和焦虑,确切原因不明,据认为与日照减少引发脑内各种激素和神经递质的反应有关)

sebaceous *adjective* (i) referring to sebum 皮脂的 (ii) which produces oil 出油的; **sebaceous cyst** = cyst which forms when a sebaceous gland is blocked 皮脂囊; **sebaceous gland** = gland in the skin which secretes sebum at the base of each hair follicle 皮脂腺 ◊ 见图 SKIN & SENSORY RECEPTORS

◇ **seborrhoea** *noun* excessive secretion of sebum by the sebaceous glands, common in young people at puberty, and sometimes linked to seborrhoeic dermatitis 皮脂溢出

◇ **seborrhoeic** *adjective* (i) caused by seborrhoea 皮脂溢出的 (ii) with an oily secretion 分泌油性的; **seborrhoeic dermatitis** *or* **seborrhoeic eczema** = type of eczema where scales form on the skin 脂溢性皮炎; **seborrhoeic rash** = rash where the skin surface is oily 脂溢性皮疹

◇ **sebum** *noun* oily substance secreted by a sebaceous gland, which makes the skin smooth; it also protects the skin against bacteria and the body against rapid evaporation of water 皮脂

second 1 *noun* unit of time equal to 1/60 of a minute 秒 2 *adjective* coming after the first 第二,次之,其次; **second intention** = healing of an infected wound *or* ulcer, which takes places lowly and leaves a prominent scar 二期愈合; **second molars** = molars at the back of the jaw, before the wisdom teeth, erupting at about 12 years of age 第二磨牙

◇ **secondary** 1 *adjective* (i) which comes after the first 继发的 (ii) (condition) which develops from another condition (the primary condition) 继发性的: ***He was showing symptoms of secondary syphilis.*** 他表现出继发性梅毒的症状。 **secondary amenorrhoea** 继发性经闭 *see*

见 AMENORRHOEA; **secondary bronchi** = air passages supplying a lobe of a lung 次级支气管; **secondary haemorrhage** = haemorrhage which occurs some time after an injury, usually due to infection of the wound 继发性出血; **secondary medical care** = specialized treatment provided by a hospital 二级医疗保健; **secondary prevention** = ways (such as screening tests) of avoiding a serious disease by detecting it early 二级预防; **secondary sexual characteristics** = sexual characteristics (such as pubic hair *or* breasts) which develop after puberty 副性征 **2** *noun* malignant tumour which metastasized from another malignant tumour 转移癌 *see also* 参见 PRIMARY

secrete *verb* (*of a gland*) to produce a substance (such as hormone *or* oil *or* enzyme)分泌

◇ **secretin** *noun* hormone secreted by the duodenum, which encourages the production of pancreatic juice 胰泌素,肠促胰液肽

◇ **secretion** *noun* (**a**) process by which a substance is produced by a gland 分泌: ***The pituitary gland stimulates the secretion of hormones by the adrenal gland.*** 垂体刺激肾上腺激素的分泌。(**b**) substance produced by a gland 分泌液: ***Sex hormones are bodily secretions.*** 性激素是身体分泌的。

◇ **secretor** *noun* person who secretes ABO blood group substances into mucous fluids in the body (such as the semen, the saliva)分泌者

◇ **secretory** *adjective* referring to *or* accompanied by *or* producing a secretion 分泌的

section *noun* (**a**) part of something 部分: ***The middle section of the aorta.*** 主动脉中部。(**b**)(i) action of cutting tissue 切开术 (ii) cut made in tissue 切口; **Caesarean section** = surgical operation to deliver a baby by cutting through the abdominal wall into the uterus 恺撒切开,帝王切开,剖宫产 (**c**) slice of tissue cut for examination under a microscope 切片 (**d**) part of a document, such as an Act of Parliament 部分: ***She was admitted under section 5 of the Mental Health Act.*** 按照精神卫生法第五部分收她住院。

sedate *verb* to calm (a patient) by giving a drug which acts on the nervous system and relieves stress *or* pain, and in larger doses makes a patient sleep 镇静: ***Elderly or confused patients may need to be sedated to prevent them wandering.*** 老人或意识不清的病人需要给镇静剂以防他们盲目走动。

◇ **sedation** *noun* calming a patient with a sedative 镇静; **under sedation** = having been given a sedative 给了镇静剂的: ***He was still under sedation, and could not be seen by the police.*** 他还处在镇静剂作用期,不能让警察问讯。

◇ **sedative** *noun & adjective* (drug) which acts on the nervous system to help a patient sleep *or* to relieve stress 镇静剂,镇静剂的: ***She was prescribed sedatives by the doctor.*** 医生给她开了镇静剂。

sedentary *adjective* sitting 静坐的,坐位的; **sedentary occupations** = jobs where the workers sit down for most of the time 常坐着工作的职业

> QUOTE: Changes in lifestyle factors have been related to the decline in mortality from ischaemic heart disease. In many studies a sedentary lifestyle has been reported as a risk factor for ischaemic heart disease.
> 引文:生活习惯的改变与缺血性心脏病死亡率的下降有关。许多研究报告显示坐位工作是缺血性心脏病的一个危险因素。
> **Journal of the American Medical Association** 美国医学会杂志

sediment *noun* solid particles, usually insoluble, which fall to the bottom of a liquid 沉淀

◇ **sedimentation** *noun* action of solid particles falling to the bottom of a liquid 沉淀作用; **erythrocyte sedimentation rate (ESR)** = test to show how fast erythrocytes settle in a sample of blood plasma, used as a diagnostic of various blood conditions 红细胞沉降率,血沉

segment *noun* part of an organ *or* piece of tissue which is clearly separate from other parts 节段

◊ **segmental** *adjective* formed of segments 节段性的: **segmental ablation** = surgical removal of part of a nail, as treatment for an ingrowing toenail 节段性摘除 *see also* 参见 BRONCHI

◊ **segmentation** *noun* movement of separate segments of the wall of the intestine to mix digestive juice with the food before it is passed along by the action of peristalsis 节段性运动

◊ **segmented** *adjective* formed of segments 由若干节段组成的

seizure *noun* fit *or* convulsion *or* sudden contraction of the muscles, especially in a heart attack *or* stroke *or* epileptic fit 抽搐

select *verb* to make a choice *or* to choose some things, but not others 选择: ***The committee is meeting to select the company which will supply kitchen equipment for the hospital service.*** 委员会正在开会选出一家公司为医院后勤提供厨房设备。***She was selected to go on a midwifery course.*** 她被选去上助产士课程。

◊ **selection** *noun* act of choosing some things, but not others 选择: ***The candidates for the post have to go through a selection process.*** 候选人必须通过选举产生。***They have begun the selection of suitable donor for a bone marrow transplant.*** 他们开始为骨髓移植选择合适的捐献者。**genetic selection** = choosing only the best examples of a genus for reproduction 基因选择

◊ **selective** *adjective* which choose only certain things, and not others 选择性的

selenium *noun* non-metallic trace element 硒 (NOTE: chemical symbol is **Se**)

self- *prefix* referring to oneself 自我

◊ **self-admitted** *adjective* (patient) who has admitted himself to hospital without being sent by a doctor 自动入院的(不是医生转诊的)

◊ **self-care** *noun* looking after yourself properly, so that you remain healthy 自我保健

◊ **self-defence** *noun* defending yourself when someone is attacking you 自卫

◊ **self-governing hospital** *noun* NHS hospital trust, a hospital which earns its revenue from services provided to the District Health Authorities and family doctors 自主管理的医院

sella turcica *noun* pituitary fossa, a hollow in the upper surface of the sphenoid bone in which the pituitary gland sits 蝶鞍

semeiology = SYMPTOMATOLOGY 症状学

semen *noun* thick pale fluid containing spermatozoa, produced by the testes and seminal vesicles, and ejaculated from the penis 精液

semi- *prefix* meaning half 半

◊ **semicircular** *adjective* shaped like half a circle 半环形的; **semicircular canals** = three canals in the inner ear filled with fluid and which regulate the sense of balance 半规管 ◊ 见图 EAR; **semicircular ducts** = ducts inside the canals in the inner ear 半规管导管

> COMMENT: The three semicircular canals are on different planes. When a person's head moves (as when he bends down), the fluid in the canals moves and this movement is communicated to the brain through the vestibular section of the auditory nerve.
>
> 注释:三个半规管分别位于不同平面。当一个人的头运动时(如低头),半规管里的液体流动,这种流动的信息经听神经的前庭支传递到脑。

◊ **semi-conscious** *adjective* half conscious *or* only partly aware of what is going on 半意识的,半清醒的: ***She was semi-conscious for most of the operation.*** 手术中大多数时间她是半清醒的。

◇ **semi-liquid** *adjective* half liquid and half solid 一半是液体一半是固体的

◇ **semilunar** *adjective* shaped like half a moon 半月形的; **semilunar cartilage** *or* **meniscus** = one of two pads of cartilage (lateral meniscus and medial meniscus) between the femur and the tibia in the knee 半月板; **semilunar valve** = one of two valves in the heart, either the pulmonary or the aortic valve, through which blood flows out of the ventricles 半月瓣

seminal *adjective* referring to semen 精液的; **seminal fluid** = fluid part of semen, formed in the epididymis and seminal vesicles 精液; **seminal vesicles** = two glands near the prostate gland which secrete fluid into the vas deferens 精囊 ◊ 见图 UROGENITAL SYSTEM (male)

◇ **seminiferous tubule** *noun* tubule in the testis which carries semen 输精管

◇ **seminoma** *noun* malignant tumour in the testis 精原细胞瘤

semipermeable membrane *noun* membrane which allows some substances in liquid solution to pass through, but not others 半透膜

◇ **semiprone** *adjective* (position) where the patient lies face downwards, with one knee and one arm bent forwards and the face turned to one side 半俯卧位的

◇ **semi-solid** *adjective* half solid and half liquid 一半是固体一半是液体的

SEN = STATE ENROLLED NURSE 国家注册护士

senescence *noun* the ageing process 衰老

◇ **senescent** *adjective* becoming old 衰老的,变老的

Sengstaken tube *noun* tube with a balloon, which is passed through the mouth into the oesophagus to stop oesophageal bleeding 森氏管,三腔管(用于食管静脉曲张出血时压迫止血)

senile *adjective* (i) referring to old age *or* to the infirmities of old age 老年的 (ii) (person) whose mental faculties have become weak because of age 衰老的; **senile cataract** = cataract which occurs in an elderly person 老年性白内障; **senile dementia** = form of mental degeneration sometimes affecting old people 老年性痴呆

◇ **senility** *noun* weakening of the mental and physical faculties in an old person 衰老

◇ **senilis** 老年性 *see* 见 ARCUS

senior *adjective* & *noun* (person) who has a more important position than others 上级,资深的: ***He is the senior anaesthetist in the hospital.*** 他是医院的资深麻醉师。***Senior members of staff are allowed to consult the staff records.*** 资深工作人员被允许看人事记录。

senna *noun* laxative made from the dried fruit and leaves of a tropical tree 番泻叶

sensation *noun* feeling *or* information about something which has been sensed by a sensory nerve and is passed to the brain 感觉; **burning sensation** = sensation similar to that of being hurt by fire 烧灼感

◇ **sense 1** *noun* one of the five faculties by which a person notices things in the outside world (sight, hearing, smell, taste and touch) 感觉: ***When he had a cold, he lost his sense of smell.*** 他感冒时嗅觉失去。***Blind people develop an acute sense of touch.*** 盲人会发展敏锐的触觉。**sense organ** = organ (such as the nose, the skin) in which there are various sensory nerves and which can detect environmental stimuli (such as scent, heat and pain) and transmit information about them to the central nervous system 感觉器官 **2** *verb* to notice something 感到: ***Teeth can sense changes in temperature.*** 牙齿可以感知温度的变化。

◇ **sensible** *adjective* which can be detected by the senses 可感知到的; **sensible perspiration** = drops of sweat which can be seen on the skin 可感知的出汗,显性出汗

◇ **sensibility** *noun* being able to detect and interpret sensations 可感知性

◇ **sensitive** *adjective* able to detect and respond to an outside stimulus 敏感的

◇ **sensitivity** *noun* (i) being able to detect and respond to an outside stimulus 敏感性(ii) rate of positive responses in a test from persons with a specific disease (a high rate of sensitivity means a low rate of false negatives) 敏感度 (NOTE: compare with **specificity**)

◇ **sensitization** *noun* (i) making a person sensitive 致敏(ii) abnormal reaction to an allergen *or* to a drug, caused by the presence of antibodies which were created when the patient was exposed to the drug *or* allergen in the past 过敏

◇ **sensitize** *verb* to make someone sensitive to a drug or allergen 过敏: **sensitized person** = person who is allergic to a drug *or* who reacts badly to a drug 对(某药)过敏的人; **sensitizing agent** = substance which, by acting as an antigen, makes the body form antibodies 过敏原

sensorineural deafness *noun* perceptive deafness, deafness caused by a disorder in the auditory nerves *or* the brain centres which receive impulses from the nerves 神经性聋

◇ **sensory** *noun* referring to the detection of sensations by nerve cells 感觉的; **sensory cortex** = term which was formerly used to refer to the area of the cerebral cortex which receives information from nerves in all parts of the body 感觉皮质; **sensory deprivation** = condition where a person becomes confused because of lacking sensations 感觉缺失; **sensory nerve** = afferent nerve which transmits impulses relating to a sensation (such as a taste *or* a smell) to the brain 感觉神经; **sensory neurone** = nerve cell which transmits impulses relating to sensations from the receptor to the central nervous system 感觉神经元; **sensory receptor** = nerve ending *or* special cell which senses a change in the surrounding environment (such as cold *or* pressure) and reacts to it by sending out an impulse through the nervous system 感受器 ◊ 见图 SKIN & SENSORY RECEPTORS

separate *verb* to move two things apart *or* to divide 分开: ***The surgeons believe it may be possible to separate the Siamese twins.*** 外科医师们相信有可能将暹逻孪生子(联体双胎)分开。***The retina has become separated from the back of the eye.*** 视网膜已经从眼球后部剥脱了。

◇ **separation** *noun* act of separating *or* dividing 分开

sepsis *noun* presence of bacteria and their toxins in the body (usually following the infection of a wound), which kill tissue and produce pus 脓毒症

◇ **sept-** *or* **septi-** *prefix* referring to sepsis 脓毒症

septa- *prefix* referring to a septum 中隔,间隔

◇ **septal** *adjective* referring to a septum 中隔的,间隔的; (**atrial** *or* **ventricular**) **septal defect** = congenital defect where a hole exists in the wall between the two atria *or* the two ventricles of the heart which allows blood to flow abnormally through the heart and lungs 房间隔缺损(室间隔缺损)

◇ **septate** *adjective* divided by a septum 分隔的

septic *adjective* referring to *or* produced by sepsis 脓毒性的

◇ **septicaemia** *noun* blood poisoning, condition where bacteria or their toxins are present in the blood, multiply rapidly and destroy tissue 败血症

◇ **septicaemic** *adjective* caused by septicaemia *or* associated with septicaemia 败血症的 *see also* 参见 PLAGUE

septo- *prefix* referring to a septum 间隔

◇ **septoplasty** *noun* operation to

straighten the cartilage in the septum 鼻中隔成形术

◇ **septum** *noun* wall between two parts of an organ (as between two parts of the heart *or* between the two sides of the nose)中隔,间隔 ◇ 见图 HEART; **interatrial septum** = membrane between the right and left atria in the heart 房间隔; **interventricular septum** = membrane between the right and left ventricles in the heart 室间隔; **nasal septum** = wall of cartilage between the two nostrils and the two parts of the nasal cavity 鼻中隔; **septum defect** = condition where a hole exists in a septum (usually the septum of the heart) 间隔缺损 (NOTE: the plural is **septa**)

sequelae *noun* disease *or* conditions which follow on from an earlier disease 后遗症: ***Kaposi's sarcoma can be a sequela of AIDS*.** 卡波西肉瘤可能是艾滋病的后遗症。***Biochemical and hormonal sequelae is the result of the eating disorders*.** 进食障碍引起生化和激素改变。(NOTE: singular is **sequela, sequel**)

sequence 1 *noun* series of things, numbers, etc., which follow each other in order 序列 **2** *verb* to put in order 排序; **to sequence amino acids** = to show how amino acids are linked together in chains to form protein 氨基酸测序

sequestrectomy *noun* surgical removal of a sequestrum 死骨切除术

◇ **sequestrum** *noun* piece of dead bone which is separated from whole bone 死骨

ser- *or* **sero-** *prefix* referring to (i) blood serum 血清 (ii) serous membrane 浆膜

sera 血清,浆液 *see* 见 SERUM

serine *noun* an amino acid in protein 丝氨酸

serious *adjective* very bad 严重的: ***He's had a serious illness*.** 他得了重病。***There was a serious accident on the motorway*.** 机动车道上出了严重的交通事故。***There is a serious shortage of plasma*.** 血浆严重短缺。

◇ **seriously** *adverb* in a serious way 严重地: ***She is seriously ill*.** 她病得很重。

serological *adjective* referring to serology 血清学的: **serological diagnosis** = diagnosis which comes from testing serum 血清学诊断; **serological type** = SEROTYPE 血清型

◇ **serology** *noun* scientific study of serum and antibodies contained in it 血清学

◇ **seronegative** *adjective* (person) who gives a negative reaction to a serological test 血清学试验阴性的

◇ **seropositivity** *noun* giving a positive reaction to a serological test 血清学试验阳性

◇ **seropositive** *adjective* (person) who gives a positive reaction to a serological test 血清学试验阳性的

◇ **seropus** *noun* mixture of serum and pus 浆液性脓

◇ **serosa** *noun* serous membrane, the membrane which lines an internal cavity which has no contact with air (such as the peritoneum)浆膜

◇ **serositis** *noun* inflammation of serous membrane 浆膜炎

◇ **serotherapy** *noun* treatment of a disease using serum from immune individuals or immunized animals 血清治疗

◇ **serotonin** *noun* compound (5-hydroxytryptamine) which exists mainly in blood platelets and is released after tissue is injured 血清素,5-羟色胺

◇ **serotype** *or* **serological type 1** *noun* (i) category of microorganisms *or* bacteria that have some antigens in common 微生物的血清型 (ii) series of common antigens which exists in microorganisms and bacteria 抗原的血清学分型 **2** *verb* to group microorganisms and bacteria according to their antigens 按抗原血清型分型

◇ **serous** *adjective* referring to serum *or* producing serum *or* like serum 血清的,浆液的; **serous membrane** *or* **serosa** = membrane which lines an internal cavity which has no contact with air (such as the peritoneum and pleura) and covers the organs in the cavity (such as the heart and lungs) 浆膜

serpens 匐行的 *see* 见 ERYTHEMA

serpiginous *adjective* (i) (ulcer *or* eruption) which creeps across the skin 匐行的 (ii) (wound *or* ulcer) with a wavy edge 锯齿状的

serrated *adjective* (wound) with a zigzag *or* saw-like edge 锯齿状的

◇ **serration** *noun* one of the points in a zigzag *or* serrated edge 锯齿形

Sertoli cells *noun* cells which support the seminiferous tubules in the testis 塞尔托利细胞(支持睾丸内输精管的细胞)

serum *noun* (**a**) **blood serum** = yellowish watery liquid which separates from (whole) blood when the blood clots 血清; **serum albumin** = major protein in blood serum 血清白蛋白; **serum globulin** = major protein in blood serum which is an antibody 血清球蛋白 (**b**) **antitoxic serum** = immunizing agent formed of serum taken from an animal which has developed antibodies to a disease and used to protect a patient from that disease 抗毒素血清(抗血清); **snake bite serum** = ANTIVENENE 抗蛇毒血清; **serum hepatitis** = HEPATITIS B 血清性肝炎,乙型肝炎; **serum sickness** = anaphylactic shock, an allergic reaction to a serum injection 血清病 *see also* 参见 ANTISERUM (NOTE: plural is **sera**, **serums**)

> COMMENT: Blood serum is plasma without the clotting agents. It contains salt and small quantities of albumin, globulin, aminoacids, fats and sugars; its main component is water. Serum used in serum therapy is taken from specially treated animals; in rare cases this can cause an allergic reaction in a patient.
> 注释:血清是去掉了凝血因子的血浆。它含有盐和小量白蛋白、球蛋白、氨基酸、脂肪和糖,它的主要成分是水。从经特殊处理的动物体内提取的血清可用于血清治疗,但在极少数病例中出现过敏反应。

service *noun* group of people working together 公共服务组织; ***the National Health Service*** = British medical system, including all doctors, nurses, dentists, hospitals, clinics, etc., which provide free or cheap treatment to patients 国家保健事业

sesamoid bone *noun* any small bony nodule in a tendon, the largest being the kneecap 籽骨

sessile *adjective* anything which has no stem (often applied to a tumour) 无柄的,无蒂的 (NOTE: the opposite is **pedunculate**)

session *noun* visit of a patient to a therapist for treatment 一次治疗: ***She has two sessions a week of physiotherapy.*** 她每周有两次理疗。***The evening session had to be cancelled because the therapist was ill.*** 晚上那次治疗不得不取消了,因为治疗师病了。

set *verb* (**a**) to put the parts of a broken bone back into their proper places and keep the bone fixed until it has mended (骨折)复位: ***The doctor set his broken arm.*** 医生将他的断臂复位。(**b**) (*of a broken bone*) to mend *or* to form a solid bone again (骨折)复位并固定: ***His arm has set very quickly.*** 他的手臂很快复位了。***Her broken wrist is setting very well.*** 她折了的腕骨复位很好。*see also* 参见 RESET

settle *verb* (*of a sediment*) to fall to the bottom of a liquid (沉淀)下沉; (*of a parasite*) (to attach itself *or* to stay in a part of the body 寄生虫在体内寄生: ***The fluke settles in the liver.*** 吸虫在肝脏寄生。

sever *verb* to cut off 切断: ***His hand was severed at the wrist.*** 他的手从腕部被切断了。***Surgeons tried to sew the severed finger back onto the patient's hand.*** 外科医师试图将断指再缝合到病人的手上去。

severe *adjective* very bad 严重的: ***The***

patient is suffering from severe bleeding. 病人严重出血。***A severe outbreak of whooping cough occurred during the winter.*** 冬天发生了严重的百日咳爆发流行。***She is suffering from severe vitamin D deficiency.*** 她严重缺乏维生素D。

◇ **severely** *adverb* very badly 严重地：***Severely handicapped children need special care.*** 严重残疾的孩子需要特殊照顾。***Her breathing was severely affected.*** 严重影响了她的呼吸。

◇ **severity** *noun* degree to which something is bad 严重性：***Treatment depends on the severity of the attack.*** 治疗依发作的严重性而定。

> QUOTE：Many severely confused patients, particularly those in advanced stages of Alzheimer's disease, do not respond to verbal communication.
> 引文：许多严重迷乱的病人，特别是那些阿尔茨海默病进展期的患者，对言语交流没有反应。
>
> **Nursing Times** 护理时代

sex *noun* (**a**) one of two groups (male and female) into which animals and plants can be divided 性别：***The sex of a baby can be identified before birth.*** 出生前就可以确定婴儿的性别。***The relative numbers of the two sexes in the population are not equal, more males being born than females.*** 人口中两性的相对数目不是相等的，出生的男性比女性多。**sex act** = act of sexual intercourse 性活动（指性交）；**sex chromatin** = Barr body, chromatin found only in female cells, which can be used to identify the sex of a baby before birth 性染色质；**sex determination** = way in which the sex of an individual organism is fixed by the number of chromosomes which make up its cell structure 性别决定；**sex organs** = organs which are associated with reproduction and sexual intercourse (such as the testes and penis in men, and the ovaries, Fallopian tubes, vagina and vulva in women) 性器官 (**b**) sexual intercourse 性交；**safe sex** = measures to reduce the possibility of catching a sexually transmitted disease, such as using a contraceptive sheath and having only one sexual partner 安全的性交

◇ **sex chromosome** *noun* chromosome which determines if a person is male or female 性染色体

> COMMENT：Out of the twenty-three pairs of chromosomes in each human cell, two are sex chromosomes which are known as X and Y. Females have a pair of X chromosomes and males have a pair consisting of one X and one Y chromosome. The sex of a baby is determined by the father's sperm. While the mother's ovum only carries X chromosomes, the father's sperm can carry either an X or a Y chromosome. If the ovum is fertilized by a sperm carrying an X chromosome, the embryo will contain the XX pair and so be female.
> 注释：每个人体细胞的23对染色体中有2个是性染色体，即我们熟知的X染色体和Y染色体。婴儿的性别是由父亲的精子决定的。母亲的卵子只携带有X染色体，而父亲的精子则携带有X或Y染色体。如果卵子与携带着X染色体的精子发生受精，胚胎含有一对X染色体，这样就是女性。

◇ **sex hormone** *noun* hormone secreted by the testis *or* ovaries, which regulates sexual development and reproductive functions 性激素

> COMMENT：The male sex hormones are androgens (testosterone and androsterone), and the female hormones are oestrogen and progesterone
> 注释：男性激素为雄激素（睾酮和雄甾酮），女性激素是雌激素和孕激素。

◇ **sex-linkage** *noun* existence of characteristics which are transmitted through the X chromosomes 性连锁

◇ **sex-linked** *adjective* (i) (genes) which are linked to X chromosomes 性连锁的，与X染色体连锁的 (ii) (characteristics, such as colour-blindness) which are transmitted through the X chromosomes 借X染色体传递的性状

◇ **sexology** *noun* study of sex and sexual behaviour 性学

◇ **sexual** *adjective* referring to sex 性别的;**sexual act** *or* **sexual intercourse** *or* **coitus** = action of inserting the man's erect penis into the woman's vagina, and releasing spermatozoa from the penis by ejaculation, which may fertilize ova from the woman's ovaries 性活动,性交;**sexual reproduction** = reproduction in which gametes from two individuals fuse together 有性生殖

◇ **sexually transmitted disease** (**STD**) *noun* any of several diseases which are transmitted from an infected person to another person during sexual intercourse 性传播疾病

> COMMENT: Among the commonest STDs are non-specific urethritis, genital herpes, hepatitis B and gonorrhoea; AIDS is also a sexually transmitted disease.
> 注释:最常见的性传播疾病有非特异性尿道炎、生殖器疱疹、乙型肝炎和淋病;艾滋病也是一种性传播疾病。

sextuplet *noun* one of six babies born to a mother at the same time 六胞胎 *see also* 参见 QUADRUPLET, QUINTUPLET, TRIPLET, TWIN

shaft *noun* (i) long central section of a long bone 骨干 (ii) main central section of the erect penis 勃起阴茎的干,阴茎体

shake *verb* to move *or* make something move with short quick movements 打颤,寒战

sharp *adjective* (**a**) which cuts easily 锋利: ***A surgeon's knife has to be kept sharp***. 外科医师的刀必须保持锋利。(**b**) acute (pain) (as opposed to dull pain) 锐(痛): ***She felt a sharp pain in her shoulder***. 她感到肩膀一阵刺痛。

◇ **sharply** *adverb* suddenly 突然地: ***His condition deteriorated sharply during the night***. 夜间他的状况突然恶化。

shave 1 *noun* cutting off hair level with the skin with a razor 刮(体毛),如剃须 **2** *verb* to cut off hair level with the skin with a razor 刮(体毛),如剃须: ***He cut himself while shaving***. 他剃须时划伤了自己。***The nurse shaved the area where the surgeon was going to make the incision***. 护士刮外科医师要做手术切口处的体毛。

sheath *noun* (**a**) layer of tissue which surrounds a muscle *or* a bundle of nerve fibres 鞘(如肌鞘,神经鞘) (**b**) (**contraceptive**) **sheath** = condom, rubber covering put over the penis before sexual intercourse as a protection against infection and also as a contraceptive 避孕套

shed 1 *verb* to lose (blood *or* tissue) 脱落,脱换: ***The lining of the uterus is shed at each menstrual period***. 子宫的内膜每次月经期都要脱换。***He was given a transfusion because he had shed a lot of blood***. 因为他失血量很大,所以给他输血。(NOTE: **sheds-shedding-shed-has shed**)

sheet) **2** *noun* large piece of cloth which is put on a bed 床单: ***The sheets must be changed each day***. 床单必须每天更换。***The soiled sheets were sent to the hospital laundry***. 脏床单被送到医院的洗衣房。*see also* 参见 DRAW-SHEET

shelf operation *noun* surgical operation to treat congenital dislocation of the hip in children, where bone tissue is grafted onto the acetabulum 支架手术,关节造顶术

sheltered accommodation *or* **sheltered housing** *noun* rooms *or* small flats provided for elderly people, with a resident supervisor or nurse 敬老院,福利院

shift *noun* (**a**) way of working, where one group of workers work for a period and are then replaced by another group 轮班;period of time worked by a group of workers 轮值时间: ***She is working on the night shift***. 她正在上夜班。***The day shift comes on duty at 6:30 in the***

***morning*.** 白班早晨六点半接班。(**b**) movement迁移,运动; **Purkinje shift** = change in colour sensitivity which takes place in the eye in low light when the eye starts using the rods in the retina because the light is too weak to stimulate the cones 普肯耶迁移(人眼在弱光下色觉敏感性改变的现象,由于视锥细胞不能被弱光激活,只有视杆细胞工作所致)

Shigella *noun* genus of bacteria which causes dysentery 志贺杆菌属

◊ **shigellosis** *noun* infestation of the digestive tract with *Shigella*, causing bacillary dysentery 志贺杆菌引起的疾病,即细菌性痢疾

shin *noun* front part of the lower leg 胫,胫部; **shin splints** = extremely sharp pains in the front of the lower leg, felt by athletes 外胫夹(运动员在趾长屈肌劳损后出现的沿胫骨疼痛)

◊ **shinbone** *noun* the tibia 胫骨

shingles = HERPES ZOSTER 带状疱疹

Shirodkar's operation *or* **Shirodkar pursestring** *noun* surgical operation to narrow the cervix of the womb in a woman who suffers from habitual abortion, to prevent another miscarriage, the suture being removed before labour starts 宫颈缩窄术(防止流产)

shiver *verb* to tremble *or* shake all over the body because of cold *or* a fever, caused by the involuntary rapid contraction and relaxation of the muscles 战栗,寒战

◊ **shivering** *noun* trembling *or* shaking all over the body because of cold *or* a fever, caused by the involuntary rapid contraction and relaxation of the muscles 颤抖

shock 1 *noun* (**a**) weakness caused by illness *or* injury, which suddenly reduces the blood pressure 休克: ***The patient went into shock*.** 病人休克了。***Several of the passengers were treated for shock*.** 几位乘客因休克而接受治疗。***A patient in shock should be kept warm and lying down, until plasma or blood transfusions can be given*.** 应让休克的病人保持温暖平卧,直到输血或血浆为止。**neurogenic shock** = state of shock caused by bad news *or* an unpleasant surprise 神经性休克(遭受精神上的打击后的休克); **traumatic shock** = state of shock caused by an injury which leads to loss of blood 创伤性休克; **shock syndrome** = group of symptoms (pale face, cold skin, low blood pressure, rapid and irregular pulse) which show that a patient is in a state of shock 休克综合征 *see also* 参见 ANAPHYLACTIC (NOTE: you say that someone is **in shock**, **in a state of shock or went into shock**) (**b**) **electric shock** = sudden pain caused by the passage of an electric current through the body 电休克; **shock therapy** *or* **shock treatment** = method of treating some mental disorders by giving the patient an electric shock to induce an epileptic convulsion 休克疗法,休克治疗 **2** *verb* to give someone an unpleasant surprise, and so put him in a state of shock 震荡: ***She was still shocked several hours after the accident*.** 事故几个小时后她还处在脑震荡状态。

shoe *noun* piece of clothing made of leather or hard material which is worn on the foot 鞋; **surgical shoe** = specially made shoe to support *or* correct a deformed foot 外科鞋

short *adjective* lacking *or* with not enough of something 短缺; **short of breath** = unable to breathe quickly enough to supply the oxygen needed 呼吸急促: ***After running up the stairs he was short of breath*.** 跑上楼之后他呼吸急促。

◊ **shortness of breath** *noun* panting, being unable to breathe quickly enough to supply oxygen needed 呼吸急促

◊ **shortsighted** = MYOPIC 近视的

◊ **shortsightedness** = MYOPIA 近视

shot *noun* (*informal* 非正式) injection 注射: ***The doctor gave him a tetanus***

shot*.** 医生给他打了破伤风针。He needed a shot of morphine to relieve the pain*.** 他需要注射一针吗啡来缓解疼痛。

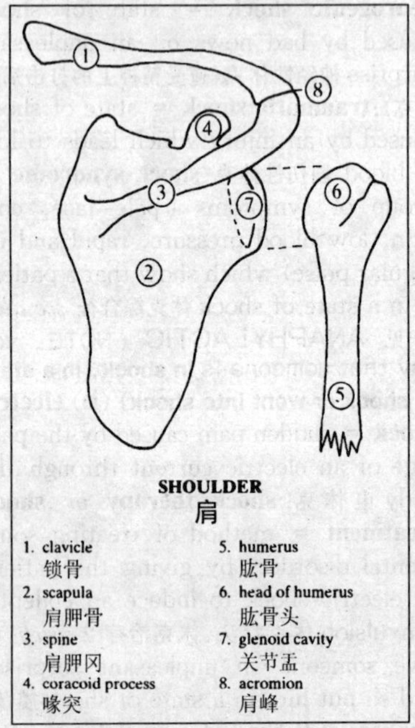

SHOULDER
肩

1. clavicle 锁骨
2. scapula 肩胛骨
3. spine 肩胛冈
4. coracoid process 喙突
5. humerus 肱骨
6. head of humerus 肱骨头
7. glenoid cavity 关节盂
8. acromion 肩峰

shoulder *noun* joint where the top of the arm joins the main part of the body 肩: ***He dislocated his shoulder*.** 他肩膀脱臼了。***She was complaining of pains in her shoulder or of shoulder pains*.** 她主诉肩膀疼。**shoulder blade** *or* **scapula** = one of two large triangular flat bones covering the top part of the back 肩胛骨; **shoulder girdle** *or* **pectoral girdle** = the shoulder bones (scapulae and clavicles) to which the arm bones are attached 肩胛带; **shoulder joint** = ball and socket joint which allows the arm to rotate and move in any direction 肩关节; **shoulder lift** = way of carrying a heavy patient where the upper part of his body rests on the shoulders of two carriers 肩扛法; **frozen shoulder** = stiffness and pain in the shoulder, after injury *or* after the shoulder has been immobile for some time, when it may be caused by inflammation of the membranes of the shoulder joint with deposits forming in the tendons 冻肩(肩关节受伤或患病后疼痛僵硬)

show *noun* first discharge of blood at the beginning of childbirth 血先露,见红

shrivel *verb* to become dry and wrinkled 皱缩

shuffling walk *or* **shuffling gait** *noun* way of walking (as in Parkinson's disease) where the feet are not lifted off the ground 拖曳步态

shunt 1 *noun* (i) passing of blood through a channel which is not the usual one 分流 (ii) channel which links two different blood vessels and carries blood from one to the other 短路; **portocaval shunt** = artificial passage made between the portal vein and the inferior vena cava to relieve pressure on the liver 门腔静脉分流术(将下腔静脉和门静脉吻合以减少肝脏的血流负荷); **right-left shunt** = defect in the heart, allowing blood to flow from the pulmonary artery to the aorta 右向左分流(心脏缺损右侧的血向左侧分流) **2** *verb* (*of blood*) to pass through a channel which is not the normal one 分流: ***As much as 5% of venous blood can be shunted unoxygenated back to the arteries*.** 有5%的静脉血未经氧化便分流回动脉。

◇ **shunting** *noun* condition where some of the deoxygenated blood in the lungs does not come into contact with air, and full gas exchange does not take place 短路分流(未氧合的血不与空气接触,未发生血氧交换的状况)

Si *chemical symbol for* silicon 硅的化学元素符号

SI *abbreviation for* (缩写) Systme International, the international system of metric measurements 国际单位制; **SI units** = international system of units for measuring physical properties (such as weight *or* speed *or* light, etc.) 国际单位

sial- *or* **sialo-** *prefix* meaning (i) saliva 唾液 (ii) a salivary gland 唾液腺

◇ **sialadenitis** *or* **sialodenitis** *or* **sialitis** *noun* inflammation of a salivary gland 唾液腺炎

◇ **sialagogue** *or* **sialogogue** *noun* substance which increases the production of saliva 促进唾液分泌的物质

◇ **sialography** *or* **ptyalography** *noun* X-ray examination of a salivary gland 唾液腺造影

◇ **sialolith** *or* **ptyalith** *noun* stone in a salivary gland 唾液腺结石

◇ **sialorrhoea** *noun* production of an excessive amount of saliva 唾液溢出

Siamese twins *or* **conjoined twins** *noun* twins who are joined together at birth 暹逻孪生子,联体双胎

COMMENT: Siamese twins are always identical twins, and can be joined at the head, chest or hip. In some cases Siamese twins can be separated by surgery, but this is not possible if they share a single important organ, such as the heart.
注释:联体双胎总是同卵双胎,可以是头部、胸部或髋部相连。有些联体双胎能够用外科手术分开,但如果他们共用一个重要脏器,如心脏,就不可能了。

sib = SIBLING 血缘的,同胞的

sibilant *adjective* (*applied to a rale*) whistling (sound)哮鸣音(罗音的一种)

sibling *noun* brother *or* sister 兄弟或姊妹

Sichuan flu *noun* (*informal* 非正式) virulent type of flu 四川流感

COMMENT: The virus was first discovered in 1987 in Sichuan, a southwestern province of China; the symptoms are the same as those of ordinary flu (fever, sore throat, aching muscles, etc.) but more pronounced.
注释:该病毒于 1987 年首先在中国四川被发现;症状与普通流感相同(发热、嗓子疼、肌肉疼痛等)但是更显著。

sick *adjective* (**a**) ill *or* not well 病了: ***He was sick for two weeks.*** 他病了两周了。***She's off sick from work.*** 工作使她病愈。**to report sick** = to say officially that you are ill and cannot work 患病证明 (**b**) wanting to vomit, having a condition where food is brought up from the stomach into the mouth 反胃,恶心: ***The patient got up this morning and felt sick.*** 病人今晨起来感到恶心。***He was given something to make him sick.*** 给他吃的东西使他感到恶心。***The little boy ate too much and was sick all over the floor.*** 小男孩吃得太多,吐得满地都是。***She had a sick feeling*** *or* ***she felt sick.*** = She felt that she wanted to vomit. 她感到恶心想吐。

◇ **sickbay** *noun* room where patients can visit a doctor for treatment in a factory *or* on a ship 医务室

◇ **sickbed** *noun* bed where a person is lying sick 病床: ***She sat for hours beside her daughter's sickbed.*** 她在女儿的病榻旁坐了好几个小时。

◇ **sick building syndrome** *noun* condition where many people working in a building feel ill or have headaches, caused by blocked air-conditioning ducts in which stale air is recycled round the building, often carrying allergenic substances or bacteria 建筑致病综合征(很多在建筑物内工作的人都有的一种不适和头疼感,是因为空调管道堵塞,腐臭的带有致敏物质或细菌的空气在建筑物内循环所致)

◇ **sicken for** *verb* (*informal* 非正式) to begin to have an illness *or* to feel the first symptoms of an illness 染病之初: ***She's looking pale - she must be sickening for something.*** 她看上去脸色苍白,一定是得了什么病。

◇ **sicklist** *noun* list of people (children in a school *or* workers in a factory) who are sick 患者名单: ***We have five members of staff on the sicklist.*** 我们有 5 名工作人员上了病号名单。

◇ **sickly** *adjective* (*usually of children*) always slightly ill *or* never completely well; weak *or* subject to frequent sickness 病病怏怏的: ***He was a sickly child, but now is a strong and healthy man.*** 他曾是个病病怏怏的孩子,但现在是个强壮健康的男子汉了。

◇ **sickness** *or* **illness** *noun* (**a**) not being well 患病,生病: ***There is a lot of sickness in the winter months.*** 冬天有许多人生病。***Many children are staying away from school because of sickness.*** 许多孩子因患病而不能上学。*see also* 参见 SEASICKNESS, TRAVEL SICKNESS (**b**) feeling of wanting to vomit 恶心,反胃

◇ **sickroom** *noun* bedroom where someone is ill 病房: ***Visitors are not allowed into the sickroom.*** 探视者不允许进入病房。

sickle cell *noun* drepanocyte, an abnormal red blood cell shaped like a sickle, due to an abnormal haemoglobin (HbS), which can cause blockage of capillaries 镰状细胞; **sickle-cell disease (SCD)** = disease caused by sickle cells in the blood 镰状细胞病; **sickle-cell anaemia** *or* **drepanocytosis** = hereditary condition where the patient develops sickle cells which block the circulation, causing anaemia and pains in the joints and abdomen 镰状细胞贫血; **sickle-cell chest syndrome** = common complication of sickle-cell disease, with chest pain, fever and leucocytosis 镰状细胞性胸部综合征(镰状细胞病常见的并发症,表现为胸痛、发热和白细胞增多)

> COMMENT: Sickle-cell anaemia is a hereditary condition which is mainly found in Africa and the West Indies.
> 注释:镰状细胞贫血是一种遗传病,主要见于非洲和西印度群岛。

> QUOTE: Children with sickle-cell anaemia are susceptible to severe bacterial infection. Even children with the milder forms of sickle-cell disease have an increased frequency of pneumococcal infection.
> 引文:镰状细胞贫血的孩子易患严重的细菌感染。即便是相对轻微的镰状细胞病患儿患肺炎球菌感染的机会也要增高。
> **Lancet** 柳叶刀

side *noun* (i) part of the body between the hips and the shoulder 肋,身体的侧面 (ii) part of an object which is not the front, back, top or bottom 侧面: ***She was lying on her side.*** 她侧躺着。***The nurse wheeled the trolley to the side of the bed.*** 护士把平车推到病床旁。**side rails** = rails at the side of a bed which can be lifted to prevent a patient falling out(病床的)侧档 *see also* 参见 BEDSIDE

◇ **side-effect** *noun* effect produced by a drug *or* treatment which is not the main effect intended 副作用: ***One of the side-effects of chemotherapy is that the patient's hair falls out.*** 化疗的副作用之一是病人脱发。***Doctors do not recommend using the drug for long periods because of the unpleasant side-effects.*** 医生们不推荐长期用这种药物,因为它引起令人不快的副作用。***The drug is being withdrawn because of its side-effects.*** 因为副作用而把这个药撤了。

> QUOTE: The treatment is not without possible side-effects, some of which can be particularly serious. The side-effects may include middle ear discomfort, claustrophobia, increased risk of epilepsy.
> 引文:治疗不可能没有副作用,有些副作用还特别严重。副作用包括中耳不适、幽闭恐怖、癫痫的危险性增加。
> **New Zealand Medical Journal**
> 新西兰医学杂志

sidero- *prefix* referring to iron 铁

◇ **sideropenia** *noun* lack of iron in the blood probably caused by insufficient iron in diet 铁缺乏症

◇ **siderophilin** *or* **transferrin** *noun* substance found in the blood, which carries iron in the bloodstream 载铁蛋白

◇ **siderosis** *noun* (i) condition where iron deposits form in tissue 铁质沉着 (ii) inflammation of the lungs caused by inhaling dust containing iron 肺铁末沉着病,铁尘肺

SIDS = SUDDEN INFANT DEATH SYNDROME 婴儿猝死综合征

sight *noun* one of the five senses, the ability to see 视觉: ***His sight is beginning to fail.*** 他的视力开始减退。***Sur-***

geons are fighting to save her sight. 外科医师们努力保住她的视力。***He lost his sight.*** = He became blind. 他失明了。

◇ **sighted** *adjective* (person) who can see 视力健全的: ***the sighted*** = people who can see 视力健全者; ***He is partially sighted and uses a white stick.*** 他的视力不全,得用马竿。

sigmoid *or* **sigmoid colon** *or* **sigmoid flexure** *noun* fourth section of the colon which joins the rectum 乙状结肠 ◇ 见图 DIGESTIVE SYSTEM

◇ **sigmoidectomy** *noun* surgical operation to remove the sigmoid colon 乙状结肠切除术

◇ **sigmoidoscope** *noun* surgical instrument with a light at the end which can be passed into the rectum so that the sigmoid colon can be examined 乙状结肠镜

◇ **sigmoidostomy** *noun* surgical operation to bring the sigmoid colon out through a hole in the abdominal wall 乙状结肠造口术

sign 1 *noun* (**a**) movement *or* mark *or* colouring *or* change which has a meaning and can be recognized by a doctor as indicating a condition 体征 (NOTE: a change in function which is also noticed by the patient is a **symptom**) (**b**) **sign language** = signs made with the fingers and hands, used to indicate words when talking to a deaf and dumb person, or when such a person wants to communicate 手语 **2** *verb* to write one's name on a form, cheque, etc. or at the end of a letter 签字: ***The doctor signed the death certificate.*** 医生签署了死亡证明。

◇ **signature** *noun* name which someone writes when he signs 签字: ***The chemist could not read the doctor's signature.*** 药剂师认不得医生的签字。***Her signature is easy to recognize.*** 她的签字易于辨认。

significant *adjective* important, worth noting 明显的: ***No significant inflammatory responses were observed.*** 未观察到明显的炎症反应。

◇ **significantly** *adverb* in an important manner, in a manner worth noting 明显地: ***He was not significantly better on the following day.*** = He was not much better. 次日他没有明显好转。

silence *noun* lack of noise *or* lack of speaking 沉默: ***The crowd waited in silence.*** 人群静静地等待。

◇ **silent** *adjective* (**a**) not making any noise *or* not talking 沉默的 (**b**) not visible *or* showing no symptoms 沉寂的,无可见症状的,隐匿的: ***Genital herpes may be silent in women.*** 女性的生殖器疱疹可以是隐匿的。***Graft occlusion is often silent with 80% of patients.*** 移植血管的阻塞在 ***80%*** 的病人是隐匿的。

silicon *noun* non-metallic chemical element 硅; **silicon dioxide** = SILICA 二氧化硅 (NOTE: chemical symbol is **Si**)

◇ **silica** *noun* silicon dioxide, mineral which forms quartz and sand 二氧化硅

◇ **silicosis** *noun* form of pneumoconiosis, disease of the lungs caused by inhaling silica dust from mining *or* stonecrushing operations 矽肺

> COMMENT: This is a serious disease which makes breathing difficult and can lead to emphysema and bronchitis.
> 注释:这是一种导致呼吸困难并能引起肺气肿和支气管炎的严重疾病。

silver *noun* white-coloured metallic element 银 (NOTE: chemical symbol is **Ag**)

◇ **silver nitrate**($AgNO_3$) *noun* salt of silver, mixed with a cream or solution, used to disinfect burns, to kill warts, etc. 硝酸银(用于消毒烧伤创面)

Silvester method *noun* method of giving artificial respiration where the patient lies on his back and the firstaider brings the patient's hands together on his chest and then moves them above the patient's head 西尔韦斯特法(一种人工呼吸方法) *see also* 参见 HOLGER-NIELSEN METHOD

Simmonds' disease *noun* condition

of women where there is lack of activity in the pituitary gland, resulting in wasting of tissue, brittle bones and premature senility, due to postpartum haemorrhage 西蒙兹病(女性垂体功能低下,导致组织废用,骨质变脆和早衰,由于产后出血造成)

simple *adjective* ordinary *or* not very complicated 简单的; **simple epithelium** = epithelium formed of a single layer of cells 单层上皮; **simple fracture** = fracture where the skin surface around the damaged bone has not been broken and the broken ends of the bone are close together 单纯骨折 *see also* 参见 TACHYCARDIA

simplex 单纯的 *see* 见 HERPES

sinew *noun* ligament, the tissue which holds together the bones at a joint; tendon *or* tissue which attaches a muscle to a bone 腱

singultus = HICCUP 1 呃逆

sino- *or* **sinu-** *prefix* referring to a sinus 窦

◇ **sinoatrial node** (**SA node**) *noun* node in the heart at the junction of the superior vena cava and the right atrium, which regulates the heartbeat 窦房结

◇ **sinogram** *noun* X-ray photograph of a sinus 窦道造影

◇ **sinography** *noun* examining a sinus by taking an X-ray photograph 窦道造影术

◇ **sinuatrial node** = SINOATRIAL NODE 窦房结

sinus *noun* (i) cavity inside the body, including the cavities inside the head behind the cheekbone, forehead and nose 鼻窦 (ii) tract *or* passage which develops between an infected place where pus has gathered and the surface of the skin 窦道 (iii) wide venous blood space 静脉窦: ***He has had sinus trouble during the winter.*** 冬天他的鼻窦爱犯毛病。***The doctor diagnosed a sinus infection.*** 医生诊断了鼻窦感染。**carotid sinus** = expanded part attached to the carotid artery which monitors blood pressure in the skull 颈动脉窦(有监测颅内血压的作用); **cavernous sinus** = one of two cavities in the skull behind the eyes, which form part of the venous drainage system 海绵窦; **coronary sinus** = vein which takes most of the venous blood from the heart muscles to the right atrium 冠状窦(入右心房前的大静脉窦); **ethmoidal sinuses** = air cells inside the ethmoid bone 筛窦; **frontal sinus** = one of two sinuses in the front of the face above the eyes and near the nose 额窦; **maxillary sinus** = one of two sinuses behind the cheekbones in the upper jaw 上颌窦; **paranasal sinus** = one of the four pairs of sinuses in the skull near the nose(the frontal, maxillary, ethmoidal and sphenoidal) 鼻旁窦; **renal sinus** = cavity in which the tubes leading into a kidney go 肾窦; **sphenoidal sinus** = one of two sinuses behind the nasal passage 蝶窦; **sinus nerve** = nerve which branches from the glossopharyngeal nerve 窦神经(舌咽神经的分支) *see also* 参见 TACHYCARDIA

◇ **sinusitis** *or* **sinus trouble** *noun* inflammation of the mucous membrane in the sinuses, especially the maxillary sinuses 鼻窦炎: ***She has sinus trouble.*** = She has an inflammation of the sinuses. 她有鼻窦炎。

◇ **sinusoid** *noun* specially shaped small blood vessel in the liver, adrenal glands and other organs 窦状的

◇ **sinus venosus** *noun* cavity in the heart of an embryo, part of which develops into the coronary sinus, and part of which is absorbed into the right atrium 静脉窦(胎心的一个腔,一部分发育成冠状窦,一部分没入右心房)

siphonage *noun* removing liquid from one place to another, with a tube, as used to empty the stomach of its contents 虹吸

Sippy diet *noun US* alkaline diet of

milk and dry biscuits as a treatment for peptic ulcers 西皮氏饮食(牛奶,饼干组成的碱性饮食,治疗消化性溃疡)

sister *noun* (**a**) female who has the same father and mother as another child 姐妹,姊妹: ***He has three sisters.*** 他有三个姐妹。***Her sister works in a children's clinic.*** 她的姐姐在儿科诊所工作。(**b**) senior nurse 资深护士; **sister in charge** *or* **ward sister** = senior nurse in charge of a hospital ward 护士长,病房护士长; **nursing sister** = sister with certain administrative duties 护理部护士长 (NOTE: sister can be used with names: **Sister Jones**)

sit up *verb* (i) to sit with your back straight 坐直了 (ii) to move from a lying to a sitting position 坐起来: ***The patient is sitting up in bed.*** 病人从床上坐起来了。(NOTE: **sits - sitting - sat - has sat**)

site 1 *noun* position of something *or* place where something happened; place where an incision is to be made in an operation 位置,切口位置: ***The X-ray showed the site of the infection.*** X线片显示了感染的位置。**2** *verb* to put something *or* to be in a particular place 位于: ***The infection is sited in the right lung.*** 感染位于右肺。

QUOTE: Arterial thrombi have a characteristic structure: platelets adhere at sites of endothelial damage and attract other platelets to form a dense aggregate.
引文:动脉血栓具有典型结构:血小板附着于上皮损坏的部位,吸引其他血小板形成一个致密的凝块。
British Journal of Hospital Medicine 英国医院医学杂志

QUOTE: The sublingual site is probably the most acceptable and convenient for taking temperature.
引文:舌下可能是最易被患者接受和最方便的试体温的位置。
Nursing Times 护理杂志

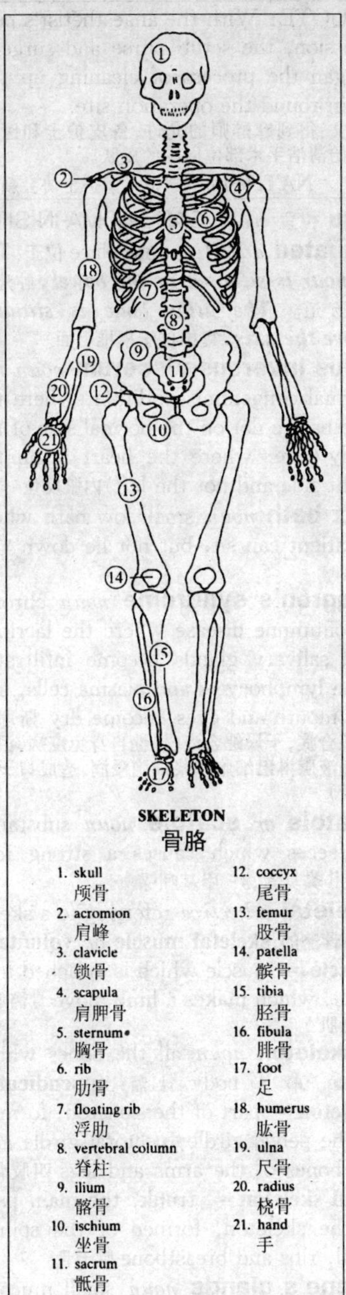

SKELETON
骨胳

1. skull 颅骨
2. acromion 肩峰
3. clavicle 锁骨
4. scapula 肩胛骨
5. sternum• 胸骨
6. rib 肋骨
7. floating rib 浮肋
8. vertebral column 脊柱
9. ilium 髂骨
10. ischium 坐骨
11. sacrum 骶骨
12. coccyx 尾骨
13. femur 股骨
14. patella 髌骨
15. tibia 胫骨
16. fibula 腓骨
17. foot 足
18. humerus 肱骨
19. ulna 尺骨
20. radius 桡骨
21. hand 手

QUOTE: With the anaesthetist's permission, the scrub nurse and surgeon began the process of cleaning up the skin round the operation site.
引文:得到麻醉师的允许,备皮护士和医生开始清洁手术部位周围的皮肤。
NATNews 全国手术室护士协会新闻

situ 位置 *see* 见 CARCINOMA-IN-SITU

situated *adjective* in a place 位于: ***The tumour is situated in the bowel.*** 肿瘤位于肠道。***The atlas bone is situated above the axis.*** 寰椎位于枢椎上面。

situs inversus viscerum *noun* abnormal congenital condition, where the organs are not on the normal side of the body (i. e. where the heart is on the right side and not the left) 内脏反位

sitz bath *noun* small low bath where a patient can sit, but not lie down 坐浴盆

Sjögren's syndrome *noun* chronic autoimmune disease where the lacrimal and salivary glands become infiltrated with lymphocytes and plasma cells, and the mouth and eyes become dry 斯耶格伦综合症,干燥综合症(慢性自身免疫病,泪腺和唾液腺淋巴细胞和浆细胞浸润,造成口干和眼干)

skatole *or* **scatole** *noun* substance in faeces which causes a strong foul smell 粪臭素,3-甲基吲哚

skeletal *adjective* referring to a skeleton 骨骼的; **skeletal muscle** *or* **voluntary muscle** = muscle which is attached to a bone, which makes a limb move 骨骼肌,随意肌

◇ **skeleton** *noun* all the bones which make up a body 骨骼; **appendicular skeleton** = part of the skeleton, formed of the pelvic girdle, pectoral girdle and the bones of the arms and legs 四肢骨; **axial skeleton** = trunk, the main part of the skeleton, formed of the spine, skull, ribs and breastbone 躯干骨

Skene's glands *noun* small mucous glands in the urethra in women 斯基恩氏腺,(女性)尿道旁腺

skia- *prefix* meaning shadow 影(尤指X线影)

◇ **skiagram** *noun* old term for X-ray photograph X线片的旧称

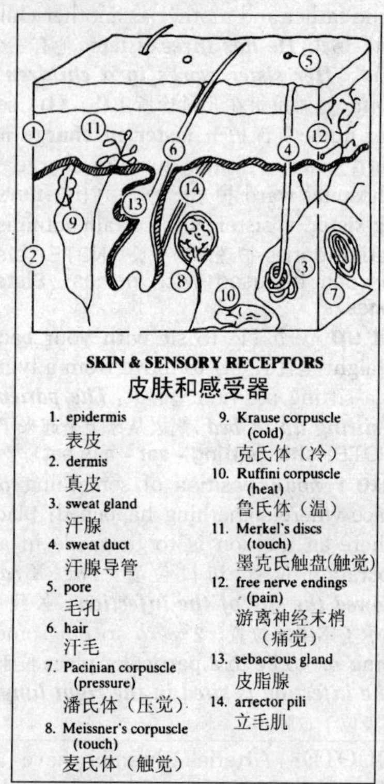

SKIN & SENSORY RECEPTORS
皮肤和感受器

1. epidermis 表皮
2. dermis 真皮
3. sweat gland 汗腺
4. sweat duct 汗腺导管
5. pore 毛孔
6. hair 汗毛
7. Pacinian corpuscle (pressure) 潘氏体(压觉)
8. Meissner's corpuscle (touch) 麦氏体(触觉)
9. Krause corpuscle (cold) 克氏体(冷)
10. Ruffini corpuscle (heat) 鲁氏体(温)
11. Merkel's discs (touch) 墨克氏触盘(触觉)
12. free nerve endings (pain) 游离神经末梢(痛觉)
13. sebaceous gland 皮脂腺
14. arrector pili 立毛肌

skill *noun* ability to do difficult work, which is acquired by training 技术: ***You need special skills to become a doctor.*** 想要成为一名医生你需要有专业技术。

◇ **skilled** *adjective* having acquired a particular skill by training 有技术的,熟练的: ***He's a skilled plastic surgeon.*** 他是一位熟练的矫形外科医师。

skin *noun* tissue (the epidermis and dermis) which forms the outside surface of the body 皮肤: ***His skin turned brown in the sun.*** 他的皮肤被阳光晒成了棕色。***After the operation she had to have a skin graft.*** 手术后,她必须进行皮肤移植。***Skin problems in adolescents may be caused by diet.*** 青少年的皮肤问题可能是饮

食引起的。***She went to see a specialist about her skin trouble.*** 她因皮肤毛病去看专家。**skin graft** = layer of skin transplanted from one part of the body to cover an area where the skin has been destroyed 皮肤移植（NOTE: for other terms referring to skin, see words beginning with **cut- or derm-**）

◇ **skinny** *adjective* (*informal* 非正式) very thin 皮包骨的

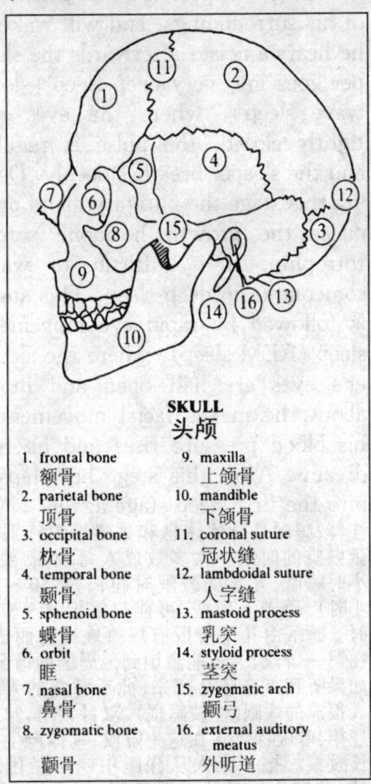

SKULL
头颅

1. frontal bone 额骨
2. parietal bone 顶骨
3. occipital bone 枕骨
4. temporal bone 颞骨
5. sphenoid bone 蝶骨
6. orbit 眶
7. nasal bone 鼻骨
8. zygomatic bone 颧骨
9. maxilla 上颌骨
10. mandible 下颌骨
11. coronal suture 冠状缝
12. lambdoidal suture 人字缝
13. mastoid process 乳突
14. styloid process 茎突
15. zygomatic arch 颧弓
16. external auditory meatus 外听道

COMMENT: The skin is the largest organ in the human body. It is formed of two layers: the epidermis is the outer layer, and includes the top layer of particles of dead skin which are continuously flaking off. Beneath the epidermis is the dermis, which is the main layer of living skin. Hairs and nails are produced by the skin, and pores in the skin secrete sweat from the sweat glands underneath the dermis. The skin is sensitive to touch and heat and cold, which are sensed by the nerve endings in the skin. The skin is a major source of vitamin D which it produces when exposed to sunlight.
注释:皮肤是人体最大的器官。它由两层组成:表皮是外层,包括不断脱落死皮碎屑的表层。上皮下面是真皮,是活皮肤主要层。毛发和指甲是皮肤里长出来的,皮肤上的毛孔分泌来自皮下汗腺的汗液。皮肤对冷热和触觉敏感,感知它们的是皮肤里的神经末梢。皮肤是维生素 D 的主要来源,这是皮肤暴露在阳光下时产生的。

skull *noun* bones which are fused *or* connected together to form the head 头骨,颅骨; **skull fracture** *or* **fracture of the skull** = condition where one of the bones in the skull has been fractured 颅骨骨折（NOTE: for other terms referring to the skull, see words beginning with **crani-**）

COMMENT: The skull is formed of eight cranial bones which make up the head, and fourteen facial bones which form the face.
注释:头颅由 8 块颅骨组成头部,14 块颜面骨构成面部。

slash 1 *noun* long cut with a knife 砍伤: ***He had bruises on his face and slashes on his hands.*** 他的脸青了,手上有砍伤。***The slash on her leg needs three stitches.*** 她腿上的刀伤需要缝 3 针。**2** *verb* (**a**) to cut with a knife *or* sharp edge 用刀砍; **to slash one's wrists** = to try to kill oneself by cutting the blood vessels in the wrists 割腕(一种自尽方式,力图割断腕部血管致死) (**b**) to cut costs *or* spending sharply 削减: ***The hospital building programme has been slashed.*** 医院建筑计划被大幅度削减了。

SLE = SYSTEMIC LUPUS ERYTHEMATOSUS 系统性红斑狼疮

sleep 1 *noun* resting (usually at night) when the eyes are closed and you are not conscious of what is happening 睡眠: ***Most people need eight hours' sleep each night.*** 大多数人每晚需要睡 8 个小时。

You need to get a good night's sleep if you have a lot of work to do tomorrow. 如果你明天有大量工作要做，晚上需要好好睡一觉。***He had a short sleep in the middle of the afternoon.*** 他下午眯了一小觉。**to get to sleep** *or* **go to sleep** = to start sleeping 入睡：***Don't make a noise, the baby is trying to go to sleep.*** 别弄出声音，婴儿正要入睡呢。*see also* 参见 RAPID EYE MOVEMENT, SLOW-WAVE **2** *verb* to be asleep *or* to rest with the eyes closed not knowing what is happening 熟睡：***He always sleeps for eight hours each night.*** 他总是每晚睡 8 个小时。Don't disturb him — he's trying to sleep. 别打搅他，他正要睡呢。(NOTE: **sleeps - sleeping - slept - has slept**)

◇ **sleeping pill** *or* **sleeping tablet** *noun* drug (usually a barbiturate) which makes a person sleep 安眠药：***She died of an overdose of sleeping tablets.*** 她死于安眠药过量。

◇ **sleeping sickness** *or* **African trypanosomiasis** *noun* African disease, spread by the tsetse fly, where trypanosomes infest the blood 昏睡病，非洲锥虫病

> COMMENT: Symptoms are headaches, lethargy and long periods of sleep. The disease is fatal if not treated.
> 注释：症状有头疼、嗜睡和长时间睡眠。这种病不治疗有生命危险。

◇ **sleeplessness** *or* **insomnia** *noun* being unable to sleep 失眠

◇ **sleepwalker** = SOMNAMBULIST 梦游症者

◇ **sleepwalking** = SOMNAMBULISM 梦游症

◇ **sleepy** *adjective* feeling ready to go to sleep 困倦的：***The children are very sleepy by 10 o'clock.*** 孩子们到十点就很困。**sleepy sickness** *or* **encephalitis lethargica** = virus infection, a form of encephalitis which occurred in epidemics in the 1920s 20 世纪睡病，昏睡性脑炎(病毒感染，20 世纪 20 年代流行的脑炎的一种) (NOTE: **sleepy - sleepier - sleepiest.** Note also that for other terms referring to sleep see words beginning with **hypn-**, **narco-**)

> COMMENT: Sleep is a period when the body rests and rebuilds tissue, especially protein. Most adults need eight hours' sleep each night. Children require more (10 to 12 hours) but old people need less, possibly only four to six hours. Sleep forms a regular pattern of stages: during the first stage the person is still conscious of his surroundings, and will wake if he hears a noise; afterwards the sleeper goes into very deep sleep (slow-wave sleep), where the eyes are tightly closed, the pulse is regular and the sleeper breathes deeply. During this stage the pituitary gland produces the growth hormone somatotrophin. It is difficult to wake someone from deep sleep. This stage is followed by rapid eye movement sleep (REM sleep), where the sleeper's eyes are half open and move about, he makes facial movements, his blood pressure rises and he has dreams. After this stage he relapses into the first sleep stage again.
> 注释：睡眠是身体休息和重建组织特别是蛋白质的时期。大多数成人每晚需 要 8 小时睡眠，儿童的睡眠时间长些(10～12 小时)，而老人短些，可能只需要 4～6 小时。睡眠由几个阶段有规律地组合而成：在第一阶段，人还能意识到他周围的情况，如果听到声音还会醒来；此后睡觉的人进入很深的睡眠(慢波睡眠)，双目紧闭，脉搏规律，呼吸深沉。在这一阶段，垂体产生生长激素。把一个人从深睡中叫醒是困难的。此期之后是快动眼睡眠，睡觉的人半闭着眼，眼球转动，面部肌肉有运动，血压升高，并做梦。此期之后，人又返回到睡眠的第一期。

slice *noun* thin flat piece of tissue which has been cut off 切片：***He examined the slice of brain tissue under the microscope.*** 他在显微镜下检查脑组织切片。

slide 1 *noun* piece of glass, on which a tissue sample is placed, to be examined under a microscope 载玻片 **2** *verb* to move along smoothly 滑动: ***The plunger slides up and down the syringe.*** 针芯在注射管内上下滑动。**sliding traction** = traction for a fracture of a femur, where weights are attached to pull the leg 滑轮牵引(股骨骨折时牵引以助复位)

slight *adjective* not very serious 轻微的: ***He has a slight fever.*** 他有点儿轻度发烧。***She had a slight accident.*** 她出了个小事故。(NOTE: **slight - slighter - slightest**)

slim 1 *adjective* pleasantly thin 苗条的: ***She has become slim again after being pregnant.*** 她怀孕后又苗条了。**2** *verb* to try to become thinner *or* to weight less 减肥: ***He stopped eating bread when he was slimming.*** 他减肥期间停止吃面包了。***She is trying to slim before she goes on holiday.*** 她力争度假前使自己瘦下来。**slimming diet** *or* **slimming food** = special diet *or* special food which is low in calories and which is supposed to stop a person getting fat 减肥饮食,减肥食品

sling *noun* triangular bandage attached round the neck, used to support an injured arm and prevent it from moving 悬带: ***She had her left arm in a sling.*** 她的左臂绑着绷带悬吊了起来。**elevation sling** = sling tied round the neck, used to hold an injured hand or arm in a high position to prevent bleeding 高位悬吊

slipped disc *noun* condition where a disc of cartilage separating two bones in the spine becomes displaced *or* where the soft centre of a disc passes through the hard cartilage outside and presses on a nerve 椎间盘脱出

slow-wave sleep *noun* period of sleep when the sleeper sleeps deeply and the eyes do not move 慢波睡眠

> COMMENT: During slow-wave sleep, the pituitary gland secretes the hormone somatotrophin.
> 注释:在慢波睡眠期垂体分泌生长激素。

slough 1 *noun* dead tissue (especially dead skin) which has separated from healthy tissue 腐痂,腐肉 **2** *verb* to lose dead skin which falls off(腐痂)脱落

small *adjective* (**a**) not large 小的: ***His chest was covered with small red spots.*** 他胸部布满小红点。***She has a small cyst in the colon.*** 她的结肠有一个小囊肿。**small intestine** = section of the intestine from the stomach to the caecum, consisting of the duodenum, jejunum and ileum 小肠; **small stomach** = stomach which is reduced in size after an operation, making the patient unable to eat large meals 小胃(胃大部切除后之残胃)(**b**) young 年轻: ***He had chickenpox when he was small.*** 他小时候出过水痘。**small children** = young children (between about 1 and 14 years of age) 小孩

◇ **small of the back** *noun* middle part of the back between and below the shoulder blades 位于肩胛骨之间及其下部的后背中部

◇ **smallpox** *noun* variola, formerly a very serious, usually fatal, contagious disease, caused by the poxvirus, with a severe rash, leaving masses of small scars on the skin 天花

> COMMENT: Vaccination has proved effective in eradicating smallpox.
> 注释:实践证明接种疫苗可有效根除天花。

> QUOTE: In 1996 it will be the 200th anniversary of Jenner's first smallpox vaccine and smallpox is now clinically extinct.
> 引文:1996 年是 Jenner 首创天花疫苗 200 周年纪念,现在,天花在临床上已经绝迹了。
> **Guardian** 卫报

smear *noun* sample of soft tissue (such as blood *or* mucus) taken from a patient and spread over a glass slide to be examined under a microscope 涂片; **cervical smear** = test for cervical cancer, where cells taken from the mucus in the cervix of the uterus are examined 宫颈涂片; **smear test** = PAP TEST 涂片检查

smegma *noun* oily secretion with an unpleasant smell, which collects on and under the foreskin of the penis 包皮垢

smell 1 *noun* one of the five senses *or* the sense which is felt through the nose 嗅觉: ***Dogs have a good sense of smell.*** 狗的嗅觉很灵敏。***The smell of flowers makes him sneeze.*** 闻到花香让他打喷嚏。**2** *verb* (**a**) to notice the smell of something through the nose 嗅，闻: ***I can smell smoke.*** 我能闻见烟味。***He can't smell anything because he's got a cold.*** 因为他得了感冒所以什么也闻不见了。(**b**) to produce a smell 散味儿: ***It smells of gas here.*** 这儿闻起来有某种气味儿。(NOTE: **smells - smelling - smelled** *or* **smelt - has smelled or has smelt**)

◊ **smelling salts** *noun* crystals of an ammonia compound, which give off a strong smell and can revive someone who has fainted 嗅盐(有强烈难闻的味儿，用于刺激癔病性晕厥的病人)

> COMMENT: The senses of smell and taste are closely connected, and together give the real taste of food. Smells are sensed by receptors in the nasal cavity which transmit impulses to the brain. When food is eaten, the smell is sensed at the same time as the taste is sensed by the taste buds, and most of what we think of as taste is in fact smell, which explains why food loses its taste when someone has a cold and a blocked nose.
> 注释:嗅觉和味觉紧密相关,一起构成食物的真正味道。嗅觉由鼻腔里的感受器感知并传递到脑的。吃东西时,味蕾感受味觉的同时嗅器官也闻到味道,我们认为是味觉的多数成分其实是嗅觉,这解释了为什么感冒鼻塞时食物失去了原有的味道。

Smith-Petersen nail *noun* metal nail used to attach the fractured neck of a femur 史密斯-彼得森钉(用于固定骨折的股骨颈)

smog *noun* pollution of the atmosphere in towns, caused by warm damp air combining with smoke and exhaust fumes from cars 烟雾

smoke 1 *noun* white, grey or black product made of small particles, given off by something which is burning 烟: ***The room was full of cigarette smoke.*** 房间里充满烟草的烟气。***Several people died from inhaling toxic smoke.*** 有几个人因吸入毒烟而死。**2** *verb* to breathe in smoke from a cigarette, cigar, pipe, etc., which is held in the lips 吸烟: ***She was smoking a cigarette.*** 她正在吸烟。***He only smokes a pipe.*** 他只吸旱烟。***Doctors are trying to persuade people to stop smoking.*** 医生们尽力劝说人们停止吸烟。***Smoking can injure your health.*** 吸烟会损害你的健康。

◊ **smokeless** *adjective* where there is no smoke *or* where smoke is not allowed 无烟的; **smokeless** *or* **smoke-free area** = part of a public place (restaurant *or* aircraft, etc.) where smoking is not allowed 无烟区,禁烟区; **smokeless fuel** = special fuel which does not make smoke when it is burnt 无烟燃料; **smokeless zone** = part of a town where open fires are not permitted 烟火管制区

◊ **smoker** *noun* person who smokes cigarettes 吸烟者，烟民; **smoker's cough** = dry asthmatic cough, often found in people who smoke large numbers of cigarettes 烟民中常见的咳嗽，喘咳

> COMMENT: The connection between smoking tobacco, especially cigarettes, and lung cancer has been proved to the satisfaction of the British government, which prints a health warning on all packets of cigarettes. Smoke from burning tobacco contains nicotine and other substances which stick in the lungs, and can in the long run cause cancer.
> 注释:吸烟,特别是吸香烟,与肺癌的关系已经被证实了,英国政府对此感到满意,并在所有烟盒上都印上了注意健康的警告。烟草的烟雾内含有尼古丁和其他可以沉积于肺的物质,长期作用会导致肺癌。

QUOTE: Three quarters of patients aged 35～64 on GPs' lists have at least one major risk factor: high cholesterol, high blood pressure or addiction

to tobacco. Of the three risk factors, smoking causes a quarter of heart disease deaths.
引文：在全科医师的病人名册上35～64岁的病人中3/4存在至少一种主要的危险因素：高胆固醇、高血压或吸烟成瘾。三个危险因素中，吸烟在心脏病致死的原因占1/4。
Health Services Journal 保健事业杂志

smooth 1 *adjective* flat *or* not rough 平滑，光滑；**smooth muscle** *or* **involuntary muscle** = muscle which moves without a person being aware of it, such as the muscle in the walls of the intestine which makes the intestine contract 平滑肌，不随意肌 *compare* 比较 STRIATED, VOLUNTARY MUSCLE (NOTE: **smooth - smoother - smoothest**) **2** *verb* to make something smooth 弄平：***She smoothed down the sheets on the bed.*** 她把床单弄平。

SMR = SUBMUCOUS RESECTION 粘膜下软骨切除

snake bite *noun* bite from a snake, especially a poisonous one 蛇咬伤（特别是毒蛇咬伤）

snare *noun* surgical instrument made of a loop of wire, used to remove growths without the need of an incision 勒除器；**diathermy snare** = snare which is heated by electrodes and burns away tissue 电烙勒除器

sneeze 1 *noun* reflex action to blow air suddenly out of the nose and mouth because of irritation in the nasal passages 喷嚏：***She gave a loud sneeze.*** 她打了个很响的喷嚏。**2** *verb* to blow air suddenly out of the nose and mouth because of irritation in the nasal passages 打喷嚏：***The smell of flowers makes him sneeze.*** 闻到花的香味使他打了个喷嚏。***He was coughing and sneezing and decided to stay in bed.*** 他又咳嗽又打喷嚏，决定卧床休息。

◇ **sneezing fit** *noun* sudden attack when the patient sneezes many times 喷嚏发作

COMMENT: A sneeze sends out a spray of droplets of liquid, which, if infectious, can then infect anyone who happens to inhale them.
注释：喷嚏喷出飞沫，如果飞沫具有感染性，碰巧吸入它们的人就可能感染。

Snellen chart *noun* chart commonly used by opticians to test eyesight 斯内伦视力表；**Snellen type** = different type sizes used on a Snellen chart 斯内伦视力表

COMMENT: The Snellen chart has rows of letters, the top row being very large, and the bottom very small, with the result that the more rows a person can read, the better his eyesight.
注释：斯内伦视力表由若干行字母组成，顶上的一行字母很大，底边的则很小，一个人检查时能读出的行越多，他的视力就越好。

sniff 1 *noun* breathing in air *or* smelling through the nose 以鼻吸气，嗅：***They gave her a sniff of smelling salts to revive her.*** 他们给她闻嗅盐让她醒来。**2** *verb* to breathe in air *or* to smell through the nose 以鼻吸气，嗅：***He was sniffing because he had a cold.*** 他感冒了，使劲用鼻子吸气。***She sniffed and said that she could smell smoke.*** 她使劲用鼻子吸吸气，说她能闻到烟味儿。***He is coughing and sniffing and should be in bed.*** 他咳嗽鼻塞，必须卧床。

◇ **sniffles** *noun* (*informal* 非正式，*used to children*) cold (when you sniff and sneeze) 感冒鼻塞：***Don't go out into the cold when you have the sniffles.*** 如果你鼻子不通气了就别到外边着凉风。

snore 1 *noun* loud noise produced in the nose and throat when asleep 鼾声 **2** *verb* to make a loud noise in your nose and throat when you are asleep 打鼾

◇ **snoring** *noun* making a series of snores 鼾声不断的

COMMENT: A snore is produced by the vibration of the soft palate at the back of the mouth, and occurs when a sleeping person breathes through both mouth and nose.
注释：打鼾是口腔后部软腭震动产生的，当睡着的人同时通过口和鼻呼吸时发生。

snot *noun* (*informal* 非正式) mucus in the nose 鼻粘膜

snow *noun* water which falls as white flakes in cold weather 雪; **snow blindness** = temporary painful blindness caused by bright sunlight shining on snow 雪盲; **carbon dioxide snow** = carbon dioxide which has been solidified at a very low temperature and is used in treating skin growths such as warts, or to preserve tissue samples 干冰(二氧化碳结成的固体,用于冷冻保存标本)

snuffles *noun* (*informal* 非正式, *used to small children*) breathing noisily through a nose which is blocked with mucus, which can sometimes be a sign of congenital syphilis 婴儿鼻塞(见于先天梅毒)

soak *verb* to put something in liquid, so that it absorbs some of it 浸泡: ***Use a compress made of cloth soaked in warm water.*** 用一种热水浸过的布制的敷料

social *adjective* referring to society *or* to groups of people 社会的,社交的; *US* **social diseases** = sexually transmitted diseases 社会病(性病); **social medicine** = medicine as applied to treatment of diseases which occur in certain social groups 社会医学; **social security** = payments made by the government to people *or* families who need money 社会保险; **social worker** = government official who works to improve living standards of groups (such as families) 社会工作者

socket *noun* hollow part in a bone, into which another bone *or* organ fits (骨头上的)窝,臼,槽: ***The tip of the femur fits into a socket in the pelvis.*** 股骨头嵌入骨盆的髋臼中。 **ball and socket joint** 杵臼关节 *see* 见 JOINT; **eye socket** *or* **orbit** = hollow bony depression in the front of the skull in which each eye is placed 眼窝,眼眶

soda 苏打 *see* 见 BICARBONATE

sodium *noun* chemical element which is the basic substance in salt 钠; **sodium balance** = balance maintained in the body between salt lost in sweat and urine and salt taken in from food, the balance is regulated by aldosterone 钠平衡; **sodium bicarbonate** ($NaHCO_3$) = sodium salt used in cooking, also as a relief for indigestion and acidity 碳酸氢钠; **sodium chloride** (NaCl) = common salt 氯化钠(即普通食盐); **sodium pump** = cellular process where sodium is immediately excreted from any cell which it enters and potassium is brought in 钠泵 (NOTE: chemical symbol is **Na**)

> COMMENT: Salt is an essential mineral and exists in the extracellular fluid of the body. Sweat and tears also contain a high proportion of sodium chloride.
> 注释:盐是重要的矿物质,存在于体内的细胞外液中。汗水和泪液都含有高比例的氯化钠。

sodokosis *or* **sodoku** *noun* form of rat-bite fever, but without swellings in the jaws(不伴有下颌肿胀的)鼠咬热

sodomy *noun* anal sexual intercourse between men 鸡奸

soft *adjective* not hard 柔软的; **soft palate** = back part of the palate, leading to the uvula 软腭; **soft sore** *or* **soft chancre** *or* **chancroid** = venereal sore with a soft base, situated in the groin or on the genitals and caused by the bacterium *Haemophilus ducreyi* 软下疳(性病之一,生殖器和腹股沟有软的肿块并疼痛,由杜克雷嗜血杆菌引起) (NOTE: **soft - softer - softest**)

◇ **soften** *verb* to make *or* become soft 软化

soil 1 *noun* earth in which plants grow 土壤 **2** *verb* to make dirty 弄脏: ***He soiled his sheets.*** 他把自己的床单弄脏了。 ***Soiled bedclothes are sent to the hospital laundry.*** 脏的床上用品被送到医院洗衣房去了。

solarium *noun* room where patients can lie under sun lamps *or* where patients can lie in the sun 日光浴室

solar plexus *noun* nerve network situated at the back of the abdomen between the adrenal glands 太阳神经丛(位于腹腔后部两肾上腺之间)

sole *noun* part under the foot 脚心: ***The soles of the feet are very sensitive.*** 脚心是很敏感的。

soleus *noun* flat muscle which goes down the calf of the leg 比目鱼肌(小腿肚上的扁平肌肉)

solid *adjective* hard *or* not liquid 坚固的,坚硬的: ***Water turns solid when it freezes.*** 冷冻时水变成固体。**solid food** *or* **solids** = food which is chewed and eaten, not drunk 固体食物: ***She is allowed some solid food*** *or* ***she is allowed to eat solids.*** 允许她吃固体食物了。

> COMMENT: Solid foods are introduced gradually to babies and to patients who have had intestinal operations.
> 注释:婴儿和肠道手术后的病人要逐渐添加固体食物。

◇ **solidify** *verb* to become solid 固化: ***Carbon dioxide solidifies at low temperatures.*** 二氧化碳在低温下变成固体。

soln *abbreviation for* (缩写) SOLUTION 溶液

soluble *adjective* which can dissolve 可溶解的;**a tablet of soluble aspirin** 一片可溶性阿司匹林;**soluble fibre** = fibre in vegetables, fruit and pulses and porridge oats, which is partly digested in the intestine and reduces the absorption of fats and sugar into the body, so lowering the level of cholesterol 可溶性纤维

◇ **solute** *noun* solid substance which is dissolved in a solvent to make a solution 溶质

◇ **solution** *noun* mixture of a solid substance dissolved in a liquid 溶液;**barium solution** = liquid solution containing barium sulphate ($BaSO_4$) which a patient drinks to increase the contrast of an X-ray of the alimentary tract 钡溶液(含硫酸钡,用作造影剂)

◇ **solvent** *noun* liquid in which a solid substance can be dissolved 溶剂;**solvent inhalation** *or* **solvent abuse** *or* **glue sniffing** = type of drug abuse where the addict inhales the toxic fumes given off by certain types of volatile chemical 吸胶毒(滥用药物的一种,对吸入挥发性化学物质成瘾)

> QUOTE: Deaths among teenagers caused by solvent abuse have reached record levels.
> 引文:因吸胶海导致青少年死亡已创记录。
> **Health Visitor** 保健访视员

soma *noun* the body (as opposed to the mind)身体(与心灵相对)(NOTE: plural is **somata or somas**)

◇ **somat-** *or* **somato-** *prefix* (i) referring to the body 身体 (ii) meaning somatic 躯体的

◇ **somatic** *adjective* referring to the body (i) as opposed to the mind 身体的 (ii) as opposed to the intestines and inner organs 躯体的;**somatic nerves** = sensory and motor nerves which control skeletal muscles 体干神经 *see also* 参见 PSYCHOSOMATIC

◇ **somatotrophic hormone** *or* **somatotrophin** *noun* growth hormone, secreted by the pituitary gland, which stimulates the growth of long bones 生长激素

-some *suffix* referring to tiny cell bodies 小体

somnambulism *or* **sleepwalking** *noun* condition affecting some people (especially children), where the person gets up and walks about while still asleep 梦游症

◇ **somnambulist** *or* **sleepwalker** *noun* person who walks in his sleep 梦游症者

◇ **somnambulistic** *adjective* referring to sleepwalking 梦游症的

◇ **somnolent** *adjective* sleepy 困倦的,嗜睡的

◇ **somnolism** *noun* trance which is induced by hypnotism 催眠状态

-somy *suffix* referring to the presence of chromosomes 染色体

son *noun* male child of a parent 儿子: ***They have two sons and one daughter.***

他们有 2 个儿子和 1 个女儿。

Sonne dysentery *noun* common form of mild dysentery in the UK, caused by *Shigella sonnei* 宋内氏痢疾

sonogram *noun* chart produced using ultrasound waves to find where something is situated in the body 超声图像

◊ **sonoplacentography** *noun* use of ultrasound waves to find how the placenta is placed in a pregnant woman 超声胎盘图像

◊ **sonotopography** *noun* use of ultrasound waves to produce a sonogram 超声图像

soothe *verb* to relieve pain 安慰,缓解疼痛: ***The calamine lotion will soothe the rash.*** 炉甘石洗剂能缓和皮疹带来的不适。

◊ **soothing** *adjective* which relieves pain *or* makes someone less tense 安慰性的,起镇痛作用的: ***They played soothing music in the dentist's waiting room.*** 他们在牙医的候诊室里放轻松的音乐。

soporific *noun* & *adjective* (drug) which makes a person go to sleep 安眠的,安眠药

sordes *noun* dry deposits round the lips of a patient suffering from fever 口垢

sore 1 *noun* small wound on any part of the skin, usually with a discharge of pus 疮,皮肤溃疡; **cold sore** *or* **herpes simplex** = burning sore, usually on the lips 感冒疮,单纯疱疹,唇疱疹; **running sore** = sore which is discharging pus 脓疡; **soft sore** = soft chancre *or* venereal sore with a soft base, situated in the groin or on the genitals and caused by the bacterium *Haemophilus ducreyi* 软下疳参见 *see also* 参见 BEDSORE **2** *adjective* rough and inflamed (skin); painful (muscle) 痛的,发炎的; **sore throat** = condition where the mucous membrane in the throat is inflamed (sometimes because the patient has been talking too much, but usually because of an infection) 咽喉炎

s.o.s. *abbreviation for* (缩写) *the Latin phrase* 'si opus sit': if necessary (written on a prescription to show that the dose should be taken once) 需要时(处方用语)

souffle *noun* soft breathing sound, heard through a stethoscope 呼吸音,吹气音,杂音

sound 1 *noun* (**a**) something which can be heard 声音: ***The doctor listened to the sounds of the patient's lungs.*** 医生听诊患者肺部。***His breathing made a whistling sound.*** 他呼吸呈哮鸣音。(**b**) long rod, used to examine *or* to dilate the inside of a cavity in the body 探子 **2** *adjective* strong and healthy 强健的: ***He has a sound constitution.*** 他体质强健。***Her heart is sound, but her lungs are congested.*** 她的心脏强健有力,但肺部充血。**3** *verb* (**a**) to make a noise 发声,出声: ***Her lungs sound as if she had pneumonia.*** 她肺里发出的声音示她可能得了肺炎。(**b**) to examine the inside of a cavity using a rod 用探子探查(体内腔、道)

sour *adjective* one of the basic tastes, not bitter, salt or sweet 酸的

source *noun* substance which produces something; place where something comes from 来源,资源,根源: ***Sugar is a source of energy.*** 糖是能量的来源。***Vegetables are important sources of vitamins.*** 蔬菜是维生素的重要来源。***The source of the allergy has been identified.*** 已经找到了过敏的根源。***The medical team has isolated the source of the infection.*** 医疗队已经隔离了传染源。

soya *noun* plant which produces edible beans which have a high protein and fat content and very little starch 大豆

space *noun* place *or* empty area between things 空间: ***An abscess formed in the space between the bone and the cartilage.*** 软骨和骨骼之间的腔隙内形成了一个脓肿。***Write your name in the space at the top of the form.*** 把你的名字写在表格顶端的空白处。**dead space** = breath in the last part of the inspiration which does not get further than the bronchial tubes 死腔

spare 1 *adjective* extra *or* which is only used in emergencies 空余的：***We have no spare beds in the hospital at the moment.*** 目前医院里没有空床。***The doctor carries a spare set of instruments in his car.*** 医生用他的汽车运一套备用设备。**spare part surgery** = surgery where parts of the body (such as bones *or* joints) are replaced by artificial pieces 置换手术 2 *verb* to be able to give *or* spend 空出，腾出：***Can you spare the time to see the next patient?*** 你能腾出时间看下一个病人吗？***We have only one bed to spare at the moment.*** 我们目前只能腾出一张病床。

sparganosis *noun* condition caused by the larvae of the worm Sparganum under the skin (it is widespread in the Far East) 裂头蚴病

spasm *noun* sudden, usually painful, involuntary contraction of a muscle (as in cramp) 痉挛：***The muscles in his leg went into spasm.*** 他腿部肌肉痉挛了。***She had painful spasms in her stomach.*** 她的胃痉挛性疼痛。**clonic spasms** = spasms which recur regularly 阵挛；**muscle spasm** = sudden sharp contraction of a muscle 肌肉痉挛；(*of a muscle*) **to go into spasm** = to begin to contract (肌肉)开始抽动

◇ **spasmo-** *prefix* referring to a spasm 痉挛

◇ **spasmodic** *adjective* (i) which occurs in spasms 痉挛的 (ii) which happens from time to time 不时的

◇ **spasmolytic** *noun* drug which relieves muscle spasms 解痉药

◇ **spasmus nutans** *noun* condition where the patient nods his head and at the same time has spasms in the neck muscles and rapid movements of the eyes 点头状痉挛

◇ **spastic** 1 *adjective* (i) with spasms *or* sudden contractions of muscles 痉挛的 (ii) referring to cerebral palsy 脑瘫的；**spastic colon** = MUCOUS COLITIS 痉挛性结肠；**spastic diplegia** *or* **Little's disease** = congenital form of cerebral palsy which affects mainly the legs 痉挛性双侧瘫；**spastic gait** = way of walking where the legs are stiff and the feet not lifted off the ground 痉挛步态；**spastic paralysis** *or* **cerebral palsy** = disorder of the brain affecting spastics, due to brain damage which has occurred before birth 痉挛性麻痹，脑瘫；**spastic paraplegia** = paralysis of one side of the body after a stroke 痉挛性截瘫 2 *noun* **a spastic** = patient suffering from cerebral palsy 脑瘫患者

◇ **spasticity** *noun* condition where a limb resists passive movement 痉挛状态，强直状态 *see also* RIGIDITY

speak *verb* to say words *or* to talk 说：***He is learning to speak again after a laryngectomy.*** 喉切除后他正在重新学习说话。(NOTE: **speaks - speaking - spoke - has spoken**)

◇ **speak up** *verb* to speak louder 大声说：***Speak up, please - I can't hear you!*** 说大点儿声，我听不见！

special *adjective* which refers to one particular thing *or* which is not ordinary 特殊的，特异性的：***He has been given a special diet to cure his allergy.*** 为治愈他的过敏，给他特殊饮食。***She wore special shoes to correct a defect in her ankles.*** 她穿上特制的鞋以矫正其踝部缺陷。**special care baby unit** = unit in a hospital which deals with premature babies *or* babies with serious disorders 婴儿特护病房；**special hospital** = hospital for dangerous mental patients 特种医院(为具有危险性的精神病人而设)；**special school** = school for children who are handicapped 特教学校

◇ **specialism** = SPECIALITY 专业

◇ **specialist** *noun* doctor who specializes in a certain branch of medicine 专家：***He is a heart specialist.*** 他是个心脏科专家。***She was referred to an ENT specialist.*** 她被转诊到肠道专家那里。

◇ **speciality** *noun* particular branch of medicine 专科

◇ **specialization** *noun* (i) act of specializing in a certain branch of medicine 专业化 (ii) particular branch of medicine which a doctor specializes in 专科

◇ **specialize in** *verb* to study *or* to treat one particular disease *or* one particular type of patient 专门研究,专攻: ***He specializes in children with breathing problems.*** 他专攻儿童呼吸问题。***She decided to specialize in haematology.*** 她决心专攻血液学

◇ **specialty** *US* = SPECIALITY 专业

species *noun* division of a genus *or* group of living things which can interbreed 物种

specific 1 *adjective* particular *or* (disease) caused by one microbe 特发的; **specific urethritis** = inflammation of the urethra caused by gonorrhoea 特发性尿道炎 *see also* 参见 NON-SPECIFIC 2 *noun* drug which is used to treat a particular disease 特效药

◇ **specificity** *noun* rate of negative responses in a test from persons free from a disease (a high specificity means a low rate of false positives) 特异性 *compare* 比较 SENSITIVITY

specimen *noun* (i) small quantity of something given for testing 标本 (ii) one item out of a group 样本: ***He was asked to bring a urine specimen.*** 要求他带一份尿样来。***We keep specimens of diseased organs for students to examine.*** 我们保留了患病器官的标本让学生检查用。

spectacles *plural noun* glasses which are worn in front of the eyes to help correct defects in vision 眼镜: ***The optician said he needed a new pair of spectacles.*** 验光师说他需要一副新眼镜。***She was wearing a pair of spectacles with gold frames.*** 她戴着一副金框眼镜。

COMMENT: Spectacles can correct defects in the focusing of the eye, such as shortsightedness, longsightedness and astigmatism. Where different lenses are required for reading, an optician may prescribe two pairs of spectacles, one for normaluse and the other reading glasses. Otherwise, spectacles can be fitted with a divided lens (bifocals).
注释:眼镜能矫正眼睛聚光的缺陷,如近视、远视和散光。若阅读需要不同的透镜,验光师可以配出两副眼镜,一个平常用,另一个阅读时用。另外,还可以使一副眼镜装配不同的透镜(双焦距透镜)。

spectrography *noun* recording of a spectrum on photographic film 摄谱术

◇ **spectroscope** *noun* instrument used to analyse a spectrum 分光镜

◇ **spectrum** *noun* (i) range of colours (from red to violet) into which white light can be split (different substances in solution have different spectra) 光谱 (ii) range of diseases which an antibiotic can be used to treat 疾病谱; **broad-spectrum antibiotic** = antibiotic used to control many types of bacteria 广谱抗生素 (NOTE: the plural is **spectra**)

> QUOTE: Narrow-spectrum compounds have a significant advantage over broad-spectrum ones in that they do not upset the body's normal flora to the same extent.
> 引文:窄谱抗生素明显优于广谱抗生素的地方在于它不干扰体内同等范围的正常菌群。
> **British Journal of Hospital Medicine**
> 英国医院医学杂志

speculum *noun* surgical instrument which is inserted into an opening in the body (such as a nostril *or* the vagina) to keep it open, and allow a doctor to examine the inside 窥器 (NOTE: plural is **specula**, **speculums**)

speech *noun* making intelligible sounds with the vocal cords 言语; **speech block** = temporary inability to speak, caused by the effect of nervous stress on the mental processes 言语阻塞; **speech impediment** = condition where a person cannot speak properly because of a deformed mouth or tongue 言语障碍; **speech therapist** = qualified person who practises speech therapy 言语治疗师; **speech therapy** = treatment to cure a speech disorder such as stammering 言语治疗,交谈疗法

spell *noun* short period 小发作: ***She has dizzy spells.*** 她眩晕发作。***He had two spells in hospital during the winter.*** 冬天他在医院里发作了两次。

sperm *noun* spermatozoon, a male sex cell 精子; **sperm bank** = place where sperm can be stored for use in artificial in semination 精子库; **sperm count** = calculation of the number of sperm in a quantity of semen 精子计数; **sperm duct** *or* **vas deferens** = tube along which sperm pass from the epididymis to the prostate gland 输精管(NOTE: no plural for sperm: **there are millions of sperm in each ejaculation**)

◇ **sperm-** *or* **spermi(o)-** *or* **spermo-** *prefix* referring to sperm and semen 精子,精液

◇ **spermat-** *or* **spermato-** *prefix* referring to (i) sperm 精子 (ii) the male reproductive system 男性生殖系统

◇ **spermatic** *adjective* referring to sperm 精子的; **spermatic artery** = artery which leads into the testes 精索动脉; **spermatic cord** = cord running from the testis to the abdomen carrying the vas deferens, the blood vessels, nerves and lymphatics of the testis 精索

◇ **spermatid** *noun* immature cell, formed from a spermatocyte, which becomes a spermatozoon 精子细胞

◇ **spermatocele** *noun* cyst which forms in the scrotum 精子囊肿

◇ **spermatocyte** *noun* early stage in the development of a spermatozoon 精母细胞

◇ **spermatogenesis** *noun* formation and development of spermatozoa in the testes 精子发生

◇ **spermatogonium** *noun* cell which forms a spermatocyte 精原细胞

◇ **spermatorrhoea** *noun* discharge of a large amount of semen frequently and without an orgasm 精液溢出

◇ **spermatozoon** *noun* sperm, a mature male sex cell, which is ejaculated from the penis and is capable of fertilizing an ovum 精子(NOTE: plural is **spermatozoa**)

◇ **spermaturia** *noun* sperm in the urine 精子尿

◇ **spermicidal** *adjective* which can kill sperm 杀精子的

◇ **spermicide** *noun* substance which kills sperm 杀精子药

> COMMENT: A human spermatozoon is very small and is formed of a head, neck and very long tail. A spermatozoon can swim by moving its tail from side to side. The sperm are formed in the testes and ejaculated through the penis. Each ejaculation may contain millions of sperm. Once a sperm has entered the female uterus, it remains viable for about three days.
> 注释:人的精子非常小,由头、颈和长长的尾巴组成。精子可以通过左右摇尾巴而游动。精子在睾丸中形成,并通过阴茎射精排出。每次射精可能含有数以百万计的精子。当精子进入女性的子宫,它能大约保持活力三天。

spheno- *prefix* referring to the sphenoid bone 蝶骨

◇ **sphenoid bone** *noun* one of two bones in the skull which form the side of the socket of the eye 蝶骨; **sphenoid sinus** *or* **sphenoidal sinus** = one of the sinuses in the skull behind the nasal passage 蝶窦

◇ **sphenopalatine ganglion** *noun* ganglion in the pterygopalatine fossa associated with maxillary sinus 蝶腭神经节

spherocyte *noun* abnormal round red blood cell 球形红细胞

◇ **spherocytosis** *noun* condition where a patient has spherocytes in his blood, causing anaemia, enlarged spleen and gallstones, as in acholuric jaundice 球形红细胞增多症

sphincter (muscle) *noun* ring of muscle at the opening of a passage in the body, which can contract to close the passage 括约肌; **anal sphincter** =

ring of muscle which closes the anus 肛门括约肌; **pyloric sphincter** = muscle which surrounds the pylorus, makes it contract and separates it from the duodenum 幽门括约肌; **sphincter pupillae muscle** = annular muscle in the iris which constricts the pupil 瞳孔括约肌

◇ **sphincterectomy** *noun* surgical operation to remove (i) a sphincter 括约肌切除术 (ii) part of the edge of the iris in the eye 虹膜部分切除

◇ **sphincteroplasty** *noun* surgery to relieve a tightened sphincter 括约肌成形术

◇ **sphincterotomy** *noun* surgical operation to make an incision into a sphincter 括约肌切开术

sphyg *noun* (*informal* 非正式) = SPHYGMOMANOMETER 血压计

◇ **sphygmo-** *prefix* referring to the pulse 脉搏

◇ **sphygmocardiograph** *noun* device which records heartbeats and pulse rate 心动脉搏记录仪

◇ **sphygmograph** *noun* device which records the pulse 脉搏记录仪

◇ **sphygmomanometer** *noun* instrument which measures blood pressure in the arteries 血压计

COMMENT: The sphygmomanometer is a rubber sleeve connected to a scale with a column of mercury, allowing the nurse to take a reading; the rubber sleeve is usually wrapped round the arm and inflated until the blood flow is stopped; the blood pressure is determined by listening to the pulse with a stethoscope placed over an artery as the pressure in the rubber sleeve is slowly reduced, and by the reading on the scale.
注释:血压计是一副橡胶袖带连着一个有标尺的水银柱,护士可以从标尺上读数;通常将橡胶袖带缠在胳膊上并充气直至血流被阻止;在慢慢减小袖带压力的同时,把听诊器放到动脉上方听脉搏,并同时读数,以此确定血压。

spica *noun* way of bandaging a joint where the bandage crisscrosses over itself like the figure 8 on the inside of the bend of the joint 人字形绷带 (NOTE: plural is **spicae** or **spicas**)

spicule *noun* small splinter of bone 骨刺

spina bifida *or* **rachischisis** *noun* serious condition where part of the spinal cord protrudes throught the spinal column 脊柱裂

COMMENT: Spina bifida takes two forms: a mild form, spina bifida occulta, where only the bone is affected, and there are no visible signs of the condition; and the serious spina bifida cystica where part of the meninges or spinal cord passes through the gap; it may result in paralysis of the legs, and mental retardation is often present where the condition is associated with hydrocephalus.
注释:脊柱裂有两种形式:轻型隐性脊柱裂,这种情况下只有椎骨受影响,而没有可见的体征;重型囊性脊柱裂,这种情况下部分脊膜和脊索从裂隙中突出,可以导致双腿瘫痪,如果并发脑积水,还经常存在精神发育迟滞。

spinal *adjective* referring to the spine 脊柱的: ***He has spinal problems.*** 他的脊柱有问题。***She suffered spinal injuries in the crash.*** 事故造成她脊柱损伤。**spinal accessory nerve** = eleventh cranial nerve which supplies the muscles in the neck and shoulders 脊髓副神经; **spinal anaesthesia** = local anaesthesia (subarachnoid *or* epidural) in which an anaesthetic is injected into the cerebrospinal fluid 脊髓麻醉(腰麻); **spinal block** = analgesia produced by injecting an analgesic solution into the space between the vertebral canal and the dura mater 脊髓阻滞(硬膜外麻醉); **spinal canal** *or* **vertebral canal** = hollow running down the back of the vertebrae, containing the spinal cord 椎管; **spinal column** = backbone *or* spine *or* vertebral column 脊柱; **spinal cord** = part of the central nervous system running from the medulla oblongata to the filum terminale, in the vertebral canal of the spine 脊髓; **spinal curvature** *or* **curvature of the spine** = abnormal bending of the spine 脊柱弯曲; **spinal fusion** = surgical operation to join two vertebrae together to make the spine more rigid 脊椎融合术; **spinal nerves** = 31 pairs of nerves which lead from the spinal cord 脊神经; **spinal puncture** *or* **lumbar puncture** *or* US **spinal tap** = surgical operation to remove a sample of cerebrospinal fluid by inserting a hollow needle into the lower part of the spinal canal 腰穿 (NOTE: for terms referring to the spinal cord, see words beginning with **myel-**, **myelo-**, **rachi-**, **rachio-**)

spindle *noun* long thin structure 梭,纺锤体; **spindle fibre** = one of the elements visible during cell division 纺锤丝; **muscle spindles** = sensory receptors which lie along striated muscle fibres 肌梭

spine *noun* (i) backbone, the series of bones (the vertebrae) linked together to form a flexible column running from the pelvis to the skull 脊柱 (ii) any sharp projecting part of a bone 嵴: ***She injured her spine*** *or* ***she had spine injuries in the crash*.** 在事故中她脊柱受伤。**spine of the scapula** = ridge on the posterior face of the scapula 肩胛冈 ◊ 见图 SHOULDER

◊ **spino-** *prefix* referring to (i) the spine 脊柱 (ii) the spinal cord 脊髓

◊ **spinocerebellar tracts** *noun* nerve fibres in the spinal cord, taking impulses to the cerebellum 脊髓小脑束

◊ **spinous process** *noun* projection on a vertebra *or* a bone, that looks like a spine 脊突 ◊ 见图 VERTEBRAL COLUMN

COMMENT: The spine is made up of twenty-four ring-shaped vertebrae, with the sacrum and coccyx, separated by discs of cartilage. The hollow canal of the spine (the spinal canal) contains the spinal cord. See also note at VERTEBRA.
注释:脊柱由 24 块环形的椎骨组成,包括骶骨和尾骨,椎骨间由软骨盘分开。脊柱中空的管道(椎管)内含有脊髓。参见椎骨中的注释。

spiral *adjective* which runs in a continuous circle upwards 螺旋的; **spiral bandage** = bandage which is wrapped round a limb, each turn overlapping the one before 螺旋绷带; **spiral ganglion** = ganglion in the eighth cranial nerve which supplies the organ of Corti 螺旋神经节; **spiral organ** = ORGAN OF CORTI 螺旋器,科蒂氏器

Spirillum *noun* one of the bacteria which cause rat-bite fever 螺菌属

spirit *noun* strong mixture of alcohol and water 烈酒; **methylated spirit(s)** = almost pure alcohol, with wood alcohol and colouring added 甲基化酒精; **surgical spirit** = ethyl alcohol with an additive giving it an unpleasant taste, used as a disinfectant *or* for cleansing the skin 外科酒精(用于消毒皮肤)

spiro- *prefix* referring to (i) a spiral 螺旋体 (ii) the respiration 呼吸

◊ **spirochaetaemia** *noun* presence of spirochaetes in the blood 螺旋体血症

◊ **spirochaete** *or* *US* **spirochete** *noun* bacterium with a spiral shape, such as that which causes syphilis 螺旋体

◊ **spirogram** *noun* record of a patient's breathing made by a spirograph 呼吸描计图

◊ **spirograph** *noun* device which records depth and rapidity of breathing 呼吸描计器

◊ **spirography** *noun* recording of a patient's breathing by use of a spirograph 呼吸描计法

◊ **spirometer** *noun* instrument which measures how much air a person inhales or exhales 肺活量测定仪

◊ **spirometry** *noun* measurement of the vital capacity of the lungs by use of a spirometer 肺活量测定法

spit 1 *noun* saliva which is sent out of the mouth 痰 2 *verb* to send liquid out of the mouth 吐痰: ***Rinse your mouth out and spit into the cup provided.*** 漱漱口,吐到准备好的痰盂里。***He spat out the medicine.*** 他把药吐了出来。(NOTE: **spits - spitting - spat - has spat**)

Spitz-Holter valve *noun* valve with a one-way system, surgically placed in the skull, and used to drain excess fluid from the brain in hydrocephalus 斯-霍氏瓣(用于单向引流脑脊液,治疗脑积水)

splanchnic *adjective* referring to viscera 内脏的; **splanchnic nerve** = any sympathetic nerve which supplies organs in the abdomen 内脏神经(支配腹腔内脏的交感神经)

◊ **splanchnology** *noun* special study of the organs in the abdominal cavity 腹腔内脏学

spleen *noun* organ in the top part of the abdominal cavity behind the stomach and below the diaphragm 脾脏 ◊ 见图 DIGESTIVE SYSTEM

◊ **splen-** *or* **spleno-** *prefix* referring to the spleen 脾

◊ **splenectomy** *noun* surgical operation to remove the spleen 脾切除术

◊ **splenic** *adjective* referring to the spleen 脾脏的; **splenic anaemia** *or* **Banti's syndrome** *or* **Banti's disease** = type of anaemia where the patient has portal hypertension, an enlarged spleen and haemorrhages, caused by cirrhosis of the liver 脾源性贫血,班替综合征,班替病(门脉高压,脾脏增大,出血所致的贫血,由肝硬化引起); **splenic flexure** = bend in the colon, where the transverse colon joins the descending colon(结肠)脾曲

◊ **splenitis** *noun* inflammation of the spleen 脾脏炎症

◊ **splenomegaly** *noun* condition where the spleen is abnormally large, associated with several disorders including malaria and some cancers 脾增大

◊ **splenorenal anastomosis** *noun* surgical operation to join the splenic vein to a renal vein, as a treatment for portal hypertension 脾肾静脉吻合术

◊ **splenovenography** *noun* X-ray examination of the spleen and the veins which are connected to it 脾静脉造影

> COMMENT: The spleen, which is the largest endocrine (ductless) gland, appears to act to remove dead blood cells and fight infection, but its functions are not fully understood and an adult can live normally after his spleen has been removed.
> 注释:脾脏是最大的内分泌腺,它的功能是清除死亡的血细胞和对抗感染,但至今我们对其全部的功能尚缺乏了解。成年人在脾切除后可正常生活。

splint *noun* (**a**) stiff support attached to a limb to prevent a broken bone from moving 夹板: ***He had to keep his arm in a splint for several weeks.*** 他的胳膊不得不带几周夹板。*see also* 参见 BRAUN'S SPLINT, DENIS BROWNE SPLINT, FAIRBANKS' SPLINT, THOMAS'S SPLINT (**b**) **shin splints** 外胫夹 *see* 见 SHIN

splinter *noun* tiny thin piece of wood *or* metal which gets under the skin and can be irritating and cause infection 碎片

split *verb* to divide 分裂

◊ **split-skin graft** *or* **Thiersch graft** *noun* type of skin graft where thin layers of skin are grafted over a wound 皮片移植

spondyl *noun* a vertebra 脊椎

◊ **spondyl-** *or* **spondylo-** *prefix* referring to the vertebrae 脊椎

◊ **spondylitis** *noun* inflammation of the vertebrae 脊椎炎; **ankylosing spondylitis** = condition with higher incidence in young men, where the vertebrae and sacroiliac joints are inflamed and become stiff 强直性脊柱炎(好发于男青年,脊椎和骶髂关节炎症导致关节僵直)

◊ **spondylolisthesis** *noun* condition where one of the lumbar vertebrae moves forward over the one beneath 脊椎前移

◊ **spondylosis** *noun* stiffness in the spine and degenerative changes in the intervertebral discs, with osteoarthritis (it is common in older people)脊椎关节强直(是一种退行性变,常见于老年人,并伴有骨关节炎); **cervical spondylosis** = degenerative change in the neck bones 颈椎关节强直

sponge *noun* piece of light absorbent material, either natural *or* synthetic, used in bathing, cleaning etc. 海绵; **contraceptive sponge** = piece of synthetic sponge impregnated with spermicide, which is inserted into the vagina before intercourse 避孕海绵球

◊ **sponge bath** *noun* washing a patient in bed, using a sponge *or* damp cloth 海绵擦浴: ***The nurse gave the old lady a sponge bath.*** 护士给这位老太太进行了海绵擦浴。

spongioblastoma = GLIOBLASTOMA 成胶质细胞瘤

spongiosum 松质的 *see* 见 CORPUS

spongy *adjective* soft and full of holes like a sponge 海绵状的; **spongy bone** = cancellous bone, light spongy bone tissue which forms the inner core of a bone and also the ends of long bones 松质骨 ◊ 见图 BONE STRUCTURE

spontaneous *adjective* which happens without any particular outside cause 自发的; **spontaneous abortion** = MISCARRIAGE 自发流产

spoon *noun* instrument with a long handle at one end and a small bowl at the other, used for taking liquid medicine 勺; ***a 5ml spoon*** 一个 5 毫升的药勺

◊ **spoonful** *noun* quantity which a spoon can hold 一勺: ***Take two 5ml spoonfuls of the medicine twice a day.*** 每次用 5 毫升药勺喝两勺,每天 2 次。

sporadic *adjective* (disease) where outbreaks occur as separate cases, not in epidemics 散发的

spore *noun* reproductive body of certain bacteria and fungi which can survive in extremely hot or cold conditions for a long time 孢子(某些细菌和真菌的生殖体,可以在很冷或很热的环境下存活)

◊ **sporicidal** *adjective* which kills spores 杀孢子的

◊ **sporicide** *noun* substance which kills bacterial spores 杀胞子药

◊ **sporotrichosis** *noun* fungus infection of the skin which causes abscesses 孢子丝菌病

◊ **Sporozoa** *noun* type of parasitic Protozoa which includes Plasmodium, the cause of malaria 孢子虫纲(寄生性原生动物的一个类型,包括疟原虫)

sport *noun* playing of games 体育运动; **sports injuries** = injuries commonly occurring when playing sports (injuries to the neck in Rugby, ligament injuries in football, etc.) 运动损伤; **sports medicine** = study of the treatment of sports injuries 运动医学

spot *noun* small round mark *or* pimple 斑点: ***The disease is marked by red spots on the chest.*** 此病的标志特征是胸部出现红色斑点。***He suddenly came out in spots on his chest.*** 他的胸部突然出了很多斑点。**black spots (in front of the eyes)** = moving black dots seen when looking at something, more noticeable when a person is tired *or* run-down, more common in shortsighted people 黑点(眼冒金星,视疲劳或近视时常见); **to break out in spots** *or* **to come out in spots** = to have a sudden rash 急疹 *see also* 参见 KOPLIK

◊ **spotted fever** *noun* meningococcal meningitis, the commonest epidemic form of meningitis, caused by a bacterial infection, where the meninges become inflamed causing headaches and fever 斑疹热(脑膜炎球菌引起的脑膜炎,是最常见的流行性脑膜炎,引起头疼和发热) *see also* 参见 ROCKY MOUNTAIN

◊ **spotty** *adjective* covered with pimples 布满小丘疹的

sprain 1 *noun* condition where the ligaments in a joint are stretched or torn because of a sudden movement 扭伤 **2** *verb* to tear the ligaments in a joint with a sudden movement 扭伤: ***She sprained her wrist when she fell*.** 她摔倒时扭伤了手腕。

spray 1 *noun* (**a**) mass of tiny drops 气雾: ***An aerosol sends out a liquid in a fine spray*.** 喷雾器喷出细小的气雾。(**b**) special liquid for spraying onto an infection 喷剂; **throat spray** *or* **nasal spray** 鼻咽喷剂 **2** *verb* to send out a liquid in fine drops 喷: ***They sprayed the room with disinfectant*.** 他们在房间里喷洒消毒剂。

spread *verb* to go out over a large area 播散, 传播: ***The infection spread right through the adult population*.** 这种感染只侵及成年人。***Sneezing in a crowded bus can spread infection*.** 在拥挤的公共汽车里打喷嚏会传染疾病。(NOTE: **spreads-spreading-spread-has spread**)

> QUOTE: Spreading infection may give rise to cellulitis of the abdominal wall and abscess formation.
> 引文:感染播散可导致腹壁蜂窝织炎和形成脓肿。
>
> **Nursing Times** 护理时代

Sprengel's deformity *or* **Sprengel's shoulder** *noun* congenitally deformed shoulder, where one scapula is smaller and higher than the other 施普伦格畸形(先天性肩胛翼状畸形,一侧肩胛骨小而高于对侧)

sprue = PSILOSIS 口炎性腹泻

spud *noun* needle used to get a piece of dust *or* other foreign body out of the eye(眼科)刮铲(用于取出眼内异物,如灰尘)

spur *noun* sharp projecting part of a bone 骨刺

sputum *or* **phlegm** *noun* mucus which is formed in the inflamed nose *or* throat *or* lungs and is coughed up 痰: ***She was coughing up bloodstained sputum*.** 她咳出了带血的痰。

squama *noun* thin piece of hard tissue, such as a thin flake of bone *or* scale on the skin 鳞片,鳞屑 (NOTE: plural is **squamae**)

◊ **squamous** *adjective* thin and hard like a scale 鳞状的; **squamous bone** = part of the temporal bone which forms the side of the skull 颞骨鳞部(片状骨); **squamous epithelium** *or* **pavement epithelium** = epithelium with flat cells like scales which forms the lining of the pericardium, the peritoneum and the pleura 鳞状上皮,扁平上皮

squint 1 *noun* strabismus, a condition where the eyes focus on different points 斜视; **convergent squint** = condition where one or both eyes look towards the nose 会聚性斜视,内斜视; **divergent squint** = condition where one or both eyes look away from the nose 分散性斜视,外斜视 **2** *verb* to have one eye or both eyes looking towards the nose 斜视,斜眼: ***Babies often appear to squint, but it is corrected as they grow older*.** 婴儿经常显出斜视的样子,但当他们长大些这种现象便会得到纠正。

Sr *chemical symbol for* strontium 锶的化学元素符号

SRN = STATE REGISTERED NURSE 国家注册护士

stab 1 *noun* (**a**) 刺; **stab wound** = deep wound made by the point of a knife 穿刺伤 (**b**) sharp pain 刺痛: ***He had a stab of pain in his right eye*.** 他右眼感到刺痛。**2** *verb* to cut by pushing the point of a knife into the flesh 刺, 戳: ***He was stabbed in the chest*.** 他被扎伤了胸部。

◊ **stabbing** *adjective* (pain) in a series of short sharp stabs 刺痛的: ***He had stabbing pains in his chest*.** 他胸口刺痛。

stabilize *verb* to make a condition stable 使稳定: ***We have succeeded in stabilizing his blood sugar level*.** 我们成功地稳定住了他的血糖水平。

stable *adjective* not changing 稳定的: ***His condition is stable*.** 他的病情稳定。**stable angina** = angina which has not changed for a long time 稳定性心绞痛

staccato speech *noun* abnormal way of speaking, with short pauses between each word 断续言语

Stacke's operation *noun* surgical

operation to remove the posterior and superior wall of the auditory meatus 斯塔克手术(鼓室乳突根治术)

stadium invasioni *noun* incubation period, the period between catching an infectious disease and the appearance of the first symptoms of the disease(感染)侵入期,侵袭期,潜伏期

staff *noun* people who work in a hospital, clinic, doctor's surgery, etc. 工作人员: ***We have 25 full-time medical staff.*** 我们有25名全日制医务人员。***The hospital is trying to recruit more nursing staff.*** 医院要招募更多的护理人员。***The clinic has a staff of 100.*** 诊所有100名工作人员。**staff midwife** = midwife who is on the permanent staff of a hospital 医院助产士; **staff nurse** = senior nurse who is employed full-time 护师 (NOTE: when used as a subject, staff takes a plural verb: **a staff of 25 but the ancillary staff work very hard**)

stage *noun* point in the development of a disease, which allows a decision to be taken about the treatment which should be given 阶段,期: ***The disease has reached a critical stage.*** 病到了关键期。***This is a symptom of the second stage of syphilis.*** 这是二期梅毒的症状之一。

> QUOTE: Memory changes are associated with early stages of the disease; in later stages, the patient is frequently incontinent, immobile and unable to communicate.
> 引文:记忆改变是疾病早期的征象;疾病后期病人经常二便失禁、不能活动并不能与人交流。
> **Nursing Times** 护理时代

stagger *verb* to move from side to side while walking *or* to walk unsteadily 蹒跚

stagnant loop syndrome 盲袢综合征 *see* 见 LOOP

stain 1 *noun* dye *or* substance used to give colour to tissues which are going to be examined under the microscope 染料 **2** *verb* to treat a piece of tissue with a dye to increase contrast before it is examined under the microscope(给切片)染色

◇ **staining** *noun* colouring of tissue *or* bacterial samples, etc., to make it possible to examine them and to identify them under the microscope 染色

> COMMENT: Some stains are designed to have an affinity only with those chemical, cellular or bacterial elements in a specimen that are of interest to a microbiologist; thus the concentration or uptake of a stain, as well as the overall picture, can be diagnostic.
> 注释:某些染料对特定的微生物学家感兴趣,因其只与标本上的化学物质、细胞或细菌的某些成分有亲和力,根据染色的浓度或对染料摄取的多少,加上整片显示,可对疾病作出诊断。

stalk *noun* stem, piece of tissue which attaches a growth to the main tissue 柄

stammer 1 *noun* speech defect, where the patient repeats parts of a word or the whole word several times *or* stops to try to pronounce a word 口吃,结巴: ***He has a bad stammer.*** 他口吃得厉害。***She is taking therapy to try to correct her stammer.*** 她在接受治疗以矫正她的口吃。**2** *verb* to speak with a stammer 口吃,结巴

◇ **stammerer** *noun* person who stammers 口吃的人

◇ **stammering** *or* **dysphemia** *noun* difficulty in speaking, where the person repeats parts of a word or the whole word several times *or* stops to try to pronounce a word 口吃 *see also* 参见 STUTTER

stamp out *verb* to remove completely 根除: ***International organizations have succeeded in stamping out smallpox.*** 国际组织成功地根除了天花。***The government is trying to stamp out waste in the hospital service.*** 政府决心清除医院服务中的浪费现象。

stand up *verb* **(a)** to get up from being on a seat 站起来: ***He tried to stand***

up*, *but did not have the strength*.**他努力想站起来,但力不从心。(**b**) to hold yourself upright 站直了:She still stands up straight at the age of ninety-two*.**她92岁还能腰板挺直地站着。

standard 1 *adjective* normal 标准的:***It is the standard practice to take the patient's temperature twice a day*.** 标准的护理是一天给病人测两次体温。**2** *noun* something which has been agreed upon and is used to measure other things by 标准:***The standard of care in hospitals has increased over the last years*.**医院护理的标准在过去的几年中提高了。***The report criticized the standards of hygiene in the clinic*.**报告批评了临床的卫生标准。

stapedectomy *noun* surgical operation to remove the stapes 镫骨切除术

◇ **stapediolysis** *or* **stapedial mobilization** *noun* surgical operation to relieve deafness by detaching an immobile stapes from the fenestra ovalis 镫骨松动术

◇ **stapes** *noun* one of the three ossicles in the middle ear, shaped like a stirrup 镫骨(三块听小骨之一);**mobilization of the stapes** = STAPEDIOLYSIS 镫骨松动术◇ 见图 EAR

> COMMENT: The stapes fills the fenestra ovalis, and is articulated with the incus, which in turn articulates with the malleus.
> 注释:镫骨盖住卵圆窗,它还与砧骨形成关节,砧骨再与锤骨形成关节。

staphylectomy *noun* surgical operation to remove the uvula 悬雍垂切除术

staphylococcal *adjective* referring to Staphylococci 葡萄球菌的;**staphylococcal poisoning** = poisoning by Staphylococci which have spread in food 葡萄球菌食物中毒

◇ **Staphylococcus** *noun* bacterium which grows in a bunch like a bunch of grapes, and causes boils and food poisoning 葡萄球菌属(NOTE: plural is **Staphylococci**)

staphyloma *noun* swelling of the cornea or the white of the eye(角膜或巩膜)葡萄肿

staphylorrhaphy = PALATORRHAPHY 软腭缝合术

staple 1 *noun* small piece of bent metal, used to attach tissues together U形钉(用于固定组织) **2** *verb* to attach tissues with staples 用U形钉固定组织

◇ **stapler** *noun* device used in surgery to attach tissues with staples, instead of suturing 钉书机式缝合器

starch *noun* usual form in which carbohydrates exist in food, especially in bread, rice and potatoes 淀粉

◇ **starchy** *adjective* (food) which contains a lot of starch 富含淀粉的:***He eats too much starchy food*.**他吃了太多的高淀粉食物。

> COMMENT: Starch is present in common foods, and is broken down by the digestive process into forms of sugar.
> 注释:普通食物中就有淀粉,经消化降解为多种形式的糖。

Starling's Law *noun* law that the contraction of the ventricles is in proportion to the length of the ventricular muscle fibres at end of diastole 斯塔林定律(心室的收缩力与心室收缩末肌纤维的长度成正比)

starvation *noun* having had very little *or* no food 饥饿,绝食;**starvation diet** = diet which contains little nourishment, and is not enough to keep a person healthy 缺乏营养饮食

◇ **starve** *verb* to have little *or* no food or nourishment 绝食,辟谷:***The parents let the baby starve to death*.**父母把婴儿饿死了。

stasis *noun* stoppage *or* slowing in the flow of a liquid (such as blood in veins *or* food in the intestine)停滞,淤滞

◇ **-stasis** *suffix* referring to stoppage in the flow of a liquid "停滞""淤滞"

> QUOTE: A decreased blood flow in the extremities has been associated with venous stasis which may precipitate vascular complications.

引文：肢体血流减少与静脉淤滞有关，这可能引发血管并发症。
British Journal of Nursing 英国护理杂志

stat. *abbreviation for*（缩写）*the Latin word* 'statim': immediately (written on prescriptions) 即刻用（处方用语）

state *noun* (**a**) the condition of something *or* of a person 状态，状况：***His state of health is getting worse.*** 他的健康状况在恶化。***The disease is in an advanced state.*** 疾病处于进展状态。(**b**) (*formerly in Britain*) **State Registered Nurse** = nurse qualified to carry out all nursing services 国家注册护士

statistics *plural noun* study of facts in the form of official figures 统计：***Population statistics show that the birth rate is slowing down.*** 人口统计显示出生率在下降。

status *Latin for* 'state' 状态；**status asthmaticus** = attack of bronchial asthma which lasts for a long time and results in exhaustion and collapse 哮喘持续状态；**status epilepticus** = repeated and prolonged epileptic seizures without recovery of consciousness between them 癫痫持续状态；**status lymphaticus** = condition where the glands in the lymphatic system are enlarged 淋巴体质

QUOTE: The main indications being inadequate fluid and volume status and need for evaluation of patients with a history of severe heart disease.
引文：主要的指征是液体量和血容量不足，并需要评估病人有无严重心脏病史。
Southern Medical Journal 南部医学杂志

QUOTE: The standard pulmonary artery catheters have four lumens from which to obtain information about the patient's haemodynamic status.
引文：标准的肺动脉导管有 4 个腔，由此获得病人血液动力学状态的信息。
RN Magazine 注册护士杂志

stay 1 *noun* time which someone spends in a place 留：***The patient is only in hospital for a short stay.*** 这个病人只是短期留院。**long stay patient** = patient who will stay in hospital for a long time 长期住院的病人；**long stay ward** = ward for patients who will stay in hospital for a long time 长期住院病房 **2** *verb* to stop in a place for some time 留：***She stayed in hospital for two weeks.*** 她在医院住了 2 周。***He's ill with flu and has to stay in bed.*** 他得了感冒，不得不卧床。

STD = SEXUALLY TRANSMITTED DISEASE 性传播疾病

steapsin *noun* enzyme produced by the pancreas, which breaks down fats in the intestine 胰脂酶

stearic acid *noun* one of the fatty acids 硬脂酸

steat- *or* **steato-** *prefix* referring to fat 脂肪

◇ **steatoma** *noun* sebaceous cyst, a cyst in a blocked sebaceous gland 脂肪瘤

◇ **steatorrhoea** *noun* condition where fat is passed in the faeces 脂肪痢

Stein-Leventhal syndrome *noun* condition in young women, where menstruation becomes rare, or never takes place, together with growth of body hair, usually due to cysts in the ovaries 斯坦因－利文撒尔综合征（女性月经稀少或闭经，体毛增生，通常由卵巢囊肿引起）

Steinmann's pin *noun* pin for attaching traction wires to a fractured bone 斯坦曼氏导钉（用于固定骨折的牵引线）

stellate *adjective* shaped like a star 星形的；**stellate fracture** = fracture of the kneecap, shaped like a star（髌骨）星形骨折；**stellate ganglion** = inferior cervical ganglion *or* group of nerve cells in the neck 星状神经节（颈部的神经节）

Stellwag's sign *noun* symptom of exophthalmic goitre, where the patient does not blink often, because the eyeball is protruding 施特耳瓦格征（突眼性甲状腺肿的眼征之一，瞬目减少）

stem *noun* thin piece of tissue which attaches an organ *or* growth to the main tissue 柄，干；**brain stem** = lower part of the brain which connects the brain to the spinal cord 脑干(脑的下半部分,与脊髓相连)

steno- *prefix* meaning (i) narrow 狭窄 (ii) constricted 缩窄

◇ **stenose** *verb* to make narrow 缩窄; **stenosed valve** = valve which has become narrow *or* constricted 狭窄的瓣膜; **stenosing condition** = condition which makes a passage narrow 缩窄状态

◇ **stenosis** *noun* condition where a passage becomes narrow 狭窄; **aortic stenosis** = condition where the aortic valve is narrow 主动脉狭窄; **mitral stenosis** = condition where the opening in the mitral valve becomes smaller because the cusps have fused (almost always the result of rheumatic endocarditis) 二尖瓣狭窄; **pulmonary stenosis** = condition where the opening to the pulmonary artery in the right ventricle becomes narrow 肺动脉狭窄

◇ **stenostomia** *or* **stenostomy** *noun* abnormal narrowing of an opening 开口狭窄

Stensen's duct *noun* duct which carries saliva from the parotid gland 斯坦森导管(腮腺导管)

stent *noun* support of artificial material often inserted in a tube *or* vessel which has been sutured 支架

step *noun* movement of the foot and the leg as in walking 步: ***He took two steps forward.*** 他向前走了两步。 ***The baby is taking his first steps.*** 婴儿正在迈出他的第一步。

◇ **step up** *verb* (*informal* 非正式) to increase 增加: ***The doctor has stepped up the dosage.*** 医生增加了药量。

sterco- *prefix* referring to faeces 粪便

◇ **stercobilin** *noun* brown pigment which colours the faeces 粪胆素

◇ **stercobilinogen** *noun* substance which is broken down from bilirubin and produces stercobilin 粪胆原

◇ **stercolith** *noun* hard ball of dried faeces in the bowel 粪石

◇ **stercoraceous** *adjective* made of faeces; similar to faeces; containing faeces 粪便的,含粪便的

stereognosis *noun* being able to tell the shape of an object in three dimensions by means of touch 实体觉

◇ **stereoscopic vision** *noun* being able to judge the distance and depth of an object by binocular vision 立体视觉(能够通过双眼判断物体的距离和深度)

◇ **stereotaxy** *or* **stereotaxic surgery** *noun* surgical procedure to identify a point in the interior of the brain, before an operation can begin, to locate exactly the area to be operated on(脑)立体定向术

◇ **stereotypy** *noun* repeating the same action *or* word again and again 刻板症

sterile *adjective* (**a**) with no microbes *or* infectious organisms 无菌的,消毒的: ***She put a sterile dressing on the wound.*** 她把无菌敷料盖在伤口上。 ***He opened a pack of sterile dressings.*** 他打开了一包无菌敷料。(**b**) infertile *or* not able to produce children 不育的,不孕的

◇ **sterility** *noun* (i) being free from germs 无菌 (ii) infertility *or* being unable to produce children 不孕

◇ **sterilization** *noun* (i) action of making instruments, etc., free from germs 消毒灭菌 (ii) action of making a person sterile 绝育

◇ **sterilize** *verb* (**a**) to make something sterile (by killing microbes *or* bacteria) 消毒灭菌: ***Surgical instruments must be sterilized before use.*** 手术器械使用前必须消毒。 ***Not using sterilized needles can cause infection.*** 不用消毒针头会造成感染。(**b**) to make a person unable to have children 绝育

◇ **sterilizer** *noun* machine for sterilizing surgical instruments by steam *or* boiling water, etc. 消毒器

COMMENT: Sterilization of a woman can be done by removing the ovaries or cutting the Fallopian tubes; sterilization of a man is

carried out by cutting the vas deferens (vasectomy).
注释:女性绝育可以切除卵巢或切断输卵管;男性绝育是通过切断输精管实现的。

sternal *adjective* referring to the breastbone胸骨的;**sternal angle** = ridge of bone where the manubrium articulates with the body of the sternum 胸骨角(胸骨与胸骨柄形成关节处的突起);**sternal puncture** = surgical operation to remove a sample of bone marrow from the breastbone for testing 胸骨穿刺(为取骨髓)

◇ **sternoclavicular angle** *noun* angle between the sternum and the clavicle 胸骨锁骨角

◇ **sternocleidomastoid muscle** *noun* muscle in the neck, running from the breastbone to the mastoid process 胸锁乳突肌

◇ **sternocostal joint** *noun* joint where the breastbone joins a rib 胸肋关节

◇ **sternohyoid muscle** *noun* muscle in the neck which runs from the breastbone into the hyoid bone 胸骨舌骨肌

◇ **sternomastoid** *adjective* referring to the breastbone and the mastoid 胸骨乳突的;**sternomastoid muscle** = STERNOCLEIDOMASTOID MUSCLE 胸锁乳突肌;**sternomastoid tumour** = benign tumour which appears in the sternomastoid muscle in newborn babies 胸骨乳突瘤(见于新生儿胸锁乳突肌的良性肿瘤)

◇ **sternotomy** *noun* surgical operation to cut through the breastbone, so as to be able to operate on the heart 胸骨切开术

◇ **sternum** *noun* the breastbone, bone in the centre of the front of the chest 胸骨

COMMENT: The sternum runs from the neck to the bottom of the diaphragm. It is formed of the manubrium (the top section), the body of the sternum, and the xiphoid process. The upper seven pairs of ribs are attached to the sternum.
注释:胸骨起自颈部,止于横膈的底部。它由胸骨柄、胸骨体和剑突组成。上7对肋骨与胸骨相连。

sternutatory *noun* substance which makes someone sneeze 催喷剂

steroid *noun* any of several chemical compounds with characteristic ring systems, including the sex hormones, which affect the body and its functions 甾体激素,类固醇

COMMENT: The word steroid is usually used to refer to corticosteroids. Synthetic steroids are used in steroid therapy, to treat arthritis, asthma and some blood disorders. They are also used by some athletes to improve their physical strength, but these are banned by athletic organizations and can have serious side-effects.
注释:类固醇一词通常指皮质类固醇。合成的类固醇用于类固醇治疗,主治关节炎、哮喘和某些血液病。有的运动员还用它来增强体力,但这是体育组织所禁止的,会引起严重的副作用。

sterol *noun* insoluble substance which belongs to the steroid alcohols such as cholesterol 甾醇,固醇(一类不可溶解的甾体醇,如胆固醇)

stertor *noun* noisy breathing sounds in an unconscious patient 鼾声

steth- *or* **stetho-** *prefix* referring to the chest 胸

◇ **stethograph** *noun* instrument which records breathing movements of the chest 呼吸描计器

◇ **stethography** *noun* recording movements of the chest 呼吸描计法

◇ **stethometer** *noun* instrument which records how far the chest expands when a person breathes in 胸围测量器

◇ **stethoscope** *noun* surgical instrument with two earpieces connected to a tube and a metal disc, used by doctors to listen to sounds made inside the body (such as the sound of the heart *or* lungs) 听诊器; **electronic stethoscope** = stethoscope with an amplifier which makes sounds louder 电子听诊器

Stevens-Johnson syndrome *noun* severe form of erythema multiforme affecting the face and genitals, caused by an allergic reaction to drugs 斯-约二氏综合征(严重的多形性红斑,侵及面部和生殖器,由对药物的过敏反应引起)

stick *verb* to attach *or* to fix together (as with glue) 粘: ***In bad cases of conjunctivitis the eyelids can stick together.*** 严重的结膜炎会使眼睑粘在一起。

◇ **sticking plaster** *noun* adhesive plaster *or* tape used to cover a small wound or to attach a pad of dressing to the skin 创可贴

◇ **sticky** *adjective* which attached like glue 粘的; **sticky eye** = condition in babies where the eyes remain closed because of conjunctivitis 眼睑粘连(婴儿结膜炎所致)

stiff *adjective* which cannot be bent *or* moved easily 僵直,僵硬: ***My knee is stiff after playing football.*** 玩完足球后我的膝盖僵直了。**stiff neck** = condition where moving the neck is painful, usually caused by a strained muscle *or* by sitting in cold draughts 颈僵硬(落枕) (NOTE: **stiff - stiffer - stiffest**)

◇ **stiffly** *adverb* in a stiff way 僵硬地: ***He is walking stiffly because of the pain in his hip.*** 他因为髋部疼痛走路僵硬。

◇ **stiffness** *noun* being stiff 僵硬: ***Arthritis accompanied by stiffness in the joints.*** 关节炎伴关节僵硬。

stigma *noun* visible symptom which shows that a patient has a certain disease 病征 (NOTE: plural is **stigmas, stigmata**)

stilet *or* **stilette** *noun* thin wire inside a catheter to make it rigid 套管针

stillbirth *noun* birth of a dead fetus, more than 28 weeks after conception 死产

◇ **stillborn** *adjective* (baby) born dead (婴儿)死产的: ***Her first child was stillborn.*** 她的第一个孩子是死产。

Still's disease *noun* arthritis affecting children, similar to rheumatoid arthritis in adults 斯蒂尔病(儿童的关节炎,与成人类风湿性关节炎相似)

stimulant *noun* & *adjective* (substance) which makes part of the body function faster 刺激,刺激物: ***Caffeine is a stimulant.*** 咖啡因是一种刺激性物质。

◇ **stimulate** *verb* to make a person *or* organ react *or* respond *or* function 刺激,使有反应: ***The drug stimulates the heart.*** 这种药对心脏有刺激作用。***The therapy should stimulate the patient into attempting to walk unaided.*** 治疗应促使病人试着不靠扶助地行走。

◇ **stimulation** *noun* action of stimulating 刺激

◇ **stimulus** *noun* something (drug, impulse, etc.) which makes part of the body react 刺激 (NOTE: plural is **stimuli**)

> COMMENT: Natural stimulants include some hormones, and drugs such as digitalis which encourage a weak heart. Drinks such as tea and coffee contain stimulants.
> 注释:自然的兴奋剂中有某些激素和药物,如地高辛有强心作用;饮料如茶和咖啡也含有刺激性物质。

sting 1 *noun* piercing of the skin by an insect which passes a toxic substance into the bloodstream (蚊虫)叮咬 **2** *verb* (*of an insect*) to make a hole in the skin and pass a toxic substance into the blood 叮咬: ***He was stung by a wasp.*** 他被黄蜂叮了。**stinging sensation** = burning sensation as if after being stung by an insect 被叮咬的感觉 (NOTE: **stings - stinging - stung**)

> COMMENT: Stings by some insects, such as the tsetse fly can transmit a bacterial infection to a person. Other insects such as bees have toxic substances which they pass into the bloodstream of the victim, causing irritating swellings. Some people are particularly allergic to insect stings.
> 注释:被某些昆虫叮咬,如采采蝇,可传给人细菌感染。其它昆虫,如蜜蜂,含有有毒物质,叮咬时注入体内引起刺激性肿胀。有些人对昆虫叮咬特别敏感。

stirrup *or* **stapes** *noun* one of the three ossicles in the middle ear 镫骨

stitch 1 *noun* (**a**) suture, a small loop of thread or gut, used to attach the sides of a wound or incision to help it to heal 缝合: ***He had three stitches in his head.*** 他头上缝了三针。***The doctor told her to come back in ten days' time to have the stitches taken out.*** 医生告诉她10天后回来拆线。(**b**) pain caused by cramp in the side of the body after running 刺痛,岔气儿: ***He had to stop running because he developed a stitch.*** 因为岔气儿他不得不停止跑步。**2** *verb* to attach with a suture 缝合: ***They tried to stitch back the finger which had been cut off in an accident.*** 他们努力想把事故中切断的手指缝合上去。

St John Ambulance Association and Brigade *noun* voluntary organization which gives training in first aid and whose members provide first aid at public events such as football matches, demonstrations, etc. 圣约翰救护协会和救护队(自愿组成的救护组织)

stock culture *noun* basic culture of bacteria, from which other cultures can be taken 原代培养

stocking *noun* close-fitting piece of clothing to cover the leg 长袜; **compression stockings** = strong elastic stockings worn to support a weak joint in the knee or to hold varicose veins tightly 弹力长袜(用于加固虚弱的关节或紧缚曲张的静脉)

Stokes-Adams syndrome *noun* loss of consciousness due to the stopping of the action of the heart because of asystole *or* fibrillation 阿-斯氏综合征,心跳骤停,心脏纤颤导致意识丧失

stoma *noun* (i) any opening into a cavity in the body 体腔的开口 (ii) the mouth 口 (iii) (*informal* 非正式) colostomy 结肠造口 (NOTE: the plural is **stomata**)

◇ **stomal** *adjective* referring to a stoma 开口的,小孔的; **stomal ulcer** = ulcer in the region of the jejunum 十二指肠溃疡(幽门口溃疡)

stomach *noun* (**a**) part of the body shaped like a bag, into which food passes after being swallowed and where the process of digestion continues 胃: ***She complained of pains in the stomach*** *or* ***of stomach pains.*** 她说她胃疼。***He has had stomach trouble for some time.*** 他得胃病有一段时间了。**acid stomach** 胃酸 *see* 见 ACIDITY; **stomach ache** = pain in the abdomen *or* stomach (caused by eating too much food *or* by an infection) 胃疼; **stomach cramp** = sharp spasm of the stomach muscles 胃痉挛; **stomach pump** = instrument for sucking out the contents of a patient's stomach, especially if he has just swallowed a poisonous substance 洗胃泵; **stomach tube** = tube passed into the stomach to wash it out or to take samples of the contents 胃管; **stomach upset** = slight infection of the stomach 胃部不适 (**b**) region of the abdomen 上腹部(对应胃的位置): ***He had been kicked in the stomach.*** 他的胃部被踢了。

◇ **stomachic** *noun* substance which increases the appetite of a person by stimulating the secretion of gastric juice by the stomach 健胃药 (NOTE: for other terms referring to the stomach, see words beginning with **gastr-**)

COMMENT: The stomach is situated in the top of the abdomen, and on the left side of the body between the oesophagus and the duodenum. Food is partly broken down by hydrochloric acid and other gastric juices secreted by the walls of the stomach and is mixed and squeezed by the action of the muscles of the stomach, before being passed on into the duodenum. The stomach continues the digestive process started in the mouth, but few substances (except alcohol and honey) are actually absorbed into the bloodstream in the stomach.

注释:胃位于上腹部的左侧,在食管和十

二指肠之间。食物被胃壁分泌的盐酸和其它胃液部分降解，并经胃平滑肌的蠕动混合、研磨，然后送入十二指肠，继续始于口腔的消化过程，除酒精和蜂蜜外没有物质在胃被吸收入血。

stomat- *or* **stomato-** *prefix* referring to the mouth 口

◊ **stomatitis** *noun* inflammation of the inside of the mouth 口炎

◊ **stomatology** *noun* branch of medicine which studies diseases of the mouth 口腔学

-stomy *or* **-ostomy** *suffix* meaning an operation to make an opening 造口

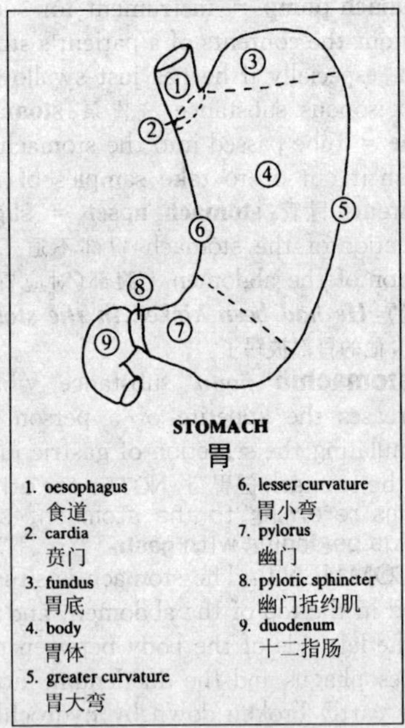

STOMACH
胃

1. oesophagus 食道
2. cardia 贲门
3. fundus 胃底
4. body 胃体
5. greater curvature 胃大弯
6. lesser curvature 胃小弯
7. pylorus 幽门
8. pyloric sphincter 幽门括约肌
9. duodenum 十二指肠

stone *noun* (**a**) calculus, a hard mass of calcium like a little piece of stone which forms inside the body 结石 *see also* 参见 GALLSTONE, KIDNEY STONE (NOTE: for other terms referring to stones, see words beginning or ending with **-lith**) (**b**) measure of weight (= 14 pounds or 6.35 kilograms)英石(合 14 磅或 6.35 千克): ***He tried to lose weight and lost three stone.*** 他在减体重，减了 3 英石。She weighs eight stone ten (i.e. 8 stone 10 pounds)她体重 122 磅。(NOTE: no plural form in this meaning: **'she weighs ten stone'**)

◊ **stone-deaf** *adjective* totally deaf 全聋的

stools *or* **faeces** *plural noun* solid waste matter passed from the bowel through the anus 粪便 (NOTE: can also be used in the singular: **'he passed an abnormal stool'**)

stop needle *noun* needle with a ring round it, so that it can only be pushed a certain distance into the body 定深针(针头上带有限制刺入深度的环)

◊ **stoppage** *noun* act of stopping the function of an organ 停止; **heart stoppage** = condition where the heart has stopped beating 心跳停止

storage disease *noun* disease where abnormal amounts of a substance accumulate in a part of the body 沉积病(某种物质在体内某处异常积聚造成的疾病)

stove-in chest *noun* result of an accident, where several ribs are broken and pushed towards the inside 炉膛状胸(事故造成几根肋骨骨折并压缩进胸腔)

strabismus *or* **squint** *noun* condition where the eyes focus on different points 斜视; **convergent strabismus** = condition where one or both eyes look towards the nose 内斜视; **divergent strabismus** = condition where one or both eyes look away from the nose 外斜视

◊ **strabismal** *adjective* cross-eyed 斜视的，斜眼的

straight *adjective* (line) with no irregularities such as bends, curves or angles 直的

◊ **straighten** *verb* to make straight 弄直，伸直: ***His arthritis is so bad that he cannot straighten his knees.*** 他的关节炎很严重以致他膝盖都伸不直。

strain 1 *noun* (**a**) condition where a muscle has been stretched *or* torn by a strong or sudden movement 拉伤，劳损; **back strain** = condition where the muscles *or* ligaments in the back have been stretched 背部劳损 (**b**) group of microorganisms which are different from others of the same type(细菌)株; ***a new strain of influenza virus*** 一株新发现的感冒病毒 (**c**) nervous tension and stress精神紧张,压力: ***Her work is causing her a lot of strain.*** 她的工作使她倍感压力。***He is suffering from nervous strain and needs to relax.*** 他罹患神经紧张,需要放松。**2** *verb* to stretch a muscle too far 拉伤: ***He strained his back lifting the table.*** 抬桌子时他拉伤了腰部。***She had to leave the game with a strained calf muscle.*** 因为小腿肌肉拉伤她不得不离开运动场。***The effort of running upstairs strained his heart.*** 跑楼梯使他的心脏不堪负荷。

strangle *verb* to kill someone by squeezing his throat so that he cannot breathe or swallow 扼杀,勒死

◊ **strangulated** *adjective* (part of the body) caught in an opening in such a way that the circulation of blood is stopped绞窄的(致血液循环不通); **strangulated hernia** = condition where part of the intestine is squeezed in a hernia and the supply of blood to it is cut 绞窄性疝气

◊ **strangulation** *noun* squeezing a passage in the body 绞窄

strangury *noun* condition where very little urine is passed, although the patient wants to pass water, caused by a bladder disorder *or* by a stone in the urethra 痛性尿淋沥

strap (up) *verb* to wrap a bandage round a limb tightly *or* to attach tightly 包扎: ***The nurses strapped up his stomach wound.*** 护士们把他上腹的伤口包扎起来。***The patient was strapped to the stretcher.*** 病人被绑缚到担架上。

◊ **strapping** *noun* wide strong bandages *or* adhesive plaster used to bandage a large part of the body 宽绷带

stratified *adjective* made of several layers 分层的; **stratified epithelium** = epithelium formed of several layers of cells 复层上皮

◊ **stratum** *noun* layer of tissue forming the epidermis 层 (NOTE: the plural is **strata**)

COMMENT: The main layers of the epidermis are: the Malpighian layer or stratum germinativum which produces the cells that are pushed up to form the stratum lucidum, a thin clear layer of dead and dying cells, and the stratum corneum, the outside layer made of dead keratinized cells.
注释:上皮主要有以下几层:表皮生发层或生发层,产生细胞,向上生长形成透明层,后者是一透明的薄层,由死细胞和垂死的细胞组成;还有角质层,是上皮的外层,由死亡的角化细胞组成。

strawberry mark *noun* naevus, a red birthmark in children, which will disappear in later life 草莓斑(胎记)

streak *noun* long thin line of a different colour 条纹

strength *noun* being strong 力气: ***After her illness she had no strength in her limbs.*** 她病后四肢无力。**full strength solution** = solution which has not been diluted 原液

◊ **strengthen** *verb* to make strong 加强

strenuous *adjective* (exercise) which involves using a lot of force 费力的,用力的: ***Avoid doing any strenuous exercise for some time while the wound heals.*** 伤口愈合期间避免所有用力的活动。

strep throat *noun* (*informal* 非正式) infection of the throat by a streptococcus 链球菌性咽喉炎

◊ **strepto-** *prefix* referring to organisms which grow in chains 链状生长的微生物

◊ **streptobacillus** *noun* type of bacterium which forms a chain 链杆菌属

◊ **streptococcus** *noun* genus of bacteria which grows in long chains, and causes fevers such as scarlet fever, tonsillitis and rheumatic fever 链球菌 (NOTE: plural is **streptococci**)

◊ **streptococcal** *adjective* (infection)

caused by a streptococcus 链球菌的

◇ **streptodornase** *noun* enzyme formed by streptococci which can make pus liquid 链道酶,链球菌脱氧核糖核酸酶

◇ **streptokinase** *noun* enzyme formed by streptococci which can break down blood clots 链激酶

◇ **streptolysin** *noun* toxin produced by streptococci in rheumatic fever, which acts to destroy red blood cells 链球菌溶血素

◇ **Streptomyces** *noun* genus of bacteria used to produce antibiotics 链霉菌属

◇ **streptomycin** *noun* antibiotic used against many types of infection, but especially tuberculosis 链霉素

stress *noun* (**a**) physical pressure 应力;**stress fracture** = fracture of a bone caused by excessive force, as in certain types of sport 应力性骨折 (**b**) condition where an outside influence changes the working of the body, used especially of mental *or* emotional stress which can affect the hormone balance 应激; **stress disorder** = disorder caused by stress 应激障碍; **stress incontinence** = condition where the sufferer is not able to retain his urine when coughing 应力性尿失禁; **stress reaction** = response to an outside stimulus which disturbs the normal physiological balance of the body 应激反应

stretch *verb* to pull out *or* to make longer 伸; **stretch reflex** = reflex reaction of a muscle which contracts after being stretched 伸反射(肌肉对牵张刺激的反射);**stretch mark** = mark on the skin of the abdomen of a pregnant woman *or* of a woman who has recently given birth 妊娠纹 *see also* 参见 STRIAE GRAVIDARUM

stretcher *noun* folding bed, with handles, on which an injured person can be carried by two people 担架: ***She was carried out of the restaurant on a stretcher.*** 她被用担架抬出了饭馆。***Some of the accident victims could walk to the ambulances, but there were several stretcher cases.*** 有些事故受害者能步行到救护车上,但也有的要用担架抬。**stretcher bearer** = person who helps to carry a stretcher 抬担架的人,担架员; **stretcher case** = person who is so ill that he has to be carried on a stretcher 病重需用担架抬的病人; **stretcher party** = group of people who carry a stretcher and look after the patient on it 担架队; **Furley stretcher** *or* **standard stretcher** = stretcher made of a folding frame with a canvas bed, with carrying poles at each side and small feet underneath 普通担架; **paraguard stretcher** *or* **Neil Robertson stretcher** = type of strong stretcher to which the injured person is attached, so that he can be carried upright (used for rescuing people from mountains or from tall buildings)加缚担架(用于在山区运送伤员,可以立起来而伤员不会掉下来); **pole and canvas stretcher** = simple stretcher made of a piece of canvas and two poles which slide into tubes at the side of the canvas 帆布双棒担架; **scoop stretcher** = stretcher in two sections which slide under the patient and can lock together 分体担架

stria *noun* pale line on skin which is stretched (as in obese people)条纹;**striae gravidarum** = stretch marks, lines on the skin of the abdomen of a pregnant woman *or* of a woman who has recently given birth 妊娠纹 (NOTE: plural is **striae**)

◇ **striated** *adjective* marked with pale lines 有条纹的;**striated muscle** = muscle which is attached to the bone which it moves 横纹肌 *compare* 比较 SMOOTH

strict *adjective* severe *or* which must not be changed 严格的: ***She has to follow a strict diet.*** 她必须遵守严格的饮食控制。***The doctor was strict with the patients who wanted to drink alcohol in the hospital.*** 医生对想在医院里喝酒的病人很严厉。

stricture *noun* narrowing of a

passage in the body 狭窄; **urethral stricture** = narrowing *or* blocking of the urethra by a growth 尿道狭窄

stridor *or* **stridulus** *noun* sharp high sound made when air passes an obstruction in the larynx 喘鸣(喉部阻塞时发出的尖利的呼吸音) *see also* 参见 LARYNGISMUS

strike-through *noun* blood absorbed right through a dressing so as to be visible on the outside 血浸透敷料

> QUOTE: If strike-through occurs, the wound dressing should be repadded, not removed.
> 引文:如果血浸透了敷料,应当在伤口再垫敷料而不是去掉浸透的敷料。
> **British Journal of Nursing** 英国护理杂志

string sign *noun* thin line which appears on the ileum, a sign of regional ileitis or Crohn's disease 线征(回肠造影见到的特殊细线,是节段性回肠炎或克隆氏病的征象)

strip 1 *noun* long thin piece of material *or* tissue 条: ***The nurse bandaged the wound with strips of gauze.*** 护士用纱布条包扎伤口。***He grafted a strip of skin over the burn.*** 在他的烧伤创面上移植了一条皮肤。**2** *verb* to take off (especially clothes) 脱(衣服): ***The patients had to strip for the medical examination.*** 为做医学检查病人必须脱去衣服。**to strip to the waist** = to take off the clothes on the top part of the body 脱去上服,暴露腰部以上

stroke 1 *noun* (**a**) sudden loss of consciousness caused by a cerebral haemorrhage or a blood clot in the brain 脑卒中,中风: ***He had a stroke and died.*** 他中风死了。***She was paralysed after a stroke.*** 中风后她瘫痪了。**stroke patient** = person who has suffered a stroke 中风病人 *see also* 参见 HEAT STROKE, SUNSTROKE (**b**) **stroke volume** = amount of blood pumped out the ventricle at each heartbeat 每搏输出量(每次心搏从心室泵出的血量) **2** *verb* to touch softly with the fingers 轻叩

> COMMENT: There are two causes of stroke: cerebral haemorrhage (haemorrhagic stroke), when an artery bursts and blood leaks into the brain, and cerebral thrombosis (occlusive stroke), where a blood clot blocks an artery.
> 注释:中风的原因有二:脑出血(出血性中风),动脉破裂,血液漏到脑组织中;脑血栓(阻塞性中风),血凝块阻塞了动脉。

> QUOTE: Stroke is the third most frequent cause of death in developed countries after ischaemic heart disease and cancer.
> 引文:在发达国家,中风是居缺血性心脏病和癌症之后造成死亡的第三大常见原因。
> **British Journal of Hospital Medicine**
> 英国医院医学杂志

> QUOTE: Raised blood pressure may account for as many as 70% of all strokes. The risk of stroke rises with both systolic and diastolic blood pressure.
> 引文:血压升高可以造成70%的中风。无论收缩压高还是舒张压高中风的危险都上升。
> **British Journal of Hospital Medicine**
> 英国医院医学杂志

stroma *noun* tissue which supports an organ, as opposed to parenchyma *or* functioning tissues in the organ 基质

Strongyloides *noun* parasitic worm which infests the intestines 类圆线虫属 ◊ **strongyloidiasis** *noun* being infested with *Strongyloides* which enters the skin and then travels to the lungs and the intestines 类圆线虫病

strontium *noun* metallic element 锶; **strontium-90** = isotope of strontium which is formed in nuclear reactions and, because it is part of the fallout of nuclear explosions, can enter the food chain, attacking in particular the bones of humans and animals ^{90}锶 (NOTE: chemical symbol is **Sr**)

structure *noun* way in which an organ *or* muscle is formed (组织)结构

struma *noun* goitre 甲状腺肿

strychnine *noun* poisonous alkaloid drug, made from the seeds of a tropical tree, and formerly used in small dose as a tonic 士的宁

student *noun* person who is studying at a college or university 学生: ***All the medical students have to spend some time in hospital.*** 所有医学生都必须在医院里度过一段时间。**student nurse** = person who is studying to become a nurse 实习护士

study 1 *noun* examining something to learn about it 学习,研究: ***He's making a study of diseases of small children.*** 他正在研究幼儿疾病。***They have finished their study of the effects of the drug on pregnant women.*** 他们已经完成了该药物对孕妇作用的研究。**2** *verb* to examine something to learn about it 学习,研究: ***He's studying pharmacy.*** 他在学习药剂学。***Doctors are studying the results of the screening programme.*** 医生们在研究筛查方案的结果。

stuffy *or* **stuffed up** *adjective* (nose) which is blocked with inflamed mucous membrane and mucus 鼻塞的

stump *noun* short piece of a limb which is left after the rest has been amputated 残肢

stun *verb* to concuss *or* to knock out by a blow to the head 打懵,打昏

stunt *verb* to stop something growing 抑制生长发育: ***The children's development was stunted by disease.*** 疾病阻滞了孩子们的发育。

stupe *noun* wet medicated dressing used as a compress 热敷布

stupor *noun* state of being semi-conscious 木僵,意识不清: ***After the party several people were found lying on the floor in a stupor.*** 聚会后发现几个人躺在地板上意识不清。

Sturge-Weber syndrome *noun* dark red mark on the skin above the eye, together with similar marks inside the brain, possibly causing epileptic fits 斯特奈-韦伯综合征(一种血管痣,位于眼睛上方,与脑内血管瘤同时发生,可能是引起癫痫的原因之一)

stutter 1 *noun* speech defect where the patient repeats the sound at the beginning of a word several times 口吃: ***He is taking therapy to try to cure his stutter.*** 他在接受治疗,想治愈自己的口吃。**2** *verb* to speak with a stutter 口吃

◊ **stuttering** *or* **dysphemia** *noun* difficulty in speaking where the person repeats parts of words *or* stops to try to pronounce words 口吃

St Vitus' dance *noun* old name for Sydenham's chorea 小舞蹈症的旧称

stye *noun* hordeolum, inflammation of the gland at the base of an eyelash 睑板腺炎,麦粒肿

stylo- *prefix* referring to the styloid process 茎突

◊ **styloglossus** *noun* muscle which links the tongue to the styloid process 茎突舌骨肌

◊ **styloid** *adjective* pointed 茎突的; **styloid process** = piece of bone which projects from the bottom of the temporal bone (颞骨)茎突 ◊ 见图 SKULL

stylus *noun* long thin instrument used for applying antiseptics *or* ointments onto the skin 药笔(用于给皮肤上药)

styptic *adjective* & *noun* (substance) which stops bleeding 止血药(的); **styptic pencil** = stick of alum, used to stop bleeding from small cuts 止血棒(明矾棒,用于小切口的止血)

sub- *prefix* meaning underneath *or* below 下面

◊ **subacute** *adjective* (condition) which is not acute but may become chronic 亚急性的; **subacute bacterial endocarditis** *or* **subacute infective endocarditis** = infection of the endocardium (the membrane covering the inner surfaces of the heart) by bacteria 亚急性细菌性心内膜炎,亚急性感染性心内膜炎; **subacute combined degeneration (of the spinal cord)** = condition (caused by vitamin B_{12} deficiency) where the sensory and motor nerves in the spinal cord become damaged and the patient has difficulty in moving 亚急性联合变性(由于缺乏维生素B_{12}使脊髓的感觉和运动神经受损,病人活动困难)

◇ **subarachnoid** *adjective* beneath the arachnoid membrane 蛛网膜下的; **subarachnoid haemorrhage** = bleeding into the cerebrospinal fluid of the subarachnoid space 蛛网膜下出血; **subarachnoid space** = space between the arachnoid membrane and the pia mater in the brain, containing cerebrospinal fluid 蛛网膜下腔

◇ **subclavian** *adjective* underneath the clavicle 锁骨下的; **subclavian artery** = one of two arteries branching from the aorta on the left, and from the innominate artery on the right, continuing into the brachial arteries and supplying blood to each arm 锁骨下动脉; **subclavian veins** = veins which continue the axillary veins into the brachiocephalic vein 锁骨下静脉

◇ **subclinical** *adjective* (disease) which is present in the body, but which has not yet developed any symptoms 亚临床的(病已在身,尚无症状)

◇ **subconscious** *adjective* & *noun* (referring to) mental processes (such as the memory) of which people are not aware all the time, but which can affect their actions 下意识的,下意识

◇ **subcortical** *adjective* beneath a cortex 皮层下的

◇ **subcostal** *adjective* below the ribs 肋骨下的; **subcostal plane** = imaginary horizontal line drawn across the front of the abdomen below the ribs 肋骨下平面(假想的低于肋骨经腹前面的平面)

◇ **subculture** *noun* culture of bacteria which is taken from a stock culture 传代培养

◇ **subculturing** *noun* taking of a bacterial culture from a stock culture 传代

◇ **subcutaneous** *adjective* under the skin 皮下的; **subcutaneous injection** = injection made just under the skin (as to administer pain-killing drugs) 皮下注射; **subcutaneous oedema** = fluid collecting under the skin, usually at the ankles 皮下水肿; **subcutaneous tissue** = fatty tissue under the skin 皮下组织

◇ **subdural** *adjective* between the dura mater and the arachnoid 硬膜下的

◇ **subinvolution** *noun* condition where a part of the body does not go back to its former size and shape after having swollen *or* stretched (as in the case of the uterus after childbirth) 复旧不全(器官肿胀或牵张后不能完全恢复到原来的大小和形状,如产后的子宫)

subject *noun* (**a**) patient *or* person suffering from a certain disease 患者: ***The hospital has developed a new treatment for arthritic subjects.*** 医院建立了一种针对关节炎病人的新疗法。(**b**) thing which is being studied *or* written about 对象,主题: ***The subject of the article is 'Rh-negative babies'.*** 这篇文章的题目是"Rh 阴性的婴儿"。

◇ **subjective** *adjective* referring to the person concerned 主观的: ***The psychiatrist gave a subjective opinion on the patient's problem.*** 精神病学家对病人的问题给出一个主观的看法。

◇ **subject to** *adverb* likely to suffer from 易患,易感: ***The patient is subject to fits.*** 这个病人易患抽搐。***After returning from the tropics he was subject to attacks of malaria.*** 从热带地区回来后,他极易染上疟疾。

sublimate 1 *noun* deposit left when a vapour condenses(物质)升华 **2** *verb* to convert violent emotion into a certain action which is not antisocial(精神)升华

◇ **sublimation** *noun* doing a certain action as an unconscious way of showing violent emotions which would otherwise be expressed in antisocial behaviour(精神)升华

subliminal *adjective* (stimulus) which is too slight to be noticed by the senses 阈值以下的,不易被感知的

sublingual *adjective* under the tongue 舌下的; **sublingual gland** = salivary gland under the tongue 舌下腺 ◊ 见图 THROAT

QUOTE: The sublingual region has a rich blood supply derived from the carotid artery and indicates changes in central body temperature more rapidly than the rectum.
引文:舌下区有来自颈动脉的丰富血供,比直肠更能提示体温的变化。
Nursing Times 护理时代

subluxation *noun* condition where a joint is partially dislocated 半脱位

◊ **submandibular gland** *or* **submaxillary gland** *noun* salivary gland on each side of the lower jaw 颌下腺(唾液腺之一) ◊ 见图 THROAT

◊ **submental** *adjective* under the chin 颏下的

◊ **submucosa** *noun* tissue under mucous membrane 粘膜下层

◊ **submucous** *adjective* under mucous membrane 粘膜下的; **submucous resection (SMR)** = removal of a bent cartilage from the septum in the nose(鼻)粘膜下鼻中隔切除术,开窗切除术

◊ **subnormal** *adjective* (patient) with a mind which has not developed fully 低于正常的,低下的; **severely subnormal** = (patient) whose mind has not developed and is incapable of looking after himself 智力严重低下

◊ **subnormality** *noun* condition where a patient's mind has not developed fully (智力)低下

◊ **suboccipital** *adjective* beneath the back of the head 枕骨下的

◊ **subphrenic** *adjective* under the diaphragm 膈下的; **subphrenic abscess** = abscess which forms between the diaphragm and the liver 膈下脓肿

subside *verb* to go down *or* to become less violent 平息,消退: ***After being given the antibiotics, his fever subsided.*** 给了抗生素后,他的烧退了。

substance *noun* chemical material 物质: ***Toxic substances released into the bloodstream.*** 有毒物质释放入血。***He became addicted to certain substances.*** 他对某些物质成瘾。

substitution *noun* replacing one thing with another 取代; **substitution therapy** = treating a condition by using a different drug from the one used before 替代治疗

substrate *noun* substance which is acted on by an enzyme 底物

QUOTE: Insulin is a protein hormone and the body's major anabolic hormone, regulating the metabolism of all body fuels and substrates.
引文:胰岛素是一种蛋白类激素,是身体主要的分解代谢激素,调节体内所有提供热量物质和底物的代谢。
Nursing 87 护理 87

subsultus *noun* twitching of the muscles and tendons, caused by fever (发热所致肌肉和肌腱的)抽动、痉挛

subtertian fever *noun* type of malaria, where the fever is present most of the time 亚间日疟

subtotal *adjective* (operation) to remove most of an organ 次全的(指手术去掉器官的大部分); **subtotal gastrectomy** = surgical removal of most of the stomach 胃次全切除术; **subtotal hysterectomy** = removal of the uterus, but not the cervix 子宫次全切除术; **subtotal thyroidectomy** = removal of most of the thyroid gland 甲状腺次全切除术

subungual *adjective* under a nail 甲下的

succeed *verb* to do well *or* to do what one was trying to do 成功: ***Scientists have succeeded in identifying the new influenza virus.*** 科学家们成功地鉴定了新的流感病毒。***They succeeded in stopping the flow of blood.*** 他们成功地止住了血。

◊ **success** *noun* **(a)** doing something well *or* doing what one was trying to do 成功: ***They tried to isolate the virus but without success.*** 他想分离病毒,但没有成功。**(b)** something which does well 成功: ***The operation was a complete*** *success*. 手术是完全成功的。

◇ **successful** *adjective* which works well 成功的: ***The operation was completely successful***. 手术完全成功了。

◇ **succession** *noun* line of things, one after the other 序列: ***She had a succession of miscarriages***. 她习惯流产。

◇ **successive** *adjective* (things) which follow one after the other 序列的, 接着的: ***She had a miscarriage with each successive pregnancy***. 她每次怀孕后都流产。

succus *noun* juice secreted by an organ(器官分泌的)汁、液; **succus entericus** = juice formed of enzymes, produced in the intestine to help the digestive process 肠液

succussion *noun* splashing sound made when there is a large amount of liquid inside a cavity in the body (as in the stomach)震水音(腹腔积水时的体征)

suck *verb* to pull liquid *or* air into the mouth *or* into a tube 吮吸: ***They applied the stomach pump to suck out the contents of the patient's stomach***. 他们安装洗胃泵来吸出病人的胃内容物。***The baby is sucking its thumb***. 婴儿正在吮吸他的手指。

◇ **suction** *noun* action of sucking 吮吸: ***The dentist hooked a suction tube into the patient's mouth***. 牙医用吮吸管钩在病人嘴里。

suckle *verb* to breastfeed a baby 哺乳

sucrase *noun* enzyme in the intestine which breaks down sucrose into glucose and fructose 蔗糖酶(消化蔗糖的酶)

◇ **sucrose** *noun* sugar found in plants, especially in sugar cane, beet and maple syrup (sucrose is formed of glucose and fructose)蔗糖

sudamen *noun* little blister caused by sweat 痱子,汗疱疹 (NOTE: plural is **sudamina**)

sudden *adjective* which happens quickly 突然; **sudden death** = death without identifiable cause *or* not preceded by an illness 猝死; **sudden infant death syndrome** (**SIDS**) = sudden death of a baby in bed, without any identifiable cause 婴儿猝死综合征

> COMMENT: Occurs in very young children, up to the age of about 12 months; the causes are still being investigated.
> 注释:发生于非常小的孩子,低于 12 个月龄;病因尚在研究中。

Sudeck's atrophy *noun* osteoporosis in the hand or foot 祖德克萎缩(手足的外伤性急性骨质疏松)

sudor *noun* sweat 汗

◇ **sudorific** *noun* drug which makes a patient sweat 发汗药

suffer *verb* (**a**) to have an illness for a long period of time 长期患病: ***She suffers from headaches***. 她患有头疼病。***He suffers from not being able to distinguish certain colours***. 他罹患不能分辨颜色的毛病。(**b**) to feel pain 受苦: ***Did she suffer much in her last illness***? 她上次得病是吃了很多苦头吗? ***He did not suffer at all and was conscious until he died***. 他一点儿也不痛苦,直至死去都是清醒的。(**c**) to receive (an injury)受伤: ***He suffered multiple injuries in the accident***. 他在事故中多处受伤。

◇ **sufferer** *noun* person who has a certain disease 患者: ***A drug to help asthma sufferers or sufferers from asthma***. 一种帮助哮喘患者的药。

◇ **suffering** *noun* feeling pain over a long period of time 苦难,煎熬: ***The doctor gave him a morphine injection to relieve his suffering***. 医生给他注射一针吗啡以缓解他的痛苦。

suffocate *verb* to make someone stop breathing by cutting off the supply of air to his nose and mouth 窒息

◇ **suffocation** *noun* making someone become unconscious by cutting off his supply of air 窒息

suffuse *verb* to spread over *or* through something 遍布,扩散

◇ **suffusion** *noun* spreading (of a red flush) over the skin 红晕

sugar *noun* any of several sweet carbohydrates 糖；**blood sugar level** = amount of glucose in the blood 血糖水平；**sugar content** = percentage of sugar in a substance *or* food 含糖量；**sugar intolerance** = diarrhoea caused by sugar which has not been absorbed 糖不耐受(糖不吸收造成的腹泻)(NOTE：for other terms referring to sugar, see words beginning with **glyc-**)

COMMENT：There are several natural forms of sugar：sucrose（in plants), lactose（in milk), fructose (in fruit), glucose and dextrose（in fruit and in body tissue). Edible sugar used in the home is a form of refined sucrose. All sugars are useful sources of energy, though excessive amounts of sugar can increase weight and cause tooth decay. Diabetes mellitus is a condition where the body is incapable of absorbing sugar from food.

注释：有几种自然形式的糖：(植物中的)蔗糖、(乳汁中的)乳糖、(水果中的)果糖及(水果和身体组织中的)葡萄糖和右旋葡萄糖。家用的食用糖是一种精炼的蔗糖。所有糖类都是能量的可用来源，然而吃糖过量可以导致体重上升和牙齿损坏。糖尿病是身体不能利用从食物吸收来的糖所致的一种疾病。

suggest *verb* to mention an idea 建议，提示：***The doctor suggested that she should stop smoking.*** 医生建议她停止吸烟。

◊ **suggestion** *noun* (**a**) idea which has been mentioned 提示，提法：***The doctor didn't agree with the suggestion that the disease had been caught in the hospital.*** 医生不同意这种病已经在医院里得到控制的提法。(**b**)(*in psychiatry*) making a person's ideas change, by suggesting different ideas which the patient can accept, such as that he is in fact cured 暗示(精神科用语)

suicidal *adjective* (person) who wants to kill himself 自杀的：***He has suicidal tendencies.*** 他有自杀倾向。

◊ **suicide** *noun* act of killing oneself 自杀；**to commit suicide** = to kill oneself 自杀：***After his wife died he committed suicide.*** 他妻子死后，他自杀了。**attempted suicide** = trying to kill oneself, but not succeeding 自杀企图，自杀未遂

sulcus *noun* groove *or* fold (especially between the gyri in the brain)(脑)沟；**Harrison's sulcus** = hollow on either side of the chest which develops in children with lung problems 哈里森沟(胸部下缘的下陷，有肺病的孩子身上可见)；**lateral sulcus and central sulcus** = two grooves which divide a cerebral hemisphere into lobes 外侧沟和中央沟(大脑分叶的主要沟)(NOTE：plural is **sulci**)

sulphate *noun* salt of sulphuric acid 硫酸盐；**barium sulphate** (**$BaSO_4$**) = salt of barium not soluble in water and which shows as opaque in X-ray photographs 硫酸钡(用作造影剂) *see also* 参见 MAGNESIUM

◊ **sulphonamide** *or* **sulpha drug** *or* **sulpha compound** *noun* bacteriostatic drug used to treat bacterial infection, especially in the intestine and urinary system 磺胺药

◊ **sulphur** *noun* yellow non-metallic chemical element which is contained in some amino acids and is used in creams to treat some skin disorders 硫 (NOTE：chemical symbol is **S**, Note also that words beginning **sulph-** are spelt **sulf-** in US English)

sun *noun* very hot star round which the earth travels and which gives light and heat 太阳

◊ **sunbathing** *noun* lying in the sun to absorb sunlight 日光浴

◊ **sun blindness** = PHOTORETINITIS 日射盲

◊ **sunburn** *noun* damage to the skin by excessive exposure to sunlight 日光灼伤

◊ **sunburnt** *adjective* (skin) made brown *or* red by exposure to sunlight 日光灼伤的

◊ **sunglasses** *plural noun* dark glasses which are worn to protect the eyes from the sun 太阳镜

◊ **sunlight** *noun* light from the sun 阳

光:*He is allergic to strong sunlight*. 他对强烈的阳光过敏。

◇ **sunstroke** *noun* serious condition caused by excessive exposure to the sun or to hot conditions, where the patient becomes dizzy and has a high body temperature but does not perspire 中暑

> COMMENT: Sunlight is essential to give the body vitamin D, but excessive exposure to sunlight will not simply turn the skin brown, but also may burn the surface of the skin so badly that it dies and pus forms beneath. Constant exposure to the sun can cause cancer of the skin.
> 注释:日光是给身体带来维生素 D 的基本要素,但过分曝晒不仅使皮肤变成棕色,而且会严重灼伤皮肤表层,以致表层死亡而形成皮下脓液,持续暴露在阳光下可引起皮肤癌。

super- *prefix* meaning (i) above 在之上 (ii) extremely 极端

◇ **superciliary** *adjective* referring to the eyebrows 眉毛的

◇ **superego** *noun* (*in psychology*) part of the mind which is the conscience *or* which is concerned with right and wrong 超我(心理学词汇,心灵中评判对错的部分,良心的部分)

◇ **superfecundation** *noun* condition where two or more ova produced at the same time are fertilized by different males 同期复孕(排卵不止一个,且不止与一个男性受孕)

◇ **superfetation** *noun* condition where an ovum is fertilized in a woman who is already pregnant 复孕

◇ **superficial** *adjective* on the surface *or* close to the surface *or* on the skin 表浅的; **superficial burn** = burn on the skin surface 表层灼伤; **superficial fascia** = membranous layers of connective tissue found just under the skin 浅筋膜; **superficial vein** = vein near the surface of the skin (as opposed to deep vein) 浅静脉

◇ **superinfection** *noun* second infection which affects the treatment of the first infection, because it is resistant to the drug used to treat the first 二重感染

superior *adjective* (*of part of the body*) higher up than another part 上面的; **superior aspect** = view of the body from above 上面观,俯瞰; **superior vena cava** = branch of the large vein into the heart, carrying blood from the head and the top part of the body 上腔静脉

◇ **superiority** *noun* being better than something *or* someone else 自尊; **superiority complex** = condition where a person feels he is better in some way than others and pays little attention to them 自尊情结,优越感 (NOTE: the opposite is **inferior, inferiority**)

supernumerary *adjective* extra; (*of teeth, etc.*) one (or more than one) more than the usual number 额外的

> QUOTE: Allocation of supernumerary students to clinical areas is for their educational needs and not for service requirements.
> 引文:安排额外学生到临床是为了他们的教育需要,而不是医疗服务的需要。
> **Nursing Times** 护理时代

supervise *verb* to manage *or* to organize something 监管,监控: ***The administration of drugs has to be supervised by a qualified person***. 必须在合格人员的监察下服用药物。***She has been appointed to supervise the transfer of patients to the new ward***. 她被委任监管运送病人到新病房。

◇ **supervision** *noun* management *or* organization 监管,监控: ***Elderly patients need constant supervision***. 年老的病人需要持续监护。***The sheltered housing is under the supervision of a full-time nurse***. 福利院由全日制护士监管。

◇ **supervisor** *noun* person who supervises 监督员: ***the supervisor of hospital catering services*** 医院膳食服务的监督员

supinate *verb* to turn (the hand) so that the palm is upwards 向后翻转,旋后

◇ **supination** *noun* turning the hand so that palm faces upwards 旋后

◇ **supinator** *noun* muscle which turns the hand so that the palm faces upwards 旋后肌

◇ **supine** *adjective* (i) lying on the back 仰卧位 (ii) with the palm of the hand facing upwards(手臂的)旋后位 (NOTE: the opposite is **pronation, prone**)

QUOTE: The patient was to remain in the supine position, therefore a pad was placed under the Achilles tendon to raise the legs.
引文:病人保持仰卧位,因此在跟腱下垫上垫子将双腿抬高。
NATNews 全国手术室护士协会新闻

supply 1 *noun* something which is provided 供应: ***The arteries provide a continuous supply of oxygenated blood to the tissues.*** 动脉持续向组织提供氧合血。***The hospital service needs a constant supply of blood for transfusion.*** 医院后勤需要不断有血液供应以备输血之用。***The government sent medical supplies to the disaster area.*** 政府向受灾地区派出了医疗救援。**2** *verb* to provide *or* to give something which is needed 供应: ***A balanced diet will supply the body with all the vitamins and trace elements it needs.*** 平衡膳食能供给身体需要的所有维生素和微量元素。***The brachial artery supplies the arm and hand.*** 臂动脉向手臂供血。

support 1 *noun* (**a**) help to keep something in place 支持: ***The bandage provides some support for the knee.*** 绷带给膝关节某些支持。***He was so weak that he had to hold onto a chair for support.*** 他太虚弱了,以致只能靠在椅子上才能站稳。(**b**) handle *or* metal rail which a person can hold 支架,托,扶手: ***There are supports at the side of the bed.*** 床的侧面有扶手。***The bath is provided with metal supports.*** 浴盆带有金属扶手。**2** *verb* to hold something *or* to keep something in place 支持: ***He wore a truss to support a hernia.*** 他戴着疝袋兜住疝气。

◇ **supportive** *adjective* (person) who helps *or* comforts someone in trouble 支持的: ***Her family were very supportive when she was in hospital.*** 她住院时家人给了她很大支持。***The local health authority has been very supportive of the hospital management.*** 地方卫生当局一直非常支持医院管理。

suppository *noun* piece of soluble material (such as glycerine jelly) containing a drug, which is placed in the rectum (to act as lubricant), or in the vagina (to treat disorders such as vaginitis) and is dissolved by the body's fluids 栓剂(纳入直肠、阴道的可溶解的药物制剂)

suppress *verb* to remove (a symptom) *or* to reduce the action of something completely *or* to stop (the release of a hormone) 抑制: ***A course of treatment which suppresses the painful irritation.*** 抑制痛性刺激的疗程。***The drug suppresses the body's natural instinct to reject the transplanted tissue.*** 这种药物抑制身体排斥移植组织的天性。***The release of adrenaline from the adrenal cortex is suppressed.*** 抑制肾上腺皮质释放肾上腺素。

◇ **suppression** *noun* act of suppressing 抑制: ***the suppression of allergic responses*** 抑制过敏反应; ***the suppression of a hormone*** 抑制某种激素

suppurate *verb* to form and discharge pus 化脓,流脓

◇ **suppurating** *or* **purulent** *adjective* containing *or* discharging pus 化脓的,流脓的

◇ **suppuration** *noun* formation and discharge of pus 化脓,流脓

supra- *prefix* meaning above *or* over 在上面,超出

◇ **supraoptic nucleus** *noun* nucleus in the hypothalamus from which nerve fibres run to the posterior pituitary gland 视上核(下丘脑的神经核团之一,神经纤维走向垂体后部)

◇ **supraorbital** *adjective* above the orbit of the eye 眶上的; **supraorbital ridge** = ridge of bone above the eye, covered by the eyebrow 眶上嵴

◇ **suprapubic** *adjective* above the pubic bone *or* pubic area 耻骨上的

◇ **suprarenal** *adjective* above the kidney 肾上的;**suprarenal area** = the area of the body above the kidney 肾上区;**suprarenal glands** *or* **suprarenals** *or* **adrenal glands** = two endocrine glands at the top of the kidneys, which secrete adrenaline and other hormones 肾上腺,位于肾脏顶端的两个内分泌腺体,分泌肾上腺素和其他激素

◇ **suprasternal** *adjective* above the sternum 胸骨上的

surface *noun* top layer of something 表面: ***The surfaces of the two membranes may rub together.*** 两层膜的表面可能会相互磨擦。

surfactant *noun* substance in the alveoli of the lungs which keeps the surfaces of the lungs wet and prevents lung collapse 表面活性物质,肺泡里的物质,保持肺泡表面湿润、防止肺萎陷。

surgeon *noun* doctor who specializes in surgery 外科医师;**eye surgeon** = surgeon who specializes in operations on eyes 眼外科医师;**heart surgeon** = surgeon who specializes in operations on hearts 心外科医师;**plastic surgeon** = surgeon who repairs defective *or* deformed parts of the body 整形外科医师;*US* **surgeon general** = government official responsible for all aspects of public health 负责公共保健的政府官员(NOTE: although surgeons are doctors, in the UK they are traditionally called '**Mr**' and not '**Dr**', so '**Dr Smith**' may be a GP, **but 'Mr Smith' is a surgeon**)

◇ **surgery** *noun* (**a**) treatment of a disease *or* disorder which requires an operation to cut into *or* to remove *or* to manipulate tissue *or* organs *or* parts 外科手术: ***The patient will need plastic surgery to remove the scars he received in the accident.*** 这个病人将需要整形外科手术来去掉车祸中留下的疤痕。***The surgical ward is for patients waiting for surgery.*** 外科病房是为等待手术的病人准备的。***Two of our patients had to have surgery.*** 我们的4个病人中有2个不得不做手术。**exploratory surgery** = surgical operations in which the aim is to discover the cause of the patient's symptoms *or* the extent of the illness 探查手术,为搞清病因或疾病范围而做的手术,本身不能起治疗作用;**major surgery** = surgical operations involving important organs in the body 大手术(涉及重要脏器的手术);**plastic surgery** *or* **reconstructive surgery** = surgery to repair defective *or* deformed parts of the body 整形手术,重建手术;**spare part surgery** = surgical operations where parts of the body (such as bones *or* joints) are replaced by artificial pieces 置换手术(如换人工关节的手术) *see also* 参见 CRYOSURGERY, MICROSURGERY (**b**) room where a doctor *or* dentist sees and examines patients 外科诊室: ***There are ten patients waiting in the surgery.*** 外科诊室里等着10个病人。***Surgery hours are from 8:30 in the morning to 6:00 at night.*** 外科门诊时间是从早上8:30到晚上6点。

◇ **surgical** *adjective* (i) referring to surgery 外科的 (ii) (disease) which can be treated by surgery(疾病)可以用外科方法治疗的: ***All surgical instruments must be sterilized.*** 所有外科器械都必须消毒。***We manage to carry out six surgical operations in an hour.*** 我们尽力在1个小时里安排6台手术。**surgical care** = looking after patients who have had surgery 外科护理;**surgical emphysema** = air bubbles in tissue, not in the lungs 外科气肿,皮下气肿;**surgical gloves** = thin plastic gloves worn by surgeons 外科手套;**surgical neck** = narrow part at the top of the humerus, where the arm can easily be broken 外科颈(肱骨上端细的部分);**surgical spirit** = ethyl alcohol with an additive which gives it an unpleasant taste, used as a disinfectant *or* for rubbing on the skin 外科酒精(用于消毒,气味难闻)(NOTE: the US English is **rubbing alcohol**);**surgical stockings** = strong elastic stockings worn to support a weak joint in the knee or to hold varicose veins tightly 外科袜(高弹性的长袜,用于稳固膝关节或束紧曲张的静脉);

surgical ward = ward in a hospital for patients who have to have operations 外科病房

◇ **surgically** *adverb* using surgery 用外科方法处理地: ***The growth can be treated surgically.*** 这个增生物可以用外科方法处理。

surrogate *adjective* taking the place of 取代的; **surrogate mother** = (i) person who takes the place of a real mother 代理母亲 (ii) woman who has a child by artificial insemination for a couple where the wife cannot bear children, with the intention of handing the child over to them when it is born 愿意让不能生育的女性借其腹怀胎的女性

surround *verb* to be all around something 围绕: ***The wound is several millimetres deep and the surrounding flesh is inflamed.*** 伤口有几毫米深,周围的肉都发炎了。

◇ **surroundings** *noun* area round something 周遭,环境: ***The cottage hospital is set in pleasant surroundings.*** 小村医院坐落在宜人的环境里。

survive *verb* to continue to live 生存,存活: ***He survived two attacks of pneumonia.*** 他2次患肺炎都活了下来。***They survived a night on the mountain without food.*** 他们在绝粮的情况下在山里熬过了一整夜。***The baby only survived for two hours.*** 婴儿只活了2个小时。

◇ **survival** *noun* continuing to live 存活: ***The survival rate of newborn babies has begun to fall.*** 新生儿存活率已经开始下降了。

◇ **survivor** *noun* person who survives 存活的人,幸存者

susceptible *adjective* likely to catch (a disease) 易感的: ***She is susceptible to colds*** *or* ***to throat infections.*** 她易患感冒或喉咙感染

◇ **susceptibility** *noun* lack of resistance to a disease 易感性

> QUOTE: Low birthweight has been associated with increased susceptibility to infection.
> 引文:出生体重低与对感染的易感性有关。
> **East African Medical Journal** 东非医学杂志

> QUOTE: Even children with the milder forms of sickle-cell disease have an increased frequency of pneumococcal infection. The reason for this susceptibility is a profound abnormality of the immune system.
> 引文:即便是镰状细胞病相当轻的孩子患肺炎球菌感染的机率也升高。易感的原因是免疫系统的严重异常。
> **Lancet** 柳叶刀

suspect 1 *noun* person who doctors believe may have a disease 可疑病人: ***They are screening all typhoid suspects.*** 他们在筛查所有可能的伤寒病人。**2** *verb* to think that someone may have a disease 怀疑: ***He is a suspected diphtheria carrier.*** 他被怀疑是白喉携带者。***Several cases of suspected meningitis have been reported.*** 报告了几例可疑的脑膜炎病例。

> QUOTE: Those affected are being nursed in five isolation wards and about forty suspected sufferers are being barrier nursed in other wards.
> 引文:被感染的人在5个隔离病房里接受护理,约40个被怀疑染病的人被羁留在其他病房。
> **Nursing Times** 护理时代

suspension *noun* liquid with solid particles in it 悬液

◇ **suspensory** *adjective* which is hanging down 悬吊的; **suspensory bandage** = bandage to hold a part of the body which hangs 吊带; **suspensory ligament** = ligament which holds a part of the body in position 悬韧带

sustain *verb* (**a**) to keep *or* to support *or* to maintain 支撑,维系: ***These bones can sustain quite heavy weights.*** 这些骨骼可以支撑很重的重量。***He is not eating enough to sustain life.*** 他吃得太少,还不足以维系生命。(**b**) to suffer (an injury) 受苦: ***He sustained a severe head injury.*** 他头部严重受伤。

sustentacular *adjective* referring to

sustentaculum 支持物的

◇ **sustentaculum** *noun* part of the body which supports another part 支柱

suture 1 *noun* (**a**) fixed joint where two bones are fused together, especially the bones in the skull 缝 ◊ 见图 SKULL 头颅; **coronal suture** = horizontal joint across the top of the skull between the parietal and frontal bones 冠状缝; **lambdoidal suture** = horizontal joint across the back of the skull between the parietal and occipital bones 人字缝; **sagittal suture** = joint along the top of the head between the two parietal bones 矢状缝 (**b**) attaching the sides of an incision *or* wound with thread, so that healing can take place 缝合 (**c**) thread used for attaching the sides of a wound so that they can heal 缝线 **2** *verb* to attach the sides of a wound *or* incision together with thread so that healing can take place 缝合

> COMMENT: Wounds are usually stitched using thread or catgut which is removed after a week or so. Sutures are either absorbable (made of a substance which is eventually absorbed into the body) or non-absorbable, in which case they need to be removed after a certain time.
> 注释:通常用线或肠线缝合伤口,过一周左右拆线。缝线可以分为可溶解的(由最终被身体吸收的物质制成)或不可吸的,如果是不可吸缝线,过一定时间后需要拆线。

swab *noun* (**a**) cotton wool pad, often attached to a small stick, used to clean a wound *or* to apply ointment *or* to take a specimen, etc. 拭子,棉签 (**b**) specimen taken with a swab 用拭子采取的标本; ***a cervical swab*** 宫颈拭子

swallow *verb* to make liquid *or* food (and sometimes air) go down from the mouth to the stomach 吞咽: ***Patients suffering from nose bleeds should try not to swallow the blood.*** 鼻子出血的病人不要把血吞咽下去。

◇ **swallowing** *or* **deglutition** *noun* action of passing food *or* liquids (sometimes also air) from the mouth into the oesophagus and down into the stomach 吞咽 *see also* 参见 AEROPHAGY

sweat 1 *noun* sudor *or* perspiration *or* salt moisture produced by the sweat glands 汗: ***Sweat was running off the end of his nose.*** 汗从他的鼻尖上流下来。***Her hands were covered with sweat.*** 她的双手沁满汗水。**sweat duct** = thin tube connecting the sweat gland with the surface of the skin 汗腺导管; **sweat gland** = gland which produces sweat, situated beneath the dermis and connected to the surface of the skin by a thin tube 汗腺; **sweat pore** = hole in the skin through which the sweat comes out 汗毛孔 ◊ 见图 SKIN & SENSORY RECEPTORS **2** *verb* to perspire *or* to produce moisture through the sweat glands and onto the skin 出汗: ***After working in the fields he was sweating.*** 由于在野外工作,他大汗淋漓。

> COMMENT: Sweat cools the body as the moisture evaporates from the skin. Sweat contains salt, and in hot countries it may be necessary to take salt tablets to replace the salt lost through the skin.
> 注释:当湿气从皮肤蒸发时,汗液起到降低体温的作用。汗液中有盐,在热带国家有必要服用盐片来补充皮肤出汗所致的盐分损失。

sweet *adjective* one of the basic tastes, not bitter, sour or salt 甜的: ***Sugar is sweet, lemons are sour.*** 糖是甜的,柠檬是酸的。

swell *verb* to become larger 肿胀,膨胀: ***The disease affects the lymph glands, making them swell.*** 这种病影响淋巴腺,使淋巴腺肿胀。***The doctor noticed that the patient had swollen glands in his neck.*** 医生注意到病人颈部肿大的腺体。***She finds her swollen ankles painful.*** 她觉得自己肿胀的脚踝疼。(NOTE: **swelling - swelled - has swollen**)

◇ **swelling** *noun* condition where fluid accumulates in tissue, making the tissue become large 肿胀: ***They applied a cold***

compress to try to reduce the swelling. 他们用冷敷来减轻肿胀。

sycosis *noun* bacterial infection of hair follicles 毛囊感染; **sycosis barbae** *or* **barber's rash** = infection of hair follicles on the sides of the face and chin 须疮

Sydenham's chorea 西登汉姆氏舞蹈病 *see* 见 CHOREA

Sylvius 西耳维厄斯 *see* 见 AQUEDUCT

symbiosis *noun* condition where two organisms exist together and help each other to survive 共生(两种生物生活在一起,在生存上有相互的帮助)

symblepharon *noun* condition where the eyelid sticks to the eyeball 睑球粘连

symbol *noun* sign *or* letter which means something 象征,符号; **chemical symbol** = letters which indicate a chemical substance 元素的化学符号: ***Na is the symbol for sodium.*** Na 是钠的符号。° is the symbol for degree. °是度的符号。

Syme's amputation *noun* surgical operation to amputate the foot above the ankle 塞姆截肢(连同踝关节截去足部)

sympathectomy *noun* surgical operation to cut part of the sympathetic nervous system, as a treatment of high blood pressure 交感神经切除术

◇ **sympathetic nervous system** *noun* part of the autonomic nervous system, which runs down the spinal column and connects with various important organs, such as the heart, the lungs, the sweat glands, etc. 交感神经系统,自主神经系统的一部分,沿脊柱下行,与多个重要脏器相连,如心脏、肺、汗腺等

◇ **sympatholytic** *noun* drug which stops the sympathetic nervous system working 交感神经阻滞剂

◇ **sympathomimetic** *adjective* (drug) which stimulates the activity of the sympathetic nervous system 拟交感作用的

symphysiectomy *noun* surgical operation to remove part of the pubic symphysis to make childbirth easier 耻骨联合部分切除术(为使分娩顺利些)

◇ **symphysiotomy** *noun* surgical operation to make an incision in the pubic symphysis to make the passage for a fetus wider 耻骨联合切开术(使产道变宽些)

◇ **symphysis** *noun* point where two bones are joined by cartilage which makes the joint rigid 联合; **pubic symphysis** *or* **symphysis pubis** *or* **interpubic joint** = piece of cartilage which joins the two sections of the pubic bone 耻骨联合; **symphysis menti** = point in the front of the lower jaw where the two halves of the jaw are fused to form the chin 颏联合

symptom *noun* change in the way the body works *or* change in the body's appearance, which shows that a disease *or* disorder is present and is noticed by the patient himself 症状,病人本人感受到的预示疾病的身体功能状态或身体形态的改变: ***The symptoms of hay fever are a running nose and eyes.*** 枯草热的症状是流涕、流泪。***A doctor must study the symptoms before making his diagnosis.*** 医生必须先研究症状再下诊断。***The patient presented all the symptoms of rheumatic fever.*** 病人具备风湿热的所有症状。(NOTE: if a symptom is noticed only by the doctor, it is a **sign**)

◇ **symptomatic** *adjective* which is a symptom 症状的: ***The rash is symptomatic of measles.*** 皮疹是麻疹的症状。

◇ **symptomatology** *or* **semeiology** *noun* branch of medicine concerned with the study of symptoms 症状学

syn- *prefix* meaning joint *or* fused 合

◇ **synalgia** *or* **referred pain** *noun* pain which is felt in one part of the body, but is caused by a condition in another part (such as pain in the groin which can be a symptom of kidney stone and pain in the right shoulder which can indicate gall bladder infection) 牵涉痛,一处有病,带得另一处疼痛,如胆囊炎时右肩痛;肾结石时腹股沟疼痛

synapse 1 *noun* point in the nervous system where the axons of neurones are in contact with the dendrites of other neurones 突触(神经元轴突与其他神经元树突的接点) 2 *verb* to link with a neurone 形成突触

◇ **synaptic** *adjective* referring to a synapse 突触的; **synaptic connection** = link between the dendrites of one neurone with another neurone 突触连接

synarthrosis *noun* joint (as in the skull) where the bones have fused together 不动关节

◇ **synchondrosis** *noun* joint, as in children, where the bones are linked by cartilage, before the cartilage has changed to bone 软骨联合

◇ **synchysis** *noun* condition where the vitreous humour in the eye becomes soft 玻璃体液化

◇ **syncope** *or* **fainting fit** *noun* becoming unconscious for a short time because of reduced flow of blood to the brain 昏厥,晕厥,由于大脑血液供应下降导致的短暂的意识丧失

◇ **syncytium** *noun* continuous length of tissue in muscle fibres 合胞体(肌纤维中连续的长组织); **respiratory syncytial virus** = virus which causes infections of the nose and throat in children 呼吸道合胞病毒

◇ **syndactyly** *noun* condition where two toes *or* fingers are joined together with tissue 并指,并趾

syndesm- *or* **syndesmo-** *prefix* referring to ligaments 韧带

◇ **syndesmology** *noun* branch of medicine which studies joints 韧带学

◇ **syndesmosis** *noun* joint where the bones are tightly linked by ligaments 韧带联合

syndrome *noun* group of symptoms and other changes in the body's functions which, when taken together, show that a particular disease is present 综合征,一组症状和其他身体功能变化同时发生,提示存在某一特殊疾病

synechia *noun* condition where the iris sticks to another part of the eye 虹膜粘连

◇ **syneresis** *noun* releasing of fluid as in a blood clot when it becomes harder 凝缩,脱水(如血块凝固时液体渗出,血块变硬)

◇ **synergism** *noun* (*of two things*) acting together in such a way that both are more effective 协同作用,两者合力大于算术相加

◇ **synergist** *noun* muscle *or* drug which acts with another and increases the effectiveness of both 协同肌,增效剂

◇ **synergy** *noun* working together, so that the combination is twice as effective 协同作用

◇ **syngraft** *or* **isograft** *noun* graft of tissue from an identical twin 同卵双生间的移植

◇ **synoptophore** *noun* instrument used to correct a squint 斜视矫正器,同视机

◇ **synostosis** *noun* fusing of two bones together by forming new bone tissue 骨性联合; (*of bones*) **synostosed** = fused together with bone tissue 骨性联合的

synovectomy *noun* surgical operation to remove the synovial membrane of a joint 滑膜切除术

◇ **synovia** = SYNOVIAL FLUID 滑液

◇ **synovial** *adjective* referring to the synovium 滑膜的; **synovial cavity** = space inside a synovial joint 滑膜腔; **synovial fluid** = fluid secreted by a synovial membrane to lubricate a joint 滑液; **synovial joint** = diarthrosis, joint which can move freely 滑膜关节; **synovial membrane** *or* **synovium** = smooth membrane which forms the inner lining of the capsule covering a joint and secretes the fluid which lubricates the joint 滑膜

◇ **synovioma** *noun* tumour in a synovial membrane 滑膜瘤

◇ **synovitis** *noun* inflammation of the synovial membrane 滑膜炎

◇ **synovium** = SYNOVIAL MEM-

BRANE 滑膜◊见图 JOINTS

> QUOTE: 70% of rheumatoid arthritis sufferers develop the condition in the metacarpophalangeal joints. The synovium produces an excess of synovial fluid which is abnormal and becomes thickened.
> 引文:70%的风湿性关节炎患者掌指关节异常。滑膜产生过多的滑液,滑液不正常并变稠。
>
> **Nursing Times** 护理时代

synthesize *verb* to make a chemical compound from its separate components 合成: ***Essential amino acids cannot be synthesized.*** 必需氨基酸是(身体)不能合成的。***The body cannot synthesize essential fatty acids and has to absorb them from food.*** 身体不能合成必需脂肪酸,必须从食物中摄取。

◊ **synthetic** *adjective* made by man *or* made artificially 人工的,合成的

◊ **synthetically** *adverb* made artificially 人造地,合成地: ***Synthetically produced hormones are used in hormone therapy.*** 合成激素用于激素治疗。

syphilide *noun* rash *or* open sore which is a symptom of the second stage of syphilis 梅毒疹

◊ **syphilis** *noun* sexually transmitted disease caused by a spirochaete *Treponema pallidum* 梅毒,由梅毒螺旋体导致的性传播疾病; **congenital syphilis** = syphilis which is passed on from a mother to her unborn child 先天性梅毒

◊ **syphilitic** *noun & adjective* (person) suffering from syphilis 梅毒的,梅毒患者

> COMMENT: Syphilis is a serious sexually transmitted disease, but it is curable with penicillin injections if the treatment is started early. Syphilis has three stages: in the first (or primary) stage, a hard sore (chancre) appears on the genitals or sometimes on the mouth; in the second (or secondary) stage about two or three months later, a rash appears, with sores round the mouth and genitals. It is at this stage that the disease is particularly infectious. After this stage, symptoms disappear for a long time, sometimes many years. The disease reappears in the third (or tertiary) stage in many different forms: blindness, brain disorders, ruptured aorta, or general paralysis leading to insanity and death. The tests for syphilis are the Wassermann test and the less reliable Kahn test.
> 注释:梅毒是严重的性传播疾病,但如果及早开始用青霉素注射治疗,还是可以治愈的。梅毒有三期:第一期,生殖器或口唇出现硬下疳;2～3个月后是第二期,皮疹出现,同时口周和生殖器周围有溃疡,在这一期,此病的传染性特别强,此期以后,症状长期消失,有时几年都没有症状;第三期,疾病再现可以呈多种不同形式:失明、脑功能障碍、主动脉破裂或导致精神失常和死亡的全身瘫痪。检查梅毒的试验是瓦氏反应和康氏反应,后者可靠性逊于前者。

syring- *or* **syringo-** *prefix* referring to tubes, especially the central canal of the spinal cord 管,脊髓的中央管

◊ **syringe 1** *noun* surgical instrument made of a tube with a plunger which slides down inside it, forcing the contents out through a needle (as in an injection) or slides up the tube, allowing a liquid to be sucked into it 注射器,清洗器 **2** *verb* to wash out (the ears) using a syringe 注射,清洗(如耳道)

◊ **syringobulbia** *noun* syringomyelia in the brain stem 延髓空洞症

◊ **syringocystadenoma** *or* **syringoma** *noun* benign tumour in sweat glands and ducts 汗腺瘤

◊ **syringomyelia** *noun* disease which forms cavities in the neck section of the spinal cord, affecting the nerves so that the patient loses his sense of touch and pain 脊髓空洞症

◊ **syringomyelocele** *noun* severe form of spina bifida where the spinal cord pushes through a hole in the spine 脊髓中央管突出(严重的脊柱裂)

◊ **syrinx** = EUSTACHIAN TUBE 咽

鼓管

system *noun* (**a**) the body as a whole 整个身体: ***Amputation of a limb gives a serious shock to the system.*** 截肢对整个身体是一个严峻的打击。(**b**) arrangement of certain parts of the body so that they work together 系统; **the alimentary system** = system of organs and tracts which digest and break down food (including the alimentary canal, the salivary glands, the liver, etc.) 消化系统; **the cardiovascular system** = system of organs and blood vessels where the blood circulates round the body (including the heart, arteries and veins) 心血管系统; **central nervous system** = the brain and spinal cord which link together all the nerves 中枢神经系统; **respiratory system** = series of organs and passages which take air into the lungs and exchange oxygen for carbon dioxide 呼吸系统; **urinary system** = system of organs and ducts which separate waste liquids from blood and excrete them as urine (including the kidneys, bladder, ureters and urethra) 泌尿系统 *see also* 参见 AUTONOMIC, PARASYMPATHETIC, PERIPHERAL, SYMPATHETIC

◊ **Systme International** 国际单位制 *see* 见 SI

◊ **systemic** *adjective* referring to the whole body 系统性的,全身的: ***Septicaemia is a systemic infection.*** 脓毒血症是全身性感染。**systemic circulation** = circulation of blood around the whole body (except the lungs), starting with the aorta and returning through the venae cavae 体循环; **systemic lupus erythematosus** (**SLE**) = one of several collagen diseases, forms of lupus, where red patches form on the skin and spread throughout the body 系统性红斑狼疮,严重胶原病的一种,形成狼疮,皮肤上红色斑片遍布全身

systole *noun* phase in the beating of the heart when it contracts as it pumps blood out(心脏)收缩期: ***The heart is in systole.*** = The heart is contracting and pumping. 心脏处在收缩期。(NOTE: often used without the : '**at systole the heart pumps blood into the arteries**')

◊ **systolic** *adjective* referring to the systole 收缩的; **systolic pressure** = blood pressure taken at the systole 收缩压 *compare* 比较 DIASTOLE, DIASTOLIC

> COMMENT: Systolic pressure is always higher than diastolic.
> 注释:收缩压总是高于舒张压。

Tt

T *symbol for* tera-太拉的符号(垓,兆兆,万亿,10^{12})

T-cell *or* **T-lymphocyte** *noun* lymphocyte produced by the thymus gland 胸腺淋巴细胞,T细胞

Ta *chemical symbol for* tantalum 钽的化学元素符号

TAB vaccine *noun* vaccine which immunizes against typhoid fever and paratyphoid A and B 伤寒及 A、B型副伤寒疫苗: ***He was given a TAB injection.*** 给他注射了 TAB 疫苗。TAB ***injections give only temporary immunity against paratyphoid.*** 注射 TAB 对副伤寒只产生暂时免疫力。

tabes *noun* wasting away 消瘦,脊髓痨; **tabes dorsalis** *or* **locomotor ataxia** = disease of the nervous system, caused by advanced syphilis, where the patient loses his sense of feeling, the control of his bladder, the ability to coordinate movements of the legs, and suffers severe pains 脊髓痨,运动性共济失调,进展型梅毒引起的神经系统疾病,病人失去感觉,不能控制膀胱和双腿的共济运动,并有剧痛; **tabes mesenterica** = wasting of glands in the abdomen 肠系膜痨,肠系膜淋巴结核 ◇ **tabetic** *adjective* which is wasting away *or* affected by tabes dorsalis 消瘦的,脊髓痨的

table *noun* piece of furniture with a flat top and legs, used to eat at *or* to work at 台子,桌子; **operating table** = special flat table on which a patient lies while undergoing an operation 手术台

tablet *noun* small flat round piece of dry drug which a patient swallows 药片,片剂: ***a bottle of aspirin tablets*** 一瓶阿司匹林片; ***The soluble tablets dissolve in water.*** 可溶性片剂溶解在水里了。***Take two tablets three times a day.*** 每天3次,每次服2片。

taboparesis *noun* final stage of syphilis where the patient has locomotor ataxia and general paralysis of the insane 脊髓痨性全身麻痹症,梅毒的终末阶段,病人局部运动共济失调和精神失常性全身麻痹

tachy- *prefix* meaning fast 快 ◇ **tachycardia** *noun* rapid beating of the heart 心动过速; **nodal tachycardia** *or* **paroxysmal tachycardia** = sudden attack of rapid heartbeats 结性心动过速,阵发性心动过速; **sinus tachycardia** *or* **simple tachycardia** = rapid heartbeats caused by stimulation of the sinoatrial node 窦性心动过速,单纯性心动过速 ◇ **tachyphrasia** *noun* rapid speaking, as in some mentally disturbed patients 言语过快 ◇ **tachyphyl(l)axis** *noun* rapid decrease of the effect of a drug 药性快速减退,快速免疫法,快速减敏 ◇ **tachypnoea** *noun* very fast breathing 呼吸急促

tactile *adjective* which can be sensed by touch 可触知的; **tactile anaesthesia** = loss of sensation of touch 触觉麻痹

taenia *noun* (**a**) long ribbon-like part of the body(身体内的)带状结构; **taenia coli** = outer band of muscle running along the large intestine 结肠带 (**b**) **Taenia** = genus of tapeworm 绦虫属 (NOTE: plural is **Taeniae**) ◇ **taeniacide** *adjective* substance which kills tapeworms 杀绦虫药 ◇ **taeniafuge** *noun* substance which makes tapeworms leave the body 驱绦虫药 ◇ **taeniasis** *noun* infestation of the intestines with tapeworms 绦虫病

> COMMENT: The various species of Taenia which affect humans are taken into the body from eating meat which has not been properly cooked. The most obvious symptom of tapeworm infestation is a sharply increased appetite, together with a loss of weight. The most serious infestation is with *Taenia solium*, found in pork, where the larvae develop in the body and can form hydatid cysts.

注释：各种影响人体的绦虫都是通过进食烹饪不当的肉食进入人体的。绦虫感染最明显的症状是突然胃口大增却体重下降。最严重的是猪肉绦虫感染，它的幼虫在人体内发育并可以形成包囊。

take 1 *noun* **on (the) take** = on duty (admitting patients to hospital) 上班 2 *verb* (**a**) to swallow *or* to drink (a medicine) 服(药)：***She has to take her tablets three times a day.*** 她不得不一天吃三次药。***The medicine should be taken in a glass of water.*** 吃这药时要喝一杯水。(**b**) to do certain actions 做：***The dentist took an X-ray of his teeth.*** 牙医给他的牙拍了一张牙片。***The patient has been allowed to take a bath.*** 病人已被允许洗澡。(**c**) (*of graft*) to be accepted by the body 接受(移植物)：***The skin graft hasn't taken.*** 移植的皮肤没有被接受。***The kidney transplant took easily.*** 肾移植很容易被接受。(NOTE **takes - taking - took - has taken**)

◇ **take after** *verb* to be like (a parent) 长得像：***He takes after his father.*** 他长得像他的父亲。

◇ **take care of** *verb* to look after *or* to attend to (a patient) 照顾：***The nurses will take care of the accident victims.*** 护士将照顾事故受伤者。

◇ **take off** *verb* to remove (especially clothes) 脱去(衣服)：***The doctor asked him to take his shirt off*** *or* ***to take off his shirt.*** 医生让他脱去衬衫。

talc *noun* soft white powder used to dust on irritated skin 滑石

◇ **talcum powder** *noun* scented talc 滑石粉

talipes *or* **club foot** *noun* congenitally deformed foot 畸形足

COMMENT: The most usual form (talipes equinovarus) is where the person walks on the toes because the foot is permanently bent forward; in other forms, the foot either turns towards the inside (talipes varus), towards the outside (talipes valgus), or upwards (talipes calcaneus) at the ankle, so that the patient cannot walk on the sole of the foot.

注释：最常见的足畸形是马蹄内翻足，病人用脚趾走路，因为脚总是向前弯的；其他形式的足畸形，脚可以向内翻(内翻足)，也可以向外翻(外翻足)或从踝部向上翻(仰趾足)，总之病人不能靠足底走路。

tall *adjective* high, usually higher than other people 高于：***He's the tallest in the family - he's taller than all his brothers.*** 他是家里最高的。***How tall is he? he's 5 foot 7 inches (5′7″) tall*** *or* **1.25 metres tall** 他有多高？他有5英尺7英寸(1.25米)高。(NOTE: **tall - taller - tallest**)

talo- *prefix* referring to the ankle bone"踝骨"

◇ **talus** *noun* ankle bone, the top bone in the tarsus which articulates with the tibia and fibula in the leg, and with the calcaneus in the heel 踝骨 ◊ 见图 FOOT

tampon *noun* (i) wad of absorbent material put into a wound to soak up blood during an operation 纱垫儿 (ii) wad of absorbent material which is inserted into the vagina to absorb menstrual flow 经期用卫生塞

◇ **tamponade** *noun* (i) putting a tampon into a wound 填塞 (ii) abnormal pressure on part of the body 压塞；**cardiac tamponade** *or* **heart tamponade** = pressure on the heart when the pericardial cavity fills with blood 心脏填塞，心包充盈时加在心脏上的压力

tan *verb* (*of skin*) to become brown (in sunlight) 晒黑：***He tans easily.*** 他容易被晒黑。***She is using a tanning lotion.*** 她用着防晒油。

◇ **tannin** *or* **tannic acid** *noun* substance found in the bark of trees and in tea and other liquids, which stains brown 鞣酸

tantalum *noun* rare metal, used to repair damaged bones 钽，稀有金属，用于修复损伤的骨；**tantalum mesh** = type of net made of tantalum wire, used to repair cranial defects 钽钢丝(用于颅骨缺损) (NOTE: chemical symbol is **Ta**)

tantrum *noun* violent attack of bad behaviour, usually in a child, where the child breaks things *or* lies on the floor and screams 发脾气

tap 1 *noun* pipe with a handle which can be turned to make a liquid *or* gas 龙头 **2** *verb* (**a**) to remove *or* drain liquid from part of the body 穿刺放液 *see also* 参见 SPINAL (**b**) to hit lightly 轻叩: ***The doctor tapped his chest with his finger.*** 医生用手指轻叩他的胸壁。

◇ **tapping** *or* **paracentesis** *noun* removing liquid from part of the body using a hollow needle 穿刺术

tape *noun* long thin flat piece of material 带子; **adhesive tape** = dressing with a sticky substance on the back so that it can stick to the skin 胶带; **tape measure** *or* **measuring tape** = tape with marks on it showing centimetres or inches 皮尺

◇ **tapeworm** *noun* parasitic worm with a small head and long body like a ribbon 绦虫

> COMMENT: Tapeworms enter the intestine when a person eats raw meat or fish. The worms attach themselves with hooks to the side of the intestine and grow longer by adding sections to their bodies. Tapeworm larvae do not develop in humans, with the exception of the pork tapeworm, *Taenia solium*.
> 注释:当一个人吃生的肉或鱼时绦虫进入肠道。虫子以钩吻附着在肠壁上并通过增加体节而变长。绦虫的幼虫不在人体中发育,猪肉绦虫例外。

tapotement *noun* type of massage where the therapist taps the patient with his hands 叩抚法(按摩的方法之一)

target *noun* place which is to be hit by something 靶子; **target cell** *or* **target organ** = (i) cell *or* organ which is affected by a drug *or* by a hormone *or* by a disease 靶细胞,靶器官 (ii) large red blood cell which shows a red spot in the middle when stained 靶形红细胞

> QUOTE: The target cells for adult myeloid leukaemia are located in the bone marrow.
> 引文:成年髓性白血病的靶细胞位于骨髓。
> **British Medical Journal** 英国医学杂志

tars(o)- *prefix* referring to (i) the ankle bones 跗骨 (ii) the edge of an eyelid 睑板

◇ **tarsal 1** *adjective* referring to the tarsus 跗骨的; **tarsal bones** = seven small bones in the ankle, including the talus (ankle bone) and calcaneus (heel bone) 跗骨; **tarsal gland** = MEIBOMIAN GLAND 睑板腺 **2** *noun* **the tarsals** = seven small bones which form the ankle 跗骨

◇ **tarsalgia** *noun* pain in the ankle 跗骨痛

◇ **tarsectomy** *noun* surgical operation to remove (i) one of the tarsal bones in the ankle 跗骨切除术 (ii) the tarsus of the eyelid 睑板切除术

◇ **tarsitis** *noun* inflammation of the edge of the eyelid 睑板炎

◇ **tarsorrhaphy** *noun* operation to join the two eyelids together to protect the eye after an operation 睑板缝合术

◇ **tarsus** *noun* (**a**) the seven small bones of the ankle 跗骨 (**b**) connective tissue which supports an eyelid 睑板 ◇ 见图 FOOT (NOTE: plural is **tarsi**)

> COMMENT: The seven bones of the tarsus are: calcaneus, cuboid, the three cuneiforms, navicular and talus.
> 注释:跗骨的7块骨头是:跟骨、骰骨、三块楔骨、舟骨和距骨。

tartar *noun* hard deposit of calcium which forms on teeth, and has to be removed by scaling 牙石

tartrazine *noun* yellow substance added to food to give it an attractive colour (although widely used, tartrazine provokes reactions in hypersensitive people and is banned in some countries) 酒石黄(加在食物中有诱人的颜色,但可以引起过敏,所以在某些国家禁用)

taste 1 *noun* one of the five senses,

where food *or* substances in the mouth are noticed through the tongue 味觉：***He doesn't like the taste of onions***.他不喜欢洋葱的味道。***He has a cold, so food seems to have lost all taste*** *or* ***seems to have no taste***.他感冒了，所以食物好像都没味儿了。**taste bud** = tiny sensory receptor in the vallate and fungiform papillae of the tongue and in part of the back of the mouth 味蕾 **2** *verb* (i) to notice the taste of something with the tongue 尝味道 (ii) to have a taste 有某种味道：***You can taste the salt in this butter***.在这块黄油中你可以尝出咸味。***This cake tastes of chocolate***.这块蛋糕尝起来有巧克力的味道。***He has a cold so he can't taste anything***.他得了感冒，什么味儿也尝不出来。

COMMENT: The taste buds can tell the difference between salt, sour, bitter and sweet tastes. The buds on the tip of the tongue identify salt and sweet tastes, those on the sides of the tongue identify sour, and those at the back of the mouth the bitter tastes. Note that most of what we think of as taste is in fact smell, and this is why when someone has a cold and a blocked nose, food seems to lose its taste. The impulses from the taste buds are received by the taste cortex in the temporal lobe of the cerebral hemisphere.
注释：味蕾可以尝出咸、酸、苦和甜的不同。舌尖的味蕾可以分辨咸和甜，舌侧的可以识别酸味，口腔后部的可以识别苦味。注意，我们所认为的许多味道实际是嗅觉，这就是为什么当一个人感冒和鼻塞时食物好像失去了味道。大脑半球颞叶的味觉皮质接受来自味蕾的冲动。

taurine *noun* amino acid which forms bile salts 牛磺酸(形成胆汁酸盐的氨基酸)

taxis *noun* pushing *or* massaging dislocated bones or hernias to make them return to their normal position 整复，将错位的骨骼或疝气复位

◇ **-taxis** *suffix* meaning manipulation 手法复位

Tay-Sachs disease *or* **amaurotic familial idiocy** *noun* inherited form of mental abnormality, where the legs are paralysed and the child becomes blind and mentally retarded 泰－萨二氏病，黑矇性家族性白痴，遗传性精神异常，双腿瘫痪，患儿变盲并精神发育迟滞

TB *abbreviation for* (缩写) TUBERCULOSIS 结核病：***He is suffering from TB***.他得了结核病。***She has been admitted to a TB sanatorium***.她被收入了结核病疗养院。

T bandage *noun* bandage shaped like the letter T, used for bandaging the area between the legs T字绷带

TBI = TOTAL BODY IRRADIATION 全身照射

t.d.s. *or* **TDS** *abbreviation for* (缩写) *the Latin phrase* 'ter in diem sumendus': three times a day (written on prescriptions)一日三次(处方用语)

tea *noun* (i) dried leaves of a plant used to make a hot drink 茶叶 (ii) hot drink made by pouring boiling water onto the dried leaves of a plant 茶水；**herb tea** = hot drink made from the leaves of a herb 草药茶：***She drank a cup of peppermint tea***.她喝了一杯薄荷茶。

teach *verb* (i) to give lessons 授课 (ii) to show someone how to do something 教：***Professor Smith teaches neurosurgery***.史密斯教授教神经外科。***She was taught first aid by her mother***.她妈妈教她如何急救。**teaching hospital** = hospital which is part of a medical school, where student doctors work and study as part of their training 教学医院，医学院附属医院(医学生在此工作和学习) (NOTE: **teaches - teaching - taught - has taught**)

team *noun* group of people who work together 队：***The heart-lung transplant was carried out by a team of surgeons***.有一组外科医师做心肺移植。

tear 1 *noun* (**a**) salty excretion which forms in the lacrimal gland when a person cries 眼泪：***Tears ran down her face***.她泪流满面。***She burst into tears***. =

She suddenly started to cry. 她泪如泉涌。 **tear gland** *or* **lacrimal gland** = gland which secretes tears 泪腺（NOTE: for other terms referring to tears, see words beginning with **dacryo-**, **lacrim-**, **lacrym-**）(**b**) a hole *or* a split in a tissue often due to over-stretching 撕裂: ***An episiotomy was needed to avoid a tear in the perineal tissue.*** 需要侧切以防会阴撕裂。**2** *verb* to make a hole *or* a split in a tissue by pulling or stretching too much 撕: ***He tore a ligament in his ankle.*** 他撕裂了踝韧带。***They carried out an operation to repair a torn ligament.*** 他们做手术修复撕裂韧带。(NOTE: **tears - tearing - tore - has torn**)

teat *noun* rubber nipple on the end of a baby's feeding bottle 奶嘴儿

technique *noun* way of doing scientific *or* medical work 技术: ***a new technique for treating osteoarthritis*** 一项治疗骨关节炎的新技术; ***She is trying out a new laboratory technique.*** 她正在试行一种新的实验室技术。

◇ **technician** *noun* qualified person who does practical work in a laboratory *or* scientific institution 技师: ***He is a laboratory technician in a laboratory attached to a teaching hospital.*** 他是在一所教学医院附属的实验室当技师。**dental technician** = qualified person who makes false teeth, plates, etc. 牙科技师

QUOTE: Few parts of the body are inaccessible to modern catheter techniques, which are all performed under local anaesthesia.
引文:身体任何部位均可在局麻下用现代导管技术插管。
British Medical Journal 英国医学杂志

QUOTE: The technique used to treat aortic stenosis is similar to that for any cardiac catheterization.
引文:用于治疗主动脉缩窄的技术与其他心导管技术相似。
Journal of the American Medical Association 美国医学学会杂志

QUOTE: Cardiac resuscitation techniques used by over half the nurses in a recent study were described as 'completely ineffective'.
引文:近期的一项研究说明半数以上的护士采用的心脏复苏技术是"完全无效的"。
Nursing Times 护理时代

tectorial membrane *noun* membrane in the inner ear which contains the hair cells which transmit impulses to the auditory nerve 耳蜗被膜

tectospinal tract *noun* tract which takes nerve impulses from the mesencephalon to the spinal cord 顶盖脊髓束（从中脑到脊髓的传导束）

teeth 牙 *see* 见 TOOTH

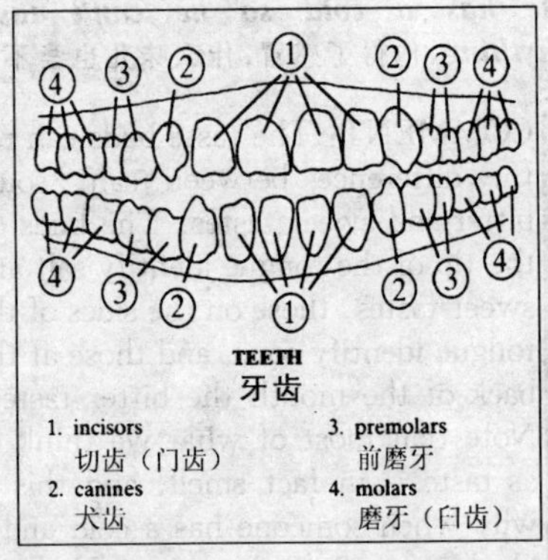

TEETH
牙齿
1. incisors 切齿（门齿）
2. canines 犬齿
3. premolars 前磨牙
4. molars 磨牙（臼齿）

◇ **teething** *noun* period when a baby's milk teeth are starting to erupt, and the baby is irritable 出牙: ***He is awake at night because he is teething.*** 他夜间醒来因为他在出牙。***She has teething trouble and won't eat.*** 她受出牙影响,不想吃东西。

tegmen *noun* covering for an organ 盖（NOTE: plural is **tegmina**）

tel- *or* **tele-** *prefix* meaning done at a distance 远距离,遥

telangiectasis *noun* small dark red spots on the skin, formed by swollen capillaries 毛细血管扩张症

teleceptor *noun* sensory receptor which receives sensations from a distance 距离感受器

telencephalon *noun* cerebrum, the main part of the brain 端脑

COMMENT: The telencephalon is the largest part of the brain, formed of two cerebral hemispheres. It controls the main mental processes, including the memory.
注释:端脑是脑最大的部分,由两个大脑半球组成。它控制着主要的精神活动,包括记忆。

teleradiography *noun* radiography where the source of the X-rays is at a distance from the patient 远距X线照相术

◇ **teleradiotherapy** *noun* radiotherapy, where the patient is some way away from the source of radiation 远距放疗

telo- *prefix* meaning end 端

◇ **telophase** *noun* final stage of mitosis, the stage in cell division after anaphase 末期(有丝分裂的最后一期)

temper *noun* (usually bad) state of mind 脾气: ***He's in a (bad) temper.*** = He is annoyed. 他在发脾气。***He lost his temper.*** = He became very angry. 他发火了。**temper tantrum** = violent attack of bad behaviour, usually in a child, where the child breaks things *or* lies on the floor and screams 脾气爆发

temperature *noun* (**a**) heat of the body *or* of the surrounding air, measured in degrees 体温: ***The doctor asked the nurse what the patient's temperature was.*** 医生问护士病人的体温是多少。***His temperature was slightly above normal.*** 他的体温略高于正常。***The thermometer showed a temperature of 99℉ (37.2℃).*** 体温计显示体温为99℉(37.2℃)。**to take a patient's temperature** = to insert a thermometer in a patient's body to see what his body temperature is 量病人的体温; ***They took his temperature every four hours.*** 他们每4小时给他测一次体温。***When her temperature was taken this morning, it was normal.*** 今天早晨给她试体温时是正常的。**central temperature** = temperature of the brain, thorax and abdomen, which is constant 体内温度,脑、喉和腹的温度,较恒定; **environmental temperature** = temperature of the air outside the body 外界温度 (**b**) illness when your body is hotter than normal 发热: ***He's in bed with a temperature.*** 他躺在床上发烧。***Her mother says she's got a temperature, and can't come to work.*** 她妈妈说她发烧了,不能来上班。

COMMENT: The normal average body temperature is about 37° Celsius or 98° Fahrenheit. This temperature may vary during the day, and can rise if a person has taken a hot bath or had a hot drink. If the environmental temperature is high, the body has to sweat to reduce the heat gained from the air around it. If the outside temperature is low, the body shivers, because rapid movement of the muscles generates heat. A fever will cause the body temperature to rise sharply, to 40℃ (103℉) or more. Hypothermia exists when the body temperature falls below about 35℃ (95℉).
注释:正常的平均体温是37℃或98℉。这一温度一天之内有所变化,人在洗了热水澡或喝了热饮后体温会上升。如果环境温度高,身体就不得不以出汗来散去从周围空气吸收的热。如果外界温度低,身体会打颤,因为肌肉的快速运动能够产热。发热会导致体温骤升到40℃(103℉)或更高。当体温降至35℃(95℉)以下时就是低体温了。

temple *noun* flat part of the side of the head between the top of the ear and the eye 颞部

◇ **temporal** *adjective* referring to the temple 颞部的; **temporal arteritis** = inflammation of the arteries in the temple 颞动脉炎; **temporal fossa** = depression at the side of the temporal bone, above the zygomatic arch 颞窝,颞骨侧面的凹陷,在颧弓之上; **temporal lobe** = lobe above the ear in each cerebral hemisphere 颞叶; **temporal lobe epilepsy** = epilepsy due to a disorder of the temporal lobe and causing impaired memory, hallucinations and automatism 颞叶癫痫

◇ **temporal bone** *noun* one the bones which form the sides and base of the cranium 颞骨 ◊ 见图 SKULL, EAR

COMMENT: The temporal bone is in two parts: the petrous part forms the base of the skull and the inner and middle ears, while the squamous part forms the side of the skull. The lower back part of the temporal bone is the mastoid process, while the part between the ear and the cheek is the zygomatic arch
注释:颞骨分为两个部分:岩部构成颅骨的底以及内耳和中耳,鳞部形成颅骨的侧面。颞骨后下部是乳突,耳和颊之间是颧弓。

◊ **temporalis (muscle)** *noun* flat muscle running down the side of the head from the temporal bone to the coronoid process, which makes the jaw move up 颞肌

temporary *adjective* which is not permanent *or* which is not final 暂时的: ***The dentist gave him a temporary filling.*** 牙医给他做了监时填充。***The accident team put a temporary bandage on the wound.*** 救护队给伤口绑缚了临时绷带。

temporo- *prefix* referring to (i) the temple 颞骨 (ii) the temporal lobe 颞叶

◊ **temporomandibular joint** *noun* joint between the jaw and the skull, in front of the ear 颞下颌关节

tenaculum *noun* surgical instrument shaped like a hook, used to pick up small pieces of tissue during an operation 持钩

tend *verb* **to tend to do something** = to do something generally *or* as a normal process 倾向,趋向: ***The prostate tends to enlarge as a man grows older.*** 男性变老时前列腺有增大的趋势。

◊ **tendency** *noun* being likely to do something 趋势: ***to have a tendency to something*** = to be likely to have something 趋向; ***There is a tendency to obesity in her family.*** 她的家族易发胖。***The children of the area show a tendency to vitamin-deficiency diseases.*** 这一地区的孩子显示出维生素缺乏病的倾向。

QUOTE: Premature babies have been shown to have a higher tendency to develop a squint during childhood.
引文:已经证实,早产儿在儿童期有较高的发生斜视的倾向。
Nursing Times 护理时代

tender *adjective* (skin *or* flesh) which is painful when touched 触痛的: ***The bruise is still tender.*** 磕青的地方一碰还疼。***Her shoulders are still tender where she got sunburnt.*** 她肩膀上被晒的地方一碰还疼。***A tender spot on the abdomen indicates that an organ is inflamed.*** 腹部有压痛点说明某一器官发炎了。

◊ **tenderness** *noun* feeling painful when touched 压痛,触痛: ***Tenderness when pressure is applied is a sign of inflammation.*** 压痛被认为是炎症的征象。

tendineae *noun* **chordae tendineae** = tiny fibrous ligaments in the heart which attach the edges of some of the valves to the walls of the ventricles 腱索,将心脏瓣膜附着于心肌的纤维韧带

◊ **tendinitis** *noun* inflammation of a tendon, especially after playing sport, and often associated with tenosynovitis 腱炎,特别是在运动之后,常与腱鞘炎一起发生

◊ **tendinous** *adjective* referring to a tendon 肌腱的

◊ **tendo calcaneus** *or* **Achilles tendon** *noun* tendon at the back of the ankle which connects the calf muscles to the heel and which acts to pull up the heel when the calf muscle is contracted 跟腱

◊ **tendon** *noun* strip of connective tissue which attaches a muscle to a bone 肌腱,使肌肉附着于骨骼的结缔组织条带; **tendon sheath** = tube of membrane which covers and protects a tendon 腱鞘

◊ **tendovaginitis** *noun* inflammation of a tendon sheath, especially in the thumb 腱鞘炎 (NOTE: for other terms referring to a tendon, see also words beginning with **teno-**)

tenens 人员 *see* 见 LOCUM

tenesmus *noun* condition where the patient feels he needs to pass faeces (or sometimes urine) but is unable to do so and experiences pain 里急后重

tennis elbow *noun* inflammation of the tendons of the extensor muscles in the hand which are attached to the bone near the elbow 网球肘,附着在肘部骨骼上的手伸肌肌腱发炎

teno- *prefix* referring to a tendon 肌腱

◇ **tenonitis** *noun* inflammation of a tendon 肌腱炎

Tenon's capsule *noun* tissue which lines the orbit of the eye 特农氏囊,眼球筋膜,眼球囊

tenoplasty *noun* surgical operation to repair a torn tendon 肌腱成形术

◇ **tenorrhaphy** *noun* surgical operation to stitch pieces of a torn tendon together 肌腱缝合术

◇ **tenosynovitis** *or* **peritendinitis** *noun* painful inflammation of the tendon sheath and the tendon inside 腱鞘炎,肌腱周围炎

◇ **tenotomy** *noun* surgical operation to cut through a tendon 肌腱切断术

◇ **tenovaginitis** *noun* inflammation of the tendon sheath, especially in the thumb 腱鞘炎(特别指拇指腱鞘炎)

tense *adjective* (**a**) (*of a muscle*) contracted (肌肉)紧张的,处于收缩的 (**b**) nervous and worried 紧张: ***The patient was very tense while he waited for the report from the laboratory.*** 病人在等待实验室报告时非常紧张。

◇ **tension** *noun* nervous stress 紧张; **tension headache** = headache all over the head, caused by worry and stress 紧张性头疼

◇ **tensor** *noun* muscle which makes a joint stretch out 张肌,使关节伸展的肌肉 *compare* 比较 EXTENSOR FLEXOR

tent *noun* small shelter put over and round a patient's bed so that gas *or* vapour can be passed inside 帐篷; **oxygen tent** = type of cover put over a patient's bed so that he can inhale oxygen 氧幕,罩在病床上给病人吸氧

tentorium cerebelli *noun* part of the dura mater which separates the cerebellum from the cerebral hemispheres 小脑幕,硬脑膜的一部分,将小脑和两个大脑半球分开

tera- *prefix* meaning 10^{12} 千京,兆兆 (NOTE: symbol is **T**)

terat- *or* **terato-** *prefix* meaning congenitally abnormal 先天异常

◇ **teratogen** *noun* substance (such as the German measles virus) which causes an abnormality to develop in an embryo 致畸物质

◇ **teratogenesis** *noun* development of abnormalities in an embryo and fetus 畸形发生

◇ **teratology** *noun* study of abnormal development of embryos and fetuses 畸胎学

◇ **teratoma** *noun* tumour which is formed of abnormal tissue, usually developing in an ovary or testis 畸胎瘤,由异常组织形成的肿瘤,通常由卵巢或睾丸发育而来

teres *noun* one of two shoulder muscles running from the shoulder blade to the top of the humerus 圆肌,肩带肌之一,从肩胛骨到肱骨顶端

> COMMENT: The larger of the two muscles, the teres major, makes the arm turn towards the inside, and the smaller, the teres minor, makes it turn towards the outside.
> 注释:两圆肌之中较大的是大圆肌,使手臂内收;较小的是小圆肌,使手臂外展。

term *noun* (**a**) length of time, especially the period from conception to childbirth 时期,特指孕期: ***she was coming near the end of her term.*** = She was near the time when she would give birth. 她正临近孕期末。(**b**) part of a college *or* school year 学期: ***The anatomy exams are at the beginning of the third term.*** 解剖考试在第三学期开始时进行。

terminal 1 *adjective* (i) referring to the last stage of a fatal illness(疾病的)终末期,晚期 (ii) referring to the end *or* being at the end of something 末端: ***The disease is in its terminal stages.*** 疾病已到晚期。***He is suffering from terminal***

***cancer*.** 他得了晚期癌症。**terminal branch** = end part of a neurone which is linked to a muscle 终末支,神经元与肌肉连接的部分 ➪ 见图 NEURONE; **terminal illness** = illness from which the patient will soon die 晚期疾病 **2** *noun* ending *or* part at the end of an electrode *or* nerve 末端

◊ **terminale**末端的 *see* 见 FILUM

◊ **terminally ill** *adjective* very ill and about to die 濒死的: ***She was admitted to a hospital for terminally ill patients*** *or* ***for the terminally ill*.** 她被收入临终关怀医院。

◊ **termination** *noun* ending 结束,终止; **termination (of pregnancy)** = abortion 流产,终止妊娠

tertian fever *noun* type of malaria where the fever returns every two days 间日疟 *see also* 参见 QUARTAN

tertiary *adjective* third *or* coming after secondary and primary 第三的; **tertiary bronchi** = air passages supplying a segment of a lung 三级支气管 *see also* 参见 SYPHILIS

test 1 *noun* short examination to see if a sample is healthy *or* if part of the body is working well 检查: ***He had an eye test this morning*.** 今天早晨他做了眼睛检查。***Laboratory tests showed that she was a meningitis carrier*.** 实验室检查发现她是脑膜炎携带者。***Tests are being carried out on swabs taken from the operating theatre*.** 正在对手术台上取下来的拭子进行检查。**blood test** = laboratory test of a blood sample to analyse its chemical composition 验血: ***The patient will have to have a blood test*.** 必须给这个病人验血。**laboratory test** = test carried out in a laboratory 实验室检查; ***The urine test was positive*.** = The examination of the urine sample showed the presence of an infection *or* a diagnostic substance. 尿检呈阳性。**2** *verb* to examine a sample of tissue to see if it is healthy *or* an organ to see if it is working well 检查,检测: ***They sent the urine sample away for testing*.** 他们把尿样送去检测。***I must have my eyes tested*.** 我必须检查一下我的眼睛。

◊ **test meal** *noun* test to test the secretion of gastric juices 检测餐

◊ **test tube** *noun* small glass tube with a rounded bottom, used in laboratories to hold samples of liquids 试管; **test-tube baby** = baby which develops after the mother's ova have been removed from the ovaries, fertilized with a man's spermatozoa in a laboratory, and returned to the mother's womb to continue developing normally 试管婴儿,将母亲的卵子从卵巢中取出,在实验室里和精子受精后再放回母亲的子宫继续让它正常发育

> COMMENT: This process of in vitro fertilization is carried out in cases where the mother is unable to conceive, though both she and the father are normally fertile.
> 注释:在父母双方都有生殖能力但母亲不能受孕时采用这种体外受精的方法。

testicle *or* **testis** *noun* one of two male sex glands in the scrotum 睾丸 (NOTE: the plural of testis is **testes**)

◊ **testicular** *adjective* referring to the testes 睾丸的: ***Testicular cancer comprises only 1% of all malignant neoplasms in the male*.** 睾丸癌占男性所有恶性肿瘤的百分之一。**testicular hormone** = testosterone 睾酮 ,睾丸激素(NOTE: for other terms referring to the testes, see words beginning with **orchi-**) ➪ 见图 UROGENITAL SYSTEM (male)

> COMMENT: The testes produce both spermatozoa and the sex hormone, testosterone. Spermatozoa are formed in the testes, and passed into the epididymis to be stored. From the epididymis they pass along the vas deferens through the prostate gland which secretes the seminal fluid, and are ejaculated through the penis.
> 注释:睾丸既产生精子也产生性激素睾丸酮。精子是在睾丸中形成的,然后被送到附睾储存。再从附睾沿输精管经分泌精液的前列腺,最终从阴茎射出。

testosterone *noun* male sex hormone, secreted by the Leydig cells in the testes, which causes physical changes (such as the development of body hair and deep voice) to take place in males as they become sexually mature 睾酮,雄性激素,由睾丸间质细胞分泌,在男性性成熟过程中引起身体的变化(如体毛生长,声调变低)。

tetanic *adjective* referring to tetanus 破伤风的

◇ **tetanus** *noun* (**a**) continuous contraction of a muscle, under repeated stimuli from a motor nerve 肌肉强直 (**b**) lockjaw, an infection caused by *Clostridium tetani* in the soil, which affects the spinal cord and causes spasms in the muscles which occur first in the jaw 破伤风,由土壤中的破伤风芽胞杆菌引起的感染,影响脊髓,导致肌肉痉挛,最先出现在下颌

> COMMENT: People who are liable to infection with tetanus, such as farm workers, should be immunized against it, though booster injections are needed from time to time.
> 注释:易感破伤风的人,如农场工人,应当针对此病进行免疫,并需要不时追加免疫。

tetany *noun* spasms of the muscles in the feet and hands, caused by a reduction in the level of calcium in the blood *or* by lack of carbon dioxide 手足搐搦,由于缺钙或体内二氧化碳缺乏导致的手足痉挛 *see* 见 PARATHYROID HORMONE

tetracycline *noun* antibiotic used to treat a wide range of bacterial diseases 四环素

> COMMENT: Because of its side-effects tetracycline should not be given to children.
> 注释:由于四环素存在某些副作用,不得用于儿童。

tetradactyly *noun* congenital deformity where a child has only four fingers or toes(先天性)四指(趾)畸形

tetralogy of Fallot *or* **Fallot's tetralogy** *noun* disorder of the heart which makes a child's skin blue 法乐四联征,先天性心脏病的一种,引起儿童紫绀 *see also* 参见 BLALOCK'S OPERATION, WATERSTON'S OPERATION

> COMMENT: The condition is formed of four disorders occurring together: the artery leading to the lungs is narrow, the right ventricle is enlarged, there is a defect in the membrane between the ventricles, and the aorta is not correctly placed.
> 注释:此病同时发生四种障碍:肺动脉狭窄、右心室肥大、室间隔缺损和主动脉错位。

tetraplegia = QUADRIPLEGIA 四肢瘫

textbook *noun* book which is used by students 教科书;**a haematology textbook** *or* **a textbook on haematology** 血液学教科书;**textbook case** = case which shows symptoms which are exactly like those described in a textbook 典型病例

thalam- *or* **thalamo-** *prefix* referring to the thalamus"丘脑"

◇ **thalamencephalon** *noun* group of structures in the brain linked to the brain stem, formed of the epithalamus, hypothalamus, and thalamus (广义的)丘脑,由上丘脑、下丘脑和丘脑组成

◇ **thalamic syndrome** *noun* condition where a patient is extremely sensitive to pain, caused by a disorder of the thalamus 丘脑综合征,病人对痛觉极端敏感,由丘脑障碍引起

◇ **thalamocortical tract** *noun* tract containing nerve fibres, running from the thalamus to the sensory cortex 丘脑皮质束,由丘脑到感觉皮质的神经纤维束

◇ **thalamotomy** *noun* surgical operation to make an incision into the thalamus to treat intractable pain 丘脑切开术,用于治疗难治性疼痛

◇ **thalamus** *noun* one of two masses of grey matter situated beneath the cerebrum where impulses from the sensory neurones are transmitted to the cerebral cortex 丘脑,位于小脑下的两个灰质团,将传来的冲动,传递到大脑皮质 ◊ 见图 BRAIN (NOTE: plural is **thalami**)

thalassaemia *or* **Cooley's anaemia** *noun* hereditary type of anaemia, found in Mediterranean countries, due to a defect in the production of haemoglobin 地中海贫血,遗传性贫血,在地中海地区发现,由血红蛋白上的缺陷造成

thaw *verb* to bring something which is frozen back to normal temperature 解冻,融化

theatre *noun* (**operating**) **theatre** *US* **operating room** = special room in a hospital where surgeons carry out operations 手术室; **theatre gown** = gown worn by a patient *or* by a surgeon *or* nurse in an operating theatre 手术衣; **theatre nurse** = nurse who is specially trained to assist in operations 手术室护士

> QUOTE: While waiting to go to theatre, parents should be encouraged to participate in play with their children.
> 引文:在等待进入手术室时,应鼓励父母和患儿玩。
> **British Journal of Nursing** 英国护理杂志

theca *noun* tissue shaped like a sheath 膜,鞘

thenar *adjective* (referring to) the palm of the hand 鱼际的,手掌的; **thenar eminence** = the ball of the thumb *or* lump of flesh in the palm of the hand below the thumb 鱼际 *compare* 比较 HYPOTHENAR

theory *noun* argument which explains a scientific fact 理论

therapeutic *adjective* (treatment *or* drug) which is given in order to cure a disorder *or* disease 治疗性的; **therapeutic abortion** = legal abortion carried out because the health of the mother is in danger 治疗性流产,由于母亲继续怀孕有危险而采取的流产

◇ **therapeutics** *noun* study of various types of treatment and their effect on patients 治疗学

◇ **therapist** *noun* person specially trained to give therapy 治疗师; ***an occupational therapist*** 职业治疗师 *see also* 参见 PSYCHOTHERAPIST

◇ **therapy** *noun* treatment of a patient to help cure a disease *or* disorder 治疗; **aversion therapy** = treatment where the patient is cured of a type of behaviour by making him develop a great dislike for it 厌恶治疗,让病人对某种不良行为产生强烈厌恶的疗法; **behaviour therapy** = psychiatric treatment where the patient learns to improve his condition 行为治疗,让病人学会改善自身状况的精神科治疗; **group therapy** = type of treatment where a group of people with the same disorder meet together with a therapist to discuss their condition and try to help each other 群体治疗,具有相同疾病的一群患者和治疗师一起探讨病情,互相帮助; **heat therapy** *or* **thermotherapy** = using heat (from infrared lamps *or* hot water) to treat certain conditions such as arthritis and bad circulation 热疗,用于治疗关节炎和循环不好; **light therapy** = treatment of a disorder by exposing the patient to light (sunlight, UV light, etc) 光疗; **occupational therapy** = work or hobbies used as a means of treatment, especially for handicapped or mentally ill patients 工娱治疗,针对残疾人或精神疾病患者采取的以工作或娱乐为手段的康复治疗; **shock therapy** = method of treating some mental disorders by giving the patient an electric shock to induce convulsions and loss of consciousness 休克疗法,用电休克导致病人抽搐和意识丧失来治疗某些精神障碍; **speech therapy** = treatment to cure a speech disorder such as stammering 言语治疗,针对言语障碍,如口吃 *see also* 参见 PSYCHOTHERAPY, RADIOTHERAPY (NOTE: both therapy and therapist are used as suffixes: **psychotherapist**, **radiotherapy**)

thermal *adjective* referring to heat 温度的; **thermal anaesthesia** = loss of feeling of heat 温度觉缺失

◇ **thermo-** *prefix* referring to (i) heat 热 (ii) temperature 温度

◇ **thermoanaesthesia** *noun* condition where the patient cannot tell the difference between hot and cold 温度觉缺失

◇ **thermocautery** *noun* removing dead tissue by heat 热烙术

◇ **thermocoagulation** *noun* removing tissue and coagulating blood by heat 热凝术
◇ **thermogram** *noun* infrared photograph of part of the body 温度分布图,身体某部位的红外线照片,可以显示不同温度
◇ **thermography** *noun* technique of photographing part of the body using infrared rays, which record the heat given off by the skin, and show variations in the blood circulating beneath the skin, used especially in screening for breast cancer 温度记录法,红外线摄片以显示温度分布的技术
◇ **thermolysis** *noun* loss of body temperature (as by sweating) 散热
◇ **thermometer** *noun* instrument for measuring temperature 温度计; **clinical thermometer** = thermometer used in a hospital *or* by a doctor for taking a patient's body temperature 临床体温计; **oral thermometer** = thermometer which is put into the mouth to take a patient's temperature 口腔温度计,口表; **rectal thermometer** = thermometer which is inserted into the patient's rectum to take the temperature 直肠温度计,肛表
◇ **thermophilic** *adjective* (organism) which needs a high temperature to grow (微生物)嗜热的,喜热的
◇ **thermoreceptor** *noun* sensory nerve which registers heat 温度感受器
◇ **thermotaxis** *noun* automatic regulation of the body's temperature 体温调节
◇ **thermotherapy** *noun* heat treatment, using heat (as in hot water *or* infrared lamps) to treat conditions such as arthritis and bad circulation 热疗
thiamine = VITAMIN B_1 维生素 B_1,硫胺
thicken *verb* (**a**) to become wider *or* larger 增厚: ***The walls of the arteries thicken under deposits of fat.*** 脂肪沉积使动脉壁变厚。(**b**) (of liquid) to become more dense and viscid and flow less easily 变浓: ***The liquid thickens as its cools.*** 冷却时液体浓缩。
Thiersch graft = SPLIT-SKIN GRAFT 蒂尔施移植物,皮片移植物
thigh *noun* top part of the leg from the knee to the groin 大腿
◇ **thighbone** *or* **femur** *noun* bone in the top part of the leg, which joins the acetabulum at the hip and the tibia at the knee 大腿骨,股骨 (NOTE: for other terms referring to the thigh, see words beginning with **femor-**)
thin *adjective* (**a**) not fat 瘦: ***His arms are very thin.*** 他的胳膊很瘦。***She's getting too thin - she should eat more.*** 她太瘦了,应当多吃点。***He became quite thin after his illness.*** 病后他瘦多了。(NOTE: **thin - thinner - thinnest**) (**b**) not thick 薄: ***They cut a thin slice of tissue for examination under the microscope.*** 为在显微镜下做检查,他们切了一片组织薄片。(**c**) (blood) which is watery (血液)稀
thirst *noun* feeling of wanting to drink 渴: ***He had a fever and a violent thirst.*** 他发烧了,渴得要命。
◇ **thirsty** *adjective* wanting to drink 渴的: ***If the patient is thirsty, give her a glass of water.*** 如果病人渴了,给她一杯水。(NOTE: **thirsty - thirstier - thirstiest**)
Thomas's splint *noun* type of splint used on a fractured femur, with a ring at the top round the thigh, and a bar under the foot at the lower end 托马斯夹板,用于股骨骨折的一种夹板
thorac(o)- *prefix* referring to the chest 胸廓,胸腔
◇ **thoracectomy** *noun* surgical operation to remove one or more ribs 胸廓部分切除术(去掉一或几根肋骨)
◇ **thoracentesis** *noun* operation where a hollow needle is inserted into the pleura to drain fluid 胸腔穿刺引流术
◇ **thoracic** *adjective* referring to the chest *or* thorax 胸廓的; **thoracic cavity** = chest cavity, containing the diaphragm, heart and lungs 胸腔; **thoracic duct** = one of the main terminal ducts in the lymphatic system, running from the abdomen to the left side of the neck

胸导管,终末淋巴导管之一,由腹部到左侧颈部;**thoracic inlet** = small opening at the top of the thorax 胸廓上口;**thoracic inlet syndrome** *or* **scalenus syndrome** = pain in an arm, caused when the scalenes press the brachial plexus against the vertebrae 胸廓上口综合征,斜角肌综合征,斜角肌将臂丛压迫到脊椎上,引起胳臂疼痛;**thoracic outlet** = large opening at the bottom of the thorax 胸廓出口,胸廓下口;**thoracic vertebrae** = the twelve vertebrae in the spine behind the chest, to which the ribs are attached 胸椎 ◊ 见图 VERTEBRAL COLUMN

◇ **thoracocentesis** *noun* operation where a hollow needle is inserted into the pleura to drain fluid 胸腔穿刺引流术

◇ **thoracoplasty** *noun* surgical operation to cut through the ribs to allow the lungs to collapse, formerly a treatment for pulmonary tuberculosis 胸廓成形术(肺萎陷术,过去用于治疗肺结核)

◇ **thoracoscope** *noun* surgical instrument, like a tube with a light at the end, used to examine the inside of the chest 胸腔镜

◇ **thoracoscopy** *noun* examination of the inside the chest, using a thoracoscope 胸腔镜检查

◇ **thoracotomy** *noun* surgical operation to make a hole in the wall of the chest 胸廓切开术

◇ **thorax** *noun* chest, the cavity in the top part of the front of the body above the abdomen, containing the diaphragm, heart and lungs, and surrounded by the ribcage 胸,胸廓

thread 1 *noun* thin piece of cotton, suture, etc. 线: ***The surgeon used strong thread to make the suture.*** 外科医师用结实的线做缝合。2 *verb* to insert a thin piece of cotton, suture, etc. through the eye of (a needle)穿针引线

◇ **threadworm** *or* **pinworm** *noun* thin parasitic worm, *Enterobius* which infests the large intestine and causes itching round the anus 蛲虫,感染大肠引起肛周瘙痒

◇ **thready** *adjective* (pulse) which is very weak and can hardly be felt 脉纤细,脉如悬丝

threonine *noun* essential amino acid 苏氨酸

threshold *noun* 阈 (i) point below which a drug has no effect 药物治疗阈 (ii) point at which a sensation is strong enough to be sensed by the sensory nerves 感觉阈: ***She has a low hearing threshold.*** 她的听觉阈值低。**pain threshold** = point at which a person cannot bear pain without crying 痛阈,能忍痛不叫的极限

> QUOTE: If intracranial pressure rises above the treatment threshold, it is imperative first to validate the reading and then to eliminate any factors exacerbating the rise in pressure.
> 引文:如果颅内压上升到治疗阈值以上,就必须首先确认读数,然后去掉加剧颅压升高的因素。
> **British Journal of Hospital Medicine**
> 英国医院医学杂志

thrill *noun* vibration which can be felt with the hands 颤抖

thrive *verb* to do well *or* to live and grow strongly 努力,茁壮成长;**failure to thrive** = wasting disease of small children who have difficulty in absorbing nutrients *or* who are suffering from malnutrition 消瘦病,使营养不良或吸收营养物质有困难的幼儿停止生长的一种消耗性疾病

throat *noun* (i) top part of the tube which goes down from the mouth to the stomach 咽喉 (ii) front part of the neck below the chin 颈前部: ***If it is cold, wrap a scarf round your throat.*** 如果天冷,在脖子前面围块围巾。***A piece of meat got stuck in his throat.*** 一块肉卡在他嗓子里了。**to clear the throat** = to give a little cough 轻咳;**sore throat** = condition where the mucous membrane in the pharynx is inflamed (sometimes because the person has been talking too much, but usually because of an infection)咽喉

痛

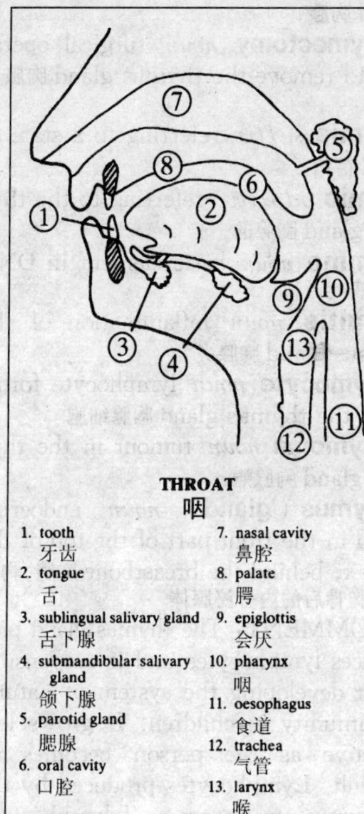

THROAT
咽

1. tooth 牙齿
2. tongue 舌
3. sublingual salivary gland 舌下腺
4. submandibular salivary gland 颌下腺
5. parotid gland 腮腺
6. oral cavity 口腔
7. nasal cavity 鼻腔
8. palate 腭
9. epiglottis 会厌
10. pharynx 咽
11. oesophagus 食道
12. trachea 气管
13. larynx 喉

COMMENT: The throat carries both food from the mouth and air from the nose and mouth. It divides into the oesophagus, which takes food to the stomach, and the trachea, which takes air into the lungs.
注释：咽喉既负责来自口腔的食物通过，也负责来自鼻腔的空气通过。它分为食管和气管，食物由食管到胃去，空气由气管进入肺。

throb *verb* to have a regular beat, like the heart 搏动: ***His head was throbbing with pain.*** 他的头一跳一跳地疼。

◇ **throbbing** *adjective* (pain) which comes again and again like a heart beat 刺痛: ***She has a throbbing pain in her finger.*** 她的手指刺痛。 ***He has a throbbing headache.*** 他的头刺痛。

thrombectomy *noun* surgical operation to remove a blood clot 血栓切除术

◇ **thrombin** *noun* substance which converts fibrinogen to fibrin and so coagulates blood 凝血酶

◇ **thrombo-** *prefix* referring to (i) blood clot 血块 (ii) thrombosis 血栓形成

◇ **thromboangiitis obliterans** *or* **Buerger's disease** *noun* disease of the arteries, where the blood vessels in a limb (usually the leg) become narrow, causing gangrene 血栓闭塞性脉管炎，肢体的动脉血管(通常是下肢)狭窄，造成坏疽

◇ **thromboarteritis** *noun* inflammation of an artery caused by thrombosis 血栓性动脉炎

◇ **thrombocyte** *or* **platelet** *noun* little blood cell which encourages the coagulation of blood 血小板

◇ **thrombocythaemia** *noun* disease where the patient has an abnormally high number of platelets in his blood 血小板增多

◇ **thrombocytopenia** *noun* condition where the patient has an abnormally low number of platelets in his blood 血小板减少

◇ **thrombocytopenic** *adjective* referring to thrombocytopenia 血小板减少的

◇ **thrombocytosis** *noun* increase in the number of platelets in a patient's blood 血小板增多症

◇ **thromboembolism** *noun* condition where a blood clot forms in one part of the body and moves through the blood vessels to block another, usually smaller, part 血栓栓塞

◇ **thromboendarterectomy** *noun* surgical operation to open an artery to remove a blood clot which is blocking it 血栓动脉内膜切除术

◇ **thromboendarteritis** *noun* inflammation of the inside of an artery, caused by thrombosis 血栓动脉内膜炎

◇ **thrombokinase** *or* **thromboplastin** *noun* substance which converts prothrombin into thrombin 凝血激酶

◇ **thrombolysis** *noun* breaking up of blood clots 溶栓

◇ **thrombolytic** *adjective* (substance) which will break up blood clots 溶栓的

◇ **thrombophlebitis** *noun* blocking of a vein by a blood clot, sometimes causing inflammation 血栓性静脉炎

◇ **thromboplastin** *or* **thrombokinase** *noun* substance which converts prothrombin into thrombin 凝血激酶

◇ **thrombopoiesis** *noun* process by which blood platelets are formed 血小板生成

◇ **thrombosis** *noun* blood clotting *or* blocking of an artery *or* vein by a mass of coagulated blood 血栓形成; **cerebral thrombosis** *or* **stroke** = condition where a blood clot enters and blocks a brain artery 脑血栓,中风; **coronary thrombosis** = blood clot which blocks one of the coronary arteries, leading to a heart attack 冠状动脉血栓形成; **deep vein thrombosis (DVT)** = blood clot in the deep veins of the leg or pelvis 深静脉血栓形成

◇ **thrombus** *noun* soft mass of coagulated blood in a vein or artery 血栓; **mural thrombus** = thrombus which forms on the wall of a vein or artery 附壁血栓 (NOTE: plural is **thrombi**)

throw up *verb* to be sick *or* to vomit 反胃: ***She threw up all over the bathroom floor.*** 她在浴室吐了一地板。***He threw up his dinner.*** 他把吃的晚饭都吐出来了。(NOTE: **throws - throwing - threw - has thrown**)

thrush *noun* infection of the mouth (or sometimes the vagina) with the bacterium *Candida albicans* 鹅口疮,真菌性口炎

thumb *noun* short thick finger, with only two phalanges, which is separated from the other four fingers on the hand 拇指: ***He hit his thumb with the hammer.*** 他被锤子砸伤了拇指。***The baby was sucking its thumb.*** 婴儿正在吮拇指。

◇ **thumb-sucking** *noun* action of sucking a thumb 吮拇指: ***Tumb-sucking tends to push the teeth forward.*** 吮拇指会使牙前突。

thym- *prefix* referring to the thymus gland 胸腺

◇ **thymectomy** *noun* surgical operation to remove the thymus gland 胸腺切除术

-thymia *suffix* referring to a state of mind 情绪

thymic *adjective* referring to the thymus gland 胸腺的

thymine *noun* basic element in DNA 胸腺嘧啶

thymitis *noun* inflammation of the thymus gland 胸腺炎

◇ **thymocyte** *noun* lymphocyte formed in the thymus gland 胸腺细胞

◇ **thymoma** *noun* tumour in the thymus gland 胸腺瘤

◇ **thymus (gland)** *noun* endocrine gland in the front part of the top of the thorax, behind the breastbone 胸腺,胸廓上部胸骨后的内分泌腺体

> COMMENT: The thymus gland produces lymphocytes and is responsible for developing the system of natural immunity in children. It grows less active as the person becomes an adult. Lymphocytes produced by the thymus are known as T-lymphocytes or T-cells.
> 注释:胸腺产生淋巴细胞并负责儿童自然免疫系统的发育。成年后,它的生长不再活跃。胸腺产生的淋巴细胞称作胸腺淋巴细胞或 T 细胞。

thyro- *prefix* referring to the thyroid gland 甲状腺

◇ **thyrocalcitonin** *or* **calcitonin** *noun* hormone, produced by the thyroid gland, which is believed to regulate the level of calcium in the blood 降钙素,甲状腺分泌,有调节血钙水平的作用

◇ **thyrocele** *noun* swelling of the thyroid gland 甲状腺肿

◇ **thyroglobulin** *noun* protein stored in the thyroid gland which is broken down into thyroxine 甲状腺球蛋白

◇ **thyroglossal** *adjective* referring to the thyroid gland and the throat 甲状舌管的; **thyroglossal cyst** = cyst in the front of the neck 甲状舌管囊肿

◇ **thyroid**1 *adjective* referring to the thyroid gland 甲状腺的; **thyroid cartilage** = large cartilage in the larynx, part of which forms the Adam's apple 甲状软骨,大的喉软骨,部分构成喉结 ◊ 见图 LUNGS; **thyroid dysfunction** = abnormal functioning of the thyroid gland 甲状腺功能失调; **thyroid extract** = substance extracted from thyroid glands of animals and used to treat hypothyroidism 甲状腺提取物,从动物甲状腺提取的物质,用于治疗甲状腺功能低下; **thyroid hormone** = hormone produced by the thyroid gland 甲状腺激素 **2** *noun* **thyroid (gland)** = endocrine gland in the neck below the larynx 甲状腺

COMMENT: The thyroid gland is activated by the pituitary gland, and produces thyroxine, a hormone which regulates the body's metabolism. The thyroid gland needs a supply of iodine in order to produce thyroxine. If the thyroid gland malfunctions, it can result in hyperthyroidism (producing too much thyroxine) leading to goitre, or in hypothyroidism producing too little thyroxine) which causes cretinism in children and myxoedema in adults.
注释:甲状腺由垂体活化,活化后产生甲状腺素,甲状腺素调节机体的代谢;甲状腺产生甲状腺素需要碘的供应,如果甲状腺功能失调,可以导致甲状腺功能亢进(产生甲状腺素过多)导致甲状腺肿,或甲状腺功能低下(甲状腺素产生过少),在儿童引起克汀病,在成人引起粘液水肿。

◇ **thyroidectomy** *noun* surgical operation to remove all *or* part of the thyroid gland 甲状腺切除术

◇ **thyroiditis** *noun* inflammation of the thyroid gland 甲状腺炎

◇ **thyroid-stimulating hormone (TSH)** *or* **thyrotrophin** *noun* hormone secreted by the pituitary gland which stimulates the thyroid gland 促甲状腺素,垂体分泌的刺激甲状腺的激素

◇ **thyrotomy** *noun* surgical opening made in the thyroid cartilage *or* the thyroid gland 甲状腺切开术,甲状软骨切开术

◇ **thyrotoxic** *adjective* referring to severe hyperthyroidism 甲状腺毒性的; **thyrotoxic crisis** = sudden illness caused by hyperthyroidism 甲状腺危象; **thyrotoxic goitre** = goitre caused by thyrotoxicosis 毒性甲状腺肿

◇ **thyrotoxicosis** *or* **Graves' disease** *or* **exophthalmic goitre** *or* **Basedow's disease** *noun* type of goitre, caused by hyperthyroidism, where the heart beats faster, the thyroid gland swells, the patient trembles and his eyes protrude 甲状腺毒症,格雷夫斯病,突眼性甲状腺肿,巴塞岛病,甲状腺肿的一种,甲状腺素分泌过多引起,出现心跳加快、甲状腺肿胀、病人震颤并有眼球突出

◇ **thyrotrophin** *or* **thyroid-stimulating hormone** *noun* hormone secreted by the pituitary gland which stimulates the thyroid gland 促甲状腺素

◇ **thyrotrophin-releasing hormone (TRH)** *noun* hormone secreted by the hypothalamus, which makes the pituitary gland release thyrotrophin, which in turn stimulates the thyroid gland 促甲状腺素释放激素(下丘脑分泌的激素,促进垂体释放促甲状腺素,后者再刺激甲状腺)

◇ **thyroxine** *noun* hormone produced by the thyroid gland which regulates the body's metabolism and conversion of food into heat 甲状腺素,调节机体代谢,将食物转化为热量

COMMENT: Synthetic thyroxine is used in treatment of hypothyroidism.
注释:人工合成的甲状腺素用于治疗甲状腺功能低下。

Ti *chemical symbol for* titanium 钛的化学元素符号

TIA = TRANSIENT ISCHAEMIC ATTACK 一过性脑缺血发作

QUOTE: Blood pressure control reduces the incidence of first stroke and aspirin appears to reduce the risk of stroke after TIAs by some 15%.

引文:控制血压可以减少初发中风的危险,而阿司匹林将一过性脑缺血后中风的危险减少15%。

British Journal of Hospital Medicine
英国医院医学杂志

tibia *noun* shinbone, the larger of the two long bones in the lower leg running from the knee to the ankle (the other, thinner, bone in the lower leg is the fibula)胫骨

◇ **tibial** *adjective* referring to the tibia 胫骨的; **tibial arteries** = two arteries which run down the front and back of the lower leg 胫动脉(兼指胫前动脉和胫后动脉)

◇ **tibialis** *noun* one of two muscles in the lower leg running from the tibia to the foot 胫骨肌

◇ **tibio-** *prefix* referring to the tibia 胫骨

◇ **tibiofibular** *adjective* referring to both the tibia and the fibula 胫骨腓骨的

tic *noun* involuntary twitching of the muscles (usually in the face) 抽搐(常用于面部抽搐); **tic douloureux** *or* **trigeminal neuralgia** = pain in the trigeminal nerve which sends intense pains shooting across the face 三叉神经痛

tick *noun* tiny parasite which sucks blood from the skin 蜱,一种吸血的小寄生虫; **tick fever** = infectious disease transmitted by bites from ticks 蜱热

t.i.d. *or* **TID** *abbreviation for* (缩写) *the Latin phrase* 'ter in die': three times a day (written on prescriptions)一日三次(处方用语)

tie *verb* to attach a thread with a knot 打结: ***The surgeon quickly tied up the stitches.*** 外科医师迅速将缝线打结。***The nurse had tied the bandage too tight.*** 护士把绷带打得太紧了。(NOTE: **ties - tying - tied - has tied**)

tight *adjective* which fits firmly *or* which is not loose 紧的: ***Make sure the bandage is not too tight.*** 保证绷带不要太紧。***The splint must be kept tight, or the bone may move.*** 必须束紧夹板,否则骨骼会移位。***Tight-fitting clothes can affect the circulation.*** 紧身衣会影响血液循环。(NOTE: **tight - tighter - tightest**)

◇ **tightly** *adverb* in a tight way 紧紧地: ***She tied the bandage tightly round his arm.*** 她紧紧地将绷带绕在他的胳膊上。

time *noun* period of hours, minutes, seconds, etc. 时间; **bleeding time** = test of clotting of a patient's blood, by timing the length of time it takes for the blood to congeal 出血时间,检验病人凝血功能的试验指标; **clotting time** *or* **coagulation time** = the time taken for blood to coagulate under normal conditions 凝血时间,正常条件下血液凝固的时间

tincture *noun* medicinal substance dissolved in alcohol 酊,酊剂; **tincture of iodine** = disinfectant made of iodine and alcohol 碘酊,即俗称的碘酒

tinea *or* **ringworm** *noun* infection by a fungus, in which the infection spreads out in a circle from a central point 癣; **tinea barbae** = ringworm in the beard 须疮; **tinea capitis** = ringworm on the scalp 头癣; **tinea pedis** = athlete's foot, fungal infection between the toes 脚癣

tingle *verb* to give a feeling like a slight electric shock 麻刺感: ***He had a tingling feeling in his fingers.*** 他的手指一阵麻刺感。

tinnitus *noun* ringing sound in the ears 耳鸣

> COMMENT: Tinnitus can sound like bells, or buzzing, or a loud roaring sound. In some cases it is caused by wax blocking the auditory canal, but it is also associated with Ménière's disease, infections of the middle ear and acoustic nerve conditions.
> 注释:耳鸣可以像铃声、蜂鸣或很响的机器声。某些病例是耳垢阻塞听小管引起的,但也可以与梅尼埃病、中耳感染和听神经障碍有关。

tipped womb *noun US* condition where the uterus slopes backwards away from its normal position 子宫后倾 (NOTE: the UK English is **retroverted uterus**)

tired *adjective* feeling sleepy *or* feeling that a person needs to rest 疲劳的: ***The patients are tired, and need to go to bed.*** 病人累了,需要上床休息。***There is something wrong with her — she's always tired.*** 她可能是病了——老是疲劳。

◇ **tired out** *adjective* feeling extremely tired *or* feeling in need of a rest 筋疲力尽: ***She is tired out after the physiotherapy.*** 理疗后她筋疲力尽。

◇ **tiredness** *noun* being tired 疲劳

tissue *noun* material made of cells, of which the parts of the body are formed 组织,由一定的细胞群组成: ***Most of the body is made up of soft tissue, with the exception of the bones and cartilage.*** 除骨骼和软骨外,身体大部分是由软组织构成的。***The main types of body tissue are connective, epithelial, muscular and nerve tissue.*** 身体的主要组织有结缔组织、上皮组织、肌肉组织和神经组织。**adipose tissue** = tissue where the cells contain fat 脂肪组织; **connective tissue** = tissue which forms the main part of bones and cartilage, ligaments and tendons, in which a large amount of fibrous material surrounds the tissue cells 结缔组织; **elastic tissue** = connective tissue as in the walls of arteries, which contains elastic fibres 弹性组织; epithelial tissue = tissue which forms the skin 上皮组织; **fibrous tissue** = strong white tissue which makes tendons and ligaments and also scar tissue 纤维组织; **lymphoid tissue** = tissue in the lymph nodes, the tonsils and the spleen, which forms lymphocytes and antibodies 淋巴组织; **muscle tissue** *or* **muscular tissue** = tissue which forms the muscles, and which can contract and expand 肌肉组织; **nerve tissue** = tissue which forms nerves, and which is able to transmit nerve impulses 神经组织; **tissue culture** = live tissue grown in a culture in a laboratory 组织培养; **tissue typing** = identifying various elements in tissue from a donor and comparing them to those of the recipient to see if a transplant is likely to be rejected (the two most important factors are the ABO blood grouping and the HLA antigen system) 组织配型 (NOTE: for other terms referring to tissue, see words beginning with **hist-**, **histo-**)

titanium *noun* light metallic element which does not corrode 钛 (NOTE: chemical symbol is **Ti**)

titration *noun* process of measuring the strength of a solution 滴定

◇ **titre** *noun* measurement of the quantity of antibodies in a serum 滴度

tobacco *noun* leaves of a plant which are dried and smoked, either in a pipe or as cigarettes or cigars 烟草

> COMMENT: Tobacco contains nicotine, which is an addictive stimulant. This is why it is difficult for a person who smokes a lot of cigarettes to give up the habit. Nicotine can enter the bloodstream and cause poisoning; tobacco smoking also causes cancer, especially of the lungs and throat.
> 释释:烟草含有尼古丁,它是一种成瘾性刺激物。这就是为什么抽烟很多的人难于戒掉吸烟的习惯。尼古丁可以进入血液并造成中毒,吸烟还会导致癌症,特别是肺癌和喉癌。

toco- *prefix* referring to childbirth 分娩

◇ **tocography** *noun* recording of the contractions of the uterus during childbirth 宫缩图

Todd's paralysis *or* **Todd's palsy** *noun* temporary paralysis of part of the body which has been the starting point of focal epilepsy 托德瘫痪,局灶性癫痫开始时的身体某部分的一过性瘫痪

toe *noun* one of the five separate parts at the end of the foot (each toe is formed of three bones *or* phalanges, except the big toe, which only has two) 趾; **big toe** *or* **great toe and little toe** = biggest and smallest of the five toes 踇趾和小趾

◇ **toenail** *noun* thin hard growth covering the end of a toe 趾甲

toilet *noun* (**a**) cleaning of the body 盥洗:***She was busy with her toilet.*** 她在忙着盥洗。(**b**) lavatory, place or room where a person can pass urine or faeces 厕所

◇ **toilet paper** *noun* special paper for wiping the anus after defecating 卫生纸

◇ **toilet roll** *noun* roll of toilet paper 卫生纸卷

◇ **toilet training** *noun* teaching a small child to pass urine *or* faeces in a toilet, so that it no longer requires nappies(对儿童)大小便训练

tolerance *noun* ability of the body to tolerate a substance *or* an action 耐受性: ***He has been taking the drug for so long that he has developed a tolerance to it.*** 他已经服用这种药很长时间了以致对它产生了耐药。**drug tolerance** = condition where a drug has been given to a patient for so long that his body no longer reacts to it, and the dosage has to be increased 耐药性,长期用药导致对药物没有反应而不得不追加剂量; **glucose tolerance test** = test for diabetes mellitus, where the patient eats glucose and his blood and urine are tested regularly 糖耐量试验,检测糖尿病的试验,病人服用葡萄糖后定期检测他的血和尿

◇ **tolerate** *verb* to accept *or* not to react to (a drug)忍受,耐受

> QUOTE: 26 patients were selected from the outpatient department on grounds of disabling breathlessness, severely limiting exercise tolerance and the performance of activities of normal daily living.
> 引文:根据气喘、严重的制动耐受及日常活动表现情况从门诊选取了26例患者。
> **Lancet** 柳叶刀

tomo- *prefix* meaning a cutting *or* section 切

◇ **tomogram** *noun* picture of part of the body taken by tomography X线断层照片

◇ **tomography** *noun* scanning of a particular part of the body using X-rays *or* ultrasound 断层扫描; **computerized axial tomography** (**CAT**) = system of scanning a patient's body, where a narrow X-ray beam, guided by a computer, can photograph a thin section of the body *or* of an organ from several angles, using the computer to build up an image of the section 计算机轴向断层扫描

◇ **tomotocia** *or* **Caesarean section** *noun* surgical operation to deliver a baby by cutting through the mother's abdominal wall into the uterus 剖宫产,剖腹产

-tomy *suffix* referring to a surgical operation 手术

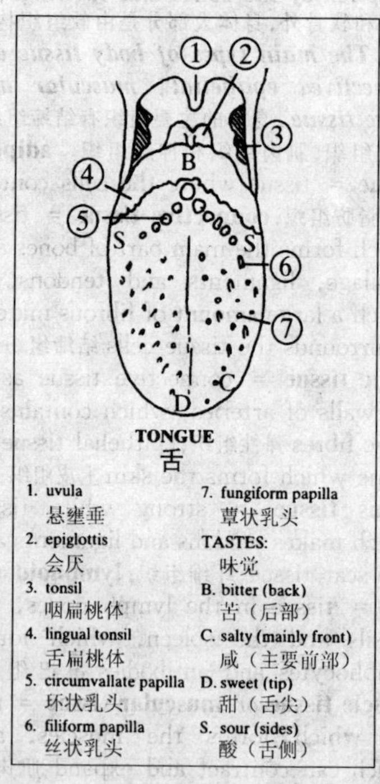

TONGUE
舌

1. uvula 悬壅垂
2. epiglottis 会厌
3. tonsil 咽扁桃体
4. lingual tonsil 舌扁桃体
5. circumvallate papilla 环状乳头
6. filiform papilla 丝状乳头
7. fungiform papilla 蕈状乳头

TASTES: 味觉
B. bitter (back) 苦(后部)
C. salty (mainly front) 咸(主要前部)
D. sweet (tip) 甜(舌尖)
S. sour (sides) 酸(舌侧)

tone *noun* tonus *or* tonicity *or* normal slightly tense state of a healthy muscle when it is not fully relaxed 肌张力,健康肌肉不完全放松的正常状态

tongue *or* **glossa** *noun* long muscular organ inside the mouth which can move and is used for tasting, swallowing and speaking 舌: ***The doctor told him to stick out his tongue and say 'Ah.'*** 医生让他伸出舌头说"啊"。(NOTE: for other terms referring to the tongue see **lingual** and words beginning with **gloss-**)

COMMENT: The top surface of the tongue is covered with papillae, some of which contain buds. The tongue is also necessary for speaking certain sounds such as 'l', 'd', 'n' and 'th'. 注释:舌的表面布满乳头,有些乳头带有味蕾。舌对于某些发音来说也是必需的,如"c"、"d"、"n"、和"th"。

tonic 1 *adjective* (muscle) which is contracted(肌肉)有张力的 **2** *noun* substance which improves the patient's general health *or* which makes a tired person stronger 强壮剂,补药: ***He is taking a course of iron tonic tablets.*** 他正在服用一疗程的补铁药片。***She asked the doctor to prescribe a tonic for her anaemia.*** 她要求医生针对她的贫血开些补药。

◇ **tonicity** *noun* tonus *or* tone *or* normal state of a healthy muscle which is not fully relaxed 肌张力

tono- *prefix* referring to pressure 压力

◇ **tonography** *noun* measurement of the pressure inside an eyeball 眼压图

◇ **tonometer** *noun* instrument which measures the pressure inside an organ, especially the eye 压力计(如眼压计)

◇ **tonometry** *noun* measurement of pressure inside an organ, especially the eye 测压(如测眼压)

tonsil *or* **palatine tonsil** *noun* area of lymphoid tissue at the back of the throat in which lymph circulates and protects the body against germs entering through the mouth 扁桃体: ***The doctor looked at her tonsils.*** 医生查看她的扁桃体。***They recommended that she should have her tonsils out.*** 他们建议她切除扁桃体。***There are red spots on his tonsils.*** 他的扁桃体上有红点。**lingual tonsil** = lymphoid tissue on the top surface of the back of the tongue 舌扁桃体; **pharyngeal tonsil** *or* **adenoidal tissue** = lymphoid tissue at the back of the throat where the passages from the nose join the pharynx 咽扁桃体 ◇ 见图 TONGUE

◇ **tonsillar** *adjective* referring to the tonsils 扁桃体的

◇ **tonsillectomy** *noun* surgical operation to remove the tonsils 扁桃体切除术

◇ **tonsillitis** *noun* inflammation of the tonsils 扁桃体炎

◇ **tonsillotome** *noun* surgical instrument used in operations on the tonsils 扁桃体刀

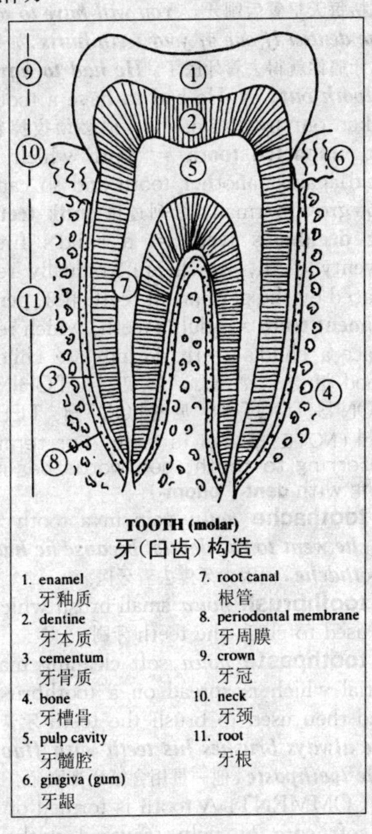

TOOTH (molar)
牙(臼齿)构造

◇ **tonsillotomy** *noun* surgical operation to make an incision into the tonsils 扁桃体切开术

COMMENT: The tonsils are larger in

children than in adults, and are more liable to infection. When infected, the tonsils become enlarged and can interfere with breathing.
注释:儿童的扁桃体比成人的大,而且更容易感染。如果感染了,扁桃体增大并可能影响呼吸。

tonus *noun* tone *or* tonicity *or* normal state of a healthy muscle which is not fully relaxed 肌张力

tooth *noun* one of a set of bones in the mouth which are used to chew food 牙齿: ***Dental hygiene involves cleaning the teeth every day after breakfast.*** 牙齿卫生包括每天早餐后刷牙。***You will have to see the dentist if one of your teeth hurts.*** 如果你牙痛你就得去看牙医了。***He had to have a tooth out.*** = He had to have a tooth taken out by the dentist. 他必须拔掉颗牙。**impacted tooth** = tooth which is held against another tooth and so cannot grow normally 牙列过挤; **milk teeth** *or* **deciduous teeth** = a child's first twenty teeth, which are gradually replaced by the permanent teeth 乳牙; **permanent teeth** = adult's teeth, which replace a child's teeth during late childhood 恒牙 *see also* 参见 HUTCHINSON'S TOOTH ◊ 见图TOOTH, TEETH (NOTE: plural is **teeth**. For terms referring to teeth, see words beginning with **dent-**, **odont-**)

◊ **toothache** *noun* pain in a tooth 牙疼: ***he went to the dentist because he had toothache.*** 他因为牙疼去看牙医。

◊ **toothbrush** *noun* small brush which is used to clean the teeth 牙刷

◊ **toothpaste** *noun* soft cleaning material which is spread on a toothbrush and then used to brush the teeth 牙膏: ***He always brushes his teeth with fluoride toothpaste.*** 他一贯用含氟牙膏刷牙。

COMMENT: A tooth is formed of a soft core of pulp, covered with a layer of hard dentine. The top part of the tooth (the crown), which can be seen above the gum, is covered with hard shiny enamel which is very hard-wearing. The lower part of the tooth (the root), which attaches the tooth to the jaw, is covered with cement, also a hard substance, but which is slightly rough and holds the periodontal ligament which links the tooth to the jaw. The milk teeth in a child appear over the first two years of childhood and consist of incisors, canines and molars. The permanent teeth which replace them are formed of eight incisors, four canines, eight premolars and twelve molars, the last four molars (the third molars or wisdom teeth), are not always present, and do not appear much before the age of twenty. Permanent teeth start to appear about the age of 5 to 6. The order of eruption of the permanent teeth is: first molars, incisors, premolars, canines, second molars, wisdom teeth.
注释:牙齿由软的牙髓外覆一层坚硬的牙本质组成。牙的顶部是牙冠,是能看见的露在牙龈外的部分,包有坚硬、有光泽的珐琅质,它非常耐磨。牙齿的下部是覆有釉质的牙根,略粗糙,通过牙周韧带将牙齿附着于下颌。儿童在 2 岁以前出乳牙,分为切齿、犬齿和臼齿。代替它们的恒牙有 8 个切牙,4 个犬齿,8 个前磨牙和 12 个磨牙组成,最后 4 个磨牙(第三磨牙或智齿)不一定人人都有,而且也不会在 20 岁前出现。恒牙 5~6 岁时开始时出现,出牙的顺序是:第一磨牙、切牙、前磨牙、犬齿、第二磨牙、智齿。

topagnosis *noun* being unable to tell which part of your body has been touched, caused by a disorder of the brain 位置觉缺失

tophus *noun* deposit of solid crystals in the skin, or in the joints, especially with gout 痛风石 (NOTE: plural is **tophi-**)

topical *adjective* referring to one particular part of the body 局部的; **topical drug** = drug which is applied to one part of the body only 局部用药

◊ **topically** *adverb* (applied) to one external part of the body only 局部地,外用地: ***The drug is applied topically.*** 这药

是外用药。

> QUOTE: One of the most common routes of neonatal poisoning is percutaneous absorption following topical administration.
> 引文:新生儿中毒最常见的途径之一是局部涂抹后经皮肤吸收。
> **Southern Medical Journal** 南部医学杂志

topographical *adjective* referring to topography 局部解剖学的
◇ **topography** *noun* description of each particular part of the body 局部解剖学
tormina *noun* colic, pain in the intestine 绞痛
torpor *noun* condition where a patient seems sleepy *or* slow to react 迟钝、不活泼
torso *noun* main part of the body, not including the arms, legs and head 躯干
torticollis *or* **wry neck** *noun* deformity of the neck, where the head is twisted to one side by contraction of the sternocleidomastoid muscle 斜颈,颈部畸形,头扭向一侧,由一侧胸锁乳突肌异常收缩引起
total *adjective* complete *or* covering the whole body 完全的,全部的: ***He has total paralysis of the lower part of the body.*** 他下半身完全瘫痪了。**total hip arthroplasty** *or* **replacement** = replacing both the head of the femur and the acetabulum with an artificial joint 全髋关节置换,将股骨头和髋臼都换成人工的
◇ **totally** *adverb* completely 完全地: ***She is totally paralysed.*** 她完全瘫痪了。***He will never totally regain the use of his left hand.*** 他永远不会完全恢复对左手的使用了。
touch *noun* one of the five senses, where sensations are felt by part of the skin, especially by the fingers and lips 触觉

> COMMENT: Touch is sensed by receptors in the skin which send impulses back to the brain. The touch receptors can tell the difference betweens hot and cold, hard and soft, wet and dry, and rough and smooth.
> 注释:触觉是皮肤内的感受器感知的,然后再将冲动传回大脑。触觉感受器可以分辨冷热、软硬、干湿以及粗糙还是平滑。

tough *adjective* solid *or* which cannot break or tear easily 坚韧: ***The meninges are covered by a layer of tough tissue, the dura mater.*** 脑膜被一层坚韧的组织覆盖着,这就是硬膜。(NOTE: **tough - tougher - toughest**)
tourniquet *noun* instrument *or* tight bandage wrapped round a limb to constrict an artery, so reducing the flow of blood and stopping bleeding from a wound 止血带
towel *noun* (**a**) piece of soft cloth which is used for drying 毛巾 (**b**) **sanitary towel** = wad of absorbent cotton placed over the vulva to absorb the menstrual flow 卫生巾
tox- *or* **toxo-** *prefix* meaning poison 毒
◇ **toxaemia** *noun* blood poisoning, presence of poisonous substances in the blood 毒血症; **toxaemia of pregnancy** = condition which can affect pregnant women towards the end of pregnancy, where the patient develops high blood pressure and passes protein in the urine 妊高症,妊娠末期孕妇高血压,尿中出现蛋白
◇ **toxic** *adjective* poisonous 有毒的; **toxic goitre** *or* **thyrotoxicosis** = type of goitre where the thyroid gland swells, the patient's limbs tremble and the eyes protrude 毒性甲状腺肿
◇ **toxicity** *noun* degree to which a substance is poisonous *or* harmful; amount of poisonous *or* harmful material in a substance 毒性: ***Scientists are measuring the toxicity of car exhaust fumes.*** 科学家在检测汽车尾气的毒性。**acute toxicity** = level of concentration of a toxic substance which makes people seriously ill *or* can cause death 急性毒性; **chronic toxicity** = exposure to harmful levels of a toxic substance over a long

period of time 慢性毒性

◇ **toxico-** *prefix* meaning poison 毒

◇ **toxicologist** *noun* scientist who specializes in the study of poisons 毒理学家

◇ **toxicology** *noun* scientific study of poisons and their effects on the human body 毒理学

◇ **toxicosis** *noun* poisoning 中毒

◇ **toxin** *noun* poisonous substance produced in the body by germs or microorganisms, and which, if injected into an animal, stimulates the production of antitoxins 毒素

◇ **toxocariasis** *or* **visceral larva migrans** *noun* infestation of the intestine with worms from a dog or cat 弓蛔虫病,一种从猫或狗传染来的肠道寄生虫病

◇ **toxoid** *noun* toxin which has been treated and is no longer poisonous, but which can still provoke the formation of antibodies 类毒素,把毒素进行处理使它不再有毒性但能引发机体形成抗毒素

> COMMENT: Toxoids are used as vaccines, and are injected into a patient to give immunity against a disease.
> 注释:类毒素可以用作疫苗,注射到病人体内使他对特定疾病有免疫力。

◇ **toxoid-antitoxin** *noun* mixture of toxoid and antitoxin, used as a vaccine 类毒素-抗毒素合剂(用作疫苗)

◇ **toxoplasmosis** *noun* **disease caused by the parasite** *Toxoplasma* which is carried by animals 由弓形体引起的寄生虫病,弓形体病; **congenital toxoplasmosis** *or* **toxoplasma encephalitis** = condition of a baby which has been infected with toxoplasmosis by its mother while still in the womb 先天性弓形体病,弓形体脑炎,胎儿在母体即感染了弓形体引起的疾病

> COMMENT: Toxoplasmosis can cause encephalitis or hydrocephalus and can be fatal.
> 注释:弓形体病可以引起脑炎和脑积水,并可能是致命的。

trabecula *noun* thin strip of stiff tissue which divides an organ *or* bone tissue into sections 小梁,把器官或骨组织分成若干部分的细小的条带,如骨小梁 (NOTE: plural is **trabeculae**)

◇ **trabeculectomy** *noun* surgical operation to treat glaucoma by cutting a channel through trabeculae to link with Schlemm's canal 小梁切除术,治疗青光眼的一种手术

trace *noun* (**a**) very small amount 痕迹量,微量: ***There are traces of the drug in the blood sample.*** 血样中有微量药物。 ***The doctor found traces of alcohol in the patient's urine.*** 医生在病人的尿样中发现了微量酒精。 **trace element** = element which is essential to the human body, but only in very small quantities 微量元素

> COMMENT: The trace elements are cobalt, chromium, copper, magnesium, manganese, molybdenum, selenium and zinc.
> 注释:微量元素有钴、铬、铜、镁、锰、钼、硒和锌。

◇ **tracer** *noun* substance (often radioactive) injected into a substance in the body, so that doctors can follow its passage round the body 示踪物质,通常是带有放射性的物质,注射进体内,医生可以随其在体内的运行观察某种物质的代谢途径。

trachea *or* **windpipe** *noun* main air passage which runs from the larynx to the lungs, where it divides into the two main bronchi 气管 ◊ 见图 LUNGS, THROAT

> COMMENT: The trachea is about 10 centimetre long, and is formed of rings of cartilage and connective tissue.
> 注释:气管有 10 厘米长,由环状软骨和结缔组织构成。

◇ **tracheal** *adjective* referring to the trachea 气管的; **tracheal tugging** = feeling that something is pulling on the windpipe when the patient breathes in, a symptom of aneurysm 气管拖曳感,病人吸气时好像什么东西在气管里拖过,是动脉瘤的症状

◇ **tracheitis** *noun* inflammation of the trachea due to an infection 气管炎

trachelorrhaphy *noun* surgical

operation to repair tears in the cervix of the uterus 宫颈缝合术

tracheobronchitis *noun* inflammation of both the trachea and the bronchi 气管及支气管炎

◇ **tracheostomy** *or* **tracheotomy** *noun* surgical operation to make a hole through the throat into the windpipe, so as to allow air to get to the lungs in cases where the trachea is blocked, as in pneumonia, poliomyelitis or diphtheria 气管切开术,为保证通气而将气管切开,用于气管阻塞时,如肺炎、脊髓灰质炎或白喉时

> COMMENT: After the operation, a tube is inserted into the hole to keep it open. The tube may be permanent if it is to bypass an obstruction, but can be removed if the condition improves.
> 注释:气管切开术后,将一根管子插入切口,使切口处于张开状态。如果要起阻塞前分流的作用,气管插管可以是永久的,但如果病情改善了,也可以去掉它。

trachoma *noun* contagious viral inflammation of the eyelids, common in tropical countries, which can cause blindness if the conjunctiva becomes scarred 沙眼,衣原体感染所致的眼睑炎症,常见于热带地区,如果结膜形成瘢痕可以致盲

tract *noun* (i) series of organs *or* tubes which allow something to pass from one part of the body to another 通道 (ii) series *or* bundle of nerve fibres connecting two areas of the nervous system and transmitting nervous impulses in one or in both directions 束; **cerebrospinal tracts** = main motor pathways in the anterior and lateral white columns of the spinal cord 大脑脊髓束,位于脊髓白质的前外侧,是主要的运动传导途径; **olfactory tract** = nerve tract which takes the olfactory nerve from the nose to the brain 嗅束,由鼻腔的嗅神经到脑的传导途径; **pyramidal tract** = tract in the brain and spinal cord carrying motor neurone fibres from the cerebral cortex 锥体束,从大脑皮质向下传导运动神经元冲动的传导束 *see also* 参见 DIGESTIVE TRACT

> QUOTE: GI fistulae are frequently associated with infection because the effluent contains bowel organisms which initially contaminate the fistula tract.
> 引文:胃肠瘘经常与感染相关,因其流出物含有结肠微生物,因此首先污染瘘道。
> **Nursing Times** 护理时代

traction *noun* pulling applied to straighten a broken or deformed limb 牵引术: ***The patient was in traction for two weeks.*** 病人做牵引已经2周了。

> COMMENT: A system of weights and pulleys is fixed over the patient's bed so that the limb can be pulled hard enough to counteract the tendency of the muscles to contract and pull it back to its original position. Traction can also be used for slipped discs and other dislocations. Other forms of traction include frames attached to the body.
> 注释:在病床上装了滑轮和重物,这样可以用足够的力度将肢体拉伸以对抗肌肉收缩的张力而把它拉回原来的位置。牵引还可用于椎间盘脱出和其它错位。还有其他的牵引方法如固着于身体的支架牵引。

tractotomy *noun* surgical operation to cut the nerve pathway taking sensations of pain to the brain, as treatment for intractable pain 神经束切断术,用于治疗难治性疼痛

tragus *noun* piece of cartilage in the outer ear which projects forward over the entrance to the auditory canal 耳屏,耳廓

training *noun* educating by giving instruction and the opportunity to practise 训练 *see also* 参见 TOILET

trait *noun* characteristic which is particular to a person 特质,特性; **physical genetic trait** = characteristic of the body of a person (such as red hair *or* big feet) which is inherited 躯体遗传特性,如红头发,大脚

trance *noun* condition where a person is in a dream, but not asleep, and seems not to be aware of what is happening round him 出神,神游: ***He walked round the room in a trance*.** 他在出神地绕着房间走。***The hypnotist waved his hand and she went into* or *came out of a trance*.** 催眠师摇了摇她的手,她进入(出了)出神状态。

tranquillizer *or* **tranquillizing drug** *noun* drug which relieves a patient's anxiety and calms him down 镇静剂: ***She's taking tranquillizers to calm her nerves*.** 她正服用镇静剂使自己平静下来。***He's been on tranquillizers ever since he started his new job*.** 自从他从事新职业以来一直用镇静剂。

> COMMENT: Tranquillizing drugs can be habit-forming.
> 注释:镇静类药物可以成瘾。

trans- *prefix* meaning through *or* across 经过; **transdiaphragmatic approach** = operation carried out through the diaphragm(手术)经膈路径

◇ **transaminase** *noun* enzyme involved in the transamination of amino acids 转氨酶

◇ **transamination** *noun* process by which amino acids are metabolized in the liver 转氨基作用

◇ **transection** *noun* (i) cutting across part of the body 断面 (ii) sample of tissue which has been taken by cutting across a part of the body 断面样本

◇ **transfer** *verb* to pass from one place to another 转移: ***The hospital records have been transferred to the computer*.** 医院病历被转输入计算机。***The patient was transferred to a special burns unit*.** 病人被转到特殊的烧伤病房。

◇ **transference** *noun* (*in psychiatry*) condition where the patient transfers to the psychoanalyst the characteristics belonging to a strong character from his past (such as a parent), and reacts to the analyst as if he were that person 移情(精神病学词汇),病人把精神分析学家当作他过去经历中的有强大影响的人物(如父母),采取对待过去生活中那个人的态度对待分析师

◇ **transferrin** *or* **siderophilin** *noun* substance found in the blood, which carries iron in the bloodstream 转铁蛋白

◇ **transfusion** *noun* transferring blood *or* saline fluids from a container into a patient's bloodstream 输血,输液; **blood transfusion** = transferring blood which has been given by another person into a patient's vein 输血; **exchange transfusion** = method of treating leukaemia *or* erythroblastosis where almost all the abnormal blood is removed from the body and replaced by normal blood 换血,治疗白血病、成红细胞增多症的一种方法,几乎将病人所有异常的血液全部换成正常血

transient *adjective* which does not last long 一过性的; **transient ischaemic attack** (**TIA**) = mild stroke caused by a short stoppage of blood supply 一过性缺血发作,轻微的中风

transillumination *noun* examination of an organ by shining a bright light through it 透照法,用强光透射器官的检查法

◇ **transitional** *adjective* which is in the process of developing into something 转变的,过渡的; **transitional epithelium** = type of epithelium found in the urethra 移行上皮,尿道的上皮

◇ **translocation** *noun* moving of part of a chromosome to a different chromosome pair which causes abnormal development of the fetus(染色体)易位,染色体上的一部分移到另一对染色体上,可造成胎儿发育异常

◇ **translumbar** *adjective* through the lumbar region 经腰部的

◇ **transmigration** *noun* movement of a cell through a membrane 移行,血细胞渗出

◇ **transmit** *verb* to pass (a message *or* a disease) 传递,传播: ***Impulses are transmitted along the neural pathways*.** 冲动是经神经通路传递的。***The disease is transmitted by lice*.** 这种病是由虱子传播的。

◇ **transparent** *adjective* which can be seen through 透明的: ***The cornea is a transparent tissue on the front of the*** *eye*. 角膜是眼睛前面的透明组织。

◇ **transplacental** *adjective* through the placenta 经胎盘的

transplant 1 *noun* (i) act of taking an organ (such as the heart *or* kidney) or tissue (such as skin) and grafting it into a patient to replace an organ *or* tissue which is diseased or not functioning properly 移植 (ii) the organ or tissue which is grafted 移植物: ***She had a heart-lung transplant***. 她做了心肺移植。***The kidney transplant was rejected***. 移植的肾被排斥了。2 *verb* to graft an organ *or* tissue onto a patient to replace an organ *or* tissue which is diseased or not functioning correctly 移植

◇ **transplantation** *noun* transplant *or* the act of transplanting 移植

> QUOTE: Bone marrow transplantation has the added complication of graft-versus-host disease.
> 引文:骨髓移植有移植物抗宿主反应的另外并发症。
> **Hospital Update** 现代化医院

transport *verb* to carry to another place 转运: ***Arterial blood transports oxygen to the tissues***. 动脉血将氧气转运到组织。

> QUOTE: Insulin's primary metabolic function is to transport glucose into muscle and fat cells, so that it can be used for energy.
> 引文:胰岛素的主要代谢功能是将葡萄糖转运到肌肉和脂肪细胞中,供其能量。
> **Nursing 87** 护理 87

transposition *noun* congenital condition where the aorta and pulmonary artery are placed on the opposite side of the body to their normal position(内脏)换位,移位术,错位,主动脉和肺动脉长到正常位置的对面,是一种先天性疾病

◇ **transpyloric plane** *noun* plane at right angles to the sagittal plane, passing midway between the suprasternal notch and the symphysis pubis 经幽门平面,与矢状面呈直角的平面,在锁骨上切迹和耻骨联合之间通过

◇ **transrectal** *adjective* through the rectum 经直肠的

◇ **transsexual** *noun & adjective* (person) who feels a desire to be a member of the opposite sex 易性癖患者,(一个人)希望成为另一性别的成员;(behaviour) showing that a person wants to be a member of the opposite sex 易性癖的,(行为)显示某人想成为另一性别的成员

◇ **transsexualism** *noun* sexual abnormality where a person wants to be a member of the opposite sex 易性癖,是一种性身份异常,表现为想成为另一性别的成员。

◇ **transtubercular plane** *noun* plane at right angles to the sagittal plane, passing through the tubercles of the iliac crests 经结节平面,与矢状平面成直角的平面,通过髂嵴结节

◇ **transudation** *noun* passing of a fluid from the body's cells outside the body 漏出,渗出

◇ **transurethral** *adjective* through the urethra 经尿道的; **transurethral prostatectomy** *or* **transurethral resection (TUR)** = surgical operation to remove the prostate gland, where the operation is carried out through the urethra 经尿道前列腺切除术,经尿道切除术

◇ **transverse** *adjective* across *or* at right angles to an organ 横的; **transverse arch** = arched structure across the sole of the foot 横弓,横跨足底的弓形结构; **transverse colon** = second section of the colon, which crosses the body below the stomach 横结肠 ◊ 见图 DIGESTIVE SYSTEM; **transverse fracture** = fracture where the bone is broken straight across 横骨折; **transverse plane** = plane at right angles to the sagittal plane, running horizontally across the body 水平面; **transverse presentation** = position of the baby in the womb, where the baby's side will appear first, normally requiring urgent manipulation *or* Caesarean section to prevent complications 横位,胎儿在子宫中的位置使它将以侧先露临产,一般需要手法转位或剖宫产以防发生并发

症;**transverse process** = part of a vertebra which protrudes at the side 横突

◇ **transvesical prostatectomy** *noun* operation to remove the prostate gland, where the operation is carried out through the bladder 经膀胱前列腺切除术

◇ **transvestite** *noun* person who dresses in the clothes of the opposite sex, as an expression of transsexualism 易装癖,穿另一性别的衣服,是易性癖的表现

trapezium *noun* one of the eight small carpal bones in the wrist 大多角骨,八块腕骨之一 ◊ 见图 HAND

◇ **trapezius** *noun* triangular muscle in the upper part of the back and the neck, which moves the shoulder blade and pulls the head back 斜方肌,上背部和后颈部的三角形肌肉,将肩胛骨和头向后拉

◇ **trapezoid(bone)** *noun* one of the eight small carpal bones in the wrist 小多角骨,八块腕骨之一 ◊ 见图 HAND

trauma *noun* (i) wound *or* injury 创伤 (ii) mental shock caused by a sudden happening which was not expected to take place 精神创伤,由毫无预见、突如其来的事件引起

◇ **traumatic** *adjective* referring to trauma *or* caused by an injury 创伤性的;**traumatic fever** = fever caused by an injury 创伤性发热;**traumatic shock** = state of general weakness caused by an injury and loss of blood 创伤性休克

◇ **traumatology** *noun* branch of surgery which deals with injuries received in accidents 创伤学

travel sickness *or* **motion sickness** *noun* illness and nausea felt when travelling 晕动病

> COMMENT: The movement of liquid inside the labyrinth of the middle ear causes motion sickness, which is particularly noticeable in vehicles which are closed , such as planes , coaches, hovercraft.
> 注释:内耳淋巴迷路液体的运动造成晕动病,在密闭的交通工具里如飞机、客车车厢、直升飞机特别明显。

tray *noun* (i) flat board for carrying plates of food for a patient to eat 盘子 (ii) flat metal plate for carrying equipment needed to a surgical intervention (such as a 'rectoscopy tray')医用弯盘

treat *verb* to look after a sick or injured person *or* to try to cure a sick person 照顾治疗患者;to try to cure a disease 治疗疾病: ***After the accident the passengers were treated in hospital for cuts.*** 事故后,乘客们在医院里对伤口进行治疗。***She has been treated with a new antibiotic.*** 她已经接受了新抗生素的治疗。***She's being treated by a specialist for heart disease.*** 她在接受心脏病专家的治疗。

◇ **treatment** *noun* way of looking after a sick *or* injured person; way of trying to cure a disease 治疗: ***This is a new treatment for heart disease.*** 这是治疗心脏病的一种新方法。***He is receiving*** *or* ***undergoing treatment for a slipped disc.*** 他在接受椎间盘脱出的治疗。***She's in hospital for treatment to her back.*** 她在医院里治疗她的后背。***We are going to try some cortisone treatment.*** 我们正准备试用可的松治疗。

trematode *noun* fluke *or* parasitic flatworm 吸虫

tremble *verb* to shake *or* shiver slightly 颤抖: ***His hands are trembling with cold.*** 他冷得手直哆嗦。***Her body trembled with fever.*** 发热使她身体打颤。

◇ **trembling** *noun* making rapid small movements of a limb or muscles 颤抖: ***Trembling of the hands is a symptom of Parkinson's disease.*** 手颤是帕金森病的症状之一。

tremens 震颤性 *see* 见 DELIRIUM

tremor *noun* shaking *or* making slight movements of a limb *or* muscle 震颤; **coarse tremor** = severe trembling 粗大震颤; **essential tremor** = involuntary slow trembling movement of the hands often seen in old people 原发性震颤(老年性震颤); **intention tremor** = trembling of the hands when a person suffering from certain brain disease makes a voluntary movement to try to touch something 意向性震颤,有意做某动作时出现或加重的震颤; **physiological tremor** = normal small movements of limbs which take place when a person tries to remain still 生理性震颤,努力想保持不动时出现的轻微抖动

trench fever *noun* fever caused by Rickettsia bacteria, similar to typhus but recurring every five days 战壕热,立克次体感染所致发热,与伤寒相像,但每5天发作一回; **trench foot** *or* **immersion foot** = condition, caused by exposure to cold and damp, where the skin of the foot becomes red and blistered and in severe cases turns black when gangrene sets in. (The condition was common among soldiers serving in the trenches during the First World War) 战壕足,浸渍足,脚泡在湿、冷的环境中,皮肤变红,起水疱,严重时坏疽变黑。(常见于第一次世界大战中战壕里的士兵); **trench mouth** 口腔溃肠 *see* 见 GINGIVITIS

Trendelenburg's position *noun* position where the patient lies on a sloping bed, with the head lower than the feet, and the knees bent (used in surgical operations to the pelvis) 特伦德伦伯格卧位,垂头仰卧位; **Trendelenburg's operation** = operation to tie a saphenous vein in the groin before removing varicose veins 特伦德伦伯格手术,隐静脉结扎术; **Trendelenburg's sign** = symptom of congenital dislocation of the hip, where the patient's pelvis is lower on the opposite side to the dislocation 特伦德伦伯格氏征,蹒跚步态,先天性髋脱臼的体征,脱臼侧较低

trepan *verb* (*formerly*) to cut a hole in the skull, as a treatment for some diseases of the head 在颅骨上钻孔

trephine *noun* surgical instrument for making a round hole in the skull *or* for removing a round piece of tissue 环钻

Treponema *noun* spirochaete which causes disease such as syphilis or yaws 密螺旋体,可以引起梅毒或雅司病

◇ **treponematosis** *noun* yaws, an infection by the bacterium *Treponema pertenue* 密螺旋体病,雅司病

TRH = THYROTROPHIN-RELEASING HORMONE 促甲状腺释放激素

triad *noun* three organs *or* symptoms which are linked together in a group 三联征

trial *noun* test 试验; **clinical trial** = trial carried out in a medical laboratory on a patient or on tissue from a patient 临床试验; **multicentric trial** = trial carried out in several centres at the same time 多中心试验

triangle *noun* flat shape which has three sides; part of the body with three sides 三角; **rectal triangle** *or* **anal triangle** = posterior part of the perineum 直肠三角,肛门三角 *see also* 参见 FEMORAL, SCARPA

◇ **triangular** *adjective* with three sides 三角的; **triangular bandage** = bandage made of a triangle of cloth, used to make a sling for the arm 三角绷带; **triangular muscle** = muscle in the shape of a triangle 三角肌

triceps *noun* muscle formed of three parts, which are joined to form one tendon 三头肌; **triceps brachii** = muscle in the back part of the upper arm which makes the forearm stretch out 肱三头肌,上臂后侧的肌肉,有伸前臂的作用

trichiasis *noun* painful condition where the eyelashes grow in towards the eye and scratch the eyeball 倒睫

◇ **trichinosis** *or* **trichiniasis** *noun* disease caused by infestation of the intestine by larvae of roundworms *or* nematodes, which pass round the body in the bloodstream and settle in muscles 旋毛虫病,旋毛虫经肠道感染人体,经血循环定位于肌肉

> COMMENT: The larvae enter the body from eating meat, especiallypork, which has not been properly cooked.
> 注释:幼虫由烹饪不熟的食肉进入人体,特别是猪肉。

◇ **trich(o)-** *prefix* (i) referring to hair 毛发 (ii) like hair 像毛发的

◇ **Trichocephalus** *noun* whipworm, thin round parasitic worm which infests the caecum 鞭虫属

◇ **trichology** *noun* study of hair and the diseases which affect it 毛发学

◇ **Trichomonas** *noun* species of long thin parasite which infests the intestines 毛滴虫属; **Trichomonas vaginalis** = parasite which infests the vagina and causes an irritating discharge 阴道滴虫

◇ **trichomoniasis** *noun* infestation of the intestine *or* vagina with Trichomonas 滴虫病,感染肠道或阴道

◇ **trichomycosis** *noun* disease of the hair caused by a corynebacterium 毛发菌病

◇ **Trichophyton** *noun* fungus which affects the skin, hair and nails 毛癣菌

◇ **trichophytosis** *noun* infection caused by Trichophyton 毛癣菌病

◇ **trichosis** *noun* abnormal condition of the hair 毛发病

◇ **trichotillomania** *noun* condition where a person pulls his hair out compulsively 拔毛狂

trichromatic *adjective* (vision) which is normal, where the person can tell the difference between the three primary colours 三色视的,色觉正常的 *compare* 比较 DICHROMATIC

◇ **trichrome stain** *noun* stain in three colours used in histology 三色染色,用三种颜色染色的组织学染色方法

trichuriasis *noun* infestation of the intestine with whipworms 鞭虫病

◇ **Trichuris** *noun* whipworm, thin round parasitic worm which infests the caecum 鞭虫属

tricuspid valve *noun* inlet valve with three cusps between the right atrium and the right ventricle in the heart 三尖瓣,右房室瓣,由三个瓣组成 ◇ 见图 HEART

trifocal lenses *or* **trifocals** *plural noun* type of glasses, where three lenses are combined in one piece of glass to give clear vision over different distances 变焦透镜 *see also* 参见 BIFOCAL

trigeminal *adjective* in three parts 三叉的; **trigeminal nerve** = fifth cranial nerve (formed of the ophthalmic nerve, the maxillary nerve, and the mandibular nerve) which controls the sensory nerves in the forehead, face and chin, and the muscles in the jaw 三叉神经,第五对颅神经,由眼神经、上颌神经和下颌神经组成,负责前额、面部和下巴的感觉,控制咀嚼肌; **trigeminal neuralgia** *or* **tic douloureux** = pain in the trigeminal nerve, which sends intense pains shooting across the face 三叉神经痛,面部放射性剧痛

trigeminy *noun* irregular heartbeat, where a normal beat is followed by two ectopic beats 三联律,不规则心律,一次正常搏动伴随两次异位搏动。

trigger *verb* to start something happening 诱发: ***It is not known what triggers the development of shingles.*** 是什么诱发了带状疱疹还不清楚。

◇ **trigger finger** *noun* condition where a finger can bend but is difficult to straighten, probably because of a nodule on the flexor tendon 扳机指,指头可弯而难伸直,可能是由于曲肌腱上长有结节

> QUOTE: The endocrine system releases hormones in response to a change in the concentration of trigger substances in the blood or other body fluids.
> 引文:血液或其他体液中激发物质浓度的变化引起内分泌系统释放激素。
> **Nursing 87** 护理 87

triglyceride *noun* substance (such as fat) which contains three fatty acids 甘油三酯

trigone *noun* triangular piece of the wall of the bladder, between the openings for the urethra and the two ureters 膀胱三角区,如膀胱三角区,三顶点分别是两个输尿管开口和尿道开口

◇ **trigonitis** *noun* inflammation of the bottom part of the wall of the bladder 三角区炎症

◇ **trigonocephalic** *adjective* (skull)

which shows signs of trigonocephaly 三角头畸形的

◇ **trigonocephaly** *noun* condition where the skull is deformed in the shape of a triangle, with points on either side of the face in front of the ears 三角头畸形

triiodothyronine *noun* hormone synthesized in the body from thyroxine secreted by the thyroid gland 三碘甲状腺原氨酸

trimester *noun* one of the three 3-month periods of a pregnancy 三个月,三月期(特指怀孕时每三个月为一阶段)

trip 1 *noun* (**a**) journey 旅途,旅行: ***He finds it too difficult to make the trip to the outpatients department twice a week.*** 他发现每周两次去门诊实在勉为其难。(**b**) trance induced by drugs 恍惚; **bad trip** = trance induced by drugs, producing a very bad reaction 吸毒产生的幻觉 **2** *verb* to fall down because of knocking the foot on something 绊倒: ***He tripped over the piece of wood.*** 他在一块木头上绊倒了。***She tripped up and fell down*** 她向前一个趔趄,然后摔倒了。

triphosphate 三磷酸盐 *see* 见 ADENOSINE TRIPHOSPHATE (ATP)

triplet *noun* one of three babies born to a mother at the same time 三胞胎之一 *see also* 参见 QUADRUPLET, QUINTUPLET, SEXTUPLET, TWIN

triploid *noun* & *adjective* (cell, organ, etc.) having 3N chromosomes *or* three times the haploid number 三倍体,有相当于三套单倍体的染色体

triquetral (bone) *or* **triquetrum** *noun* one of the eight small carpal bones in the wrist 三角骨,八块腕骨之一 ◊ 见图 HAND

trismus *noun* lockjaw, spasm in the lower jaw, which makes it difficult to open the mouth, a symptom of tetanus 牙关紧闭,破伤风的症状

trisomic *adjective* referring to Down's syndrome 三体的

◇ **trisomy** *noun* condition where a patient has three chromosomes instead of a pair 染色体三体,正常情况是两两成对; **trisomy 21** = DOWN'S SYNDROME 21-三体型综合征

tritanopia *noun* rare form of colour blindness, a defect in vision where the patient cannot see blue 第三色盲,蓝色盲 *compare* 比较 DALTONISM, DEUTERANOPIA

trocar *noun* surgical instrument *or* pointed rod which slides inside a cannula to make a hole in tissue to drain off fluid 套针,用于穿刺组织以便引流

trochanter *noun* two bony lumps on either side of the top end of the femur where muscles are attached 转子,股骨顶端两侧附着肌肉的骨性突起

> COMMENT: The lump on the outer side is the greater trochanter, and that on the inner side is the lesser trochanter.
> 注释:外侧的突起是大转子,内侧的是小转子。

trochlea *noun* any part of the body shaped like a pulley, especially (i) part of the lower end of the humerus, which articulates with the ulna 滑车,肱骨下端与尺骨形成关节的部分 (ii) curved bone in the frontal bone through which one of the eye muscles passes 额骨上弯曲的有一束眼肌通过的部分 (NOTE: plural is **trochleae**)

◇ **trochlear** *adjective* referring to a ring in a bone 滑车的; **trochlear nerve** = fourth cranial nerve, which controls the muscles of the eyeball 滑车神经,第四对颅神经,控制眼球运动的神经之一

trochoid joint *or* **pivot joint** *noun* joint where a bone can rotate freely about a central axis as in the neck, where the atlas articulates with the axis 滑车关节

trolley *noun* wheeled table *or* cupboard, which can be pushed from place to place 推车: ***She takes newspapers and books round the wards on a trolley.*** 他在推车上放着报纸和书籍推着转病房。***The patient was placed on a trolley to be taken to the operating theatre.*** 把病人放在平车

上推到手术室。(NOTE: the US English is **cart**)

troph(o)- *prefix* referring to food *or* nutrition 营养

◇ **trophoblast** *noun* tissue which forms the wall of a blastocyst 滋养层

◇ **-trophy** *suffix* meaning (i) nourishment 营养 (ii) development of an organ 生长

-tropic *suffix* meaning (i) turning towards 趋向 (ii) which influences 影响

◇ **tropics** *plural noun* hot areas of the world *or* countries near the equator 热带: ***He lives in the tropics.*** 他居住在热带地区。***disease which is endemic in the tropics*** 热带地区的地方病

◇ **tropical** *adjective* referring to the tropics 热带的: ***The disease is carried by a tropical insect.*** 这种病由热带昆虫携带。**tropical countries** = the tropics, countries near the equator 热带地区: ***disease which is endemic in tropical countries*** 热带地区的地方病; **tropical disease** = disease which is found in tropical countries, such as malaria, dengue, Lassa fever 热带病,见于热带地区的病,如疟疾、登革热、拉沙热; **tropical medicine** = branch of medicine which deals with tropical diseases 热带病医学; **tropical ulcer** *or* **Naga sore** = large area of infection which forms round a wound, especially in tropical countries 热带溃疡,伤口周围大面积感染,特别见于热带地区

trouble *noun* any type of illness *or* disorder 毛病: ***He has had stomach trouble for the last few months.*** 最近几个月他一直患胃病。***She is undergoing treatment for back trouble.*** 她在治疗后背的毛病。***His bladder is giving him some trouble.*** 他的膀胱有病。***What seems to be the trouble?*** = What are your symptoms *or* what are you suffering from? 你怎么了?

Trousseau's sign *noun* spasm in the muscles in the forearm, causing the index and middle fingers to extend, when a tourniquet is applied to the upper arm, a sign of latent tetany, showing that the blood contains too little calcium 特鲁索征,前臂肌肉痉挛,造成敲击上臂时食指和中指伸指运动,是潜在搐搦的征象,说明血钙含量过低。

true *adjective* correct *or* right 真实的; **true ribs** = top seven pairs of ribs which are attached to the breastbone 真肋

truncus *noun* main blood vessel in a fetus, which develops into the aorta and pulmonary artery 血管干,胎儿的主要血管,发育成主动脉和肺动脉。

trunk *noun* main part of the body, without the head, arms and legs 躯干 *see also* 参见 BRONCHOMEDIASTINAL, COELIAC

truss *noun* belt worn round the waist, with pads to hold a hernia in place 疝带,系在腰部的带子,有一个小垫托住疝气

trust *noun* **trust status** = position of a hospital which is a self-governing trust 信托地位,医院有自我管理责任的地位; **hospital trust** = self-governing hospital, a hospital which earns its revenue from services provided to the District Health Authorities and family doctors 自我管理医院

Trypanosoma *or* **trypanosome** *noun* genus of parasite which causes sleeping sickness and Chagas' disease 锥虫属

◇ **trypanocide** *noun* drug which kills trypanosomes 杀锥虫药

◇ **trypanosomiasis** *noun* disease, spread by insect bites, where trypanosomes infest the blood 锥虫病,由昆虫叮咬传播

> COMMENT: Symptoms are pains in the head, general lethargy and long periods of sleep. In Africa, sleeping sickness, and in South America, Chagas' disease, are both caused by trypanosomes.
> 注释:症状有头疼、普遍性嗜睡和长时间睡眠。非洲的昏睡病和南美的恰加斯病,都是锥虫引起的。

trypsin *noun* enzyme converted from trypsinogen by the duodenum and secreted into the digestive system where it absorbs protein 胰蛋白酶

◇ **trypsinogen** *noun* enzyme secreted by the pancreas into the duodenum 胰蛋白酶原

tryptophan *noun* essential amino acid 色氨酸,必需氨基酸之一

tsetse fly *noun* African insect which passes trypanosomes into the human bloodstream, causing sleeping sickness 采采蝇,非洲的一种昆虫,将锥虫病传入人的血液

TSH = THYROID-STIMULATING HORMONE 促甲状腺素

tsutsugamushi disease *or* **scrub typhus** *noun* form of typhus caused by the Rickettsia bacteria, passed to humans by mites (found in South East Asia)恙虫病,立克次体感染所致疾病,由昆虫叮咬传给人,发现于东南亚

tubal *adjective* referring to a tube 试管的,管子的;**tubal pregnancy** = the most common form of ectopic pregnancy, where the fetus develops in a Fallopian tube instead of the uterus 输卵管妊娠,最常见的异位妊娠,胚胎在输卵管内发育

◇ **tube** *noun* (**a**) long hollow passage in the body, like a pipe 管道 *see also* 参见 EUSTACHIAN, FALLOPIAN (**b**) soft flexible pipe for carrying liquid or gas 软管:***The tube leading to the colostomy bag had become detached.*** 通向结肠造口袋的管子脱落了。(**c**) soft plastic *or* metal pipe, sealed at one end and with a lid at the other, used to dispense a paste *or* gel 牙膏管:***a tube of eye ointment*** 一管眼膏; ***an empty tube of toothpaste*** 一个空牙膏管

tuber *noun* swollen *or* raised area 结节;**tuber cinereum** = part of the brain to which the stalk of the pituitary gland is connected 灰结节,脑的一部分,与垂体干相连

◇ **tubercle** *noun* (**a**) small bony projection (as on a rib)(骨)结节,粗隆 (**b**) small infected lump characteristic of tuberculosis, where tissue is destroyed and pus forms 结核结节,内部组织被破坏形成脓肿;**primary tubercle** = first infected spot where tuberculosis starts to infect a lung 原发性结核

◇ **tubercular** *adjective* (i) which causes *or* refers to tuberculosis 结核的 (ii) (patient) suffering from tuberculosis 结核病人 (iii) with small lumps, though not always due to tuberculosis 有结节的

◇ **tuberculid(e)** *noun* skin wound caused by tuberculosis 结核疹

◇ **tuberculin** *noun* substance which is derived from the culture of the tuberculosis bacillus and is used to test patients for the presence of tuberculosis 结核菌素,结核菌培养基中的衍生物,用于检测病人是否患有结核;**tuberculin test** *or* **Mantoux test** = test to see if someone has tuberculosis, where the patient is given an intracutaneous injection of tuberculin and the reaction of the skin is noted 结核菌素试验,皮内注射结核菌素,注意皮肤反应,以此判断是否有结核病 *see also* 参见 PATCH TEST

◇ **tuberculosis (TB)** *noun* infectious disease caused by the tuberculosis bacillus, where infected lumps form in the tissue 结核病,结核菌引起的感染性疾病,在组织中形成感染灶;**miliary tuberculosis** = form of tuberculosis which occurs as little nodes in many parts of the body, including the meninges of the brain and spinal cord 粟粒性结核,结核病的一种形式,身体许多部分有小结节,可以侵及脑膜和脊髓;**post-primary tuberculosis** = reappearance of tuberculosis in a patient who has been infected before 再发性结核;**primary tuberculosis** = infection with tuberculosis for the first time 原发性结核;**pulmonary tuberculosis** = tuberculosis in the lungs, which makes the patient lose weight, cough blood and have a fever 肺结核,病人体重下降、咯血并发热

◇ **tuberculous** *adjective* referring to tuberculosis 结核病的

> COMMENT: Tuberculosis can take many forms: the commonest form is infection of the lungs (pulmonary tuberculosis), but it can also attack the

bones (Pott's disease), the skin (lupus), or the lymph nodes (scrofula). Tuberculosis is caught by breathing in germs or by eating contaminated food, especially unpasteurized milk; it can be passed from one person to another, and the carrier sometimes shows no signs of the disease. Tuberculosis can be cured by treatment with antibiotics, and can be prevented by inoculation with BCG vaccine. The tests for the presence of TB are the Mantoux test and patch test; it can also be detected by X-ray screening.
注释:结核有多种形式:最常见的形式是肺部感染(肺结核),但也可以侵及骨骼(波特病),皮肤(狼疮),或淋巴结(瘰疬)。结核是由吸入病菌或进食被污染的食物,特别是未经巴斯德法灭菌的牛奶引起的;可由一个人传给另一个人,而携带者有时没有病征。结核病可以用抗生素治疗,可以通过接种卡介苗来预防。检测是否有结核病的试验有结核菌素试验和斑贴试验;还可以经 X 线扫描发现结核。

tuberose *adjective* with lumps *or* nodules 有结节的,结节状的;**tuberose sclerosis** *or* **epiloia** = hereditary disease of the brain, where a child is mentally retarded, suffers from epilepsy and many little tumours appear on the skin and on the brain 结节硬化,遗传性脑病,患儿精神发育迟滞,患有癫痫,皮肤和脑内有许多小肿瘤

◇ **tuberosity** *noun* large lump on a bone 粗隆;**deltoid tuberosity** = raised part of the humerus to which the deltoid muscle is attached 三角肌粗隆,肱骨上隆起的部分,三角肌附着的地方

◇ **tuberous** *adjective* with lumps *or* nodules 有结节的,结节状的

tubo- *prefix* referring to a Fallopian tube *or* the auditory meatus 输卵管或听小管

◇ **tuboabdominal** *adjective* referring to a Fallopian tube and the abdomen 输卵管腹腔的

◇ **tubo-ovarian** *adjective* referring to a Fallopian tube and an ovary 输卵管卵巢的

◇ **tubotympanal** *adjective* referring to the Eustachian tube and the tympanum 咽鼓管鼓室的

◇ **tubular** *adjective* (i) shaped like a tube 管状的 (ii) referring to a tubule 小管的;**tubular bandage** = bandage made of a tube of elastic cloth 管状绷带;**tubular reabsorption** = process where some substances filtered into the kidney are reabsorbed into the bloodstream 肾小管重吸收,肾小球滤过的物质经肾小管重吸收入血的过程;**tubular secretion** = secretion of substances by the tubules of a kidney into the urine 肾小管分泌

◇ **tubule** *noun* small tube in the body 小管;**renal tubule** = small tube in the kidney, part of the nephron 肾小管

tuft *noun* small group of hairs *or* of blood vessels 丛,如血管丛、神经丛;**glomerular tuft** = group of blood vessels in the kidney which filters the blood 肾小球血管丛

tugging 牵引感 *see* 见 TRACHEAL

tularaemia *or* **rabbit fever** *noun* disease of rabbits, caused by the bacterium *Pasteurella or* Brucella tularensis, which can be passed to humans 土拉菌病,兔热病,兔子的疾病,由细菌引起,可以传染给人

COMMENT: In humans, the symptoms are headaches, fever and swollen lymph nodes.
注释:人患病的症状有头疼、发热和淋巴结肿大。

tulle gras *noun* dressing made of open gauze covered with soft paraffin wax which prevents sticking 润肤细布,敷伤巾

tumefaction *noun* oedema, swelling of tissue caused by liquid which accumulates underneath 水肿

◇ **tumescence** *noun* oedema, swollen tissue where liquid has accumulated underneath 水肿

◇ **tumid** *adjective* swollen 水肿的

tumoral *or* **tumorous** *adjective* referring to a tumour 肿瘤的

◇ **tumour** *US* 肿瘤

◇ **tumor** *noun* abnormal swelling *or* growth of new cells 肿瘤: ***The X-ray showed a tumour in the breast.*** X线发现乳腺肿瘤。***She died of a brain tumour.*** 她死于脑肿瘤。***The doctors diagnosed a tumour in the liver.*** 医生诊断肝脏有肿瘤。**benign tumour** = tumour which is not cancerous, and which will not grow again *or* spread to other parts of the body if is is removed surgically 良性肿瘤,如果手术切除不会再长,也不会播散到身体其他部位。**malignant tumour** = tumour which is cancerous and can grow again *or* spread into other parts of the body, even if removed surgically 恶性肿瘤,即便手术切除后仍会再长,播散到身体其他部分(NOTE: for other terms referring to tumours, see words beginning with **onco-**)

tummy *noun* (*informal* 非正式) child's word for stomach *or* abdomen 肚,儿童对胃和腹部的称呼; **tummy ache** = child's expression for stomach pain 肚疼,儿童对腹痛的表达 *see also* 参见 GIPPY

tunica *noun* layer of tissue which covers an organ 被膜; **tunica albuginea** = white fibrous membrane covering the testes and the ovaries 白膜,被覆睾丸和卵巢的纤维白色膜; **tunica vaginalis** = membrane covering the testes and epididymis 鞘膜

> COMMENT: The wall of a blood vessel is made up of several layers: the outer layer (tunica adventitia); the inner layer (tunica intima), and in between the central layer (tunica media).
> 注释:血管壁由几层组成:外层(外膜),内层(内膜)和中间层(中膜)。

tuning fork *noun* special metal fork which, if hit, gives out a perfect note, used in hearing tests, such as Rinne's test 音叉,能发出特定音阶声音的金属叉,用于听力检测

tunnel vision *noun* field of vision which is restricted to the area directly in front of the eye 管状视野,视野局限于眼前的区域

TUR = TRANSURETHRAL RESECTION 经尿道切除术

turbinal bones *or* **turbinate bones** *or* **nasal conchae** *plural noun* three little bones which form the sides of the nasal cavity 鼻甲骨,形成鼻腔的三块小骨头

◇ **turbinectomy** *noun* surgical operation to remove a turbinate bone 鼻甲切除术

turbulent flow *noun* rushing *or* uneven flow of blood in a vessel, usually caused by a partial obstruction 湍流,血管内血流不平稳,通常由血管部分阻塞引起

turcica 蝶 *see* 见 SELLA

turgescence *noun* swelling of tissue, when fluid accumulates underneath 肿胀

◇ **turgid** *adjective* swollen with blood 胀满的,充血的

◇ **turgor** *noun* being swollen 充盈,充满,胀满

turn 1 *noun* (*informal* 非正式) slight illness *or* attack of dizziness 小病,头晕发作: ***She had one of her turns on the bus.*** 她在公共汽车上晕了一阵。***He had a bad turn at the office and had to be taken to hospital.*** 他在办公室好难受了一阵,不得不被人送到医院。**2** *verb* (**a**) to move the head *or* body to face in another direction 转: ***He turned to look at the camera.*** 他转头看着相机。***She has difficulty in turning her head.*** 她转头有困难。(**b**) to change into something different 转变: ***The solution is turned blue by the reagent.*** 放入试剂后溶液变蓝。***His hair has turned grey.*** 他的头发花白了。

◇ **turn away** *verb* to send people away 送走: ***The casualty ward is closed, so we have had to turn the accident victims away.*** 事故病房关闭了,所以我们不得不将事故受害者转走。

Turner's syndrome *noun* congenital condition of females, where sexual development is retarded and no ovaries develop 特纳综合征,女性的先天疾病,性发育迟滞,卵巢不发育

COMMENT: The condition is caused by the absence of one of the pair of X chromosomes.
注释:这种病是由于少了一个 X 染色体。

turricephaly = OXYCEPHALY 尖头畸形

tussis *noun* coughing 咳嗽

tutor *noun* teacher *or* person who teaches small groups of students 导师; **nurse tutor** = experienced nurse who teaches student nurses 护理导师

tweezers *noun* instrument shaped like small scissors, with ends which pinch, and do not cut, used to pull out or pick up small objects 镊子: ***She pulled out the splinter with her tweezers.*** 她用镊子拉出括约肌。***He removed the swab with a pair of tweezers.*** 他用镊子夹出棉签。

twenty-twenty vision *noun* perfect normal vision 视力极佳(眼科写作视力20/20)

twilight *noun* time of day when the light is changing from daylight to night 黄昏; **twilight myopia** = condition of the eyes, where the patient has difficulty in seeing in dim light 黄昏近视; **twilight state** = condition (of epileptics and alcoholics) where the patient can do certain automatic actions, but is not conscious of what he is doing 意识朦胧状态,病人可以做某些自主动作,但不能意识到他在做什么,如癫痫和酒中毒状态时; **twilight sleep** = type of anaesthetic sleep, where the patient is semi-conscious but cannot feel any pain 朦胧睡眠,麻醉性睡眠的一种形式,病人意识半清醒,但不会感到疼痛

COMMENT: Twilight state is induced at childbirth, by introducing anaesthetics into the rectum.
注释:分娩时通过直肠给麻醉药诱导出意识朦胧状态。

twin *noun* one of two babies born to a mother at the same time 双胞胎之一; **fraternal** *or* **dizygotic twins** = twins who are not identical because they come from two different ova fertilized at the same time 异卵双胞胎,两个卵子同时受孕发育成的双胞胎; **identical** *or* **monozygotic twins** = twins who are exactly the same in appearance because they developed from the same ovum 同卵双胞胎,由同一个受精卵发育来的双胞胎 *see also* 参见 QUADRUPLET, QUINTUPLET, SEXTUPLET, SIAMESE, TRIPLET

COMMENT: Twins are relatively frequent (about one birth in eighty) and are often found in the same family, where the tendency to have twins is passed through females.
注释:双胞胎是相对常见的(1/80),而且经常见于同一个家族,怀双胞胎的倾向是通过母系遗传的。

twinge *noun* sudden feeling of sharp pain 刺痛: ***He sometimes has a twinge in his right shoulder.*** 他的右肩有时刺痛。***She complained of having twinges in the knee.*** 她说她膝盖刺痛。

twist *verb* to turn *or* bend a joint in a wrong way 扭转: ***He twisted his ankle.*** = He hurt it by bending it in an odd direction. 他扭伤了踝部。

twitch *verb* to make small movements of the muscles 抽搐: ***The side of his face was twitching.*** 他一侧面部在抽搐。

◇ **twitching** *noun* small movements of the muscles in the face *or* hands 抽搐,面部,手的肌肉颤动

tylosis *noun* development of a callus 胼胝形成

tympan(o)- *prefix* referring to the eardrum 鼓膜

◇ **tympanic** *adjective* referring to the eardrum 鼓膜的,鼓室的; **tympanic cavity** *or* **middle ear** = section of the ear between the eardrum and the inner ear, containing the three ossicles 鼓室,中耳,鼓膜和内耳之间的部分,有三块听小骨; **tympanic membrane** *or* **tympanum** *or* **eardrum** = membrane at the inner end of the external auditory meatus which vibrates with sound and passes the vibrations on to the ossicles in the middle ear 鼓膜,外耳道深处尽头的膜,随声音震动并将震动传到中耳的听小骨

◇ **tympanites** *or* **meteorism** *noun* expansion of the stomach with gas 胃胀

气

◇ **tympanitis** *or* **otitis** *noun* middle ear infection 鼓室炎,中耳炎

◇ **tympanoplasty** *or* **myringoplasty** *noun* surgical operation to correct a defect in the eardrum 鼓室成形术

◇ **tympanotomy** *or* **myringotomy** *noun* surgical operation to make an opening in the eardrum to allow fluid to escape 鼓膜切开术,为引流中耳积液

◇ **tympanum** *noun* (**a**) eardrum, the membrane at the inner end of the external auditory meatus leading from the outer ear, which vibrates with sound and passes the vibrations on to the ossicles in the middle ear 鼓膜,外耳道深处尽头的膜,随声音震动并将震动传到中耳的听小骨 ◇ 见图 EAR (**b**) the tympanic cavity, the section of the ear between the eardrum and the inner ear, containing the three ossicles 鼓室,鼓膜和内耳之间的部分,有三块听小骨

typhlitis *noun* inflammation of the caecum (large intestine) 盲肠炎

typhoid fever *noun* infection of the intestine caused by *Salmonella typhi* in food and water 伤寒,伤寒沙门菌感染

> COMMENT: Typhoid fever gives a fever, diarrhoea and the patient may pass blood in the faeces. It can be fatal if not treated; patients who have had the disease may become carriers, and the Widal test is used to detect the presence of typhoid fever in the blood.
> 注释:伤寒表现发烧、腹泻,而且病人还可能有血便,如果不治疗是可以致命的。得过此病的人可以成为携带者,用肥达反应来检测是否患有伤寒。

typhus *noun* one of several fevers caused by the Rickettsia bacterium, transmitted by fleas and lice 斑疹伤寒,立克次体感染所致发热性疾病之一,由跳蚤和虱子传播; **endemic typhus** = fever transmitted by fleas from rats 地方性斑疹伤寒,由跳蚤从老鼠传给人的发热性疾病; **epidemic typhus** = fever with headaches, mental disturbance and a rash, caused by lice which come from other humans 流行性斑疹伤寒,发热、头痛,精神紊乱,出皮疹,经虱子从别的人那儿传染而来 *see also* 参见 SCRUB TYPHUS

> COMMENT: Typhus victims have a fever, feel extremely weak and develop a dark rash on the skin. The test for typhus is Weil-Felix reaction.
> 注释:斑疹伤寒患者出现发热,感到极端虚弱,皮肤出现暗色皮疹。检测斑疹伤寒的试验是外-斐氏反应。

typical *adjective* showing the usual symptoms of a condition 典型的: ***His gait was typical of a patient suffering from Parkinson's disease.*** 他的步态是典型帕金森病患者的步态。

◇ **typically** *adverb* in a typical way 典型地: ***The anorexia patient is typically an adolescent or young woman, who is suffering from stress.*** 典型情况下,厌食症患者是处于压力下的青少年或年轻女性。

tyramine *noun* enzyme found in cheese, beans, tinned fish, red wine and yeast extract, which can cause high blood pressure if found in excessive quantities in the brain 酪胺,存在于乳酪、豆类、罐装鱼、红葡萄酒和酵母提取物中的酶,如果脑内含量过高可以引起高血压 *see also* 参见 MONOAMINE OXIDASE

tyrosine *noun* amino acid in protein which is a component of thyroxine 酪氨酸,一种氨基酸,是形成甲状腺素的原料物质

◇ **tyrosinosis** *noun* condition caused by abnormal metabolism of tyrosine 酪氨酸代谢病

Uu

UKCC = UNITED KINGDOM CENTRAL COUNCIL 联合王国中央委员会

ulcer *noun* open sore in the skin *or* in mucous membrane, which is inflamed and difficult to heal 溃疡,皮肤或粘膜上开放发炎并难以愈合的创面: ***He is on a special diet because of his stomach ulcers.*** 由于胃溃疡他正司特殊饮食。**aphthous ulcer** = little ulcer in the mouth 口疮性溃疡; **decubitus ulcer** *or* **bedsore** = inflamed patch of skin on a bony part of the body (usually found on the shoulder blades, buttocks, base of the back or heels), which develops into an ulcer, caused by pressure of the part of the body against the mattress 褥疮,身体压在床垫上的部位(如肩,臀,后背及脚跟)由于压迫造成的溃疡; **dendritic ulcer** = branching ulcer on the cornea, caused by herpesvirus 树状(角膜)溃疡,由疱疹病毒引起; **duodenal ulcer** = ulcer in the duodenum 十二指肠溃疡; **gastric ulcer** = ulcer in the stomach 胃溃疡; **peptic ulcer** = benign ulcer in the stomach or duodenum 消化性溃疡; **trophic ulcer** = ulcer caused by lack of blood (such as a bedsore) 缺血性溃疡; **varicose ulcer** = ulcer in the leg as a result of bad circulation and varicose veins 静脉曲张性溃疡 *see also* 参见 RODENT

◇ **ulcerated** *adjective* covered with ulcers 有溃疡的

◇ **ulcerating** *adjective* which is developing into an ulcer 形成溃疡的

◇ **ulceration** *noun* (i) condition where ulcers develop 溃疡 (ii) the development of an ulcer 溃疡形成

◇ **ulcerative** *adjective* referring to ulcers *or* characterized by ulcers 溃疡的; **ulcerative colitis** = severe pain in the colon, with diarrhoea and ulcers in the rectum, possibly with a psychosomatic cause 溃疡性结肠炎,严重的结肠疼痛,伴有腹泻和直肠溃疡,可能由心身原因引起

◇ **ulceromembranous gingivitis** *noun* inflammation of the gums, which can also affect the mucous membrane in the mouth 膜溃疡性龈炎

◇ **ulcerous** *adjective* (i) referring to an ulcer 溃疡的 (ii) like an ulcer 溃疡性的

ulitis *noun* inflammation of the gums 牙龈炎

ulna *noun* the longer and inner of the two bones in the forearm between the elbow and the wrist (the other, outer bone, is the radius) 尺骨,前臂两根长骨中较长的靠内侧的一根 ◇ 见图 HAND

◇ **ulnar** *adjective* referring to the ulna 尺骨的; **ulnar artery** = artery which branches from the brachial artery at the elbow and runs down the inside of the forearm to join the radial artery in the palm of the hand 尺动脉,肱动脉在肘部的分支,沿尺骨下行,在手掌与桡动脉汇合; **ulnar nerve** = nerve which runs from the neck to the elbow and controls the muscles in the forearm and some of the fingers (and passes near the surface of the skin at the elbow, where it can easily be hit, giving the effect of the 'funny bone') 尺神经,从颈部下行至肘的神经,控制前臂和部分手指(肘部近于皮下,容易被撞击,造成"麻筋"现象); **ulnar pulse** = secondary pulse in the wrist, taken near the inner edge of the forearm 尺侧脉搏

> QUOTE: The whole joint becomes disorganised, causing ulnar deviation of the fingers resulting in the typical deformity of the rheumatoid arthritic hand.
> 引文:整个关节变形,引起手指向尺侧偏移,导致典型的类风湿关节炎手畸形。
> **Nursing Times** 护理时代

ultra- *prefix* meaning (i) further than 超 (ii) extremely 极端地

◇ **ultrafiltration** *noun* filtering of the blood where tiny particles are removed, as when the blood is filtered by the kidney 超滤作用,过滤血液,去掉小颗粒,如肾脏对血液的滤过

◇ **ultramicroscopic** *adjective* so small that it cannot be seen using a normal microscope 超微的,一般显微镜看不到的

◇ **ultrasonic** *adjective* referring to ultrasound 超声的

◇ **ultrasonics** *noun* study of ultrasound and its use in medical treatments 超声学

◇ **ultrasonograph** *noun* machine which takes pictures of internal organs, using ultrasound 超声仪

◇ **ultrasonography** *noun* passing ultrasound waves through the body and recording echoes which show details of internal organs 超声检查

◇ **ultrasonotomography** *noun* making pictures of organs which are placed at different depths inside the body, using ultrasound 超声图像

◇ **ultrasound** *or* **ultrasonic waves** *noun* 超声,超声波;very high frequency sound wave 很高频率的声波: ***The nature of the tissue may be made clear on ultrasound examination.*** 组织的性质可以在超声检查中清晰地显示。***Ultrasound scanning provides a picture of the ovary and the eggs inside it.*** 超声扫描提供了卵巢和卵子的图像。**Ultrasound treatment.** = treatment of soft tissue inflammation using ultrasound waves 超声治疗,用超声波治疗软组织炎症 (NOTE: no plural for **ultrasound**)

COMMENT: The very high frequency waves of ultrasound can be used to detect and record organs or growths inside the body (in a similar way to the use of X-rays), by recording the differences in echoes sent back from different tissues. Ultrasound is used to treat some conditions such as internal bruising and can also destroy bacteria and calculi.
注释:因不同组织回声不同,超声的高频波可用来探测和记录体内的器官或新生物(与利用 X 线的方式相似)。超声还可用来治疗某些疾病,如内部的淤血,也可以用来破坏细菌和结石。

◇ **ultraviolet rays** (**UV rays**) *noun* invisible rays of light, which have very short wavelengths and are beyond the violet end of the spectrum, and form the tanning and burning element in sunlight 紫外线,不可见光,波长很短,在光谱紫色一端之外,是阳光中使人晒黑和灼伤的因素;**ultraviolet lamp** = lamp which gives off ultraviolet rays which tan the skin, help the skin produce Vitamin D, and kill bacteria 紫外灯,发射紫外线的灯,可以用来照射皮肤,增加皮肤合成维生素 D,还可以用来杀菌

umbilical *adjective* referring to the navel 脐带的; **umbilical circulation** = circulation of blood from the mother's bloodstream through the umbilical cord into the fetus 脐循环,母亲血流经脐带进入胎儿的循环; **umbilical hernia** *or* **exomphalos** = hernia which bulges at the navel, mainly in young children 脐疝,主要见于儿童; **umbilical region** = central part of the abdomen, lower than the epigastrium 脐部

◇ **umbilical cord** *noun* cord containing two arteries and one vein which links the fetus inside the womb to the placenta 脐带,内有两根动脉和一根静脉,将子宫内胎儿与胎盘相连

COMMENT: The arteries carry the blood and nutrients from the placenta to the fetus and the vein carries the waste from the fetus back to the placenta. When the baby is born, the umbilical cord is cut and the end tied in a knot. After a few days, this drops off, leaving the navel marking the place where the cord was originally attached.
注释:动脉将血液和营养从胎盘带给胎儿,而静脉把胎儿的废物带回胎盘。当婴儿出生后,脐带被剪断并将末端打个结。几天后,这个结脱落,只留下肚脐标志着脐带原来附着的部位。

◇ **umbilicated** *adjective* with a small depression, like a navel, in the centre 脐形的,凹陷的

◇ **umbilicus** *or* **navel** *or* **omphalus**

noun scar with a depression in the middle of the abdomen where the umbilical cord was attached to the fetus 脐

umbo *noun* projecting part in the middle of the outer side of the eardrum(鼓膜)凸,鼓膜外侧中间突起的部分

un- *prefix* meaning not 不,非

◇ **unaided** *adjective* without any help 不需帮助的: ***Two days after the operation, he was able to walk un aided across the ward.*** 手术两天后,他不需要扶助就能在病房里走动了。

◇ **unblock** *verb* to remove something which is blocking 去掉阻塞,疏通: ***This operation is to unblock an artery.*** 这是个疏通动脉的手术。***If you swallow it will unblock your ears.*** 吞咽可使咽鼓管疏通。

◇ **unboiled** *adjective* which has not been boiled 未沸腾的: ***In some areas, it is dangerous to drink unboiled water.*** 在某些地区,喝没烧开的水是危险的。

◇ **unborn** *adjective* not yet born 未出生的: ***a pregnant woman and her unborn child*** 孕妇和她未出生的孩子

unciform bone *noun* hamate bone, one of the eight small carpal bones in the wrist, shaped like a hook 钩骨,形状像钩子,是 8 块腕骨之一 ◊ 见图 HAND

uncinate *adjective* shaped like a hook 钩状的; **uncinate epilepsy** = type of temporal lobe epilepsy, where the patient has hallucinations of smell and taste 钩回性癫痫,颞叶癫痫的一种,病人有幻嗅和幻味

unconscious 1 *adjective* not conscious *or* not aware of what is happening 无意识的: ***He was found unconscious in the street.*** 人们发现他丧失了意识,躺在街上。***The nurses tried to revive the unconscious accident victims.*** 护士们试图救活丧失意识的事故受害者。***She was unconscious for two days after the accident.*** 事故之后,她有两天都处在无意识状态。***She became unconscious and did not revive.*** 她意识丧失,而且再没恢复过来。**2** *noun* (*in psychology*) **the unconscious** = the part of the mind which stores feelings *or* memories *or* desires, which the patient cannot consciously call up, but which influence his actions 潜意识,心灵中贮存感受、记忆、期望的所在,而病人本人并不能有意识地唤起它们,但它们却影响着他的行动 *see also* 参见 SEMI-CONSCIOUS, SUBCONSCIOUS

◇ **unconsciousness** *noun* being unconscious (it may be the result of lack of oxygen or some other external cause such as a blow on the head) 意识丧失: ***He relapsed into unconsciousness, and never became conscious again.*** 他又进入意识丧失状态,并且再也没有恢复意识。

uncontrollable *adjective* which cannot be controlled 不能控制的: ***She has an uncontrollable desire to drink alcohol.*** 她有一种不能控制的饮酒欲望。***There is an uncontrollable spread of the disease through the population.*** 无法控制疾病在人群中流行。

◇ **uncoordinated** *adjective* not joined together *or* not working together 不协调: ***His finger movements are completely uncoordinated.*** 他的手指运动完全不协调。***The symptoms are uncoordinated movements of the arms and legs.*** 症状是胳臂和腿的运动不协调。

uncus *noun* projecting part of the cerebral hemisphere, shaped like a hook 钩回

under- *prefix* meaning less than *or* not as strong as 下,次; **underactivity** = less activity than usual 活动过少; **underhydration** = having too little water in the body 脱水; **undernourished** = having too little food 营养不良; **underproduction** = producing less than normal 产出不足,减产

◇ **undergo(surgery)** *verb* to have (an operation) 做(手术): ***He underwent an appendicectomy.*** 他做了阑尾切除术。***She will probably have to undergo another operation.*** 她将不得不再做另一个手术。***There are six patients undergoing physiotherapy.*** 有 6 个病人在做理疗。

◇ **undertake** *verb* to carry out (a surgical operation) 进行(手术): ***Replacement***

***of the joint is mainly undertaken to relieve pain*.** 进行关节置换术是为了缓解疼痛。

◇ **underweight** *adjective* too thin *or* not heavy enough 体重过低: ***He is several pounds underweight for his age*.** 按他的年龄,他体重轻了几磅。

undescended testis *noun* condition where a testis has not descended into the scrotum 睾丸未降

undigested *adjective* (food) which is not digested in the body 未消化的

undine *noun* glass container for a solution to bathe the eyes 洗眼壶

undress *verb* to take off all *or* most of your clothes 脱(衣): ***The doctor asked the patient to undress or to get undressed*.** 医生让病人脱去衣服。

undulant fever = BRUCELLOSIS 波浪热,布氏杆菌病

unfertilized *adjective* which has not been fertilized 未受精的: ***Unfertilized ova are produced in the ovaries and can be fertilized by spermatozoa*.** 卵巢产生未受精的卵子,能和精子发生受精。

◇ **unfit** *adjective* not fit *or* not healthy 不舒服,不健康: ***She used to play a lot of tennis, but she became unfit during the winter*.** 她过去常打网球,但今冬她不太舒服。

ungual *adjective* referring to the fingernails *or* toenails 指(趾)甲的

unguent *noun* ointment *or* smooth oily medicinal substance which can be spread on the skin to soothe irritations 软膏

◇ **unguentum** *noun* (*in pharmacy*) ointment 软膏

unguis = NAIL 指(趾)甲

unhealthy *adjective* not healthy *or* which does not make someone healthy 不健康的,使不健康的: ***The children have a very unhealthy diet*.** 这些孩子的饮食很不健康。 ***Not taking any exercise is an unhealthy way of living*.** 不做任何锻炼是一种不健康的生活方式。 ***The office is an unhealthy place, and everyone always feels ill there*.** 办公室是一个不健康的地方,每个人在那都感到不舒服。

◇ **unhygienic** *adjective* which is not hygienic 不卫生的: ***The conditions in the hospital laundry have been criticized as unhygienic*.** 医院洗衣房因卫生状况不好而受到批评。

uni- *prefix* meaning one 一

◇ **unicellular** *adjective* (organism) formed of one cell 单细胞生物的

◇ **uniform 1** *noun* special clothes worn by a group of people, such as the nurses in a hospital 制服: ***The nurses' uniform does not include a cap*.** 护士的工作服不包括帽子。 ***He was wearing the uniform of the St John Ambulance Brigade*.** 他穿着圣约翰救护队的制服。 **2** *adjective* the same *or* similar 一样的,相似的: ***Healthy red blood cells are of a uniform shape and size*.** 健康的红细胞有一样的形状和大小。

◇ **unigravida** = PRIMIGRAVIDA 初孕妇

◇ **unilateral** *adjective* affecting one side of the body only 单侧的; **unilateral oophorectomy** = surgical removal of one ovary 单侧卵巢切除术

union *noun* joining together of two parts of a fractured bone 联合 *see also* 参见 MALUNION (NOTE: opposite is **non-union**)

uniovular twins *noun* monozygotic twins, twins who are identical in appearance because they developed from a single ovum 单卵双胞胎

◇ **unipara** = PRIMIPARA 初产妇

◇ **unipolar** *adjective* (neurone) with a single process 单极的,(神经元)只有一个树突的 *compare* 比较 BIPOLAR, MULTIPOLAR; **unipolar lead** = electric lead to a single electrode 单极导线

unit *noun* (**a**) single part (as of a series of numbers) 单位; **SI units** = international system of measurement for physical properties 国际单位: ***Lumen is the SI unit of illumination*.** 流明是光度的国际单位。(**b**) specialized section of a hospital 部门,病房: ***She is in the mater-***

nity unit*.**她住产科病房。He was rushed to the intensive care unit*.**他被急送进监护病房。***The burns unit was full after the plane accident*.**飞机失事后烧伤病房满了。

> QUOTE: The blood loss caused his haemoglobin to drop dangerously low, necessitating two units of RBCs and one unit of fresh frozen plasma.
> 引文:失血使他的血红蛋白下降到危险的程度,需要两个单位的红细胞和一个单位的新鲜冷冻血浆。
> **RN Magazine** 注册护士杂志

United Kingdom Central Council (for Nursing, Midwifery and Health Visiting) (UKCC) *noun* official body which regulates and registers nurses, midwives and health visitors 联合王国(护理、助产和保健访视)中央委员会

univalent *adjective* = MONOVALENT 单价的

unmedicated dressing *noun* sterile dressing with no antiseptic or other medication on it 未用药物处理的敷料

◇ **unpasteurized** *adjective* which has not been pasteurized 未经灭菌的: ***Unpasteurized milk can carry bacilli*.**未经灭菌的牛奶可能含有杆菌。

◇ **unprofessional conduct** *noun* action by a professional person (a doctor *or* nurse, etc.) which is considered wrong by the body which regulates the profession 违反职业道德的行为,专业人员(医生,护士)行为中被专业管理机构认定为错误的

> QUOTE: Refusing to care for someone with HIV-related disease may well result in disciplinary procedure for unprofessional conduct.
> 引文:拒绝照顾患人类免疫缺陷病毒相关疾病患者可能会以违反职业道德而受到纪律处罚。
> **Nursing Times** 护理时代

unqualified *adjective* (person) who has no qualifications *or* who has no licence to practise 不合格的,未经认证的: ***The hospital is employing unqualified nursing staff*.**这家医院雇佣不合格的护理人员。

◇ **unsaturated fat** *noun* fat which does not have a large amount of hydrogen, and so can be broken down more easily 不饱和脂肪,含氢不多的脂肪,易于降解 *see also* 参见 FAT, SATURATED

◇ **unstable** *adjective* not stable *or* which may change easily 不稳定的: ***The patient was showing signs of an unstable mental condition*.**病人表现出精神状态不稳定的征象。**unstable angina** = angina which has suddenly become worse 不稳定心绞痛,突然加重的心绞痛

◇ **unsteady** *adjective* likely to fall down when walking 行走不稳的: ***He is still very unsteady on his legs*.**他双腿还非常不稳。

◇ **unsterilized** *adjective* which has not been sterilized 未经消毒的: ***He had to carry out the operation using unsterilized equipment*.**他不得不用未经消毒的器械进行手术。

◇ **unsuitable** *adjective* not suitable 不合适的: ***Radiotherapy is unsuitable in this case*.**这个病人不适合放疗。

◇ **untreated** *adjective* which has not been treated 未经治疗的: ***The disease is fatal if left untreated*.**如果不治疗,这种疾病是致命的。

◇ **unwanted** *adjective* which is not wanted 多余的,讨厌的: ***a cream to remove unwanted facial hair*** 一种去掉讨厌的面部软毛的霜剂

◇ **unwashed** *adjective* which has not been washed 没洗过的: ***Dysentery can be caused by eating unwashed fruit*.**吃没洗过的水果可以引起痢疾。

unwell *adjective* sick *or* not well 不适的,病的: ***She felt unwell and had to go home*.**她感觉不适,不得不回家了。(NOTE: not used before a noun: **a sick woman but the woman was unwell**)

upper *adjective* at the top *or* higher 上面的;**the upper limbs** = the arms 上肢;**upper arm** = part of the arm from the shoulder to the elbow 上臂,从肩到肘: ***He had a rash on his right upper arm*.**

他右上臂出了一个皮疹。**upper respiratory infection** = infection of the upper part of the respiratory system 上呼吸道感染 *see also* 参见 NEURONE (NOTE: opposite is **lower**)

upright *adjective & adverb* in a vertical position *or* standing 直立的,挺直的: ***He became dizzy as soon as he stood upright.*** 他刚一站直就感到头晕目眩。

upset 1 *noun* slight illness 不舒服,小病;**stomach upset** = slight infection of the stomach 轻度胃炎: ***She is in bed with a stomach upset.*** 她的胃有点儿小病,躺在床上歇着。2 *adjective* slightly ill 不舒服的,闹小病的: ***She is in bed with an upset stomach.*** 她的胃有点儿小病,躺在床上歇着。

upside down *adverb* with the top turned to the bottom 颠倒地; *US* **upside-down stomach** = DIAPHRAGMATIC HERNIA 膈疝

uraemia *noun* disorder caused by kidney failure, where urea is retained in the blood, and the patient develops nausea, convulsions and in severe cases goes into a coma 尿毒症,肾衰竭造成的障碍,尿素滞留在血液中,病人恶心、痉挛,严重时可以昏迷

◇ **uraemic** *adjective* referring to and suffering from uraemia 尿毒症的

uran- *prefix* referring to the palate 腭

◇ **uraniscorrhaphy** = PALATORRHAPHY 腭修补术

urataemia *noun* condition where urates are present in the blood, as in gout 尿酸盐血症,发生在痛风时

◇ **urate** *noun* salt of uric acid found in urine 尿酸盐

◇ **uraturia** *noun* presence of excessive amounts of urates in the urine, as in gout 尿酸盐尿,尿中尿酸含量过高,发生在痛风时

urea *noun* substance produced in the liver from excess amino acids, and excreted by the kidneys into the urine 尿素,氨基酸在肝代谢的产物,经肾分泌入尿液

◇ **urease** *noun* enzyme which converts urea into ammonia and carbon dioxide 尿素酶,将尿素转化成氨和二氧化碳的酶

◇ **urecchysis** *noun* condition where uric acid leaves the blood and enters connective tissue 尿酸浸润,尿酸离开血液进入结缔组织

◇ **uresis** *noun* passing urine 排尿

ureter *noun* one of two tubes which take urine from the kidneys to the urinary bladder 输尿管,由肾到膀胱的两根输送尿液的管道 ◇ 见图 KIDNEY

◇ **ureter-** *or* **uretero-** *prefix* referring to the ureters 输尿管

◇ **ureteral** *or* **ureteric** *adjective* referring to the ureters 输尿管的;**ureteric calculus** = kidney stone in the ureter 输尿管结石;**ureteric catheter** = catheter passed through the ureter to the kidney, to inject an opaque solution into the kidney before taking an X-ray 输尿管导管,经输尿管插到肾脏的导管,在X线肾造影前用此法注射不透射线的溶液到肾脏 *see also* 参见 IMPACTED

◇ **ureterectomy** *noun* surgical removal of a ureter 输尿管切除术

◇ **ureteritis** *noun* inflammation of a ureter 输尿管炎

◇ **ureterocele** *noun* swelling in a ureter caused by narrowing of the opening where the ureter enters the bladder 输尿管疝,输尿管进入膀胱处的开口狭窄造成输尿管肿胀

◇ **ureterocolostomy** *noun* surgical operation to implant the ureter into the sigmoid colon, so as to bypass the bladder 结肠代膀胱术,输尿管结肠吻合术

◇ **ureteroenterostomy** *noun* artificially formed passage between the ureter and the intestine 输尿管肠吻合术

◇ **ureterolith** *noun* calculus *or* stone in a ureter 输尿管结石

◇ **ureterolithotomy** *noun* surgical removal of a stone from the ureter 输尿管结石切除术

◇ **ureteronephrectomy** *or* **nephroureterectomy** *noun* surgical removal of a kidney and the ureter attached to it 肾输尿管切除术

◇ **ureteroplasty** *noun* surgical operation to repair a ureter 输尿管成形术

◇ **ureteropyelonephritis** *noun* inflammation of the ureter and the pelvis of the kidney to which it is attached 输尿管肾盂肾炎

◇ **ureterosigmoidostomy** = URETEROCOLOSTOMY 输尿管乙状结肠吻合术

◇ **ureterostomy** *noun* surgical operation to make an artificial opening for the ureter into the abdominal wall, so that urine can be passed directly out of the body 输尿管造口术

◇ **ureterotomy** *noun* surgical operation to make an incision into the ureter mainly to remove a stone 输尿管切开术

◇ **ureterovaginal** *adjective* referring to the ureter and the vagina 输尿管阴道的

urethr- *or* **urethro-** *prefix* referring to the urethra 尿道

◇ **urethra** *noun* tube which takes urine from the bladder to be passed out of the body 尿道,将尿液从膀胱排出体外的管道 ◇ 见图 UROGENITAL SYSTEM; **penile urethra** = channel in the penis through which both urine and semen pass 尿道阴茎部; **prostatic urethra** = section of the urethra which passes through the prostate 尿道前列腺部

> COMMENT: In males, the urethra serves two purposes: the discharge of both urine and semen. The male urethra is about 20cm long; in women it is shorter, about 3cm and this relative shortness is one of the reasons for the predominance of bladder infection and inflammation (cystitis) in women. The urethra has sphincter muscles at either end which help control the flow of urine.
>
> 注释:男性尿道有两个作用:排除尿液和排出精液。男性尿道有 20 厘米长,女性的要短些,约 3 厘米长;女性尿道短是膀胱感染和炎症主要见于女性的原因之一。尿道两端都有括约肌,帮助控制尿流的排出。

◇ **urethral** *adjective* referring to the urethra 尿道的; **urethral catheter** = catheter passed up the urethra to allow urine to flow out of the bladder, used to empty the bladder before an abdominal operation 导尿管,插入尿道使尿液流出膀胱,用于腹部手术前排空膀胱; **urethral stricture** = URETHROSTENOSIS 尿道狭窄

◇ **urethritis** *noun* inflammation of the urethra 尿道炎; **specific urethritis** = inflammation of the urethra caused by gonorrhoea 特异性尿道炎,淋病性尿道炎 *see also* 参见 NON-SPECIFIC URETHRITIS

◇ **urethrocele** *noun* (i) swelling formed in a weak part of the wall of the urethra 尿道憩室 (ii) prolapse of the urethra in a woman 尿道突出

◇ **urethrogram** *noun* X-ray photograph of the urethra 尿道造影

◇ **urethrography** *noun* X-ray examination of the urethra after an opaque substance has been introduced into it 尿道造影检查,向尿道内注射不透射线物质后用 X 线进行检查

◇ **urethroplasty** *noun* surgical operation to repair a urethra 尿道成形术

◇ **urethrorrhaphy** *noun* surgical operation to repair a torn urethra 尿道缝合术

◇ **urethrorrhoea** *noun* discharge of fluid from the urethra, usually associated with urethritis 尿道溢液

◇ **urethroscope** *noun* surgical instrument, used to examine the interior of a man's urethra 尿道镜,外科仪器,用于检查男性尿道前部

◇ **urethroscopy** *noun* examination of the inside of a man's urethra with a urethroscope 尿道镜检查

◇ **urethrostenosis** *or* **urethral stricture** *noun* narrowing *or* blocking of the urethra by a growth 尿道狭窄

◇ **urethrostomy** *noun* surgical operation to make an opening for a man's urethra between the scrotum and the anus 尿道造口术,在阴囊和肛门之间为男性尿道造一个出口

◇ **urethrotomy** *noun* surgical

operation to open a blocked *or* narrowed urethra 尿道切开术

urge *noun* strong need to do something 急迫: ***He was given drugs to reduce his sexual urge.*** 给他药以减轻他的早泄。

urgent *adjective* which has to be done quickly 急迫的: ***He had an urgent message to go to the hospital.*** 他得到紧急消息让他去医院。***Urgent cases are referred to the accident unit.*** 急诊病例被转诊到意外事故病房。***She had an urgent operation for strangulated hernia.*** 她因为绞窄性疝做了急诊手术。

◇ **urgently** *adverb* immediately 急迫地: ***The relief team urgently requires more medical supplies.*** 救援队急需更多的医疗支援。

-uria *suffix* meaning (i) a condition of the urine 尿的性状 (ii) a disease characterized by a condition of the urine 伴有尿性状改变的病

uric acid *noun* chemical compound which is formed from nitrogen in waste products from the body and which also forms crystals in the joints of patients suffering from gout 尿酸,含氮废物代谢中形成的化合物,可以在病人关节结晶,形成痛风 *see also* 参见 LITHAEMIA

◇ **uricosuric(drug)** *noun* drug which increases the amount of uric acid excreted in the urine 促尿酸排泄药

uridrosis *noun* condition where excessive urea forms in the sweat 尿汗症,汗液中尿素过多

urin- *or* **urino-** *prefix* referring to urine 尿

◇ **urinalysis** *noun* analysis of a patient's urine, to detect diseases such as diabetes mellitus 尿液分析,对病人尿液进行分析,以探察某些疾病如糖尿病

◇ **urinary** *adjective* referring to urine 尿的; **urinary bladder** = sac where the urine collects from the kidneys through the ureters, before being passed out of the body through the urethra 膀胱,从肾脏及输尿管收集尿液的囊,经尿道排出体外前存在此囊中 ◊ 见图 KIDNEY, UROGENITAL SYSTEM; **urinary catheter** = catheter passed up the urethra to allow urine to flow out of the bladder, used to empty the bladder before an abdominal operation 导尿管,插入尿道使尿液流出膀胱,用于腹部手术前排空膀胱; **urinary duct** *or* **ureter** = one of two tubes which take urine from the kidneys to the bladder 输尿管; **urinary obstruction** = blockage of the urethra which prevents urine being passed 尿道梗阻; **urinary system** = system of organs and ducts which separates waste liquids from the blood and excretes them as urine (including the kidneys, urinary bladder, ureters and urethra) 泌尿系统,将血液中的废液分离出来并分泌到尿液中去的器官和管道所组成的系统(包括肾脏、膀胱、输尿管和尿道); **urinary tract** = tubes down which the urine passes from the kidneys to the bladder and from the bladder out of the body 尿路,从肾到膀胱,从膀胱到排出体外的尿液通道; **urinary trouble** = disorder of the urinary tract 尿路疾病

◇ **urinate** *verb* to pass urine from the body 排尿: ***The patient has difficulty in urinating.*** 病人排尿困难。***He urinated twice this morning.*** 他今天早晨排了两次尿。

◇ **urination** *or* **micturition** *noun* passing of urine out of the body 排尿

◇ **urine** *noun* yellowish liquid, containing water and waste products (mainly salt and urea), which is excreted by the kidneys and passed out of the body through the ureters, bladder and urethra 尿液

◇ **uriniferous** *adjective* which carries urine 输送尿液的; **uriniferous tubule** *or* **renal tubule** = tiny tube which is part of a nephron 肾小管

◇ **urinogenital** *or* **urogenital** *adjective* referring to the urinary and genital systems 泌尿生殖系统的

◇ **urinometer** *noun* instrument which measures the specific gravity of urine 尿比重计

urobilin *noun* yellow pigment formed when urobilinogen comes into contact

with air 尿胆素,尿胆原接触空气后产生的黄色色素

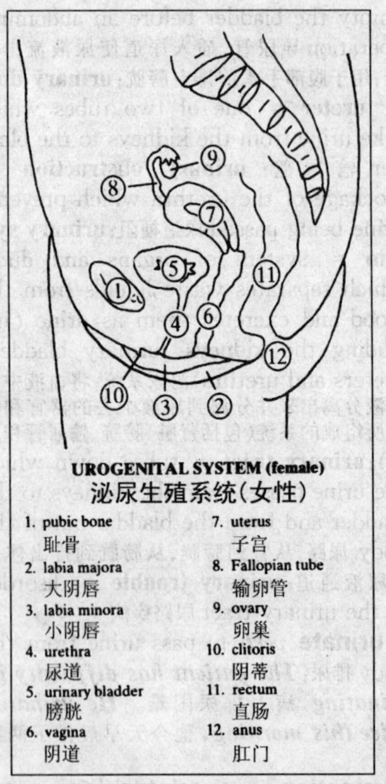

UROGENITAL SYSTEM (female)
泌尿生殖系统(女性)

1. pubic bone 耻骨
2. labia majora 大阴唇
3. labia minora 小阴唇
4. urethra 尿道
5. urinary bladder 膀胱
6. vagina 阴道
7. uterus 子宫
8. Fallopian tube 输卵管
9. ovary 卵巢
10. clitoris 阴蒂
11. rectum 直肠
12. anus 肛门

◇ **urobilinogen** *noun* colourless pigment formed when bilirubin is reduced to stercobilinogen in the intestines 尿胆原,胆红素在肠道还原成粪胆原时形成的无色物质

◇ **urocele** *noun* swelling in the scrotum which contains urine 阴囊积尿

◇ **urochesia** *noun* passing of urine through the rectum, due to injury of the urinary system 直肠尿瘘

◇ **urochrome** *adjective* pigment which colours the urine yellow 尿色素

urogenital *adjective* referring to the urinary and genital systems 泌尿生殖系统的;**urogenital diaphragm** = layer of fibrous tissue beneath the prostate gland, through which the urethra passes 泌尿生殖隔,前列腺下的纤维组织层,尿道从此穿过;**urogenital system** = the whole of the urinary tract and reproductive system 泌尿生殖系统

urography *noun* X-ray examination of part of the urinary system after injection of radio-opaque dye 尿路造影

◇ **urokinase** *noun* enzyme formed in the kidneys, which begins the process of breaking down blood clots 尿激酶,肾脏产生的一种酶,发动血块溶解过程

◇ **urolith** *noun* stone in the urinary system 尿路结石

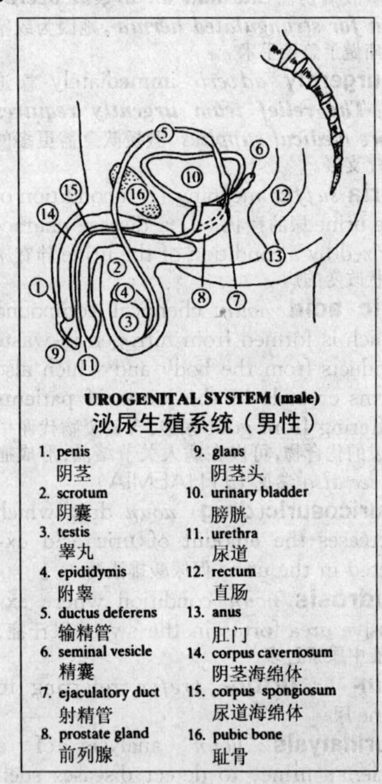

UROGENITAL SYSTEM (male)
泌尿生殖系统(男性)

1. penis 阴茎
2. scrotum 阴囊
3. testis 睾丸
4. epididymis 附睾
5. ductus deferens 输精管
6. seminal vesicle 精囊
7. ejaculatory duct 射精管
8. prostate gland 前列腺
9. glans 阴茎头
10. urinary bladder 膀胱
11. urethra 尿道
12. rectum 直肠
13. anus 肛门
14. corpus cavernosum 阴茎海绵体
15. corpus spongiosum 尿道海绵体
16. pubic bone 耻骨

◇ **urological** *adjective* referring to urology 泌尿学的

◇ **urologist** *noun* doctor who specializes in urology 泌尿科医师,泌尿学家

◇ **urology** *noun* scientific study of the urinary system and its diseases 泌尿学

urticaria *noun* allergic reaction (to injections *or* to certain foods) where the skin forms irritating reddish patches (also called 'hives' *or* 'nettlerash') 荨麻疹,皮肤过敏反应,形成很多有刺激性的红色斑片

USP = UNITED STATES PHARMACOPEIA 美国药典 *see* 见 PHARMACOPOEIA

uter- *or* **utero-** *prefix* referring to the uterus 子宫

◇ **uterine** *adjective* referring to the uterus 子宫的: ***The fertilized ovum becomes implanted in the uterine wall.*** 受精卵在子宫壁着床。**uterine cavity** = the inside of the uterus 子宫腔; **uterine fibroma** *or* **fibroid** = benign tumour in the muscle fibres of the uterus 子宫肌瘤; **uterine subinvolution** = condition where the uterus does not go back to its normal size after childbirth 子宫复旧不全; **uterine tube** = FALLOPIAN TUBE 输卵管 *see also* 参见 INTRAUTERINE; **uterine procidentia** *or* **uterine prolapse** = condition where part of the uterus has passed through the vagina (usually after childbirth) 子宫脱垂,子宫部分从阴道脱出

> COMMENT: Uterine prolapse has three stages of severity: in the first the cervix descends into the vagina, in the second the cervix is outside the vagina, but part of the uterus is still inside, and in the third stage, the whole uterus passes outside the vagina.
> 注释:子宫脱垂的严重程度分三级:一级,宫颈下降入阴道;二级,宫颈脱出阴道,但子宫仍有部分留在体内;三级,整个子宫脱出阴道。

◇ **uterocele** *or* **hysterocele** *noun* hernia of the uterus 子宫疝

◇ **uterogestation** *noun* normal pregnancy, where the fetus develops in the uterus 宫内孕即正常怀孕,胎儿在子宫中发育

◇ **uterography** *noun* X-ray examination of the uterus 子宫造影

◇ **utero-ovarian** *adjective* referring to the uterus and the ovaries 子宫卵巢的

◇ **uterosalpingography** = HYSTEROSALPINGOGRAPHY 子宫输卵管造影术

◇ **uterovesical** *adjective* referring to the uterus and the bladder 子宫膀胱的

◇ **uterus** *or* **womb** *noun* hollow organ in a woman's pelvic cavity, behind the bladder and in front of the rectum 子宫,女性盆腔里的空腔脏器,位于膀胱之后,直肠之前 ◇ 见图 UROGENITAL SYSTEM (female); **double uterus** = condition where the uterus is divided into two sections by a membrane 双子宫,子宫被一层膜分成两部分 *see also* 参见 DIMETRIA (NOTE: for other terms referring to the uterus, see words beginning with **hyster-, metr-**)

> COMMENT: The top of the uterus is joined to the Fallopian tubes which link it to the ovaries, and the lower end (cervix uteri or neck of the uterus) opens into the vagina. When an ovum is fertilized it becomes implanted in the wall of the uterus and develops into an embryo inside it. If fertilization and pregnancy do not take place, the lining of the uterus (endometrium) is shed during menstruation. At childbirth, strong contractions of the wall of the uterus (myometrium) help push the baby out through the vagina.
> 注释:子宫的顶部与输卵管相连,输卵管又连接着卵巢,子宫的下端(子宫颈)开口于阴道。当卵子受精后,它种植于子宫壁并在子宫里发育成一个胚胎。如果没有发生受精和受孕,子宫的覆膜(子宫内膜)在月经中脱落。分娩时,子宫壁(肌层)的强烈收缩帮助把婴儿娩出阴道。

utricle *or* **utriculus** *noun* (**a**) large sac inside the vestibule of the ear, which relates information about the upright position of the head to the brain 椭圆囊,内耳前庭内的囊,将头部上下的位置觉传给脑 (**b**) **prostatic utricle** = sac branching off the urethra as it passes through the prostate gland 前列腺囊,尿道经过前列腺时分出的一个小囊

UV = ULTRAVIOLET 紫外线

uvea *noun* layer of organs in the eye

beneath the sclera, formed of the iris, the ciliary body and the choroid 葡萄膜,眼色素层,眼睛内巩膜下的一层器官,由虹膜、睫状体和脉络膜组成

◇ **uveal** *adjective* referring to the uvea 葡萄膜的;**uveal tract** = layer of organs in the eye beneath the sclera, containing the iris, the ciliary body and choroid 眼色素层,眼睛内巩膜下的一层器官,由虹膜、睫状体和脉络膜组成

◇ **uveitis** *noun* inflammation of any part of the uvea 色素层炎

◇ **uveoparotid fever** *or* **syndrome** *noun* inflammation of the uvea and of the parotid gland 眼色素膜腮腺热,眼色素膜腮腺综合征,眼色素膜和腮腺的炎症

uvula *noun* piece of soft tissue which hangs down from the back of the the soft palate 悬雍垂,软腭后部悬垂下去的软组织小片

◇ **uvular** *adjective* referring to the uvula悬雍垂的

◇ **uvulectomy** *noun* surgical removal of the uvula 悬雍垂切除术

◇ **uvulitis** *noun* inflammation of the uvula悬雍垂炎 ◊ 见图 TONGUE

Vv

vaccinate *verb* to use a vaccine to give a person immunization against a specific disease 免疫接种：***She was vaccinated against smallpox as a child.*** 小时候她接种了天花疫苗。(NOTE: you vaccinate someone **against**)

◇ **vaccination** *noun* action of vaccinating 免疫接种

◇ **vaccine** *noun* substance which contains the germs of a disease, used to inoculate or vaccinate 疫苗：***The hospital is waiting for a new batch of vaccine to come from the laboratory.*** 医院等着来自实验室的一批新疫苗。***New vaccines are being developed all the time.*** 每时每刻都有新的疫苗产生。***MMR vaccine is given to control measles, mumps and rubella.*** MMR疫苗是控制麻疹、腮腺炎和风疹的。***There is, as yet, no vaccine for meningococcal meningitis.*** 现在还没有针对脑膜炎球菌的疫苗。

◇ **vaccinia** = COWPOX 牛痘

◇ **vaccinotherapy** *noun* treatment of a disease with a vaccine 疫苗接种治疗 (NOTE: Originally the words **vaccine** and **vaccination** applied only to smallpox immunization, but they are now used for immunization against any disease)

COMMENT: A vaccine contains the germs of the disease, sometimes alive and sometimes dead, and this is injected into the patient so that his body will develop immunity to the disease. The vaccine contains antigens, and these provoke the body to produce antibodies, some of which remain in the bloodstream for a very long time and react against the same antigens if they enter the body naturally at a later date when the patient is exposed to the disease. Vaccination is mainly given against cholera, diphtheria, rabies, smallpox, tuberculosis, and typhoid.
注解：疫苗含有致病的病原体，有时是活的，有时是死的，把疫苗注射到病人体内，他的身体会对此病产生免疫。疫苗含有抗原，引起身体产生抗体，有些抗体在体内血液中保留很长时间并在以后病人暴露于疾病，抗原自然进入人体时对同样的抗原起反应。免疫接种主要针对霍乱、白喉、狂犬病、天花、结核病和伤寒。

vacuole *noun* space in a fold of a cell membrane 空泡，细胞膜的皱褶里的空隙。

vacuum extractor *noun* surgical instrument formed of a rubber suction cup which is used in vacuum extraction *or* pulling on the head of the baby during childbirth 真空胎头吸引器，用于分娩时胎吸助产

vagal *adjective* referring to the vagus nerve 迷走神经的；**vagal tone** = action of the vagus nerve to slow the beat of the SA node 迷走张力，迷走神经降低窦房结搏动发放的神经活动

vain(o)- *prefix* referring to the vagina 阴道

◇ **vagina** *noun* passage in a woman's reproductive tract between the entrance to the uterus (the cervix) and the vulva, able to stretch enough to allow a baby to pass through during childbirth 阴道，从外阴到子宫入口的女性生殖道，分娩时能伸展到足以使胎儿娩出

◇ **vaginal** *adjective* referring to the vagina 阴道的；**vaginal bleeding** = bleeding from the vagina 阴道出血；**vaginal diaphragm** = contraceptive device, inserted into the woman's vagina and placed over the neck of the uterus 阴道隔，避孕工具，放入阴道盖住宫颈；**vaginal discharge** = flow of liquid from the vagina 阴道分泌物；**vaginal douche** = (i) washing out of the vagina 阴道冲洗 (ii) the device used to wash out the vagina 阴道冲洗器 *see also* 参见 DOUCHE；**vaginal examination** = checking the vagina for signs of disease or growth 阴道检查；**vaginal orifice** = opening leading from the vulva to the uterus 阴道开口 ◇ 见图 UROGENITAL SYSTEM (female) (NOTE: for other terms referring to the vagina, see words beginning with **colp-**)

◇ **vaginalis** 鞘、阴 道 *see* 见 TRICHOMONAS, TUNICA

◇ **vaginectomy** *noun* surgical operation to remove the vagina or part of it 阴道切除术

◇ **vaginismus** *noun* painful contraction of the vagina which prevents sexual intercourse 阴道痉挛,阴道疼痛性收缩,造成性交不能

◇ **vaginitis** *noun* inflammation of the vagina which is mainly caused by the bacterium *Trichomonas vaginalis* or by a fungus *Candida albicans* 阴道炎

◇ **vaginography** *noun* X-ray examination of the vagina 阴道 X 线检查

◇ **vaginoplasty** *noun* surgical operation to graft tissue on to the vagina 阴道成形术

◇ **vaginoscope** *or* **colposcope** *noun* surgical instrument inserted into the vagina to inspect the inside of it 阴道镜,放入阴道进行阴道内检查的外科仪器

vago- *prefix* referring to the vagus nerve 迷走神经

◇ **vagotomy** *noun* surgical operation to cut through the vagus nerve which controls the nerves in the stomach, as a treatment for peptic ulcers 迷走神经切断术,切断控制胃的迷走神经,治疗消化性溃疡

◇ **vagus nerve** *noun* tenth cranial nerve, which controls swallowing and the nerve fibres in the heart, stomach and lungs 迷走神经,第十对颅神经,控制吞咽和支配心脏、胃和肺的神经纤维

valency *or* **valence** *noun* number of atoms with which any single atom will combine chemically 化合价

valgus *noun* type of deformity where the foot *or* hand bends away from the centre of the body 足外翻,手外偏; **genu valgum** = knock knee, state where the knees touch and the feet are apart when a person is standing straight 膝外翻; **hallux valgus** = condition of the foot, where the big toe turns towards the other toes and a bunion is formed 拇趾外翻 *compare* 比较 VARUS

valine *noun* essential amino acid 缬氨酸

vallate papillae *noun* large papillae which form a line towards the back of the tongue and contain taste buds 杯状乳头,舌背侧形成一线的大乳头,含有味蕾 ◊ 见图 TONGUE

vallecula *noun* natural depression *or* fissure in an organ as between the hemispheres of the brain 谷,器官上自然的凹陷或裂隙,如两大脑半球之间的裂 (NOTE: plural is **valleculae**)

value *noun* quantity shown as a number 价值; **calorific value** = number of calories which a certain amount of a certain food contains 热量价,某种食物所含的热量的数值; **energy value** = amount of energy produced by a certain amount of a certain food 能量价,某种特定食物所能产生的能量

valve *noun* flap, mainly in the heart *or* blood vessels *or* lymphatic vessels but also in other organs, which opens and closes to allow liquid to pass in one direction only 瓣膜,,心脏、血管和淋巴管或其它组织内的活瓣,其开闭控制液体的单向流动; **aortic valve** = valve with three flaps at the opening into the aorta 主动脉瓣; **bicuspid (mitral) valve** = valve in the heart which allows blood to flow from the left atrium to the left ventricle but not in the opposite direction 二尖瓣(僧帽瓣),保证血流从左心房流向左心室而不反流的瓣膜; **ileocaecal valve** = valve at the end of the ileum, which allows food to pass from the ileum into the caecum 回盲瓣,回肠末端保证肠内容物进入盲肠的瓣膜; **pulmonary valve** = valve at the opening of the pulmonary artery 肺动脉瓣; **semilunar valve** = one of two valves in the heart, either the aortic valve or pulmonary valve 半月瓣,指主动脉瓣或肺动脉瓣之一; **tricuspid valve** = inlet valve with three cusps between the right atrium and the right ventricle in the heart 三尖瓣,右心房和右心室之间的三个瓣片组成的瓣膜

◇ **valvotomy** *or* **valvulotomy** *noun* surgical operation to cut into a valve to make it open wider 瓣膜切开术; **mitral valvotomy** = surgical operation to separate the cusps of the mitral valve in mitral stenosis 二尖瓣切开术,用于二尖瓣狭窄时分离两瓣膜

◇ **valvula** *noun* small valve 小的瓣或瓣膜 (NOTE: plural is **valvulae**)

◇ **valvular** *adjective* referring to a valve 瓣膜的; **valvular disease of the heart** (**VDH**) = inflammation of the membrane which lines the valves of the heart 心脏瓣膜病,,覆盖在瓣膜上的生物膜的炎症

◇ **valvulitis** *noun* inflammation of a valve in the heart 瓣膜炎

◇ **valvuloplasty** *noun* surgery to repair valves in the heart without opening the heart 瓣膜成形术

> QUOTE: In percutaneous balloon valvuloplasty a catheter introduced through the femoral vein is placed across the aortic valve and into the left ventricle; the catheter is removed and a valve-dilating catheter bearing a 15mm balloon is placed across the valve.
> 引文:经皮球囊瓣膜成形术是用一根导管从股动脉插入,经主动脉瓣进入左心室;以带有15毫米球囊的瓣膜扩张管取代原来的导管,跨在瓣膜上。
> **Journal of the American Medical Association** 美国医学会杂志

van den Bergh test *noun* test of blood serum to see if a case of jaundice is caused by an obstruction in the liver or by haemolysis of red blood cells 范登伯试验,检查黄疸是由肝内阻塞还是由溶血引起的血清试验

vapour *or US* **vapor** *noun* substance in the form of gas 蒸气; medicinal oil in steam 吸入剂,吸剂

◇ **vaporize** *verb* to turn a liquid into a vapour 蒸发

◇ **vaporizer** *noun* device which warms a liquid to which medicinal oil has been added, so that it provides a vapour which a patient can inhale 雾化器,汽化器

Vaquez-Osler disease = POLYCYTHAEMIA VERA 真性红细胞增多症

vara 内翻的 *see* 见 VARUS

variation *noun* change from one level to another 变异,变化: ***There is a noticeable variation in his pulse rate.*** 他的脉率变异很明显。***The chart shows the variations in the patient's temperature over a twenty-four hour period.*** 体温曲线图显示病人24小时的体温变化。

varicectomy *noun* surgical operation to remove a vein *or* part of a vein 曲张静脉切除术

varicella = CHICKENPOX 水痘

varices 脉管曲张 *see* 见 VARIX

varicocele *noun* swelling of a vein in the spermatic cord and which can be corrected by surgery 精索静脉曲张

◇ **varicose veins** *plural noun* veins, usually in the legs, which become twisted and swollen 曲张静脉: ***She wears special stockings to support her varicose veins.*** 她穿着特殊弹力袜以控制静脉曲张。 **varicose eczema** = form of eczema which develops on the legs, caused by bad circulation 静脉曲张性湿疹,由循环不良所致。 **varicose ulcer** = ulcer in the leg as a result of varicose veins 静脉曲张性溃疡

◇ **varicosity** *noun* (*of veins*) being swollen and twisted 静脉曲张

◇ **varicotomy** *noun* surgical operation to make a cut into a varicose vein 曲张静脉切开(除)术

variola = SMALLPOX 天花

◇ **varioloid** *noun* type of mild smallpox which affects patients who have already had smallpox *or* have been vaccinated against it 轻天花或变形天花,已得过天花或接受过免疫接种者所患的一种轻型天花

varix *noun* swollen blood vessel, especially a swollen vein in the leg 血管曲张(尤其是腿部静脉曲张) (NOTE: plural is **varices**)

Varolii 脑的 *see* 见 PONS (b)

varus *noun* deformity where the foot or hand bends in towards the centre of the body 足内翻，手内偏；**coxa vara** = deformity of the hip bone, making the legs bow 髋内翻，；**genu varum** = bow legs, state where the ankles touch and the knees are apart when a person is standing straight 膝内翻，站直时踝相并而膝相远，俗称弓形退 *compare* 比较 VALGUS

vary *verb* to change *or* to try different actions 变化：***The dosage varies according to the age of the patient.*** 剂量随病人年龄而有所不同。***The patient was recommended to change to a more varied diet.*** 建议病人采用花样更多的饮食。

vas- *prefix* referring to (i) a blood vessel 血管 (ii) the vas deferens 输精管

vas *noun* tube in the body 管；**vasa vasorum** = tiny blood vessels in the walls of larger blood vessels 血管滋养管

◊ **vas deferens** *or* **ductus deferens** *or* **sperm duct** *noun* one of two tubes along which sperm passes from the epididymis to the prostate gland for ejaculation 输精管，从附睾到前列腺的输送精子的管道 ◊ 见图 UROGENITAL SYSTEM (male)

◊ **vas efferens** *noun* one of many tiny tubes which take the spermatozoa from the testis to the epididymis 精子输出管，输送精子从睾丸到附睾的小管 (NOTE: plurals are **vasa**, **vasa deferentia**, **vasa efferentia**)

vascular *adjective* referring to blood vessels 血管的；**peripheral vascular disease** = disease affecting the blood vessels which supply the arms and legs 外周血管病，供应肢体血管的疾病；**vascular lesion** = damage to a blood vessel 血管损伤；**vascular system** = series of vessels such as veins, arteries and capillaries, carrying blood around the body 血管系统

◊ **vascularization** *noun* development of new blood vessels 血管生成

◊ **vasculitis** *noun* inflammation of a blood vessel 血管炎

vasectomy *noun* surgical operation to cut a vas deferens, to prevent sperm travelling from the epididymis up the duct 输精管切除术；**bilateral vasectomy** = surgical operation to cut both vasa deferentia and so make the patient sterile. 双侧输精管切除术，是一种男性绝育手段

COMMENT: Bilateral vasectomy is a safe method of male contraception.
注释：双侧输精管切除术是一种安全的男性避孕手段。

vaso- *prefix* referring to (i) a blood vessel 血管 (ii) the vas deferens 输精管

◊ **vasoactive** *adjective* (agent) which has an effect on the blood vessels (especially one which constricts the arteries) 血管活性的(物质，尤其指可收缩动脉者)

◊ **vasoconstriction** *noun* contraction of blood vessels which makes them narrower 血管收缩

◊ **vasoconstrictor** *noun* chemical substance which makes blood vessels become narrower, so that blood pressure rises 血管收缩药

◊ **vasodilatation** *noun* relaxation of blood vessels which makes them wider 血管扩张

◊ **vasodilator** *noun* chemical substance which makes blood vessels become wider, so that blood flows more easily and blood pressure falls 血管扩张药；**peripheral vasodilator** = chemical substance which acts to widen the blood vessels in the arms and legs, and so helps bad circulation as in Raynaud's disease 周围血管扩张剂，扩张四肢血管的药物，用于治疗雷诺病等周围循环不好的疾病

QUOTE: Volatile anaesthetic agents are potent vasodilators and facilitate blood flow to the skin
.引文：吸入性麻醉剂是强力血管扩张剂，可使皮肤血流增多。
British Journal of Nursing 英国护理杂志

◊ **vasoligation** *nou* surgical operation to tie the vasa deferentia to prevent infection entering the epididymis from the urinary system 输精管结扎术，结扎输精管，以防止感染从泌尿系统进入附睾

◇ **vasomotion** *noun* vasoconstriction *or vasodilatation* 血管舒缩，指血管收缩和扩张

◇ **vasomotor** *adjective* which makes blood vessels narrower *or* wider 血管舒缩的；**vasomotor centre** = nerve centre in the brain which changes the rate of heartbeat and the diameter of blood vessels and so regulates blood pressure 血管舒缩中枢，脑内的神经中枢，调节心率和血管直径，由此起到调节血压的作用；**vasomotor nerve** = nerve in the wall of a blood vessel which affects the diameter of the vessel 血管舒缩神经

◇ **vasopressin** *or* **antidiuretic hormone**（**ADH**）*noun* hormone secreted by the pituitary gland which acts on the kidneys to regulate the quantity of salt in body fluids and the amount of urine excreted by the kidneys 加压素或抗利尿激素，垂体分泌的激素，作用于肾脏，调节体液的含盐量和肾的泌尿量

◇ **vasopressor** *noun* substance which increases blood pressure by narrowing the blood vessels 升压药

◇ **vasospasm** *or* **Raynaud's disease** *noun* condition where the fingers become cold, white and numb 血管痉挛或雷诺病，表现为手指发冷、变白并麻木

◇ **vasovagal** *adjective* referring to the vagus nerve and its effect on the heartbeat and blood circulation 血管迷走神经的；**vasovagal attack** = fainting fit (following a slowing down of the heartbeats caused by the vagus nerve) 血管迷走神经昏厥

◇ **vasovasostomy** *noun* surgical operation to reverse a vasectomy 输精管吻合术

◇ **vasovesiculitis** *noun* inflammation of the seminal vesicles and a vas deferens 输精管精囊炎

vastus intermedius *or* **vastus medialis** *or* **vastus lateralis** *noun* three of the four parts of the quadriceps femoris *or* muscle of the thigh 股中间肌、股内侧肌、股外侧肌

VD = VENEREAL DISEASE 性病；**VD clinic** = clinic specializing in the diagnosis and treatment of venereal diseases 性病门诊：***He is attending a VD clinic.*** 他在看性病门诊。***The treatment for VD takes several weeks*** 治疗性病要几周时间。

VDH = VALVULAR DISEASE OF THE HEART 心脏瓣膜病

vectis *noun* curved surgical instrument used in childbirth 助产杠杆

vector *noun* insect, an animal which carries a disease and can pass it to humans 媒介，将疾病从动物传染给人的昆虫：***The tsetse fly is a vector of sleeping sickness.*** 采采蝇是非洲锥虫病的传播媒介。

vegan *noun & adjective* strict vegetarian *or* (person) who does not eat meat, dairy produce, eggs or fish and eats only vegetables and fruit 绝对素食者，只吃蔬菜和水果，不吃肉、乳制品、鸡蛋或鱼的严格的素食者 *compare* 比较 LACTOVEGETARIAN, VEGETARIAN

vegetable *noun* plant grown for food, not usually sweet 蔬菜：***Green vegetables are a source of dietary fibre.*** 绿色蔬菜是食用纤维的来源之一。

◇ **vegetarian** *noun & adjective* (person) who does not eat meat, but eats mainly vegetables and fruit and sometimes dairy produce, eggs or fish 素食者，不吃肉类，主要吃蔬菜、水果，有时也吃些乳制品，鸡蛋和鱼的人：***He is on a vegetarian diet.*** 他在吃素食。***She is a vegetarian.*** 她是个素食者。*compare* 比较 LACTOVEGETARIAN, VEGAN

vegetation *noun* growth on a membrane (as on the cusps of valves in the heart) 赘生物

◇ **vegetative** *adjective* (i) referring to growth of tissue *or* organs 增殖的 (ii) (state) after brain damage, where a person is alive and breathing but shows no responses 植物人的；**permanent vegetative state** (**PVS**) = condition where a patient is alive and breathes, but shows no brain activity, and will never recover consciousness 永久植物人状态

vehicle *noun* liquid in which a dose of a drug is put 药水

vein *noun* blood vessel which takes deoxygenated blood containing waste carbon dioxide from the tissues back to the heart 静脉,含有去氧血液,将废物和二氧化碳从组织带回心脏的血管; **azygos vein** = vein which brings blood back into the vena cava from the abdomen 奇静脉,将腹部血液带回腔静脉的血管; **basilic vein** = large vein running along the inside of the arm 头臂静脉,沿上肢内侧走行的大静脉; **deep vein** = vein which is deep in tissue, near the bones 深静脉,组织深部的静脉,靠近骨骼; **hepatic vein** = vein which carries blood from the liver to the vena cava 肝静脉,从肝输送血液到腔静脉的血管; **lingual vein** = vein which takes blood away from the tongue 舌静脉,运送舌部血液的静脉; **portal vein** = vein which takes blood from the stomach, pancreas, intestines and spleen to the liver 门静脉,从胃、胰、肠和脾输送血液到肝脏的静脉; **pulmonary vein** = vein which carries oxygenated blood from the lungs back to the left atrium of the heart (it is the only vein which carries oxygenated blood) 肺静脉,从肺输送氧合血液到左心房的血管(是唯一运送氧合血液的静脉); **superficial vein** = vein which is near the surface of the skin 表浅静脉,位于皮肤表层的静脉 (NOTE: for other terms referring to the veins, see words beginning with **phleb-**)

vena cava *noun* one of two large veins which take deoxygenated blood from all the other veins into the right atrium of the heart 腔静脉,将所有静脉的去氧血液输送回右心房的大静脉,分上腔静脉和下腔静脉 ◊ 见图 HEART, KIDNEY (NOTE: plural is **venae cavae**)

> COMMENT: The superior vena cava brings blood from the head and the top part of the body, while the inferior vena cava brings blood from the abdomen and legs.
> 注释:上腔静脉回收来自头部和身体上部的血液,而下腔静脉回收来自腹部和双腿的血液。

vene- *or* **veno-** *prefix* referring to veins 静脉

venene *noun* mixture of different venoms, used to produce antivenene 蛇毒,多种蛇毒的混合物,用于制备抗蛇毒血清

venepuncture *or* **venipuncture** *noun* puncturing a vein either to inject a drug *or* to take a blood sample 静脉穿刺

venereal disease (**VD**) *noun* disease which is passed from one person to another during sexual intercourse 性病

> COMMENT: Now usually called sexually transmitted diseases (STDs), the main types of venereal disease are syphilis, gonorrhoea, AIDS, non-specific urethritis, genital herpes and chancroid. The spread of sexually transmitted diseases can be limited by use of condoms. Other forms of contraceptive offer no protection against the spread of disease.
> 注释:现在通常叫做性传播疾病,主要的性病有梅毒、淋病、艾滋病、非特异性尿道炎、生殖器疱疹和软下疳。性传播疾病的传播可以通过使用避孕套得以控制。其他形式的避孕方法对性病的传播没有保护作用。

venereologist *noun* doctor who specializes in the study of venereal diseases 性病专家

◊ **venereology** *noun* scientific study of venereal diseases 性病学

◊ **venereum** 性病性 *see* 见 LYMPHOGRANULOMA

◊ **veneris** 阴道的 *see* 见 MONS

venesection *noun* operation where a vein is cut so that blood can be removed (as when taking blood from a donor) 静脉切开术

venoclysis *noun* introducing slowly a saline *or* other solution into a vein 静脉输液

◊ **venogram** = PHLEBOGRAM 静脉造影片

◊ **venography** = PHLEBOGRAPHY 静脉造影术

venom *noun* poison in the bite of a

snake *or* insect 毒液，蛇或昆虫叮咬的毒汁

> COMMENT: Depending on the source of the bite, venom can have a wide range of effects, from a light irritating spot after a mosquito sting, to death from a scorpion. Antivenene will counteract the effects of venom, but is only effective if the animal which gave the bite can be correctly identified.
> 注释：依叮咬的来源不同，毒液具有很宽的作用谱，从蚊子咬后轻微的刺激性小点，到蝎子蛰后致死。抗毒血清可以对抗毒液的作用，但只有在能正确认明咬人的动物的前提下才能发挥作用。

◇ **venomous** *adjective* (animal) which has poison in its bite 分泌毒液的，毒的：***The cobra is a venomous snake.*** 眼镜蛇是一种毒蛇。***He was bitten by a venomous spider.*** 他被毒蜘蛛咬了。

venosus 静脉的 *see* 见 DUCTUS

venous *adjective* referring to the veins 静脉的；**venous bleeding** = bleeding from a vein 静脉出血；**venous blood** = deoxygenated blood, from which most of the oxygen has been removed by the tissues and is darker than oxygenated arterial blood (it is carried by all the veins except for the pulmonary vein which carries oxygenated blood) 静脉血，去氧合的血液，因为多数氧已经被组织吸收了，所以静脉血颜色比氧合的动脉血暗(除了肺静脉血是氧合血外，其他静脉的血液都是去氧合血)；**venous system** = system of veins which bring blood back to the heart from the tissues 静脉系统；**venous thrombosis** = blocking of a vein by a blood clot 静脉血栓；**venous ulcer** = ulcer in the leg, caused by varicose veins or by a blood clot 静脉曲张性溃疡，腿上因静脉曲张或血栓阻塞所致的溃疡；**central venous pressure** = blood pressure in the right atrium, which can be measured by means of a catheter 中心静脉压，右心房的血压，通过插入导管测得。

> QUOTE: Venous air embolism is a potentially fatal complication of percutaneous venous catheterization.
> 引文：静脉空气栓塞是经皮静脉导管插入术潜在的致命性并发症。
> **Southern Medical Journal** 南部医学杂志

> QUOTE: A pad was placed under the Achilles tendon to raise the legs, thus aiding venous return and preventing deep vein thrombosis.
> 引文：在跟腱下垫一个垫子抬高双腿，这样能辅助静脉回流，预防深静脉血栓形成。
> **NATNews** 全国手术室护士协会新闻

ventilation *noun* breathing air in or out of the lungs, so removing waste products from the blood in exchange for oxygen 通气，肺吸入空气，呼出血氧交换产生的废气 *see also* 参见 DEAD SPACE；**artificial ventilation** = breathing which is assisted *or* controlled by a machine 人工通气，用机器辅助或控制通气；**mouth-to-mouth ventilation** = making a patient start to breathe again by blowing air through his mouth into his lungs 口对口通气

◇ **ventilator** *or* **respirator** *noun* machine which pumps air into and out of the lungs of a patient who has difficulty in breathing 呼吸机：***The newborn baby was put on a ventilator.*** 给这个新生儿上了呼吸机。

◇ **ventilatory failure** *noun* failure of the lungs to oxygenate the blood correctly 呼吸衰竭

ventral *adjective* referring to (i) the abdomen 腹部的 (ii) the front of the body 身体前面的 (NOTE: the opposite is **dorsal**)

ventricle *noun* cavity in an organ, especially in the heart or brain 室，器官里的空腔，特别是心室和脑室 ◇ 见图 HEART

> COMMENT: There are two ventricles in the heart: the left ventricle takes oxygenated blood from the pulmonary vein through the left atrium, and pumps it into the aorta to circulate round the body; the right ventricle takes blood from the veins through the right atrium, and pumps

it in to the pulmonary artery to be passed to the lungs to be oxygenated. There are four ventricles in the brain, each containing cerebrospinal fluid. The two lateral ventricles in the cerebral hemispheres contain the choroid processes which produce cerebrospinal fluid. The third ventricle lies in the midline between the two thalami. The fourth ventricle is part of the central canal of the hindbrain.
注释:心脏有两个心室:左心室接受经左心房来的肺静脉氧合血液,并将它们泵入主动脉而后周流全身;右心室接受来自右心房的静脉血,并将它们泵入肺动脉,进而入肺进行氧合。脑内有 4 个脑室,都含有脑脊液。两大脑半球内的侧脑室含有脉络膜颗粒能产生脑脊液;第三脑室位于中线部位,两丘脑之间;第四脑室是后脑中央管的一部分。

◇ **ventricul(o)-** *prefix* referring to a ventricle in the brain *or* heart 心室,脑室

◇ **ventricular** *adjective* referring to the ventricles 脑室的,心室的; **ventricular fibrillation** = serious heart condition where the ventricular muscles flutter and the heart no longer beats 心室纤颤,严重的心律失常,心室肌扑动而心脏不再跳动; **ventricular folds** *or* **vocal cords** = two folds in the larynx which can be brought together to make sounds as air passes between them 声带

ventriculitis *noun* inflammation of the brain ventricles 脑室炎

◇ **ventriculoatriostomy** *noun* operation to relieve pressure caused by excessive quantities of cerebrospinal fluid in the brain ventricles 脑室心房造口术

◇ **ventriculogram** *noun* X-ray picture of the brain ventricles 脑室造影片

◇ **ventriculography** *noun* method of taking X-ray pictures of the ventricles of the brain after air has been introduced to replace the cerebrospinal fluid 脑室造影，以气体取代脑脊液进行气脑造影

◇ **ventriculoscopy** *noun* examination of the brain using an endoscope 脑室镜检查

◇ **ventriculostomy** *noun* surgical operation to pass a hollow needle into a brain ventricle so as to reduce pressure *or* take a sample of fluid 脑室(造口)引流术

ventro- *prefix* (i) meaning ventral 腹侧 (ii) referring to the abdomen 腹部

◇ **ventrofixation** *noun* surgical operation to treat retroversion of the uterus by attaching the uterus to the wall of the abdomen 子宫固定术,治疗子宫后倾时将它固定在腹壁上的手术方法

◇ **ventrosuspension** *noun* surgical operation to treat retroversion of the uterus 子宫悬吊术,治疗子宫后倾的手术方法

venule *noun* small vein *or* vessel leading from tissue to a larger vein 小静脉

vera 生 *see* 见 DECIDUA

verbigeration *noun* condition seen in mental patients, where the patient keeps saying the same words over and over again 言语重复,见于精神科病人,一遍又一遍说同一句话

vermicide *noun* substance which kills worms in the intestine 杀蠕虫药,杀死肠道寄生虫的药物

◇ **vermiform** *adjective* shaped like a worm 蠕虫样的; **vermiform appendix** = small tube attached to the caecum which serves no function, but can become infected, causing appendicitis 阑尾,与盲肠连接的细小的管状器官,已无功能,但可以感染,引起阑尾炎

◇ **vermifuge** *noun* & *adjective* (substance) which removes worms from the intestine 驱蠕虫的,驱蠕虫药

◇ **vermix** *noun* vermiform appendix 阑尾

vermil(l)ion border *noun* external red parts of the lips 唇线

vermis *noun* central part of the cerebellum, which forms the top of the fourth ventricle 小脑蚓部,小脑的中央部分,形成第四脑室的顶

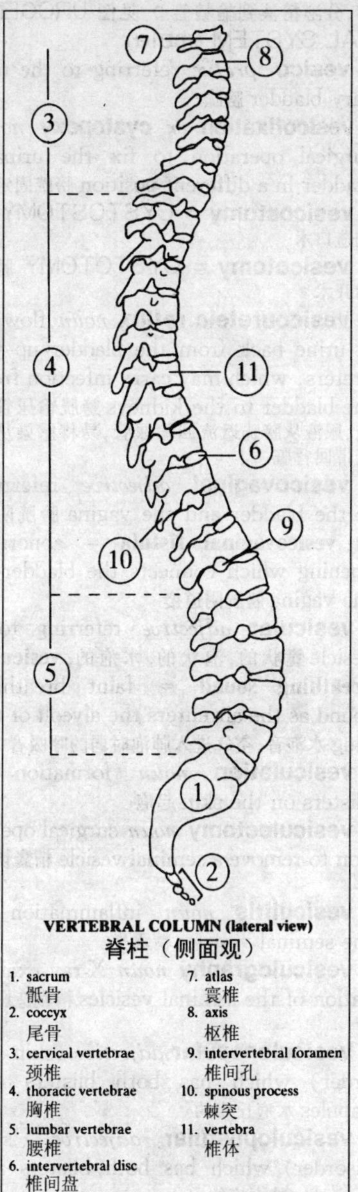

VERTEBRAL COLUMN (lateral view)
脊柱（侧面观）

1. sacrum 骶骨
2. coccyx 尾骨
3. cervical vertebrae 颈椎
4. thoracic vertebrae 胸椎
5. lumbar vertebrae 腰椎
6. intervertebral disc 椎间盘
7. atlas 寰椎
8. axis 枢椎
9. intervertebral foramen 椎间孔
10. spinous process 棘突
11. vertebra 椎体

vernix caseosa *noun* oily substance which covers a baby's skin at birth 胎儿皮脂,出生时覆盖在婴儿皮肤上的油性物质

verruca *noun* wart, small hard benign growth on the skin, caused by a virus 疣,俗称瘊子,是皮肤上小的良性赘生物,由病毒引起 (NOTE: plural is **verrucae**)

version *noun* turning the fetus in a womb so as to put it in a better position for birth 倒转术,使子宫内的胎儿转到一个较利于分娩的位置; **cephalic version** = turning a wrongly positioned fetus round in the uterus, so that the head will appear first at birth 胎头倒转术,使胎位不正的胎儿在分娩时头先露; **pelvic version** = version performed by moving the buttocks of the fetus 胎臀倒转术; **podalic version** = turning a fetus in the womb so that the baby will be born feet first 胎足倒转术,通过转位使分娩时足先露; **spontaneous version** = movement of a fetus to take up another position in the womb, caused by the contractions of the womb during childbirth *or* by movements of the baby itself before birth 自发转位,由于分娩时子宫收缩或出生前胎儿自己的运动,使胎儿由一个胎位转到另一个胎位

vertebra *noun* one of twenty-four ring-shaped bones which link together to form the backbone 椎骨,形成脊柱的24个环状骨之一 (NOTE: plural is **vertebrae**)

◇ **vertebral** *adjective* referring to the vertebrae 椎骨的; **vertebral arteries** = two arteries which go up the back of the neck into the brain 椎动脉,沿脊柱两侧上行至项部的两支动脉; **vertebral canal** = channel formed of the holes in the centre of each vertebra, through which the spinal cord passes 椎管,椎骨的中间孔形成的腔道,脊髓从中通过; **vertebral column** = backbone, series of bones and discs linked together to form a flexible column running from the base of the skull to the pelvis 脊柱; **vertebral disc** *or* **intervertebral disc** = thick piece of cartilage which lies between two vertebrae and acts as a cushion 椎间盘,两椎骨之间厚的软骨垫,有缓冲作用; **vertebral foramen** = hole in the centre of a vertebra which links with others to form the vertebral canal 椎孔,椎骨中央的空洞,串起来形成椎管(NOTE: the vertebrae are referred to by numbers and letters: **C6** = the sixth cervical vertebra; **T11** = the eleventh thoracic vertebra, and so on)

COMMENT: The top vertebra (the atlas) supports the skull; the first seven vertebrae in the neck are the cervical vertebrae; then follow the twelve thoracic or dorsal vertebrae which are behind the chest and five lumbar vertebrae in the lower part of the back. The sacrum and coccyx are formed of five sacral vertebrae and four coccygeal vertebrae which have fused together.
注释:最上的椎骨(寰椎)支撑着颅骨,颈部的头 7 个椎骨是颈椎,其后是 12 个胸椎,它们位于胸部水平的后背;后腰下部是 5 个腰椎。5 块骶骨和 4 块尾骨融合在一起,形成骶椎和尾椎。

vertex *noun* top of the skull 头顶;**vertex delivery** = normal birth of a baby, where the head appears first 头位分娩,正常分娩,头先露。

vertigo *noun* (**a**) dizziness *or* giddiness *or* loss of balance where the patient feels that everything is rushing round him, caused by a malfunction of the sense of balance 眩晕 (**b**) fear of heights *or* sensation of dizziness which is felt when high up (especially on a tall building) 晕高: ***He won't sit near the window — he suffers from vertigo.*** 他不能坐在窗户附近,他晕高。

vesical *adjective* referring to the bladder 膀胱的

◊ **vesicant** *or* **epispastic** *noun* substance which makes the skin blister 起疱剂

◊ **vesicle** *noun* (**a**) small blister on the skin (such as those caused by eczema) 小疱,皮肤上的小水疱 (**b**) sac which contains liquid 小囊泡; **seminal vesicles** = two organs near the prostate gland which secrete seminal fluid into the vas deferens 精囊,前列腺附近的两个器官,分泌精液到输精管 ◊ 见图 UROGENITAL SYSTEM (male)

◊ **vesico-** *prefix* referring to the urinary bladder 膀胱

◊ **vesicofixation** *or* **cystopexy** *noun* surgical operation to fix the urinary bladder in a different position 膀胱固定术

◊ **vesicostomy** = CYSTOSTOMY 膀胱造口术

◊ **vesicotomy** = CYSTOTOMY 膀胱切开术

◊ **vesicoureteic reflux** *noun* flowing of urine back from the bladder up the ureters, which may carry infection from the bladder to the kidneys 膀胱输尿管返流,尿液从膀胱返流回输尿管,易将感染从膀胱带回肾脏

◊ **vesicovaginal** *adjective* referring to the bladder and the vagina 膀胱阴道的; **vesicovaginal fistula** = abnormal opening which connects the bladder to the vagina 膀胱阴道瘘

◊ **vesicular** *adjective* referring to a vesicle 囊状的,泡状的,水疱的; **vesicular breathing sound** = faint breathing sound as the air enters the alveoli of the lung 水泡音,空气进入肺泡时弱的呼吸音

◊ **vesiculation** *noun* formation of blisters on the skin 起疱

◊ **vesiculectomy** *noun* surgical operation to remove a seminal vesicle 精囊切除术

◊ **vesiculitis** *noun* inflammation of the seminal vesicles 精囊炎

◊ **vesiculography** *noun* X-ray examination of the seminal vesicles 精囊造影检查

◊ **vesiculopapular** *adjective* (skin disorder) which has both blisters and papules 水疱丘疹的

◊ **vesiculopustular** *adjective* (skin disorder) which has both blisters and pustules 脓水疱的

vessel *noun* tube in the body along which liquid flows, especially a blood vessel 管; **afferent vessel** = tube which brings lymph to a gland 淋巴输入管; **blood vessel** = any tube (artery *or* vein *or* capillary) which carries blood round the body 血管; **efferent vessel** = tube which drains lymph from a gland 淋巴输出管; **lymphatic vessel** = tube which carries lymph round the body 淋巴管 (NOTE: for other terms referring to vessels, see words beginning with vasc-, vaso-)

vestibular *adjective* referring to a vestibule, especially the vestibule of the inner ear 前庭的,特别是内耳前庭; **vestibular folds** = folds in the larynx, above the vocal cords 前庭褶,声带上方,咽部的皱褶; **vestibular glands** = glands at the point where the vagina and vulva join, which secrete a lubricating substance 前庭腺,阴道和外阴交汇处的腺体,分泌润滑物质; **greater vestibular gland** *or* **Bartholin's gland** = the more posterior of the vestibular glands 前庭大腺,前庭腺体中靠后的一个; **lesser vestibular gland** = the more anterior of the vestibular glands 前庭小腺,前庭腺体中靠前的一个; **vestibular nerve** = part of the auditory nerve which carries information about balance to the brain 前庭神经,听神经的一部分,传递平衡信息到脑

◇ **vestibule** *noun* cavity in the body at the entrance to an organ especially 前庭,体内进入某一脏器入口处的空腔,特别是 (i) the first cavity in the inner ear 内耳的第一空腔 (ii) the space in the larynx above the vocal cords 咽部声带上方的空间 (iii) a nostril 鼻孔

◇ **vestibuli**前庭的 *see* 见 FENESTRA

◇ **vestibulocochlear nerve** *or* **acoustic nerve** *or* **auditory nerve** *noun* eighth cranial nerve which governs hearing and balance 前庭耳蜗神经或听神经,第八对颅神经,负责听觉和平衡

vestigial *adjective* which exists in a rudimentary form 残迹的,剩余的: ***The coccyx is a vestigial tail.*** 尾骨是尾巴的残迹。

viable *adjective* (fetus) which can survive if born(胎儿)生后可存活的: ***A fetus is viable by about the 28th week of pregnancy.*** 妊娠满 28 周,胎儿就可以存活。

◇ **viability** *noun* being viable 活力,生机: ***The viability of the fetus before the 22nd week is doubtful.*** 怀孕满 22 周以前出世的胎儿能否存活还有疑问。

vibrate *verb* to move rapidly and continuously 震动

◇ **vibration** *noun* rapid and continuous movement 震动: ***Speech is formed by the vibrations of the vocal cords.*** 语音是声带震动发出的。***Sounds make the eardrum vibrate and the vibrations are sent to the brain as nervous impulses.*** 声音使鼓膜震动,这震动以神经冲动的形式传递到脑。 **vibration white finger** = condition caused by using a chain saw *or* pneumatic drill, which affects the circulation in the fingers 震动病白指,使用链锯或气钻影响手指血液循环所致

◇ **vibrator** *noun* device to producevibrations, which may be used for massages 震荡器,产生震动的装置,可用于按摩

Vibrio *noun* genus of Gram-negative bacteria which are found in water and cause cholera 霍乱弧菌,水中的革兰氏阴性细菌,可引起霍乱

vibrissae *plural noun* hairs in the nostrils *or* ears 鼻毛,耳毛

vicarious *adjective* (done by one organ *or* agent) in place of another 代偿的; **vicarious menstruation** = discharge of blood other than by the vagina during menstrual periods 代偿性月经,月经期间没有阴道出血,身体其他部位反而出血

victim *noun* person who is injured in an accident *or* who has caught a disease 受害者: ***The victims of the rail crash were taken to the local hospital.*** 火车相撞事故的受害者被送到地方医院。***Half the people eating at the restaurant fell victim to salmonella poisoning.*** 在这家饭馆吃饭的人有一半成了沙门氏菌中毒的受害者。***The health authority is planning a special hospital for AIDS victims.*** 卫生当局正计划为艾滋病受害者开办一家专科医院。

vigour *or US* **vigor** 活力、健壮 *see* 见 HYBRID

villus *noun* tiny projection like a finger on the surface of mucous membrane

绒毛，粘膜上长的状如手指的细小突起；**arachnoid villi** = villi in the arachnoid membrane which absorb cerebrospinal fluid 蛛网膜绒毛，有吸收脑脊液的作用；**chorionic villi** = tiny folds in the membrane covering the fertilized ovum 绒膜绒毛，被覆受精卵的膜上的细小皱褶；**intestinal villi** = projections on the walls of the intestine which help in the digestion of food 小肠绒毛 (NOTE: plural is **villi**)

◇ **villous** *adjective* shaped like a villus *or* formed of villi 绒毛的，绒毛状的

Vincent's angina = ULCERATIVE GINGIVITIS 奋森氏咽峡炎，溃疡性咽峡炎，膜溃疡性龈炎

vinculum *noun* thin connecting band of tissue 纽，组织之间纤细的连接带 (NOTE: plural is **vincula**)

violent *adjective* very strong *or* very severe 强烈的，剧烈的：***He had a violent headache***. 他一阵剧烈头疼。***Her reaction to the injection was violent***. 她对注射反应剧烈。

◇ **violently** *adverb* in a strong way 强烈地：***He reacted violently to the antihistamine***. 他对抗组胺药反应强烈。

violet *noun* dark, purplish blue colour at the end of the visible spectrum 紫色 *see also* 参见 CRYSTAL, GENTIAN

viraemia *noun* virus in the blood 病毒血症

◇ **viral** *adjective* caused by a virus *or* referring to a virus 病毒的：***He caught viral pneumonia on a plane***. 他在飞机上得了病毒性肺炎。

virgin *noun* female who has not experienced sexual intercourse 处女，无性交经历的女子

◇ **virginity** *noun* condition of a female who has not experienced sexual intercourse 童贞

virile *adjective* like a man *or* with strong male characteristics 男性的，有男性特征的

◇ **virilism** *noun* male characteristics (such as body hair *or* deep voice) in a woman 男性化，妇女具有男性特征

◇ **virilization** *noun* development of male characteristics in a woman, caused by a hormone defect *or* therapy 男性化，妇女发生男性性征，由激素缺陷或雄激素治疗引起

virology *noun* scientific study of viruses 病毒学

virulence *noun* (i) ability of a microbe to cause a disease 毒力 (ii) violent effect (of a disease)(疾病)破坏力

◇ **virulent** *adjective* (i) (microbe) which can cause a disease(微生物)有毒力的，可致病的 (ii) (disease) which has violent effects and develops rapidly(疾病)具有破坏力的

virus *noun* tiny germ cell which can only develop in other cells, and often destroys them 病毒，只能生活在其它细胞中的一种微生物，往往破坏宿主细胞：***Scientists have isolated a new flu virus***. 科学家们分离出了新的流感病毒株。***Shingles is caused by the same virus as chickenpox***. 带状疱疹和水痘是同一种病毒引起的。**infectious virus hepatitis** = hepatitis transmitted by a carrier through food or drink 传染性病毒性肝炎；**virus pneumonia** = inflammation of the lungs caused by a virus 病毒性肺炎

> COMMENT: Many common diseases such as measles or the common cold are caused by viruses; viral diseases cannot be treated with antibiotics.
> 注释：许多常见病如麻疹或普通感冒是病毒引起的，病毒性疾病不能用抗生素治疗。

viscera *plural noun* internal organs (such as the heart, lungs, stomach, intestines) 内脏；**abdominal viscera** = the organs inside the abdomen 腹部内脏 (NOTE: the singular (rarely used) is **viscus**)

◇ **visceral** *adjective* referring to the internal organs 内脏的；**viscera larva migrans** = toxocariasis, infestation of the intestine with worms from a dog or cat 弓蛔虫病，由猫狗身上的蠕虫传给人导致的肠道传染病；**visceral muscle** *or* **smooth muscle** = muscle in the wall of the intestine which makes the intestine contract 内脏肌肉，平滑肌；**visceral pericar-**

dium = inner layer of serous pericardium attached to the wall of the heart 脏层心包; **visceral peritoneum** = part of the peritoneum which covers the organs in the abdominal cavity 脏层腹膜; **visceral pleura** = inner pleura, membrane attached to the surface of a lung 脏层胸膜; **visceral pouch** = PHARYNGEAL POUCH 咽囊

◇ **visceromotor** *adjective* (reflex, etc.) which controls the movement of viscera 内脏运动的

◇ **visceroptosis** *noun* movement of an internal organ downwards from its usual position 内脏下垂

◇ **visceroreceptor** *noun* receptor cell which reacts to stimuli from organs such as the stomach, heart and lungs 内脏感受器,对来自内脏刺激起反应的感受器

viscid *adjective* sticky *or* slow-moving (liquid) 粘的

◇ **viscosity** *noun* state of a liquid which moves slowly 粘性

◇ **viscous** *adjective* thick *or* slow-moving (liquid) 粘滞的

viscus 内脏 *see* 见 VISCERA

visible *adjective* which can be seen 可见的,明显的: ***There were no visible symptoms of the disease.*** 此病尚无明显症状。

vision *noun* ability to see *or* eyesight 视力: ***After the age of 50, many people's vision begins to fail.*** 50岁以后,多数人视力开始下降。**binocular vision** = ability to see with both eyes at the same time, which gives a stereoscopic effect and allows a person to judge distances 双眼视觉,两眼同时视物的能力,可产生立体视觉,让人能判断远近; **blurred vision** = condition where the patient does not see objects clearly 视力模糊; **field of vision** = area which can be seen without moving the eye 视野,不转动眼睛所能看到的区域; **impaired vision** = eyesight which is not fully clear 视力缺陷; **monocular vision** = seeing with one eye only, so that the sense of distance is impaired 单眼视觉,只用一只眼看,判断距离的感觉会有缺陷; **partial vision** = being able to see only part of the total field of vision 部分视野; **stereoscopic vision** = being able to judge how far something is from you, because of seeing it with both eyes at the same time 立体视觉; **tunnel vision** = field of vision which is restricted to the area immediately in front of the eye 管状视野,只能看到眼睛正前方的区域; **twenty-twenty vision** *or* **20/20 vision** = perfect normal vision 视力20/20,视力极佳

visit 1 *noun* (**a**) short stay with someone (especially to comfort a patient) 看望: ***The patient is too weak to have any visits.*** 病人身体太弱不宜探视。***He is allowed visits of ten minutes only.*** 他只允许10分钟的探视。(**b**) short stay with a professional person 看(病): ***They had a visit from the district nurse.*** 地区护士察看了他们的病情。***She paid a visit to the chiropodist.*** 她花钱看了一次足疗师。***On the patient's last visit to the physiotherapy unit, nurses noticed a great improvement in her walking.*** 病人最后一次到理疗病房看病时,护士们注意到她的行走有了很大进步。**2** *verb* to stay a short time with someone 看望,探访: ***I am going to visit my brother in hospital.*** 我要去看我住院的兄弟。***She was visited by the health visitor.*** 保健访视员看望了她。**visiting times** = times of day when friends are allowed into a hospital to visit patients 探视时间,允许到医院看望病人的时间

◇ **visitor** *noun* person who visits 探视者: ***Visitors are allowed into the hospital on Sunday afternoons.*** 星期天下午允许探视病人。***How many visitors did you have this week?*** 这周有多少人来看你? **health visitor** = registered nurse with qualifications in midwifery or obstetrics and preventive medicine, who visits mothers and babies, and sick people in their homes and advises on treatment 保健访视员,有助产、产科或预防医学资格的注册护士,他们到家中访视母婴和病人,提出治疗建议

visual *adjective* referring to sight *or*

vision 视觉的; **visual acuity** = being able to see objects clearly 视敏度; **visual axis** = the line between the object on which the eye focuses, and the fovea 视轴,所注视物体和眼球中央凹之间的连线; **visual cortex** = part of the cerebral cortex which receives information about sight 视觉皮质; **visual field** = field of vision, the area which can be seen without moving the eye 视野,不转动眼睛所能看到的区域; **visual purple** *or* **rhodopsin** = purple pigment in the rods of the retina which makes it possible to see in bad light 视紫红质,视网膜视杆细胞内的紫色色素,使人在弱光下能看见

vitae 活的 *see* 见 ARBOR

vital *adjective* most important for life 性命攸关的: ***If circulation is stopped, vital nerve cells begin to die in a few minutes.*** 如果循环停止了,几分钟内重要的神经细胞便开始死亡。***Oxygen is vital to the human system.*** 氧对人体系统来说是至关重要的。**vital capacity** = largest amount of air which a person can exhale 肺活量,人能呼出的最大气体量; **vital centre** = group of nerve cells in the brain which govern a particular function of the body (such as the five senses) 生命中枢,脑内的一群神经细胞,掌握着特殊的身体功能(如五种感觉); **vital organs** = the most important organs in the body, without which a human being cannot live (such as the heart, lungs, brain) 生命器官,少了它人就活不了的器官(如心、肺、脑); **vital signs** = measurement of pulse, breathing and temperature 生命体征,包括脉搏、呼吸和体温; **vital statistics** = official statistics relating to the population of a place (such as the percentage of live births per thousand, the incidence of a certain disease, the numbers of births and deaths) 生命统计,一个地区的官方人口统计(如每千例分娩的活产数、某病的发病率、出生率和死亡率)

vitamin *noun* essential substance not synthesized in the body, but found in most foods, and needed for good health 维生素,身体不能合成的必需物质,但可以在大多数食物中找到,是身体健康所需的; **vitamin deficiency** = lack of necessary vitamins 维生素缺乏: ***He is suffering from Vitamin A deficiency.*** 他患了维生素 A 缺乏症。***Vitamin C deficiency causes scurvy.*** 维生素 C 缺乏引起坏血病。

vitellus *noun* yolk of an egg (ovum) 卵黄

◇ **vitelline sac** *noun* sac attached to an embryo, where the blood cells first form 卵黄囊,胚胎中的一个囊,是血液细胞最初形成的地方

vitiligo *noun* leucoderma, condition where white patches appear on the skin 白斑,皮肤出现的白色斑片

vitreous body *or* **vitreous humour** *noun* transparent jelly which fills the main cavity behind the lens in the eye 玻璃体,眼球中晶状体后面的透明胨状结构

vitro 试管 *see* 见 IN VITRO

Vitus 维特斯 *see* 见 ST VITUS

viviparous *adjective* (animal) which bears live young (such as humans, as opposed to birds and reptiles which lay eggs) 胎生的

◇ **vivisection** *noun* dissecting a living animal as an experiment 活体解剖,解剖活的动物做试验

vocal *adjective* referring to the voice 声音的; **vocal cords** *or* **vocal folds** 声带 *see* 见 CORD; **vocal fremitus** = vibration of the chest as a patient speaks *or* coughs 语颤,说话或咳嗽时胸部的震动; **vocal ligament** = ligament in the centre of the vocal cords 声韧带,声带中央的韧带; **vocal resonance** = sound heard by a doctor when he listens through a stethoscope while a patient is speaking 语颤,病人说话时医生用听诊器听到的声音

voice *noun* sound made when a person speaks *or* sings 嗓音: ***The doctor has a quiet and comforting voice.*** 医生嗓音平静而柔和。***I didn't recognize your voice over the phone.*** 在电话里我听不出你的声音了。**to lose one's voice** = not to be able to speak because of a throat infection失声,因咽喉感染而发不出声音; ***His voice has broken.*** = His voice has become deeper and adult, with the onset of puberty.他的嗓子劈了,变声。

◇ **voice box** *or* **larynx** *noun* organ at the back of the throat which produces sounds 喉

> COMMENT: The voice box is a hollow organ containing the vocal cords, situated behind the Adam's apple.
> 注释:喉是一个中空器官,内含声带,位于喉结的后面。

volar *adjective* referring to the palm of the hand *or* sole of the foot 掌(侧)的,跖(侧)的

volatile *adjective* (liquid) which turns into gas at normal room temperature 挥发的,正常室温下由液体变成气体; **volatile oils** = concentrated oils from plants used in cosmetics and as antiseptics 挥发油,浓缩的植物油,用于化妆和消毒

volitantes 飞的 *see* 见 MUSCAE

volition *noun* ability to use the will 意志

Volkmann's canal *noun* canal running horizontally through compact bone, carrying blood to the Haversian systems 福尔克曼管,骨膜下容纳血管的小管

◇ **Volkmann's contracture** 福尔克曼氏挛缩 *see* 见 CONTRACTURE

volsella *or* **vulsella** *noun* type of forceps with hooks at the end of each arm 双爪钳

volume *noun* amount of a substance 容量; **blood volume** = total amount of blood in the body 血容量; **stroke volume** = amount of blood pumped out of a ventricle at each heartbeat 每搏输出量,每次心跳泵出的血量

voluntary *adjective* not forced *or* (action) done because one wishes to do it 自主的,随意的; **voluntary admission** = admitting a patient into a psychiatric hospital with the consent of the patient 自愿住院,在病人同意下收其入精神病院; **voluntary movement** = movement (such as walking *or* speaking) directed by the person's willpower, using voluntary muscles 随意肌运动; **voluntary muscles** = muscles which are moved by the willpower of the person acting through the brain 随意肌

> COMMENT: Voluntary muscles work in pairs, where one contracts and pulls, while the other relaxes to allow the bone to move.
> 注释:随意肌成对地工作,一个收缩牵拉而另一个放松使骨骼得以运动。

◇ **volunteer 1** *noun* person who offers to do something freely *or* without being paid 志愿者: ***The hospital relies on volunteers to help with sports for handicapped children.*** 医院依赖志愿者帮助残疾儿童运动。 ***They are asking for volunteers to test the new cold cure.*** 他们征求志愿者以便试用新的抗感冒治疗。 **2** *verb* to offer to do something freely 志愿: ***The research team volunteered to test the new drug on themselves.*** 研究小组志愿在自己身上试用新药。

volvulus *noun* condition where a loop of intestine is twisted and blocked, so cutting off its blood supply 肠扭转,肠襻扭曲阻塞,使自己的血运中断

vomer *noun* thin flat vertical bone in the septum of the nose 犁骨,鼻中隔上垂直的薄片状骨头

vomica *noun* (**a**) cavity in the lungs containing pus 肺脓腔 (**b**) vomiting pus from the throat or lungs 脓痰

vomit 1 *noun* vomitus, partly digested food which has been brought up into the mouth from the stomach 呕吐物: ***His bed was covered with vomit.*** 他的床上尽是呕吐物。 ***She died after choking on her own vomit.*** 她被自己的呕吐物噎死了。 **2** *verb* to bring up partly digested food from the stomach into the mouth 呕吐: ***He had a fever, and then started to vomit.*** 他发烧了,然后开始呕吐。 ***She vomited her breakfast.*** 她把早餐给吐出来了。

◇ **vomiting** *or* **emesis** *noun* being sick *or* bringing up vomit into the mouth 呕吐

◇ **vomitus** *noun* vomit 呕吐物

von Hippel-Lindau syndrome *noun* disease in which angiomas of the brain are related to angiomas and cysts in other parts of the body 冯希佩尔－井道综合征,脑视网膜血管瘤病

von Recklinghausen's disease *noun* 冯·雷克林霍曾氏病(**a**) = NEUROFIBROMATOSIS 神经纤维瘤病(**b**) osteitis fibrosa, weakness of the bones caused by excessive activity of the thyroid gland 纤维性骨炎

von Willebrand's disease *noun* hereditary blood disease (occurring in both sexes) where the mucous membrane starts to bleed without any apparent reason (involving a deficiency of a clotting factor in the blood, called 'von Willebrand's factor') von 冯·维勒布兰德氏病,遗传性血液病(两性均可患病),表现为粘膜自发性出血(血液中凝血因子即冯·维勒布兰德氏因子缺乏)

voyeurism *noun* condition where a person experiences sexual pleasure by watching others having intercourse 窥淫癖,以偷看别人性交而获得性快感

vu 相识 *see* 见 DEJA VU

vulgaris 寻常的 *see* 见 ACNE, LUPUS

vulnerable *adjective* likely to catch (a disease) because of being in a weakened state 易感的: ***Premature babies are especially vulnerable to infection*.** 早产儿特别容易感染传染病。

vulsella = VOLSELLA 双爪钳

vulv(o)- *prefix* referring to the vulva 外阴

◇ **vulva** *noun* a woman's external sexual organs, at the opening leading to the vagina 外阴 *see also* 参见 KRAUROSIS

> COMMENT: The vulva is formed of folds (the labia), surrounding the clitoris and the entrance to the vagina.
> 注释:外阴由皱褶(阴唇)形成,环绕着阴蒂和阴道口。

◇ **vulvectomy** *noun* surgical operation to remove the vulva 外阴切除术

◇ **vulvitis** *noun* inflammation of the vulva, causing intense irritation 外阴炎

◇ **vulvovaginitis** *noun* inflammation of the vulva and vagina 外阴阴道炎 (NOTE: for other terms referring to the vulva, see words beginning with **episio-**)

Ww

wad *noun* pad of material used to put on a wound 敷料垫: ***The nurse put a wad of absorbent cotton over the sore.*** 护士在伤口上敷了一块吸收力强的棉垫。

◇ **wadding** *noun* material used to make a wad 用来做敷料垫的棉垫: ***Put a layer of cotton wadding over the eye.*** 在眼睛上盖了一层棉垫。

waist *noun* narrow part of the body below the chest and above the buttocks 腰: ***He measures 85 centimetres around the waist.*** 他腰围 85 厘米。

wait *verb* to stay somewhere until something happens *or* someone arrives 等待: ***He has been waiting for his operation for six months.*** 他等待做手术已经 6 个月了。***There are ten patients waiting to see Dr Smith.*** 有 10 个病人等着史密斯医生看病。**waiting list** = list of patients waiting for admission to hospital usually for treatment of non-urgent disorders 待诊名单, 通常列的是非急诊的病人: ***The length of waiting lists for non-emergency surgery varies enormously from one region to another.*** 等待非急诊手术名单的长度因地区不同而差异很大。***It is hoped that hospital waiting lists will get shorter.*** 希望医院的待诊名单能够短点儿。**waiting room** = room at a doctor's *or* dentist's surgery where patients wait 候诊室, 等待手术的病人呆的房间: ***Please sit in the waiting room - the doctor will see you in ten minutes.*** 请坐在候诊室里, 10 分钟后医生会来看你。**waiting time** = period between the time when the name of a patient has been put on the waiting list and his admission into hospital 待入院时间, 从列入待诊名单到被收入院的时间

wake *verb* (i) to interrupt someone's sleep 唤醒 (ii) to stop sleeping 醒来: ***The nurse woke the patient*** *or* ***the patients was woken by the nurse.*** 护士叫醒了病人或病人被护士叫醒了。***The patient had to be woken to have his injection.*** 必须把病人叫醒才能给他注射。(NOTE: **wakes - waking - woke - has woken**)

◇ **wake up** *verb* to stop sleeping 醒来: ***The old man woke up in the middle of the night and started calling for the nurse.*** 老先生半夜醒来了, 并开始叫护士。

◇ **wakeful** *adjective* being wide awake *or* not wanting to sleep 醒着的

◇ **wakefulness** *noun* being wide awake 清醒, 无眠

Waldeyer's ring *noun* ring of lymphoid tissue made by the tonsils 瓦尔代尔扁桃体环

walk *verb* to go on foot 行走: ***The baby is learning to walk.*** 婴儿正在学走路。***He walked when he was only eleven months old.*** 他只有 11 个月大时就能走了。She can walk a few steps with a Zimmer. 她可以靠齐默拐的帮助走几步路了。

◇ **walking frame** *or* **walker** *noun* metal frame which is used to support someone who has difficulty in walking 助行拐

wall *noun* side part of an organ *or* a passage in the body 壁: ***An ulcer formed in the wall of the duodenum.*** 十二指肠壁形成了一个溃疡。***The doctor made an incision in the abdominal wall.*** 医生在腹壁上做了一个切口。***They removed a fibroma from the wall of the uterus*** *or* ***from the uterine wall.*** 他们从子宫壁里取掉了一个纤维瘤。

◇ **wall eye** *noun* eye which is very pale *or* eye which is squinting so strongly that only the white sclera is visible 白眼, 斜视很厉害只能见到眼白

Wangensteen tube *noun* tube which is passed into the stomach to remove the stomach's contents by suction 旺根斯滕管(通过吸引清除胃内容物)

ward *noun* room or set of rooms in a hospital, with beds for the patients 病房: ***He is in Ward 8B.*** 他在 8B 病房。***The children's ward is at the end of the corridor.*** 儿童病房在走廊的顶头。**ward sister** = senior nurse in charge of a ward 病房护士长;**accident ward** *or* **casualty ward** = ward for urgent accident victims 意外事故病房;**emergency ward** = ward for patients who require urgent attention 急诊病房;**geriatric ward** = ward for the treatment of geriatric patients 老年病房;**isolation ward** = special ward where patients suffering from dangerous infectious diseases can be kept isolated from other patients 隔离病房,隔离危险传染病人的特殊病房;**medical ward** = ward for patients who are not undergoing surgery 内科病房;**surgical ward** = ward for patients who have undergone surgery 外科病房

warm *adjective* quite hot *or* pleasantly hot 温暖的:***The patients need to be kept warm in cold weather.*** 寒冷的天气病人需要保暖。(NOTE: **warm - warmer - warmest**)

warn *verb* to tell someone that a danger is possible 警告:***The children were warned about the dangers of solvent abuse.*** 警告孩子们乱用溶剂的危险性。***The doctors warned her that her husband would not live more than a few weeks.*** 医生警告她,她丈夫活不了几周了。

◇ **warning** *noun* telling someone about a danger 警告:***There's a warning on the bottle of medicine, saying that it should be kept away from children.*** 药瓶上的警告说应远离儿童保存。***Each packet of cigarettes has a government health warning printed on it.*** 每个烟盒上都印有政府的健康警告。***The health department has given out warnings about the danger of hypothermia.*** 卫生部门已就低温的危险发出了警告。

wart *noun* verruca, a small hard benign growth on the skin 疣,皮肤上小而坚硬的良性赘生物;**common wart** = wart which appears mainly on the hands 寻常疣,主要长在手上,俗称瘊子;**plantar wart** = wart on the sole of the foot 跖疣,长在脚心的疣;**venereal wart** = wart on the genitals or in the urogenital area 性病湿疣或尖锐湿疣,长在生殖器或泌尿生殖区的疣

COMMENT: Warts are caused by a virus, and usually occur on the hands, feet or face.
注释:疣是病毒引起的,常发生于手、足或脸部。

washbasin *noun* bowl in a kitchen or bathroom where you can wash your hands 洗手池

Wassermann reaction (**WR**) *or* **Wassermann test** *noun* blood serum test to see if a patient has syphilis 瓦氏反应,用于检验梅毒感染的血清试验

waste 1 *adjective* (material *or* matter) which is useless *or* which has no use 无用的,废的:***The veins take blood containing waste carbon dioxide back into the lungs.*** 静脉血将废弃的二氧化碳运回肺。***Waste matter is excreted in the faeces or urine.*** 废物由粪便或尿排出体外。**waste product** = substance which is not needed in the body (and is excreted in urine *or* faeces) 废物,身体不再需要的物质(从尿和粪便中排出体外) **2** *verb* to use more than is needed 浪费:***The hospital kitchens waste a lot of food.*** 医院厨房浪费了大量食物。

◇ **waste away** *verb* to become thinner *or* to lose flesh 消瘦:***When he caught the disease he simply wasted away.*** 他患此病时,身体立刻就消瘦了。

◇ **wasting** *noun* condition where a person *or* a limb loses weight and becomes thin 消瘦,废用,人或肢体因不能正常活动而变瘦;**wasting disease** = disease which causes severe loss of weight *or* reduction in size (of an organ) 消瘦病

water 1 *noun* (**a**) common liquid which forms rain, rivers, the sea etc., and which makes up a large part of the body 水:***Can I have a glass of water please?*** 可以给我杯水吗?***They suffered dehydration from lack of water.*** 由于缺水他们脱水了。**water balance** = state where the water lost by the body (in urine *or* perspiration, etc.) is balanced by water absorbed from food and drink 水平衡,身体吸收的水和排出的水保持平衡;**water on the knee** = fluid in the knee joint under the kneecap, caused by a blow on the knee 膝关节积水 (**b**) urine 尿: ***He passed a lot of water during the night*** 他晚上尿了很多尿。***She noticed blood streaks in her water.*** 她在自己的尿中发现了血丝。***The nurse asked him to give a sample of his water.*** 护士让他留个尿样。(**c**) **the waters** = amniotic fluid, the fluid in the amnion in which a fetus floats 羊水 **2** *verb* to fill with tears *or* saliva 水汪汪, 泪汪汪: ***Onions made his eyes water.*** 洋葱弄得他眼泪汪汪。***Her mouth watered when she saw the ice cream.*** 她一见冰激淋就流口水。**watering eye** = eye which fills with tears because of an irritation 眼泪汪汪

◇ **water bed** *noun* mattress made of a large sack filled with water, used to prevent bedsores 水床, 用于防止褥疮

◇ **waterbrash** *noun* condition caused by dyspepsia, where there is a burning feeling in the stomach and the mouth suddenly fills with acid saliva 返胃

◇ **waterproof** *adjective* which will not let water through 防水的: ***Put a waterproof sheet on the baby's bed.*** 在婴儿床上放一个防水床单。

◇ **water sac** *or* **bag of waters** = AMNION 羊膜

◇ **waterworks** *noun* (*informal* 非正式) the urinary system 泌尿系统: ***There's nothing wrong with his waterworks.*** 他的泌尿系统没什么问题。

◇ **watery** *adjective* liquid, like water 水样的: ***He passed some watery stools.*** 他排了水样便。(NOTE: for other terms referring to water, see words beginning with **hydr-**)

> COMMENT: Since the body is formed of about 50% water, a normal adult needs to drink about 2.5 litres (5 pints) of fluid each day. Water taken into the body is passed out again as urine or sweat.
> 注释: 因为身体有 50% 是水分, 正常成人每天需要喝 2.5 升(5 品脱)水。摄入体内的水又以尿或汗的形式排出体外。

Waterhouse-Friderichsen syndrome *noun* condition caused by blood poisoning with meningococci, where the tissues of the adrenal glands die and haemorrhage 沃特豪斯-弗里德里希森综合征(暴发性脑膜炎球菌血症)。

Waterston's operation *noun* surgical operation to treat Fallot's tetralogy, where the right pulmonary artery is joined to the ascending aorta 华特斯顿手术, 治疗法四联症的手术, 将右肺动脉与升主动脉连接起来。

Watson knife *noun* type of very sharp surgical knife for skin transplants 沃森刀, 用于皮肤移植的很锋利的外科用刀

wax *noun* (**a**) soft yellow substance produced by bees *or* made from petroleum 蜡; **hot wax treatment** = treatment for arthritis in which the joints are painted with hot liquid wax 热蜡治疗, 在关节处涂热的液体蜡治疗关节炎 (**b**) **ear wax** *or* **cerumen** = wax which forms in the ear 耵聍, 耳垢

WBC = WHITE BLOOD CELL 白细胞

weak *adjective* not strong 弱的: ***After his illness he was very weak.*** 病后他很虚弱。***She is too weak to dress herself.*** 她虚弱得不能自己穿上衣服。***He is allowed to drink weak tea or coffee.*** 他被允许喝淡茶或咖啡。**weak pulse** = pulse which is not strong *or* which is not easy to feel 脉弱 (NOTE: **weak - weaker - weakest**)

◇ **weaken** *verb* to make something *or* someone weak; to become weak 削弱: ***He was weakened by the disease and could not resist further infection.*** 疾病使他的身体变弱了, 抵抗不了再次的感染。***The swelling is caused by a weakening of the wall of the artery.*** 膨出是由于动脉壁变弱造成的。

◇ **weakness** *noun* not being strong 弱: ***The doctor noticed the weakness of the patient's pulse.*** 医生注意到病人脉搏微弱。

weal *or* **wheal** *noun* small area of skin which swells because of a sharp blow *or* an insect bite 风团或风疹块, 皮肤小片肿胀, 由寒风刺激或昆虫叮咬引起

wean *verb* (i) to make a baby start to eat solid food after having only had liquids to drink 断奶 (ii) to make a baby start to drink from a bottle and start eating solid food after having been only breastfed 断奶后改用奶瓶并吃固体食物: ***The baby was breastfed for two months and then was gradually weaned onto the bottle.*** 给这个婴儿母乳喂养 2 个月后,渐渐改用奶瓶。

wear *verb* to become damaged through being used 磨损: ***The cartilage of the knee was worn from too much exercise.*** 膝关节的软骨因为运动过度而磨损了。(NOTE: **wears - wearing - wore - has worn**)

◇ **wear and tear** *noun* normal use which affects an organ 损耗, 消耗: ***A heart has to stand a lot of wear and tear.*** 心脏要经受很大的损耗。***The wear and tear of a strenuous job has begun to affect his heart.*** 高强度的工作已经开始影响他的心脏的健康了。

◇ **wear off** *verb* to disappear gradually 消散, 逐渐消失: ***The effect of the painkiller will wear off after a few hours.*** 镇痛药的作用几个小时后会逐渐消失。***He started to open his eyes, as the anaesthetic wore off.*** 当麻醉药的作用渐渐消失时,他开始睁开眼睛。

◇ **worn out** *adjective* very tired 筋疲力尽: ***He came home worn out after working all day in the hospital.*** 在医院工作了一整天后,他筋疲力尽地回到了家。***She was worn out by looking after all the children.*** 照看所有的孩子使她筋疲力尽。

Weber-Christian disease *noun* type of panniculitis where the liver and spleen become enlarged 韦-克氏病,结节性非化脓性脂膜炎,伴有肝脾增大

Weber's test *noun* test to see if both ears hear correctly, where a tuning fork is struck and the end placed on the head 韦伯试验,检测双耳听力是否都完好,击打音叉然后将柄放到额头上

Wegener's granulomatosis *noun* disease of connective tissue, where the nasal passages, lungs and kidneys are inflamed and ulcerated, with formation of granulomas; it is usually fatal 韦格纳芽肿病,一种结缔组织病,鼻腔、肺和肾发炎、溃疡,形成肉牙肿,通常是致命的

weigh *verb* (i) to measure how heavy something is 称重 (ii) to have a certain weight 重: ***The nurse weighed the baby on the scales.*** 护士在秤上称婴儿的体重。***She weighed seven pounds (3.5 kilos) at birth.*** 她出生时重 7 磅。*A woman weighs less than a man of similar height.* 身高差不多时女性比男性轻些。*The doctor asked him how much he weighed.* 医生问他有多重。*I weigh 120 pounds or **I weigh 54 kilos**.* 我重 120 磅(54 千克)。

◇ **weight** *noun* (**a**) how heavy a person is 体重: ***What's the patient's weight?*** 病人的体重是多少? ***Her weight is only 105 pounds.*** = She weighs only 105 pounds. 她的体重只有 105 磅。**to lose weight** = to get thinner 体重下降: ***She's trying to lose weight before she goes on holiday.*** 度假前她试图减轻体重。**to put on weight** = to become fatter 增重: ***He's put on a lot of weight in the last few months.*** 最近几个月他体重长了不少。**weight gain** *or* **gain in weight** = becoming fatter *or* heavier 增重, 长膘; **weight loss** = action of losing weight *or* of becoming thinner 体重下降: ***Weight loss can be a symptom of certain types of cancer.*** 体重下降可以是某些癌症的症状。(**b**) something which is heavy 重物: ***Don't lift heavy weights, you may hurt your back.*** 不要抬重物,会伤着你的背。

◇ **weightlessness** *noun* state where the body seems to weigh nothing (as experienced by astronauts) 失重状态,身体似乎没什么分量(如宇航员所经历的失重)

Weil-Felix reaction *or* **Weil-Felix test** *noun* test to see if the patient has typhus, where the patient's serum is tested for antibodies against *Proteus vulgaris* 外-斐氏反应(试验),通过检查病人血清里的抗普通变形菌抗体检测病人是否有斑疹伤寒

Weil's disease = LEPTOSPIROSIS 韦尔氏病,钩端螺旋体病

welder's flash *noun* condition where the eye is badly damaged by very bright light 电光性眼炎

welfare *noun* (**a**) good health *or* good living conditions 健康: ***They look after the welfare of the old people in the town.*** 他们在镇上照料老人们的健康。(**b**) money paid by the government to people who need it 福利: ***He exists on welfare payments.*** 他靠福利费生存。

well *adjective* healthy 健康的: ***He's not a well man.*** 他不是个健康的人。***You're looking very well after your holiday.*** 你度完假后看上去很健康。***He's quite well again after his flu.*** 感冒后他的身体又很好了。***He's not very well, and has had to stay in bed.*** 他身体不太好,不得不卧床休息。**well-woman clinic** = clinic which specializes in preventive medicine for women (such as breast screening and cervical smear tests) and gives advice on pregnancy, contraception, the menopause, etc. 妇女保健所,为妇女特设的预防医学诊所(如做乳腺扫描和宫颈涂片检查)并对怀孕、避孕及绝经等做健康咨询

◊ **wellbeing** *noun* being in good health *or* in good living conditions 健康: ***She is responsible for the wellbeing of the patients under her care.*** 她对自己护理的病人健康负责。

wen *noun* cyst which forms in a sebaceous gland 皮脂腺囊肿

Wernicke's encephalopathy *noun* condition caused by lack of vitamin B (often in alcoholics), where the patient is delirious, moves his eyes about rapidly (nystagmus), walks unsteadily and is subject to constant vomiting 韦尼克脑病,缺乏维生素 B 引起,常见于慢性酒精中毒的患者,病人谵妄,眼球快速运动(眼震),步态不稳并持续呕吐

Wertheim's operation *noun* type of hysterectomy *or* surgical operation to remove the womb, the lymph nodes which are next to it, and most of the vagina, the ovaries and the tubes, as treatment for cancer of the womb 韦特海姆手术、根治性子宫切除术,将子宫、子宫旁淋巴结、阴道的大部分和卵巢及输卵管全部切除,用于治疗子宫癌

wet 1 *adjective* not dry *or* covered in liquid 湿的: ***He got wet waiting for the bus in the rain and caught a cold.*** 他在雨中等公共汽车淋了个透湿,感冒了。***The baby has nappy rash from wearing a wet nappy.*** 婴儿因为湿尿布而得了尿布疹。**wet burn** = scald, an injury to the skin caused by touching a very hot liquid *or* steam 湿性烫伤,接触热的液体或蒸汽而烫伤 (NOTE: **wet - wetter - wettest**) 2 *verb* to urinate (in bed) 尿床: ***He is eight years old and he still wets his bed every night.*** 他 8 岁了,还每天晚上尿床。*see also* 参见 BEDWETTING

◊ **wet dressing** *noun* 湿敷料 *see* 见 COMPRESS

Wharton's duct *noun* duct which takes saliva into the mouth from the salivary glands under the lower jaw *or* submandibular salivary glands 沃顿管,下颌唾液腺通向口腔的导管

Wharton's jelly *noun* jelly-like tissue in the umbilical cord 沃顿胶,脐带里的胶样组织

wheal = WEAL 轮

wheel *verb* to push along something which has wheels 推(车,轮椅): ***The orderly wheeled the trolley into the operating theatre.*** 护理员推着平车进了手术室

◊ **wheelchair** *noun* chair with wheels in which an invalid can sit and move around 轮椅: ***He manages to get around in a wheelchair.*** 他在轮椅里转了个身。***She has been confined to a wheelchair since her accident.*** 事故后她一直不能离开轮椅。

Wheelhouse's operation *or* **urethrotomy** *noun* surgical operation to relieve blockage of the urethra by making an incision into the urethra 惠尔豪斯手术,尿道切开术

wheeze 1 *noun* whistling noise in the bronchi 喘鸣音: ***The doctor listened to his wheezes.*** 医生在听他的喘鸣音。2 *verb* to make a whistling sound when breathing 发出喘鸣: ***When she has an attack of asthma, she wheezes and has difficulty in breathing.*** 当她哮喘发作时,她发出喘鸣音,而且呼吸困难。

◇ **wheezing** *noun* whistling noise in the bronchi when breathing 喘鸣

◇ **wheezy** *adjective* making a whistling sound when breathing 喘鸣的: ***He was quite wheezy when he stopped running.*** 他跑步停下后喘得很厉害。

> COMMENT: Wheezing is often found in asthmatic patients and is also associated with bronchitis and heart disease.
> 注释:喘鸣常发生于哮喘病人,也可出现于支气管炎和心脏病患者。

whiplash injury *noun* injury to the vertebrae in the neck, caused when the head jerks backwards, often occurring in a car that is struck from behind 甩鞭伤,颈部猛的向后甩造成颈椎受伤,常发生于汽车被从后面撞击时。

Whipple's disease *noun* disease where the patient has difficulty in absorbing nutrients and passes fat in the faeces, where the joints are inflamed and the lymph glands enlarged 惠普尔病或脂肪泻,病人不能吸收脂肪所致,还有关节发炎和淋巴腺肿大

Whipple's operation = PANCREATECTOMY 惠普尔手术,胰腺切除术

whipworm *noun* *Trichuris*, thin round parasitic worm which infests the caecum 鞭虫,感染盲肠的扁圆的寄生虫

whisper 1 *noun* speaking very quietly 轻声说,耳语: ***She has a sore throat and can only speak in a whisper.*** 她嗓子疼,只能轻声说话。**2** *verb* to speak in a very quiet voice 悄声说,耳语: ***He whispered to the nurse that he wanted something to drink.*** 他悄声对护士说他想要点儿喝的。

white 1 *adjective & noun* of a colour like snow or milk 白色,白色的: ***White patches developed on his skin.*** 他的皮肤出现白色斑片。***Her hair has turned quite white.*** 她的头发变白了不少。**white blood cell (WBC)** *or* **leucocyte** = blood cell which contains a nucleus, is formed in bone marrow, and creates antibodies 白细胞,骨髓生成的血细胞,可以产生抗体; **white commissure** = part of the white matter in the spinal cord near the central canal 白质联合,脊髓中央管周围的白质; **white leg** *or* **milk leg** *or* **phlegmasia alba dolens** = acute oedema of the leg, a condition which affects women after childbirth, where a leg becomes pale and inflamed as a result of lymphatic obstruction 股白肿,腿部急性水肿,侵及产妇,由淋巴阻塞导致腿苍白发炎; **white matter** = nerve tissue in the central nervous system which contains more myelin than grey matter 白质,中枢神经系统中的神经组织,比灰质含有的髓鞘多 (NOTE: **white - whiter - whitest**) **2** *noun* main part of the eye which is white 眼白: ***The whites of his eyes turned yellow when he developed jaundice.*** 他发生黄疸时眼白变黄 *see also* 参见 LEUCORRHOEA

whitlow *or* **felon** *noun* inflammation caused by infection, near the nail in the fleshy part of the tip of a finger 瘭疽,化脓性指头炎,指尖近指甲的皮肉部分感染所致的炎症 *see also* 参见 PARONYCHIA

WHO = WORLD HEALTH ORGANIZATION 世界卫生组织

whoop *noun* loud noise made when inhaling by a person suffering from whooping cough 哮咳,患百日咳时吸气发出的很响的声音

◇ **whooping cough** *or* **pertussis** *noun* infectious disease caused by *Bordetella pertussis* affecting the bronchial tubes, common in children, and sometimes very serious 百日咳,百日咳球杆菌引起的感染性疾病,侵及支气管,常见于儿童,有时十分严重

> COMMENT: The patient coughs very badly and makes a characteristic 'whoop' when he breathes in after a coughing fit. Whooping cough can lead to pneumonia, and is treated with antibiotics. Vaccination against whooping cough is given to infants.
> 注释:病人咳得很厉害,咳嗽发作后吸气时

呈典型的哮咳。百日咳可导致肺炎,可用抗生素治疗。要给婴儿注射预防百日咳的疫苗。

Widal reaction *or* **Widal test** *noun* test to detect typhoid fever 肥达反应(试验),检测伤寒热的试验

COMMENT: A sample of the patient's blood is put into a solution containing typhoid bacilli or anti-typhoid serum is added to a sample of bacilli from the patient's faeces. If the bacilli agglutinate (i.e. form into groups) this indicates that the patient is suffering from typhoid fever.
注释:把病人的血放入含有伤寒杆菌的溶液中或将抗伤寒血清加入病人粪便中,如果杆菌凝集(即成群)说明病人患有伤寒。

widen *verb* to make wider 扩宽: ***This is an operation to widen the blood vessels near the heart.*** 这是一次扩张心脏附近血管的手术

◊ **widespread** *adjective* affecting a large area *or* a large number of people 广泛传播的: ***The government advised widespread immunization.*** 政府倡导大面积免疫。***Glaucoma is widespread in the northern part of the country.*** 青光眼是这个国家北部广泛流行的一种病。

will *noun* power of the mind to decide to do something 意愿

◊ **willpower** *noun* having a strong will 毅力: ***The patient showed the willpower to start walking again unaided.*** 病人表现出想要重新独立行走的毅力。

Willis 威利斯 *see* 见 CIRCLE OF WILLIS

Wilms' tumour = NEPHROBLASTOMA 维尔姆斯瘤,肾母细胞瘤

Wilson's disease *noun* hepatolenticular degeneration, hereditary disease where copper deposits accumulate in the liver and the brain, causing cirrhosis 威尔逊病,肝豆状核变性,为遗传性疾病,因铜在肝脏和脑内沉积造成肝硬化

wind *noun* (i) flatus, gas which forms in the digestive system 胃肠气 (ii) flatulence, accumulation of gas in the digestive system 胃肠胀气: ***The baby is suffering from wind.*** 婴儿胃肠胀气。***He has pains in the stomach caused by wind.*** 他因为胃肠胀气而胃疼。**to break wind** = to bring up gas from the stomach *or* to let gas escape from the anus 嗳气或排气

◊ **windchill factor** *noun* way of calculating the risk of exposure in cold weather by adding the speed of the wind to the number of degrees of temperature below zero 风寒指数,将风速与低于零度的气温相加,用于计算暴露于寒冷天气下的危险度

◊ **windpipe** *or* **trachea** *noun* main air passage from the nose and mouth to the lungs 气管

window *noun* small opening in the ear 窗,此处特指内耳螺旋管上的小窗; **oval window** *or* **fenestra ovalis** = oval-shaped opening between the middle ear and the inner ear, closed by a membrane and covered by the base of the stapes 卵圆窗,内耳和中耳之间的卵圆形的开口,由一层膜封闭并被镫骨底覆盖; **round window** *or* **fenestra rotunda** = round opening closed by a membrane, between the middle ear and the cochlea 圆窗,中耳和耳蜗之间的圆形开口,由一层膜封闭着 ◊ 见图 EAR

wink *verb* to close one eye and open it again rapidly 眨眼

wisdom tooth *noun* third molar, one of the four teeth in the back of the jaw, which only appears at about the age of 20 and sometimes does not appear at all 智齿,第三磨牙,共有 4 颗,在颌骨后部,只有到 20 岁左右才出现,有的人根本不出 ◊ 见图 TEETH

witch hazel *or* **hamamelis** *noun* lotion made from the bark of a tree, used to check bleeding and harden inflamed tissue and bruises 北美金缕梅,树皮中提出的洗剂

withdraw *verb* (**a**) to stop being interested in the world *or* to become isolated 退缩: ***The patient withdrew into himself and refused to eat.*** 病人自闭,且拒绝进食。(**b**) to remove (a drug) *or* to stop (a treatment) 停药,撤药: ***The doctor decided to withdraw the drug from the patient.*** 医生决定给这个病人停药。(NOTE: **withdrawing- withdrew- has withdrawn**)

◇ **withdrawal** *noun* (i) removing of interest *or* becoming isolated 退缩 (ii) removal of a drug *or* treatment 停药,撤药; **withdrawal symptom** = unpleasant physical condition (vomiting *or* headaches *or* fever) which occurs when a patient stops taking an addictive drug 戒断症状,病人停用一种成瘾性药物后发生的身体不适(呕吐、头疼、发热)

> QUOTE: She was in the early stages of physical withdrawal from heroin and showed classic symptoms: sweating, fever, sleeplessness and anxiety.
> 引文:她处在停用海洛因的戒断早期,表现出典型的症状:出汗、发热、失眠和焦虑。
> **Nursing Times** 护理时代

woman *noun* female adult person 妇女: ***It is a common disease of women of 45 to 60 years of age.*** 这是40岁到60岁女性的常见病。 ***On average, women live longer than men.*** 女性平均寿命比男性长。 **women's ward** *or* **women's hospital** = ward *or* hospital for female patients 妇科病房,妇科医院 *see also* 参见 WELL-WOMAN CLINIC (NOTE: plural is **women.** Note also that for other terms referring to women, see words beginning with **gyn-**)

womb *noun* uterus, hollow organ in a woman's pelvic cavity in which a fertilized ovum develops into a fetus 子宫,女性盆腔里的空腔脏器,受精卵在其中发育成胚胎(NOTE: for other terms referring to the womb, see words beginning with **hyster-, hystero-, metr-, metro-, utero-**)

wood *noun* material that comes from trees 木头; **wood alcohol** = methyl alcohol, a poisonous alcohol used as fuel 木醇或甲醇,用作燃料,有毒

Wood's lamp *noun* lamp which allows a doctor to see fluorescence in the hair of a patient suffering from fungal infection 伍德灯,用于检查毛发真菌感染的荧光灯

woolsorter's disease *noun* form of anthrax which affects the lungs 拣毛工病,肺炭疽病

word *noun* separate piece of language, in writing and speech, not joined to other separate pieces 词语: ***There are seven words in this sentence.*** 这句话中有7个词。

◇ **word blindness** 字盲 *see* 见 ALEXIA

World Health Organization (WHO) *noun* organization (part of the United Nations Organization) which aims to improve health in the world by teaching *or* publishing information, etc. 世界卫生组织,联合国的机构之一,旨在通过教育、发布信息促进全世界健康水平的提高

worm *noun* long thin animal with no legs or backbone, which can infest the human body, especially the intestines 蠕虫,细长无腿,无脊柱的动物,可感染人体尤其是肠道 *compare* 比较 RINGWORM *see also* 参见 FLATWORM, HOOKWORM, ROUNDWORM, TAPEWORM, WHIPWORM

wound 1 *noun* damage to external tissue which allows blood to escape 创伤,伤口: ***He had a knife wound in his leg.*** 他的腿上有刀伤。 ***The doctors sutured the wound in his chest.*** 医生缝合了他胸部的伤口。 **contused wound** = wound caused by a blow, where the skin is bruised, torn and bleeding 挫伤,打击造成皮肤青肿、撕裂并出血; **gunshot wound** = wound caused by a pellet *or* bullet from a gun 枪伤; **incised wound** = wound with clear edges, caused by a sharp knife or razor 切割伤; **lacerated wound** = wound where the skin is torn 撕裂伤; **puncture wound** = wound made by a sharp point which makes a hole in the flesh 穿刺伤 2 *verb* to harm someone by making a hole in the tissue of the body 弄伤: ***He was wounded three times in the head.*** 他的头受过伤三次。

WR = WASSERMANN REACTION 瓦氏反应(检测梅毒)

wrinkle *noun* fold in the skin 皱褶,皱纹:***Old people have wrinkles on the neck.*** 老人颈部有皱褶。***She had a face lift to remove wrinkles.*** 她仰起脸以拉平皱纹。

◊ **wrinkled** *adjective* covered with wrinkles 有皱褶的,有皱纹的

wrist *noun* joint between the hand and forearm 腕部:***He sprained his wrist and can't play tennis tomorrow.*** 他扭伤了手腕,明天不能打网球了。**wrist drop** = paralysis of the wrist muscles, where the hand hangs limp, caused by damage to the radial nerve in the upper arm 腕下垂,上肢桡神经受损导致的腕部肌肉瘫痪,手从胳膊上垂下来 (NOTE: for other terms referring to the wrist, see words beginning with **carp-**) ◊ 见图 HAND

COMMENT: The wrist is formed of eight small bones in the hand which articulate with the bones in the forearm. The joint allows the hand to rotate and move downwards and sideways. The joint is easily fractured or sprained.
注释:腕部由8块小骨头组成,它们与前臂的骨骼形成腕关节。腕关节使手可以旋转,向下和向侧面运动。腕关节容易骨折或扭伤。

writer's cramp *noun* painful spasm of the muscles in the forearm and hand which comes from writing too much 书写痉挛,由于写字太多造成前臂和手部肌肉疼痛性痉挛

writhe *verb* 扭动;**to writhe in pain** = to twist and turn because the pain is very severe 因疼痛扭动

wry neck *or* **wryneck** *noun* torticollis, deformity of the neck, where the head is twisted to one side by contraction of the sternocleidomastoid muscle 斜颈,由于胸锁乳突肌收缩造成头部扭向一侧,是一种颈部畸形

Wuchereria *noun* type of tiny nematode worm which infests the lymph system, causing elephantiasis 吴策线虫,侵及淋巴系统造成象皮肿

Xx

xanth- *or* **xantho-** *prefix* meaning yellow 黄色

◇ **xanthaemia** = CAROTENAEMIA 胡萝卜素血(症)

◇ **xanthelasma** *noun* formation of little yellow fatty tumours on the eyelids 黄斑瘤,眼睑上小的黄色脂肪瘤

◇ **xanthochromia** *noun* yellow colour of the skin as in jaundice 黄变,黄染,如黄疸时的皮肤黄染

◇ **xanthoma** *noun* yellow fatty mass (often on the eyelids and hands), found in patients with a high level of cholesterol in the blood 黄瘤,黄色的脂肪团(常见于眼睑和手),血液中胆固醇水平高的病人中可见此症 (NOTE: plural is **xanthomata**)

◇ **xanthomatosis** *noun* condition where several small masses of yellow fatty substance appear in the skin or some internal organs, caused by an excess of fat in the body 黄瘤病,皮肤或内脏多处出现小的黄色脂肪团,由体内脂肪过多引起。

◇ **xanthopsia** *noun* disorder of the eyes, making everything appear yellow 黄视症,看什么都是黄色的,是眼病造成的

◇ **xanthosis** *noun* yellow colouring of the skin, caused by eating too much food containing carotene 黄皮症,进食太多的胡萝卜素所致

X chromosome *noun* sex chromosome X染色体,性染色体的一种

> COMMENT: Every person has a series of pairs of chromosomes, one of which is always an X chromosome; a normal female has one pair of XX chromosomes, while a male has one XY pair. Defective chromosomes affect sexual development: a person with an XO chromosome pair (i. e. one X chromosome alone) has Turner's syndrome; a person with an extra X chromosome (making an XXY set) has Klinefelter's syndrome. Haemophilia is a disorder linked to the X chromosome.
> 注释:每个人都有一套成对染色体,其中总有一对中含有X染色体;正常女性有一对XX染色体,正常男性有一对XY染色体。染色体缺陷影响性发育:只有一个X染色体的人得特纳综合征;多出一个X染色体(XXY)者得Klinefelter综合征。血友病是与X染色体连锁性疾病。

xeno- *prefix* meaning different 不同

◇ **xenograft** *or* **heterograft** *noun* tissue taken from an individual of one species and grafted on an individual of another species 异种移植 (NOTE: the opposite is **homograft** *or* **allograft**)

xero- *prefix* meaning dry 干燥

◇ **xeroderma** *noun* skin disorder where dry scales form on the skin 干皮病

◇ **xerophthalmia** *noun* condition of the eye, where the cornea and conjunctiva become dry because of lack of Vitamin 干眼病,角膜和结膜干燥,由于缺乏维生素A引起

◇ **xeroradiography** *noun* X-ray technique used in producing mammograms on selenium plates 干板X线照相术,利用硒板使乳腺显影的一种X线技术

◇ **xerosis** *noun* abnormally dry condition (of skin *or* mucous membrane) 干燥(病)

◇ **xerostomia** *noun* dryness of the mouth, caused by lack of saliva 口腔干燥

xiphisternum *or* **xiphoid process** *or* **xiphoid cartilage** *noun* bottom part of the breastbone *or* sternum, which in young people is formed of cartilage and becomes bone only by middle age 剑突,胸骨下端的部分,年轻时是软骨的,到中年变成骨性的。

◇ **xiphisternal plane** *noun* imaginary horizontal line across the middle of the chest at the point where the xiphoid process starts 剑突平面,想象中的与剑突开始处水平的平面

X-ray 1 *noun* (**a**) ray with a very short wavelength, which is invisible, but can go through soft tissue and register as a photograph on a film 伦琴射线，X线，一种不可见的，波长很短的射线，可以穿透软组织并在胶片上留下影像：***The X-ray examination showed the presence of a tumour in the colon.*** ***X*** 线检查显示结肠内有肿瘤。***The X-ray department is closed for lunch.*** 放射科午餐时关闭。(**b**) photograph taken using X-rays X线摄影：***The dentist took some X-rays of the patient's teeth.*** 牙医给病人的牙齿照了 ***X*** 线片。***He pinned the X-rays to the light screen.*** 他把 ***X*** 线片别到看片灯上。***All the staff had to have chest X-rays.*** 所有工作人员都得照胸片。**2** *verb* to take an X-ray photograph of a patient 照(X线片)：***There are six patients waiting to be X-rayed.*** 有6个病人等着照 *X* 线片。

COMMENT: Because X-rays go through soft tissue, it is sometimes necessary to make internal organs opaque so that they will show up on the film. In the case of stomach X-rays, patients take a barium meal before being photographed (contrast radiography); in other cases, such as kidney X-rays, radioactive substances are injected into the bloodstream or into the organ itself. X-rays are used not only in radiography for diagnosis but as a treatment in radiotherapy. Excessive exposure to X-rays, either as a patient being treated, or as a radiographer, can cause radiation sickness.

注释：因为X线可以通过软组织，有时必须使内脏器官变成不透射线以便在胶片上显影。如果是胃，病人照相前服钡餐(增强对比X线片)；其它情况下，如给肾脏照X线片，则向血液或直接向器官中注射放射性物质。X线不仅因摄片用于诊断目的，还可以用于放射治疗。过多地暴露于X线，不管是作为接受治疗的病人还是放射科医师，都可以导致放射病。

xylose *noun* pentose which has not been metabolized 木糖，未代谢的戊糖

Yy

yawn **1** *noun* reflex action when tired *or* sleepy, where the mouth is opened wide and after a deep intake of air, the breath exhaled slowly 打哈欠: ***His yawns made everyone feel sleepy.*** 他一打哈欠使每个人都感到困了。**2** *verb* to open the mouth wide and breathe in deeply and then breathe out slowly 打哈欠

> COMMENT: Yawning can be caused by tiredness as the body prepares for sleep, but it can have other causes, such as a hot room, or even can be started by unconsciously imitating someone who is yawning near you.
> 注释:当身体准备睡觉时,出于疲乏可 以引起打哈欠,但也可以是其他原因引起的,如屋里热,甚至可以是出于无意识地模仿旁边打哈欠的人。

yaws *noun* framboesia *or* pian, a tropical disease caused by the spirochaete *Treponema pertenue* 雅司病,雅司螺旋体引起的热带病

> COMMENT: Symptoms include fever with raspberry-like swellings on the skin, followed in later stages by bone deformation.
> 注释:症状包括发热,伴有山莓样皮肤肿胀,后期出现骨骼变形。

Y chromosome *noun* male chromosome Y染色体,雄性染色体

> COMMENT: The Y chromosome has male characteristics and does not form part of the female genetic structure. A normal male has an XY pair of chromosomes. See also the note at X CHROMOSOME.
> 注释:Y染色体具有男性性征,不是女性基因结构的组成部分。正常男性具有一对XY染色体。参见 X CHROMOSOME。

yeast *noun* fungus which is used in the fermentation of alcohol and in making bread 酵母菌,用于酒精和面包发酵的真菌

> COMMENT: Yeast is a good source of Vitamin B and can be taken in dried form in tablets.
> 注释:酵母菌是维生素B的优良来源,可以制成干的片剂。

yellow *adjective* & *noun* of a colour like that of the sun or of gold 黄色,黄色的: ***His skin turned yellow when he had hepatitis.*** 他得肝炎时皮肤变成黄色。***The whites of the eyes become yellow as a symptom of jaundice.*** 眼白变成黄色是黄疸的症状。**yellow atrophy** = old name for severe damage to the liver 黄色萎缩,严重肝坏死的旧称; **yellow fibres** *or* **elastic fibres** = fibres made of elastin, which can expand easily and are found in the skin and in the walls of arteries or the lungs 黄色纤维,弹力纤维,弹性蛋白组成的纤维,易于拉伸,见于皮肤、动脉壁或肺; **yellow spot** *or* **macula lutea** = yellow patch on the retina of the eye around the fovea 黄斑,视网膜中央凹周围的黄色斑片

◊ **yellow fever** *noun* infectious disease, found especially in Africa and South America, caused by an arbovirus carried by the mosquito *Aedes aegypti* 黄热病,非洲和南美洲的一种传染病,由虫媒病毒引起,经埃及伊蚊传播

> COMMENT: The fever affects the liver and causes jaundice. There is no known cure for yellow fever and it can be fatal, but vaccination can prevent it.
> 注释:发热影响肝脏病造成黄疸。黄热病现无有效的疗法,此病可以是致命的,但注射疫苗可以起到预防作用。

Yersinia pestis *noun* bacterium which causes plague 鼠疫耶尔森菌,引起鼠疫的细菌

yolk sac = VITELLINE SAC 卵黄囊

yuppie flu *noun* (*informal* 非正式) = MYALGIC ENCEPHALOMYELITIS 肌痛性脑脊髓炎

Zz

Zadik's operation *noun* surgical operation to remove the whole of an ingrowing toenail Zadik 手术，去掉整个嵌甲的手术

zidovudine *noun* azidothymidine *or* AZT, a drug used in the treatment of AIDS 齐多夫定，一种治疗艾滋病的药物

COMMENT: There is no cure for AIDS but this drug may help to slow its progress.
注释：目前没有治愈艾滋病的药物，但此药可以起到帮助减缓疾病的进程。

Zimmer (frame) *noun* trade mark for a metal frame used by patients who have difficulty in walking 齐默尔拐，给行走困难者设计的一种金属拐的商品名：***She managed to walk some steps with a Zimmer.*** 她试着靠齐默尔拐走了几步。

zinc *noun* white metallic trace element 锌 (NOTE: chemical symbol is **Zn**)

◊ **zinc ointment** *noun* soothing ointment made of zinc oxide and oil 氧化锌软膏

◊ **zinc oxide (ZnO)** *noun* compound of zinc and oxygen, which forms a soft white soothing powder used in creams and lotions 氧化锌白色粉末，可制成软膏和洗剂，外用于皮肤病

Z line *noun* part of the pattern of muscle tissue, a dark line seen in the light I band *Z* 带，肌肉组织中的暗色线

Zn *chemical symbol for* zinc 锌的化学元素符号

Zollinger-Ellison syndrome *noun* condition where tumours are formed in the islet cells of the pancreas together with peptic ulcers 革-艾二氏综合征，胰岛细胞瘤伴发消化性溃疡

zona *noun* (**a**) = HERPES ZOSTER 带状疱疹 (**b**) zone *or* area 带，区；**zona pellucida** = membrane which forms around an ovum 透明带，卵子周围的膜

zone *noun* area of the body 区域；**erogenous zone** = part of the body which, if stimulated, produces sexual arousal (such as the penis *or* clitoris *or* nipples) 性欲发生区，受刺激时能引起性唤起的身体部位，如阴茎、阴蒂、乳头

zonula *or* **zonule** *noun* small area of the body 小带；**zonule of Zinn** = suspensory ligament of the lens of the eye 秦氏小带，睫状小带，晶状体的悬韧带

◊ **zonulolysis** *noun* removal of a zonule by dissolving it 睫状小带松解术

zoonosis *noun* disease which a human can catch from an animal 动物源性疾病，人从动物身上传染来的病 (NOTE: plural is **zoonoses**)

zoster 带状疱疹 *see* 见 HERPES ZOSTER

zygoma *noun* (i) zygomatic arch 颧弓 (ii) zygomatic bone *or* cheekbone 颧骨 (NOTE: the plural is **zygomata**)

◊ **zygomatic** *adjective* referring to the zygoma 颧骨的，颧弓的；**zygomatic arch** *or* **zygoma** = ridge of bone across the temporal bone, running between the ear and the bottom of the eye socket 颧弓；从耳到眼窝底的骨性嵴，跨在颞骨上；**zygomatic bone** = cheekbone *or* malar bone *or* bone which forms the prominent part of the cheek and the lower part of the eye socket 颧骨；**zygomatic process** = one of the bony projections which form the zygomatic arch 颧突形成颧弓的骨性突起 ◊ 见图 SKULL

zygomycosis *noun* disease caused by a fungus which infests the blood vessels in the lungs 接合菌病，真菌感染肺血管所致的疾病

zygote *noun* fertilized ovum, the first stage of development of an embryo 合子，受精卵

zym(o)- *prefix* meaning (i) enzymes 酶 (ii) fermentation 发酵

◊ **zymogen** = PROENZYME 前酶，酶原

◊ **zymosis** *noun* fermentation, the process where carbohydrates are broken down by enzymes and produce alcohol 发酵，碳水化合物被酶分解产生酒精的过程

◊ **zymotic** *adjective* referring to zymosis 发酵的

SUPPLEMENT

附　　录

ANATOMICAL TERMS

The body is always described as if standing upright with the palms of the hands facing forward. There is only one central vertical plane, termed the *median* or *sagittal* plane, and this passes through the body from front to back. Planes parallel to this on either side are *parasagittal* or *paramedian* planes. Vertical planes at right angles to the median are called *coronal* planes. The term horizontal (or *transverse*) plane speaks for itself. Two specific horizontal planes are (a) the *transpyloric*, midway between the suprasternal notch and the symphysis pubis, and (b) the *transtubercular* or *intratubercular* plane, which passes through the tubercles of the iliac crests. Many other planes are named from the structures they pass through.

Views of the body from some different points are shown on the diagram; a view of the body from above is called the *superior aspect*, and that from below is the *inferior aspect*.

Cephalic means toward the head; *caudal* refers to positions (or in a direction) towards the tail. *Proximal* and *distal* refer to positions respectively closer to and further from the centre of the body in any direction, while *lateral* and *medial* relate more specifically to relative sideways positions, and also refer to movements. *Ventral* refers to the abdomen, front or anterior, while *dorsal* relates to the back of a part or organ. The hand has a *dorsal* and a *palmar* surface, and the foot a *dorsal* and a *plantar* surface.

Note that *flexion of the thigh* moves it forward while *flexion of the leg* moves it backwards; the movements of *extension* are similarly reversed. Movement and rotation of limbs can be *medial*, which is with the front moving towards the centre line, or *lateral*, which is in the opposite direction. Specific terms for limb movements are *adduction*, towards the centre line, and *abduction*, which is away from the centre line. Other specific terms are *supination* and *pronation* for the hand, and *inversion* and *eversion* for the foot.

解剖学术语

描述人体时通常取身体直立,手掌向前的姿势。此时所见的横贯身体前后,位于正中的垂直平面称为正中面或矢状面。与此面平行,位于两侧的是旁矢状面或旁正中面。与正中面呈直角的垂直平面称为冠状面。水平面(横断面)顾名思义就是与水平面平行的平面,有两个比较重要的水平面分别是(1)经幽门水平面,经胸骨上切迹的平面;(2)经结节(结节间)水平面,穿过髂嵴结节的平面。同理,根据平面所穿过的人体结构还可命名许多不同的水平面。

图例还绘出了从不同角度的观察所见。从上往下看人体称为上面观,从下往上看称下面观。

头端指朝向头部,尾端指位于或朝向尾部。近端或远端用来指某位置在任何方向上是相对靠近还是远离身体的中心,而外侧或内侧则多专门用来描述处于两侧的位置,也可用来描述运动方向。腹面指前面,背面指某一部分或器官的后面。手有背面和掌面,脚有背面和跖面。

注意,大腿屈曲是向前,而小腿屈曲是向后,伸展则恰与此相反。肢体运动或旋转时面朝前向躯体的中线称为向内侧,反之为向外侧。描述肢体运动的专用术语有内收和外展,分别指朝向或远离躯体中线。另外还有描述手部运动的旋前、旋后,以及脚的内翻,外翻。

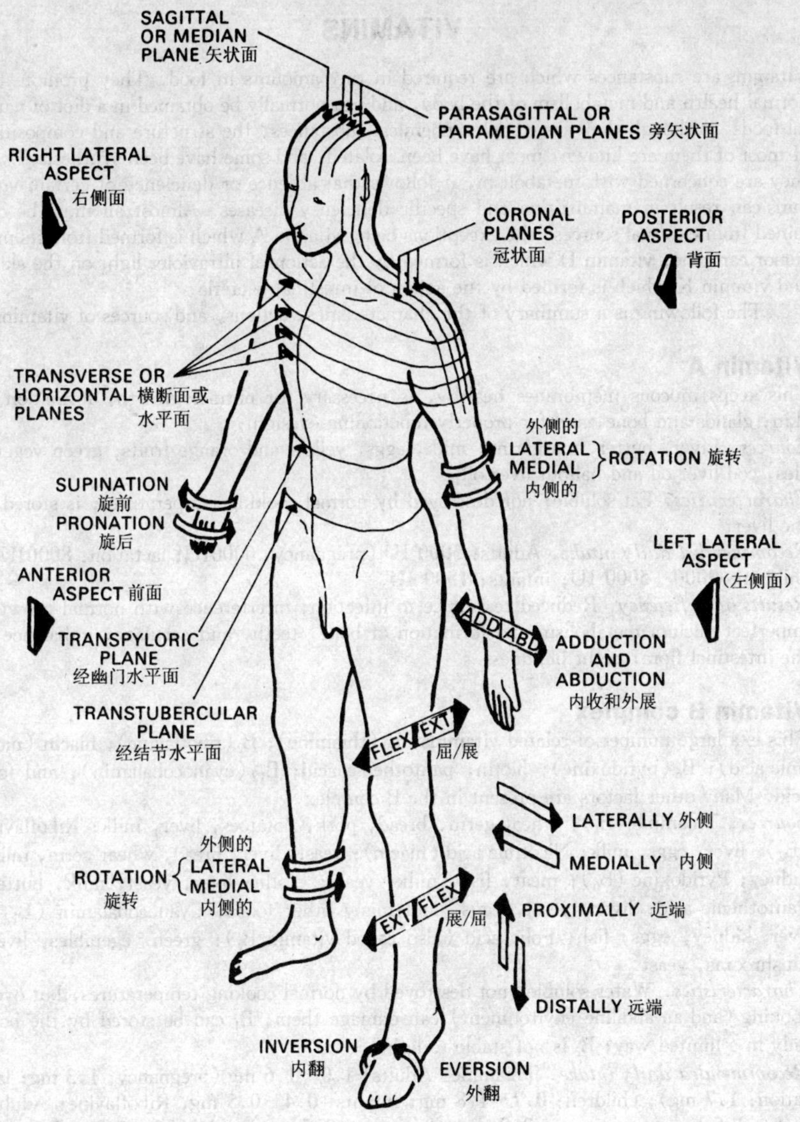
SAGITTAL OR MEDIAN PLANE 矢状面
PARASAGITTAL OR PARAMEDIAN PLANES 旁矢状面
RIGHT LATERAL ASPECT 右侧面
CORONAL PLANES 冠状面
POSTERIOR ASPECT 背面
TRANSVERSE OR HORIZONTAL PLANES 横断面或水平面
外侧的 LATERAL
MEDIAL 内侧的
ROTATION 旋转
SUPINATION 旋前
PRONATION 旋后
LEFT LATERAL ASPECT (左侧面)
ANTERIOR ASPECT 前面
ADD
ABD
TRANSPYLORIC PLANE 经幽门水平面
ADDUCTION AND ABDUCTION 内收和外展
TRANSTUBERCULAR PLANE 经结节水平面
FLEX
EXT
屈/展
LATERALLY 外侧
ROTATION 旋转
外侧的 LATERAL
MEDIAL 内侧的
MEDIALLY 内侧
EXT
FLEX
展/屈
PROXIMALLY 近端
DISTALLY 远端
INVERSION 内翻
EVERSION 外翻

VITAMINS

Vitamins are substances which are required in tiny amounts in food. They promote the normal health and metabolism of the body, and can normally be obtained in a diet of natural foods. Although they are complex chemical substances, the structure and composition of most of them are known, most have been isolated, and some have been synthesized. As they are concerned with metabolism, it follows that absence or deficiency of certain vitamins can result in malnutrition and specific deficiency diseases. Almost all must be obtained from external sources, the exceptions being vitamin A which is formed from its precursor carotene, vitamin D which is formed by the action of ultraviolet light on the skin, and vitamin K which is formed by the action of intestinal bacteria.

The following is a summary of the characteristics, actions, and sources of vitamins:

Vitamin A

This keeps mucous membranes healthy, is necessary for normal growth, formation of skin, glands and bone, and for properly functioning eyesight.
Sources. Liver, butter, margarine, milk, eggs, yellow and orange fruits, green vegetables, cod liver oil and halibut liver oil.
Characteristics. Fat soluble; not destroyed by normal cooking temperatures; is stored in the liver.
Recommended daily intake. Adults: 5000 IU (pregnancy: 6000IU; lactation: 8000IU); children: 2000 – 5000 IU; infants: 1500 IU.
Results of deficiency. Reduced resistance to infection; interference with normal growth; imperfect calcium metabolism and formation of bone, teeth, and cartilage; imbalance of the intestinal flora; night blindness.

Vitamin B complex

This is a large number of related vitamins: B_1 (thiamine); B_2 (riboflavine); niacin (nicotinic acid); B_6 (pyridoxine); biotin; pantothenic acid; B_{12} (cyanocobalamin); and folic acid. Many other factors are present in the B complex.
Sources. Thiamine (B_1): wheat germ, bread, pork, potatoes, liver, milk; Riboflavine (B_2): liver, eggs, milk; Nicotinic acid (niacin): yeast, liver, bread, wheat germ, milk, kidney; Pyridoxine (B_6): meat, fish, milk, yeast; Biotin: liver, yeast, milk, butter; Pantothenic acid: liver, yeast, eggs, and many other foods; Cyanocobalamin (B_{12}): liver, kidney, eggs, fish; Folic acid (also called vitamin B_c): green vegetables, liver, mushrooms, yeast.
Characteristics. Water soluble; not destroyed by normal cooking temperatures, but overcooking (and an alkaline environment) can damage them; B_1 can be stored by the body only in a limited way; B_2 is not stable to light.
Recommended daily intake. Thiamine: Adults: 1.0 – 1.6 mg (pregnancy: 1.3 mg; lactation: 1.7 mg); children: 0.7 – 1.8 mg; infants: 0.4 – 0.5 mg. Riboflavine: Adults: 1.4 – 2.5 mg (pregnancy: 2.0 mg; lactation: 2.5 mg); children: 1.0 – 2.0 mg; infants: 0.4 – 0.9 mg. Niacin: Adults: 17 – 21 mg (pregnancy: 15 mg; lactation: 15 mg); children: 8 – 21 mg; infants: 6 – 7 mg.
Results of deficiency. Generally, B complex vitamin deficiency results in loss of appetite, impaired digestion of starches, constipation and diarrhoea; severe deficiency results in various nervous disorders, loss of co-ordinating power of muscles, and beriberi. More specifically, B_2 deficiency results in cheilosis, weakness, and impaired growth; niacin deficiency results in pellagra, gastrointestinal disturbances, and mental disturbance. Cyanocobalamin deficiency results in anaemia (cyanocobalamin is used in the treatment of pernicious

anaemia, sprue, nutritional anaemia, and macrocytic anaemias of infancy and pregnancy).

Vitamin C (Ascorbic acid)

This increases resistance to infection and keeps the skin in a healthy condition. It improves the circulation and the condition of the gums and other body tissues, and promotes healing of wounds.
Sources. Citrus fruits, rose-hip syrup, blackcurrants, fresh vegetables, tomatoes.
Characteristics. Water soluble; easily destroyed by overcooking; storage reduces efficacy unless canned or frozen; stored in the body only to a limited extent.
Recommended daily intake. Adults: 70 mg (pregnancy: 100 mg; lactation: 150 mg); children: 35 – 100 mg; infants: 30 mg.
Results of deficiency. Lowered vitality; joint tenderness; dental caries; lowered resistance to infection; fibrous tissue abnormalities. Severe deficiency results in haemorrhage, anaemia, and scurvy.

Vitamin D

This vitamin is essential for the proper utilization of calcium and phosphorus, and thus directly influences the structure of bones and teeth. It affects the blood chemistry.
Sources. Butter, egg yolk, fish liver oils and oily fish, yeast. As mentioned, the vitamin can be synthesized by the skin under the stimulus of sunlight or ultraviolet light.
Characteristics. Fat soluble; can be stored in the liver.
Recommended daily intake. The adult can generally synthesize sufficient of this vitamin, but deficiencies have occurred in dark-skinned individuals or elderly people who live in temperate areas where the sunlight they receive is insufficient. In pregnancy: 400 IU; lactation: 400 IU; children: 400 IU; infants: 400 IU.
Results of deficiency. Interference with calcium and phosphorous metabolism; weakness and irritability. Severe deficiency results in rickets in children and osteomalacia in adults.

Vitamin E

Little is known about the physiological activity of this vitamin, but animal experiments suggest that it is concerned with the reproductive cycle and fertility; it may also have an effect on the ageing process. It is present in most foods, particularly in green vegetables.

Vitamin K

This is responsible for the biosynthesis of prothrombin and for maintaining plasma prothrombin levels.
Sources. Green leafy vegetables, liver.
Characteristics. Fat soluble; not destroyed by cooking.
Recommended daily intake. Not known, but children should receive 1 mg.

维生素

维生素是人体必需的饮食中含量极低的物质,它维持机体健康,促进新陈代谢,正常情况下可以从食物中获取。尽管维生素是一类复杂的化学物质,但其中绝大部分的化学结构和组成已被了解,且大部分已经被分离出来,有一些甚至可以合成。因为维生素参与新陈代谢,所以某些维生素缺失或缺少可以引起营养不良及相关疾病。几乎所有维生素都需从外界摄取,但也有例外,如维生素 A 是由前体物质胡萝卜素转化而来的,维生素 D 是皮肤经紫外线照射而合成的,维生素 K 则由肠道的细菌合成。
下面总结了维生素的特性、作用和来源:

维生素 A
作用:维持粘膜的正常状态,是皮肤、腺体和骨骼形成、生长以及维持正常的视觉所必需的物质。
来源:肝、黄油、人造黄油、牛奶、鸡蛋、黄色或橘黄色的水果、绿色蔬菜、鳕鱼和比目鱼的鱼肝油。
特性:脂溶性维生素,一般的烹饪温度不会破坏,储存于肝脏。
每日所需量:成人 5000IU (妊娠 6000 IU; 哺乳 8000 IU); 儿童 2000-5000 IU; 婴儿 1500 IU。
缺乏症:对感染的抵抗力下降,影响生长,钙代谢紊乱,骨骼、牙及软骨形成不良,肠道菌群紊乱和夜盲症。

维生素 B 族
这是一大类相关的维生素,包括:B_1(硫胺素)、B_2(核黄素)、烟酸(尼克酸)、B_6(吡哆醇)、生物素、泛酸、B_{12}(氰钴胺素)、叶酸以及其它许多因子。
来源:硫胺素(B_1):麦芽、面包、猪肉、土豆、肝和牛奶;核黄素(B_2):肝、鸡蛋和牛奶;尼克酸(烟酸):酵母、肝、面包、麦芽、牛奶和肾;吡哆醇(B_6):肉、鱼、牛奶和酵母;生物素:肝、酵母、牛奶和黄油;泛酸:肝、酵母、鸡蛋和许多其它食物;氰钴胺酸(B_{12}):肝、肾、鸡蛋和鱼;叶酸(维生素 B_c):绿色蔬菜、肝、菌类和酵母。
特性:水溶性维生素,一般的烹饪温度不会破坏,但过度烹饪(和碱性环境)可以使之破坏。B_1 在体内的储存量很少,B_2 对光不稳定。
每日所需量:硫胺素:成人 1.0-1.6mg (妊娠 1.3 mg, 哺乳 1.7 mg), 儿童 0.7-1.8 mg, 婴儿 0.4-0.5 mg。核黄素:成人 1.4-2.5mg (妊娠 2.0 mg, 哺乳 2.5 mg), 儿童 1.0-2.0mg, 婴儿 0.4-0.9 mg。烟酸:成人 17-21mg (妊娠 15 mg, 哺乳 15mg), 儿童 8-21mg, 婴儿 6-7mg。
缺乏症:缺乏维生素 B 族通常引起食欲不振,对淀粉类食物消化不良,便秘和腹泻。严重缺乏可导致各种神经系统疾病,肌肉协调能力丧失和脚气病。具体地说,缺乏 B_2可引起唇干裂、虚弱和生长发育不良。烟酸缺乏可引起糙皮病、胃肠功能紊乱和精神症状。氰钴胺酸缺乏可引起贫血(氰钴胺酸可用于治疗恶性贫血、口炎性腹泻、营养不良性贫血和婴儿期、妊娠期的大细胞性贫血)。

维生素 C(抗坏血酸)
作用:增强机体的抗感染能力,保持皮肤健康。促进循环,改善牙龈和其它器官的状况,加速伤口的愈合。
来源:柑橘类水果、蔷薇果汁、黑醋栗、新鲜蔬菜和西红柿。
特性:水溶性维生素,极易被过度烹饪破坏;除非罐装或冷冻,否则一般储藏容易丧失有效成分,机体内的储存量有限。
每日所需量:成人 70mg (妊娠 100mg; 哺乳 150 mg); 儿童 35-100mg; 婴儿 30 mg。
缺乏症:精力下降,关节疼痛,龋齿,对感染的抵抗力降低,纤维组织异常,严重缺乏可引起出血、贫血和坏血病。

维生素 D
作用:维生素 D 是机体利用钙、磷过程中所必需的物质,直接影响骨骼和牙齿的结构,对血液的化学组成也有影响。
来源:黄油、蛋黄、鱼肝油、鱼油和酵母。前面已经说过,维生素 D 还可由皮肤经阳光或紫外线照射而合成。
特性:脂溶性维生素,储存于肝脏。
每日所需量:由机体合成的维生素 D 就可满足成人所需,但肤色暗黑的人种或生活于温带地区的老年人因日晒不足会发生缺乏。妊娠期:400IU; 哺乳期:400IU; 儿童 400IU; 婴儿 400IU。
缺乏症:钙磷代谢紊乱,虚弱,易怒。严重缺乏在儿童可引起佝偻病,成人出现软骨病。

维生素 E

对于维生素 E 的生理功能了解很少,但动物研究显示它与生殖周期和受孕有关,对于衰老也可能有影响。大多数食物中都含有维生素 E,尤其是绿色蔬菜。

维生素 K

作用:参与凝血酶原的合成,维持血浆中凝血酶原的含量。
来源:绿叶蔬菜和肝脏。
特性:脂溶性维生素,不会被烹饪所破坏。
每日所需量:不清楚,但儿童每日需摄取 1mg。

CALORIE REQUIREMENTS

The calorie requirements of the human body depend upon age and activity. Children need a greater energy input for their weight than adults, as they are building up their body tissues.

A 'calorie' is, in the context of dietetics, a 'kilocalorie' (kcal); it is a unit of energy, and is the amount of heat required to raise 1 000 g of water by 1° Celsius. The term kilojoule (kJ) is sometimes preferred; a kilocalorie is approximately 4.2 kilojoules.

The following is a list of approximate daily calorie requirements for varying ages and activities.

人体每日所需热量

人体所需的热量随年龄、活动量的变化而变化。儿童因为生长发育需要,其单位体重所需的热量要大于成人。

1大卡在本书特指1千卡(kcal),作为热量单位,1千卡是使1千克水提高1摄氏度所需的热量。热量单位有时也用千焦(kJ),1千卡约等于4.2千焦。

下表列出了人体在不同年龄和活动量情况下每日大约所需的热量。

Children 儿童

Age (*years*)年龄(岁)	*Daily kcal* 日需量	*kJ* 千焦
≤1	800	3 360
1 - 2	1 200	5 040
2 - 3	1 400	5 880
3 - 5	1 600	6 720
5 - 7	1 800	7 560
7 - 9	2 100	8 820

boys 男孩	*kcal* 千卡	*kJ* 千焦	Girls 女孩	*kcal* 千卡	*kJ* 千焦
9 - 12	2 500	10 500	9 - 12	2 300	9 660
12 - 15	2 800	11 760	12 - 1	2 300	9 660
15 - 18	3 000	12 600	15 - 18	2 300	9 660

Men 男性

Age(years)年龄(岁)	*Activity* 活 动 度	*kcal* 千卡	*kJ* 千焦
18 - 35	sedentary 安静状态	2 700	11 340
	moderately active 轻度活动	3 000	12 600
	very active 剧烈活动	3 600	15 120
35 - 65	sedentary 安静状态	2 600	10 920
	moderately active 轻度活动	2 900	12 180
	very active 剧烈活动	3 600	15 120
65 - 75	sedentary 安静状态	2 300	9 660
>75	sedentary 安静状态	2 100	8 820

Women 女性

Age(years)年龄(岁)	*Activity* 活 动 度	*kcal* 千卡	*kJ* 千焦
18 – 35	moderately active 轻度活动	2 200	9 240
	very active 剧烈活动	2 500	10 500
	pregnant 妊娠	2 400	10 080
	lactating 哺乳	2 700	11 340
35 – 65	moderately active 轻度活动	2 200	9 240
65 – 75	sedentary 安静状态	2 050	8 610
>75	sedentary 安静状态	1 900	7 980

CALORIE CONTENT OF FOODS

食物热量表

Because the average portion of foods varies so much, both by custom and by personal preference, the following list shows the calorific value of various foods per 30 gram portion.
由于食物的平均重量相差很大,根据习惯和个人偏好,下表列出了每 30 克各种食物所含的热量。

		Per 30 gram portion 每 30 克食物	
Meat (cooked)	*肉类(熟食)*	*kcal* 千卡	*kJ* 千焦
Bacon	咸肉	160	672
Beef (roast)	牛肉(烤)	108	454
(steak)	(煎)	86	361
(corned)	(腌)	66	277
Ham	火腿	125	525
Kidney	肾	46	193
Liver (fried)	肝(油炸)	80	336
Lamb (chop)	小羊肉(羊排)	36	151
(roast leg)	(烤羊腿)	83	349
Luncheon meat	午餐肉	96	403
Pork (roast)	猪肉(烤)	90	378
Sausages	香肠	90	378
Tripe	牛肚	30	126
Veal (roast)	小牛肉(烤)	66	277
Poultry (cooked)	*禽类(熟食)*		
Chicken (roast)	鸡肉(烤)	55	232
Duck (roast)	鸭肉(烤)	90	378
Turkey (roast)	火鸡肉(烤)	56	236
Fish (cooked)	*鱼类(熟食)*		
Cod (steamed)	鳕鱼(蒸)	24	101
Haddock	黑线鳕鱼	28	118
Hake	鳕鱼类	30	126
Halibut	大比目鱼	37	156
Herring	鲱鱼	55	230
Kippers	腌鱼	57	239
Lemon sole	板鱼	26	108
Mackerel	鲭鱼	53	223
Plaice	欧蝶鱼	26	108
Salmon (canned)	鲑鱼(罐装)	39	164
(fresh)	(新鲜)	57	239
Sardines (canned)	沙丁鱼(罐装)	83	350
Sole	鳎鱼	25	105

		Per 30 gram portion 每 30 克食物	
		kcal 千卡	kJ 千焦
Shellfish	贝类		
Crab	螃蟹	36	151
Lobster	龙虾	34	143
Oysters	牡蛎	14	59
Prawns	对虾	30	126
Shrimps	小虾	32	134
Vegetables	蔬菜		
Beans (runner)	(架豆)	3	13
(broad)	(蚕豆)	12	50
(butter)	(利马豆)	26	109
(haricot)	(扁豆)	25	105
(French)	(菜豆)	3	13
Beetroot	甜菜根	13	55
Broccoli	椰菜	4	17
Brussels sprouts	芽甘蓝	5	21
Cabbage (raw)	卷心菜(生)	7	29
(cooked)	(熟)	2	8
Carrots (raw)	胡萝卜(生)	6	25
(cooked)	(熟)	5	21
Cauliflower	花椰菜	3	13
Celery (raw)	芹菜(生)	3	13
Cucumber	黄瓜	3	13
Lettuce	莴苣	3	13
Onions	洋葱	4	17
Peas (raw)	豌豆(生)	18	76
(cooked)	(熟)	28	118
Potatoes (new)	土豆(新鲜)	21	88
(old)	(老的)	23	97
(chips)	(油煎土豆片)	68	286
(crisps)	(油炸土豆片)	160	672
Spinach	菠菜	7	29
Spring green	绿牙菜	3	13
Swedes	焦青甘蓝	5	21
Tomatoes	西红柿	4	17
Turnips	芜箐	3	13
Watercress	豆瓣菜	4	17
Fruit	果类		
Apples	苹果	13	55
Apricots (raw)	杏(生)	3	34
(dried)	(杏干)	52	218
Bananas	香蕉	22	92
Blackcurrants	黑醋栗	8	34
Grapes (black)	葡萄(紫葡萄)	17	71

(white)	(白葡萄)	18	76
Grapefruit	釉子	6	25
Lemons	柠檬	4	17
Melon	西瓜	7	29
Orange	柑橘	10	42
Peaches	桃	11	46
Pears	梨	12	50
Plums	李子	11	46
Prunes	梅子	46	193
Raisins	葡萄干	71	298
Raspberries	覆盆子	7	29
Rhubarb	大黄	1	4
Strawberries (raw)	草莓	5	21
		Per 30 gram portion 每 30 克食物	
Sultanas	无核葡萄干	72	302
Dairy Products	*乳制品*		
Butter	黄油	225	945
Cheese (Cheddar)	干酪(黄色干酪)	118	496
(Cottage)	(松软干酪)	30	126
(Curd)	(凝乳)	40	168
(Blue)	(上等的带蓝纹的奶酪)	105	441
(Edam)	(依顿干酪)	88	370
(Gruyere)	(瑞士格里尔干酪)	130	546
Cream (double)	奶油 (浓)	130	546
(single)	(稀)	62	260
Eggs	鸡蛋	46	193
Margarine	人造黄油	225	946
Milk (Whole fresh)	牛奶(鲜奶)	19	80
(skimmed)	(脱脂的)	10	42
(evaporated)	(炼乳)	45	125
(condensed)	(浓缩的)	95	400
Oil (cooking)	油(食用)	250	1 050
Yoghurt (low fat)	酸乳酪(低脂的)	15	63
Preserves and Sugar	蜜饯与糖		
Chocolate (milk)	巧克力(奶油)	170	714
(plain)	(黑巧克力)	156	655
		Per 30 gram portion 每 30 克食物	
Honey	蜂蜜	95	399
Ice cream	冰淇凌	56	235
Jam	果酱	74	311
Marmalade	橘子酱	75	315
Sugar (brown or white)	糖(红糖或白糖)	111	466

Syrup (golden)	糖浆(优质)	90	378
Treacle	糖蜜	74	311
Cereals	谷类		
Bread (white, browm, or wholemeal)	面包(白面包,黑面包,全麦面包)	70	294
Cornflakes	玉米片	105	441
Cornflour	玉米面	100	420
Crispbread	面包脆	100	420
Flour (white, wholemeal)	面粉(富强粉,营养粉)	100	420
Macaroni (boiled)	通心粉(煮)	30	126
Porridge (oatmeal)	粥(燕麦片)	14	59
Rice	稻米	35	147
Sago	西米	100	420
Semolina	粗面粉	100	420
Spaghetti	意大利式细面条	106	445
Tapioca	木薯	102	428
Nuts (shelled)	*坚果(有壳的)*		
Almonds	杏仁	170	714
Brazils	巴西胡桃	182	764
Chestnuts	栗子	50	210
Coconut	椰子	180	756
Peanuts	花生	170	714
Walnuts	胡桃	154	647

LIST OF EPONYMOUS TERMS
人名术语一览表

An eponym, in medicine, is a disease, procedure or anatomical structure that bears a person's name or the name of a place. It is usually the name of the person who discovered or first described it. The following is a list of the *eponymous* terms in this dictionary.
医学中的人名名词指用人名或地名来命名的某种疾病、手术过程或解剖结构。通常采用发现或首先描述它的人的名字。下面是本词典中出现的人名术语。

Addison's disease 阿狄森氏病
Albee's operation 阿尔比氏手术
Alzheimer's disease 阿尔茨海默氏病
Apgar score 阿普伽新生儿评分
Arnold-Chiari malformation 阿-希氏畸形
Auerbach's plexus 奥尔巴赫神经丛
Babinski reflex *or* **Babinski test** 巴宾斯基反射(试验)
Baker's cyst 贝克氏囊肿
Bankart's operation 拜恩卡特手术
Banti's syndrome 班替氏综合症
Barlow's disease 巴洛氏病,婴儿坏血病
Barr body 巴氏小体,性染色体
Basedow's disease 巴塞多氏病,突眼性甲状腺肿
Bazin's disease 巴赞氏病,硬红斑
Beer's knife 贝尔刀
Behcet's syndrome 贝切特综合症
Bellocq's cannula 贝洛克氏套管
Bell's mania 贝耳氏躁狂
Bell's palsy 贝耳氏麻痹
Bence Jones protein 本-周氏蛋白
Benedict's test 本尼迪特试验
Bennett's fracture 贝奈特骨折
Besnier's prurigo 贝尼埃氏痒疹
Billroth's operation 毕罗特手术
Binet's test 比内氏测验
Bitot's spots 比托斑
Blalock's operation 布氏手术
Boeck's sarcoid 伯克氏肉样瘤
Bonney's blue 邦尼蓝,用于消毒的染料
Bowman's capsule 鲍曼氏囊
Braille 点字法
Braun's splint *or* **frame** 布朗氏支架
Bright's disease 布赖特肾病
Broadbent's sign 布罗德本征

Broca's area 布罗卡氏区
Brodie's abscess 布罗迪氏脓肿
Brown-Séquard syndrome 布朗·塞卡综合征
Brunner's glands 布伦内氏腺,十二指肠腺
Budd-Chiari symdrome 布－希综合征
Buerger's disease 伯格氏病,血栓闭塞性脉管炎
Burkitt's tumour 伯基特氏瘤
Caldwell-Luc operation 考－路二氏手术
Celsius 摄氏度
Chagas'd disease 恰加斯氏病
Charcot's joints 夏科氏关节
Cheyne-Stokes respiration 陈－施呼吸
Christmas disease 克里斯马斯病
Clutton's joints 克莱顿关节
Cooley's anaemia 库利贫血
Coombs' test 库姆斯试验
Corti (organ of) 科蒂器
Cowper's glands 库珀腺
Coxsackie virus 柯萨奇病毒
Credé's method 克勒德氏法
Crohn's disease 克隆氏病
Cushing's disease 柯兴氏病
Da Costa's syndrome 达科斯塔氏综合征
Daltonism 红色盲
Denis Browne splint 丹尼斯－布朗支架
Dercum's disease 德尔肯氏病
Descemet's membrane 德斯密氏膜
Devic's disease 德维克氏病
Dick test 狄克试验
Dietl's crisis 迪特耳危象
Döderlein's bacillus 德得莱因氏杆菌
Down's syndrome 道恩综合征
Duchenne muscular dystrophy 杜兴氏肌营养不良
Ducrey's bacillus 杜克雷氏杆菌
Dupuytren's contracture 杜普依特伦氏挛缩
Eisenmenger complex 艾森门格氏综合症
Epstein-Barr virus E-B 病毒
Erb's palsy 欧勃氏麻痹
Esmarch's bandage 埃斯马赫氏绷带
Eustachian tube 咽鼓管
Ewing's tumour 尤文氏瘤
Fallopian tube 法娄皮欧氏管,输卵管
Fallot's tetralogy 法乐氏四联征
Fanconi syndrome 范康尼氏综合征
Fehling's solution 费林氏溶液

Felty's syndrome 费耳提氏综合征
Frei test 弗莱氏试验
Freiberg's disease 弗莱伯氏病
Friedlander's bacillus 弗里德兰德氏杆菌
Friedreich's ataxia 弗里德赖希氏共济失调
Fröhlich's syndrome 弗勒利氏综合征
Gallie's operation 加利氏手术
Ganser's state 甘塞氏状态
Gasserian ganglion 加塞神经节
Gaucher's disease 戈谢氏病
Geiger counter 盖革尔计数器
Ghon's focus 冈氏病灶
Gilliam's operation 吉列姆氏手术
Girdlestone's operation 格德尔斯通手术
Golgi apparatus 高尔基体
Goodpasture's syndrome 古德帕斯特氏综合征
Graefe's knife 格雷费氏刀
Gram stain 革兰氏染色
Graves' disease 格雷夫斯氏病
Grawitz tumour 格腊维茨氏瘤
Guillain-Barré syndrome 格林巴利综合征
Hand-Schüller-Christian disease 汗－许－克三氏病
Hansen's bacillus 汉森氏杆菌(麻风分枝杆菌)
Harrison's sulcus 郝氏沟
Hartmann's solution 哈特曼氏溶液
Hartnup disease 海特那普病
Hashimoto's disease 桥本氏病
Haversian canals 哈弗管
Heberden's node 希伯登氏结节
Hegar's sign 黑加氏征
Henle (loop of) 亨利袢
Henoch purpura 神经性紫癜
Hering-Breuer reflex 赫－布二氏反射
Higginson's syringe 希京森氏注射器
Highmore (antrum of) 海墨尔氏窦
Hirschsprung's disease 赫希施普龙氏病
His (bundle of) 希氏束
Hodgkin's disease 何杰金氏病
Homans' sign 霍氏征
Horner's syndrome 霍纳氏综合征
Horton's headache 霍顿氏头痛
Huhner's test 胡讷氏试验
Huntington's chorea 亨廷顿氏舞蹈病
Hurler's syndrome 胡尔勒氏综合征
Jacksonian epilepsy 杰克逊癫痫

Jacquemier's sign 惹克米埃氏征
Kahn test 康瓦氏试验
Kaposi's sarcoma 卡波西肉瘤
Kayser-Fleischer rings 凯－费氏环
Keller's operation 凯勒氏手术
Kernig's sign 克氏征
Killian's operation 基利安氏手术
Kimmelstiel-Wilson disease 基－威二氏病
Kirschner wire 基施纳氏钢丝
Klebs-Loeffler bacillus 克－吕氏杆菌(白喉杆菌)
Klinefelter's syndrome 克莱恩费尔特氏综合征
Klumpke's paralysis 克隆普克氏麻痹
Koch's bacillus 郭霍氏杆菌(结核杆菌)
Köhler's disease 科勒氏病
Koplik's spots 科波力克氏斑
Korsakoff's syndrome *or* **pschosis** 科罗特科夫氏综合征或精神病
Krause corpuscles 克劳泽氏小体
Krebs cycle 克雷布氏循环
Krukenberg tumour 克鲁肯伯格氏瘤
Kuntscher nail 金彻氏钉
Kupffer's cells 枯否氏细胞
Kveim test 科维姆试验,检查结节病的皮肤试验
Laennec's cirrhosis 拉埃奈克氏肝硬化
Landry's paralysis 兰德里氏麻痹
Lange test 郎格试验
Langerhans (islets of) 郎格罕氏小岛
Lassa fever 拉沙热
Lassar's paste 拉萨尔糊剂
Legg-Calve-Perthes disease 累－卡－佩三氏病
Lembert's suture 郎贝尔缝术
Leydig cells 莱迪氏细胞
Lieberkuhn's glands 利贝昆氏腺
Little's disease 李特尔氏病
Ludwig's angina 路德维希氏咽峡炎
Magendie's foramen 马让迪氏孔
Mallory-Weiss tears 马－魏氏撕裂,食管和胃交界处粘膜撕裂
Malpighian body 马耳皮基氏小体
Mantoux test 芒图氏试验
Marfan's syndrome 马凡氏综合征
McBurney's point 麦氏点
Meckel's diverticulum 麦克尔憩室
Meissner's plexus 麦氏丛
Mendel's laws 孟德尔定律
Mendelson's syndrome 门德尔森氏综合征
Ménière's disease 美尼尔氏病

Merkel's disc 默克氏触盘
Michel's clips 密歇尔氏夹
Milroy's disease 米耳罗伊病
Mönckeberg's arteriosclerosis 门克伯氏动脉硬化
Montgomery's glands 蒙哥马利氏腺
Mooren's ulcer 莫伦氏溃疡
Moro reflex 莫罗氏反射
Müllerian duct 苗勒管
Münchhausen's syndrome 闵希豪生综合征
Murphy's sign 墨菲氏征
Negri bodies 内格里小体
Nissl bodies 尼斯尔体
Ortolani's sign 奥氏征
Osler's nodes 奥司勒结节
Pacinian corpuscles 帕西尼氏小体
Paget's disease 佩吉特病
Papanicolaou test 帕氏涂片检查
Parkinson's disease 帕金森氏病
Paschen body 帕兴氏小体
Pasteurization 巴斯德消毒法
Paul-Bunnell reaction 保罗－邦内氏反应
Paul's tube 保罗氏管
Pel-Ebstein fever 佩－埃二氏热
Pellegrini-Stieda disease 佩－施二氏病
Peyer's patches 派依尔氏淋巴结
Peyronie's disease 佩罗尼氏病
Placido's disk 普拉西多氏盘
Plummer-Vinson syndrome 普－文二氏综合征
Politzer bag 波利泽尔咽鼓管吹气袋
Pott's disease 波特氏病
Poupart's ligament 普帕尔韧带
Purkinje cells 浦肯耶细胞
Queckenstedt's test 奎肯斯提试验
Quick test 魁克试验
Ramstedt's operation 幽门切除术
Raynaud's disease 雷诺氏病
Reiter's syndrome 莱特尔氏综合征
Rinne's test 林内氏试验
Roentgen 伦琴(X线单位)
Romberg's sign 罗姆伯格征
Rorschach test 洛夏克测验
Roth spot 罗特斑
Rothera's test 罗瑟雷试验
Rovsing's sign 罗符辛氏征
Rubin's test 鲁宾试验

Ruffini corpuscles 鲁菲尼氏小体
Russell traction 拉塞尔牵引
Ryle's tube 赖氏管
Sabin vaccine 萨宾疫苗
Salk vaccine 索尔克疫苗
Sayre's jacket 塞尔背心
Scarpa's triangle 斯卡帕三角
Scheuermann's disease 绍依尔曼氏病
Schick test 锡克试验
Schilling test 希林试验
Schlatter's disease 施莱特病
Schlemm (canal of) 施雷姆氏管
Schönlein purpura 过敏性紫癜
Schönlein-Henoch purpura 舍－亨二氏紫癜
Schwann cells 雪旺氏细胞
Schwartze's operation 施瓦茨手术
Sengstaken tube 森氏管
Sertoli cells 塞尔托利细胞
Simmonds's disease 西蒙兹病
Sippy diet 西皮氏饮食
Skene's glands 斯基恩氏腺
Smith-Petersen nail 史密斯－彼得森氏钉
Snellen chart 斯内伦视力表
Sonne dysentery 宋内氏痢疾
Sprengel's deformity 施普伦格畸形
Stacke's operation 斯塔克手术
Stein-Leventhal syndrome 斯坦因－利文撒尔综合征
Steinmann's pin 斯坦曼氏导钉
Stellwag's sign 施特耳瓦格征
Stensen's duct 斯坦森导管
Stevens-Johnson syndrome 斯－约二氏综合征
Still's disease 斯蒂尔病
Stokes-Adams syndrome 阿－斯综合征
Sudeck's atrophy 祖德克萎缩
Sydenham's chorea 西登汉姆氏舞蹈病
Syme's amputation 塞姆截肢
Tay-Sachs disease 泰－萨二氏病
Tenon's capsule 特农氏囊
Thiersch's graft 蒂尔施移植物
Thomas's splint 托马斯夹板
Trendelenburg operation, position, sign 特伦德伦伯格氏手术/卧位/征
Trousseau's signs 特鲁索征
Turner's syndrome 特纳综合征
Vincent's angina 奋森氏咽峡炎
Von Recklinghausen's disease 冯·雷克林霍曾氏病

Von Willebrand's disease 冯·维勒布兰德氏病
Waldeyer's ring 瓦尔代尔扁桃体环
Wangensteen tube 旺根斯滕管
Wassermann reaction/test 瓦氏反应/试验
Waterhouse-Friderichsen syndrome 沃特豪斯－弗里德里希森综合征
Waterston's operation 华特斯顿手术
Weber-Christian disease 韦－克氏病
Weber's test 韦伯试验
Weil-Felix reaction, test 外－斐氏反应/试验
Weil's disease 韦尔氏病
Wernicke's encephalopathy 韦尼克脑病
Wertheim's operation 韦特海姆手术
Wharton's duct; Wharton's jelly 沃顿管/胶
Wheelhouse's operation 惠耳豪斯手术
Whipple's disease 惠普尔病
Widal reaction 肥达反应
Willis, circle of 威利斯环
Wilms' tumour 维尔姆斯瘤
Wilson's disease 威尔逊病
Wood's lamp 伍德灯
Zollinger-Ellison syndrome 卓－艾二氏综合征

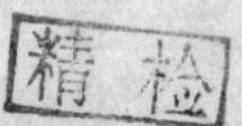